DUNCAN'S DICTIONARY FOR NURSES
2nd edition

DUNCAN'S DICTIONARY for NURSES

2nd edition

Helen A. Duncan, R.N., M.A.

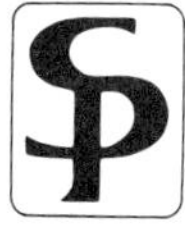

SPRINGER PUBLISHING COMPANY/NEW YORK

Springer Publishing Company, Inc.
536 Broadway
New York, NY 10012

89 90 91 92 / 5 4 3 2 1

LIBRARY OF CONGRESS
Library of Congress Cataloging-in-Publication Data

Duncan, Helen A.
[Dictionary for nurses]
Duncan's dictionary for nurses / Helen A. Duncan.—2nd ed.
p. cm.
ISBN 0-8261-6200-2
1. Nursing—Dictionaries. I. Title. II. Title: Dictionary for nurses.
[DNLM: 1. Dictionaries, Medical. 2. Nursing—dictionaries. WY 13 D911d]
RT21.D85 1988
610'.3'21—dc19
DNLM/DLC
for Library of Congress 88-15914
CIP

Printed in the United States of America

Illustration for the Cross section of the heart reprinted by permission of the author, Rita K. Chow, *Cardiosurgical Nursing Care*. New York: Springer Publishing Co., 1976.

Illustration of the larynx and trachea reprinted with permission from Sweetwood, Hannelore. *Nursing in the Intensive Respiratory Care Unit, Second Edition*. New York, Springer Publishing Co., 1979.

Photo and information detailing the intrauterine copper contraceptive courtesy of the Population Council, New York, NY.

Illustrations for the facial nerve and larynx with vocal cords are reprinted with permission from Riley, Mary Ann K., *Nursing Care of the Client with Ear, Nose, and Throat Disorders*. New York: Springer Publishing Co., 1987.

Contents

Preface

The positive reception of the first edition of *Duncan's Dictionary for Nurses,* prepared by a nurse and for nurses, prompted the preparation of this completely revised and greatly enlarged edition. Again, the definitions were chosen with nurses in active practice and student nurses chiefly in mind. The unique feature of this dictionary is that it is not an abbreviated medical dictionary; it was designed specifically for nurses. The constantly expanding role of the professional nurse and the accompanying increase in nursing functions, activities, and responsibilities require that a reference source meet the needs created by these changes. Consequently, the entries reflect extensive research in current literature, both textbooks and periodicals, in addition to conferences with many nurses in active practice. Our thanks go to the library staff of the American Journal of Nursing, to the editorial staff of Springer Publishing Company, and to the many nurse associates and authorities who gave valuable help and advice. It is our hope that this updated edition will prove to be a useful companion and tool for student and practicing nurses and their co-workers in the field of nursing.

H.A.D.

Pronunciation Key

The system of pronunciation used has deliberately been kept simple. Words that the nurse might have difficulty pronouncing are broken down into their component syllables and, when necessary, respelled phonetically. The accented syllables are indicated by a slanting mark at their terminations (′).

Vowels

Vowels are usually pronounced long or short, and are given the ordinary English pronunciation. When short, they are unmarked and are pronounced as follows:

a as in fast or father
e as in bed
i as in fit
o as in for or hot
oo as in tool
u as in but

When long, they are given a long mark and are pronounced as follows:

ā as in tame
ē as in he
ī as in time
ō as in over
ū as in use

The final syllables of words that end with *a* may be pronounced as though the word ended with *ah*. Those that end with *y* are usually pronounced as though they ended with a short *i*, as, for example, chemistry (kem′-is-tri).

Consonants

Consonants ordinarily take the common English language pronunciation. When this is not the case, the word is respelled phonetically, for example:

c may be pronounced as *s* or *k* as in cicatrix (sik′-a-triks)
ch is usually pronounced as *k* as in psychosis (sī-kō′-sis)
g may be pronounced as *j* as in pharyngeal (far-in′-jē-al)
ph may be pronounced as *f* as in physical (fiz′-i-kal)
psy may be pronounced as sī as in psyche (sī′-kē) or as si as in psychiatry (si-kī′-a-tri)

Abbreviations Used in Definitions

adj.	adjective
adv.	adverb
cf.	compare (Latin, *confer*)
e.g.	for example (Latin, *exempli gratia*)
F.	French
i.e.	that is (Latin, *id est*)
L.	Latin
n.	noun
opp.	opposite to
pl.	plural
q.v.	which see (Latin, *quod vide*)
sing.	singular
syn.	synonym
U.S.	United States
v.	verb

A

A: Chemical symbol for argon.

Å: Abbreviation for Angstrom unit (*q.v.*).

A_2: Abbreviation for aortic second sound.

a.: Abbreviation for 1. Accommodation; 2. Anode; 3. Axial.

α: Abbreviation for the Greek *alpha;* denotes the first in a series. For words beginning with alpha, see the specific terms.

a-; an-: Prefixes denoting absence, separation, away, away from, without, not, less, lacking, lack of; a- when used before a consonant; an- when before a vowel.

AA: Abbreviation for: 1. Achievement age. 2. Alcoholics Anonymous. 3. Administration on Aging.

$\overline{aa}$: Abbreviation for *ana* [G.]; sign used for "of each" in prescription writing.

Ab: Abbreviation for antibody.

ab-: Prefix denoting absent, away from, off, negative, separation, departure from, outside, deviating from.

abacterial (ā-bak-tē′-ri-al): Without bacteria; free from bacteria. **A. MENINGITIS,** aseptic meningitis; see under meningitis.

abaissement (a-bās′-mon): A lowering, depressing, or falling.

abalienation (ab-āl-yen-ā′-shun): Term formerly used for mental derangement.

abaragnosis (a-bar-og-nō′-sis): Lack or loss of the conscious perception of weight, or of the ability to estimate weight.

abarthrosis (ab-ar-thrō′-sis): Diarthrosis (*q.v.*).

abarticular (ab-ar-tik′-ū-lar): Not involving or affecting a joint. **A. GOUT,** a form of gout that affects structures other than the joints.

abarticulation (ab′-ar-tik-ū-lā′-shun): 1. The dislocation of a joint. 2. A synovial or freely movable joint; *e.g.*, the hip. See diarthrosis.

abasia (a-bā′-zi-a): Inability to walk, or unsteadiness of gait, due to motor incoordination. **ASTASIA A.,** see under astasia.—abasic, abatic, adj.

abatement (a-bāt′-ment): A decrease or lessening of a symptom or of pain.—abate, v.

abaxial (ab-ak′-si-al): Refers to a position away from the axial line of a structure.

Abbott-Miller tube: A long double-lumen intestinal tube with an inflatable balloon attached to the distal end; used in certain diagnostic tests, to treat an obstruction in the small intestine, and to relieve distention of the intestine.

ABCs: In emergency medicine, refers to *a*irway, *b*reathing, and *c*irculation in regard to priority of care.

Abd: Abbreviation for abdomen.

abdomen (ab′-do-men, ab-dō′-): The belly. The largest body cavity; lies between the thorax, from which it is separated by the diaphragm, and the pelvis; is enclosed by a wall made up of muscles, the vertebral column and the two ilia; contains the stomach, small and large intestine, liver, gallbladder, pancreas, spleen, the descending aorta and inferior vena cava, and (behind the peritoneum) the kidneys and ureters. It is lined with a serous membrane, the peritoneum, which is also reflected over most of the organs as a cover. **ACUTE A.,** term for a pathological condition within the belly that requires immediate surgery. **PENDULOUS A.,** that which occurs when the anterior wall relaxes and the abdomen sags or hangs down. **SCAPHOID A.,** an **A.** in which the anterior wall "caves in."—abdominal, adj. See regions, abdominal.

abdomin-, abdomino-: Combining forms denoting the abdomen.

abdominal (ab-dom′-i-nal): Pertaining to the abdomen. **A. AORTA,** the part of the descending aorta that passes down through the abdomen. **A. BREATHING,** breathing in which the abdominal muscles and diaphragm are active; the abdomen moves outward during inspiration and inward during expiration. Also called diaphragmatic breathing. **A. CAVITY,** the space in the trunk of the body between the diaphragm and the pelvic floor; contains the abdominal organs. **A. DELIVERY,** delivery of an infant through an abdominal incision. **A. DROPSY,** ascites (*q.v.*). **A. FISTULA,** an artificial opening from an abdominal organ to the surface, *e.g.*, a colostomy. **A. GESTATION,** see ectopic g., under ectopic. **A. HERNIA,** a hernia of a loop of intestine through the muscles of the abdominal wall. **A. HYSTERECTOMY,** removal of the uterus through an abdominal incision. **A. PREGNANCY,** ectopic pregnancy; see under ectopic. **A. REGIONS,** see under region. **A. SECTION,** an incision into the abdominal wall for surgical purposes. **A. PARACENTESIS,** removal of fluid from the abdominal cavity by means of a trocar; also called abdominocentesis and abdominal tap.

abdominal thrust: An emergency procedure used when a patient's airway is obstructed; may be executed with the patient prone or standing; consists of giving several quick upward thrusts against the patient's abdomen between the xiphoid process and the umbilicus. If the patient is standing, the rescuer stands behind the patient and grasps one fist in the other and gives the thrust; if the patient is prone, the rescuer may be either beside or bestride the patient and makes the thrust with one hand on the heel of the other. Four thrusts are given in fairly rapid succession.

abdominalgia (ab-dom-in-al′-ji-a): Pain in the belly.

abdominoanterior (ab-dom′-i-nō-an-tē′-ri-or): Pertaining to a position with the abdomen forward; usually referring to the position of the fetus in utero.

abdominocentesis (ab-dom′-i-nō-sen-tē′-sis): Surgical puncture of the abdominal wall for the aspiration of fluid from the abdominal cavity; paracentesis.

abdominocyesis (ab-dom′-i-nō-sī-ē′-sis): Abdominal pregnancy; see under abdominal.

abdominocystic (ab-dom′-i-nō-sis′-tik): Pertaining to 1) the abdomen and the gallbladder; 2) the abdomen and the urinary bladder.

abdominohysterectomy (ab-dom′-i-nō-his-ter-ek′-to-mi): Operation for the removal of the uterus through an incision in the abdominal wall.

abdominopelvic (ab-dom-i-nō-pel′-vik): Pertaining to the abdomen and pelvis or pelvic cavity.

abdominoperineal (ab-dom′-i-nō-per-in-ē′-al): Pertaining to the abdomen and the perineum. **A. RESECTION OF THE RECTUM,** an operation in which the proximal end of the bowel is brought out onto the abdominal wall as a permanent colostomy, and the growth is removed via the perineum.

abdominoposterior (ab-dom′-i-nō-pos-tē′-ri-or): Pertaining to a position with the abdomen turned backward; usually referring to the position of the fetus in utero.

abdominoscopy (ab-dom-i-nos′-ko-pi): Examination or inspection of the abdomen and/or its viscera, either with or without the use of an endoscope.

abdominothoracic (ab-dom′-i-nō-thō-ras′-ik): Pertaining to the abdomen and the thorax.

abdominous (ab-dom′-i-nus): Having a protruding or prominent abdomen.

abdominovaginal (ab-dom′-i-nō-vaj′-i-nal): Pertaining to the abdomen and the vagina.

abdominovesical (ab-dom′-i-nō-ves′-ik'l): Pertaining to the abdomen and the urinary bladder.

abduce (ab-dūs′): Abduct (*q.v.*).

abducens (ab-dū′-senz): Term applied to structures that draw a part away from the median line of the body, or that cause this to happen. **A. NERVE,** the sixth cranial nerve; supplies the muscle that moves the eyeball outward.

abducent (ab-dū′-sent): Drawing away from; abducting.

abduct (ab-dukt′): To draw away from the median line of the body or from an adjoining part. Abduce. Opp. to adduct.—abduction, n.

abduction (ab-duk′-shun): 1. The drawing away of a part from the midline of the body or of one part from an adjoining part, or the result of such action. Opp. of adduction. 2. The act of turning outward. 3. A position away from the midline. 4. The result of movement away from the midline. 5. In ophthalmology, rotation of the eye outwardly.

abductor (ab-duk′-tor): A muscle that draws a part away from the median line of the body; or a nerve supplying such a muscle. Opp. to adductor.

ABE: Abbreviation for acute bacterial endocarditis; see under endocarditis.

aberrant (ab-er′-ant): Deviating or wandering from the normal or expected in some way, as in structure, shape, or course.—aberrancy, n.

aberration (ab-e-rā′-shun): A deviation from normal. **MENTAL A.,** a mild mental abnormality. **OPTICAL A.,** any imperfection in the refraction of a lens of the eye. **SPHERICAL A.,** imperfect focus of light rays by a lens.

abetalipoproteinemia (a-bā′-ta-lip′-ō-prō-tē-in-ē′-mi-a): A rare hereditary disorder characterized by almost complete lack of lipoprotein in the blood and malabsorption of fat, and later, by retinitis, ataxia, and muscular atrophy; usually manifested early in infancy.

abeyance (a-bā′-ans): 1. Cessation of a function or an activity. 2. A state of suspended or temporary abolition of function.

ABG: Abbreviation for arterial blood gases.

abient (ab′-i-ent): Having a tendency to move away from a stimulus or the source of a stimulus.

abiogenesis (ab′-i-ō-jen′-e-sis): The obsolete theory of a spontaneous generation of living things from nonliving matter.

abiosis (ab-i-ō′-sis): 1. Without life; lifeless. 2. The condition of nonviability.—abiotic, adj.

abiotrophy (ab-i-ot′-rō-fi): A general term denoting loss of vitality, death of cells, or degeneration of tissues that is not associated with infection or poisoning.

abirritant (ab-ir′-rit-ant): 1. Relieving or lessening irritation. 2. An agent that relieves or lessens irritation.

abirritation (ab′-ir-ri-tā′-shun): Asthenia, atony, or any other condition that is characterized by diminution of tissue irritability or abolition of reflexes.—abirritative, adj.; abirritate, v.

ablactation (ab-lak-tā′-shun): 1. Cessation of the flow of milk. 2. Weaning an infant.

ablate (a-blāt′): To excise or amputate a body part completely.

ablatio (ab-lā′-shē-ō): Ablation; detachment.

A. PLACENTAE, premature detachment of the placenta. **A. RETINAE,** detachment of the retina.

ablation (ab-lā′-shun): Removal; detachment. In surgery, the removal or amputation of a part of the body.—ablative, adj.

ablepharia (a-blef-ā′-ri-a): Congenital absence of the eyelids; may be total or partial.—ablepharous, adj.

ablepsia (ab-lep′-si-a): Blindness.

abluent (ab′-lū-ent): 1. Having a detergent or cleansing action. 2. A cleansing agent such as soap.

ablution (ab-lū′-shun): 1. Washing or cleansing, especially of the body. 2. The pouring of water over the body or part of it as a therapeutic measure.

ablutomania (ab-lū′tō-mān′-i-a): Abnormal interest in washing, bathing, or cleansing oneself.

abneural (ab-nū′-ral): Away from or remote from the central nervous system.

abnormal (ab-nor′-mal): Not normal; irregular; different from the usual.—abnormality, n.

abnormal psychology: The study that deals with maladaptive behavior and deviations in mental functioning, including neuroses and psychoses, whether they occur in people of subnormal, normal, or superior intellect.

ABO: Abbreviation for the international (Landsteiner) classification of human blood types. Blood is typed according to compatibility of the ABO factors in transfusion as A, B, AB, and O. **ABO INCOMPATIBILITY,** a condition usually caused by the mother having O type blood (which has naturally occurring anti-A and anti-B antibodies) and the fetus having either A or B blood; symptoms in infants include those seen in mild anemia, hyperbilirubinemia, hepatosplenomegaly, spherocytosis, reticulocytosis. See blood groups.

abocclusion (ab-ō-kloo′-zhun): Descriptive of dentition in which the upper and lower teeth do not meet.

aboiement (a-bwah-mon′): The involuntary uttering of abnormal sounds, usually barking.

aboral (ab-ō′-ral): Away from or opposite to the mouth.

abort (a-bort′): 1. To terminate before full development. 2. To check a disease process in its early stages. 3. To terminate a pregnancy before the fetus is viable.

aborticide (a-bor′-ti-sīd): 1. The intentional destruction of the fetus in the uterus. **FAILED A.,** a rare occurrence when a pregnancy persists after incomplete loss of the products of conception. 2. A drug or agent that is capable of destroying a fetus in the uterus.

abortifacient (a-bor-ti-fā′-shent): 1. Causing abortion. 2. A drug or agent that causes expulsion of a nonviable fetus.

abortigenic (a-bor-ti-jen′-ik): Causing abortion or an agent that causes abortion.

abortion (a-bor′-shun): 1. Abrupt termination of a process. 2. Expulsion from the uterus of products of conception before the fetus is viable, *i.e.*, approximately before the end of the 28th week. **ACCIDENTAL A.,** one due to an accident. **ARTIFICIAL A.,** one brought on intentionally. **COMPLETE A.,** one in which the entire contents of the uterus are expelled. **CRIMINAL A.,** the illegal intentional evacuation of the uterus. **FAILED A.,** a rare occurrence when a pregnancy persists after incomplete loss of the products of conception. **HABITUAL A.,** repeated successive abortions; preferable term is recurrent abortion. **INCOMPLETE A.,** one in which part of the fetus or placenta is retained within the uterus. **INDUCED A., INTENTIONAL A.,** produced by mechanical or medical means. **INEVITABLE A.,** one that has advanced to a stage where termination of the pregnancy cannot be prevented. **JUSTIFIABLE A.,** one performed to save the life of the mother. **MISSED A.,** one in which early signs and symptoms of pregnancy disappear and the fetus dies but is not expelled for some time; see carneous mole. **SALINE A., A.** induced by injecting saline solution into the amniotic cavity, causing dehydration and death of the fetus; then oxytocic drugs are given intravenously, labor begins, and the fetus is expelled. Is usually done after the 12th week of pregnancy. Does not require a general anesthetic and hospitalization is short. **SEPTIC A.,** one associated with acute infection of the endometrium and myometrium and high fever; evacuation of the uterus is the usual life-saving procedure. **SPONTANEOUS A.,** unexpected expulsion of the products of conception before the 20th week of gestation. **THERAPEUTIC A.,** intentional termination of a pregnancy that is a threat to the mother's life. **THREATENED A.,** one with slight blood loss vaginally while the cervix remains undilated. **TUBAL A.,** tubal pregnancy in which the conceptus dies and is expelled from the fimbriated end of the fallopian tube.

abortionist (a-bor′-shun-ist): One who performs illegal abortions.

abortus (a-bor′-tus): 1. An aborted fetus; usually defined as one of less than 20 weeks gestation (139 days) calculated from the first day of the last menstrual period. The term is also used for uterine content that is expelled or extracted when it consists of only the placenta or part of it and membranes, and there is no identifiable fetus. 2. Any or all of the products of abortion.—**A. FEVER,** brucellosis (*q.v.*).

aboulia (a-boo′-li-a): Abulia (*q.v.*).

abrachia (a-brā′-ki-a): Congenital armlessness.

abrachiocephalia (a-brā′-ki-ō-sē-fā′-li-a): A malformed fetus that has neither head nor arms.

abrade (a-brād′): To rub, scrape away, wear

away, or roughen the skin or a mucous membrane.

abrasion (a-brā′-zhun): Superficial wound to the skin or mucous membrane caused by rubbing, scraping, or erosion; excoriation.—abrade, v., abrasive, adj.; abrasive, n.

abrasive (a-brā′-siv): 1. Causing abrasion. 2. An agent that erodes, scrapes off, or rubs off the surface or layer of a substance.

abreaction (ab-rē-ak′-shun): In psychoanalysis, a therapeutic reaction resulting from recall of a repressed idea or a traumatic experience or memory; may come about from gaining insight by talking to the analyst or under the influence of light anesthesia. See narcoanalysis. Syn., catharsis.

abrosia (a-brō′-zi-a): Starvation or abstinence from eating.

abruptio (ab-rup′-shē-ō): A tearing away; separation. A. PLACENTAE, a relatively rare occurrence usually happening prior to the third stage of labor in which there is separation of the placenta accompanied by vaginal bleeding in amounts depending on the degree of separation that occurs.

ABS: Acute brain syndrome. Any acute confusional or delirious state; usually of brief duration. Affects old and young and is reversible.

abscess (ab′-ses): Severe localized inflammation within a tissue or organ, acute or chronic, with formation of a cavity containing pus and debris from destruction of tissue by pyogenic organisms. ACUTE A., one characterized by heat, redness, swelling, pain, and pus formation ALVEOLAR A., one at the root of a tooth. ANORECTAL A., one in the tissues around the anus and rectum. APPENDICEAL A., one resulting from the perforation of an inflamed appendix. BLIND A., one with no external opening. BRAIN A., an intracranial A. involving the brain or its meninges; usually arising secondarily to infection elsewhere in the body, especially the ear or frontal sinus; characterized by headache, vomiting, delirium. BREAST A., one involving tissue of the mammary gland. BONE A., osteomyelitis (*q.v.*). BRODIE'S A., chronic osteomyelitis, usually occurring in the long bones and without an acute phase; most often seen in young adults. CEREBRAL A., brain A. CHRONIC A., one occurring in the course of a chronic inflammation; usually tuberculous; slow-growing with pus formation but slight or no inflammation. COLD A., chronic A. DRY A., one that dries up without breaking and draining. EPIDURAL A., one outside the dura but inside the cranium or spinal canal. HEPATIC A., one in the liver. HOT A., acute A. LUNG A., pulmonary A. LYMPHATIC A., one forming in a lymph node. MAMMARY A., breast A. METASTATIC A., a secondary A. forming at a distance from the source of infection. PELVIC A., one of the pelvic peritoneum, often involving the rectouterine pouch. PERINEPHRIC A., one in the kidney cortex or in the tissues surrounding the kidney. PERIODONTAL A., one arising in the periodontium. PERIPROCTIC A., one arising in the tissues around the rectum and anus. PERITONEAL A., one within the peritoneal cavity, frequently following peritonitis. PERITONSILLAR A., one that forms behind the tonsil as an extention of an infection of the tonsil; also called quinsy. PRIMARY A., one forming at the site of infection. PSOAS A., one in the psoas muscle, often resulting from tuberculosis of the lower lumbar vertebrae. PULMONARY A., nontuberculous A. of the lung with necrosis of tissue resulting in cavitation. RETROCECAL A., one posterior to the cecum, often resulting from a ruptured postcecal appendix. RETROPHARYNGEAL A., one involving the lymph nodes of the lateral and posterior walls of the pharynx. SECONDARY A., an embolic A. STERILE A., one that contains no culturable material. STITCH A., one that forms at the site of a suture. STREPTOCOCCAL A., one caused by a streptococcal organism. SUBDIAPHRAGMATIC A., one beneath the diaphragm, usually on the right side near or involving the liver. SUBDURAL A., one just under the dura mater. SUBPERIOSTEAL A., one forming under the periosteum. SUBPHRENIC A., subdiaphragmatic A. SUBUNGUAL A., one under the fingernail. SUDORIPAROUS A., one forming in a sweat gland. TONSILLAR A., acute suppurative tonsillitis. TUBERCULOUS A., one due to infection with the tubercle bacillus. TOOTH A., alveolar A.

abscission (ab-sish′-un): The cutting off of a body part or growth by surgery.

absentmindedness (ab-sent-mīnd′-ed-nes): Preoccupation or concentration so intense that one becomes detached from the surroundings.

absolute (ab-sō-lūt): Unlimited, unconditional. A. ALCOHOL, alcohol that contains less than 1 percent of water. A. REFRACTORY PERIOD, in electrocardiology, the period following depolarization of the heart muscle cells when they cannot respond to another stimulus regardless of its strength. A. THRESHOLD, the smallest amount of stimulus that can be detected by an organism.

absorb (ab-sorb′): 1. To suck up, draw up, take in, or imbibe other material, as a gas or fluid. 2. To take in, through the skin, as medicinal agents or certain rays. 3. The incorporation by body cells or tissues of substances from the blood or lymph.

absorbable (ab-sorb′-a-b′l): Capable of being absorbed. See a. ligature under ligature.

absorbefacient (ab-sor-be-fā′-shent): Causing absorption; an agent or medication that promotes or causes absorption.

absorbent (ab-sor′-bent): 1. Having the capability to absorb. 2. Any agent or substance that has the capability to absorb.

absorption (ab-sorp′-shun): 1. The assimilation, incorporation, or taking up of one substance by another, *e.g.*, liquids by solids, or gases by liquids or solids. 2. The passage of water and/or a dissolved substance through a body surface or membrane into the body fluids, tissues, or cells. 3. The taking up of heat by the body. 4. In nutrition, the taking up by the mucous membrane of the digestive tract of certain nutrients resulting from digestion, *i.e.*, water, glucose, alcohol, and certain drugs are taken up by the stomach, as well as calcium if protein and vitamin D are also present; water, electrolytes, carbohydrate, amino acids from proteins, fats, iron, and calcium—if vitamin D and protein are also present—are taken up by the small intestine; water and electrolytes are taken up by the large intestine while feces are being held awaiting evacuation. 5. In pharmacology, the process by which a drug is taken into the bloodstream; the speed and degree to which this is accomplished vary greatly and have a determining influence on the effect of a dose of a particular drug.

absorptive (ab-sorp′-tiv): Having the power or capability of absorption; absorbent.

abstinence (ab′-stin-ens): Voluntarily denying oneself some experience or substance that has provided gratification in the past, often something to which one has become habituated or addicted; especially certain drugs, food, alcohol, sexual intercourse.

abstract (ab′-strakt): In pharmacology, a preparation made from the soluble principle of a drug, or its fluidextract (*q.v.*), evaporated to twice the original strength of the drug. **A. THINKING,** the use of concepts and ideas independent of concrete objects.

abstraction (ab-strak′-shun): 1. The withdrawal of one or more constitutents of a compound or mixture. 2. The mental process of formulating abstract ideas. 3. A state of inattention resembling absentmindedness.

abtortion (ab-tor′-shun): The outward turning of both eyes simultaneously.

abulia (a-bōō′-li-a): Abnormal lack of ability to exercise will power; indecision or hesitancy in making decisions or performing voluntary acts; characteristic of certain psychoses and neuroses.

abulomania (a-bū′-lō-mā′-ni-a): A mental disorder characterized by indecision and loss of will power.

abused child: A child who has suffered repeated physical or psychological injury, sexual abuse, negligence, or maltreatment inflicted by a parent or parent surrogate. The abuse is often precipitated by minor irritations, family instability, or poverty, and may consist of fractures; burns; bruises; verbal or sexual abuse; failure to provide adequate food, housing, medical care, or emotional support.

AC: Alternating current, *i.e.*, an electrical current that reverses direction of flow periodically, usually many times a second.

Ac: Chemical symbol for actinium, a radioactive element found in uranium ore.

a.c.: Abbreviation for *ante cibum* [L.], meaning before meals.

acacia (a-kā′-sha): The dried exudate of various species of Acacia, a large woody plant found in warm climates. Used as an emollient and demulcent and sometimes intravenously in treatment of shock.

acalcicosis (a-kal-si-kō′-sis): A condition caused by prolonged deficiency in intake of calcium.

acalculia (a-kal-kū′-li-a): Loss or impairment of ability to do mathematical calculations; usually the result of a brain injury.

acampsia (a-kamp′-si-a): Loss or lack of flexibility or movement of a joint; see **ankylosis.**

acanth-, acantho-: Combining forms denoting spine, sharp, thorn, spinous.

acanthaceus (a-kan-thā′-shus): Having spikes or prickles, *e.g.*, prickle cells (*q.v.*).

acanthesthesia (a-kan-thes-thē′-zi-a): The abnormal sensation of being pricked with a sharp point or with needles.

acanthoameloblastoma (a-kan′-thō-a-mel-ō-blas-tō′-ma): An ameloblastoma (*q.v.*) composed of prickle type cells.

Acanthocephalus (a-kan-thō-sef′-a-lus): A genus of thorny- or spiny-headed worms, occasionally parasitic in man.

acanthocyte (a-kan′-thō-sīt): A misshapen erythrocyte with many protoplasmic projections giving it a horny appearance; may be hereditary; seen in such conditions as abetalipoproteinemia, severe rheumatic disease, gastric carcinoma, bleeding gastric ulcer.

acanthocytosis (a-kan′-thō-sī-tō′sis): The presence of acanthocytes in the blood; a characteristic of congenital abetalipoproteinemia.

acanthoid (a-kan′-thoid): 1. Resembling a spine. 2. Thorny.

acanthokeratodermia (a-kan′-thō-ker-a-tō-der′-mi-a): Thickening of the horny layer of the skin, particularly that of the hands and feet.

acantholysis (a-kan-thol′-i-sis): Separation of the layers of the skin, due to loss or lack of cohesion of the prickle cell layer to the layer above it.

acanthoma (a-kan-thō′-ma): 1. An inherited condition in which a nodule, or nodules, arises in the prickle cells of the epidermis. 2. A squamous cell tumor.

acanthosis (a-kan-thō′-sis): Thickening of the prickle-cell layer in the *stratum germinativum* of the epidermis, as occurs in psoriasis. **A.**

NIGRICANS, diffuse **A.** with gray to black hyperpigmentation, chiefly in the skin folds, especially of the axilla and groin.

acapnia (a-kap′-ni-a): A condition of diminished carbon dioxide content of the blood; sometimes used when hypocapnia is meant.—acapnial, adj.

acapsular (a-kap′-sū-lar): Without a capsule.

acarbia (a-kar′-bi-a): A decrease in the amount of bicarbonate in the blood.

acardia (a-kar′-di-a): Congenital absence of the heart.

acardiacus (a-kar-dī′-a-kus): Having no heart; usually refers to an underdeveloped member of a pair of twins.

acardiotrophia (a-kar′-di-ō-trō′-fi-a): Atrophy of the heart.

acariasis (ak-a-rī′-a-sis): Any disease caused by an infestation with mites; also called acarinosis.

acaricide (a-kar′-i-sīd): An agent that kills mites.

acarid (ak′-a-rid): A mite, tick, or other member of the order *Acarina* (*q.v.*).

Acarina (ak-a-rī′-na): A large order of the class Arachnida including the mites and ticks, some of which are vectors of important diseases.

acarinosis (a-kar-i-nō′-sis): Any disease caused by a mite.

acarodermatitis (ak′-ar-ō-der′-ma-tī′-tis): Inflammation of the skin, with urticaria and pruritus, caused by the bite of mites, often due to handling mite-infested plants.

acarophobia (ak′-ar-ō-fō′-bi-a): 1. Morbid dread of small organisms such as mites, ticks. 2. The delusion that the skin is infested with worms, mites, ticks or other small crawling organisms.

Acarus (ak′-ar-us): A genus of the arthropods, including many species of ticks and mites. The term is often loosely used to designate any mite. **A. SCABIEI** (*Sarcoptes scabiei*) or itch mite, a human parasite that causes scabies (*q.v.*).

acaryote (a-kar′-i-ōt): Non-nucleated, referring usually to cells; also spelled akaryote.

acatalasemia (a-kat′-a-lā-sē′-mi-a): A deficiency of the enzyme catalase in the blood; may be associated with ulceration and gangrene of the oral tissues.

acatalasia (a-kat-ā-lā′-zi-a): Absence of the enzyme catalase in the body cells, a rare congenital condition that predisposes the individual to recurrent infections of the gingiva and associated structures in the mouth.

acatalepsy, acatalepsia (a-kat′-a-lep-sē, -si-a): 1. Lack of understanding or comprehension; dementia; impairment of the mental processes. 2. A state of uncertainty of diagnosis.

acatamathesia (a-kat′-a-ma-thē′-zi-a): Lack or loss of ability to understand or comprehend, particularly speech; usually due to a central nervous system lesion.

acataphasia (a-kat-a-fā′-zi-a): Lack of power to express connected thought or to formulate sentences correctly; due to a brain lesion.

acataposis (a-kat-a-pō′-sis): Difficulty in swallowing; dysphagia.

acathexia (ak-a-thek′-si-a): Inability to retain bodily secretions or excretions.

acceleration (ak-sel-er-ā′-shun): 1. Increased speed or velocity of action, motion, or rate. 2. Change in velocity. 3. Advancement beyond normal in either physical or intellectual growth. 4. An increase in the rate of a chemical reaction.

acceleration-deceleration injury: One that occurs when the brain is thrown forward against the skull and then back against the opposite side of the skull; the injury at the first site is called "coup"and that at the second site "contrecoup."

accelerator (ak-sel′-e-rāt-or): 1. An agent, machine, or device that speeds up something, as a function or process. 2. A nerve or muscle that speeds up the performance of a bodily function.

accelerin (ak-sel′-er-in): Coagulation factor VI.

accelerometer (ak-sel-er-om′-e-ter): An instrument for measuring the velocity of an object, including both acceleration and deceleration; used by physical and rehabilitation therapists in treatment of diseased or weakened muscles, and to measure hand tremor.

accessory (ak-ses′-or-i): Supplementary; complementary; concomitant. **A. NERVES**, the 11th pair of cranial nerves.

accident (ak′-si-dent): A sudden, unforseen event that produces unintended injury, death, or property damage. **CEREBROVASCULAR A.**, one that occurs within the cerebrum, *e.g.*, cerebral hemmorrhage; abbrev. CVA. **ACCIDENT-PRONE**, said of one who appears to be more susceptible to accidents than the average person. **ACCIDENT-REPETITIVENESS**, having repeated accidents due to inexperience, age, or maladjustment to the environment; to be differentiated from accident-proneness.

acclimatization (a-klī′-ma-tī-zā′-shun): 1. The process of becoming accustomed to a new environment, especially to change in temperature and altitude. 2. Structural and physiologic changes, such as ventricular enlargement and pulmonary hypertension, which occur in people born and living in high altitudes but which do not interfere with normal activities as long as the person remains in the high altitude.

accommodation (a-kom-mō-dā′-shun): Adjustment or adaptation of an organ or a part to changing circumstances, particularly the automatic adjustment of the lens of the eye so that a distinct image is always obtained, regardless of the nearness or distance of the object being viewed

accouchement (a-koosh-mon′): Delivery in childbirth. Confinement.

accoucheur (a-koo-sher′): A male obstetrician (*q.v.*).

accoucheuse (a-koo-shuz′): A midwife or female obstetrician.

accountability (a-kown-ta-bil′-i-ti): In nursing, the obligation of answering for the results or outcomes of one's actions, as differentiated from responsibility which refers to what one *ought* to do. Traditionally, nurses have been accountable to the institution or physician employing them, but nurses now in expanding roles are also accountable to the patient just as hospitals and physicians are. See primary care nurse under nurse.

accreditation (a-kred-i-tā′-shun): In health care, a voluntary procedure of peer evaluation whereby an educational or health care facility and its program are regularly appraised and recognized as meeting the preset criteria of one or more accrediting agencies; not a legal procedure but often has the force of law, since graduation from an accredited school is often required for licensure to practice. The process involves setting standards, periodic inspections to determine whether the standards have been met, and official approval by the accrediting agency. Hospital and other health care facilities are accredited by the Joint Commission on Accreditation of Hospitals (*q.v.*); hospital accreditation remains in force for two years. The National League for Nursing accredits all nursing programs that award baccalaureate or higher degrees in nursing. The American Nurses'Association accredits continuing education programs for adult, pediatric, gerontologic, family nurse practitioners and several other nurse specialists. Some of the specialty organizations also accredit programs for nurse practitioners, *e.g.*, the National Association of Pediatric Nurse Associates and Practitioners.

accretion (a-krē′-shun): 1. An increase in substance or deposit around a central object. 2. Accumulation of foreign matter in a space or cavity. 3. Adherence or growing together of parts normally separate.

Ace bandage: See bandage.

acenesthesia (a-se-nes-thē′-zi-a): Lack or loss of awareness of one's physical existence, or of one's sense of well-being.

acentric (a-sen′-trik): 1. Not centrally located. 2. Having no center.

acephalia (a-se-fā′-li-a): A congenital anomaly with absence of the head. Acephaly.—acephalic, adj.

acephalobrachia (a-sef′-a-lō-brā′-ki-a): A congenital anomaly with absence of the head and arms.

acephalocardia (a-sef′-a-lō-kar′-di-a): A congenital anomaly with absence of the head and heart.

acephalocheiria (a-sef′-a-lō-kī′-ri-a): A congenital anomaly with absence of the head and hands.

acephalopodia (a-sef′-a-lō-pō′-di-a): A congenital anomaly with absence of the head and feet.

acephalorachia (a-sef′-a-lō-rā′-ki-a): A congenital anomaly with absence of the head and vertebral column.

acephalothoracia (a-sef′-a-lō-thō-rā′-si-a): A congenital anomaly with absence of the head and thorax.

acephalous (a-sef′-a-lus): Without a head.

acerbity (a-sur′-bi-ti): Acidity combined with astringency.

acerola (as-e-rō′-la): A West Indian shrub that produces a cherry rich in vitamin C.

acescence (a-ses′-ens): Sourness, tartness, or the process of becoming sour.

acescent (a-ses′-ent): Somewhat sour, tart, or acidulous.

acetabular (as-e-tab′ū-lar): Pertaining to the acetabulum (*q.v.*). **A. LIP**, a fibrocartilaginous ring that surrounds the acetabulum. Also called the glenoid labrum and labrum acetabulare.

acetabulectomy (as′-e-tab-ū-lek′-to-mi): Surgical removal of the acetabulum.

acetabuloplasty (as′-e-tab′-ū-lō-plas-ti): An operation to improve the shape and depth of the acetabulum, sometimes necessary to correct congenital dislocation of the hip, or to relieve osteoarthritis.

acetabulum (as-et-ab′-ū-lum): A cup-like socket on the external aspect of the innominate bone, into which the head of the femur fits to form the hip joint.—acetabula, pl.; acetabular, adj.

acetaldehyde (a-sēt-al′-dē-hīd): A colorless liquid with a pungent odor, resulting from oxidation of ethyl alcohol or from reduction of acetic acid; used in the manufacture of acetic acid, flavorings, and perfumes; produces profound narcosis and is extremely irritating to mucous membranes.

acetate (as′-e-tāt): Any salt of acetic acid.

acetic (a-sē′-tik): 1. Pertaining to acetic acid or vinegar. 2. Sour.

acetic acid (a-sē′-tik): The acid present in vinegar. In weak solution, serves as an antidote for alkaline poisons. Has several other uses in medicine.

acetification (a-sē′-ti-fi-kā′-shun): The production of acetic acid by the process of fermentation.

acetimeter (as-e-tim′-e-ter): An instrument for

measuring the amount of acetic acid in a solution.

acetoacetic acid (as-ē′-tō-as-ē′-tik as′-id): One of the ketone bodies formed in the body during the metabolism of fats. In some metabolic disturbances, *e.g.*, acidosis or diabetes mellitus, it is present in the blood in excessive amounts and appears in the urine; the excess in the blood may produce coma. Syn., diacetic acid.

Acetobacter (a-sē-tō-bak′-ter): A genus of aerobic, rod-shaped bacteria, important in the production of vinegar.

acetone (as′-e-tōn): An acrid, colorless, volatile, inflammable liquid with a sweetish odor; found in minute amounts in normal urine and in larger amounts in diabetic urine; used commercially as a solvent. **A. BODIES,** intermediate products in metabolism of fats that become greatly increased in the blood in diabetes mellitus, starvation, pregnancy, after anesthesia, and other conditions of disturbed metabolism. Also called ketone bodies. **A. BREATH,** breath with a fruity odor; usually refers to that of diabetic patients in a state of ketoacidosis.

acetonemia (as-e-tō-nē′-mi-a): The presence of large amounts of acetone bodies in the blood. Now usually called ketonemia.

acetonuria (as-e-tō-nū′-ri-a): Excess acetone bodies in the urine that give it a peculiar, sweet smell. Occurs in diabetes, carcinoma, fevers and some digestive disorders. Now usually called ketonuria.—acetonuric, adj.

acetous (a-sē′-tus, as′-e-tus): 1. Resembling acetic acid. 2. Sour tasting.

acetum (a-sē′-tum): Vinegar.

acetyl (a-sē′-til, as′-e-til): The monovalent radical, CH_3CO, of acetic acid.

acetylcholine (as′-e-til-kō′-lēn), a-sē′-til): A chemical substance normally present in various body tissues and organs; has several important physiological actions; is released from parasympathetic and voluntary nerve endings to activate muscle, secretory glands and nerve cells. Important in the transmission of nerve impulses across the synapse between one nerve fiber and another. The fibers that release this chemical are described as cholinergic.

acetylcholinesterase (as′-e-til-kō-lin-es′-ter-ās, a-se′-til-): An enzyme found in red blood cells, nervous tissue, and muscle; it is a catalyst in the hydrolysis of acetylcholine to choline and acetic acid.

acetylene (a-set′-a-lēn): A colorless gas with an unpleasant odor; combustible, it burns with a brilliant smoky flame; has been used as a general anesthetic and has some other uses in medicine.

acetylsalicylic acid (a-sē′-til-sal-i-sil′-ik, as′-e-til-): An odorless white crystalline powder, soluble in water; readily absorbed from mucous membranes, commonly used in medicine to reduce fever, relieve pain, and as an antirheumatic agent. Aspirin.

ACH: Abbreviation for adrenocortical hormone (*q.v.*).

achalasia (ak-a-lā′-zi-a): Failure to relax; often referring to sphincter muscles. **CARDIAC A.,** failure of the cardiac sphincter and lower part of the esophagus to relax to permit food to pass into the stomach, resulting in dilatation of the esophagus.

Achard–Thiers syndrome: A disorder of women, originating in the adrenal cortex; characterized by masculinization and menstrual disorders; also seen in women with glycosuria associated with diabetes mellitus.

ache (āk): A dull, continuous pain as differentiated from one that is sudden, spasmodic or intermittent; may be described according to severity, ranging from dull to severe, or according to location; *e.g.*, headache.

acheilia (a-kī′-li-a): Congenital absence of the lips.

acheiria (a-kī′-rē-a): 1. Congenital absence of one or both hands. 2. Inability to recognize which side of the body is being touched.

acheiropodia (a-kī-rō-pō′-di-a): Congenital absence of the hands and feet.

achievement (a-chēv′-ment): Accomplishment. **A. AGE.,** a figure obtained by testing; expresses the level of an individual's educational achievement as compared to that of the average child of the same chronological age. **A. QUOTIENT,** the ratio of a person's achieved educational age to his mental age. **A. TEST,** a standardized test used to measure a person's skill or knowledge in one or more fields of work or study.

Achilles (a-kil′-ēz): Mythical Greek warrior whose entire body was considered invulnerable to injury except the heel by which his mother held him when she immersed him in the river Styx. **A. BURSA,** the bursa between the tendon of Achilles and the calcaneus. **A. BURSITIS,** inflammation of the bursa between the tendon of Achilles and the posterior surface of the calcaneus. **A. REFLEX,** the knee jerk **R.,** see also under reflex. **A. TENDON,** the powerful tendon that attaches the gastrocnemius and soleus muscles to the posterior surface of the calcaneus; also called tendo calcaneus and calcaneal tendon.

achillobursitis (a-kil′-ō-bur-sī′-tis): Inflammation and swelling of the bursae around the tendon of Achilles.

achillodynia (a-kil-ō-din′-i-a): Pain in the Achilles tendon or its bursae.

achillorrhaphy (a-kil-or′-a-fi): A suturing operation on the tendon of Achilles.

achillotomy (a-kil-ot′-o-mi): Surgical division

of the Achilles tendon. Also called achillotenotomy.

achlorhydria (a-klor-hī′-dri-a): The absence of free hydrochloric acid in the gastric juice. Occurs in pernicious anemia, iron-deficiency anemia, gastric cancer, gastritis, pellagra, and sprue.—achlorhydric, adj.

achloropsia (a-klō-rop′-si-a): Color blindness for the color green.

acholia (a-kō′-li-a): 1. Lack or absence of bile. 2. Any condition that interferes with the flow of bile into the small intestine.

acholuria (a-kō-lū′-ri-a): Absence of bile pigments from the urine. See jaundice.—acholuric, adj.

achondroplasia (a-kon-drō-plā′-zi-a): A congenital, often familial, condition involving disordered chondrification and ossification at the ends of long bones, resulting in dwarfism; the arms and legs are short but the head and body are normal size; the intellect is not usually impaired. Syn., fetal rickets.—achondroplastic, adj.

achor (ā′-kor): 1. An eruption of small pustules, confined chiefly to hairy parts of the body. 2. A scaly eruption, occurring chiefly on the skin of the face and/or scalp of infants.

achoresis (ak-ō-rē′-sis): Permanent diminution of the capacity of a hollow organ, such as the stomach or bladder.

achro-: A combining form denoting colorless.

achroacyte (a-krō′-a-sīt): A colorless cell; a lymphocyte.

achroma (a-krō′-ma): Absence of color.

achromachia (a-krō-mak′-i-a): Grayness or whiteness of the hair.

achromacyte (a-krō′-ma-sīt): An erythrocyte that has lost its hemoglobin and hence is colorless.

achromasia (a-krō-mā′-si-a): 1. Lack of normal skin pigmentation. 2. Absence of normal staining reaction in cells or tissue. 3. Lack of pigmentation of the iris.

achromate (a-krō′-māt, ak′-rō-): A colorblind person.

achromatic (a-krō-mat′-ik): 1. Free from color. 2. Lacking normal pigment. 3. Not readily colored by staining agents.

achromatin (a-krō′-ma-tin): The faintly staining karyoplasm of a cell nucleus.

achromatism (a-krō′-ma-tizm): Color blindness.

achromatophil (a-krō-mat′-ō-fil): A cell or tissue that is not easily stainable.

achromatophilia (a-krō′-mat-ō-fil′-i-a): The property of resisting coloring by stains.

achromatopia (a-krō-ma-tō′-pi-a): Deficient color vision.

achromatopsia (a-krō-ma-top′-si-a): Complete color blindness

achromatosis (a-krō-ma-tō′-sis): Absence or deficiency of natural pigmentation, as in the iris or the skin.

achromatous (a-krō′-ma-tus): Colorless; nonpigmented.

achromaturia (a-krō-ma-tū′-ri-a): The voiding of very pale or colorless urine.

achromia (a-krō′-mi-a): Absence of color. Also achroma.

achromic (a-krō′-mik): Deficient in color.

achromoderma (a-krō-mō-der′-ma): A colorless state of the skin. Leukoderma.

achromotrichia (a-krō-mō-trik′-i-a): The absence or loss of hair color.

achromous (a-krō′-mus): Deficient in color; achromic.

achylia (a-kī′li-a): Absence of chyle (*q.v.*).—achylic, adj.

achylous (a-kī′-lus): 1. Lacking gastric and other digestive juices. 2. Deficiency or lack of chyle.

achymia (a-kī′-mi-a): Deficiency, or imperfect formation, of chyme.

acicular (a-sik′ū-lar): Shaped like a needle.

acid (as′-id): Any of a group of compounds which, in solution, has a pH of less than 7, turns blue litmus paper red, furnishes hydrogen ions when combined with a metal, and combines with a base to form a salt and water; may also be corrosive. In popular usage any substance with a sour, sharp, or biting taste.

acid intoxication: Severe acidosis causing a toxic condition of the body. May be due to accumulation of acid products resulting from faulty or incomplete oxidation of fats, or by acids introduced into the body from without.

acid phosphatase (fos′-fa-tās): An enzyme found in many tissues and fluids of the body, including the liver, spleen, pancreas, kidney, blood plasma, red blood cells, seminal fluid. In cancer of the prostate gland the serum A.P. is elevated.

acid rain: The cause of atmospheric pollution by sulphur dioxide contained in smoke from coal-burning power plants and smelters, and from nitrogen oxide coming from industrial sources and motor vehicles. It is transported through the atmosphere where it is changed chemically and falls as acidic rain, snow, fog or dust; destroys freshwater fish life, damages forests, crops, and buildings and may contaminate drinking water.

acid resistant: Not readily stained by acid dyes.

acid stomach: Lay term for a condition due to the formation of excessive acid in the stomach or to an acid residue left in the stomach by certain foods; marked by heartburn, belching, and pain in the upper part of the abdomen.

acidaminuria (as′-id-am-i-nū′-ri-a): The presence of an excess of amino acids in the urine.

acid-ash: Refers to foods that predominantly produce an acid ash when metabolized, including eggs, meat, fish, poultry, bread, cereals, pastries, puddings, cranberries, plums, prunes.

acid-base: 1. **ACID-BASE BALANCE,** a normal equilibrium or ratio between the acid and base elements of blood and body fluids. It is influenced by the level of hydrogen ion concentration in the blood. When the blood is in acid-base balance, the pH of the serum remains at 7.35 to 7.45, which is maintained by the regulating systems of the kidney, lungs, skin, adrenal gland and pituitary, and by the buffer system of the blood. 2. **ACID-BASE IMBALANCE,** the condition resulting from loss of the normal balance between the acidity and alkalinity of the blood and body fluids; it occurs in metabolic disturbances that accompany starvation, gastrointestinal diseases, diabetes mellitus, respiratory and renal diseases, toxemias; correction involves the buffer system of the blood and respiratory and renal regulatory actions.

acidemia (as-i-dē′-mi-a): Abnormal acidity of the blood, with a below normal pH. Cf. acidosis.

acid-fast: A bacteriological term describing a bacterium that stains with a basic dye and resists discoloration when treated with an acidic solution, *e.g.*, the *Mycobacterium tuberculosis*.

acidic (a-sid′-ik): Pertaining to or having the characteristics of an acid.

acidification (a-sid′-i-fi-kā′-shun): 1. The addition of acid to another substance. 2. Conversion of a substance or combination of substances into an acid.

acidifier (a-sid′-i-fī-er): 1. An agent that causes a substance to become acid in reaction. 2. An agent given to increase gastric acidity.

acidify (a-sid′-i-fī): 1. To become acid. 2. To render acid.

acidity (a-sid′-i-ti): The state or quality of being acid or sour and of being able to unite with basic substances. Sourness.

acidocyte (a-sid′-ō-sīt): A cell that takes acid stains easily. An eosinophil.

acidogenic (as-i-dō-jen′-ik): Producing acid, particularly in the urine.

acidophilic (as-id-ō-fil′-ik): Said of microorganisms taking acid stains readily or growing well in highly acid media.

acidophil(e) (as-id′-ō-fil, -fīl): 1. A cell or tissue that stains readily with an acid dye such as eosin. 2. A microorganism that grows well in an acid medium.

acidophilus milk (as-i-dof′-i-lus): Milk that has been fermented by *Lactobacillus acidophilus;* sometimes used to change intestinal flora.

acidosis (as-i-dō′-sis): A disturbance in the acid-base balance in the body, with a depletion of the alkali reserve, accumulation of acid, and lowering of the blood serum pH to below 7.35. May be secondary to some other condition; seen in diabetes mellitus, epilepsy, starvation, cyclic vomiting, diarrhea, and toxemias. Acidemia. **COMPENSATED A.,** results from changes in pulmonary or renal function that restore the normal pH of the blood. **DIABETIC A.,** produced by the accumulation of ketones (*q.v.*) in the blood of patients with uncontrolled diabetes; marked by a sweet fruity breath odor. **LACTIC ACID A.,** an accumulation of lactic acid in the tissues; may occur in circulatory failure, hypotension, malignancies, leukemia, or lymphoma; when severe it may be life threatening. **METABOLIC A.,** an increase in the pH of the blood, which may be the result of ingestion of acids, retention of acid products of metabolism, excessive loss of bicarbonate from the body, or excessive elimination of carbon dioxide from the lungs through hyperventilation. **MIXED A., A.** having a mixed cause, such as when shock and ventilatory failure occur simultaneously, producing both metabolic and respiratory **A. RENAL TUBULAR A.,** a syndrome characterized by inability to secrete acid urine, by low serum carbonate levels, and by high chloride levels; may occur in osteomalacia or nephrosclerosis. **RESPIRATORY A., A.** associated with a decrease in the exhalation of carbon dioxide and a consequent increase in the pCO_2 of the bloodstream; occurs in asthma, emphysema, pneumonia, and some other conditions that interfere with normal breathing.

acidosteophyte (as-i-dos′-tē-ō-fīt): A sharp pointed projection or outgrowth of bone.

acidotic (as-i-dot′-ik): Pertaining to or suffering from acidosis.

acidulate (a-sid′-ū-lāt): To render a substance more acid.

acidulent (a-sid′-ū-lent): Somewhat acid in taste or character.

acidulous (a-sid′-ū-lus): Moderately sour or acid.

aciduria (as-i-dū′-ri-a): The excretion of an acid urine.

aciduric (as-i-dū′-rik): 1. Capable of growing in strongly acid media. 2. Pertaining to aciduria.

acinar (as′-i-nar): Pertaining to an acinus or to acini.

Acinetobacter (as-i-nē′-tō-bak′-ter): A genus of aerobic, non-motile, non-spore forming bacteria which may appear as cocci or as short rods; often seen in clinical specimens. **A. CALCOACETICUS,** an opportunistic pathogenic organism sometimes seen in specimens from the genitourinary tract.

acini (as′-in-ī): Minute saccules or alveoli lined

or filled with secreting cells, found in various glands and organs; they cluster around a narrow lumen like grapes on a stem; several **A.** combine to form a lobule. Term commonly applied to the saclike termini of the small tubular passages in the lungs; sometimes used as a synonym for alveoli.—acinus, sing.; acinous, acinar, adj.

aciniform (a-sin′-i-form): Grapelike in structure

acinitis (as-i-nī′-tis): Inflammation of an acinus or the acini of a gland.

acinous (as′-i-nus): Made up of minute sacules or resembling a bunch of grapes.

ackee fruit poisoning (ah′-kē): Poisoning from eating the seeds or uncooked fruit of the ackee tree, commonly found in Jamaica. Also akee.

aclasis (ak′-la-sis): Extension of a structure, as a bone, by the growth of pathological tissue that arises from normal tissue. **DIAPHYSEAL A.,** a congenital affection marked by the formation of multiple exostoses at the metaphysial end of a long bone, sometimes causing deformity and reduction in longitudinal growth.

acleistocardia (a-klīs-tō-kar′-di-a): A condition in which the foramen ovale remains unclosed.

acme (ak′-me): 1. In illness, the time of greatest intensity of a symptom or symptoms. 2. The crisis or critical stage of a disease.

acmesthesia (ak-mes-thē′-zi-a): The sensation of pins pricking the skin.

acne (ak′-nē): A self-limiting inflammatory condition of the sebaceous glands, common in both sexes during adolescence. **A. CONGLOBATA,** severe, long-lasting **A.,** occurring mostly in males during late adolescence; characterized by burrowing abscesses and cysts, draining sinus tracts, severe scarring; systemic signs include elevated temperature, malaise, and arthralgia; lesions often form on the lower back, buttocks, and thighs as well as on the face. **A. MILIARIS,** a form in which many small white milia appear on the face. **A. PAPULOSA,** a form characterized by inflammatory papular lesions. **A. RHINOPHYMA,** a form of **A.** roseacea affecting chiefly the nose; often called whiskynose. **A. ROSACEA,** a pronounced erythema of the brow, cheeks and nose, resulting from dilatation of subcutaneous capillary vessels; seen mostly in adults and is aggravated by hot drinks, alcoholic drinks, and rich or fried food. **A. VULGARIS,** the most common form, which occurs chiefly in adolescents; comedones which develop into papules, and pustules appear on the face, neck and upper part of the trunk.

acnegenic (ak-ne-jen′-ik): Pertaining to substances thought to promote the development of acne vulgaris.

acneiform (ak-nē′-i-form): Resembling acne.

acnemia (ak-nē′-mi-a): 1. Congenital absence of the legs. 2. Atrophy of the muscles of the calves of the legs.

acognosia (ak-og-nō′-si-a): The science or knowledge of remedies, medical or surgical.

acolasia (ak-ō-lā′-zi-a): Morbid intemperance; lustfulness; self indulgence.

acolous (a-kō′-lus): Having neither upper or lower extremities.

acomia (a-kō′-mi-a): Baldness.

aconite (ak′-ō-nīt): A bitter tasting poisonous substance obtained from the dried rhizome of the *Aconitum napellus,* formerly much used in medicine as a local anesthetic, counterirritant, depressant, and diaphoretic.

acoprosis (ak-ō-prō′-sis): Absence or near absence of fecal matter in the intestine.

acorea (ah-kō-rē′-a): Congenital absence of the pupil.

acoria (a-kō′-ri-a): Continual hunger due to loss of the sensation of satiety; the appetite may not be large but the patient never feels that he has had enough to eat.

Acosta's disease: See altitude sickness.

acouesthesia (a-koo-es-thē′-zi-a): 1. The sense of hearing; acoustic sensibility. 2. Normal acuity of hearing.

acousma (a-kooz′-ma): An auditory hallucination in which one hears such nonverbal sounds as buzzing, ringing, hissing.

acousmatagnosis (a-kooz-ma-tag-nō′-sis): Inability to recognize spoken words. Also called mind deafness and auditory agnosia.

acousmatamnesia (a-kooz-ma-tam-nē′-zi-a): Lack or loss of the ability to remember sounds.

acoustic (a-koos′-tik): Pertaining to 1) the sense or organs of hearing, or 2) the science of sound. **A. NERVE,** the eighth cranial nerve, composed of the cochlear nerve, which is concerned with hearing, and the vestibular nerve, which is concerned with balance and equilibrium; also called vestibulocochlear n. **A. NEUROMA,** see under neuroma.

acoustics (a-koos′-tiks): The branch of physics that deals with sound and sound waves, their production, transmission, and reception, and with the phenomena of hearing and the perception of sounds.

acquired (a-kwīrd′): Not inherited; resulting from learning, experience, or other influences originating outside the organism after birth. **A. IMMUNITY,** any type of immunity that is not inherited. See immunity. **A. REFLEX,** same as conditioned reflex (*q.v.*).

acquired immunodeficiency syndrome (AIDS): A serious worldwide communicable disease in which the body's cellular immune system is suppressed leaving it defenseless against invasion by bacteria, viruses, fungi, parasites and tumors; introduced into the U.S. (possibly from Africa) in the early 1980s; caused by one of the retrovirus group of viruses. AIDS is transmitted by sexual contact between homosexual and bisexual men; by unsterilized needles and syringes used by drug addicts; and by contaminated blood used in transfusions (said to account for about one case in 100,000 transfusions). In addition, sexually active heterosexuals may transmit the disease (men may transmit it to women and vice versa); and mothers may transmit it to unborn fetuses. The disease has also occurred in aged persons and other sexually inactive debilitated individuals. The causative virus has been found in both saliva and tears but these secretions are probably not of any significance in transmission of the disease; blood and semen are the means of transmission in almost all cases. The risk of contracting AIDS through one exposure is thought to be minimal; repeated exposure appears to be necessary. When the disease is transmitted sexually, the virus most often enters the body through small breaks or tears in the mucous membrane of the rectum or vagina. The incubation period varies from several months to five or more years. Symptoms include fever, enlarged lymph glands, anorexia, severe weight loss, and diarrhea. The disease appears to be invariably fatal. A large number of deaths have resulted from pneumocystosis caused by the organism *Pneumocystis carinii* or from the development of Kaposi's sarcoma (*q.v.*).

acr-, acro-: Combining forms denoting: 1. An extremity of the body. 2. A tip end. 3. Extreme.

acral (ak′-ral): 1. Pertaining to an apex. 2. Pertaining to or affecting the peripheral parts of the body, *e.g.*, the ears, fingers, toes.

acrania (a-krā′-ni-a): Congenital absence of the skull or part of it.

acrasia (a-krā′-zi-a): Excess; intemperance; lack of self-control.

acratia (a-krā′-shi-a): 1. Loss of power or strength. 2. Impotence. 3. Incontinence.

acraturesis (a-krat-ū-rē′-sis): Inability to urinate normally, due to atony of the urinary bladder or obstruction in the urethra; may result in incontinence or slow dribbling of urine.

acrid (ak′-rid): Bitter, burning, irritating, pungent.

acritical (a-krit′-i-kal): Having no crisis, or not associated with a crisis, *e.g.*, an illness that resolves by lysis rather than crisis.

acroanesthesia (ak′-rō-an-es-thē′-zi-a): Lack or loss of sensation in the extremities, mostly in the hands and feet; often due to a pathological condition but may also follow general anesthesia.

acroarthritis (ak′-rō-ar-thrī′-tis): Inflammation of the joints of the hands and/or feet.

acroasphyxia (ak′-rō-as-fik′-si-a): Episodes of cyanosis, pallor, and red or blue mottling of the skin of the extremities, due to interference with the circulation; may follow exposure to cold or an emotional disturbance; associated with Raynaud's disease. Also called acrocyanosis.

acroataxia (ak′-rō-a-tak′-si-a): Lack of coordination of the muscles in the fingers and toes.

acrobrachycephaly (ak′-rō-brak-i-sef′-a-li): A congenital deformity of the skull which is abnormally high with a flattened top resulting in a shortened anterior-posterior dimension of the head.

acrocentric (ak-rō-sen′-trik): Usually refers to a chromosome in which the centrosome is located close to one end rather than being in the center.

acrocephalosyndactyly (ak′-rō-sef′-a-lō-sin-dak′-ti-li): A congenital condition characterized by acrocephaly, unnatural facies, webbing of the fingers and toes, obesity, underdeveloped genitalia, and, sometimes, mental retardation. Also called acrocephalosyndactylism and Apert's syndrome.

acrocephaly (ak-rō-sef′-a-li): A congenital malformation whereby the top of the head is more or less pointed, due to premature closure of the coronal, sagittal, and lambdoid sutures. Also called acrocephalia and oxycephaly.—acrocephalic, acrocephalous, adj.

acrochordon (ak-rō-kor′-don): A small, soft, pedunculated and usually benign skin growth, seen mostly on the eyelids, neck, groin, and axillae of older people, women in particular. Cutaneous tag.

acrocontracture (ak′-rō-kon-trak′-chur): Contracture of muscles and supportive tissues around a joint or joints of hand or foot, causing deformity.

acrocyanosis (ak′-rō-sī-a-nō′-sis): Cyanosis of the extremities. Often associated with chilblains when the skin may be bluish or reddish and mottled; usually due to a vaso-motor disturbance. In infants, the extremities are blue and cold while the cheeks and trunk are pink; usually due to faulty cardiopulmonary function; tends to clear with warmth. Also called acroasphyxia.—acrocyanotic, adj.

acrodermatitis (ak′-rō-der-ma-tī′-tis): Any inflammation of the skin of the arms and hands or of the legs and feet.

acrodolichomelia (ak′-rō-dol′-i-kō-me′-li-a): Disproportionately long or large hands and feet.

acrodynia (ak-rō-din′-i-a): A disorder seen mostly in infants and young children, characterized by irritability alternating with apathy;

pinkness of hands, feet, tip of nose, and cheeks; photophobia, diaphoresis, hypotonia, stomatitis, and insomnia. Also called pink disease and erythredema polyneuropathy.

acroedema (ak′-rō-ē-dē′-ma): Longstanding edema of the hands and feet.

acroesthesia (ak′-rō-es-thē′-zi-a): 1. Pain in the hands or feet. 2. Increased sensitiveness of the hands or feet.

acrogeria (ak-rō-jer′-i-a): Premature aging of the skin of the hands and legs with dryness, thinning, loosening, and wrinkling; tends to run in families.

acrognosis (ak-rog-nō′-sis): Sensory recognition of the presence of a limb, and of the relationship of various parts of the limbs to each other. Opp. of acragnosis (*q.v.*).

acrohyperhidrosis (ak′-rō-hī-per-hī-drō′-sis): Excessive sweating of the hands or feet, or both.

acrokeratosis (ak′-rō-ker-a-tō′-sis): A condition of the skin of the extremities, especially of the hands and feet, marked by the development of numerous horny growths.

acrolein (ak-rō′-lē-in): A volatile pungent liquid formed by the decomposition of glycerin; irritating to the gastrointestinal mucosa and the eyes. Used in chemical warfare.

acromacria (ak-rō-mak′-ri-a): "Spider" fingers; arachnodactyly (*q.v.*).

acromania (ak-rō-mā′-ni-a): A severe form of mania characterized by excessive motor activity and sometimes by muteness.

acromastitis (ak-rō-mas-tī′-tis): Inflammation of the nipple.

acromegaly (ak-rō-meg′-a-li): A fairly common chronic metabolic disorder, characterized by enlargement of the bones of the hands, face, and feet, and of the viscera. Occurs in adult life and is due to prolonged overproduction of growth-stimulating hormone by the pituitary gland.—acromegalic, adj.

acromelalgia (ak-rō-mel-al′-ji-a): Dilatation of the peripheral blood vessels of the hands and feet, causing headache; vomiting; redness, mottling, and burning pain in the palms and/or soles and then in the entire extremity; swelling of the toes and fingers. Also called erythromelalgia.

acromial (a-krō′-mi-al): Of or pertaining to the acromion.

acromicria (ak-rō-mik′-ri-a): A condition marked by smallness and delicacy of body extremities—fingers, toes, nose, jaws—and of the skull, as compared with the rest of the body; the antithesis of acromegaly; thought to be due to undersecretion of the growth hormone by the pituitary gland; may be hereditary.

acromioclavicular (ak-rō′-mi-ō-kla-vik′-ū-lar): Pertaining to the acromion process of the scapula and the clavicle.

acromiohumeral (ak-rō′-mi-ō-hū′-mer-al): Pertaining to the acromion and the humerus.

acromion (ak-rō′-mi-on): The point or summit of the shoulder; the triangular process at the extreme outer end of the spine of the scapula. It articulates with the clavicle. Also called acromial process.—acromial, adj.

acromphalus (a-krom′-fa-lus): 1. The center of the navel. 2. Undue projection of the navel.

acromyotonia (ak′-rō-mī-ō-tō′-ni-a): Myotonia (*q.v.*) of the hand or foot resulting in spastic deformity.

acroneuropathy (ak′-rō-nū-rop′-a-thi): Any nervous system disorder affecting primarily the distal parts of the body.

acronyx (ak′-rō-niks): An ingrowing nail.

acro-osteolysis (ak′-rō-os-tē-ol′-i-sis): Loss of bone substance from the ends of the fingers and sometimes the toes; may be familial in origin but may also be an occupational disease caused by exposure to vinyl chloride.

acropachyderma (ak′-rō-pak-i-der′-ma): A condition marked by thickening of the skin, especially that of the face, scalp, and extremities, along with clubbing of the fingers and other skeletal deformities usually associated with acromegaly; due to hypopituitarism.

acroparalysis (ak′-rō-pa-ral′-i-sis): Paralysis of the extremities.

acroparesthesia (ak′-rō-par-es-thē′-zi-a): A condition characterized by attacks of tingling, numbness, or stiffness of one or more of the extremities, particularly the hands and feet, often following sleep; occurs in women more often than men; additional symptoms include pain, pallor, cyanosis.

acropathy (ak-rop′-a-thi): Any disease or disorder of the extremities.

acropetal (a-krop′e-tal): Tending to rise upward toward a summit; said of certain infections.

acrophobia (ak-rō-fō′-bi-a): Morbid fear of being at a height.

acroposthitis (ak′-rō-pos-thī′-tis): Inflammation of the prepuce.

acrosclerosis (ak′-rō-sklē-rō′-sis): Hardening and thickening of the skin of the extremities, usually symmetrical, affecting chiefly the distal parts of the extremities as well as the neck and face, the nose especially; combined with features of Raynaud's disease (*q.v.*); occurs most often in women.

acrosome (ak′rō-sōm): The dense crescent-shaped body at the anterior tip of the spermatid (which becomes a spermatazoon).

acrospora (ak-rō-spō′-ra): In fungi, a spore that forms at the outer tip of a hypha (*q.v.*).

acrostealgia (ak-ros-tē-al′-ji-a): Pain in a bone; may refer to apophysitis in one or more bones of the extremities.

acrotic (a-krot′-ik): 1. Pertaining to the surface, especially to the glands of the skin. 2. Pertaining to a weak or absent pulse.

acrotism (ak′-rō-tizm): Extreme weakness or absence of the pulse.

acrotrophodynia (ak′-rō-trōf-ō-din′-i-a): Neuritis and paresthesia of the extremities resulting from prolonged exposure to cold and moisture. See trench foot under trench.

acrylic (a-kril′-ik): Pertaining to a type of cement used for anchoring prosthetic devices or metallic implants to the skeleton.

acrylic resin (a-kril′-ik rez′-in): Any of a group of several thermoplastic substances derived from acrylic acid; has many commercial uses including the manufacture of prosthetic devices including contact lenses.

ACTH: Abbreviation for adrenocorticotrophic hormone (*q.v.*).

actin (ak′-tin): A protein in the filaments of muscle fibers which, along with myosin particles, acts to cause contraction and relaxation of muscles.

acting out: 1. Coping with one's feelings and expressing them in action rather than words. In psychiatry, the expression of anxiety or emotional conflict in undesirable, possibly dangerous, behavior, *e.g.*, stealing or arson. 2. Dramatization or play therapy, in which individuals are encouraged to freely express their emotional conflicts as part of a therapeutic regimen.

actinic (ak-tin′-ik): Pertaining to radiation, particularly that which produces a chemical effect such as that from x ray or the light rays beyond the violet end of the spectrum. **A. CARCINOMA,** basal cell carcinoma occurring on exposed body surfaces as a result of prolonged exposure to x ray or sunlight. **A. DERMATITIS,** dermatitis resulting from exposure to sunlight, ultraviolet rays, or x rays. **A. KERATOCONJUNCTIVITIS,** see under keratoconjunctivitis. **A. KERATOSIS,** see under keratosis.

actinobiology (ak′-ti-nō-bī-ol′-o-ji): The study of the effects of radiation on living organisms.

actinochemistry (ak′-ti-nō-kem′-is-tri): The branch of chemistry concerned with the reaction produced by actinic radiation. Also called radiochemistry.

actinodermatitis (ak′-ti-nō-der-ma-tī′-tis): Inflammation of the skin resulting from exposure to the sun, ultraviolet light, or x rays.

actinogen (ak-tin′-ō-jen): Any substance that has the property of producing rays, especially actinic rays.—actinogenesis, n.; actinogenic, adj.

actinolite (ak-tin′-ō-līt): 1. Any substance that undergoes marked change when exposed to light. 2. A greenish mineral.

actinometer (ak-ti-nom′-e-ter): An instrument for measuring the intensity and penetrating power of actinic rays.

Actinomyces (ak′-ti-nō-mī′-sēz): A genus of gram-positive microorganisms of the order *Actinomycetales* that grow in long branching filaments; consists of several species; parasitic in man and some animals. **A. ISRAELI,** the species of **A.** that causes actinomycosis in man.

Actinomycetaceae (ak′-ti-nō-mī′-sē-tā′-se-ē): A family of *Schizomycetes* (*q.v.*) consisting of a group of aerobic forms called *Nocardia* and a group of anaerobic forms called *Actinomadura*.

Actinomycetales (ak′-ti-nō-mī′-se-tā′-lēs): An order of *Schizomycetes* which includes the families *Actinomycetaceae, Mycobacteriaceae, Streptomycetaceae,* and *Actinoplanaceae*.

actinomycete (ak-ti-nō-mī′-sēt): Any organism of the order *Actinomycetales*.

actinomycoma (ak′-ti-nō-mī-kō′-ma): A swelling or tumor due to actinomycosis (*q.v.*):

actinomycosis (ak′-ti-nō-mī-kō′-sis): An infrequent, subacute or chronic systemic disease of man and some animals, caused by a species of the genus Actinomyces. In man, the disease is caused by *Actinomyces israeli,* normally found in the mouth, tonsillar crypts and intestine, and which may be the cause of actinomycosis following tooth extraction, gum infection, inhalation of the organism into the bronchi, or an inflammatory condition of the stomach or intestine. Man may also become infected by handling infected animals or through a human bite. The disease is characterized by the formation of deep subcutaneous nodules or tumors that are first livid and hard, then suppurate and rupture, forming fistulous tracts that discharge an oily pus containing yellow granules. Sites most often affected are the jaw, lung, brain, and intestine.—actinomycotic, adj.

actinon (ak′-ti-non): A short-lived radioactive isotope of radon; radon-219.

actinoneuritis (ak′-ti-nō-nū-rī′-tis): Neuritis resulting from repeated or prolonged exposure to x rays or radium. Radioneuritis.

antinophage (ak-tin′-ō-fāj): Any virus that destroys actinomycetes.

actinotherapy (ak′-tin-ō-ther′-a-pi): Treatment by rays of light such as ultraviolet or infrared rays.

actinotoxemia (ak′-ti-nō-tok-sē′-mi-a): Toxemia resulting from the use of radiation; radiation sickness.

action: The performance of an activity or function by any part of the body or by the whole body. **ANTAGONISTIC A.,** 1) in physiology, the action of a muscle or group of muscles that limits the action of an opposing muscle or muscles; 2) in pharmacology, a drug action that opposes the effect of another drug. **BUFFER A.,**

the prevention, by certain chemical substances, of change in a body system or function, as in pH or blood pressure. **COMPULSIVE A.**, one performed independently of one's will or conscious motivation. **CUMULATIVE A.**, sudden increase in intensity of the action of a drug following repeated doses. **REFLEX A.**, an involuntary **A.** in response to a sensory stimulus. **SYNERGISTIC A.**, 1) the working together of two or more muscles to accomplish what one muscle could not do alone, or 2) the **A.** of one drug in increasing the effect of another drug.

action potential: The complete cycle of changes in the self-propagating electric impulses set up in the cell membrane of a nerve or muscle cell, or other excitable tissue, in response to a stimulus during which depolarization and repolarization of the nerve or muscle fiber takes place.

activation (ak-ti-vā'-shun): The process of rendering active or activating, as the action of a pre-enzyme on an enzyme. In nuclear physics, the process of bombarding a material with nuclear particles to make it radioactive.

activator (ak'-ti-vā-tor): A substance that renders something else active or one that converts an inactive substance into an active one.

active: Energetic; working; moving; functioning or capable of functioning. Not passive. **A. IMMUNITY,** that acquired naturally by having the disease or artificially by vaccination. **A. MOVEMENTS,** those consciously produced by the individual. **A. PRINCIPLE,** the constituent of a compound or drug that gives it its chief value or characteristic. **A. TRANSPORT,** in physiology, the energy-expending process of moving a substance across a membrane between two areas of differing concentration. **A. TREATMENT,** vigorous medical or surgical treatment, with the objective of curing the illness, not just allaying the symptoms.

activism (ak'-ti-vizm): In health care, refers to practice that emphasizes direct action in seeking cures rather than employing palliative treatment for illness. **THERAPEUTIC A.**, the extent to which a physician will intervene to attempt a cure.

activities of daily living: The activities performed by an individual for himself in the course of a normal day, *e.g.*, eating, dressing, toileting, bathing, exercising, etc. Abbreviated ADL.

activity (ak-tiv'-i-ti): The quality or state of being active; alertness. **A. THERAPY,** the therapeutic use of a variety of activities, *e.g.*, physical, social, diversional. **A. THEORY,** a theory of aging that holds that the more older people continue to engage in the activities they enjoyed earlier in life, the better off they will be both physically and mentally.

actomyosin (ak-tō-mī'-ō-sin): A complex network of actin and myosin in the muscle fibrils which contract when stimulated and thus are responsible for the contraction and relaxation of muscles.

acuity (a-kū'-i-ti): Sharpness, clearness, keenness, distinctness. **AUDITORY A.**, ability to hear clearly and distinctly. Tests include the use of tuning fork, whispered voice and audiometer. In infants, simple sounds, *e.g.*, bells, rattles, cup and spoon are utilized. **VISUAL A.**, extent of visual perception; dependent on the clarity of retinal focus, integrity of nervous elements and cerebral interpretation of the stimulus. Usually tested by Snellen's letters. See **Snellen's test type.**

acuminate (a-kū'-mi-nāt): Having a sharp point; or having a conical shape that tapers to a fine point.

acupoint (ak'-ū-poynt): Specific sensitive points on the surface of the body which are precisely described in the Chinese explanation of the theoretical foundation for acupuncture, acupressure, and moxibustion as being located on "conduits of energy." Stimulation at these points may affect the function or sensitivity of a specific area or body part. Also called acupuncture points.

acupressure (ak'-ū-presh-ur): 1. Pressure on a small surface area of the body by the fingertips or pointed object. 2. Pressure on a bleeding blood vessel to control hemorrhage by the insertion of needles into the tissues surrounding the vessel.

acupuncture (ak'-ū-pungk-chur): 1. The practice of inserting needles or fine hollow tubes at precisely located points of the body and then rapidly twirling them to produce counterirritation, to withdraw fluid as a therapeutic measure, or to produce anesthesia. Based on the Chinese theory that all body organs are connected through a system of subcutaneous pathways through which the essence of life flows, that an excess or deficiency in the flow to a body part results in pain and disease, and that needles inserted at specific points along the line of flow will correct the condition. 2. A vaccination method that utilizes a device that makes multiple small punctures in the skin.

acus (ā'-kūs): 1. A needle, particularly a surgical needle. 2. A sharp needle-like process.

acusector (ak'-ū-sek-tor): A surgical needle that operates on a high frequency current; used for cutting tissue.

acusis (a-kū'-sis): Normal perception of sound. Also acousis.

acute (a-kūt'): Short, sharp, severe, with definite symptoms, and of sudden onset. **A. ABDOMEN,** term for a serious condition that may be due to inflammation, ulceration, obstruction, or perforation of an abdominal organ, or some other pathological condition; requires immediate surgery. **A. BRAIN SYNDROME,** an acute state of delirium or confusion, assumed to be of structural origin; affects individuals of all ages; may be brief and reversible, or may progress to chronic brain syndrome. **A. HEART FAILURE,** serious impairment or failure of heart function in an individual not previously diagnosed as having heart disease. **A. RENAL FAILURE,** sudden decrease in output of urine resulting in rapid accumulation of metabolic waste products in the body; may be a postoperative complication or due to ingestion of toxic material. **A. YELLOW ATROPHY,** diffuse necrosis of the liver, often a result of viral hepatitis. **A. RESPIRATORY DISTRESS SYNDROME,** see under respiratory distress syndrome.

acute care (a-kūt'): Care rendered to a person whose illness is characterized by sudden onset and brief duration. **ACUTE CARE FACILITY,** a hospital department or medical center for diagnosis and management of short-term illnesses and emergency health problems.

acute compartment syndrome: A condition occcurring in a compartment of the hand, forearm, shoulder, buttock, thigh, or leg, most often in the leg; usually follows trauma caused by fracture or surgery that results in swelling of the muscle tissue that causes constriction of a nerve or tendon and severe ischemia and pain that increases when the person is at rest or on passive stretch of the part.

acyanopsia (a-sī-a-nop'-si-a): Inability to perceive or distinguish the color blue.

acyanotic (a-sī-a-not'-ik): Without cyanosis.

acyesis (a-sī-ē'-sis): 1. Absence of pregnancy. 2. Sterility in the female. 3. Inability of a woman to have a normal delivery.—acyetic, adj.

acystia (a-sis'-ti-a): Congenital absence of the urinary bladder.—acystic, adj.

acystinervia (a-sis-ti-ner'-vi-a): Paralysis of the bladder due to defective nervous tone.

Acystosporidia (a-sis'-tō-spō-rid'-i-a): An order of parasitic sporozoa that includes the genus *Plasmodium,* the causative organism in malaria.

a. d.: Abbreviation for *auris dextra* (L), meaning right ear. Also written A.D.

ad-: Prefix denoting to, toward, before, near, adjacent. May change to ac- before c, k, or q; af- before f; ag- before g; al- before l; ap- before p; as- before s; at- before t.

-ad: Suffix denoting toward, in the direction of.

ad lib: Abbreviation for *ad libitum* [L.], meaning at pleasure, without restraint, as much as desired.

ad nauseam (ad naw'-sē-am): To the point of nausea or of producing nausea.

adacrya (a-dak'-ri-a): The absence of tears.

adactylia (a-dak-til'-i-a): A congenital anomaly characterized by absence of fingers or toes, or both. Also adactylism, adactyly.—adactylous, adj.

adamantine (ad-a-man'-tin): 1. Pertaining to a hard, unbreakable substance. 2. Pertaining to dental enamel.

adamantinoma (ad'-a-man-ti-nō'-ma): See ameloblastoma.

Adams-Stokes disease, syndrome, or **syncope:** A disease condition characterized by sudden attacks of unconsciousness or convulsions, due to inadequate blood flow to the cerebrum; often associated with heart block.

Adam's apple: Common name for the laryngeal prominence in the front of the neck, especially in the adult male, formed by the junction of the two wings of the thyroid cartilage.

adaptability (ad-ap-ta-bil'-i-ti): The ability to adjust mentally and physically to new or changed circumstances.

adaptation (ad-ap-tā'-shun): 1. Mental and physical change that results in adjustment to a situation or condition in the environment. 2. Any beneficial change made to meet environmental change. 3. The ways in which the body counteracts stress. 4. The action of the eye in adjusting to variations in the intensity of light. 5. The decline in receptivity of a receptor when a stimulus is delivered constantly. 6. The development, in microorganisms, of resistance to antibiotic agents. **DARK A.,** the adaptation of the eye to vision in conditions of darkness; see rhodopsin.

adapter (a-dap'-ter): 1. A device that makes it possible to fit two instruments or pieces of apparatus together. 2. A device that converts electric current from one form to a different form, required by certain electrical appliances.

adaptive (a-dap'-tiv): Having a tendency toward, or the capacity for adaptation.

adaxial (ad-ak'-si-al): Directed toward or lying alongside an axis.

addicologist (ad-i-kol'-o-jist): A physician who specializes in the study and treatment of addictions.

addict (ad'-ikt, ad-ikt'): 1. One who is physically dependent on, or unable to resist indulgence in some practice or habit, such as the use of alcohol. 2. To devote oneself to something obsessively, *e.g.,* gambling, or to cause someone else to become addicted to a practice or habit.—addiction, n.; addictive, adj.

addiction (a-dik'-shun): The condition of having established the practice of yielding to something that is habit forming to the extent that discontinuing the practice causes severe physiological and psychological symptoms. In health care, a state in which therapeutic use of an addictive drug to control such symptoms as intractable pain has created a dependence wherein discontinuing the drug would result in severe distress symptoms. **ENDEMIC A.,** occurs in groups wherein addiction to certain substances is socially acceptable. **EPIDEMIC A.**, refers to a situation in which a high rate of **A.** occurs at a specific time and place. **IATROGENIC A.**, results from the regular use of drugs for the relief of severe or intractable pain. **POLYSURGICAL A.**, the habitual seeking of surgical treatment.

Addis count method: A laboratory method of counting the red and white blood cells, epithelial cells, casts, and protein content in a specific amount of a 12-hour urine specimen; useful in making diagnoses and in assessing prognoses and treatment.

addisonian (ad-i-sō′-ni-an): Pertaining to Addison's disease. **A. ANEMIA**, see under anemia. **A. CRISIS**, adrenal crisis; see under adrenal.

addisonism (ad′-i-son-izm): 1. A symptom complex sometimes seen in persons with pulmonary tuberculosis; includes weight loss, weakness, pigmentation of the skin, but not due to disease of the adrenal gland and not severe enough to be classified as Addison's disease. 2. Temporary dysfunction of the adrenal cortex.

Addison's anemia: Pernicious anemia. See anemia.

Addison's disease: Chronic adrenocortical insufficiency; characterized by reduced adrenal steroid production resulting from slowly progressive destruction of the adrenal cortex which may occur as a sequel to tuberculosis or some other systemic infection or disorder, or it may be idiopathic in origin. Characteristic symptoms include electrolytic upset, diminution of blood volume, hypotension, marked anemia, high serum potassium, bronze-like pigmentation of the skin, anorexia, gastrointestinal upsets, weight loss with emaciation, weakness, fatigability, decreased tolerance to cold, emotional disturbances, depression. [Thomas Addison, English physician, diagnostician, teacher. 1763-1860.]

additive (ad′-i-tiv): Any substance added to another to strengthen, improve, or diversify its action.

adduct (ad-dukt′): To draw toward the midline of the body or toward a neighboring part. Opp. to abduct. In optics, to turn the eyes inward.

adduction (ad-duk′-shun): 1. The drawing of a part of the body toward the midline, or of a part toward an adjacent part, or the result of such motion. Opp. to abduction. 2. The act of turning inward. 3. In optics, the turning of the eyes inwardly; may be a voluntary act or occur unconsciously as in accommodation.—adduction, n., adductent, adj.

adductor (ad-duk′-tor): Any muscle that moves a part toward the median axis of the body. Opp. to abductor.

aden-, adeno-: Combing form denoting gland or glands.

adenalgia (ad-e-nal′-ji-a): Pain in a gland.

adenasthenia (ad′-en-as-thē′-ni-a): Weakness or deficiency in the functioning of a gland.

adendritic (a-den-drit′-ik): Pertaining to a cell that has no dendrites.

adenectomy (ad-e-nek′-to-mi): 1. Surgical removal of a gland or lymph node. 2. Surgical removal of an adenoid growth.

adenemphraxis (ad′-e-nem-frak′-sis): Obstruction of the duct of a gland by whatever cause.

adenitis (ad-e-nī′-tis): Inflammation of a gland or lymph node. **CERVICAL A.**, inflammation of lymph nodes in the neck. **HILAR A.**, inflammation of bronchial lymph nodes. **MESENTERIC A.**, inflammation of lymph nodes in the mesenteric portion of the peritoneum; symptoms include pain resembling that of appendicitis but is less localized. **TUBERCULOUS A.**, swelling and induration of lymph nodes, usually cervical and most often painless; occurs in children more often than adults; caused by certain strains of the tubercle bacillus; may result in a chronic draining fistula.

adenocarcinoma (ad′-e-nō-kar-sin-ō′-ma): A malignant growth of glandular tissue. **ENDOMETRIAL A., A.** of the lining of the uterus; fairly common in women 55–65 years of age and those who have had few or no children. **VAGINAL A.**, usually an extension of cervical or endometrial carcinoma; has been found in young women whose mothers were treated with diethylstilbesterol for threatened abortion; extensive involvement of the lymphatics often results in death in about 5 years.—adenocarcinomatous, adj.; adenocarcinomata, pl.

adenocele (ad′-e-nō-sēl): A benign cyst-like tumor of glandular origin.

adenocellulitis (ad′-e-nō-sel-ū-lī′-tis): Inflammation of a gland and surrounding tissue.

adenochondroma (ad′-e-nō-kon-drō′-ma): A mixed tumor made up of both glandular and chondromatous tissue, as sometimes occurs in a salivary gland.

adenocystoma (ad′-e-nō-sis-tō′-ma): A benign epithelial gland-like tumor with cysts.

adenodynia (ad′-e-nō-din′-i-a): Pain in a gland.

adenoepithelioma (ad′-e-nō-ep-i-thē-li-ō′-ma): A tumor composed of glandular and epithelial cells.

adenofibroma (ad′-e-nō-fī-brō′-ma): A tumor composed of fibrous connective tissue and some glandular elements.

adenogenous (ad-e-noj′-e-nus): Of glandular origin.

adenohypersthenia (ad′-e-nō-hī′-per-sthē′-ni-a): Overactivity of a gland or glands.

adenohypophysis (ad′-e-nō-hī-pof′-i-sis): The anterior lobe of the pituitary gland. It secretes several important hormones: growth hormone, which helps control the metabolism of proteins, fats, and carbohydrates, and influences normal growth; thyrotropin, which stimulates thyroid activity; adrenocorticotropic hormone, which stimulates activity of the adrenal cortex; and the gonadotropic hormones including 1) the follicle-stimulating hormone; 2) the luteinizing hormone, and 3) the lactogenic hormone; all of which help control the development and functioning of the sex glands.

adenoid (ad′-e-noid): 1. Resembling a gland. 2. In the plural, refers to overgrowth of lymphoid tissue (the pharyngeal tonsil) in the nasopharynx. **A. FACIES,** the facial expression characteristic of a person with enlarged adenoids; the mouth is open, the nose appears pinched due to interference with nasal breathing.

adenoidectomy (ad′-e-noyd-ek′-to-mi): Surgical removal of adenoid tissue from the nasopharynx.

adenoiditis (ad′-e-noyd-ī′-tis): Inflammation of the nasopharyngeal adenoid tissue.

adenolipoma (ad′-e-nō-lī-po′-ma): A tumor having the characteristics of both an adenoma and a lipoma.

adenolymphitis (ad′-e-nō-lim-fī′-tis): Inflammation of the lymph glands. Lymphadenitis.

adenolymphocele (ad′-en-ō-lim′-fō-sēl): A cyst developing in a lymph node.

adenolymphoma (ad′-e-nō-lim-fō′-ma): An adenoma of a gland, particularly of a salivary gland.

adenoma (ad-e-nō′-ma): A tumor of glandular epithelial tissue; usually benign, but when occurring in the thyroid gland may be associated with carcinoma. **ADRENAL CORTICAL A.**, a benign tumor of adrenal cortical cells; may be associated with Cushing's disease or be symptomless. **BRONCHIAL A.**, a circumscribed **A.** occurring in the submucosal tissue of the large bronchi; now considered to be a low-grade malignancy. **EOSINOPHILIC A.**, a tumor of the anterior lobe of the pituitary gland; it results in acromegaly and gigantism; associated with bone weakness and sterility. **HEPATIC A.**, a benign neoplasm of the liver, sometimes seen in the newborn; associated with the use of oral contraceptives; because the tumor is highly vascular, there is danger of rupture of the liver and hemoperitoneum. **A. SEBACEUM**, a manifestation of tuberous sclerosis in the facial skin, chiefly of the fibrovascular tissue. **VILLOUS A.**, a large polyp (*q.v.*) on the mucosa of the large intestine.—adenomatoid, adj.

adenomalacia (ad′-e-nō-ma-lā′-shi-a): Abnormal softness of a gland.

adenomatoid (ad-e-nō′-ma-toyd): Resembling or pertaining to an adenoma.

adenomatosis (ad′-e-nō-ma-tō′-sis): A condition marked by the development of multiple granular adenomatous growths within an organ or in the organs of a system, *e.g.*, the endocrine system.

adenomatous (ad-en-ō′-ma-tus): Pertains to an adenoma or a nodular overgrowth of a gland.

adenomyofibroma (ad′-e-nō-mī′-ō-fī-brō′-ma): A fibroma that contains elements of both glandular and muscular tissue.

adenomyoma (ad′-en-ō-mī-ō′-ma): A tumor, usually benign, composed of muscle and glandular elements of the endometrium of the uterus.—adenomyomatous, adj., adenomyomata, pl.

adenomyosarcoma (ad′-e-nō-mī′-ō-sar-kō′-ma): A malignant tumor of glandular tissue that contains striated muscle tissue.

adenomyosis (ad′-en-ō-mī-ō′-sis): The benign overgrowth of glands and muscular tissue. **A. UTERI**, a general enlargement of the uterus due to overgrowth of the myometrium.

adenomyositis (ad′-e-nō-mī-ō-sī′-tis): Endometriosis (*q.v.*).

adenomyxoma (ad′-e-nō-mik-sō′-ma): A benign tumor that contains adenomatous and mucous elements, *e.g.*, a mixed tumor of the salivary glands.

adenoncus (ad-e-nong′-kus): An enlargement of a gland or a mass composed of large glands.

adenopathy (ad-e-nop′-a-thi): Any disorder of a gland, especially a lymphatic gland, that is characterized by swelling or enlargement.

adenopharyngitis (ad′-e-nō-far-in-jī′-tis): Inflammation of the adenoids and pharynx most often including the tonsils.

adenosarcoma (ad′-e-nō-sar-kō′-ma): An adenoma with elements of sarcoma.

adenosclerosis (ad′-e-nō-sklē-rō′-sis): Hardening of a gland with or without swelling, usually due to replacement by fibrous tissue or calcification.—adenosclerotic, adj.

adenose (ad′-e-nōs): Pertaining to or resembling a gland.

adenosine (a-den′-ō-sēn): A nucleoside derived from nucleic acid by the process of hydrolysis. **A. MONOPHOSPHATE,** an ester that has important influence on the release of energy by cells for muscular activity; abbreviated AMP. **A. DIPHOSPHATE,** a compound derived from adenosine triphosphate; a necessary substance for the production of energy by cells and needed for a variety of physical processes; abbreviated ADP. **A. TRIPHOSPHATE,** coenzyme produced by cells and used by cells to produce energy for a variety of energy-requiring activities, chiefly muscular activities; abbreviated ATP.

adenosis (ad-e-nō′-sis): 1. Any disease of a gland, especially of a lymph gland. 2. Development of an unusually large number of glandular elements without formation of a tumor.

adenotome (ad′-e-nō-tōm): A scissors-like instrument for removing the adenoids.

adenotomy (ad-e-not′-o-mi): The incision or dissection of a gland.

adenotonsillectomy (ad′-en-ō-ton-sil-ek′-to-mi): Surgical removal of the adenoids and tonsils.

adenovirus (ad′-e-nō-vī′-rus): Many types have been isolated. Some cause upper respiratory infection, others pneumonia, others tumors, still others epidemic keratoconjunctivitis.

adeps (ad′-eps): Lard or animal fat. Formerly used as a base in ointments.

adermia (a-der′-mi-a): 1. Congenital absence of skin. 2. A defect in the skin.

ADH: Abbreviation for antidiuretic hormone. See under antidiuretic.

adhesion (ad-hē′-zhun): 1. The holding together, or adhering of two substances that may be of similar or dissimilar nature. 2. In physics, the force exerted between the molecules of two substances that are in contact. 3. The joining together by fibrous tissue of bodily parts or tissues that are normally separate. 4. A band of fibrous tissue that holds together two body tissues or surfaces that are not normally in contact. 5. In the pleural, the fibrous bands that may develop following surgery or inflammation; in the abdomen they may cause obstruction; in the joints they cause restriction of movement.—adherent, adj.; adherence, n.; adhere, v.

adhesiotomy (ad-hē-zi-ot′-o-mi): The surgical division or removal of adhesions.

adhesive (ad-hē′-siv): 1. A substance that causes two substances or materials to adhere to each other. 2. Sticky. 3. Tending to cling or stick together. **A. TAPE,** tape with a sticky substance on one side; has many uses including holding bandages and dressings in place.

adiadochokinesia (a-dī′-ō-dō-kō-kī-nē′-zi-a): Inability to perform fine coordinated movements in rapid succession, *e.g.*, pronation and supination of the hand. Usually indicates cerebellar disturbance.

adiaphoresis (a′-dī-a-for-ē′-sis): Deficiency of visible perspiration.—adiaphoretic, adj.

adiaphoretic (a′-dī-a-for-et′-ik): 1. Pertaining to or characterized by absence or deficiency of visible perspiration. 2. An agent that causes reduction of or prevents sweating.—adiaphoresis, n.

Adie's syndrome: A condition in which one pupil reacts more slowly than the opposite one, and only after prolonged stimulation. Also called Adie's tonic pupil, Adie's pupil, and pseudo-Argyll-Robertson pupil. [W.J. Adie, English physician. 1886-1935.]

adipectomy (ad-i-pek′-to-mi): The surgical removal of adipose tissue. Lipectomy.

adipo-: A combining form denoting fat, fatty tissue.

adipocele (ad′-i-po-sēl): A hernia in which the sac contains only fat or fatty tissue. Lipocele.

adipocyte (ad′-i-pō-sīt): A specialized cell for the storage of fat. Syn., adipocyte; lipocyte.

adipofibroma (ad′-i-pō-fī-brō′-ma): A lipoma that contains some fibrous elements.

adipogenous (ad-i-poj′-e-nus): Producing fat.

adipokinin (ad′-i-pō-kī′-nin): A hormone secreted by the anterior pituitary that mobilizes fat, causing an increase in the serum level of fatty acids.

adipoma (ad-i-pō′-ma): A tumor made up of fat or fatty tissue. Lipoma.

adiponecrosis (ad′-i-pō-nē-krō′-sis): The necrosis of fatty tissue.

adipose (ad′-i-pōz): 1. Pertaining to fat. 2. Fat, fatty, or of a fatty nature. **A. TISSUE,** connective or areolar tissue containing masses of stored fat cells.

adiposis (ad-i-pō′-sis): Obesity; corpulence; fatness; abnormal deposit of fat in the body as a whole or in any of its parts.

adipositis (ad′-i-pō-sī′-tis): Inflammation of the fatty tissue under the skin.

adiposity (ad-i-pos′-i-ti): A condition in which the proportion of fat to the body weight is excessive, although the total weight may not be more than normal for the individual's body build.

adiposogenital dystrophy (ad′-i-pō-sō-jen′-i-tal dis′-trō-fi): A syndrome in which there is an increase in body fat, especially around the torso, hips, and thighs; underdevelopment of genital organs and changes in secondary sex characteristics; loss of hair; and metabolic disturbances. May be caused by disorder or dysfunction of the pituitary and hypothalamus, or by trauma, tumor, or encephalitis. Affects primarily adolescent boys. Syn., Froelich's syndrome; adiposogenital syndrome.

adiposuria (ad-i-pō-sū′-ri-a): The presence of fat in the urine.

adipsia (a-dip′-si-a): Absence of the sensation of thirst; avoidance of taking fluid by mouth.

aditus (ad′-it-us): In anatomy, an entrance or opening to an organ or part.

adjunct (ad′-junkt): Something attached to another thing but in a dependent or helping position; may be a procedure, a substance such as a drug, or a treatment mode.—adjunctive, adj.

adjustment: 1. The mechanism by which the tube of a microscope is raised or lowered thus bringing the object into focus. 2. In psychology, the alteration or accommodation by which an individual adapts himself and his actions to the environment.

adjuvant (ad′-joo-vant): That which aids, assists, or supports. In pharmacology, a substance included in a prescription that enhances the action of the principal constituent. **A. THERAPY,** therapy that utilizes supportive measures or substances that enhance the effects of the main treatment.

ADL: Abbreviation for activities of daily living.

Adler's theory: Holds that neuroses arise as a result of the individual's drive to overcome feelings of inferiority, either social or physical, through compensation.

Administration on Aging (AOA): A federal agency established under the former Department of Health, Education and Welfare. The principal organization designed to carry out the provisions of the Older Americans Act of 1965. Functions within the Department of Health and Human Services. Activities are concerned with programs for the elderly; also serves as a national clearing house and source of educational materials on aging, including statistics, books, pamphlets, and a monthly news magazine. Address: Office of Human Development, U.S. Department of Health and Human Services, Washington, DC 20402

ADN: Abbreviation for Associate Degree in Nursing (*q.v.*).

adnasal (ad-nā′-zal): Toward the nose, or situated near the nose.

adnexa (ad-nek′-sa): Body structures that are in close proximity to a part; appendages or accessory parts. **A. OCULI,** the lacrimal apparatus and other appendages of the eye. **A. UTERI,** the ovaries, uterine tubes, and uterine ligaments.—adnexae, pl.; adnexal, adj.

adnexitis (ad-nek-sī′-tis): Inflammation of adnexa, the adnexa uteri in particular.

adnexopexy (ad-nek′-sō-pek-si): The surgical fixation of the fallopian tube and ovary.

adolescence (ad-ō-les′-sens): The age that begins with puberty, extends through the years of physical and psychological maturation and ends with the completion of bone growth; often referred to as the teens.—adolescent, adj.

adolescent (ad-ō-les′-ent): 1. A person in the period between childhood and adulthood, who has reached puberty but has not fully matured; usually referred to as a teenager. 2. Pertaining to adolescence.

adoral (ad-or′-al): Situated near the mouth or directed toward the mouth.

adorbital (ad-or′-bi-tal): Toward or near the orbit of the eye.

ADP: Abbreviation for adenosine diphosphate.

adrenal (ad-rē′-nal): 1. Near the kidney. 2. One of two small triangular hormone-secreting glands that lie on the superior surface of each kidney, consisting of two parts: a) the medulla, the inner part, which secretes epinephrine and norepinephrine; and b) an outer part, the cortex, which secretes cortisone, aldosterone and testosterone. The cortical secretions have important actions in the control of many body functions including growth and weight changes, basal metabolism regulation, neuromuscular activity, gastrointestinal function, maintenance of body fluid balance, reproduction. Functionally, the **A.** glands are closely related to the pituitary and other endocrine glands. **A. INSUFFICIENCY,** hypofunction of the adrenal gland; Addison's disease (*q.v.*). **A. CRISIS,** acute adrenal failure, *e.g.*, a severe exacerbation of Addison's disease. **A. STEROIDS,** hormones secreted by the adrenal cortex. See also epinephrine, norepinephrine, cortisone, aldosterone, testosterone.

adrenal cortical hyperplasia: See adrenogenital syndrome.

adrenal cortical insufficiency: Failure of secretion of glucocorticoid and mineralocorticoid hormones by the adrenal cortex.

adrenalectomy (ad-rē-na-lek′-to mi): Surgical removal of all or part of one or both adrenal glands for treatment of Cushing's syndrome, pheochromocytoma, hypertension, malignant disease of the breast, or other adrenal disorder; if bilateral, requires replacement administration of cortical hormones.

Adrenalin: Trade name for epinephrine (*q.v.*).

adrenaline (a-dren′-a-lēn): British designation for epinephrine.

adrenalinemia (a-dren′-a-lin-ē′-mi-a): The appearance of epinephrine in the blood.

adrenalinuria (a-dren′-a-lin-ū′-ri-a): The presence of epinephrine in the urine.

adrenalism (a-dren′-a-lizm): Any pathologic condition due to dysfunction of the adrenal glands.

adrenalitis (a-drē-na-lī′-tis): Inflammation of one or both adrenal glands.

adrenarche (ad-ren-ar′-kē): 1. Increased activity of the adrenal cortex which induces menstruation and other physical signs of puberty. 2. The physiologic changes that occur at puberty due to the secretion of androgenic hormones by the adrenal cortex.

adrenergic (ad-re-ner′-jik): Pertains to 1) sympathetic nerve fibers that release epinephrine at their endings when stimulated, or 2) the chemical activity characteristic of epinephrine and like substances on nerve endings. **A. BLOCKING AGENTS,** compounds that inhibit responses to adrenergic nerve activity and to norepinephrine and like substances; classified according to their selective activity as alpha and beta, the beta group being in most common use. **A. CRISIS,** a condition characterized by overactivity of the part of the sympathetic system that is activated by epinephrine, causing epinephrine intoxication with symptoms of arrhythmia, tachycardia, hypertension, anxiety, dilated pupils, and often psychotic behavior.

adrenocortical (ad-rē′-nō-kor′-ti-kal): Pertaining to or originating in the adrenal cortex.

adrenocorticoid (ad-rē′-nō-kor′-ti-koyd): 1. Pertaining to the adrenal cortex or its hormonal secretion. 2. An adrenal cortical hormone. **A. STEROIDS,** endocrine secretions of the adrenal cortex; see **aldosterone, cortisone, deoxycorticosterone.**

adrenocorticosteroid (ad-rē′-nō-kor′-ti-kō-stē′-roid): A hormone that is elaborated in the cortex of the adrenal gland. See **corticosteroid.**

adrenocorticotropic (ad-rē′-nō-kor′-ti-kō-trōp′-ik): Having a hormonic effect on the cortex of the adrenal gland. See **corticotropin.** Also adrenocorticotrophic.

adrenocorticotropic hormone (ad-rē′-nō-kor′-ti-kō-trōp′-ik hor′-mōn): A secretion of the anterior lobe of the pituitary gland; it stimulates the release of the corticoid steroids from the adrenal cortex. Abbreviated ACTH. Syn., adrenocorticotropin.

adrenogenic (a-drē-nō-jen′-ik): Produced or originating in the adrenal glands.

adrenogenital syndrome (ad-rē′-nō-jen′-i-tal sin′-drōm): A congenital or acquired condition resulting from overproduction of androgenic hormones by the adrenal cortex; may be due to hyperplasia or tumor. In female children it is usually evident at birth by pseudohermaphrodism; in male children it is not usually evident until the child is three or four years old and is represented by precocious sexual development. In adults the syndrome is characterized by masculinization in women and feminization in men.

adrenoleukodystrophy (ad-rē′-nō-lū′-kō-dis′-tro-fi): A progressive, inherited, metabolic disorder of children; characterized by bronzing of the skin, adrenal insufficiency, and degeneration of the white matter in various parts of the central nervous system.

adrenolytic (ad′-ren-ō-lit′-ik): 1. Inhibiting or antagonizing the action or secretion of epinephrine. 2. Having a depressing effect on sympathetic (adrenergic) nerve fibers.

adrenomedullary (ad′-ren-ō-med′-ū-lar-i): Pertaining to the adrenal medulla.

adrenomegaly (ad-ren-ō-meg′-a-li): Enlargement of the adrenal glands.

adrenopathy (ad-ren-op′-a-thi): Any disease of the adrenal glands.

adrenosterone (ad-rēn-os′-ter-ōn): A male sex hormone present in the adrenal cortex.

adrenotropic (ad-ren-ō-trō′-pik): Pertaining to the adrenal gland, or having an effect on it; said particularly of the cortex.

Adson maneuver: A test for scalenus anticus syndrome (*q.v.*). The limb to be tested is kept hanging down while the head is rotated toward the ipsilateral shoulder; the test is positive if the radial pulse is obliterated.

adsorb (ad-sorb′): To attract or collect on its surface the molecules of a gas, liquid, or other substance.

adsorbate (ad-sor′-bāt): A substance that adheres to the surface of another substance by adsorption.

adsorbent (ad-sorb′-ent): 1. Having the quality of adsorption (*q.v.*). 2. An agent that has the quality of adsorption, *e.g.*, charcoal, which adsorbs gases and acts as a deodorant.

adsorption (ad-sorp′-shun): The process by which a gas, liquid, or other substance is collected and concentrated at the surface of another substance.

adtorsion (ad-tor′-shun): Inward turning of both eyes simultaneously.

adult (ad′-ult, a-dult′): 1. A person who is fully developed and mature. 2. A person who has reached legal age. 3. Pertaining to persons who are fully developed and mature. 4. Having attained full growth, maturity, and reproductive ability.

adult day care: May be given in a day care hospital or in a health care program sponsored by a community service organization; the aim is to save costs of hospitalization and to promote rehabilitation. The patients are transported to the facility for the day and taken home for the night.

adult respiratory distress syndrome (ARDS): See under **respiratory distress syndrome.**

adulterant (a-dul′-ter-ant): Any substance that when added to another substance renders it impure, imperfect, cheapened, or changed in some way.

adulteration (a-dul-ter-ā′-shun): The addition of an impure, cheap, or inferior substance to another substance with a deliberate attempt to alter that substance and to deceive the user; the usual implication is that the original substance is thereby rendered less effective, less desirable, weaker, or cheaper.—adulterant, n.

adulthood (a-dult′hood): The state of being fully developed, mature, and capable of reproduction.

advancement: In surgery, an operation in which a muscle or tendon is severed and reattached farther forward. Specifically, the operation to remedy strabismus; the muscle tendon opposite to the direction of the squint is detached and sutured to the sclera at a point farther from its origin.

adventitia (ad-ven-tish′-i-a): The external coat of an organ or structure, especially that of an artery or vein.—adventitiae, pl.; adventitious, adj.

adventitious (ad-ven-tish′-us): 1. Coming from the outside; external; not inherent. 2. Appearing sporadically in other than the usual location. 3. Pertaining to adventitia. **A. SOUNDS,** abnormal sounds, as in the lungs, *e.g.*, rales, rhonchi.

advocate (ad′-vō-kāt): A person who acts for or defends the rights of, another person who is unable or unwilling to act for himself. **PATIENT A.,** the primary nurse becomes the patient's advocate through her responsibilities for meeting the patient's needs through nursing activities done for the patient and/or his family.

adynamia (a-di-nā′-mi-a): Lack or loss of normal vitality or vigor; asthenia. **A. EPISODICA HEREDITARIA,** a form of periodic paralysis, usually accompanied by hyperkalemia and minor degrees of myotonia; also called Gamstorp's disease.—adynamic, adj.

Aëdes (a-ē′-dēz): A large genus of mosquitoes, many of which are vectors of important human diseases. **A. AEGYPTI,** the principal vector of yellow fever and dengue.

AEG: Abbreviation for air encephalography. See pneumoencephalography.

AEIOU TIPS: An acronym useful in assessing seizure disorders; refers to *a*lcoholism, *e*pilepsy, *i*nsulin, *o*verdose, *u*nderdose, *t*rauma or *t*umor, *i*nfection, *p*sychiatric, and *s*troke.

-aemia: See -emia.

aer-, aero-: Combining form denoting relationship to: 1. Air or atmosphere. 2. Gas. 3. Aviation.

aerate (ā′er-at): 1. To charge a substance with air or a gas such as carbon dioxide or oxygen. 2. To supply the blood with oxygen, by respiration, or by artificial ventilation.—aerated, adj.

aeration (ā′er-a′-shun): 1. Exposing to or supplying with air. 2. Charging a fluid with gas or air. 3. The process, which occurs within the lungs, whereby the CO_2 in the blood is exchanged for O_2.—aerate, v.; aerated, adj.

aeremia (ā′er-ē′mi-a): An air embolism.

Aerobacter aerogenes: Enterobacter aerogens; see under Enterobacter.

aerobe (ā′-er-ōb): A microorganism that requires oxygen for growth and life. **FACULTATIVE A.,** a microorganism that can grow and live either with or without oxygen. **OBLIGATE A.,** a microorganism that can grow and live only in the presence of free oxygen.—aerobic, adj.

aerobic (a′-er-ō′-bik): 1. Pertaining to an aerobe(s). 2. Pertaining to the utilization or requirement of oxygen in order to live and grow. **A. EXERCISE,** steady, continuous movement of the arms, legs, and trunk which forces a continuous flow of blood (and oxygen) through the heart and muscles but which is not vigorous enough or continued long enough to produce metabolic acidosis; includes jogging, walking, dancing, swimming, bicycling. See anaerobic exercise under anaerobic.

aerobiology (ā′er-ō-bī-ol′-ō-ji): The branch of biology that deals with the distribution by the air of fungus spores, microorganisms, minute insects, and pollen particles as well as smoke, dust, and other polluting substances.

aerocele (ā′er-ō-sēl): A tumor or swelling consisting of air that has collected in an abnormally formed sac or pouch, most often occurring in the trachea or larynx. **INTRACRANIAL A.,** an **A.** formed in the cranium; may occur following compound fracture of the skull.

aerocolpos (ā′er-ō-kol′-pos): Distention of the vagina with gas or air.

aerocoly (ā′er-ok′-o-li): Distention of the colon by gas.

aerocystoscopy (ā′-er-ō-sis–tos′-ko-pi): Examination of the urinary bladder with a cystoscope after the bladder has been distended with air.

aerodermectasia (ā′er-ō-der-mek-tā′-zi-a): Subcutaneous emphysema; see emphysema.

aerodynamics (ā′er-ō-dī-nam′-iks): The science and study of air and gases in motion.

aeroembolism (ā′er-ō-em′-bō-lizm): A condition that occurs particularly in aviators, when it is caused by rapid ascent to great heights, and in deep sea divers when returning to the surface from great depths. Nitrogen bubbles form in body tissues and fluids, causing symptoms that include rash, pain in the joints and lungs, itching, neuritis, paresthesia, sometimes paralysis and coma. Patients having head, neck, or heart surgery may also exhibit these symptoms.

aerogastrocolia (ā′-er-ō-gas-trō-kō′-li-a): Air or gas in the stomach and colon.

aerogen (ā′-er-ō-jen): Any gas-producing microorganism.

aerogenesis (a′-er-ō-jen′-e-sis): The production of gas.—aerogenic, adj.

aerogenous (a′-er-oj′-e-nus): 1. Gas producing. 2. Descriptive of organisms that produce gas; *e.g.*, Welch's bacillus (*q.v.*).

aerogram (ā′-er-ō-gram): An x ray of a hollow organ or structure after it has been filled with air or gas.

aerohydrotherapy (ā′-er-ō-hī-drō-ther′-a-pi): The use of air and water in therapeutics.

aeromammography (a′-er-ō-ma-mog′-ra-fi): X ray of mammary gland after it has been injected with air or a gas.

aeromedicine (a′-er-ō-med′-i-sin): Aviation medicine (*q.v.*).

aeroneurosis (a′-er-ō-nū-rō′-sis): A chronic functional psychoneurosis, occurs in aviators; caused by prolonged periods of anoxia and stress; characterized by gastric distress, insomnia, worry, loss of self-confidence, and various other physical and emotional symptoms.

aero-otitis media (ā′-er-ō-ō-tī′-tis mē′-di-a): Inflammation of the middle ear due to trauma caused by the difference between atmospheric and intratympanic pressure that develops when an aircraft descends rapidly from a high altitude.

aeropathy (ā′-er-op′-a-thi): Any pathological condition caused by change in atmospheric pressure, *e.g.*, decompression sickness, commonly called "the bends."

aerophagia (ā′-er-ō-fā′-ji-a): Air swallowing followed by belching and distention of the stomach and colon; a habit associated with nervous or digestive disorders. Syn., aerophagy.

aerophil (ā′-er-ō-fil): An organism that requires air or oxygen for growth and life. Also said of an individual who loves to be in the open air.

aerophobia (ā′-er-ō-fō′-bi-a): Abnormal dread of air, particularly fresh air, drafts of air, or bad air. 2. Abnormal dread of being up in the air, as of flying.

aerophyte (a′-er-ō-fīt): An organism that lives on air or oxygen.

Aeroplast: A spray-on dressing for burns, wounds, surface lesions.

aeroplethysmograph (a′-er-ō-ple-thiz′-mo-graf): An apparatus for measuring and registering the amount of air inspired and expired.

aerosinusitis (a′-er-ō-sī-nus-ī′-tis): See barosinusitis.

aerosol (a′-er-ō-sol): A suspension of atomized solid or liquid particles in air or a gas which is dispensed in a fine mist. Aerosols containing drugs are used in inhalation therapy for several pulmonary conditions. Bactericidal aerosols are sprayed into a room as a disinfectant. Aerosols containing chemicals are used in mosquito and insect control projects, and as deodorants. **A. SEAL,** plastic resin dissolved in ether; when sprayed onto a wound it forms a flexible adhesive seal. **A. THERAPY,** the use of aerosol or of a nebulizer that creates a vapor containing particles of a drug in a gas stream to help liquefy secretions and aid in their removal from the bronchial tree.

aerosol sniffing: The inhalation of hair spray, deodorants, household cleansers or other aerosol sprays by spraying them into a paper bag which is held over the head or face to be inhaled; causes a strange floating kind of high; has been known to cause death from cardiac arrest; most victims are teenagers.

aerosolization (ā′-er-ō-sol-ī-zā′-shun): The production or dissemination of something by spraying it in a fine mist. In bacteriology, the introduction of microorganisms into the atmosphere from contaminated articles, *e.g.*, by shaking out bed linen.—aerosolize, adj.

aerotitis (ā′-er-ō-tī′-tis): See barotitis. **A. MEDIA,** inflammation of the middle ear, caused by the difference between the atmospheric pressure and the air pressure in the middle ear, or by rapid descent in an airplane.

aerotonometer (ā′-er-ō-tō-nom′-e-ter): An apparatus for determining the tension of gases in the circulating blood.

Aesculapius (es-kū-lā′-pē-us): The Roman name for the mythological Greek god of medicine and healing, the son of Apollo and father of Hygeia, the goddess of health, and of Panakeia (Panacea), the goddess of "all healing." The main seat of his worship and his healing temple were in Epidauras. Also spelled Asclepius, Asclepios. **STAFF OF AESCULAPIUS,** the symbol of medicine and healing; consists of a rod or staff with a snake entwined about it; the insignia of several medical societies including the American Medical Association.

aesthesio-: See esthesio-

AF: Abbreviation for atrial fibrillation.

AFB: Abbreviation for acid-fast bacillus. See acid-fast.

afebrile (a-feb′-ril): Without fever.

affect (af′-ekt): The outward manifestation of a feeling or mood evoked by a stimulus; may be directed toward anything. In psychiatry, that aspect of the mind that is concerned with emotions, mood, or the external representation of mood. The term is often used interchangeably with emotion or feeling.—affective, adj.

affection (a-fek′-shun): 1. An emotional or feeling state. 2. Any disease or disorder, physical or mental. See affect.

affective (a-fek′-tiv): Pertaining to affect.

affective disorders: Categorized as neurotic, this group includes as the major affective disorders the bipolar disorders mixed, manic, and depressed (*q.v.*), as well as **MAJOR DEPRESSION,** both single episodic and recurrent. The specific affective disorder group includes **CYCLOTHYMIC DISORDER** which is characterized by periods of hypomania and depression which may be mixed or alternating, and **DYSTHYMIC DISORDER** in which there is a chronic depressed mood that may be persistent or intermittent. The atypical affective disorder group includes **ATYPICAL BIPOLAR DISORDER** in which the manic features cannot be classified under bipolar disorder or cyclothymic disorder, and **ATYPICAL DEPRESSION** in which the individual has depressive symptoms that cannot be classified under other affective disorders.

afferent (af′ - er-ent): Conveying a fluid or impulse to or toward a center; term used to designate nerves, blood vessels and lymphatics that perform this function. **A. NERVE,** a bundle of nerve fibers that carry impulses from the periphery to the central nervous system; receptors connect directly to them. Often synonymous with sensory nerve. **A. PATHWAYS,** neural structures that conduct information from the periphery to the central nervous system. Cf. efferent.

affinity (a-fin′ -i-ti): Attraction, or a common inherent relationship. In chemistry, the attractive force between two substances. In immunology, the attractive force between antibody and antigen.

afflux (af′ -luks): The rush of blood or other body fluid to a part, causing congestion.

affusion (a-fū′ -zhun): The act of pouring water on the body or a part of it; usually to reduce fever or nervousness.

afibrinogenemia (a-fī′ -brin-ō-jen-ē′ -mi-a): A rare congenital or acquired blood disorder characterized by a deficiency or absence of fibrinogen in the blood plasma. More correctly, hypofibrinogenemia.—afibrinogenemic, adj.

AFP: Abbreviation for alpha-fetoprotein.

African trypanosomiasis (trip′ an-ō-sō-mī′ -a-sis): An acute, infectious, highly fatal disease, particularly of tropical Africa; caused by the *Trypanosoma gambiense;* transmitted to man by the bite of a tsetse fly which has become infected by having previously bitten an infected man or animal. Often called African sleeping sickness and Gambian trypanosomiasis.

afterbirth: The placenta, umbilical cord, and fetal membranes that are expelled from the uterus following the birth of a child.

aftercare: Care, including but not confined to medical care, that is given during and after convalescence and rehabilitation. **AFTERCARE CLINIC,** a health care facility that continues, in modified form, treatment begun in a hospital or other facility; assists the patient in preparing to return to community life and serves as a protection should a new crisis occur during convalescence.

afterhearing: The persistence of the sensation of sound after the cessation of whatever stimulus produced the sound; may be a sympton of a nervous system disorder.

afterimage: The continued retinal impression of an object that persists after the object has been removed. Called positive **A.** when the image is seen in its natural bright colors, negative **A.** when the bright parts become dark while the dark parts become light.

afterloading (af-ter-lō-ding): The placing of a needle or applicator within a patient during surgery and later loading it with radioactive material.

afterpains: The cramp-like pains felt during the first few days following childbirth and the expulsion of the afterbirth; due to contraction of the uterine muscle fibers.

aftersensation (af-ter-sen-sā′ -shun): The persistence of a sensation after cessation or removal of the stimulus that caused it.

aftertaste (af′ -ter-tāst): Persistence of the sensation of taste after cessation of the stimulus that initiated it.

afunctional (ā-funk′ -shun-al): Without function or lacking normal function.

Ag: Chemical symbol for silver.

A/G ratio: See albumin-globulin ratio.

agalactia (a-ga-lak′ -shi-a): Lack of secretion, or imperfect secretion of milk following childbirth.—agalactic, adj.

agalorrhea (a-gal-ō-rē′ -a): Absence or arrest of the flow of milk.

agammaglobulinemia (a-gam′ -a-glob′ -ū-lin-ē′ -mi-a): A rare congenital or acquired disorder in which there is an absence or serious deficiency of gamma globulin in the blood plasma, resulting in inability of the body to produce immunity to infection.—agammaglobulinemic, adj.

aganglionosis (a-gang-gli-on-ō′ -sis): Congenital absence of parasympathetic ganglion cells, as occurs in congenital megacolon; see Hirschprung's disease; megacolon.

agar, agar-agar (ahg′ -ar): A gelatinous substance obtained from certain marine algae. It is used as a bulk-increasing laxative, a bacterial culture medium, and a suspending agent in emulsions. **A. STREAK SLANT,** agar slanted in a test tube on which bacteria are planted for culture. **BLOOD AGAR,** nutrient agar to which blood has been added. **CHOCOLATE AGAR,** agar or a nutrient boullion to which heated blood is added, turning the blood brown; it does not contain chocolate. **NUTRIENT AGAR,** a straw-colored culture medium composed of peptone, meat extract, sodium chloride, and agar.

agastria (a-gas′ -tri-a): Having no stomach.

age: 1. The amount of time that has passed since an individual was born, as measured in time units. 2. A particular period of life, *e.g.*, middle age. 3. To produce, artificially, the effects of age. 4. To grow old. **AGE OF CONSENT,** the age at which one is presumed to be capable of giving consent; refers particularly to marriage or to giving voluntary consent for sexual intercourse; usually considered to be between 13 and 19 years. **ACHIEVEMENT A.,** the expression, in years, of a child's intellectual development as compared with his chronological age; determined by proficiency tests. **ANATOMICAL A.,** one's age as expressed in the chronological age of an average person showing the same body development. **BIOLOGICAL A.,** the estimate of a person's physical status with respect to his potential life span; determined by x rays of the bones. **CHRONOLOGICAL A.,** the actual number of years a person has lived. **DEVELOPMENTAL A.,** a person's age as estimated from his anatomical development. **EMOTIONAL A.,** one's age as estimated when compared with the chronological age of an average person with the same degree of emotional maturity. **FUNCTIONAL A.,** the expression of the combined physical, emotional, and chronological ages of an individual. **MENTAL A.,** the figure which expresses the mental ability of an individual as compared with that of the average child of the same chronological age; it is determined by standardized tests. **PHYSIOLOGICAL A.,** the term applied to **A.** as assessed from appearance and behavior and measured by the amount of wear and tear on the body. **PSYCHOLOGICAL A.,** age as estimated through an assessment of the adaptive responses the individual has made to changes in environmental demands as compared to those of the average person in his peer group. **SOCIAL A.,** the social roles and habits of an individual as compared with those of the average person in one's peer group.

age spot: Senile lentigo; see under **lentigo**.

aged (ā′jed): 1. Pertaining to a person of old age. 2. Persons of old age.

ageism (ā′jizm): 1. The tendency to draw conclusions or formulate beliefs about a person on the basis of his chronological age alone. 2. The systematic discrimination and negative stereotyping of the elderly as being unhealthy, helpless, mentally confused, and in need of supportive services. This approach ignores the mental and physical potentialities of the elderly and often results in irreversible mutual withdrawal, the development of poor interrelationships, and eccentricities in older people.

agenesis (a-jen′-e-sis): 1. Incomplete and imperfect development of a body organ or part. 2. Congenital absence of a body organ or part. 3. Impotence or sterility due to lack of gonadal development. Also agenesia.

agenitalism (a-jen′-i-tal-izm): A symptom complex that develops in the absence of normal secretion of the ovaries or testes.

agent: A person, substance, or force that acts, or is capable of acting on something else, thereby producing an effect. **CATALYTIC A.,** a substance that enhances or speeds a reaction without itself being affected.

agerasia (a-jer-ā′-si-a): 1. Term used to describe the older person who is unusually healthy, vigorous, and active. 2. A deceptively youthful appearance of an older person.

ageusia (a-gū′-si-a): Impairment or loss of the sense of taste.

agglutination (a-gloo-ti-nā′-shun): 1. A phenomenon characterized by the clumping together of insoluble particles (bacteria or cells) distributed in a fluid, which is effected by specific immune antibodies (agglutinins) that develop in the blood of a previously infected or sensitized person. 2. The clumping together of blood cells when incompatible bloods are mixed in transfusion. 3. The joining together of surfaces in the healing of wounds.—agglutinate, v.

agglutinins (a-gloo′-ti-ninz): Specific substances (antibodies) that are formed in blood serum in the presence of particular invading bacteria or other cells causing them to adhere to one another forming a clump. **COLD A., A.** that will act only at low temperatures (0° to 20°C.).

agglutinogen (a-gloo-tin′-ō-jen): A protein substance that stimulates the production of a specific agglutinin when introduced into the body, *e.g.*, dead bacteria in a vaccine.

aggregate (ag′-grē-gāt): 1. To clump, gather, or crowd together in a mass. 2. The mass formed by substances or cells clumping together.

aggressin (a-gres′-in): A metabolic substance believed to be produced by certain bacteria; promotes infection by enhancing aggressive action of the bacteria against the host. Also called virulin.

aggression (a-gresh′-un): An attitude of animosity or hostility, or an assaultive action, usually resulting from frustration, fear, or a threatening situation. May be justified and self-protective. May be directed outward toward the environment and expressed in explosive actions, or inward toward the self, as occurs in depression.

aging: In the human, the gradual physical and psychological changes in the body and mind that are not due to disease or accident, and do not proceed at the same rate in all, but which are universal and inevitable and eventually terminate in death. **TIME-CLOCK THEORY OF AGING,** the theory that nature endows every individual with a time clock (the aging process) set to run down so that everyone is programmed to self-destruct.

agitation (aj-i-tā′-shun): Excessive chronic restlessness, with constant purposeless physical activity, distractibility, limited concentration, sometimes with mental disturbances and intellectual ineffectiveness; usually due to feelings of apprehension; seen in patients with severe depressive states, presenile dementia, or as a sequela of brain injury.

agitographia (aj′-i-tō-graf′-i-a): Writing with excessive speed and unconsciously omitting words or parts of words; often associated with agitophasia.

agitophasia (aj′-i-tō-fā′-zē-a): Speaking extremely rapidly and unconsciously omitting, slurring, or distorting words or parts of words.

aglaucopsia (a-glaw-kop′-si-a): Inability to distinguish the color green.

aglossia (a-glos′-i-a): Congenital absence of the tongue.

aglutition (ag-loo-tish′-un): See **dysphagia**.

aglycemia (a-glī-sē′-mi-a): Absence of sugar from the blood.

aglycosuria (a-glī-kō-sū′-rē-a): Absence of glucose from the urine.

agnail (ag′-nāl): 1. A hangnail. 2. A felon (*q.v.*).

agnathia (ag-nā′-thē-a): A developmental anomaly characterized by absence or imperfect development of the lower jaw.—agnathus, agnathy, n.; agnathous, adj.

agnogenic (ag-nō-jen′-ik): Of unknown source, cause, or origin; idiopathic (*q.v.*).

agnosia (as-nō′-si-a): Inability to recognize certain sensory impressions although recognition of other impressions is normal. Several types are distinguished, according to the sense organ(s) involved, *e.g.*, visual, auditory, gustatory, tactile. **TIME A.**, loss of comprehension of the passage of time. See also astereognosis.—agnostic, adj.

-agog, -agogue: Combining form denoting an agent that leads, incites, induces, or produces.

agomphious (a-gom′-fi-us): Toothless.

agonad (a-gō′-nad): An individual who has no sex glands.

agonal (ag′-o-nal): 1. Pertaining to or associated with agony, particularly the death agony or struggle. 2. Occurring at the time of death or just preceding it.

agonist (ag′-on-ist): 1. A muscle which contracts and shortens to perform a movement that opposes the action of another muscle which is in a state of relaxation at the same time; see **antagonist**. 2. A drug or other agent that can interact with receptors to produce an effect or response.

agony (ag′-o-ni): 1. Intense pain of mind or body. 2. Anguish, distress, or torture. 3. A violent struggle. 4. The death struggle.

agophany (a-gof′-a-ni): Speech which has a bleating or telephonic quality; may be due to consolidation of the lung, which interferes with transmission of sound frequencies.

agoraphobia (ag-ō-ra-fō′-bi-a): Morbid fear of being alone in large open spaces; of being away from home; of lakes and oceans; of crowds, stores, tunnels, bridges, theatres, or public transportation vehicles from which it might be difficult to escape.

agranular (a-gran′-ū-lar): Without granules; often refers to certain leukocytes.

agranulocyte (a-gran′-ū-lō-sīt): A leukocyte in which the cytoplasm contains no granules.

agranulocytosis (a-gran′-ū-lō-sī-tō′-sis): An acute, serious condition, characterized by sudden marked reduction or complete absence of granulocytes or polymorphonuclear leucocytes, fever, and ulceration of mucous membranes, especially those of the mouth, gastrointestinal tract, and vagina. May be idiopathic, or may result from the use of certain drugs, chemicals, or radiation therapy.

agraphia (a-graf′-i-a): Partial or total loss of the ability to express one's thoughts coherently in writing; writing is characterized by omission or repetition of words or parts of words, incorrect usage, faulty grammar; due to pathology or injury to the cerebral cortex.—agraphic, adj.

agromania (ag-rō-mā′ni-a): Abnormal desire to live in isolation or in the country.

ague (ā′-gū): Old name for malaria or a malarial type of fever.

agyria (a-jī′-ri-a): Congenital absence of convolutions in the cerebral cortex.

AHF: Abbreviation for antihemophilic factor (*q.v.*).

ahypnia (a-hip′-ni-a): Insomnia.

AI: Abbreviation for: 1. Aortic insufficiency. 2. Artificial insemination.

AID: Abbreviation for *a*rtificial *i*nsemination *d*onor.

aid: 1. Help given by one person to another. 2. Any of the various objects and appliances that help a handicapped person to walk, hear, see, etc. **FIRST AID**, care or treatment given to a person who has been injured or become suddenly ill pending further medical or surgical treatment.

aide (ād): In health care, a nonprofessional person who acts as assistant to a professional care giver.

AIDS: Abbreviation for acquired immunodeficiency syndrome (*q.v.*).

AIH: Abbreviation for *a*rtificial *i*msemination with the *h*usband's semen.

ailment (āl′-ment): A complaint, infirmity, or sickness. The term is usually applied to a physical or mental disorder of a mild nature.

ailurophilia (ī-lū-rō-fil′-i-a): Abnormal fondness for cats.

ailurophobia (i-lū-rō-fō′-bi-a): Abnormal fear of cats.

ainhum (ī′-yoom): Dyctylosis spontanea. A tropical disease of unknown cause; affects particularly Negro males; marked by the development of a constricting ring of fibrous tissue around a toe which causes the digit to be slowly amputated.

air: The colorless, odorless, tasteless gaseous mixture which surrounds the earth. It consists of approximately 4 parts of nitrogen by volume to one part of oxygen, and small amounts of such other substances as carbon dioxide, hydrogen, helium, ozone, neon, argon, krypton, xenon, ammonia, and varying amounts of water vapor. Also called atmosphere. **A. BATH,** see under bath. **A. BED,** a rubber mattress inflated with air. **A. BOOT,** a pneumatic splint or prosthesis for the lower extremity; reaches from the ankle to the knee; used to eliminate pressure by holding the foot off the bed. **A. EMBOLUS,** a bubble of air obstructing a blood vessel. **A. ENCEPHALOGRAPHY,** see pneumoencephalography. **A. HUNGER,** shortness of breath, with inspiratory and expiratory distress; characterized by rapid breathing, sighing, and gasping; due to anoxia. **A. MATTRESS,** one filled with air; supports the body uniformly with a minimum amount of pressure on the skin. **A. RING,** an inflated rubber or plastic ring, covered with bandage and placed under pressure points to prevent development of decubiti. **A. SAC,** an alveolus in the lung. **A. SICKNESS,** motion sickness occurring in airplane flights; symptoms include nausea, vomiting, dizziness. **A. SWALLOWING,** aerophagia (*q.v.*). **COMPLEMENTAL A.,** the extra air, over and above the volume of tidal air, that can be drawn into the lungs by the deepest possible inspiration. **RESIDUAL A.,** that which remains in the lungs after the fullest possible forced expiration. **STATIONARY A.,** that which remains in the lungs after normal expiration. **SUPPLEMENTAL A.,** the expiratory reserve volume; see under expiratory. **TIDAL A.,** that which passes in and out of the lungs in normal breathing.

airborne (ār′-born): In microbiology, refers to the transmission of infection from one person to another by means of droplets of moisture that contain the causative organism.

airway (ār′-way): 1. The natural passageway for air into and out of the lungs. 2. Any of several kinds of devices for maintaining a clear and unobstructed passageway for air to enter and leave the lungs. The most common types of artificial airway are: 1) **OROPHARYNGEAL,** in which a rubber or plastic tube is inserted through the mouth into the pharynx to prevent the tongue from forming an obstruction in the pharynx; 2) **ENDOTRACHEAL A.,** in which a rubber or plastic tube is inserted through the mouth or nose and passed through the larynx into the trachea; used for the administration of anesthesia and for prevention and treatment of acute respiratory failure in patients with pulmonary disease; also provides a route for ventilation with a respirator; 3) **TRACHEOSTOMY,** in which a tube is inserted into the trachea below the larynx through an incision in the neck; used when there is an obstruction in the upper respiratory tract, or to prevent aspiration of secretions from the bronchial tract, or to provide a route for mechanical ventilation.

A.K.: Abbreviation for above the knee; usually refers to the site of amputation.

akaryocyte (a-kar′-i-ō-sīt): 1. A cell that has no nucleus. 2. Erythrocyte.

akathisia (ak-a-thiz′-i-a): Inability to sit still or to lie quietly; a state in which the individual feels an inner restlessness that results in motor restlessness; may be due to an emotional disturbance or be a side effect of certain drugs, particularly the antipsychotic drugs.

akeratosis (a-ker-a-tō′-sis): A deficiency of horny tissue, of the nails in particular.

akinesia (a-kī-nē′-si-a): Inability to initiate or sustain voluntary muscular action; may be due to the side effects of certain drugs; also sometimes seen in post-encephalitic parkinsonism.—akinesic; akinetic, adj.

akinetic (a-kī-net′-ik): Without movement. **A. EPILEPSY,** a form of epilepsy in which the individual remains limp throughout the period of unconsciousness. **A. CATATONIA,** occurs in schizophrenia; see catatonia. **A. MUTISM,** a state in which the individual appears to be relaxed and asleep, makes no movements or sounds, and can be roused only with difficulty; due to a neurological or psychological disturbance.

akr-, akro-: See acr-.

Al: Chemical symbol for aluminum.

-al: A suffix denoting connection with, *e.g.*, nasal.

ala (ā′-la): Any wing-like process or structure. **A. NASI,** the cartilaginous outer flaring side of the nostril.—alae, pl.; alar, adj.

alalia (a-lā′-li-a): Lack of the power of speech; may be caused by impairment of the organs of speech or by a central lesion, or it may be of psychic origin.

alanine (al′-a-nēn): A constituent of many proteins; classified as nonessential; manufactured within the body.

Al-Anon: A world-wide self-help group for relatives and friends of alcoholics; based on the principles of Alcoholics Anonymous and adapted for non-alcoholics. Address: Al-Anon Family Group Headquarters, Madison Square Station, New York, NY 10159.

alar (ā′-lar): Wing-like. In anatomy, pertaining to 1) a wing-like bone or part of a structure; 2) the axilla.

alaryngeal (a-la-rin′-jē-al): Without a larynx. **A. SPEECH,** usually refers to esophageal speech developed following total laryngectomy.

alastrim (al-as′-trim): A tropical disease believed to be a less virulent form of smallpox; may be confused with chickenpox. Variola minor.

Alateen: A fellowship similar to Al-Anon for those aged 12 to 20 who are living with alcoholics.

alb-, alba-: A combining form meaning white, whitish.

alba (al′-ba): White.

albedo (al-bē′-dō): 1. Whiteness or paleness. 2. Reflected light from any surface. **A. RETINAE**, paleness of the retina due to edema.

Albers-Schönberg disease: A rare inherited condition in which there is spotty calcification of the bones, which fracture spontaneously; osteopetrosis. [Heinrich Ernst Albers-Schönberg, German surgeon. 1865–1921.]

albicans (al′-bi-kans): White or whitish.

albiduria (al-bi-dū′-ri-a): The voiding of very pale, low-gravity urine; albinuria.

albinism (al′-bi-nizm): A recessive genetic condition in which the inability to produce melanin results in lack of normal pigmentation of the skin, hair, and eyes. **OCULAR A.**, absence of pigmentation in the tissues of the eye. **PARTIAL A.**, lack of pigmentation in a local area only. **TOTAL A.**, lack of any pigmentation in the skin, hair, and eyes; often accompanied by photophobia, astigmatism, and nystagmus. In negroid persons the skin is tan or cream colored, sometimes freckled, the hair is brownish-yellow; the eye symptoms are similar to those in whites.

albino (al-bī′-nō): A person affected with albinism (*q.v.*); strictly speaking, a male person so affected.—albinotic, adj.

Albright's syndrome: A group of symptoms including overgrowth of several parts of the skeleton with formation of multiple cysts, the appearance of dark pigmented spots on the skin tending to occur on one side of the body, and, in females, sexual precocity. [Fuller Albright, American physician. 1900–1969]

albugo (al-bū′-gō): An opaque white spot that develops on the cornea.

albumen (al-bū′-men): 1. Egg white; composed chiefly of albumin. 2. Former spelling of albumin.

albumin (al-bū′-min): A variety of protein found in all animal tissues and in many vegetable tissues; is soluble in water and coagulates on heating. **SERUM A.**, the chief protein in blood plasma and other serous fluids.—albuminous; albuminoid, adj.

albuminemia (al-bū-mi-nē′-mi-a): The presence of an abnormal amount of albumin in the blood plasma.

albumin-globulin ratio (al-bū′-min-glob′-ū-lin): The ratio of albumin to globulin in the blood serum. Normally the ratio is from 1:3 to 1:8; lower ratios usually indicate the presence of pathology. Abbreviated A/G ratio.

albuminocholia (al-bū′-mi-nō-kō′-li-a): The presence of albumin in the bile.

albuminoid (al-bū′-mi-noyd): 1. Having the characteristics of albumin. 2. A protein. 3. Any of a group of proteins that are not soluble in aqueous solutions and which have a structural or protective function in the body, *e.g.*, collagen, keratin, or elastin; found in hair, nails, cartilage, and the lens of the eye.

albuminometer (al-bū-mi-nom′-e-ter): An instrument used for estimating the proportion of albumin in a fluid.

albuminorrhea (al-bū-min-ō-rē′-a): The excretion of an excessive amount of albumin in the urine.

albuminous (al-bū′-mi-nus): Resembling, pertaining to, or containing albumin.

albuminuretic (al-bū′-mi-nū-ret′-ik): 1. Pertaining to or promoting albuminuria. 2. An agent that promotes albuminuria.

albuminuria (al-bū′-mi-nū′-ri-a): The presence of albumin in the urine. Temporary albuminuria may occur in fevers, pregnancy, or after exercise; it usually clears up completely after the cause is removed. It may also be the result of renal impairment caused by kidney disorders, malignant hypertension, congestive heart failure. **CHRONIC A.** leads to hypoproteinemia (*q.v.*). **ORTHOSTATIC** or **POSTURAL A.**, occurs only when the person is standing; is absent during sleep; not due to renal disease.

alcaptonuria: See alkaptonuria.

alcohol (al′-ko-hol): A colorless, volatile, flammable liquid produced by fermentation of carbohydrates by yeast. The principal constituent of wine and spirits. Taken in small quantities it is a nervous system stimulant; in larger quantities it is a nervous system depressant. It enhances the action of barbiturates and tranquilizers. Medicinal uses include local application as an antiseptic or astringent; internal use as a cardiac stimulant and for its euphoric effect; as a base for tinctures and extracts; to preserve anatomical specimens. As a food, alcohol furnishes about 100 calories of heat per ounce. **ABSOLUTE A.**, contains at least 99 percent pure alcohol and is free of water and any impurities; sometimes used by injection for relief of trigeminal neuralgia and other intractable pain. **BENZYL A.**, used as a local anesthetic. **DENATURED A.**, has had some substance added to it to make it unfit for internal use; used externally on the skin as a cooling agent and disinfectant. **ETHYL A.**, ordinary **A.**, the main ingredient of alcoholic beverages; made from grain; sometimes used to stimulate appetite. **ISOPROPYL A.**, used externally for rubbing and as a disinfectant; not used internally. **METHYL A.**, made by distilling wood; for external use only. **WOOD A.**, methyl **A. A. PSYCHOSIS**, see Korsakoff's syndrome.

Alcohol, Drug Abuse, and Mental Health Administration (ADAMHA): A unit in the federal Department of Health and Human Services. Supports the development of knowledge, treatment, rehabilitation, and research activities in the areas of mental health and of alcohol and drug abuse through three agencies—the National Institute on Alcohol Abuse and Alcoholism, the National Institute on Drug Abuse, and the National Institute of Mental Health. Address: 5600 Fishers Lane, Rockville, MD 20857

alcohol withdrawal: The diagnosis now given for the condition occurring when alcohol is withdrawn after one has been drinking alcohol for several days or longer; symptoms include coarse tremor of the hands, tongue, and eyelids, nausea and vomiting, malaise, anxiety, and depression. Symptoms usually disappear within a week unless alcohol withdrawal delirium develops.

alcohol withdrawal delirium: Delirium following recent reduction or cessation of alcohol consumption. Symptoms include tachycardia, sweating, elevated blood pressure, delusions, agitated behavior, and hallucinations. Has been referred to as delirium tremens.

alcoholemia (al-kō-hol-ē′-mi-a): The presence of alcohol in the blood.

alcohol-fast: A bacteriological term describing a stained bacterium that resists discoloration by alcohol.

alcoholic (al-kō-hol′-ik): 1. Pertaining to or containing alcohol. 2. A person who habitually uses alcoholic beverages to excess. **A. AMNESTIC SYNDROME,** Korsakoff's syndrome. **A. PSYCHOSIS,** any of a group of mental disorders caused by excessive use of alcohol; associated with brain damage; symptoms include delirium tremens and hallucinosis. **A. DEMENTIA,** a nonhallucinatory dementia associated with alcoholism but not having the features of Korsakoff's syndrome. **A. HALLUCINOSIS,** a psychosis characterized by anxiety, restlessness, hallucinations of voices uttering threats, etc.; may be a withdrawal symptom in persons who have been heavy drinkers. **A. PARANOIA,** chronic paranoid psychosis characterized by delusional jealousy, delusions of persecution, and aggressive violent behavior.

Alcoholics Anonymous: A fellowship of alcoholics and former alcoholics who seek to control their compulsive urge to drink and to help others to do likewise through the group process. Address: 468 Park Ave. South, New York, NY 10016

alcoholism (al′-kō-hol-izm): 1. Alcohol poisoning. 2. Physical dependence on alcohol and its uncontrollable overuse; now recognized as a disease with physiologic, psychologic, and sociologic aspects; may be acute or chronic.

alcoholometer (al-kō-hol-om′-e-ter): An instrument for determining the amount of alcohol in a liquid.

alcoholophilia (al′-kō-hol-ō-fil′-i-a): An intense craving for alcoholic drinks or other intoxicants.

alcoholuria (al-ko-hol-ū′-ri-a): Alcohol in the urine. Basis of one test for fitness to drive a car after drinking alcohol.

aldehyde (al′-de-hīd): Any of a large class of substances that are formed by the oxidation of alcohol and that contain the chemical group CHO.

aldolase (al′-dō-lās): An enzyme found in muscle extract that acts as a catalyst in the reversible breakdown of fructose.

aldosterone (al-dō-ster′-ōn): A potent adrenocortical hormone that has an electrolyte-regulating function; it enhances the reabsorption of sodium by the kidney tubules and functions in the metabolism of sodium, chloride, and potassium; is described as a mineralocorticoid.

aldosteronism (al-dō-ster′-ō-nizm): A condition of electrolyte imbalance caused by excessive secretion of aldosterone; may be called primary when it is associated with tumor of the adrenal cortex, or secondary when it is associated with hypertension or edema, as occur in hepatic disease and kidney or cardiac failure.

Aldrich's syndrome: See Wiskott-Aldrich syndrome.

Aleppo boil: Cutaneous leishmaniasis; see under leishmaniasis.

alethia (a-lē′-thi-a): A constant dwelling on past events; inability to forget.

aleukemia (a-lū-kē′-mi-a): Lowered proportion of white blood cells in the circulating blood; aleukemic leukemia.—aleukemic, adj.

aleukia (a-lū′-ki-a): Lack of or abnormal decrease in the number of white blood cells, or of blood platelets.

alexia (a-leks′-i-a): Word blindness; a type of aphasia with loss of ability to interpret the significance of printed or written words, but without loss of visual power or intelligence. Due to a lesion in the central nervous system.—alexic, adj.

ALG: Abbreviation for antilymphocytic globulin.

algae (al′-jē): A large group of simple, unicellular marine plants, containing chlorophyll, including seaweed and fresh water plants, varying in size from microscopic to many feet in length. Some are useful as food, others in the preparation of medicinal substances. Algae collect on the top of sand filters and are effective in screening out bacteria, thus helping in the purification of water.—alga, sing.

alge-, algesi-, algo: Combining forms denoting relationship to pain.

algesia (al-jē′zi-a): Hyperesthesia; excessive sensitivity to pain. Opp. of analgesia.—algesic, adj.

algesimeter (al-je-sim′-e-ter): An instrument used for determining the degree of sensitivity to pain by pricking the skin with a sharp point.

algesthesia (al-jes-thē′-zi-a): Perception of pain.

-algia: Combining form denoting pain.

algicide (al′-ji-sīd): An agent that is destructive to algae.

algid (al′-jid): 1. Cold. 2. Condition after a severe attack of fever, especially malaria, with collapse, extreme coldness of the body, suggesting a fatal termination. During this stage the rectal temperature may be high.

alginates (al′-jin-ātz): Seaweed derivatives which, when applied locally, encourage the clotting of blood. They are available in solution and in specially impregnated gauze used in making surgical dressings. Also used for making dental impressions after being converted into a gel by combination with certain chemicals.

alginic acid (al-jin′-ik): An acid derived from several species of algae; when water is added to the salt of the acid, a clear mucilage is formed; used as a suspending agent in pharmacy and for making dental impressions.

algogenesis (al-gō-jen′-e-sis): The origin of pain.

algogenic (al-gō-jen′-ik): 1. Producing pain. 2. Producing cold. 3. Lowering the body temperature.

algolagnia (al-gō-lag′-ni-a): A sexual perversion in which the person achieves sexual gratification from inflicting or experiencing pain; masochism; sadism.

algophily (al-gof′-i-li): Sexual perversion characterized by a morbid love of inflicting, experiencing, or thinking about pain.

algophobia (al-gō-fō′-bi-a): Morbid dread of witnessing or experiencing pain.

algor (al′-gor): Coldness; rigor; a chill. **A. MORTIS,** the gradual cooling of the body after death.

algorithms (al′-gō-rith-ems): In health care, sets of step-by-step procedure guides to assist care givers in making informed decisions regarding the diagnosis and treatment of disease.

algospasm (al′-gō-spazm): A painful spasm or sudden cramp.

alienation (āl-yen-ā′-shun): 1. In psychology, the term is used in several ways: a) to express feelings of unreality or strangeness; b) the fear felt when one views a situation as foreign or unpredictable; c) the inability to think that a meaningful life is possible. 2. Insanity, 3. Mental illness. 4. In physiology, the state of a muscle that has been paralyzed and has regained some but not all of its ability to contract.

alienia (a-lī-ē′-ni-a): Congenital absence of the spleen.

alienist (al′-yen-ist): 1. A psychiatrist (obsolete). 2. In legal medicine, one who is quaified to testify in court as an expert concerning mental responsibility.

aliform (āl′-i-form): Wing-shaped.

alignment (a-līn′-ment): Arrangement in a straight line, as bones after a fracture. Also alinement.

aliment (al′-i-ment): Food.

alimentary (al-i-men′-tar-i): Pertaining to food. **A. CANAL** or **TRACT,** the passage down which the food goes during the process of digestion; it begins at the mouth and ends at the anus; the structures forming it are the mouth, pharynx, esophagus, stomach, small intestine, colon and rectum. **A. SYSTEM,** the alimentary canal and those organs connected with it that are concerned with digestion and absorption of food and the elimination of residual waste. **A. TUBE, A.** tract or canal.

alimentation (al′-i-men-tā′-shun): The act of providing or receiving nourishment; feeding. **ARTIFICIAL A.,** providing nourishment in some way other than normal, usually referring to intravenous feeding. **FORCED A.,** forced feeding of a person against his will. **PARENTERAL A.,** providing nourishment intravenously when the individual cannot take food orally. **PERIPHERAL A.,** utilizing peripheral veins for feeding intravenously. **RECTAL A.,** providing nourishment by injection into the rectum. **TOTAL PARENTERAL A.,** providing nutrients through a large central vein, *e.g.*, the subclavian.

alimentology (al′-i-men-tol′-o-ji): The science of nutrition.

aliphatic (al-i-fat′-ik): Pertaining to an oil or fat. Fatty. **A. ACIDS,** the so-called fatty acids, including acetic, butyric, and proprionic acids.

aliquot (al′-i-kwat): 1. A number that will divide evenly into a larger number. 2. A fraction of a larger sample used for analysis; in urinalysis the sample is taken from a 24-hour urine specimen.

alkalemia (al-ka-lē′-mi-a): An increase in the alkalinity of the blood. See alkalosis.—alkalemic, adj.

alkali (al′-ka-lī): Any one of a class of soluble bases that neutralize acids to form salts, combine with fatty acids to form soaps, and have a pH above 7; many are corrosive. Alkaline solutions turn red litmus blue. **ALKALI RESERVE,** a biochemical term denoting the amount of buffered alkali (normally bicarbonate) available in the blood for the neutralization of acids formed in or introduced into the body. When the alkali reserve falls, acidosis results; when it rises above normal, alkalosis results.

alkaline (al′-ka-līn): 1. Possessing the properties or reactions of an alkali. 2. Containing an alkali.

alkaline ash diet: A diet consisting of foods

that produce an alkaline ash when metabolized; includes fruits, vegetables, milk and some milk products, some nuts, fish, poultry.

alkalinity (al-ka-lin′-i-ti): The quality or condition of being alkaline.

alkalinization (al′-ka-lin-ī-zā′-shun): The process of rendering something alkaline.

alkalinuria (al-ka-lin-ū′-ri-a): Alkalinity of the urine.—alkalinuric, adj.

alkalitherapy (al-ka-lī-ther′-a-pi): The use of alkaline agents in the treatment of disease, *e.g.*, peptic ulcer.

alkalizer (al′-kalī-zer): 1. An agent that causes alkalinization. 2. An agent that neutralizes acids.

alkaloid (al′-ka-loyd): 1. Resembles an alkali. 2. Any of a large group of nitrogenous bases obtained from the leaves, seeds, bark or other part of certain plants; characteristically, alkaloids have a bitter taste and important physiological actions; those widely used in medicine include morphine, atropine, caffeine, and quinine. Some alkaloids are also produced synthetically.

alkalosis (al-ka-lō′-sis): A pathological condition in which the alkalinity of the body tends to increase; results from an excess of alkali intake or reduction of acid in the body. **METABOLIC A.**, often results from loss of body acid through vomiting and diarrhea, and is associated with an increase in pCO_2 in the blood. **RESPIRATORY A.**, usually results from hyperventilation and is associated with a decrease in pCO_2 in the blood.

alkapton (al-kap′-ton): Homogentisic acid (*q.v.*).

alkaptonuria (al-kap-tō-nū′-ri-a): A rare hereditary condition characterized by excessive secretion of homogentisic acid in the urine; results from only partial oxidation of phenylalanine and tyrosine. The urine turns brown on standing; other signs and symptoms, which occur chiefly in the middle-aged, include brown discoloration of connective tissues and degenerative changes in the intervertebral disks, joints, and cartilage.

alkylation (al-ka-lā′-shun): In organic chemistry, the substitution of an alkyl group (a radical that is formed when certain hydrocarbons lose one hydrogen atom) for an active hydrogen atom in an organic compound.

alkylating agents (al′-ka-lā-ting): Compounds containing two or more alkyl groups (see under alkylation) that readily combine with other molecules, their chief action being damage to the DNA in the nucleus of cells; includes the nitrogen mustards used in chemotherapeutic treatment of cancer.

ALL: Abbreviation for acute lymphocytic leukemia. See under leukemia.

allantiasis (al-an-tī′-a-sis): Sausage poisoning; botulism.

allantoid (a-lan′-toyd): 1. Pertaining to or resembling the allantois (*q.v.*). 2. Having a shape like a sausage.

allantois (al-an′-tō-is): A tubular diverticulum of the posterior part of the yolk sac of the embryo, passing into the body stalk, thus taking part in the formation of the umbilical cord and, later, the placenta.—allantoic, allantoid, adj.

allay (a-lā′): 1. To lessen or relieve. 2. To calm or pacify.

allele (a-lēl′): One of two or more variants of a gene that occur at the same position on homologous chromosomes; alleles account for the inheritance of particular traits.

allelomorph (a-lē′-lō-morf): See allele.

Allen's test: A test to determine whether the radial artery is suitable for use in intra-arterial monitoring. With both the radial and ulnar arteries compressed, the patient makes a fist and then rapidly opens and closes it causing a blanching of the skin of the hand; then the pressure on the ulnar artery is released and, if good color does not return to the hand, the radial artery is not suitable and another one must be selected.

allergen (al′-er-jen): Any substance capable of inducing an allergic state, *e.g.*, foods, drugs, animal fur or hair, feathers, pollens, smoke, dust, fungi, bacteria, viruses, animal parasites.—allergenic, adj.; allergenicity, n.

allergic (al-er′-jik): 1. Pertaining to or associated with an allergy. 2. Being affected with an allergy. **A. ASTHMA**, see under asthma. **A. DERMATITIS**, see dermatitis, contact. **A. REACTION**, see allergy. **A. RHINITIS**, rhinitis caused by an inhalant such as pollen.

allergist (al′-er-jist): A physician who specializes in diagnosing and treating allergies.

allergology (al-er-gol′-o-ji): The branch of medicine devoted to the study of allergy.

allergy (al′-er-ji): A hypersensitive reaction to a particular allergen (*q.v.*) or a foreign substance (which is harmless to the great majority of individuals), following initial sensitizing contact, as in hay fever, asthma, urticaria, vasomotor rhinitis, reactions to certain drugs or foods, contact dermatitis. It is due to an antigen-antibody reaction, though the antibody formed is not always demonstrable. **ALLERGY SKIN TESTING**, see sensitivity tests. See also anaphylaxis, sensitivity, sensitization.

allesthesia (al-es-thē′-zi-a): A disorder of the discriminatory sense in which the person perceives a stimulus at a point far removed from the point that is stimulated; usually indicative of a lesion in the parietal lobe.

alleviate (a-lē′-vē-āt): To lessen, mitigate, or make it easier to endure.

Allied Health Manpower: Refers to any or all of the aids, assistants, and technicians whose work and activities in the health-care field supplement that of the nurses, physicians, dentists, and other professional health-care personnel.

Allis's sign: Relaxation of the fascia between the crest of the ilium and the greater trochanter of the femur, so that a finger can be sunk into the space between the greater trochanter and the iliac crest; a positive test for fracture of the neck of the femur.

alloarthroplasty (al-lō-arth′-rō-plas-ti): The surgical creation of a new joint using materials from sources other than the human body.

allocheiria (al-ō-kī′-ri-a): A disorder of the tactile sense wherein the individual responds to a stimulus in a part of the body opposite to that where the stimulus was applied; often associated with a lesion of the parietal lobe. Also allochiria.

allochezia (al-ō-kē′-zi-a): 1. The elimination of feces through an abnormal opening in the body. 2. The elimination of non-fecal matter through the anus.

allochromasia (al-ō-krō-mā′-zi-a): Change in skin or hair color.

allocortex (al-ō-kor′-teks): Name given to several regions of the cerebral cortex; includes the olfactory cortex and the hippocampus. See neocortex.

allodromy (a-lod′-ro-mi): A disturbance in the rhythm of the heartbeat.

allograft (al′-ō-graft): Homograft; a graft of tissue from one individual to another of the same species but of a different genotype.

allolalia (al-ō-lā′-li-a): Any speech defect that has its origin in the central nervous system.

allomorphism (al-ō-mor′-fizm): The existence of a substance in more than one form with the chemical composition being the same.

allopathy (al-lop′-a-thi): A system of medical treatment in which the therapies used are intended to produce a condition that is different from or incompatible with the existing pathological condition. Opp. of homeopathy.—allopathic, adj.

alloplasty (al′-lō-plas-ti): In plastic surgery, the use of non-human material, *e.g.*, stainless steel. In psychiatry, a process of fitting one's inner needs to the external environment through adaptation involving alteration in that environment.

allopurinol (al-ō-pū′-ri-nol): A pharmaceutical substance that inhibits the production of uric acid and reduces the level of uric acid in the blood and urine: frequently used in treatment of gout.

allorhythmia (al-ō-rith′-mi-a): Irregularity of the pulse beat.

all-or-none law: States that when a nerve fiber or muscle fiber is stimulated it responds to its fullest extent or not at all.

allotherm (al′-ō-therm): An organism whose body temperature changes as the temperature of the environment changes.

allotrioguestia (a-lot′-ri-ō-gūs′-ti-a): A perverted or abnormal sense of taste or appetite.

allotriophagy (a-lot-ri-of′-a-ji): The eating of injurious substances or substances not fit for food. Pica.

allotropism (a-lot′-rō-pizm): The existence of an element in more than one form with each form having its individual characteristics and properties.

alloxuremia (al-oks-ū-rē′-mi-a): The presence of purine bodies in the blood.

alloxuria (al-oks-ū′-ri-a): The presence of purine bodies in the urine.

aloe (al′-ō): The dried juice from the leaves of several species of *Aloe*, a tropical plant; a powerful purgative with a very bitter taste.

alogia (a-lō′-ji-a): Inability to speak; may be physical or psychological in origin; usually due to a lesion in the central nervous system.

alopecia (al-ō-pē′-shi-a): Complete or partial baldness which may be congenital, premature, or due to the aging process; may be localized or general and result from systemic disease, febrile disease, extensive surgery, use of certain drugs, hormonal changes, emotional stress, radiotherapy. **A. AREATA,** a patchy baldness affecting primarily the scalp or beard but may also affect the eyebrows and lashes; cause unknown, but shock and anxiety may be precipitating factors; exclamation point hairs are diagnostic. **A. CICATRISATA,** progressive, permanent **A.** of the scalp associated with scarring and in which tufts of normal hair occur between many circular bald patches. **A. SENILIS,** baldness in the elderly, resulting from the gradual loss of hair. **A. SYPHILITICA,** transient baldness occurring in the secondary or tertiary stage of syphilis; bald patches occur chiefly over the temporoparietal area giving the individual's head a "motheaten" appearance. **A. TOTALIS,** complete baldness of the scalp. **A. UNIVERSALIS,** loss of hair from all parts of the body.

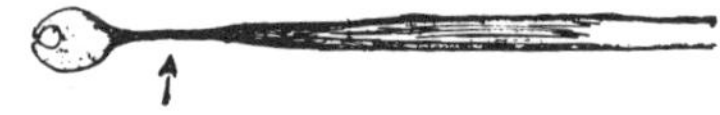

Exclamation mark hair

alpha (al′-fa): First letter of the Greek alphabet; often used as part of a chemical name to indicate the first of a series of compounds. **A. CELLS,** found in the islands of Langerhans; they secrete glucogen which stimulates glycogenolysis in the liver. **A. RAYS,** see under ray. **A. RECEPTOR,** see alpha-adrenergic receptor.

A. RHYTHM, see under rhythm. **A. TEST**, designed for use by the U.S. Army in World War I; consists of a series of intelligence tests that can be given to large groups and scored quickly; used to determine the subjects' ability to read and write. **A. WAVE**, see under wave.

alpha-adrenergic receptor: See under receptor.

alpha-antitrypsin (al'-fa-an-tī-trip'-sin): A protein found in blood plasma that inhibits the action of trypsin; deficiency of this protein is an inherited defect associated with liver disease and pulmonary emphysema.

alphafetoprotein (al'-fa-fē-tō-prō'-tē-in): A protein found in elevated amounts in the amniotic fluid in the second trimester of pregnancy if the fetus has an open neural defect such as anencephaly or spina bifida; can be detected and measured by amniocentesis. Also sometimes appears in elevated amounts in the sera of adult individuals with certain malignant conditions.

Alpha Tau Delta Nursing Fraternity (ATD): A national fraternity with chapters only in schools that offer baccalaureate or higher degrees in nursing; founded in 1921. Membership open to students of all races and creeds of high scholarship and character. Purpose: to promote high educational standards and develop leadership qualities in its members.

Alport's syndrome: Progressive hereditary glomerulonephritis marked by progressive nerve deafness and visual defects.

ALS: Abbreviation for: 1. Amyotrophic lateral sclerosis. 2. Antilymphocytic serum.

alt. dieb.: Abbreviation for *alternis diebus* [L.], meaning every other day.

alt. hor.: Abbreviation for *alternis horis* [L.] meaning every other hour.

alter ego (awl-ter-ē'-gō): 1. An individual so close to one's own character as to seem a second self. 2. Another side of oneself. 3. An intimate friend or constant inseparable companion.

alteregoism (awl-ter-ē'-go-izm): Having an interest only in those persons whose situation is similar to one's own.

alternans (al'-ter-nans): Alternating. **AUSCULTATORY A.**, occurs when the heartbeats are heard to alternate in intensity. **PULSUS A.**, occurs when the pulse alternates in strength but remains regular; may indicate myocardial disease.

alternating pressure mattress: See pulsating mattress.

alternating pressure pad: A segmented inflatable pad with an electrically operated pressure system that changes the thickness of the various segments at regular intervals; fits over a regular mattress; used to prevent decubitus ulcers.

altitude sickness: 1. **ACUTE A.S.**, occurs during airplane flights or other ascent to high altitudes, due to lessened oxygen pressure; symptoms include incapacitating headache, dyspnea, lassitude, weakness, fatigue, breathlessness, palpitation, anorexia, nausea, vomiting, nosebleed, abdominal pains, diarrhea, disturbances of vision, mental confusion, sometimes depression. Also called acute mountain sickness, hypobarism, Acosta's syndrome. 2. **CHRONIC A.S.**, occurs in people who remain in altitudes of 15,000 feet and over, the Andean region in particular; the main symptom is secondary polycythemia which results in viscosity of the blood, cyanosis, abdominal tumor, hepatomegaly, heart failure, pulmonary disorders such as emphysema or chronic bronchitis, ulceration and hemorrhage of the gastrointestinal mucosa, obesity; the symptoms are usually relieved when the individual is moved to a lower altitude. Also called chronic mountain sickness, Monge's disease, or Andes disease.

altricious (al-trish'-us): Referring to a person who requires a long period of nursing care.

alum (al'-um): A colorless crystalline or white powder substance used topically as a styptic or hemostatic and sometimes as an emetic.

aluminum (a-loo'-mi-num): An element occuring freely in nature in the form of a silvery white, light, malleable metal. Used medicinally in various forms and preparations as an astringent, styptic, demulcent, protective, antiperspirant, antacid; also for making surgical instruments and dental prostheses. **A. ACETATE**, a compound containing **A.** in solution; has mild astringent and antiseptic action on the skin; also called Burow's solution. **A. HYDROXIDE**, a mildly astringent white, tasteless powder, used externally as a dusting powder and internally for its antacid properties. **A. HYDROXIDE GEL**, a preparation of **A.** used to reduce stomach acidity and in treatment of peptic ulcer.

alveoalgia (al'-vē-ō-al'-ji-a): Pain in the alveolus of a tooth; may occur when the clot that forms following extraction of a tooth is dislodged causing a "dry socket"with exposure of the bone. Also called alveolalgia.

alveolar (al-ve'-ō-lar): Pertaining to an alveolus. **A. DUCT**, any of the minute passages which branch from the terminal bronchioles to the **A.** sacs. **A. SAC**, any of the sac-like structures at the terminus of the **A.** ducts; they are surrounded by a network of capillaries in which the exchange of oxygen in the alveoli and the carbon dioxide in the blood takes place. **A. PROCESS**, a bony ridge in the maxillae and mandibles which contain the alveoli of the teeth. **A. VENTILATION**, the exchange of gases between the inspired air and the blood in the alveoli of the lung.

alveolitis (al-vē-ō-lī'-tis): Inflammation of an

alveolus or alveoli. **EXTRINSIC ALLERGIC A.**, an occupational disease due to inhalation of organic particles; as occurs in bagassosis and farmers' lung. Characterized by a feeling of tightness in the chest, fever, chills, malaise, headache, cough, tachypnea, occurring soon after exposure; later symptoms include dyspnea, cyanosis, clubbing, thickened alveolar walls. **ALVEOLITIS SICCA DOLOROSA,** dry socket; see **alveoalgia.**

alveolotomy (al-vē-ō-lot′-o-mi): The surgical incision of a dental alveolus for treatment and drainage.

alveolus (al-vē′-ō-lus): In anatomy, a term used to designate: 1. A small cavity or sac-like dilatation. 2. The termination of a bronchiole in a microscopic sac-like vesicle of the lung where the exchange of oxygen and carbon dioxide takes place. 3. A gland follicle or acinus. 4. A tooth socket.

alymphia (a-lim′-fi-a): Lack or absence of lymph.

alymphocytosis (a-lim′-fō-sī-tō′-sis): A deficiency or complete absence of lymphocytes from the circulating blood.

alymphoplasia (a-limf′-ō-plā′-zi-a): Imperfect development or failure of development of lymphoid tissues; may be due to incomplete or imperfect development or functioning of the thymus gland.

Alzheimer's disease: Now categorized under Primary Degenerative Dementia of the Alzheimer type (see Appendix VI). A progressive form of dementia caused by destruction of nerve cells deep in the cerebrum, particularly in the frontal and occipital lobes; usually begins in persons between 40 and 50 years of age; often but not necessarily accompanied by senility. Characterized by personality changes, disorientation in time and place, depression, loss of memory, errors of judgment, decreased sociability, agnosia, speech disturbances, voice changes, abrupt onset, and fluctuating course. There is no known cure. [Alois Alzheimer, German neurologist. 1864–1915.]

A.M.: Abbreviation for *ante meridian* [L.] meaning before noon.

AMA: Abbreviation for: 1. American Medical Association, 2. Against medical advice.

amalgam (a-mal′-gam): 1. A combination, mixture, blend. 2. Dental amalgam, an alloy of mercury containing silver and tin; used for fillings.

amarilla (am-a-ril′-a): The international term for yellow fever.

amasesis (am-a-sē′-sis): Inability to chew food, for any reason.

amastia (a-mas′-ti-a): Absence of the breasts; may be a congenital condition, or due to surgical removal, or to an endocrine disturbance that inhibits development.

amaurosis (am-aw-rō′-sis): Partial or total blindness, particularly that which occurs without apparent disease or lesion of the eye; often temporary. **A. FUGAX,** sudden transient partial or complete blindness in one eye; may occur in transient ischemic attack, alcoholic poisoning, emotional shock, or from sudden acceleration as in an airplane flight.

amaurotic familial iodiocy: See **cerebral sphingolipidosis,** under **sphingolipidosis.**

ambi-: A prefix denoting both, or on both sides.

ambidexter (am-bi-dek′-ster): A person who can use either hand equally well.

ambidextrous (am-bi-deks′-trus): Ability to use both hands with equal facility.

ambient (am′-bi-ent): Surrounding; encompassing; present everywhere; moving freely or circulating, as **A.** air.

ambilateral (am-bi-lat′-er-al): Pertaining to both right and left sides, or affecting both sides.

ambiopia (am-bi-ō′-pi-a): Diplopia (*q.v.*).

ambisexuality (am′-bi-seks-ū-al′-i-ti): Having characteristics common to both sexes.

ambivalence (am-biv′-a-lens): 1. The coexistence of conflicting attitudes and feelings toward a particular situation, object, or person, *e.g.*, love and hate.

ambivalent (am-biv′-a-lent): 1. Pertaining to ambivalence. 2. Pertaining to a type of personality that has both introversive and extroversive characteristics.

ambivert (am′-bi-vert): One who is neither an extrovert nor an introvert; a person between these two extremes.

amblyacousia (am-bli-a-koo′-si-a): Dullness of the sense of hearing.

amblygeustia (am-bli-gūs-′ti-a): Temporary or permanent dullness of the sense of taste.

Amblyomma: A genus of ticks, many species of which are vectors of disease-producing organisms, including that for Rocky Mountain spotted fever.

amblyopia (am-bli-ō′-pi-a): Defective vision or dimness of vision when there is no detectable disease of the eye or error of refraction. **A. EX ANOPSIA,** results from nonuse or misuse of the eye; usually affects one eye only; in cases of strabismus may lead to monocular blindness; see **anopsia.** Also called suppression amblyopia. **TOXIC A.,** partial or complete loss of vision as a result of acute or chronic toxemia caused by uremia, diabetes, malaria, beri beri, or the excessive use of tobacco or alcohol.

Ambu bag: A hand operated resuscitator which delivers about 40 percent oxygen.

ambulance (am′-bu-lans): A vehicle used for transporting the sick or injured.

ambulant (am′-bu-lant): Able to walk and move about; not confined to bed.

ambulate (am'bū-lāt): To walk or move from place to place.

ambulation (am-bū-lā'-shun): The act of walking or moving about.

ambulatory (am'-bū-la-tor-i): Mobile. Able to walk. **A. HEALTH CARE,** care given to a person who is not a patient occupying a hospital bed, *e.g.*, care given at a health department or neighborhood health care center, outpatient department, clinic or emergency department of a hospital, occupational or school health department, or community mental health center. **A. TREATMENT, T.** in which the patient is kept on his feet as much as possible.

ameba (a-mē'-ba): A microscopic, elementary, one-celled protozoan of the genus *Amoeba* that moves by extruding pseudopodia (*q.v.*), is capable of ingestion, absorption, respiration, excretion, and reproduction by simple fission. Many species are pathogenic to man, especially *Entamoeba histolytica,* the causative organism of amebic dysentery. Also amoeba.—amebae; amebas; amoebae, pl.; amebic; ameboid; amoebic, adj.

amebiasis (am-ē-bī'-a-sis): Infestation with *Entamoeba histolytica* affecting chiefly the mucosa of the large intestine but also often involving the liver; the organism enters the body in food or water that is contaminated by feces. Symptoms include acute abdominal pain, anorexia, severe diarrhea with stools containing mucus and, sometimes, flecks of blood, jaundice, emaciation. Particularly serious in infants, older people, and the debilitated. Diagnosis is confirmed by isolating the causative organism in the stools.

amebic (a-mē'-bik): Pertaining to, resembling, or caused by an ameba. Also amoebic.

amebicide (a-mē'-bi-sīd): An agent that destroys amebae.—amebicidal, adj.

amebocyte (a-mē'-bō-sīt): Any cell having ameboid characteristics, *e.g.*, a leukocyte.

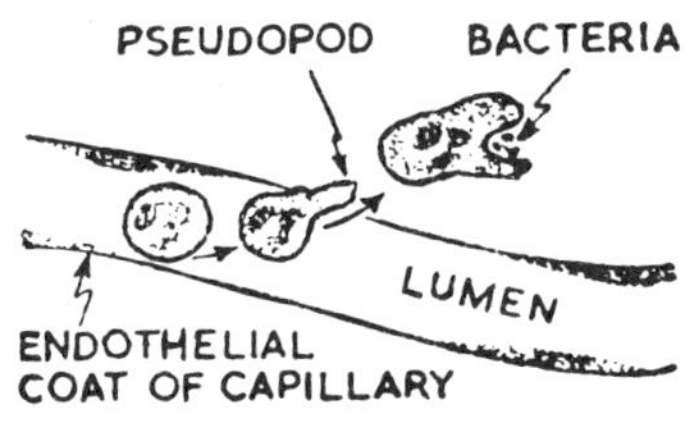

Ameboid movement of white blood cells

ameboid (a-mē'-boyd): Resembling an ameba in shape or mode of movement, *e.g.*, white blood cells. **A. MOVEMENT, M.** that progresses by diapedesis, *i.e.*, the alternate projection and retraction into the cell of "legs" of cytoplasm called pseudopodia.

ameburia (am-ē-bū'-ri-a): The presence of amebae in the urine.

amelanotic (a-mel-a-not'-ik): Without pigment.

amelia (a-mē'-li-a): A congenital anomaly characterized by the absence of a limb or limbs. **COMPLETE A.,** absence of both arms and legs.

amelioration (a-mē-li-or-ā'-shun): Reduction of the severity of symptoms. Improvement in the general condition.

ameloblast (a-mel'-ō-blast): An epithelial cell that has a function in the production of dental enamel.

ameloblastoma (a-mel'-ō-blas-tō'-ma): A rapidly growing, aggressive tumor of the jaw, usually in the molar region; begins in the epithelium at the origin of the teeth; apt to be recurrent; may cause dysphagia and blockage of the airway; hemorrhage due to erosion of blood vessels may result in death. Seen chiefly in certain areas of Africa and Asia.

amelogenesis (am-e-lō-jen'-e-sis): The formation of dental enamel. **A. IMPERFECTA,** an inherited condition in which there is deficient or imperfect development of tooth enamel resulting in brownish discoloration and friability of the teeth.

amelus (am'-e-lus): A person with congenital absence of all four extremities.

amenorrhea (a-men-ō'-rē'-a): Abnormal absence or cessation of the menses. **PRIMARY A.,** failure of menstruation to become established at puberty. **SECONDARY A.,** absence of the menses after they have once commenced; occurs in some women after they cease taking contraceptive pills.

amenorrhea-galactorrhea syndrome: Amenorrhea accompanied by milk formation in the breasts; may be due to excessive production of prolactin (*q.v.*).

ament (am'-ent): A person with severe subnormal mentality; an idiot.

amentia (a-men'-shi-a): Congenital lifelong mental subnormality; feeblemindedness; to be distinguished from dementia. **NEVOID A.,** Sturge-Weber syndrome (*q.v.*). **SENILE A., A.** due to development of excessive fibrous tissue in the brain.

American Academy of Nursing (AAN): An honorary organization, founded in 1973, under the aegis of the American Nurses' Association. Purpose is to identify and explore health issues and other topics of interest and concern to nurses and nursing; and to examine the dynamics within nursing and the interrelationship among nurses as these affect the development of the nursing process. Sponsors workshops and conducts research. As of 1980, the number of fellows was limited to 500; criteria for selection of Fellows includes membershiip in the American Nurses' Association, five years experience as a professional Registered Nurse, evidence of outstanding contribution to nursing, and evidence of potential for contribution to nursing. Address: 2420 Pershing Road, Kansas City, MO 64108

American Hospital Association (AHA): Founded in 1898. Devoted chiefly to promoting and maintaining high standards of care in hospitals in the United States. Composed of both health care institutions and individual members. Carries out research and education projects in such areas as hospital administration and economics; represents hospitals as national spokesman for legislation. *Hospitals* is its official publication. Address: 840 N. Lake Shore Drive, Chicago, IL 60611.

American Indian signs: A system of signs and signals based on gestures used by American Indians; used by individuals who have lost the power of oral speech through surgery or a pathological condition.

American Journal of Nursing Company: Since October 1900 has published the *American Journal of Nursing* as the official organ of the American Nurses' Association; at first owned by a group of nurse shareholders, it has been owned entirely by the Association since 1912. The company also publishes *Geriatric Nursing, MCN* (the *Journal of Maternal and Child Nursing*), *Nursing Research,* and (in cooperation with the National Library of Medicine) the *International Nursing Index*. Address: 555 West 55th St., New York, NY 10019

American Medical Association: Organized in 1847. Membership includes state and local groups and individuals. Purposes include dissemination of scientific information to members and the public; cooperation in setting standards for medical schools, hospitals, residency programs, and continuing education programs; offers placement service; maintains a national directory of physicians practicing in the U.S.; operates a large lending library; publishes a variety of journals, books, and pamphlets. Address: 535 N. Dearborn Streett, Chicago, IL 60610.

American Nurses' Association (ANA): The professional organization for registered nurses in the U.S.; a federation of the 50 State Nurses' Associations and the nursing organizations of Guam, the Virgin Islands, and the District of Columbia; founded 1912 after 12 years of affiliation with Canadian nurses. Purposes are to promote the professional and educational advancement of nurses; to bring nurses into contact with each other; to disseminate information about nursing; and to improve health care in the U.S. The ANA establishes standards for professional conduct and performance; provides a credentialing service and licensure system; promotes continuing education and research in nursing; sponsors American Nurses Foundation, and Nurses Coalition for Political Action; maintaiins Hall of Fame. Is represented in international nursing by membership in the International Council of Nurses. Its professional publication is *The American Journal of Nursing;* its official newspaper is *The American Nurse,* published at tthe Association headquarters, 2420 Pershing Road, Kansas City, MO 64108.

American Nurses' Association Council of Nurse Researchers: A subdivision of the American Nurses' Association; membership includes nurses who hold a masters or a higher degree and who are engaged in nursing research; promotes research activities and provides information about funding for research. Address: American Nurses' Association, Department of Research, Grants, and Contracts, 2420 Pershing Road, Kansas City, MO 64108

American Nurses' Foundation (ANF): An organization founded by the American Nurses' Association in 1955 to meet the continuing need for a program devoted primarily to nursing research. The tax exempt Foundation supports basic and applied research and scholarships through grants to individual nurse researchers, and related program activities. Address: 2420 Pershing Road, Kansas City, MO 64108.

American Public Health Association: A national organization, with over 50 affiliated groups, for professional public health workers including physicians, nurses, and others representing 45 disciplines in health care; founded in 1872. Promotes education and research; sets standards for public health care. Publishes a variety of materials on public health issues and legislation, including the *Journal of Public Health, The Nation's Health,* and *Washington News Letter*. Address: 1015 Eighteenth St., NW, Washington, D.CC. 20036.

American Red Cross (ARC): Founded 1881. Serves members of the armed forces, veterans and their families; aids disaster victims; conducts blood service; sponsors training of volunteers for hospital and other community agencies. Publishes many books and pamphlets on health promotion and preservation. Address: 17th & D Sts., N.W., Washington, D.C. 20006

American spotted fever: Rocky Mountain spotted fever (*q.v.*).

Ameslan: Acronym for American Sign Language, a method of communication with and among the deaf.

ametria (a-mē′-tri-a): Congenital absence of the uterus.

ametropia (am-ē-trō′-pi-a): Defective vision

due to imperfect refractive power of the eye that prevents proper focusing of parallel rays on the retina, and which results in such conditions as myopia, hyperopia, and astigmatism.

amianthinopsy (am-i-an′-thi-nop′-si): Inability to see the color violet.

amide (am′-īd): An organic compound derived from ammonia by chemical reaction in which an acid radical is substituted for one of the hydrogen atoms.

amidone (am′-i-dōn): Methadone.

amines (am′-ēns): Name given to organic compounds that contain the amino group (NH_2). They are derived from ammonia; important in biochemistry.

amino-: Prefix denoting a compound that contains the radical group $-NH_2$.

amino acids (am-′i-nō, a-mē′-no): Organic acids that contain one or more amine groups (NH_2) and a carboxyl group (CO_2H); the structural units of protein, occurring naturally in animal and plant foods. In the body they are the end products of protein hydrolysis and from these the body resynthesizes its protein. Classified as 1) endogenous, those amino acids that are made within the body; and 2) exogenous, those found in sources outside the body. Also classified as 1) essential, those amino acids that cannot be made within the body (exogenous) and must come from the outside; these include arginine, histidine, isoleucine, leucine, lysine, methionine, phenylalanine, threonine, tryptophan, and valine; and 2) non-essential (endogenous); these include alanine, aspartic acid, cysteine, cystine, glutamic acid, glutamine. Foods that contain large amounts of amino acids are known as complete proteins, *e.g.*, meat, fish, eggs, milk; and those that contain lesser amounts are known as incomplete proteins, *e.g.*, vegetables such as peas and beans, and wheat.

amino group (am′-i-nō, a-mē′-nō): The NH_2 group in a protein compound; it is a portion of all amino acids and is the basic building block of proteins. Also called the amino acid radical.

aminoacidemia (am′-in-ō-as-id-ē′-mi-a): An excess of amino acids in the blood.

aminoacidopathy (am′-in-ō-as-i-dop′-a-thi): Any disorder involving an imbalance of amino acids in the body.

aminoaciduria (am′-i-nō-as-i-dū′-ri-a): An excess of amino acids in the urine.

aminocaproic acid (am′-i-nō-kā-prō′-ik): An agent used as an antifibrinolytic to control excessive bleeding in hemophilia and in certain post-surgical patients.

aminoglycoside (am′-i-nō-glī′-ko-sīde): Any of the bacterial antibiotics which act by inhibiting protein synthesis; includes streptomycin, neomycin, kanamycin, gentamycin, tobramycin.

aminosis (am-i-nō′-sis): The production of excess amino acids in the body.

aminuria (am-i-nū′-ri-a): The presence of excess amino acids in the urine.

amitosis (am-ī-tō′-sis): Multiplication of a cell by direct fission, without change in either the nucleus or the protoplasm.

AML: Abbreviation for acute myelogenous leukemia. See under leukemia.

ammeter (am′-mē-ter): An instrument for measuring the amperage or intensity of an electric current.

ammoaciduria (am′-ō-as-i-dū′-ri-a): The presence of an excess of both amino acids and ammonia in the urine.

ammonia (a-mō′-ni-a): A colorless, volatile, alkaline gas with a penetrating pungent odor, formed by decomposition of nitrogenous matter; contains hydrogen and nitrogen. Highly soluble in water; widely used in industry and as a detergent. **AROMATIC SPIRIT OF A.**, solution of ammonia, water and aromatic oils; has fleeting action as a circulatory and respiratory stimulant; used in cases of fainting.

ammoniacal (am-ō-nī′-a-kal): 1. Pertaining to ammonia. 2. Containing, or having the characteristics of ammonia.

ammoniated mercury: A compound containing ammonia and mercury in ointment form; applied externally to the skin primarily but also used in treating ophthalmic conditions.

ammoniemia (a-mō-ni-ē′-mi-a): The presence of ammonia or ammonia compounds in the blood.

ammonium chloride: A white crystalline or powdery substance with hygroscopic properties and a salty taste; used as an expectorant, as a diuretic, or to acidify urine or correct acid-base imbalance.

Ammon's horn: See hippocampus.

amnalgesia (am-nal-jē′-zi-a): The abolition of pain or the memory of pain; may be brought about by the use of certain drugs or by hypnosis.

amnemonic (am-nē-mon′-ik): Pertaining to or causing impairment of memory.

amnesia (am-nē′-zi-a): Partial or complete loss of memory and of the ability to recall one's identity. May be caused by concussion, electroshock, dementia, hysteria, senility, alcoholism; or it may be a defense mechanism against anxiety-provoking situations. **ANTEROGRADE A.**, loss of memory for recent events, especially for events since the accident causing the A. **CIRCUMSCRIBED A.**, loss of memory for a limited time; may occur after an epileptic or hysterical episode; memory before and after the episode is intact. **NEUROTIC A.**, occurs when a person consciously or unconsciously wishes to forget his or her memories and does not wish to recover them. **POSTTRAUMATIC A.**, A. for a short time following severe head injury. **RETROGRADE A.**, loss of memory for events that occurred before an accident which caused amnesia. **TRAUMATIC A.**, occurs after a sudden injury. **VERBAL A.**, loss of memory for words. **VISUAL A.**, inability to recognize familiar objects.—amnesic, adj.

amnesic (am-nē′-zik): 1. Pertaining to or suffering from amnesia. 2. A drug that causes loss of memory for pain.

amniocentesis (am′-ni-ō-sen-tē′-sis): Removal of a small amount of fluid from the amniotic sac by aspiration through the abdominal wall for diagnostic purposes; usually done during or after the 15th week of pregnancy. Analysis of the chromosomes or enzyme production of the fetal cells can determine certain structural disorders and many disorders of the fetus's body chemistry that may lead to mental or physical retardation and sometimes death, *e.g.*, mongolism, or the presence of a deforming virus infection such as German measles. The fluid contains increased hemoglobin products in cases of Rhesus incompatibility.

amniogenesis (am-ni-ō-jen′-e-sis): The formation of the amnion.

amniography (am-ni-og′-ra-fi): X ray of the gravid uterus after injection of the amniotic sac with an opaque medium; it outlines the amniotic cavity, the fetus, and the umbilical cord and placenta; a diagnostic procedure when placenta previa hydatidiform mole, or choriocarcinoma is suspected.—amniogram, n.; amniographical, adj.; amniographically, adv.

amnion (am′-ni-on): The innermost of the fetal membranes; a thin transparent sac that holds the fetus suspended in the liquor amnion (amniotic fluid); commonly called the bag of waters.—amnionic, amniotic, adj.

amniorrhea (am-ni-ō-rē′-a): Escape of amniotic fluid prematurely.

amniorrhexis (am-ni-ō-rek′-sis): Rupture of the amnion.

amnioscopy (am-ni-os′-ko-pi): Direct observation of the amniotic sac, the fetus, and the color and amount of amniotic fluid through the intact membrane using a specially designed optical instrument inserted through the uterine cervix; is usually done during the last trimester of pregnancy. **TRANSABDOMINAL A.**, direct examination of the fetus and amniotic fluid through the abdominal wall; usually done during the second trimester of pregnancy.

amniotic (am-ni-ot′-ik): Of or pertaining to the amnion (*q.v.*). **A. CAVITY**, the fluid-filled amnion. **A. FLUID**, the transparent fluid that is secreted rapidly and resorbed by the amniotic sac; composed of water, urea, albumin, cells, and various salts. **A. FLUID EMBOLISM**, occurs when an embolus forms in the amniotic sac, enters the maternal circulation and is transported to the mother's lung or brain; a rare occurrence; happens after the membranes rupture. **A. FLUID INFUSION**, the escape of amniotic fluid into the maternal circulation. **A. SAC**, the sac formed by the amnion; contains amniotic fluid.

amniotitis (am-ni-ō-tī′-tis): Inflammation of the amnion (*q.v.*).

amniotome (am′-ni-ō-tōm): An instrument for rupturing the fetal membranes to induce or hasten labor.

amniotomy (am-ni-ot′-o-mi): Surgical rupture of the fetal membranes to induce or expedite labor.

amok (a-mok′): A wild, frenzied, maniacal manner of behavior that threatens harm to others.

amorph (a′-morph): An inactive gene; one which has no action at all.—amorphic, adj.

amorphous (a-mor′-fus): Having no definite structure; formless—amorphia, amorphism, n.

AMP: Abbreviation for adenosine monophosphate. See under **adenosine**.

amp: Abbreviation for: 1. Ampere. 2. Ampule.

ampere (am′-per): The standard unit of intensity of an eletric current. It describes the exact number of electrons flowing past a given point against resistance of one ohm.—amperage, n.

amph-, amphi-: Prefixes denoting around; on both sides; both.

amphetamine (am-fet′-a-mēn): Any of a group of chemical substances in the form of a white crystalline powder, odorless and tasteless, used as a nervous system stimulant; highly addictive. Used therapeutically in treatment of narcolepsy, depression, low blood pressure, obesity. Often misused by both adolescents and adults to produce euphoria and control fatigue. Also called speed (slang).

amphiarthrosis (am′-fi-arth-rō′-sis): A slightly movable joint. The articulating surfaces are separated by fibrocartilage or ligaments that permit only slight movement, as between the vertebrae.—amphiarthroses, pl.

amphibolic (am-fi-bol′-ik): Uncertain as to outcome or diagnosis; ambiguous.

amphichromic (am-fi-krō′-mik): Affecting both red and blue litmus paper.

amphicrania (am-fi-krā′-ni-a): Headache or pain involving both sides of the head.

amphigenesis (am-fi-jen′-e-sis): Sexual reproduction. Syn., amphigony.

amphigonadism (am-fi-gon′-ad-izm): Hermaphrodism; the condition of having both testicular and ovarian tissue.

amphithymia (am-fi-thī′-mi-a): An emotional state in which periods of depression and elation alternate.

amphitrichate (am-fi-trī′-kāt): Descriptive of a microorganism that has a flagellum or flagella at both ends.

amphodiplopia (am′-fō-di-plō′-pi-a): Double vision in both eyes.

amphophilic (am-fō-fil′-ik): Pertaining to cells that stain with either acid or basic dyes.

amphoric (am-for′-ik): Descriptive of a sound resembling that produced by blowing across the top of an empty bottle; heard when auscultating over a pneumothorax or over a pulmonary cavity.

amphoteric (am-fō-ter′-ik): Having two opposite characteristics; said especially of a substance that reacts as either an acid or a base.

ampule (am′-pūl): A small, hermetically sealed glass vial containing a single dose of a drug. Also spelled ampul, ampoule.

ampulla (am-poo′-la): Any flask-like dilatation. In anatomy, a flask-like dilatation of a tubal structure. **A. OF THE BREAST,** a widened portion of a lactiferous duct near its opening on the nipple. **A. OF THE FALLOPIAN TUBE,** a widened area of the tube where fertilization is thought to occur. **A. OF VATER,** the enlargement formed by the union of the common bile duct with the pancreatic duct where they enter the duodenum. [Abraham Vater, German anatomist. 1684–1751.]—ampullae, pl.; ampullar, ampullary, ampullate, adj.

amputation (am-pū-tā′-tion): 1. Removal of an appending part by surgery, *e.g.*, a breast, or limb. 2. Lack or loss of a limb or limbs due to heredity or trauma, or occurring spontaneously as a result of gangrene.

amputee (am-pū-tē′): A person who has lost a limb or limbs or had one or more limbs amputated by surgery.

amt.: Abbreviation for amount.

amuck (a-muk′): See amok.

amusia (a-mū′-zi- a): Lack of ability to identify musical sounds or to reproduce musical sounds, vocally or otherwise.

amydriasis (am-i-drī′ a-sis): Contraction of the pupil.

amyelia (a-mī-ē′-li-a): A congenital anomaly marked by the absence of the spinal cord.

amyelus (a-mī′-e-lus): A fetal monster that has no spinal cord.

amygdala (a-mig′-da-la): 1. An almond-shaped mass of gray matter in the lateral ventricle of the brain. 2. A tonsil. 3. An almond.

amygdaloid (a-mig′-da-loyd): 1. Almond-shaped. 2. Resembling an almond or a tonsil.

amygdalolith (a-mig′-da-lō-lith): A stone or a concretion in a tonsillar crypt.

amygdalotomy (a-mig-da-lot′-o-mi): Surgical destruction of the amygdala; sometimes done to control aggression or olfactory hallucinations.

amylaceous (am-i-lā′-shē-us): Starchy. Containing or resembling starch.

amylase (am′-i-lās): An enzyme of the saliva (ptyalin), pancreatic juice (amylase), or intestinal juice that converts starches into sugars. **A. TEST,** a test to determine the amount of starch in the urine; less than normal indicates a disorder of kidney function. **SERUM A. TEST,** test to measure the amount of amylase in the circulating blood; it is elevated notably in pancreatitis.

amylogenesis (am′-i-lō-jen′-e-sis): The formation of starch.

amyloid (am′-i-loyd): 1. Starch-like. 2. A starchy food or substance. 3. A wax-like protein complex that has some starch-like qualities; may be deposited in tissues in certain pathological states. See amyloidosis.

amyloidosis (am-i-loy-dō′-sis): A relatively rare disease in which amyloid is formed and deposited in various body tissues and organs. Degeneration of organs is progressive with slowed metabolism; gastrointestinal symptoms; emaciation; arrhythmias; congestive heart failure; muscle weakness; paresthesias; pain; papules, plaques, and nodules in the skin. **LICHEN A.,** a localized cutaneous form usually seen in the legs. **PRIMARY A.,** occurs when there is no coexisting disease; depositions are chiefly in the mesodermal tissues, including the cardiovascular system. **SECONDARY A.,** occurs in the terminal phase of such chronic disorders as osteomyelitis and tuberculosis. **SENILE A.,** commonly seen in very old people in a mild form affecting primarily the heart.

amylolysis (am-i-lol′-is-is): The conversion of starch to sugar by the action of enzymes during digestion.

amylopectinosis (am′-i-lō-pek-ti-nō′-sis): Glycogenosis (*q.v.*). Also called Anderson's disease and glycogen storage disease, type IV.

amylopsin (am-i-lop′-sin): A pancreatic enzyme that acts to convert insoluble starch into soluble maltose.

amylose (am′-i-lōs): Any polysaccharide (*q.v.*).

amylum (am′-i-lum): 1. Starch. 2. Corn starch.

amyluria (am-i-lū′-ri-a): The presence of an excess of starch in the urine.

amyoplasia (a-mī-ō-plā′-zi-a): Lack of formation and development of muscle tissue. **A. CONGENITA,** see arthrogryposis.

amyostasia (a-mī-ō-stā′-zi-a): Nervous shaking or tremor of the muscles with incoordination, which makes standing difficult; often seen in locomotor ataxia.

amyotonia (a-mī-ō-tō′-ni-a): Myatona. Lack or loss of muscle tone. **A. CONGENITA,** any one of several congenital conditions of infants that are characterized by pronounced muscular weakness and flaccidity; also called floppy-infant syndrome and Oppenheim's disease.

amyotrophic lateral sclerosis (a-mī-ō-trōf′-ik lat′-er-al sklē-rō′-sis): A progressive degenerative disease that affects the motor system; cause unknown. Usually occurs in the fifth to seven decade with death in about three years. Chief symptom is muscular wasting with associated weakness and difficulty in swallowing and talking. Also called Lou Gehrig's disease. See **sclerosis**.

amyotrophy (a-mi-ot′-rō-fi): Progressive muscle wasting or atrophy. Also amyotrophia.—amyotrophic, adj.

amyxia (a-mik′-si-a): Deficiency or absence of mucus.

ANA: Abbreviation for American Nurses' Association (*q.v.*).

ana: An equal quantity of each; same as $\overline{aa}$.

ana-: Prefix denoting up, upward, back, backward, excessive, again, throughout.

anabasis (a-nab′-a-sis): A phase of worsening or progression in a disease.

anabolic (an-a-bol′-ik): Pertaining to or promoting anabolism. **A. COMPOUND**, a chemical substance that causes a synthesis of body protein.

anabolism (an-ab′-ō-lizm): The constructive phase of metabolism during which foods are converted into complex body substances such as hormones, enzymes, cell glycogen and cell protein; the reverse of catabolism.—anabolic, anabolistic, adj.

anacatharsis (an-a-ka-thar′-sis): Violent prolonged vomiting.

anachlorhydria (an-a-klor-hī′-dri-a): Lack of hydrochloric acid in the gastric juice.

anacholia (an-a-kō′-li-a): Decrease in the secretion of bile.

anacidity (an-a-sid′-i-ti): Lack of or deficiency in normal acidity, especially of hydrochloric acid in gastric juice.

anaclitic (an-a-klit′-ik): Being psychologically dependent on others; refers especially to the infant. **A. DEPRESSION**, that which occurs in all aspects of an infant's development following sudden separation from its mother or mother surrogate. **A. THERAPY**, in psychiatry, a therapy that fosters dependency needs and nurtures the relationship between patient and therapist; used to reduce feelings of anxiety and guilt.

anacroasia (an-a-krō-ā′-zi-a): Inability to understand language; auditory aphasia.

anacrotism (a-nak′-rō-tizm): An oscillation in the ascending curve of a sphygmographic pulse tracing, indicating an anomaly of the pulse beat.—anacrotic, adj.

anacusis (an-a-kū′-sis): Absence or total loss of hearing. Also anacusia, anacousia, anakusis.

anadenia (an-a-dē′-ni-a): 1. Absence of glands. 2. Defective functioning of glands.

anadipsia (an-a-dip′-si-a): Excessive thirst.

anadrenalism (an-a-drē′-nal-izm): Absence of or defective function of the adrenal glands.

anaerobe (an′-er-ob): A microorganism that grows and thrives best in an oxygen-free enviroment. When this strictly so, the organism is termed obligatory. Most pathogens will flourish in either the presence or absence of oxygen and are, therefore, termed facultative.

anaerobic (an-er-ō′-bik): 1. Without oxygen. 2. Able to grow and thrive in the absence of oxygen. **A. EXERCISE**, steady vigorous exercise that is continued long enough to produce metabolic acidosis. See **aerobic exercise** under **aerobic**.

anagen (an′-a-jen): The early phase in the production of hair by the hair follicle. See **telogen**.

anagenesis (an-a-jen′-e-sis): Regeneration or repair of tissue or structure.

anagnosasthenia (an′-ag-nōs-as-thē′-ni-a): Inability to read because of a neurosis, which may occur in the absence of organic disease of the eye.

anakastia (an-a-kas′-ti-a): Any psychopathological disorder that causes the individual to act compulsively or to react emotionally against his will.—anakastic, adj.

anakatesthesia (an′-a-kat-es-thē′-zi-a): A hovering or smothering sensation.

anal (ā′-nal): Pertaining to or near the anus. **A. CANAL**, the lower end of the digestive tube; extends from the rectum to the anus. **A. CHARACTER**, a personality characterized by persistence of the erotic traits of the anal phase of childhood into adult life and behavior. **A. CRYPT**, one of the small cul-de-sacs between the folds of mucous membrane in the anal canal. **A. EROTICISM**, deriving sexual pleasure from anal functions. **A. FISSURE**, a crack or slit in the mucous membrane at the margin of the anus. **A. FISTULA**, an abnormal opening into the skin or mucous membrane near the anus. **A. PHASE** or **STAGE**, the period in a child's development, usually from one to three years of age, when he is intensely interested in the process and products of defecation. **A. SPHINCTER**, either the external or internal sphincter muscle of the anus. See **sphincter**.

analagous (a-nal′-a-gus): Similar in function and/or appearance, but not in structure.—analogue, n.

analbuminemia (an′-al-bū-min-ē′-mi-a): A deficiency or absence of serum albumins in the blood.

analeptic (an-a-lep′-tik): 1. Having restorative properties. 2. A drug that acts as a restorative by stimulating the central nervous system; often used in medicine to counteract drowsiness or the effects of barbiturates.

analgesia (an-al-jē′zi-a): Lack of sensitivity to pain without loss of consciousness; may be produced by a drug or occur as a symptom of a nervous disorder. **HYPNOTIC A.**, the production of analgesia through hypnosis; sometimes used in treatment of severe burns, migraine headache, and asthma. **WAKING IMAGED A.,** a psychological technique whereby the patient is asked to think and talk about an earlier experience that was pleasurable; sometimes succeeds in reducing moderate pain.

analgesic (an-al-jē′-zik): 1. Insensible to pain. 2. Alleviating pain. 3. A drug that relieves pain.—Syn., anodyne.

analgia (an-al′-ji-a): Without pain.—analgic, adj.

analogue (an′-a-log): An organ or part that serves the same function as another but has a different structure. In chemistry, a compound that has a structure similar to that of another but with one component that is different.

analysand (a-nal′-i-sand): That which is being analyzed or one who is under psychoanalysis.

analysis (a-nal′-a-sis): 1. The separation of substances into their components for examination and determination of their properties. 2. In chemistry, a term used to describe the procedure for determining the composition and properties of the components of a compound. 3. In psychiatry, psychoanalysis (*q.v.*).—analyses, pl.; analytic, adj.

analyst (an′-a-list): A person experienced in performing analyses. In psychiatry, a psychoanalyst (*q.v.*) **"LAY" A.,** a person outside of the medical profession who has undergone training in analysis in preparation for performing analyses.

anamnesis (an-am-nē′-sis): 1. The act of remembering or recalling to mind. 2. That which is recollected. 3. A patient's medical history, particularly that part recalled by the patient and others. 4. In immunology, a rapid and unexpectedly strong antibody response in an individual to the administration of what was assumed to be an initial dose of an antigen.

anamnestic (an-am-nes′-tik): 1. Pertaining to amnesia. 2. Helpful to the memory. 3. Pertaining to a heightened immunologic response.

ananabasia (an-an-a-bā′-zi-a): The inability to ascend to heights because of intense fear.

ananabolic (an-an-a-bol′-ik): Lack of anabolism (*q.v.*)

ananastasia (an-an-a-stā′-zi-a): Lack or loss of ability to stand up or to arise from a sitting position; due to abulia (*q.v.*)

anandria (an-an′-dri-a): Absence or loss of virility or masculinity. Impotence.

anaphase (an′-a-fāz): A phase in mitosis (*q.v.*), when the divided chromosomes are drawn apart and collected at the opposite poles of the cell to form two separate nuclei.

anaphia (an-af′-i-a): Loss or absence of the sense of touch.

anaphoresis (an-a-fō-rē′-sis): Absence or reduction of secretion of sweat.

anaphrodisia (an-af-rō-diz′-i-a): Absence or reduction of the sexual impulse.

anaphrodisiac (an-af-rō-diz′-i-ak): 1. Lessening sexual desire. 2. A drug that lessens sexual desire.

anaphylactic (an-a-fi-lak′-tik): Pertaining to anaphylaxis. **A. SHOCK,** a condition of extreme hypersensitivity to a foreign protein or other substance induced in a person who has had a previous exposure to the same substance; an emergency condition requiring immediate medical attention. Symptoms include breathlessness, dyspnea, cyanosis, pallor, weakness, fever, vascular collapse, sometimes convulsions and unconsciousness.

anaphylactogen (an-a-fi-lak′-tō-jen): A substance that induces a state of anaphylaxis.

anaphylaxis (an-a-fi-lak′-sis): Extreme hypersensitivity reaction to a foreign protein after a previous exposure to the same substance; symptoms are as for anaphylactic shock; see anaphylactic.

anaplasia (an-a-plā′-zi-a): Loss of the distinctive characteristics of a cell, with reversion to a more primitive type, often associated with proliferative activity as in cancer.—anaplastic, adj.

anaptic (an-ap′-tik): Pertaining to the loss of the sense of touch.

anarithmia (an-a-rith′-mi-a): Loss of ability to count and/or use numbers correctly, thought to be due to a brain lesion.

anarthria (an-ar′-thri-a): Loss of ability to pronounce words distinctly, due to muscle dysfunction; thought to result from a brain lesion.—anarthric, adj.

anasarca (an-a-sark′-a): Serous infiltration of the subcutaneous connective tissue and serous cavities; generalized edema; dropsy. May be associated with renal, cardiac, or liver disease.—anasarcous, adj.

anasognosia (an-a-sog-nōz′-ē-a): Inability of a hemiplegic patient to recognize his disability; or his denial of it.

anastalsis (an-a-stawl′-sis): Antiperistalsis (*q.v.*).

anastomosis (a-nas-tō-mō′-sis): 1. The joining together of two hollow organs or of two or more arteries or veins, *e.g.*, the two vertebral arteries join to form the basilar artery. 2. The surgical establishment of an artificial connection between two hollow organs, nerves, or blood vessels; may be done to bypass a vascular obstruction or aneurysm—anastomoses, pl.; anastomotic, adj., anastomose, v.

anat.: Abbreviation for anatomy.

anatherapeusis (an′-a-ther-a-pū′-sis): Treatment by steadily increasing doses of a medication.

anatomic (an-a-tom′-ik): Pertaining to the structure of the body or a body part. **ANATOMIC**

SNUFF BOX, the hollow triangular space at the base of the metacarpal of the extended thumb.

anatomical (an-a-tom′-i-kal): Pertaining to the anatomy or structure of the body. **A. NECK,** often refers to the constricted part of the humerus just below the head. **A. POSITION,** see under position.

anatomist (a-nat′-o-mist): One who specializes in the study of anatomy or who performs dissections.

anatomy (a-nat′-o-mi): The science that deals with the structure and composition of the body; it is largely based on dissection.—anatomical, adj.; anatomically, adv.

anatoxin (an-a-toks′-in): Syn., toxoid (*q.v.*).

anatripsis (an-a-trip′-sis): The use of rubbing or friction as a treatment. May or may not include the simultaneous application of a medicament.

anatriptic (an-a-trip′-tik): 1. Pertaining to anatripsis. 2. The application of an ointment or a medication by rubbing it into the skin.

anatrophic (an-a-trof′-ik): Impeding or correcting atrophy; nourishing.

anatropia (an-a-trō′-pi-a): The tendency for the eyeballs to turn upward when the individual is at rest.

anazoturia (an-ā-zō-tū′-ri-a): Less than the normal amount of nitrogenous substances in the urine.

anchylo-: See ankylo-.

ancillary (an′-si-ler-i): Auxiliary; supplementary.

ancon (ang′-kon): The elbow joint.—ancones, pl.; anconoid, adj.

anconad (an′-kō-nad): Toward the elbow.

anconal (an′-kō-nal): Pertaining to the elbow.

anconeus (an-kō′-nē-us): The small triangular muscle at the back of the elbow; it is an extensor muscle of the forearm.

anconitis (an-kō-nī′-tis): Inflammation of the elbow joint.

anconoid (an′-kō-noyd): Pertaining to or resembling the elbow.

ancyl-: See ankylo-.

Ancylostoma (an-si-los′-tō-ma): A genus of nematodes, including the hookworms. **A. DUODENALE,** the Old World hookworm of man, a species found chiefly in temperate areas in contrast to the species *Necator Americanus,* the New World hookworm which is found chiefly in tropical areas.

ancylostomiasis (an′-si-los-tō-mī′-a-sis): Hookworm disease (*q.v.*).

Anderson's disease: See glycogen storage disease, type IV; amylopectinosis.

andr-, andro-: Combining forms denoting man, male, having the characteristics of a man.

andriatrics (an-dri-at′-riks): The branch of medicine that deals with the diseases of men, the genitalia in particular.

andrin (an′-drin): Any of the androgens found in the testes.

androblastoma (an′-drō-blas-to′-ma): A tumor of the ovary or testis, composed of stromal cells; may cause development of feminization or masculinization.

androcentrism (an-drō-sen′-trizm): Domination by males or by masculine interests.

androgalactozemia (an′-drō-ga-lak′-tō-zē′-mi-a): The escape or oozing of milk from the male breast.

androgen (an′-drō-jen): Any substance that stimulates and preserves the secondary male characteristics and structure; usually a hormone secreted by the testes or adrenal cortex, also prepared synthetically. When given to a female these substances have a masculinizing effect.—androgenic, adj.

androgogy (an′-drō-gō-ji): The teaching of adults as opposed to pedagogy (the teaching of children).

androgyne (an′-drō-jīn): A person in whom the female characteristics are most prominent; a female pseudohermaphrodite.

androgyny (a-droj′-i-ni): 1. Hermaphroditism. 2. Female hermaphroditism.

android (an′-droyd): Resembling a man. **A. PELVIS,** see under pelvis.

andrologist (an-drol′-ō-jist): A specialist in the treatment of male infertility.

andrology (an-drol′-ō-ji): The study of the diseases of men, especially of the male organs of generation.

andromania (an-drō-mā′-ni-a): Nymphomania (*q.v.*).

andromorphous (an-drō-mor′-fus): Having the form or appearance of a male individual.

androphobia (an-drō-fō′-bi-a): A morbid dislike of men or fear and dislike of the male sex.—androphobic, adj.

androsterone (an-dros′-ter-on): An androgenic hormone secreted in the urine; derived from testosterone metabolism; also produced synthetically; influences the development of secondary male sex characteristics.

anemia (a-nē′-mi-a): Term applied to a large group of disorders that result from deficiency in the number of red blood cells or their hemoglobin content, or both, or the volume of packed red blood cells. Types are differentiated on the basis of cause, hereditary factors, size, shape and hemoglobin content of the red blood cells, response to therapy, etc. Also classified as primary when due to disease of the blood or blood-producing organs; secondary when it is the result of another pathological condition such as cancer, bleeding ulcers, etc. Clinical features include pallor, easy fatigue, breathlessness on exertion, giddiness, palpitation, loss of appetite, gastrointestinal disorders and amenorrhea. **ADDISONIAN A.**, pernicious **A.** **ANAPLASTIC A.**, secondary **A.**, may follow use of certain chemicals, x ray or other ionizing radiation, infection, or metastatic bone cancer; the bone marrow is replaced by fibrous tissue which results in pancytopenia. **APLASTIC A.**, **A.** from failure of the bone marrow to produce blood cells; usually fatal. **CONGENITAL HEMOLYTIC A.**, usually not recognized until late in life; may follow transient jaundice; cholelithiasis often present; may require splenectomy to prevent hemolytic crisis. **COOLEY'S A.**, thalassemia (*q.v.*). **FOLIC ACID A.**, an anaplastic **A.** due to deficiency of folic acid in the diet. **GENETIC ANEMIAS**, include sickle cell **A.**, thalassemia, and congenital hemolytic **A.** **HEMOLYTIC A.**, a type characterized by excessive destruction of red blood cells; see **acholuric jaundice**. **HYPERCHROMATIC A.**, characterized by red cells that are deeply colored. **HYPOCHROMIC A.**, characterized by low hemoglobin content of red blood cells. **HYPOCHROMIC MICROCYTIC A.**, hypochromic **A.** in which the red cells are small and the hemoglobin content reduced. **IRON DEFICIENCY A.**, the commonest type of **A.**, due to poor uptake of iron resulting from inadequate or ill balanced diet, poor absorption, increased bodily needs as in pregnancy, or to excessive blood loss. **MACROCYTIC A.**, a group of **ANEMIAS** characterized by very large blood cells and splenomegaly. **MEGALOBLASTIC A.**, **A.** characterized by the presence of megaloblasts in the blood. **MICROANGIOPATHIC A.**, hemolytic **A.** **MICROCYTIC A.**, characterized by the formation of abnormally small red blood cells. **MYELOPATHIC A.**, myelophthisic **A.** **MYELOPHTHISIC A.**, occurs in association with space-occupying disorders of the bone marrow. **NORMOCYTIC A.**, **A.** in which the red blood cells are of normal size and hemoglobin content. **NUTRITIONAL A.**, due to faulty nutrition, especially poor protein intake. **PERNICIOUS A.**, a chronic disorder primarily of middle and old age, and especially in blue-eyed, fair-haired, prematurely grayed people; the red blood cells are enlarged and often of bizarre shapes; symptoms include enlargement of the liver and spleen, icterus, glossitis, tachycardia, and such neurological symptoms as confusion, numbness, loss of muscle coordination and position sense; caused by atrophy of the stomach mucosa and its consequent failure to produce the intrinsic factor necessary for absorption of vitamin B_{12}; treated by lifelong injections of the vitamin. **POSTHEMORRHAGIC A.**, **A.** which follows a hemorrhage. **SICKLE CELL A.**, a hereditary and familial type of **A.**, peculiar to blacks; the red blood cells have a short life span, acquire a characteristic crescent or sickle shape, and tend to clog the small capillaries causing clots. Children become barrel-chested with protruding abdomens; most die before three years of age. **SIDEROBLASTIC A.**, may be hereditary or acquired; often develops from use of certain drugs; marked by elevated serum level of iron due to a derangement of heme synthesis. **SPHEROCYTIC A.**, hereditary spherocytosis; see **spherocytosis**.

anemic (a-nē'-mik): Pertaining to, affected with, or characteristic of anemia.

anemophobia (an'-e-mō-fō'-bi-a): Abnormal fear of wind or draughts of air.

anencephalohemia (an'-en-sef'-a-lō-hē'-mi-a): Lack of sufficient blood supply to the brain.

anencephaly (an-en-sef'-a-li): A congenital anomaly in which there is an absence of the flat bones of the skull and absence of the brain and spinal cord; the condition is incompatible with life. Also anencephalia.—anencephalous, anencephalic, adj.

anenzymia (an-en-zī'-mi-a): Lack of sufficient secretion, or the absence of, an enzyme in the body.

anephric (a-nef'-rik): 1. Refers to a person who lacks both kidneys, either as a congenital defect or because of surgical removal. 2. A person who has lost all kidney function due either to surgical removal or nephritic pathology.

anepia (a-nē'-pi-a): Lack of ability to speak.

anergy (an'-er-ji): 1. Lethargy; inactivity; sluggishness; lack of energy. 2. Decreased or absence of sensitivity to specific antigens. Also anergia.—anergic, adj.

anerythrocyte (an-ē-rith'-rō-sīt): A red blood cell containing no hemoglobin.

anerythroplasia (an-ē-rith'-rō-plā'-zi-a): Incomplete or inadequate formation of erythrocytes.

anerythropsia (an-er-i-throp'-si-a): Inability to distinguish the color red.

anesthekinesis (an-es'-thē-ki-nē'zi-a): Sensory and motor paralysis occurring together.

anesthesia (an-es-thē'-zi-a): Absence of feeling or sensation in a part of the body or the whole of it. May be induced by a drug, trauma, disease, or hypnosis. **BASAL A.**, a preliminary anesthesia, usually not complete, often produced by narcosis and requiring supplementation to produce surgical anesthesia. **CAUDAL A.**, produced by injection of an anesthetic into the space outside the dura mater between the fifth sacral vertebra and the coccyx or between the first and third lumbar vertebrae; used chiefly in childbirth. **CUTANEOUS A.**, produced by spraying an anesthetic into or onto the skin in a particular area. **DISSOCIATED ANESTHESIA**, loss of sensation for pain and temperature but without loss of touch sensation or proprioception; occurs in patients with syringomyelia. **ENDO-**

BRONCHIAL A., produced by administering a gaseous mixture through a slender tube into a large bronchus of one lung to exclude the anesthetic from one lung during thoracic surgery. **ENDOTRACHEAL A., A.** administered through an endotracheal tube. **EPIDURAL A.**, see epidural block. **GENERAL A.**, loss of sensation with loss of consciousness. **GLOVE-AND-STOCKING A.**, lessening or loss of sensation in areas of the hands and feet corresponding to areas covered by gloves or stockings; may be a sign of peripheral nerve disease; occasionally a hysterical phenomenon. **INFILTRATION A.**, local anesthesia induced by injection of an anesthetic solution directly into the tissues to be anesthetized. **INHALATION A.**, the oldest and most common form of administration; any one of, or a combination of, several gases and vapors is introduced through the nose, endotracheal tube, or tracheostomy tube. **INTRAVENOUS A.**, produced by the introduction of an **A.** into a vein to induce general **A. LOCAL A.**, produced by nerve blocking to prevent impulses from a limited area from reaching the brain. **NERVE-BLOCK A.**, injection of an anesthetic drug into a nerve or nerve root to anesthetize a specific area. **ORAL A., A.** produced by drugs and administered by mouth. **RECTAL A., A.** produced by injection of an anesthetic drug into the rectum. **REFRIGERATION A.**, produced by use of ethyl chloride spray or cracked ice locally for several hours to produce anesthesia of an extremity in amputation cases. **REGIONAL A., A.** producing insensitivity over a certain area by injection of an anesthetic into tissues in the immediate vicinity of the nerve to be blocked; it affects the smallest area necessary to accomplish the particular procedure. **SADDLE-BLOCK A., A.** limited to the buttocks, perineum, and inner surfaces of the thighs. **SPINAL A.**, produced by injection of an anesthetic into the spinal subarachnoid space; may also be produced by a lesion in the spinal cord. **SUBARACHNOID A.**, spinal **A. SURFACE A.**, produced by the application of an anesthetic to a particular body surface, as with a swab. **TACTILE A.**, see under tactile. **TOPICAL A.**, produced by applying a local anesthetic directly to the area to be operated on, *e.g.*, the cornea, mucous membrane or the skin.

anesthesimeter (an-es′-the-sim′-e-ter): An instrument used to regulate and measure the amount of an anesthetic being administered.

anesthesiologist (an′-es-thē-zi-ol′-ō-jist): A physician who specializes in anesthesiology and the care of the patient under anesthesia.

anesthesiology (an′-es-thē-zi-ol′-ō-ji): The medical science concerned with the uses, administration, and effects of anesthetic agents, and the care of the patient under anesthesia.

anesthetic (an-es-thet′-ik): 1. Pertaining to anesthesia. 2. An agent that produces loss of sensibility to pain and/or loss of consciousness. **GENERAL A.**, a drug or agent that produces unconsciousness. **LOCAL A.**, a drug or agent that produces local insensitivity to pain when injected into the tissues or applied topically.

anesthetist (a-nes′-the-tist): A health care professional who is skilled in the administration of anesthetic agents; may or may not be a physician. **NURSE A.**, a professional nurse who has completed an approved course in anesthesiology and is certified by the American Association of Nurse Anesthetists; responsible for administering anesthesia and for monitoring patients under anesthesia.

anesthetization (a-nes′-the-tī-zā′-shun): The act of producing insensibility to pain through the administration of an anesthetic (*q.v.*).—anesthetize, v.

aneuploid (an′-ū-ployd): Having an abnormal number of diploid chromosomes.

aneuria (a-nū′-ri-a): A condition of diminished nervous energy.

aneurin (e) hydrochloride (an′-ū-rin hī-drō-klō′-rīd): Thiamine hydrochloride; see thiamin. Also called vitamin B_1.

aneurysm (an′-ū-rizm): Permanent, abnormal, local dilatation or ballooning out of a blood vessel wall, most commonly in the aorta; the result of a congenital defect or of degeneration and weakening of the wall due to injury or disease which produces a pulsating swelling over which a murmur may be heard. **ABDOMINAL AORTIC A.**, common in the elderly; usually associated with degenerative atherosclerosis. **ARTERIAL A.**, an **A.** in an artery; may be due to a congenital defect or to hypertensive atherosclerosis. **ARTERIOVENOUS A.**, an abnormal direct connection between an artery and a vein, often follows an injury. **ARTERIOSCLEROTIC A.**, the commonest type of abdominal **A.**; occurs chiefly in the elderly, due to atherosclerosis. **BERRY A.**, a small thin-walled **A.** often occurring at the junction of a cerebral artery; likely to rupture causing hemorrhage into the subarachnoid space. **CARDIAC A.**, thinning and bulging of a weakened ventricular wall, usually the result of a myocardial infarction. **CEREBRAL A., BERRY A., CHARCOT-BOUCHARD A.**, a small **A.** of an artery or arteriole; may be the cause of a massive cerebral hemorrhage. **CIRCOID A.**, a tangled mass of pulsating blood vessels, appearing as a subcutaneous tumor, often of the scalp. **DISSECTING A.**, one that is formed by a longitudinal tear or break in the intima, usually of the aorta, which allows blood to collect between the intima and the other layers of the vessel wall. **FALSE A.**, one in which all the coats of the vessel rupture and the blood is retained by the surrounding tissue. **FUSIFORM A.**, an elongated spindle-shaped **A.** that involves the entire circumference of the arterial wall. **INTRACRANIAL A.**, one within the cranium. **MYCOTIC A.**, an **A.** produced by the growth of microorganisms in the vessel wall; often a sequela of bacterial endocarditis; syn., bacterial aneurysm. **POSTERIOR-COMMUNICATING A.**, an **A.** in the artery that passes from the internal carotid to the posterior cerebral artery. **SACCULAR A.**, a localized outpouching of an artery that does not affect the entire circumference of the artery, often occurring in an artery of the Circle of Willis; does not usually produce symptoms unless it ruptures. **THORACIC AORTIC A.**, an **A.** in the thoracic aorta that develops slowly and is less apt to rupture than an abdominal aortic **A.**; usually seen in the elderly.

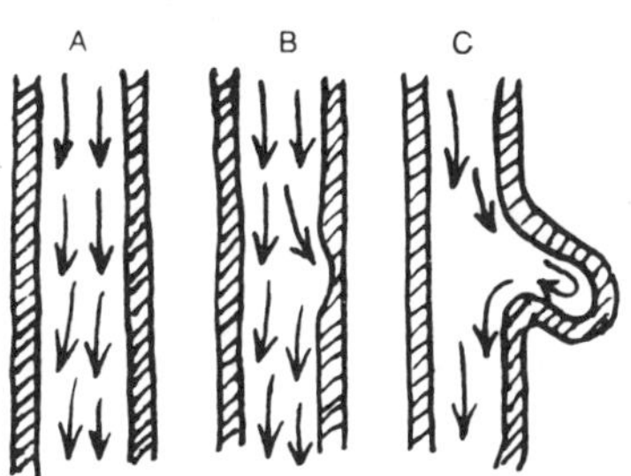

Development of aneurysm A. normal B. weakness in wall of artery C. aneurysm

aneurysmal (an-ū-riz′-mal): Pertaining to an aneurysm.

aneurysmectomy (an-ū-riz-mek′-to-mi): The surgical removal of the sac of an aneurysm.

aneurysmoplasty (an-ū-riz′-mō-plas-ti): Plastic repair of an artery damaged by an aneurysm.

aneurysmorrhaphy (an-ū-riz-mor′-a-fi): Suturing of a blood vessel damaged by an aneurysm.

aneuthanasia (an-ū′-tha-nā′-zi-a): A painful agonizing death.

ANF: Abbreviation for the American Nurses' Foundation (*q.v.*).

ANF (antinuclear factor) test: A screening test for the presence of antibodies against the cell nuclear material (DNA). A positive reaction is indicative of lupus erythematosus.

angi-. angio-: Combining forms denoting a vessel(s), particularly a blood or lymph vessel.

angiectasis (an-ji-ek′-ta-sis): Abnormal dilatation of blood vessels; seen mostly in older people as red or purplish areas usually on the chest or trunk. See **telangiectasis**.—angiectatic, adj.

angiectomy (an-ji-ek′-tō-mi): Surgical excision of part or all of a blood or lymph vessel.

angiitis (an-ji-ī′-tis): Inflammation of a blood or lymph vessel.—angiitic, adj.

angina (an-jī′-na): A sense of suffocation, choking, or constriction; or a disease characterized by spasmodic suffocative attacks. **A. DECUBITUS**, attacks of **A.** occurring when the person is sleeping or in the recumbent position. **INTESTINAL A.**, cramping pains in the abdomen following a meal; caused by ischemia of the musculature of the intestine. **LUDWIG'S A.**, a severe, acute, purulent infection of the floor of the mouth, particularly around the submaxillary gland, usually caused by streptococcus; may originate with a dental infection; see **cellulitis**. **A. PECTORIS**, severe but temporary paroxysmal attack of cardiac pain which may radiate to the shoulder, arm, or epigastrium; accompanied by a feeling of suffocation and impending death; caused by inadequate supply of oxygen to the heart muscle; may be precipitated by exercise or emotional stress. **PREINFARCTION A.**, **A.** characterized by severe abrupt onset of chest pain that lasts longer than usual anginal pain; may be precipitated by situations of minimal stress; symptoms include severe dyspnea and, unless the patient is treated, heart failure may ensue. **PRINZMETAL'S A.**, a type of **A.** that is caused by spasm of one of the large coronary vessels; may occur during normal activity or during rest; tends to occur at one time of day and the pain is severe and long-lasting; sudden death may occur as a result of severe dysrhythmia. **VINCENT'S A.**, a bacterial infection of the mucous membranes of the mouth, especially of the gums but may extend to the tonsils and pharynx, with necrosis of the gingivae, causing bleeding, tenderness, offensive breath, fever, swelling of the cervical lymph glands; seen mostly in adolescents. Also called trench mouth.—anginal, anginoid, adj.

angina pectoris (an-jī′-na pek′-tor-is): See under **ANGINA. INTRACTABLE A.P.**, can become quite crippling; treatment includes use of antihypertensives if indicated and eliminating stressors as much as possible as well as giving up smoking. **STABLE A.P.**, the causes, frequency, and severity of attacks are all predictable. **STATUS ANGIOSUS**, a type of **A.P.** in which the pain lasts an hour; due to coronary insufficiency.

angioblast (an′-ji-ō-blast): 1. The embryonic tissue from which the blood vessels and the blood cells in the early embryo develop. 2. A blood vessel-forming cell.

angioblastoma (an′-ji-ō-blas-tō′-ma): A tumor arising in a blood vessel of the meninges of the brain or spinal cord; angioblastic meningioma.

angiocardiogram (an-ji-ō-kar′-di-ō-gram): An x-ray film of the heart and great vessels after the intravenous injection of an opaque medium.

angiocardiography (an′ji-ō-kar-di-og′-ra-fi): A radiographic procedure for demonstrating the chambers of the heart and the great blood vessels after injecton of a radiopaque medium.—angiocardiographic, adj.; angiocardiographically, adv.

angiocardiopathy (an′-ji-ō-kar-di-op′-a-thi): Any disease or disorder of the heart and blood vessels.

angiocarditis (an′-ji-ō-kar-dī′-tis): Inflammation of the great vessels and the heart.

angiocatheter (an-ji-ō-cath′-e-ter): A device consisting of a soft flexible catheter surrounding a venipuncture needle; after the vein has been punctured, the needle is withdrawn leaving the catheter in place in the vein.

angiocholecystitis (an′-ji-ō-kō-le-sis-tī′-tis): Inflammation of the bile ducts and the gallbladder.

angiochondroma (an′-ji-ō-kon-drō′-ma): A benign tumor containing both vascular and cartilaginous tissue; sometimes referred to as hamartoma.

angiodermatitis (an′-ji-ō-der-ma-tī′-tis): Inflammation of the blood vessels of the skin.

angioectasia (an′-ji-ō-ek-tā′-zi-a): Dilated tufts of skin capillaries; seen chiefly in the elderly as red or purplish spots on the trunk.

angioedema (an′-ji-ō-ē-dē′-ma): Angioneurotic edema (*q.v.*).

angioendothelioma (an′-ji-ō-en′-dō-thē-li-ō′-ma): Ewing's tumor (*q.v.*).

angiofibroma (an′-ji-ō-fī-brō′-ma): A fibroma that contains numerous blood vessels: often appears as a skin tag.

angioglioma (an′-ji-ō-gli-ō′-ma): A glioma (*q.v.*) that contains numerous blood vessels.

angiogram (an′-ji-ō-gram): A series of x-ray pictures of blood vessels, especially arteries, after injection of a radiopaque medium.

angiography (an-ji-og′-ra-fi): Radiography of the blood vessels following the injection of a radiopaque material.—angiogram, n.; angiographic, adj.; angiographically, adv.

angiokeratoma (an′-ji-ō-ker-a-tō′-ma): A skin disease with thickening of the epidermis and the appearance of small wart-like elevations on the skin. **A. CORPORIS DIFFUSUM**, see Fabry's disease.

angiolipoma (an′-ji-ō-lip-ō′-ma): A lipoma containing numerous prominent blood vessels; occurs mostly in subcutaneous tissue.

angiolith (an′ji-ō-lith): A calculus in the wall of a blood vessel.

angiology (an-ji-ol′-ō-ji): The science dealing with the lymphatic and blood vessel systems.—angiological, adj.

angiolupoid (an-ji-ō-loo′-poyd): Cutaneous sarcoidosis in which bluish-red nodules and telangiectasia appear, chiefly on the nose and the skin around it.

angiolymphitis (an′-ji-ō-lim-fī′-tis): Lymphangitis (*q.v.*).

angiolysis (an-ji-ol′-i-sis): A condition that may be hereditary or may occur at any age, characterized by progressive fibrosis of blood vessel walls resulting in scar formation causing obliteration of the vessel.

angioma (an-ji-ō′-ma): An innocent tumor formed of blood vessels. See hemangioma; lymphangioma. **CAVERNOUS A.**, a benign tumor present at birth, consisting of a spongy, bluish red mass made up of many large cavernous spaces filled with blood and blood vessels. **CHERRY A.**, raised bright red vascular papules containing many vascular loops, usually appearing on the trunk; often seen in the middle aged and elderly. **SPIDER A.**, spider nevus; characterized by a small central elevated red dot from which tiny blood vessels radiate like a spider's web; usually appear on the face, neck, arms, and upper trunk. **STRAWBERRY A.**, a cavernous **A.** the size and color of a strawberry.—angiomata, angiomas, pl.; angiomatous, adj.

angiomalacia (an′-ji-ō-ma-lā′-shi-a): Softening of the blood vessel walls.

angiomatosis (an′-ji-ō′-ma-tō′-sis): A condition characterized by the multiple formation of angiomas.

angiomegaly (an-ji-ō-meg′-a-li): Enlargement of one or more blood vessels, particularly when it occurs in the eyelid.

angiomyolipoma (an′-ji-ō-mī′-ō-lī-pō′-ma): A benign tumor having vascular and adipose tissue elements.

angiomyoma (an′-ji-ō-mi-ō′ma): An angioma combined with a myoma.

angiomyoneuroma (an′ji-ō-mī′-ō-nū-rō′-ma): A glomus tumor; see under glomus.

angiomyopathy (an′-ji-ō-mī-op′-a-thi): Any disorder of the muscular walls of the blood vessels.

angioneuroma (an′-ji-ō-nū-rō′-ma): A benign tumor containing elements of vascular and nerve fiber tissue.

angioneurosis (an′-ji-ō-nū-rō′-sis): A condition caused by injury or disease of the nerves of the vasomotor system.

angioneurotic edema (an′-ji-ō-nū-rot′-ik ē-dē′-ma): An acute condition characterized by the sudden development of large painless, localized, edematous, itchy lesions; may involve the face, lips, larynx, neck, hands, feet, or genitalia; is accompanied by swelling of subcutaneous and submucous tissues; edema of the glottis may be fatal; may be caused by an allergy, usually a food allergy, or by infection, emotional stress, insect bites, parasitic infestation; may also be a congenital conditon.

angiopathy (an-ji-op′-a-thi): Any disease of the blood vessels or lymph vessels.—angiopathic, adj.

angiophakomatosis (an′-ji-ō-fak′-ō-ma-tō′-sis): Angiomatosis of the retina associated with angiomatosis of the cerebellum and angiomata in other viscera; von Hippel-Landau disease.

angiophilia (an-ji-ō-fil′-i-a): Hemophilia, with bleeding from the skin and mucous membranes, a conditon characterized by increased bleeding time and low activity of Factor VIII (*q.v.*).

angioplacentography (an′-ji-ō-pla-sen-tog′-ra-fi): Radiography of the blood vessels of the placenta after the injection of a radiopaque dye.

angioplasty (an′-ji-ō-plas-ti): 1. Plastic surgery of blood vessels. 2. A surgical procedure to restore blood flow in an artery by threading a balloon-tipped catheter into the vessel and then inflating it, thus pressing the atherosclerotic plaque causing the obstruction against the walls of the vessel, thus widening its lumen.

angiopoiesis (an′-ji-ō-poy-ē′-sis): The process of developing blood vessels in new tissue.

angioretinography (an′-ji-ō-ret-i-nog′-ra-fi): Visualization of the blood vessels of the retina after injection of a radiopaque or fluorescent material.

angiorrhaphy (an-ji-or′-a-fi): Suturing of a blood vessel.

angiorrhexis (an′-ji-ō-rek′-sis): Rupture of a blood vessel.

angiosarcoma (an′-ji-ō-sar-kō′-ma): Hemangiosarcoma (*q.v.*).

angiosclerosis (an′-ji-ō-sklē-rō′-sis): Hardening and thickening of the blood vessel walls.

angioscotoma (an′-ji-ō-skō-tō′-ma): Defective vision caused by shadows cast on the retina by the blood vessels.

angiosialitis (an′-ji-ō-sī-a-lī′-tis): Inflammation of the excretory duct of one of the salivary glands.

angiospasm (an′-ji-ō-spazm): Local, intermittent constriction of the walls of a blood vessel.

angiostaxis (an-ji-ō-stak′-sis): The oozing of blood from capillaries as may occur in hemophilia.

angiostenosis (an′-ji-ō-stē-nō′-sis): Narrowing of the lumen of a vessel; usually refers to a blood vessel.

angiosteosis (an′-ji-os-tē-ō′-sis): Ossification of blood vessel walls.

angiostrongyliasis (an′-ji-ō-stron-ji-lī′-a-sis): Infestation with nematodes of the genus *Angiostrongylus cantonensis*.

Angiostrongylus (an′-ji-ō-stron′-ji-lus): A parasitic nematode found in certain areas of the Pacific and Asia.

angiotelectasis (an′-ji-ō-te-lek′-ta-sis): Dilatation of one or more blood vessels; usually refers to the arterioles and smaller vessels.

angiotensin (an-ji-ō-ten′-sin): A polypeptide formed in the blood plasma by the action of the enzyme renin on a globulin in the plasma; a potent vasoconstrictor; stimulates release of aldosterone from the kidney cortex.

angiotitis (an-ji-ō-tī′-tis): Inflammation of the blood vessels of the ear.

angiotomy (an-ji-ot′-o-mi): Surgical excision into a blood or lymph vessel, or the severing of a vessel.

angiotonin (an-ji-ō-tō′-nin): Angiotensin (*q.v.*)

angle of Louis: A landmark on the anterior chest wall; it is a projection formed at the junction of the manubrium and the body of the sternum at the level of the fifth thoracic vertebra.

angor (ang′-or): A feeling of extreme distress or anguish. Angina (*q.v.*). **A. ANIMI,** a deep sense of impending doom or disaster, common in angina pectoris.

Angstrom unit: An internationally adopted unit of measurement; used primarily to express electromagnetic wavelengths. Equals one ten thousandth of a micron; one tenth of a millimicron; one ten millionth of a millimeter; one hundred millionth of a centimeter; or 1/254,000,000 of an inch. Ten million angstroms equal 39.37 inches.

angulation (ang-ū-lā′-shun): 1. The bending of a hollow structure to form an abnormal angle, as may occur in the intestine or ureter; may become the site of an obstruction. 2. A deviation from the normal axis of a structure, as may occur in fracture of a long bone.

anhaphia (an-hā′-fi-a): Anaphia (*q.v.*).

anhedonia (an-hē-dō′-ni-a): Lack of the capacity to enjoy normally enjoyable experiences.

anhematopoieses (an-hē′-ma-tō-poy-ē′-sis): Defective or deficient formation of blood.

anhemolytic (an-hē-mō-lit′-ik): Not destructive to red blood cells by lysis; opp. of hemolytic.

anhidrosis (an-hī-drō′-sis): Absence or deficiency of sweat secretion.—anhidrotic, adj.

anhidrotic (an-hī-drot′-ik): 1. Reducing or inhibiting perspiration. 2. An agent that reduces perspiration.

anhydrase (an-hī′-dras): An enzyme that acts as a catalyst in removing water from a compound.

anhydration (an-hī-drā′-shun): Dehydration. The condition of being without water.

anhydremia (an-hī-drē′-mi-a): Decreased fluid content of the blood.—anhydremic, adj.

anhydride (an-hī′-drid): A chemical compound that results when water is removed from a substance, particularly from an acid, base, or alcohol.

anhydrochloria (an-hī-drō-klō′-ri-a): Deficiency or absence of hydrochloric acid in the gastric secretion. Achlorhydria.

anhydromyelia (an-hī′-drō-mī-ē′-li-a): Deficiency of cerebrospinal fluid.

anhydrous (an-hī′-drus): Entirely without water; dry.

anhypnosis (an-hip-nō′-sis): Sleeplessness.

anicteric (ak-ik′-ter-ik): Without jaundice.

anile (an′-il, ā′-nīl): Weak; infirm; old womanish; doddering, imbecilic, senile.—anility, adj.

aniline (an′-i-lin): An oily compound obtained from the dry distillation of coal and much used in the preparation of dyes for medical as well as industrial uses.

anima (an′-i-ma): In Jungian psychiatry, the soul, inner being, or personality as contrasted with the persona or outer character of a person.

animate (an′-i-mat): Having life.

animation (an-i-mā′-shun): The quality of being alive. **SUSPENDED A.**, a temporary condition marked by suspension of normal vital functions.

animia (a-nim′-i-a): Loss of the ability to mimic or to imitate gestures and to communicate by gestures; due to damage or disorder of the language center in the cortex.

animism (an′-i-mizm): 1. The tendency to ascribe qualities of life to inanimate objects; occurs normally in children. 2. The belief that all animals and inanimate objects possess souls; basic to many primitive religions. 3. An ancient doctrine which, among other theories, held that the soul is the vital principle governing all life phenomena, both normal and abnormal.

animus (an′-i-mus): 1. A feeling of hostility or hatred. 2. In Jungian psychology, the masculine as compared to the feminine aspect of the inner self.

anion (an′-ī-on): A negatively charged ion that is attracted to and moves toward the positively charged anode during electrolysis (*q.v.*). In physiological chemistry, the important ions are bicarbonate, chloride, and phosphate. **A. GAP**, the difference between the serum sodium concentrates and the sum of the bicarbonate and chloride concentrates.

aniridia (an-i-rid′-i-a): Lack or defect of the iris; usually congenital and usually bilateral. Also called irideremia.

anis-, aniso-: Combining forms denoting irregular or unequal.

anisakiasis (an-i-sak-ī′-a-sis): An infection caused by a parasitic worm that thrives on salt-water fish; is not communicable; occurs in those who eat raw infected fish; causes severe acute abdominal symptoms resembling those of appendicitis or intestinal blockage. The parasite, which is found in flounder, cod and haddock sold in the United States, survives smoking but is killed by heat and freezing. Also called herring worm disease.

anischuria (an-is-kū′-ri-a): Incontinence of urine.

anise (an′-is): An extract derived from the seeds of a plant of the parsley family; used in medicine as an expectorant, carminitive, and antiflatulent.

aniseikonia (an′-ī-sī-kō′-ni-a): A visual defect in which the retinal image of an object is different in the two eyes.

anisochromatic (an-ī′-sō-krō-mat′ ik): Not of uniform color throughout.

anisochromia (an-ī′-sō-krō-mi-a): A condition in which the color or staining intensity of red blood cells varies due to unequal distribution of hemoglobin among the red blood cells.

anisocoria (an-ī′-sō-kō′-ri-a): Inequality in the diameter of the pupils, frequently seen in older people and those with nervous system disorders or head trauma.

anisocytosis (an-ī′-so-sī-tō′-sis): Inequality in the size of cells that are normally uniform, especially red blood cells.

anisodactyly (an-ī′-sō-dak′-ti-li): Unequal length in corresponding digits.—anisodactylous, adj.

anisodont (an-ī′-sō-dont): Having teeth that are irregular or uneven in length, shape, or spacing.

anisognathous (an-ī-sog′-na-thus): Having jaws of unequal size, with the upper one usually being the larger.

anisoleukocytosis (an-ī′-sō-lū′-kō-sī-tō′-sis): Abnormality in the ratio of the various forms of leukocytes in the blood.

anisomastia (an-ī′-sō-mas′-ti-a): Inequality in the size of the breasts.

anisomelia (an-ī′-sō-mē′-li-a): A condition of inequality between two paired limbs or right and left parts, as digits.

anisometropia (an-i′-sō-mē-trō′-pi-a): A condition in which light rays are refracted differently in the two eyes; usually correctable by ordinary lenses.

anisopiesis (an-ī-sō-pī-ē′-sis): Inequality of arterial blood pressure in different or paired parts of the body as registered by a sphygmomanometer.

anisosphygmia (an-ī-sō-sfig′-mi-a): Unequal pulse beat in two corresponding arteries, *e.g.*,the right and left temporal arteries.

anisuria (an-i-sū′-ri-a): A condition marked by changes in the amount of urine excreted, alternating between polyuria and oliguria.

ankle (ang′-kl): A synovial hinge joint, the distal ends of the tibia and fibula articulating with the talus (astragalus); the joint between the lower leg and the foot. **A. CLONUS**, a series of rapid muscular contractions of the calf muscle when the foot is dorsiflexed by pressure upon the sole. **A. JERK,** contraction of calf muscles causing extension of the foot, elicited by tapping the tendon of Achilles.

ankyl-, ankylo-: Combining forms denoting 1) crooked, curved; 2) stiff, immobile, constricted or closed because of adhesion.

ankyloblepharon (ang′-ki-lō-blef′-a-ron): Adhesion of the eyelids to each other at the ciliary edges.

ankylocolpos (ang′-ki-lō-kol′-pos): Imperforation of the vagina due to adhesion of the vaginal walls.

ankylodactylia (ang′-ki-lō-dak-til′i-a): A deformity in which two or more fingers or toes are in adhesion with each other; a fairly common congenital anomaly.

ankyloglossia (ang′-ki-lō-glos′-i-a): Tongue-tie.

ankyloproctia (ang′-ki-lō-prok′-shi-a): Stricture or imperforation of the anus.

ankylosing spondylitis (ang′ki-lō-sing spon-di-lī′-tis): See **spondylitis.**

ankylosis (ang′-ki-lō′-sis): Immobility or fixation of a joint; may result from trauma or a pathological condition, or be produced by surgery.

Ankylostoma: Ancylostoma (*q.v.*).

ankylostomiasis: Ancylostomiasis (*q.v.*).

ankylotia (ang-ki-lō′-shi-a): Closure or occlusion of the external auditory canal.

ankyroid (ang′-ki-royd): Hook-shaped.

"anniversary" phenomenon: The occurrence or deepening of depression, associated with an exacerbation of any physical symptoms, coinciding with the anniversary of the death or loss of a loved one; commonly seen in the elderly.

annular (an′-ū-lar): Ring-shaped. **A. LIGAMENTS,** surround adjoining parts and bind them together; *e.g.,* **A. L.** of the wrist and of the ankle.

annuloplasty (an′-ū-lō-plas-ti): Plastic surgery on an annular structure, *e.g.,* an annulus surrounding a cardiac valve.

annulotomy (an-ū-lot′-o-mi): The surgical division of a ring-like structure; often refers to the annulus of a cardiac valve.

annulus, anulus (an′-ū-lus): A ring, ring-like or encircling structure, *e.g.,* the tough fibrocartilaginous ring that joins the borders of the vertebra and holds them together, or the dense fibrous rings around the four major orifices of the heart. **A. OF ZINN,** the circular fibrous ligament at the back of the orbit that gives rise to the extraocular muscles.

ano-: Combining form denoting: 1. Anus. 2. Upper or upward.

anochromia (an-ō-krō′-mi-a): The concentration of the hemoglobin of the erythrocytes around the edges of the cells, leaving the centers pale; occurs in certain types of anemia.

anoci-association (a-nō′-si-a-sō-si-ā′-shun): A method of preventing or minimizing surgical shock by allaying the patient's anxiety, fear, or apprehension through the use of sedatives and hypnotics previous to anesthesia, and by measures that reduce postoperative discomfort.

anococcygeal (ā-nō-kok-sij′-ē′-al): Pertaining to the anus and the coccyx.

anocutaneous (ā-nō-kū-tā′-nē-us): Pertaining to the anus and the skin around it.

anode (an′-ōd): The positive pole or terminus of an electric source such as the galvanic battery.—anodal, anodic, adj.

anodermous (ā-nō-der′-mus): Without skin.

anodmia (an-od′-mi-a): Anosmia (*q.v.*).

anodontia (an-ō-don′-shi-a): Absence of some or all of the teeth; may be congenital and affect both the deciduous and permanent teeth, or may occur in an older person who has had teeth extracted.

anodyne (an′-ō-dīn): An agent that relieves pain. Analgesic.

anodynia (an-ō-din′-i-a): The state of being free from pain.

anoesia (an-ō-ē′-zi-a): Idiocy; severe mental retardation.—anoetic, adj.

anogenital (ā-nō-jen′-i-tal): Pertaining to the anal and genital regions.

anomaloscope (a-nom′-a-lō-skōp): An instrument used in testing for color blindness, especially the red-green color defect.

anomalous (a-nom′-a-lus): Abnormal, irregular; out of the ordinary.

anomaly (a-nom′-a-li): That which is unusual, abnormal or unconforming; that in which there is marked deviation from the normal in form, structure, or location.—anomalous, adj.

anomia (an-ō′-mi-a): Inability to name objects or persons. Same as nominal aphasia.—anomic, adj.

anomie (an′-ō-mē): In society, refers to a state characterized by lack or loss of normative standards of conduct. In individuals, refers to a person who lacks normal standards of conduct, is disoriented, anxious, isolated, and cannot relate to others.

anonychia (an-ō-nik′-i-a): Absence of a nail or nails.

anoopsia (an-ō-op′-si-a): Strabismus, accompanied by a tendency for one eye to turn upward.

anopelvic (ā-nō-pel′-vik): Pertaining to the anus and the pelvis.

anoperineal (ā′-nō-per-i-nē′-al): Pertaining to the anus and perineum.

Anopheles (a-nof′-e-lēz): A genus of mosquitoes; many of the several species are vectors of disease, *e.g.,* malaria, dengue, filariasis.

The females are the vectors of the malarial parasite, and their bite is the means of transmitting the disease to man.

anophoria (an-o-fō′-ri-a): The condition in which one eye turns upward because its visual axis rises above that of the other eye which is normal. Also anopia, anotropia, hyperphoria.

anophthalmia (an-of-thal′-mi-a): A congenital anomaly characterized by the absence of one or both eyes. Also anophthalmos.

anophthalmos (en-of-thal′-mus): Retraction of the eyeball within its orbit.

anoplasty (ā′-nō-plas-ti): Plastic repair or correction of an abnormality of the anus or anal canal.

anopsia (an-op′-si-a): Suppression of or inability to use the vision; may result from failure to use the eyes due to long confinement in a dark place, from cataract, or from refractive errors of high degree.

anorchid (an-or′-kid): A male with congenital absence of testes in the scrotum, or with cryptorchism; may be unilateral or bilateral.

anorchism (an-or′-kizm): Congenital absence of one or both testes.

anorchous (an-or′-kus): Having no testes or the condition of the testes not having descended into the scrotum.

anorectal (ā-nō-rek′-tal): Pertaining to the anus and rectum, as a fissure (*q.v.*). **A. AGENESIS**, lack of normal development of the anus and rectum.

anorectic (a′-nō-rek′-tik): 1. An appetite depressant. 2. Pertaining to anorexia.

anorectocolonic (ā′-nō-rek′-tō-kō-lon′-ik): Pertaining to the anus, rectum, and colon.

anorexia (an-ō-rek′-si-a): Loss or lack of appetite for food. **A. NERVOSA**, a psychosomatic disorder characterized by an aversion to food leading to atrophy of the stomach, emaciation and, in women, amenorrhea; willful starvation.—anorexic, anorectic, adj.

anorexigenic (an′-ō-rek-si-jen′-ik): 1. Producing anorexia. 2. An agent that dimishes the appetite.

anorgasmy (an-or-gaz′-mi): Failure to reach orgasm during normal sexual intercourse. Also called anorgasmia.

anorthography (an-or-thog′-ra-fi): Loss or impairment of ability to express oneself correctly in writing; agraphia (*q.v.*).

anorthopia (an-or-thō′-pi-a): A distortion of vision in which straight lines appear as bent or curved lines.

anoscope (ā′-nō-skōp): An endoscope (*q.v.*) for direct visualization of the anal canal and the lower end of the rectum.

anoscopy (ā-nos′-ko-pi): Examination of the lower rectum and the anus by means of an anoscope.—anoscopic, adj.

anosmia (an-oz′-mi-a): Absence or impairment of the sense of smell; may result from a lesion of the olfactory nerve, an obstruction in the nasal passages, cerebral disease involving the olfactory center, or there may be no apparent cause.—anosmic, anosmatic, anosmous, adj.

anosognosia (an-ō-sog-nō′-zi-a): Inability to recognize, denial of, or unawareness of loss or defect of a physical function; seen most often in patients with a lesion of the left hemisphere but may occur in those with other brain lesions also.

anostosis (an-os-tō′-sis): Defective formation or ossification of bone.

anotia (a-nō′-shi-a): Congenital absence of the auricles of the ears.

anovaginal (ā-nō-vaj′-i-nal): Pertaining to the anus and the vagina.

anovesical (ā-nō-ves′-i-kal): Pertaining to both the anus and the urinary bladder.

anovular (an-ov′-ū-lar): Not pertaining to, associated with, or coincidental with ovulation. **A. BLEEDING** is uterine bleeding that has not been preceded by ovulation. Also anovulatory.

anovulation (an-ov-ū-lā′-shun): Cessation or absence of ovulation.

anoxemia (an-ok-sē′-mi-a): Literally, no oxygen in the blood. More correctly, hypoxemia (*q.v.*); less than the physiologically normal amount of oxygen in the blood.—anoxemic, adj.

anoxia (a-nok′-si-a): Literally, no oxygen in the tissues, which occurs when the blood supply to a part is cut off; results in injury or death of the tissues involved. More frequently used to refer to a condition in which there is less than the normal amount of oxygen in red blood cells, consequently, reduced amounts in tissues and organs; or failure of tissues to utilize sufficient oxygen. May be due to impaired lung function, lack of hemoglobin, or circulatory disorders.—anoxic. adj.

ANS: Abbreviation for autonomic nervous system.

ansa (an′-sa): A loop-like anatomical structure. **A. CERVICALIS**, a nerve loop in the neck, consisting of fibers that innervate the infrahyoid muscles.

ansiform (an′-si-form): Loop-shaped.

-ant: An adjective-forming suffix denoting 1) a thing or agent that enhances a specific action; 2) a thing or substance that is acted upon in a specific manner.

Antabuse (an′-ta-būs): Disulfiram. A drug used in the treatment of alcoholism; produces intense discomfort if one takes alcohol while on this medication.

antacid (ant-as′-id): 1. Neutralizing or counteracting an acid. 2. Any substance that neutralizes or counteracts acidity, *e.g.*, that of the gastric juice.

antagonism (an-tag′-ō-nizm): A state of mutual opposition or force between like things that is characteristic of some muscles, drugs, and organisms. In pharmacotherapeutics, refers to a situation in which two drugs given together produce an action that is less intense than that of either of the drugs given alone.

antagonist (an-tag′-ō-nist): 1. A muscle that relaxes to allow its agonist (*q.v.*) to perform a movement. 2. Any agent that opposes or nullifies the action of another agent. 3. A drug that reduces or counteracts the effects of another drug.

antalgesic (ant-al-jē′-sik): Analgesic.

antalgic (ant-al′-jik): 1. Countering pain. 2. Pertaining to a position, motion, or posture taken to avoid pain; often used to describe a gait.

antaphrodisiac (ant′-af-rō-diz′-i-ak): An agent that diminishes sexual desire.

ante-: Prefix denoting before, with reference to time or place.

ante cibum (an′-tē sī′-bum): Before meals. [L.] Abbreviated a.c.

ante mortem (an′-tē mor′-tem): Before death. Opp. to post mortem.—antemortem, adj.

anteaural (an-tē-aw′-ral): Located in front of the ear

antebrachium (an-tē-brā′-kē-um): The part of the arm between the elbow and the wrist; the forearm.

antecedent (an-te-sē′-dent): 1. A preceding event, cause, or condition. 2. Prior in time or cause.

antecubital (an-tē-kū′-bit-al): Situated in front of the elbow. **A. FOSSA** or **SPACE,** the depression on the inner aspect of the elbow.

anteflexion (an-tē-flek′-shun): The abnormal bending forward of an organ. Commonly applied to the position of the uterus. Opp. to retroflexion.

antegrade (an′-tē-grād): Extending or moving forward. Also anterograde.

antehypophysis (an′-tē-hī-pof′-i-sis): The anterior lobe of the pituitary body.

antemetic (ant-ē-met′-ik): Antiemetic (*q.v.*).

antenatal (an-tē-nā′-tal): Pertaining to any event or condition that occurs or exists in the embryo or the mother during the period between conception and delivery of the infant.

antepartal (an-tē-par′-tal): Occurring before childbirth.

antepartum (an-te-par′-tum): In obstetrics, before parturition; generally refers to the three months preceding full-term delivery.

antepyretic (an-tē-pī-ret′-ik): Before the onset of fever. (Not to be confused with antipyretic.)

anteriad (an-tē′-ri-ad): Forward; toward the anterior. In anatomy, located on or at the anterior aspect of the body.

anterior (an-tē′-ri-or): In front of; the front surface of; ventral. **A. CHAMBER OF THE EYE,** the space between the posterior surface of the cornea and the anterior surface of the iris; contains aqueous humor (*q.v.*). **A. PITUITARY,** refers to the anterior lobe of the pituitary gland.

anterior poliomyelitis: Poliomyelitis (*q.v.*).

anterior spinal cord syndrome: Results from a flexion injury that damages the anterior spinal artery or the anterior aspect of the cord; marked by paralysis and loss of pain, temperature, and touch sensations; position and proprioception are retained.

anterior tibial compartment syndrome: A condition characterized by rapid swelling of the anterior tibial compartment, accompanied by pain in the leg, necrosis of the compartment muscle, edema, erythema over the area; may result from local injury due to excessive exertion or arterial occlusion.

antero-: Prefix denoting before; in front of.

anteroexternal (an′-ter-ō-eks-ter′-nal): Situated at the front and on the outside.

anterograde (an′ter-ō-grād): Proceeding or extending forward. **A. AMNESIA,** see **amnesia.**

anteroinferior (an′-ter-ō-in-fē′-ri-or): Situated in front and below.

anterointerior (an′-te-rō-in-tē′-ri-or): Situated in front and internally.

anterointernal (an′-ter-ō-in-ter′-nal): Situated in front and toward the inner side.

anterolateral (an′-ter-ō-lat′-er-al): 1. Pertaining to the front and one side. 2. Situated in front and to one side.

anteromedian (an′-ter-ō-mē′-di-an): Situated in front of and toward or on the midline.

anteroposterior (an′-ter-ō-pos-tē′-ri-or): 1. Passing from the front to the back of the body. 2. Relating to both front and back.

anterosuperior (an′-ter-ō-sūp-ēr′-i-or): Situated in front and above.

anteversion (an-tē-ver′-zhun): The forward tilting or displacement forward, without bending, of the whole of an organ or part. Opp. to retroversion.—anteverted, adj.; antevert, v.

anthelix (ant-hē′-liks): The cartilaginous semicircular ridge on the auricle of the ear below and in front of the helix (*q.v.*). Also called antihelix.

anthelmintic (ant-hel-min′-tik): 1. Destructive to intestinal worms. 2. Any remedy for the destruction or elimination of intestinal worms.

anthracemia (an-thra-sē′-mi-a): Anthrax septicemia; the presence of *Bacillus anthracis* in the blood stream.—anthracemic, adj.

anthracia (an-thrā′-shi-a): A condition characterized by the formation of carbuncles.

anthracoid (an′-thra-koyd): Resembling anthrax.

anthracometer (an-thra-kom′-e-ter): An instrument for measuring the amount of carbon dioxide in the air.

anthracosilicosis (an′-thra-kō-sil-i-kō′-sis): A disease of the lungs caused by inhalation of coal dust and particles of silica; often an occupational disease; symptoms are those of both anthrocosis and silicosis.

anthracosis (an-thra-kō′-sis): Black pigmentation of the lung due to inhalation of coal dust; when large amounts of coal dust are inhaled, as occurs in coal miners, pneumoconiosis may develop.

anthrax (an′-thrax): An acute infectious disease of animals, cattle and sheep especially, caused by the *Bacillus anthracis,* a spore-forming organism found in soil and directly transmissible to man through an abrasion in the skin or by inhalation or ingestion of airborne spores. An occupational disease occurring particularly in people who handle wool, fleece, hides, hair, or other animal tissues; characterized by the formation, at the site of infection, of a papule which becomes vesicular and ulcerates producing a tenacious, thick, black crust with the underlying and surrounding tissues becoming very swollen and edematous; may occur in the tongue and throat, intestine, and lung in addition to the skin. Other symptoms include headache, fever, malaise, pruritus; the acute form may be rapidly fatal. Protective measures include prophylactic immunization of cattle and man. Also called woolsorter's disease.

anthro-, anthrop-, anthropo-: Combining forms denoting man or human being.

anthropogeny (an-thro-poj′-e-ni): The study of the evolution of man.

anthropoid (an′-thro-poyd): Manlike. **A. PELVIS,** see under **pelvis**.

anthropology (an-thrō-pol′-o-ji): The study of mankind in all its aspects including man's origins, physical, social, and cultural development and behavior, racial characteristics, customs and beliefs.

anthropometer (an-thrō-pom′-e-ter): An instrument designed for measuring the various dimensions of the trunk and extremities of the human body.

anthropometry (an-thrō-pom′-e-tri): The science dealing with measurements of the human body and its parts, especially when done on a comparative basis; a basic technique in physical anthropology.—anthropometric, adj.

anthropomorphic (an′-thrō-pō-mor′-fik): Having a human form.

anthropophobia (an′-thrō-pō-fō′-bi-a): A morbid dread of human society or companionship.

anthropozoonosis (an′-thrō-pō-zō′-ō-nō′-sis): A disease which may affect either animal or man and may be transmitted from one species to the other.

anti-: Prefix denoting against, effective against, opposed to, counter.

antiabortifacient (an′-ti-a-bor-ti-fā′-shent): 1. An agent that prevents abortion or promotes normal gestation. 2. Tending to prevent abortion.

antiacid (an-ti-as′-id): See **antacid**.

antiadrenergic (an′-ti-ad-ren-er′-jik): Counteracting or modifying adrenergic action.

antiagglutinin (an-ti-ag-gloo′-tin-in): A specific antibody that has the power of neutralizing or destroying the action of the corresponding agglutinin.

antiallergic (an-ti-a-ler′-jik): 1. Tending to prevent or lessen an allergic reaction. 2. A substance or drug that prevents or lessens allergic reactions.

antiamebic (an-ti-a-mē′-bik): 1. An agent that retards or prevents the growth of amebas. 2. Tending to prevent or retard the growth of amebas.

antiamylase (an-ti-am′-i-las): A substance that combats the action of the enzyme amylase.

antianaphylaxis (an′-ti-an-a-fī-lak′-sis): A state of insusceptibility or immunity. A state in which anaphylaxis is avoided by injecting small but progressively increasing amounts of antigen to which the subject is sensitive.

antiandrogen (an-ti-an′-drō-jen): A substance that inhibits or in some other way affects the activity of androgen.

antianemic (an-ti-a-nē′-mik): 1. Any agent that prevents or relieves anemia. 2. Relieving or preventing anemia. **A. FACTOR,** vitamin B_{12} (cyanocobalamin) found in liver, fish meal, eggs, and some other natural products; for absorption in the body it must combine with hydrochloric acid and an intrinsic factor produced by the lining of the stomach; it is essential for proper development of red blood cells in the bone marrow.

antianginal (an-ti-an-jī′-nal): Tending to prevent or relieve angina pectoris.

antiantibody (an′-ti-an′-ti-bod-i): A substance that is formed in the body after the injection of an antibody which the substance is intended to counteract.

antianxiety (an′-ti-ang-zī′-e-ti): **A. AGENT,** a drug that depresses the activity of the central nervous system through its sedative and hypnotic actions and thus reduces anxiety.

antiarrhythmic (an′-ti-a-rith′-mik): 1. Preventing or correcting cardiac arrhythmia (*q.v.*). 2. An agent that prevents or corrects arrhythmia.

antiarthritic (an′ti-ar-thrit′-ik): 1. Relieving

arthritis or gout. 2. An agent that relieves arthritis or gout.

antibacterial (an′-ti-bak-tēr′-i-al): 1. An agent that destroys bacteria or prevents their growth and reproduction. 2. Tending to destroy bacteria or prevent their growth and reproduction.

antibecic an′-ti-bek′-ik): 1. An agent that relieves cough. 2. Tending to relieve cough.

antibiosis (an′-ti-bī-ō′-sis): An association between organisms of different species that is harmful to one of them. Opp. to symbiosis.—antibiotic, adj.

antibiotic (an′-tī-bī-ot′-ik): 1. Pertaining to antibiosis. 2. Destructive to life. 3. Any of a group of antibacterial chemical compounds originally derived from fungi, molds, or bacteria; many are now produced synthetically; used extensively in medicine. Some are active against only certain bacteria, fungi, or viruses; others are active against a wider range of microorganisms. Some are effective when given by injection or orally; others are rarely used internally because of their high toxicity but are effective applied topically. **BROAD-SPECTRUM A.**, one which is effective against many different microorganisms. **A. RESISTANT,** a condition that exists when an antibiotic is given in too low doses or is not continued long enough; the offending organism survives and its descendents have the ability to resist the antibiotic.

antiblennorrhagic (an′-ti-blen-ō-raj′-ik): 1. Preventing gonorrhea or relieving its symptoms.

antibodies (an′-ti-bod′-ēz): A class of specific protein substances in the blood that destroy or render inactive certain foreign substances, particularly bacteria and their products. May be developed naturally or in response to a specific antigen that has been introduced into the body parenterally or otherwise; may be transferred to the fetus in utero; may develop as a result of a subclinical infection with the specific agent, thus producing immunity to the specific disease. They cause agglutination, flocculation, inactivvation or lysis of the antigen. **A.** include agglutinins, amboceptors, antienzymes, antitoxins, bacteriolysins, cytotoxins, hemolysins, opsonins and precipitins.

antibrachium (an-ti-brā′-ki-um): The forearm. Also antebrachium.

antibromic (an-ti-bro′-mik): 1. Counteracting unpleasant odors. 2. A deodorizer.

anticachectic (an′-ti-ka-kek′-tik): 1. An agent that prevents or relieves cachexia. 2. Tending to prevent or relieve cachexia.

anticarcinogen (an′-ti-kar-sin′-ō-jen): An agent that opposes the action of carcinogens.

anticardium (an′-ti-kar′-di-um): The precordium (*q.v.*).

anticariogenic (an′-ti-kar-i-ō-jen′-ik): Having the effect of retarding decay, dental decay in particular.

anticathexis (an′-ti-ka-thek′-sis): The outward expression of an emotional impulse that is the complete opposite of the emotion actually felt, *e.g.*, the expression of unconscious hate as conscious love.

anticheirotonus (an-ti-kī-rot′-o-nus): A spasmodic flexion of the thumb, often seen before or during an epileptic seizure.

anticholagogue (an-ti-kōl′-a-gog): Any agent or process that interferes with the secretion of bile by the liver.

anticholesterolemic (an′-ti-kōl-es′-te-rō-lē′-mik): A substance that acts to lower the cholesterol levels of the blood.

anticholinergic (an′-ti-kō-lin-er′-jik): 1. Tending to inhibit the action of a parasympathetic nerve by interfering with the action of acetylcholine, a chemical by which such a nerve transmits its impulses at neural or myoneural junctions. 2. An agent that blocks the transmission of impulses across the parasympathetic ganglia or blocks the effect of acetylcholine, *e.g.*, atropine.

anticholinesterase (an′-ti-kō-lin-es′-ter-ās): A substance that lessens or inhibits the enzymatic activity of cholinesterase.

anticipatory grief: A stage of bereavement engaged in by relatives who have accepted the fact that death of a loved one is inevitable.

anticoagulant (an′-ti-kō-ag′-ū-lant): An agent that suppresses, prevents, or retards the clotting of blood. 2. Having the effect of suppressing, preventing or retarding the clotting of blood. **A. THERAPY,** the administration of an anticoagulant to prevent intravascular clotting in the treatment of coronary thrombosis, phlebothrombosis, and similar disorders.

anticonceptive (an′-ti-kon-sep′-tiv): Contraceptive.

anticonvulsant (an′-ti-kon-vul′-sant): 1. An agent that stops or prevents convulsions. 2. Tending to prevent or relieve the severity of convulsions.

anticus (an-tī′-kus): Anterior; in front of. **A. SIGN,** dorsiflexion of the ankle in response to percussion of the tibialis anterior muscle; indicative of central nervous system disease.

anticytotoxin (an-ti-sī′-tō-tok′-sin): A substance that counteracts the action of cytotoxin.

anti-D immunoglobulin (an′-ti dē′ im-mū-nō-glob′-ū-lin): an immune globulin specific for the D antigen; it is administered to Rh negative women within 72 hours of delivery to destroy any Rh positive cells that the mother may have received from the fetal blood during delivery; done to prevent formation of antibodies that would affect future pregnancies.

antidepressant (an′-ti-dē-pres′-ant): An

agent or procedure that inhibits or alleviates depression.

antidiabetic (an′-ti-dī-a-bet′-ik): Literally, "against diabetes." Used to describe therapeutic measures in diabetes mellitus, *e.g.*, use of the hormone insulin (*q.v.*).

antidiarrheal (an′-ti-dī-a-rē′-al): 1. An agent that prevents or checks diarrhea. 2. Tending to prevent or alleviate diarrhea. Also diarrheic.

antidinic (an-ti-din′-ik): 1. An agent that relieves dizziness. 2. Tending to relieve dizziness.

antidiphtheritic (an′-tī-dif-ther-it′-ik): Against diphtheria; referring to such preventive measures as immunization.

antidiuresis (an′-ti-dī-ū-rē′-sis): Reduction in the amount of urine excreted.

antidiuretic (an′-ti-dī-ū-ret′-ik): 1. An agent that reduces the volume of urine secreted. 2. Tending to reduce the secretion of urine.

antidiuretic hormone (ADH): A hormone made and stored in the posterior pituitary gland, and released as required to suppress diuresis. It stimulates reabsorption of water in the kidney tubules and thus helps to regulate fluid balance. Too small an amount results in diabetes insipidus; too large an amount results in oliguria and excessive fluid retention. See **diabetes**. Also called vasopressin.

antidotal (an-ti-dō′-tal): Pertaining to or acting as an antidote.

antidote (an′-ti-dōt): An agent that counteracts or neutralizes the action of a poison.

antidysenteric (an′-ti-dis-en-ter′-ik): An agent that counteracts, relieves, or prevents dysentery.

antidysthanasia (an′-ti-dis-tha-nā′-zi-a): Descriptive of a belief or commitment not to utilize extraordinary measures to prolong life in a patient who faces a long and agonizing death.

antiedemic (an′-ti-ē-dē′-mik): 1. An agent that prevents or helps to relieve edema. 2. Tending to prevent edema.

antiembolism stockings: Tight fitting elastic stockings that compress the superficial veins; prescribed for immobilized patients to promote the flow of blood in the leg veins and decrease the possibility of embolus formation and other circulatory problems.

antiemetic (an′-ti-ē-met′-ik): 1. Against emesis (*q.v.*). 2. Any agent that prevents nausea and vomiting.

antienzyme (an-ti-en′-zīm): A substance that exerts a specific inhibiting effect on an enzyme. In the digestive tract they prevent digestion of the digestive tube lining; in the blood they act as antibodies (*q.v.*).

antiepileptic (an′-tī-ep-i-lep′-tik): An agent that reduces the frequency and/or the severity of epileptic attacks.

antifebrile (an-ti-feb′-ril): 1. Reducing or abolishing fever. 2. Any agent that reduces or allays fever.

antifibrinolytic (an′-ti-fī-brin-ō-lit′-ik): Any substance that inhibits or retards the proteolytic action of fibrinolysin.

antiflatulent (an-ti-flat′-ū-lent): 1. Tending to prevent and relieve flatulence. 2. A drug that tends to prevent and relieve flatulence.

antifungal (an-ti-fung′-gal): Any agent that destroys or inhibits the growth of fungi or is effective against fungal infections.

antigalactic (an-ti-ga-lak′-tik): 1. Any drug or agent that tends to diminish the secretion of milk. 2. Tending to reduce the secretion of milk.

antigen (an′-ti-jen): Any substance, usually a protein, which can stimulate the production of antibodies and react specifically with those antibodies; may be a bacterium, pollen, grain, etc.; each type requires a different antibody to neutralize it. **AUSTRALIAN A.**, an **A.** found in the serum of patients with acute serum hepatitis and in normal inhabitants of southeast Asia and the tropics. Now called hepatitis B surface antigen (*q.v.*) in the U.S.

antigen-antibody reaction: The specific reaction of an antibody to an antigen; occurs when the antigen provokes an immunologic response and antibodies are produced which try to neutralize the antigen that stimulated their production.

antigenicity (an′-ti-jen-is′-i-ti): The ability to promote antibody formation.

antigoitrogenic (an′-ti-goy-trō-jen′-ik): 1. An agent that inhibits the development of goiter. 2. Tending to inhibit the development of goiter.

antigravity (an-ti-grav′-i-ti): Against or opposing the force of gravity. **A. MUSCLES**, the muscles of the limbs which support the body in the upright position, chiefly the extensor muscles. **A. POSTURE**, the upright position; the ability to achieve and maintain this position is usually learned by the end of the first year of life.

antihelix (an-ti-hē′-liks): Anthelix (*q.v.*).

antihemolysin (an′-ti-hē-mol′-i-sin): An agent that prevents or inhibits hemolysis.

antihemophilic (an′-ti-hē-mō-fil′-ik): An agent that counteracts the bleeding tendency in hemophilia.

antihemophilic factor (an′-ti-hē-mō-fil′-ik fak′-tor): Factor VIII, required for the formation of a blood clot. Deficiency of this inherited factor causes classic hemophilia. Also called antihemophilic globulin (AHG) and thromboplastinogen. Abbreviated AHF.

antihemorrhagic (an′-ti-hem-ō-raj′-ik): 1. Any drug or agent that prevents hemorrhage. 2. Tending to prevent hemorrhage. **A. VITAMIN**, vitamin K (*q.v.*).

antihidrotic (an′-ti-hī-drot′-ik): Anhidrotic (*q.v.*).

antihistamines (an-ti-hist′-a-mēnz): Drugs that suppress some of the effects of released histamine (*q.v.*); widely used in treatment of hay fever, urticaria, angioneurotic edema, and some forms of pruritus. Because of their antiemetic properties, are used to prevent motion and radiation sickness. Side effects include drowsiness.—antihistaminic, adj. and n.

antihuman globulin (antī-hū′-man glob′-ū-lin): Any natural or artificially produced substance which reacts with globulin that has been prepared by immunizing an animal with purified human gamma globulin. Also called antiglobulin and Boombs serum.

antihypercholesterolemic (an′-ti-hī-per-kō-les′-ter-o-lē′-mik): 1. Tending to prevent or relieve hypercholesterolemia. 2. An agent that prevents or relieves hypercholesterolemia.

antihyperglycemic (an′-ti-hī-per-glī-sē′-mik): 1. An agent that acts to reduce high levels of glucose in the blood. 2. Reducing high glucose levels in the blood.

antihypertensive (an′-ti-hī-per-ten′-siv): 1. Any drug or agent that lowers blood pressure in hypertensive patients. 2. Tending to counteract hypertension.

antihypnotic (an′-ti-hip-not′-ik): 1. An agent that prevents or hinders sleep. 2. Tending to prevent sleep.

antihypotensive (an′-ti-hī-pō-ten′-siv): 1. Counteracting abnormally low blood pressure. 2. An agent that counteracts abnormally low blood pressure.

antihysteric (an′-ti-his-ter′-ik): 1. An agent that prevents or counteracts hysteria. 2. Tending to relieve hysteria.

anti-icteric (an-ti-ik′-ter-ik): 1. An agent that relieves jaundice. 2. Tending to relieve jaundice.

anti-immune (an′-ti-i-mūn′): Preventing the development of immunity.

anti-infective (an′-ti-in-fek′-tiv): 1. Counteracting infection. 2. Any agent that counteracts or prevents infection. See **vitamin A**.

anti-inflammatory (an′-ti-in-flam′-a-tō-ri): 1. Counteracting or preventing inflammation. 2. An agent that counteracts or suppresses inflammation.

antiketogenic (an′-ti-kē-tō-jen′-ik): Inhibiting the formation of ketone bodies.

antilepsis (an-ti-lep′-sis): Treatment of a disease by application of a remedy to a healthy part; called treatment by derivation or revulsion.

antilethargic (an′-ti-le-thar′-jik): 1. An agent that counteracts lethargy. 2. Tending to prevent or hinder sleep.

antileukemic (an′-ti-lū-kē′-mik): 1. An agent that controls or suppresses the symptoms of leukemia. 2. Tending to suppress, inhibit, or diminish the symptoms of leukemia.

antilithic (an-ti-lith′-ik): 1. Tending to counteract the formation of stones or calculi. 2. An agent that helps prevent the formation of stones or calculi, or that aids in their dissolution.

antiluetic (an′-ti-loo-et′-ik): See **antisyphilitic**.

antilymphocyte globulin (an′-tī-limf′-ō-sit glob′-u-lin): The globulin fraction of antilymphocyte serum prepared by injecting the individual's lymphocytes into a different species; a powerful immunosuppressive agent used in combating the rejection reaction in persons who have had an organ transplant.

antilysin (an-ti-lī′-sin): An antibody that opposes the activity of a lysin thereby protecting cells against lysis.

antilysis (an-ti-lī′-sis): The prevention or inhibition of lysis (*q.v.*).

antilyssic (an-ti-lis′-ik): Effective in preventing or checking rabies; antirabic.

antilytic (an-ti-lit′-ik): 1. Pertaining to an antilysin. 2. Destroying a lysin or interfering with its action. 3. An agent that destroys a lysin or interferes with its action.

antimalarial (an-ti-ma-lā′-ri-al): 1. Having the effect of preventing or suppressing malaria. 2. Any drug or measure taken to prevent or suppress malaria, or to destroy the causative agent in malaria.

antimetabolite (an′-tī-me-tab′-ō-līt): A drug or other agent that is similar in constituents to the chemicals needed by a cell for formation of nucleoproteins, and which interferes with cell metabolism of essential metabolites, thereby preventing further development of the cell.

antimetropia (an′-ti-me-trō′-pi-a): An ocular condition in which the two eyes present different refractive errors: *e.g.*, one eye may be myopic and the other hypermetropic.

antimitotic (an′-ti-mī-tot′-ik): 1. Pertaining to the inhibition of mitosis. 2. An agent that inhibits or prevents reproduction of a cell by mitosis.

antimony (an′-ti-mō-ni): A crystalline metallic element; resembles arsenic in action but is less toxic. Once quite widely used in medicine; now sometimes used for its expectorant and diaphoretic properties and as an emetic.

antimycotic (an′-ti-mī-kot′-ik): 1. Preventing or suppressing the growth of fungi. 2. An agent or measure that destroys or suppresses the growth of fungi.

antinarcotic (an′-ti-nar-kot′-ik): 1. Preventing or relieving the effects of a narcotic drug (*q.v.*). 2. A drug or agent that counteracts the stupor produced by a narcotic drug.

antinauseant (an′-ti-naw′-sē-ant): 1. Tending

to relieve or counteract nausea. 2. An agent that relieves or counteracts nausea.

antineoplastic (an′-ti-nē-ō-plas′-tik): 1. Having the effect of inhibiting or preventing the development and proliferation of malignant cells. 2. Referring to a chemically produced substance that inhibits or controls the growth of certain malignant cells.

antinephritic (an′-ti-ne-frit′-ik): 1. Effective against nephritis. 2. An agent that relieves or prevents nephritis.

antineuralgic (an′-ti-nū-ral′-jik): 1. Alleviating neuralgic pain. 2. An agent or procedure that alleviates neuralgic pain.

antineuritic (an′-ti-nū-rit′-ik): An agent that relieves or prevents neuritis; applied especially to vitamin B complex (*q.v.*).

antinuclear antibody: An antibody found in persons with any of several connective tissue disorders; its action is directed at the components of the cell nucleus.

antiodontalgic (an′-ti-ō-don-tal′-jik): An agent that relieves or prevents toothache.

antiotomy (an′-ti-ot′-o-mi): Surgical removal of the tonsils.

antiovulatory (an′-ti-ov′-ū-la-tō-ri): Suppressing or inhibiting ovulation.

antioxidant (an′-tī-oks′-i-dant): Any of several substances, synthetic or natural, that prevent deterioration by the action of oxygen; commonly used in the preparation of foods for marketing, *e.g.*, vegetable oils and fats.

antiparasitic (an′-ti-par-a-sit′-ik): 1. Destructive to parasites. 2. Any agent that destroys parasites or inhibits their growth.

antiparkinsonian (an′-ti-park-in-sōn′-i-an): Effective against the symptoms of parkinsonism; said especially of certain drugs.

antipathy (an-tip′-a-thi): Incompatability; aversion; distaste; dislike. In medicine, the mutual antagonism between two diseases.—antipathic, adj.

antipellagra (an′-ti-pe-lag′-ra): 1. Against pellagra. 2. Pertaining to the nicotinic acid portion of vitamin B complex (*q.v.*).

antiperiodic (an′-ti-pē-ri-od′-ik): Any agent or measure that prevents the periodic recurrence of symptoms of disease, *e.g.*, the use of quinine in malaria.

antiperistalsis (an′-ti-per-i-stal′-sis): A reversal of the normal peristaltic action, *i.e.*, beginning in the lower ileum the peristaltic wave proceeds from below upward preventing the passage of intestinal contents into the cecum.—antiperistaltic, adj.

antiperistaltic (an′-ti-per-i-stal′-tik): 1. Inhibiting or diminishing peristalsis. 2. A substance that inhibits or diminishes peristalsis.

antiperspirant (an′-ti-per′-spi-rant): An agent having an inhibitory action on the secretion of sweat.

antiphlogistic (an′-ti-flō-jis′-tik): 1. Effective in relieving or reducing inflammation. 2. Any agent that relieves or reduces inflammation.

antiplastic (an-ti-plas′-tik): Unfavorable to the healing process, especially to granulation and scar formation.

antiplatelet (an-ti-plāt′-let): A substance that acts to lyse or agglutinate blood platelets and thus inhibits or destroys their normal action.

antipodal (an-tip′-ō-dal): Situated exactly opposite.

antiprothrombin (an′-ti-prō-throm′-bin): An anticoagulant present in the blood or an agent that acts to prevent conversion of prothrombin into thrombin.

antipruritic (an′-ti-proo-rit′-ik): 1. Any procedure or agent that relieves or prevents itching. 2. Having the action of preventing or relieving itching.

anti-psychiatry: Term used to describe a movement to denigrate psychiatry, modern psychiatric treatments, and the conduct of institutions for the care of psychiatric patients.

antipsychotic (an′-ti-sī-kot′-ik): Usually pertains to an agent that reduces psychomotor activity; a neuroleptic agent.

antipyic (an-ti-pī′-ik): 1. An agent that prevents or inhibits the formation of pus. 2. Preventing or inhibiting suppuration.

antipyogenic (an′-ti-pī-ō-jen′-ik): Antipyic (*q.v.*).

antipyretic (an′-ti-pī-ret′-ik): 1. Effective in reducing or relieving fever. 2. Any agent that reduces or relieves fever.—antipyresis, n.

antipyrotic (an′-ti-pī-rot′-ik): 1. Effective in relieving pain and promoting healing of burns. 2. An agent used to allay pain and promote healing of burns.

antirabic (an-ti-rā′-bik): 1. Preventive of rabies. 2. Any agent that prevents rabies or is used therapeutically in the treatment of rabies.

antirachitic (an′-ti-ra-kit′-ik): 1. Having the effect of preventing rickets. 2. An agent used to prevent rickets. 3. Pertaining to vitamin D (*q.v.*).

antirickettsial (an′-ti-ri-ket′-si-al): 1. Effective against rickettsiae. 2. Any agent that is effective against rickettsiae.

antiscorbutic (an′-ti-skor-bū′-tik): 1. Having the effect of preventing scurvy. 2. Any agent that prevents scurvy. 3. Pertaining to vitamin C. See **ascorbic acid**.

antisecretory (an′-ti-sē-kre′-to-ri): 1. Having the effect of preventing or inhibiting glandular secretion. 2. Any agent that prevents or inhibits glandular secretion.

antisepsis (an-ti-sep′-sis): 1. The prevention

of sepsis (*q.v.*) by any or all of the following actions: destroying the microorganisms that produce infection; preventing their access to the site of potential infection; or inhibiting their growth and multiplication. Introduced into surgery in 1880 by Lord Lister who used carbolic acid to prevent sepsis. 2. The use of specific procedures or agents to prevent the development of sepsis.

antiseptic (an-ti-sep′-tik): 1. Tending to prevent or inhibit the growth and multiplication of microorganisms and viruses that produce disease. 2. Any agent that inhibits or prevents the growth and multiplication of microorganisms that produce disease.

antisepticism (an-ti-sep′-ti-sizm): The systematic use of agents or methods to prevent the development of sepsis (*q.v.*).—antisepticize, v.

antiserum (an′-ti-sē′-rum): A serum (from man or animal) that contains specific antibody or antibodies against a specific bacterium or other antigenic agent; the specific antibodies may be produced by infection with the specific bacterium or toxin, or by immunization through repeated injection of the specific bacterium or toxin into the tissues or blood. Useful in creating passive immunity (*q.v.*) or in treating such diseases as diphtheria, tetanus, meningitis.—antisera, pl.

antishock trousers: See military antishock trousers.

antisialagogue (an′-ti-sī-al′-a-gog): An agent that inhibits or checks the secretion of saliva.

antisialic (an′-ti-sī-al′-ik): 1. Antisialagogue (*q.v.*). 2. Having the effect of checking the flow of saliva.

antisocial (an-ti-sō′-shal): Against society. A term used to denote a psychopathic state in which the individual cannot accept the obligations and restraints imposed by a community on its members and, consequently, is in frequent conflict with society. The individual develops behavior patterns characterized by callous indifference to the effect of his actions on others, and irresponsibility. **A. PERSONALITY,** see under personality disorders.

antispasmodic (an′-ti-spaz-mod′-ik): 1. Tending to prevent spasm of smooth muscle. 2. Any agent or measure used to prevent smooth muscle spasm.

antispastic (an-ti-spas′-tik): 1. Tending to prevent or relieve skeletal muscle spasm. 2. An agent or therapeutic measure that tends to prevent or relieve skeletal muscle spasm.

antistalsis (an-ti-stal′-sis): Reversed peristalsis (*q.v.*).

antistatic (an-ti-stat′-ik): Any measure taken to prevent or deal with the collection of static electricity.

antisterility (an′-ti-ste-ril′-i-ti): 1. Tending to combat sterility. 2. Pertaining to vitamin E (*q.v.*).

antistreptolysin (an′-ti-strep-tol′-i-sin): An inhibitor of the streptolysin on group A hemolytic streptococci (see blood groups); a raised titer of **A.** in the blood is indicative of recent streptococcal infection.

antisudorific (an′-ti-sū-dō-rif′-ik): 1. Acting to inhibit or reduce secretion of sweat. 2. An agent that inhibits or reduces the secretion of sweat.

antisyphilitic (an′-ti-sif-i-lit′-ik): 1. Any measures taken or agent used to combat or treat syphilis. 2. Effective against syphilis.

antitabetic (an-ti-ta-bet′-ik): 1. Counteracting or preventing tabes dorsalis. 2. An agent effective in lessening the symptoms of tabes dorsalis (*q.v.*).

antithermic (an-ti-ther′-mik): 1. Cooling; acting to reduce body temperature. 2. An agent that lowers the body temperature. Syn., antipyretic (*q.v.*).

antithrombin (an-ti-throm′-bin): Any substance that occurs naturally in the blood, *e.g.*, heparin, or is given therapeutically to inhibit clotting of blood and the formation of thrombi.

antithromboplastin (an′-ti-throm-bō-plas′-tin): A substance that interferes with the action of thromboplastin and thus inhibits normal coagulation of blood.

antithrombotic (an′-ti-throm-bot′-ik): Any measure that helps to prevent or relieve thrombosis.

antithyroid (an-ti-thī′-roid): 1. Any agent or drug used to reduce the activity of the thyroid gland; *e.g.*, thiouracil. 2. Capable of counteracting the influence of the thyroid gland.

antitoxic (an-ti-tok′-sik): 1. Pertaining to an antitoxin. 2. Antidotal; counteracting or neutralizing the action of a toxin. **ANTITOXIC SERA,** the serum of horses which have been immunized by injections of pathogenic bacterial toxins, such as tetanus and gas gangrene. Such serum contains antibodies or antitoxins, and after injection into humans confers a temporary immunity against the original toxin.

antitoxin (an-ti-tok′-sin): An antibody that neutralizes a given toxin. It is elaborated in the body in direct response to the invasion of a bacteria or a toxin. Antitoxins may be prepared from the blood serum of animals or humans that have been immunized against specific toxins, and used therapeutically.

antitoxinogen (an′-ti-tok-sin′-ō-jen): Any antigen that stimulates the formation of an antitoxin in the body.

antitrismus (an-ti-triz′-mus): Inability to close the mouth due to tonic muscle spasm.

antitrypsin (an-ti-trip′-sin): A substance that inhibits the physiologic action of trypsin.

antituberculin (an-ti-tū-ber′-kū-lin): An antibody developed within the body after the injection of tuberculin (*q.v.*).

antituberculotic (an′-ti-tū-ber-kū-lot′-ik): 1. Effective against tuberculosis. 2. An agent that is effective against the spread of tuberculosis.

antitumorigenic (an′-ti-tū-mor-i-jen′-ik): 1. Capable of preventing or inhibiting the growth of a tumor. 2. An agent that prevents or inhibits the growth of a tumor.

antitumorigenesis (an′-ti-tū-mor-i-jen′-e-sis): Inhibition of the growth of a neoplasm.

antitussive (an-ti-tus′-iv): 1. Effective in relieving or suppressing cough. 2. Any measure or agent that suppresses cough.

antivenin (an-ti-ven′-in): An antiserum (*q.v.*) obtained from an animal immunized against the venom of a particular snake or insect and containing antitoxin to that venom. Used as an antidote in first aid treatment of poisoning by snake bite.

antiviral (an-ti-vī′-ral): 1. Destructive to viruses and inhibiting their replication. 2. An agent that is active against viruses and inhibits their replication.

antivitamin (an-ti-vī′-ta-min): A substance that interferes with the absorption or normal functioning of a vitamin.

antivivisection (an′-ti-viv-i-sek′-shun): Opposition to the use of living animals for experimentation or medical research.

Anton's syndrome or symptom: A condition in which bilateral infarction of the occipital lobe of the brain has caused blindness which the patient tries to deny by elaborate confabulations.

antrectomy (an-trek′-to-mi): Excision of the walls of an antrum, especially the mastoid or the pyloric antrum.

antritis (an-trī′-tis): Inflammation of an antrum, particularly the antrum of Highmore.

antrobuccal (an-trō-buk′-al): Pertaining to the maxillary antrum and the mouth. **A. FISTULA** can occur after extraction of an upper molar tooth, the root of which has protruded into the floor of the antrum.

antroscope (an′-trō-skōp): An instrument, usually having a light-bulb attachment, used for visual examination of an antrum, the maxillary antrum particularly.

antrostomy (an-tros′-to-mi): An incision into an antrum to provide for drainage.

antrotomy (an-trot′-o-mi): The operation of cutting into an antrum.

antrum (an′-trum): A closed or nearly closed cavity, especially in a bone, *e.g.*, the antrum of Highmore in the superior maxillary bone. [Nathaniel Highmore, British physician. 1613–1685.] The term is also used to describe the pyloric end of the stomach when it is partially shut off from the fundus, during digestion, by the contraction of the pyloric sphincter.—antra, pl.; antral, adj.

anuclear (a-nū′-klē-ar): Having no nucleus; said particularly of erythrocytes.

anulus (an′-ū-lus): See **annulus.**

anuresis (an-ū-rē′-sis): Failure to excrete urine. May be due to either lack of secretion or obstruction in the urinary passages.—aneuretic, adj.

anuria (a-nū′-ri-a): Cessation of the production and excretion of urine. See **suppression.**—anuric, adj.

anus (ā′-nus): The opening at the end of the alimentary canal; the extreme termination of the rectum; formed of a sphincter muscle which relaxes to allow fecal matter to pass through. **IMPERFORATE A.,** a congenital anomaly in which there is no opening at the terminus of the alimentary canal.

anvil (an′-vil): The middle of the three ossicles of the middle ear which conduct sound waves from the tympanum to the inner ear; likened to an anvil in shape; also called the incus.

anxiety (ang-zī′-e-ti): A condition of disturbed mood and behavior, characterized by feelings of fear, apprehension, nervousness, inadequacy, tension, and dread; usually associated with a real or imagined threat to one's security. Signs and symptoms include increased heart rate and muscle tone, restlessness, perspiration, and agitation. **ANXIETY NEUROSIS,** or **STATE,** see under **neurosis. CASTRATION A.,** castration complex; see under **complex. FREE FLOATING A., A.** without any apparent or conscious cause. **SEPARATION A.,** a state usually seen in infants from six to ten months of age; marked by apprehension when the mother or mother surrogate is not present; may continue into later life when the person is separated from his normal environment or from persons who are significant to him.

anxiolytic (ang-zi-ō-lit′-ik): An agent that helps to dispel anxiety.

anydremia (an-i-drē′-mi-a): Anhydremia (*q.v.*).

AOBS: Abbreviation for acute organic brain syndrome.

aorta (ā-or′-ta): The main trunk of the arterial system of the body; it arises in the left ventricle, carries oxygenated blood away from the heart, and, along with its branches, forms the arterial system of the body. Anatomically, the aorta is divided into three main parts: 1) the **ASCENDING A.,** that portion that arises in the left ventricle of the heart and, passing upward, joins the heart to the arch of the aorta; 2) **ARCH OF THE AORTA,** the part that passes anteroposteriorally over the base of the heart, and joins the ascending aorta to the descending aorta; 3) the **DESCENDING A.,** extends downward from the arch to the level of the fourth lumbar vertebra where it divides into the right and left iliac arteries. The portion of the descending **A.** that lies above the diaphragm is called the **THORACIC A.**, and the portion below the diaphragm is called the **ABDOMINAL A.**—aortal, aortic, adj.

aortalgia (ā-or-tal′-ji-a): Pain in the area of the aorta.

aortarctia (ā-or-tark′-shi-a): Narrowing or stenosis of the aorta.

aortectasia (ā-or-tek-tā′-zi-a): Dilatation of the aorta.

aortic (ā-ōr′-tik): Pertaining to the aorta. **A. ARCH,** see under aorta. **A. BODIES,** small neurovascular chemoreceptive structures on both sides of the aorta near the arch; they have a function in regulating respiration by responding to changes in concentrations of oxygen, carbon dioxide, and hydrogen in the blood. **A. HIATUS,** the opening in the diaphragm through which the aorta passes from the thorax into the abdominal cavity. **A. INSUFFICIENCY** or **INCOMPETENCE,** improper closing of the valve between the left ventricle and the aorta permitting the backflow of blood. **A. MURMUR,** an abnormal sound heard as blood flows through a diseased aorta or aortic valve. **A. PLEXUS,** important network of sympathetic nerves, extending from the celiac (solar) plexus over the anterolateral aspect of the aorta and downward to the hypogastric plexus. **A. SINUS,** one of the sac-like dilatations of the aorta opposite the semilunar valve cusps. **A. STENOSIS,** see under stenosis. **A. VALVE,** a tricuspid valve at the junction of the left ventricle and the aorta.

aortitis (ā-or-tī′-tis): Inflammation of the aorta.

aortogram (a-or′-tō-gram): An x-ray picture of the aorta made by aortography.

aortography (ā-or-tog′-ra-fi): Roentgenography of the aorta utilizing a radiopaque medium. See also arteriography.

aortoiliac (ā-or′-tō-il′-i-ak): Pertaining to the abdominal aorta and the iliac arteries.

aortolith (ā-or′-tō-lith): A stone or concretion in the aorta.

aortomalacia (ā-or-tō-mal-ā′-shi-a): Softening of the walls of the aorta.

aortopathy (ā-or-top′-a-thi): Any pathologic condition of the aorta.

aortorrhaphy (ā-or-tor′-a-fi): A suturing of the aorta.

aortosclerosis (ā-or′-tō-sklē-rō′-sis): Sclerosis of the aorta.

aortostenosis (ā-or′-tō-sten-ō′-sis): Narrowing of the aorta.

aortotomy (ā-or-tot′-o-mi): Incision into the aorta.

AP: Abbreviation for: 1. Arterial pressure. 2. Anterior-posterior; also written A-P.

ap-, apo-: Prefixes denoting: 1. Away from, detached from, separate. 2. Related to.

A. P. test: Alkaline phosphatase test to determine the level of this substance in the blood serum. Elevated levels occur in hyperthyroidism, hyperparathyroidism, Paget's disease, leukemias, various types of carcinoma, osteogenesis imperfecta, osteitis deformans, Gaucher's disease, rickets, liver and kidney diseases. May also occur following intake of large amounts of vitamin D.

apandria (ap-an′-dri-a): Morbid aversion to males.

apareunia (a-pa-roo′-nē-a): Inability to practice sexual intercourse; usually because of an obstruction in the vagina, or an atresic vagina.

apastia (a-pas′-ti-a): Abstention from food when it occurs as a symptom of neurological or psychological disorder.

apathism (ap′-a-thizm): Indifference or sluggishness of reaction.

apathy (ap′-a-thi): Want of feeling, emotion, or concern; indifference, insensibility. Seen in patients with depression, dementia, schizophrenia, and certain organic disorders.—apathetic, apathic, adj.

APC: Abbreviation for: 1. Atrial premature contraction. 2. Aspirin, phenacetin, and caffeine.

apepsia (a-pep′-si-a): 1. Lack of pepsin in the gastric juice. 2. Incomplete or imperfect digestion of food.

apepsinia (a-pep-sin′-i-a): Absence of pepsin or pepsinogen in the gastric juice.

aperient (a-pē′-ri-ent): A mild laxative.

aperistalsis (a-per-i-stal′-sis): Absence of the normal contractions of the intestines as occurs *e.g.*, in paralytic ileus.—aperistaltic, adj.

aperture (ap′-er-chur): An opening or orifice in an anatomical structure.

Apert's syndrome: Acrocephalosyndactyly (*q.v.*).

apex (ā′-peks): In anatomy, a term used to designate the top or the tip of an organ or body, or the pointed end of a cone-shaped or pyramidal structure, *e.g.*, the heart or lungs. Also applied to the end of a tooth. **A. BEAT,** see under beat. **A. OF THE HEART,** the blunt narrow end enclosing mainly the left ventricle; it rests on the diaphragm. **A. OF THE LUNG,** that portion nearest the shoulder level.—apical, adj.; apices, pl.

apexcardiogram (ā′-peks-kar′-di-ō-gram): The graphic recording produced by apexcardiography.

apexcardiography (ā′-peks-kar-di-og′-ra-fi): Roentgenography of the chest wall movements produced by the apical heartbeat.

Apgar score: The numerical expression of a newborn infant's well-being and ability to survive; consists of the sum of points from zero to

10, based on five signs ranked in order of importance, with assessments being made at one minute and five minutes after birth. Included are 1) heart rate; 2) respiratory effort as demonstrated by the infant's cry; 3) muscle tone, checked by flexion and response of the extremities; 4) reflex irritability, checked by flicking the sole of the foot or tickling the nostril with a wisp of cotton and noting foot or facial changes; 5) color, check for presence or absence of cyanosis and general body color. [Virginia Apgar, American anesthesiologist. 1909–1974].

APHA: Abbreviation for American Public Health Association.

aphagia (a-fā'ji-a): Inability or refusal to swallow.—aphagic, adj.

aphakia (a-fā'-ki-a): Absence of all or part of the crystalline lens.—aphakic, adj.

aphalangia (a-fa-lan'-ji-a): Congenital absence of one or more of the fingers or toes.

aphasia (a-fā'-zi-a): Loss of ability to use language normally; usually due to damage to the cortex of the dominant cerebral hemisphere that results from disease or trauma. May involve impairment of ability to express ideas by speech, writing, or signs, or of the ability to comprehend spoken or written language. Many types are recognized, depending on the area of the brain that has been damaged. **AMNESIC A.**, inability to name a familiar object. **ATAXIC A.**, see motor **A. AUDITORY A.**, word deafness in which the person hears spoken words but does not understand them. **BROCA'S A.**, **A.** in which the person cannot speak or write although he understands spoken and written language. **EXPRESSIVE A.**, Broca's **A. GLOBAL A.**, complete loss of all functions of communication even when hearing is normal. **JARGON A.**, repetition of unfamiliar words that the person appears to understand. **MIXED A.**, loss of voluntary speech and ability to write, and difficulty in understanding speech. **MOTOR A.**, inability to articulate speech or to communicate by writing, gestures, or signs, although understanding remains intact. **NOMINAL A.**, amnesic **A. OPTIC A.**, inability to recognize and name a familiar object. **SENSORY A.**, loss of power to recognize the meaning of written or spoken words or phrases, gestures, or signs. **WERNICKE'S A.**, loss of ability to comprehend language; accompanied by inappropriate use of language.—aphasic, adj.

aphemia (a-fē'-mi-a): Motor aphasia (*q.v.*). Loss of ability to articulate words.

aphephobia (af-e-fō'-bi-a): Morbid dread of physical contact with other persons or of being touched by another.

aphlexia (a-flek'-si-a): 1. Absentmindedness. 2. Daydreaming.

aphonia (a-fō'-ni-a): Loss of voice from a cause other than a cerebral lesion. May be due to organic causes such as disease or injury of the larynx, or to psychic causes. **CONVERSION A.**, a voice disorder caused by anxiety, stress, or depression and used by a patient to meet an uncomfortable situation. **HYSTERICAL A.**, loss of voice associated with a functional disorder; more common in women than men.

aphonogelia (a-fō-nō-jē'-li-a): Inability to laugh out loud.

aphrasia (a-frā'-zi-a): Inability to speak or to use connected phrases in speaking. **A. PARANOICA**, voluntary and stubborn silence in the mentally ill.

aphrenia (a-frē'-ni-a): Dementia.

aphrodisiac (af-rō-diz'-i-ak): 1. Tending to arouse the sexual impulse. 2. A drug or agent that stimulates or arouses the sexual impulse.

aphrodisiomania (af-rō-diz'-i-ō-mā'-ni-a): Excessive and abnormal sexual interest. Erotomania.

aphronesia (a-frō-nē'-si-a): Dementia; silliness; foolishness.

aphthae (af'-thē): Small whitish or grayish ulcerous areas, usually surrounded by a ring of erythema, found on mucous membrane of the mouth, sometimes also of the gastrointestinal tract. Caused by various fungi and bacteria. Characteristic of such diseases as thrush, sprue, aphthous stomatitis (*q.v.*). **BEDNAR'S A.**, whitish ulcerous spots on the posterior part of the hard palate, seen in young children. **CACHECTIC A.**, an often fatal disease characterized by lesions under the tongue and such severe constitutional symptoms as enlargement and degeneration of liver and spleen.—aptha, sing.; aphthous, adj.

aphthous (af'-thus): Pertaining to or characterized by apthae. **A. FEVER**, see foot-and-mouth disease. **A. STOMATITIS**, inflammation of the mucous membrane of the mouth with the formation of small painful ulcerations.

apical (ā'-pi-kal): Pertaining to or located at the apex of a structure. **A. BEAT**, heart rate taken over the apex of the heart. **A. PULSE**, **A.** beat.

apicitis (ā-pi-sī'-tis): Inflammation at 1) the apex of a lung, or 2) the apex of a tooth.

apicoectomy (ap-i-kō-ek'-to-mi): Excision of the root of a tooth.

apicolysis (ap-i-kol'-i-sis): The operation of stripping the parietal pleura from the upper anterior chest wall to ensure collapse of the lung apex to obliterate a cavity in the apex; formerly frequently done in treatment of pulmonary tuberculosis.

aplasia (a-plā'-zi-a): 1. Incomplete development of an organ or tissue. 2. Defective cell formation. 3. Absence of growth.

aplastic (a-plas'-tik): 1. Pertaining to aplasia. 2. Incapable of forming new tissue. **A. ANEMIA**, see under anemia. **A. CRISIS**, a type of sickle cell crisis in which the production of red cells is diminished, causing the patient to become pale, listless and dyspneic due to lack of sufficient oxygen in the circulating blood.

Apley: 1. **A. TEST,** a test for torn meniscus of the knee joint; is positive when the prone patient's knee is rotated laterally and produces pain at the lateral tibial condyles. 2. **A. SCRATCH TEST,** used in evaluating external rotation and abduction of the arm as the patient reaches around the chest to the opposite shoulder.

apnea (ap'-nē-a): Temporary cessation of breathing, as seen, *e.g.*, in Cheyne-Stokes respiration.—apneic, adj.

apneumia (ap-nū'-mi-a): A congenital anomaly characterized by absence of the lungs.

apneusis (ap-nū'-sis): Continued contraction of the muscles of inspiration for an abnormally prolonged period of time; usually occurs after surgery for removal of part of the pons.

apneustic (ap-nū'-stik): Pertaining to or exhibiting apneusis. **A. BREATHING,** breathing that is characterized by long inspirations, short inefficient expirations, and long pauses between breaths; the respiratory rate may become very slow and finally fade into apnea. **A. CENTER,** located in the pons; assists in controlling inspiration.

apnoea: See apnea.

apo-: Combining form denoting away from or derived from.

apocamnosis (ap-ō-kam-nō'-sis): Abnormally easy fatigability, as seen in patients with myasthenia. Also apokamnosis.

apocarteresis (ap'-ō-kar-te-rē'-sis): Suicide by voluntary starvation.

apocleisis (ap-ō-klī'-sis): Aversion to food or eating.

apocrine (ap'-ō-krin): Designating a type of glandular secretion that contains some of the protoplasm of the cells that elaborate it. **A. GLANDS,** modified sweat glands, especially in the axillae, genital, mammary and perineal regions; they produce both sweat and a solution that, after puberty, is responsible for body odor.

apodal (a-pō'-dal): Without feet.

apodemialgia (ap'-ō-dē-mi-al'-ji-a): A morbid longing to leave one's home; wanderlust.

apodia (a-pō'-di-a): Congenital absence of one or both feet.—apodal, adj.

apogee (ap'-ō-jē): The climax or crisis of a disease, or the period of greatest severity of a disease.

apolepsis (ap-ō-lep'-sis): Deficiency or cessation of the production of a natural secretion.

Apollo cover: A tent-like covering placed over the bed to maintain a satisfactory environmental temperature while allowing the severely burned patient to remain unclothed and uncovered.

apomorphine (ap-ō-mor'-fēn): A derivative of morphine; used in medicine as a powerful emetic.

aponeurectomy (ap'-ō-nū-rek'-tō-mi): The surgical removal of the aponeurosis of a muscle.

aponeurorrhaphy (ap'-ō-nū-ror'-a-fi): The suturing of an aponeurosis.

aponeurosis (ap'-ō-nū-rō'-sis): A broad glistening sheet of tendon-like tissue that serves to invest and attach muscles to each other, and also to the parts which they move.—aponeuroses, pl.; aponeurotic, adj.

aponeurositis (ap'-ō-nū-rō-sī'-tis): Inflammation of an aponeurosis.

aponeurotomy (ap'-ō-nū-rot'-ō-mi): An incision into an aponeurosis.

apophyseal (a-pō-fiz'-ē-al): Of or pertaining to a hypophysis.

apophysis (a-pof'-i-sis): A projection, protuberance, or outgrowth, usually from a bone to which it remains attached.—apophyses, pl.; apophyseal, apophysial, adj.

apophysitis (a-pof-i-sī'-tis): Inflammation of an apophysis.

apoplexy (ap'-ō-pleks-i): Term formerly used to designate stroke. A sudden hemorrhage of blood into an organ, often into the brain after the rupture of an intracranial vessel. Signs include stertorous breathing, unconsciousness, incontinence of urine and feces, and usually some degree of hemiplegia.—apoplectic, adj.

aposia (a-pō'-zi-a): 1. Absence of the sensation of thirst. 2. Reluctance to taking fluid by mouth.

apositia (ap-ō-sish'-i-a): Disgust for and aversion to food.

apostasis (a-pos'-ta-sis): 1. An abscess. 2. The termination by crisis of a disease or attack.

aposthia (a-pos'-thi-a): Congenital absence of the prepuce.

apothecaries' system (a-poth'-e-kā-rēz): A system of weights and measures in which weights are given in grains, scruples, drams, ounces and pounds. Capacity is given in minims, fluidrams, fluidounces, gills, pints, and quarts.

apothecary (a-poth'-e-kā-ri): 1. A pharmacist. 2. A pharmacy.

apotripsis (ap-ō-trip'-sis): The surgical removal of an opacity from the cornea.

appendage (a-pen'-dij): A subordinate attached or suspended part of an organ or structure; usually less important in function and smaller than the main structure.

appendectomy (a-pen-dek'-to-mi): 1. Surgical removal of the vermiform appendix (*q.v.*). 2. Surgical removal of an appendage.

appendicectomy (a-pen-di-sek'-tō-mi): Surgical removal of the vermiform appendix. Appendectomy.

appendices epiploicae (a-pen′-di-sēz-ep-i-plō′-i-sē): Peritoneum-covered tabs of fat that are attached to the tenia (*q.v.*) of the colon.

appendicitis (a-pen-di-sī′-tis): Inflammation of the vermiform appendix (*q.v.*), chronic or acute; usually sudden in onset with pain over the entire abdomen but which later localizes in the lower right side. **RETROCECAL A.**, presents with the usual signs of appendicitis, except that the anterior abdominal signs are lacking due to the location of the appendix at the back of the cecum.

appendicolithiasis (a-pen′-di-kō-li-thī′-a-sis): A condition marked by the presence of stones in the vermiform appendix. Also called appendolithiasis.

appendicostomy (a-pen-di-kos′-to-mi): An operation in which the appendix is brought to the surface and an opening made into it so that a catheter can be inserted for the purpose of irrigating and/or draining the large bowel.

appendicular (a-pen-dik′-ū-lar): 1. Pertaining to an appendage. 2. Pertaining to the upper and lower extremities of the body. **A. SKELETON**, the arms and legs.

appendix (a-pen′-diks): An appendage. **A. VERMIFORMIS**, a worm-like appendage of the cecum; about the thickness of a pencil and may be from two to six inches long, ending in a blind extremity. Usually extends downward in the right iliac region but its position is variable. Apparently functionless. Frequently referred to as the vermiform appendix.—appendices, pl.; appendiceal, appendicular, adj.

apperception (ap-er-sep′-shun): 1. Clear perception of a sensory stimulus, particularly when there is identification or recognition. 2. Perception as modified by one's own emotions, memories, and experiences.—apperceptive, adj.

appestat (ap′-e-stat): The center in the hypothalamus that probably controls the appetite.

appetite (ap′-e-tīt): A normal desire to satisfy a natural physical or mental need; specifically, the desire to eat.

applanation (ap-la-nā′-shun): Undue flatness as sometimes seen in the cornea.

appliance (a-plī′-ans): Any device to assist an individual in the performance of a basic function.

applicator (ap′-li-kā-tor): An instrument for applying local remedies, often consisting of a slender rod of wood or metal to which a cotton pledget has been attached.

appose (a-pōz′): To juxtapose or to place next to one another.

apposition (ap-ō-zish′-un): 1. The bringing of two adjacent surfaces or edges together so they are in contact. 2. Side by side.

apprehension (ap-rē-hen′-shun): Fear; anxiety, dread.

approximate (a-prok′-si-māt): To bring close together or into apposition, as the teeth in the human jaw.—approximation, n., approximal, adj.

apraxia (a-prak′-si-a): Loss of the ability to perform learned or purposeful movements, to maintain posture, to make proper use of objects, or to execute acts that are normally automatic, when there is no sensory loss or paralysis; many variations are described. **CONSTRUCTIONAL A., A.** in which the person apparently understands directions but cannot copy simple drawings or use building blocks to construct simple patterns. **IDEATIONAL A.**, characterized by extreme absentmindedness and lack of purpose of various actions; thought to be due to an affection of the ideation area of the cortex. **IDEOMOTOR A.**, inability to execute ideas; thought to be due to disconnection between the two motor areas of the cortex. **SPEECH** or **VERBAL A.**, impairment of the ability to control the positioning and sequence of the speech muscles and their movements, resulting in incorrect formation of sounds; may be due to brain injury.

aproctia (a-prok′ shi-a): Absence or imperforation of the anus; a congenital anomaly.

aprosexia (a-prō-sek′-si-a): Inability to fix the attention or to concentrate, arising from such causes as mental deficiency or deficient hearing or vision.

aprosody (a-prōs′-o-di): The absence, in one's speech, of the normal rhythm, pitch, and variations in stress and tone.

apsychia (a-sī′-ki-a): Temporary loss of consciousness, *e.g.*, fainting.

APT: Alum-precipitated diphtheria toxoid; a diphtheria prophylactic used mainly for immunization of children.

aptitude (ap′-ti-tūd): Natural ability or acquired facility in performing certain tasks, either mental or physical. In psychology, potential rather than developed ability or facility for learning a certain kind of performance; *e.g.*, musical aptitude. **A. TEST**, one which permits evaluation of one's potential for learning certain skills or for performing tasks which may or may not have similarity to the test tasks, or for success in a particular field or profession.

aptyalia (ap-tī-ā′-li-a): Absence or diminished secretion of saliva. Also aptyalism.

APUD cells: So called because of their capability of *a*mine *p*recursor *u*ptake *d*ecarboxylation; refers to epithelial cells found in the pancreas, bile ducts, gastrointestinal tract, and bronchi, and which are capable of synthesizing and secreting polypeptide hormones such as gastrin and glucagon.

apudoma (ā-pū-dō′-ma): A benign or malignant tumor composed of APUD cells (*q.v.*). Also called APUD tumor.

apus (ā′-pus): An individual without feet, or without lower extremities entirely.

apyogenous (a-pī-oj′-e-nus): 1. Not characterized by the presence of pus. 2. Not caused by pus.

apyrexia (a-pī-rek′-si-a): Absence of fever.—apyrexial, apyretic, adj.

apyrogenic (a-pī-rō-jen′-ik): Not acting to produce fever.

AQ: Abbreviation for achievement quotient (*q.v.*).

aq: Abbreviation for *aqua* [L.], meaning water.

aqua (ak′-wa): Water. **A. AMNII,** amniotic fluid. **A. DESTILLATA,** distilled water. **A. FORTIS,** a solution of nitric acid. **A. MENTHAE PIPERITAE,** peppermint water. **A. OCULI.,** the aqueous humor of the eye. **A. PURA,** pure water. **A. ROSEA,** rose water.

aquapuncture (ak-wa-pungk′-tūr): The hypodermic injection of water as a placebo, for counterirritation, or for any other purpose.

aqueduct (ak′-we-dukt): A canal in an organ or structure for the passage of fluid. **A. OF SYLVIUS,** the canal connecting the 3rd and 4th ventricles of the brain; aqueductus cerebri. [Francois Sylvius de la Boe, French anatomist. 1614–1672.]

aqueous (ā′-kwē-us): Watery. **A. HUMOR,** the clear watery fluid that fills the anterior and posterior chambers of the eye.

arachidonic acid (ar-ak-i-don′-ik as′-id): A polyunsaturated fatty acid; essential in nutrition. Found in small amounts in human and animal liver and organ fats; also synthesized from linoleic acid.

Arachnida (a-rak′-ni-da): A class of Arthropoda, comprising mites, ticks, spiders, scorpions.

arachnidism (a-rak′-ni-dizm): Systemic poisoning resulting from the bite of a spider.

arachnitis (ar-ak-nī′-tis): Arachnoiditis (*q.v.*).

arachnodactyly (a-rak-nō-dak′-ti-li): A congenital abnormality marked by long, slender, curved fingers, often called "spider" fingers, as seen in Marfan's syndrome. Toes are also sometimes affected.

arachnoid (a-rak′-noyd): Resembling a spider's web. **A. MEMBRANE,** a delicate membrane enveloping the brain and spinal cord, lying between the pia mater internally and the dura mater externally; the middle serous membrane of the meninges.

arachnoidea (a-rak-noyd′-ē-a): The arachnoid membrane; see under **arachnoid.**

arachnoidism (a-rak′-noyd-izm): Poisoning caused by a spider bite.

arachnoiditis (a-rak′-noy-dī′-tis): Inflammation of the arachnoid. **OPTICOCHIASMATIC A.,** chronic inflammation around the optic chiasm and optic nerves; may be due to syphilis; results in impairment of vision and optic atrophy. **CHRONIC ADHESIVE A.,** thickening and adhesion of the pia mater and arachnoid membranes; may result from trauma or meningitis and cause obliteration of the subarachnoid space; symptoms vary.

arachnophobia (a-rak-nō-fō′-bi-a): Morbid fear of spiders.

Aran-Duchenne disease: A chronic, progressive wasting and atrophy of muscles beginning in the extremities, usually bilateral, and gradually progressing to other parts of the body; may be familial in origin or due to infection, avitaminosis, or toxins; also known as pseudohypertrophic muscular dystrophy or progressive spinal muscular atrophy.

arbor: In anatomy, a structure or part that is tree-like in appearance. **A. ALVEOLARIS,** the branched terminal end of an air passage in the lung. **A. VITAE,** 1) the tree-like outline of white substance seen on section of the cerebellum; 2) the pattern of folds and ridges seen in the mucous membrane of the uterine cervix.

arborescent (ar-bō-res′-ent): Having branches, like a tree.

arborization (ar-bor-ī-zā′-shun): A treelike formation or structure or the forming of such a structure; a characteristic of both ends of a neuron.

arboviruses (ar′-bō-vī′ rus-es): Any of a great number of viruses transmitted by bloodsucking arthropods, including mosquitoes, sandflies, fleas, ticks; the causative agent of yellow fever, plague, dengue, Rift Valley fever, sandfly fever, viral encephalitis, Rocky Mountain spotted fever.

arc (ark): **REFLEX A.,** in anatomy, the pathway over which a nerve impulse travels in producing a reflex action; *i.e.,* the afferent nerve that carries the impulse to a nerve center, the nerve center, the efferent nerve that carries the impulse to a peripheral organ or structure, and the organ or structure that produces the reflex action.

arcate (ar′-kāt): Curved. In anatomy, an arch-like structure.

arch: A curve or loop; a curved or bow-like structure. **A. OF THE AORTA,** the curved part between the ascending and descending aorta. **A. OF THE FOOT,** 1) transverse, along the line of the tarsometatarsal joints; 2) inner longitudinal, formed by the calcaneus, talus, navicular, three cuneiform bones, and the first three toes; 3) outer longitudinal, formed by the calcaneus and cuboid bones and the fourth and fifth toes. **GLOSSOPHARYNGEAL A.,** the posterior of two folds of mucous membrane that connect with the soft palate at either side of the oropharynx; the palatine tonsil is located between it and the palatoglossal **A. PALATOGLOSSAL A.,** the more forward of the two folds of mucous membrane that connect with the soft palate at either side of the oropharynx. **PALMAR A.**, the **A.** formed by the union of the radial and ulnar arteries in the palm. **PLANTAR A.**, that formed by the anastomosis of the plantar and dorsalis pedis arteries in the foot. **PUBIC A.**, that formed by the convergence of the rami of the ischium and pubis on each side; it is immediately below the symphysis pubis. **ZYGOMATIC A.**, that formed by the malar and temporal bones.

archetype (ar′-ke-tīp): 1. The original model or pattern on which all things of the same type are copied. 2. In Jungian psychology, an inherited mode of thought, derived from the experiences of the race, which is present in the unconsciousness of the individual.

archiform (ar′-ki-form): Refers to lesions that appear in circles, arcs, or irregular combinations of both forms.

Archimedes' principle: A submerged or floating body is kept buoyed up in the water by a force equal to its weight.

architis (ar-kī′-tis): Proctitis; inflammation of the anus.

archoptosis (ar-kō-tō′-sis): Prolapse of the rectum.

archorrhagia (ar-kō-rā′-jē-a): Hemorrhage from the rectum.

archorrhea (ar-kō-rē′ a): A discharge of purulent liquid from the rectum.

arcuate (ar′-kū-āt): Bow-shaped or arched.

arcus (ar′-kus): A curved, bow-like structure or ring. **A. SENILIS,** an opaque grayish white ring around the edge of the cornea; usually bilateral; does not interfere with vision; seen in the elderly.

ARDS: Adult respiratory distress syndrome. See under respiratory distress syndrome. Also called shock lung.

areflexia (a-rē-flek′-si-a): The state of being without reflexes.—areflexic, adj.

Arenavirus (ar-ē′-na-vī′-rus): Any of a family of RNA viruses that are characterized by the presence of fine granules in their virions; choriomeningitis is an example of diseases caused by a member of this group of viruses. Lassa fever, seen chiefly in Africa, and Argentinian and Bolivian hemorrhagic fevers, seen chiefly in Latin America, are other examples.

areocystoscopy (ar-ē-ō-sis-tos′-ko-pi): Examination of the urinary bladder with a cystoscope after the bladder has been distended with air.

areola (ar-ē′-o-la): 1. The pigmented area around a part, *e.g.*, the nipple; or around an area, *e.g.*, around certain lesions on the skin. 2. The part of the iris immediately surrounding the pupil. 3. A minute interstice or space in a tissue. **A. MAMMAE,** the darkened ring that surrounds the nipple. **SECONDARY A.**, a dark circle of pigmentation that surrounds the primary areola of the nipple in pregnancy.—areolar, adj.

areolitis (ar-ē-ō-lī′-tis): Inflammation of the areola of the nipple.

ARF: Abbreviation for: 1. Acute renal failure. 2. Acute respiratory failure.

argent-: A combining form meaning silver.

argentaffin (ar-jen′-ta-fin): Having an affinity for silver salts or chromium salts. **A. CELLS,** cells that are capable of being stained by silver salts.

argentaffinoma (ar′-jen-taf-i-nō′-ma): A tumor originating in argentaffin cells; usually occurs in the terminal part of the ileum or the vermiform appendix. May be benign or malignant when it is referred to as carcinoid syndrome. Seen chiefly in the middle-aged and elderly.

argentum (ar-jen′-tum): Silver. Chemical symbol is Ag.

arginase (ar′-ji-nās): An enzyme found in the liver, kidney and spleen. It splits arginine into ornithine and urea.

arginine (ar′-ji-nin): One of the essential amino acids (*q.v.*). It is obtained from animal and vegetable proteins and must be supplied in the diet. Also prepared synthetically.

argininosuccinic acid (ar′-ji-nin-ō-suk-sin′-ik): A substance formed during the process of urea formation in the liver; not normally found in the urine.

argininosuccinicaciduria (ar′-ji-nin-ō-suk-sin′-ik-as-i-dū′-ri-a): The presence of argininosuccinic acid in the urine; occurs rarely as an inborn error of metabolism; associated with mental retardation.

argon (ar′-gon): An inert, gaseous element present in small quantity, 0.94 per cent, in the atmosphere.

Argonz-Del Castillo syndrome: Galactorrhea, amenorrhea, and low production of the follicle-stimulating hormone; cause unknown; may be due to overproduction of prolactin or the presence of a pituitary tumor.

Argyll Robertson pupil: A pupil that is small and does not react when a light is shone in it but contracts when shown a near object; usually bilateral; seen chiefly in diseases of the nervous system. (Douglas Argyll Robertson, Scottish ophthalmologist, 1837–1909.)

argyria (ar-jir′-i-a): A permanent grayish or bluish discoloration of tissues resulting from long administration of silver preparations. Also called argyrosis, argyrism.

argyrophilic (ar-ji-rō-fil′-ik): Said of tissues that are capable of binding silver salts which may later, under the influence of light, make a black deposit of silver.

arhinia (a-rin′-ē-a): A congenital anomaly with the absence of a nose. Also arrhinia.

ariboflavinosis (a-rī′-bō-flā-vin-ō′-sis): A deficiency state caused by lack of sufficient riboflavin in the diet; characterized by cheilosis, seborrheic dermatitis, angular stomatitis, glossitis, and photophobia.

arm: In common usage, the upper extremity from the shoulder to the wrist. In anatomy, the part of the upper extremity from the shoulder to the elbow, as distinguished from the forearm.

arm board: A piece of firm, flat, padded material used to keep the arm straight, usually to keep the arm extended while the patient is receiving intravenous infusion.

armamentarium (ar-ma-men-tā′-rē-um): Word used to describe the entire equipment of a medical practitioner or institution; includes instruments, books, medicines, appliances, etc.

armpit: The axilla.

Army alpha intelligence test: A set of mental tests used to measure the general intelligence of World War I army recruits who could read and write. Also called alpha test and alpha intelligence test.

Arnold-Chiari malformation: A congenital abnormality in which parts of the cerebellum and medulla oblongata herniate through the foramen magnum into the upper part of the cervical vertebral canal; may or may not be associated with spina bifida or meningomyelocele.

aromatherapy (a-rō-ma-ther′-a-pi): The use of odors for their effect on emotions in the treatment of tense, emotionally disturbed patients.

aromatic (ar-ō-mat′-ik): 1. Having a fragrant, spicy, or pungent odor. 2. A medicinal substance having a fragrant, spicy aroma; often of vegetable origin and used as a stimulant.—aromatic, adj.

arousal (a-row′-sal): The state of being responsive to stimuli; wakefulness.

arrector (a-rek′-tor): Refers to the minute smooth muscles of the skin that are attached to the hair follicles. See arectores pilorum.

arrectores pilorum (a-rek-tō′-rēz pī-lō′-rum): Any of the minute internal, plain, involuntary muscles of the skin which are attached to hair follicles and which, under the stimulus of fright or cold, contract and thus erect the hair follicles causing "goose-flesh."—a. pili, pl.

arrest: The sudden stoppage or cessation of a physiological function or of the course of a disease. **CARDIAC A.**, complete cessation of mechanical action of the heart, *i.e.*, the heartbeat. **EPIPHYSEAL A.**, arrest of the growth of long bones by premature fusion of the diaphysis and epiphysis.

arrhenoblastoma (a-rē′-nō-blas-tō′-ma): A relatively rare malignant tumor of the ovary that may result in production of androgen and consequent masculinization.

arrhythmia (a-rith′-mi-a): In physiology, any deviation from the normal rhythm of the heartbeat. **ATRIAL A.**, A. that originates in any part of the atrium except the sinoatrial node. **SINUS A.**, A. that originates in the sinoatrial node; the rhythm of the heartbeat varies, being slower during expiration and more rapid during inspiration; fairly common in children in whom it appears to be normal, and in the elderly. **VENTRICULAR A.**, A. originating in an ectopic focus in the ventricle.

arrhythmogenic (a-rith-mō-jen′-ik): Producing or capable of producing arrthythmia.

ARS: Abbreviation for antirabies serum (equine). See HRIG.

arsenic (ar′-sen-ik): A metallic element. Formerly widely used in medicine; now largely replaced by penicillin. Its toxic potential is high; poisoning is recognized by the garlic odor of the breath; industrial exposure is likely to put one at risk to bronchial carcinoma. **A.** contained in weed and rat poisons and in insecticides is a frequent cause of poisoning.

art therapy: The use of various art forms in therapy—drawing, painting, sculpture, music, dancing, writing.

arteri-, arterio-: Combining forms denoting artery or arteries.

arterial (ar-tē′-rē-al): Pertaining to an artery (ies). **A. ANEURYSM**, an aneurysm occurring in an artery; may be due to a congenital defect; also caused by hypertensive atherosclerosis. **A. BLOOD**, blood that has been oxygenated in the lungs and passes to the left side of the heart from which it is distributed throughout the body. **A. BLOOD GASES**, gases dissolved in the liquid part of the blood, specifically oxygen, carbon dioxide, and nitrogen. **A. THROMBOSIS**, the development of a thrombus in an artery; usually a slow process causing paresthesias with coldness of the part, paralysis of muscles, and absence of pulses below the obstruction; may break away and become an embolus.

arterialgia (ar-tēr-i-al′-ji-a): Pain in or emanating from an inflamed artery.

arteriarctia (ar-tēr-i-ark′-shi-a): Vasoconstriction; reducing the caliber of an artery or arteries.

arteriectasia (ar-tēr-i-ek-tā′-si-a): Vasodilation; increasing the caliber of an artery or arteries. Also arteriectasis.

arteriectomy (ar-tēr-i-ek′-tō-mi): Excision of a segment of an artery. Also arterectomy.

arteriogram (ar-tē′r-i-ō-gram): X ray of an artery or arteries after injection of an opaque medium.

arteriography (ar-tēr′-i-og′-ra-fi): 1. Roentgenography of the arteries after the intravenous administration of a radiopaque substance. 2. Sphygmography (*q.v.*). **COMPUTERIZED INTRAVENOUS A.**, direct visualization of the arterial system following injection of a contrast medium into a peripheral vein.

arteriolar (ar-tēr-i-ō′-lar): Pertaining to an arteriole. **A. SCLEROSIS,** arteriosclerosis (*q.v.*).

arteriole (ar-tēr′-i-ōl): A small artery, particularly one joining an artery to a capillary.

arteriolith (ar-tēr′-i-ō-lith): A calculus in an arterial wall or in a thrombus.

arteriolitis (ar-tēr′-i-ō-lī′-tis): Inflammation of an arteriole or of several arterioles.

arteriolonecrosis (ar-tēr′-i-ō-lō-nē-krō′-sis): Necrosis of arterioles resulting from degeneration.

arteriomalacia (ar-tēr′-i-ō-ma-lā′ shi-a): Softening of the walls of an artery or arteries.

arterionephrosclerosis (ar-tēr′-i-ō-nef-rō-skle-rō′-sis): Gradual narrowing of the larger branches of the renal artery with hardening of the kidney, occurring in the elderly; may be due to hypertension; may also cause hypertension. Also called arterial nephrosclerosis and senile nephrosclerosis.

arteriopathy (ar-tēr′-i-op′-a-thi): Any disease of an artery or arteries.—arteriopathic, adj.

arterioplasty (ar-tēr′-i-ō-plas′-ti): Plastic surgery applied to an artery. Term often used to denote an operation for the reconstruction of an artery after an aneurysm.—arterioplastic, adj.

arteriopuncture (ar-tēr′-i-ō-pungk′-tur): The insertion of needle into an artery, usually for the purpose of withdrawing blood.

arteriorrhagia (ar-tēr′-i-ō-rā′-ji-a): Hemorrhage from an artery.

arteriorrhaphy (ar-tēr′-i-or′-a-fi): 1. Suture of an artery. 2. A plastic procedure on an artery, such as obliteration of an aneurysm.

arteriorrhexis (ar-tēr′-i-ō-rek′-sis): Rupture of an artery.

arteriosclerosis (ar-tēr′-i-ō-skle-rō′-sis): Name given to a group of common disorders characterized by degenerative changes in the arteries, primarily thickening and hardening of the walls with loss of elasticity and narrowing of the lumen which leads to decreased blood supply, chiefly to the brain and extremities. Although the specific cause of **A.** is usually unknown, it is often associated with high blood pressure, lipidemia, kidney disease and diabetes. The usual signs and symptoms include headache, intermittent claudication, bruits over the artery. **ARTERIOLAR A., A.** that affects the arterioles. **A. OBLITERANS, A.** in which the lumen of the artery is obliterated by thickening of the intima; usually affects the smaller vessels. **CEREBRAL A., A.** involving the arteries of the brain; most often seen in men and those over 50 years of age; patients are usually also hypertensive. **CORONARY A., A.** that involves the coronary arteries. **MÖNCKEBERG'S A., A.** characterized by calcification and thickening of the medial (muscular) coat in arteries, affecting especially the extremities; may lead to intermittent claudication or gangrene; also called medial **A. SENILE A.**, occurs as a natural process during aging. See also **atherosclerosis; Buerger's disease.**—arteriosclerotic, adj.

arteriosclerotic (ar-tēr′-i-ō-skle-rot′-ik): Pertaining to or associated with arteriosclerosis. **A. DEMENTIA,** impairment of mental functions, due to occlusion of blood vessels in the brain, and ischemic infarction. **A. HEART DISEASE,** common in the elderly; characterized by arrhythmias, angina pectoris, infarction, sudden death.

arteriostenosis (ar-tēr′-i-ō-stē-nō′-sis): A temporary or permanent decrease in the size of the lumen of an artery or arteries.

arteriotomy (ar-tēr′-i-ot′-o-mi): The surgical opening of an artery.

arteriovenous (ar-tēr′-i-ō-vē′-nus): Pertaining to both an artery and a vein. **A. FISTULA,** an abnormal direct connection between an arteriole and a venule. **A. SHUNT,** see under **shunt.**

arterioversion (ar-tēr′-i-ō-ver′-shun): A turning back or eversion of the walls of the cut end of an artery to arrest hemorrhage.

arteritis (ar-te-rī′-tis): A general term for inflammation of one or more of the arterial coats. May be secondary to some underlying condition, or primary. **GIANT-CELL A.**, affects particularly the temporal and cranial arteries; characterized by headache, fever, pain, and neurological disturbances including blindness; occurs mostly in the elderly. Also called Takayasu's **A.**; pulseless disease.—arteritides, pl.

artery (ar′-ter-i): A large vessel carrying blood from the heart to supply the various organs and tissues of the body. With the exception of the pulmonary artery, the arteries carry blood that has been oxygenated in the lungs. Arteries are tubular structures with three coats: 1) the internal endothelial lining (tunica intima) which provides a smooth surface to prevent clotting of blood; 2) the middle layer of plain muscle fibers (tunica media) which allows for distension as blood is pumped from the heart; and 3) the outer, mainly connective tissue layer (tunica adventitia), which prevents overdistension. The lumen is largest near the heart; it gradually decreases in size —arterial, adj.

arthr-, arthro-: Combining forms denoting joint(s).

arthragra (ar-thrag′-ra): Gouty pain in a joint or joints.

arthral (ar′-thral): Relating or pertaining to a joint.

arthralgia (ar-thral′-ji-a): Pain in a joint, especially when there is no inflammation. Syn., arthrodynia.—arthralgic, adj.

arthrectomy (ar-threk′-to-mi): Excision of a joint.

arthritic (ar-thrit′-ik): 1. Pertaining to or affected by arthritis. 2. An individual suffering from arthritis.

arthritis (ar-thrī′-tis): Inflammation of a joint, often accompanied by pain, swelling, stiffness, and structural changes. May be caused by a variety of factors including infection, neurological disorders, metabolic disturbances, neoplasms, bursitis, acromegaly, trauma. **ACUTE A.**, marked by pain, heat, redness, swelling; may be due to gout, rheumatism, gonorrheal infection, trauma; may occur after surgical procedures, particularly parathyroidectomy. **ACUTE RHEUMATIC A.**, rheumatic fever. **ACUTE SEPTIC A.**, may follow the same course as acute osteomyelitis. **A. DEFORMANS**, rheumatoid **A.**, usually begins in the fingers and is progressive, resulting in deformity. **A. DEFORMANS JUVENILIS**, Still's disease (*q.v.*); see also Perthes' disease. **A. DEFORMANS NEOPLASTICA**, osteitis fibrosa (*q.v.*). **A. NODOSA (A. URATICA)**, gout. **DEGENERATIVE A.**, osteoarthritis (*q.v.*). **GONOCOCCAL A.**, severe pain and swelling of the joints resulting from an infection with the *Neisseria gonorrhoeae* organism. **GOUTY A., A.** in which uric acid salts are deposited in cartilage, bursae, and ligaments. **INFECTIOUS** or **INFECTIVE A., A.** in which microorganisms enter the joint from the bloodstream, or from a wound, or from osteomyelitis already present; acute or insidious onset; marked by acute or chronic inflammation of a joint or joints; organisms involved are usually staphylococcus, streptococcus, gonococcus, or meningococcus; most often affects joints already damaged by osteoarthritis, but may attack normal joints. **NEUROPATHIC A.**, a condition that may accompany neurologic disorders that interfere with deep pain impulses; the joints become disorganized from repeated minor injuries. **POLYARTICULAR A., A.** affecting several joints. **PSORIATIC A.**, rheumatoid **A.** associated with psoriasis, affecting chiefly the distal interphalangeal joints. **PYOGENIC A.**, caused by infection of a joint with pyogenic bacteria; characterized by severe pain on movement, swelling, and fever; may result in ankylosis. **RHEUMATOID A.**, chronic, mild, nonbacterial **A.**; usually affects several joints at one time; occurs chiefly in young adults: see under rheumatoid. **SEPTIC A.**, pyogenic **A. TUBERCULOUS A.**, caused by infection of a joint with tubercle bacilli from a focal infection elsewhere; affects mostly the intervertebral, hip, and knee joints; causes erosion of cartilage and bone with formation of cold abscess which may rupture and create a tuberculous fistula; occurs most often in children and young adults. See osteoarthritis.

arthrocele (ar′-thrō-sēl): 1. A swollen joint. 2. A hernia of the synovial membrane into the joint capsule.

arthrocentesis (ar′-thrō-sen-tē′-sis): A puncture through a joint capsule into a joint cavity for the purpose of removing fluid.

arthrochalasis (ar-thrō-kal′-a-sis): Unusual looseness or flaccidity of a joint.

arthrochondritis (ar′ thrō-kon-drī′-tis): Inflammation of the cartilages within and around a joint. Also called osteochrondritis.

arthroclasia (ar-thrō-klā′-zi-a): Breaking down of an ankylosed joint to produce a wider range of movement. Arthroclasis.

arthrodesis (ar-throd′-e-sis): The fixation or stiffening of a joint by surgical means.

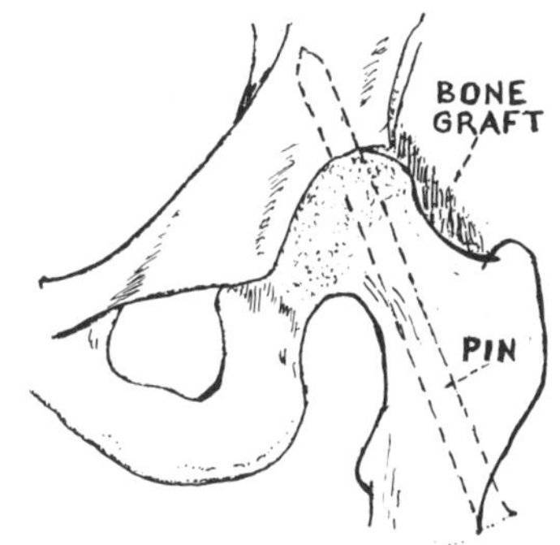

Arthrodesis of hip

arthrodia (ar-thrō′-di-a): A joint permitting gliding movement.—arthrodial, adj.

arthrodynia (ar-thrō-din′-i-a): Pain in a joint. See arthralgia.—arthrodynic, adj.

arthrodysplasia (ar′-thrō-dis-plā′-zi-a): Hereditary deformity of various joints; the patella is usually affected and the nails are absent; also called nail patella syndrome.

arthroempyesis (ar′-thrō-em-pī-ē′-sis): Infection of a joint, with suppuration.

arthroendoscopy (ar′-thrō-en-dos′-kō-pi): Visualization of the interior of a joint using an endoscope (*q.v.*).—arthroendoscopic, adj.; arthroendoscopically, adv.

arthrogram (ar′-thrō-gram): A roentgenogram of a joint, often after injection of a contrast material, which demonstrates the internal structure of the joint.

arthrography (ar-throg′-raf-i): X ray of a joint, sometimes after injection of air or radiopaque material.—arthrographic, adj.; arthrographically, adv.

arthrogryposis (ar′-thrō-grī-pō′-sis): The permanent retention of a joint in a flexed position as a result of muscular contractions and adhesions about the joint capsule. **A. MULTIPLEX CONGENITA,** a congenital syndrome characterized by contractures, ankylosis, deformities of many joints, limitation of motion, and lack of muscle development.

arthrokatadysis (ar′-thrō-ka-tad′-i-sis): Limitation of hip motion caused by a sinking in of the floor of the acetabulum, which allows the head of the femur to protrude through it into the pelvic cavity.

arthrolith (ar′-thrō-lith): A calculus or "stone" within a joint.

arthrology (ar-throl′-o-ji): The science that deals with joints, their diseases and treatment.

arthrolysis (ar-throl′-i-sis): The operation of restoring mobility to an ankylosed joint by breaking up adhesions.

arthrometer (ar-throm′-e-ter): An instrument that can measure and record the extent and degree of motion that can be produced by a joint; a type of goniometer (*q.v.*).

arthroncus (ar-throng′-kus): Swelling or a tumor of a joint.

arthroneuralgia (ar′-thrō-nū-ral′-ji-a): Neuralgia of a joint.

arthropathy (ar-throp′-a-thi): Any joint disease. **NEUROGENIC** and **NEUROPATHIC A.,** chronic degenerative joint disease seen in persons with neurologic disease, particularly tabes dorsalis; characterized by loss of sensation and joint fusion; see also Charcot's joint. **OSTEOPULMONARY A.,** clubbing of fingers and toes and enlargement of ends of long bones; usually occurs in persons with chronic cardiac or pulmonary disease. **PSORIATIC A.,** see under arthritis. **TABETIC A.,** neuropathic **A.**

arthroplasty (ar′-thrō-plas-ti): Plastic surgery on a joint; the repair, reconstruction, reformation, or replacement of a diseased or damaged joint. **CUP A.,** plastic surgery on a ball and socket joint, now usually consists of replacement of the ends of the articulating bones with an inert prosthesis; most often used for repair of hip and knee joints.

arthropod (ar′-thrō-pod): Any of the many invertebrate organisms of the family *Arthropoda* (*q.v.*).

Arthropoda (ar-throp′-o-da): A large group of invertebrate animals (over 700,000 species) whose members are characterized by segmented bodies, a hard outer shell, and paired jointed appendages. Includes crustaceans (crabs and lobsters); mites; ticks; spiders; and insects. Many species are important in medicine because they are parasites, vectors of disease, or troublesome pests whose bites and stings produce varying physiological reactions.

arthropyosis (ar′-thrō-pī-ō′-sis): The production of pus in a joint cavity; arthropyesis.

arthrosclerosis (ar′-thrō-sklē-rō′-sis): Stiffening of a joint(s), particularly in the aged.

arthroscope (ar′-thrō-skōp): A self-illuminating and magnifying endoscope for visualizing the interior of a joint cavity.—See endoscope.—arthroscopic, adj.

arthroscopy (ar-thros′-kō-pi): The act of visualizing the interior of a joint with an arthroscope.—arthroscopic, adj.

arthrosis (ar-thrō′-sis): 1. A joint or articulation. 2. Degeneration or disease of a joint. See amphiarthrosis, diarthrosis, pseudoarthrosis, synarthrosis, synchondrosis.—arthroses, pl.

arthrosteitis (ar-thros-tē-ī′-tis): Inflammation of the bony parts of a joint.

arthrostomy (ar-thros′-tō-mi): The surgical establishment of an opening into a joint, usually for the purpose of drainage.

arthrosynovitis (ar′-thrō-sin-ō-vī′-tis): Inflammation of the synovial membrane of a joint.

arthrotomy (ar-throt′-o-mi): Incision into a joint.

Arthu's reaction: A severe hypersensitive reaction with inflammation and edema at the site of repeated injections of an antigen, but may also present as a generalized anaphylactic reaction. Also called Arthu's phenomenon.

articular (ar-tik′-ū-lar): Pertaining to a joint or articulation. Applied to cartilage, surface, capsule, disk, fracture, process, etc.

articulate (ar-tik′-ū-lāt): 1. To join together, as in a joint. 2. Articulated; jointed. 3. To enunciate words and sentences distinctly. 4. In dentistry, to adjust teeth so they are in correct relationship to each other.

articulated (ar-tik′-ū-lāt-ed): The state of being joined together. In anatomy, the connection of separate parts in such a way as to permit motion.

articulation (ar-tik-ū-lā′-shun): 1. The junction of two or more bones; a joint. 2. Enunciation of speech.—articular, adj.

articulo mortis (ar-tik′-ū-lō mor′-tis): At the moment or instant of death.

articulus (ar-tik′-ū-lus): 1. A joint. 2. A knuckle.

artifact (ar′-ti-fakt): 1. Any artificial product resulting from a physical or chemical agency. 2. An unnatural change in a structure or tissue. 3. In electrocardiography, any wave or mark on the electrocardiograph tracing that does not represent part of the cardiac cycle; caused by the technique used. Also artefact.

artificial (ar-ti-fish′-al): 1. Imitated by art; not natural; made, invented, or performed by man. 2. Pertaining to an apparatus designed to take over the function of a diseased organ such as the eye, kidney, larynx, or heart, or of a disordered function such as feeding or respiration. **A. INSEMINATION,** see under insemination. **A.**

PACEMAKER, see under pacemaker. **A. RESPIRATION**, see under respiration.

aryepiglottic (ar′-i-ep-i-glot′-ik): Pertaining to the arytenoid cartilage and the epiglottis. **A. FOLDS**, folds of mucous membrane in the lateral walls at both sides of the entrance to the larynx; they extend from the arytenoid cartilage to the epiglottis.

aryl hydrocarbon hydroxylase (ar′-il hī-drō-kar′-bon hī-droks′-i-lās): An enzyme that is believed to act within the lung to convert carcinogenic substances in tobacco smoke or in the environmental air into active carcinogens.

arytenoid (ar-i-tē′-noyd): Shaped like a funnel or the mouth of a pitcher. **A. CARTILAGE**, see under cartilage.

arytenoidectomy (ar′-i-tē-noyd-ek′-to-mi): Surgical removal of an arytenoid cartilage.

arytenoiditis (ar′-i-tē-noyd-ī′-tis): Inflammation of the arytenoid muscles or the arytenoid cartilage.

A.S.: Abbreviation for *auris sinistra* [L.], meaning left ear.

As: Chemical symbol for arsenic.

ASAP: Abbreviation for as soon as possible.

asaphia (a-saf′-i-a): Indistinct speech or pronunciation as occurs particularly in patients with cleft palate.

asbestos (as-bes′-tōs): A fibrous, incombustible, mineral substance of magnesium and calcium silicone; has many uses in industry. Small spicules may cause keratotic papules on hands of industrial workers. Inhalation of asbestos dust or spicules is a serious occupational hazard, and for the same reason, the use of asbestos as fireproofing in the construction of schools and public buildings is an important public health issue.

asbestosis (as-bes-tō′-sis): A form of chronic lung disease resulting from prolonged inhalation of fine asbestos dust and fibrils. Manifested in several forms and may be related to lung cancer, particularly diffuse malignant mesothelioma; sometimes occurs in more than one form in the same individual. Asbestos miners and workers are most often affected, but school children and others exposed to asbestos building materials are also at risk.

ascariasis (as-ka-rī′-a-sis): Infestation with worms of the genus *Ascaris* (*q.v.*). The bowel is most often affected, but in the case of round worms, infestation may spread to the stomach, liver, and lungs. Also ascaridiasis, ascaridosis, ascariosis.

ascaricide (as-kar′-i-sīd): An agent that is lethal to worms of the genus *Ascaris*.

Ascaris (as′-kar-is): A genus of nematode worms which includes the round worm (*Ascaris lumbricoides*) and the threadworm (*Enterobius vermicularis*).—ascarides, pl.

ascending: Rising; taking an upward course. In the nervous system refers to impulses that move from the periphery up the spinal cord to the central nervous system via the afferent fibers. **A. AORTA**, the first part of the aorta between its origin at the heart and its arch. **A. COLON**, the part of the large intestine between the cecum and the hepatic flexure. **A. PARALYSIS**, Guillain-Barré syndrome (*q.v.*). **A. POLIOMYELITIS**, see under poliomyelitis.

Aschoff: A'S. BODIES, a group of cells and leukocytes appearing as nodules in the interstitial tissues of the heart in patients with rheumatic myocarditis; also called A.'s nodules. **A'S. NODE**, a flat white microscopic mass of Purkinje fibers found beneath the endocardium of the right atrium of all mammalian hearts and continuous with the muscle fibers of the atrium and the atrioventricular bundle of His. [Ludwig Aschoff, German pathologist. 1866–1942.]

ascites (as-sī′-tēz): Accumulation of excess free serous fluid in the peritoneal cavity. Causes include cirrhosis of the liver, tumor, tuberculous peritonitis, interference in venous circulation, cardiac or renal failure. **MALIGNANT A.**, a condition sometimes occurring in the end stage of cancer with metastasis to the peritoneum; treatment may consist of peritoneovenous shunt (see under shunt).—Syn., hydroperitoneum, abdominal dropsy.

Ascomycetes (as′-kō-mī-sē′-tēz): A group of fungi; includes yeasts, blue molds, mildews, ergot, truffles.

ascorbemia (as-kor-bē′-mi-a): The presence of ascorbic acid in the blood.

ascorbic acid (as-kor′-bik): Vitamin C (*q.v.*). Essential element of diet; not stored in the body so needs to be supplied regularly. Occurs naturally in citrus fruits, green leafy vegetables, tomatoes, potatoes, berries; also prepared synthetically. Used in treatment of anemia and to promote healing.

ascus (as′-kus): A sac-like structure that is the spore case for certain fungi.—asci, pl.

ASD: Abbreviation for arterial septal defect.

-ase: Suffix denoting: 1. An enzyme. 2. A destroying substance.

asemasia (as-e-mā′-zi-a): Inability to communicate by the usual means; *i.e.*, the patient cannot produce or comprehend spoken or written language, signs, etc. A form of aphasia. Syn., asymbolia.—asemic, adj.

asepsis (a-sep′-sis): The state of being free from living pathogenic microorganisms. **MEDICAL A.**, reduction in the number and possibility of transfer of pathogenic organisms in a particular area or environment; involves proper handwashing, and use of clean articles such as gowns, masks, gloves, etc. **SURGICAL A.**, the elimination of all microorganisms from a particular field or area; involves the use of sterile gloves, gowns, masks, etc., and use of proper methods to protect the sterile area or field.—aseptic, adj.; asepticize, v.

aseptic (a-sep′-tik): Pertaining to asepsis. **A. MENINGITIS,** a condition usually caused by a virus with the spinal fluid showing an increase in white blood cells but being bacteriologically sterile. **A. NECROSIS,** necrosis that occurs without infection. **A. TECHNIQUE,** a precautionary method used in any procedure in which there is a possibility of introducing pathogenic organisms into the patient's body; every article used must have been sterilized.

asexual (a-seks′-ū-al): Without sex or without reference to sex. **A. REPRODUCTION,** reproduction without sexual union.

asexualization (a-seks′-ū-al-ī-zā′-shun): Castration or sterilization of an individual.

Asherman's syndrome: Adhesions within the endometrial cavity; a frequent cause of amenorrhea and infertility.

Ashman's phenomenon: In the electrocardiogram, an aberrant beat of the ventricle at the end of a short cycle that follows a long cycle; seen in atrial fibrillation and some other arrhythmias.

asialia (a-sī-ā′-li-a): A deficiency or lack of secretion of saliva.

asiderosis (a-sid-er-ō′-sis): A deficiency in the body's iron reserve.

ASIS: Abbreviation for anterior superior iliac spine.

-asis: Suffix denoting: 1. Affected with; state or condition. 2. Action; process.

ASO: Abbreviation for antistreptolysin O.

asocial (a-sō′-shul): Unable or unwilling to conform to the social demands of the environment; selfish; indifferent, withdrawn from normal social intercourse.

asparaginase (as-par′-a-jin-āse): An enzyme present in liver and other animal tissues, yeast, and some bacteria; has some antileukemic activity and may be used in chemotherapeutic treatment of acute lymphoblastic leukemia.

aspartic acid (as-par′-tik as′-id): One of the non-essential amino acids; found in certain animals and plants, especially in molasses from sugarcane and sugarbeets.

aspergilloma (as-per-jil-ō′-ma): A tumor-like mass that forms in a bronchus or a pulmonary cavity; caused by the fungus *Aspergillus*.

aspergillosis (as-per-jil-ō′-sis): Infection caused by any species of the fungus *Aspergillus* (*q.v.*), characterized by formation of granulomatous tumor-like lesions in the skin, ear, sinuses, lungs, and sometimes in the meninges and bones. Likely to occur as an allergic condition in people who handle grain or seeds. See bronchomycosis. **BRONCHOPULMONARY A.,** infection of the bronchi and lungs with *Aspergillus*.

Aspergillus (as-per-jil′-us): A genus of fungi, found in soil, manure, and on various grains; includes many species of molds, some of which are pathogenic. *Aspergillis fumigatus* is the species most commonly pathogenic to plants, animals, and birds; the source of the antibacterial substance fumigasin, and may be the cause of certain nosocomial infections.

aspermia (a-sperm′-i-a): Inability to form or to ejaculate semen, or absence of sperm in the semen.

aspersion (as-per′-shun): The sprinkling of water on the body or on an affected part; a procedure used in hydrotherapy.

aspheric (a-sfēr′-ik): In anatomy, refers to a structure that varies slightly from complete roundness; usually refers to lenses of the eyes.

asphyxia (as-fik′-si-a): Suffocation, local or systemic lack of oxygen and increase in carbon dioxide in the blood as a result of interruption in breathing. This occurs when not enough oxygen is taken in or when the tissues are unable to utilize what is taken in; *e.g.*, in drowning, electric shock, chest injury, poisoning by a gas such as carbon monoxide, or by a substance such as cyanide. **A. NEONATORUM, A.** occurring in the newborn; among the causes are prolapsed cord, immaturity, intracranial damage, blockage of an airway. **BLUE A.** or **A. LIVIDA,** a condition of the newborn when the skin color is deep blue but there is good muscle tone and responsiveness to stimuli. **SECONDARY A., A.** caused by hemorrhage or edema of the lung, pneumothorax, narcotic drugs, tumor, aspiration of vomitus or a foreign body. **WHITE A.,** or **A. PALLIDA,** a serious condition of the newborn; the skin is pale and there is flaccidity and unresponsiveness to stimili.

asphyxiant (as-fik′-si-ant): Producing asphyxia or an agent that is capable of producing asphyxia.

asphyxiate (as-fik′-si-āt): To deprive the body of oxygen and thus cause asphyxiation.

asphyxiation (as-fik′-si-ā′-shun): Suffocation.

aspirate (as′-pi-rāt): 1. To remove gas or fluid by suction or negative pressure. 2. Fluid drawn off from a body cavity by means of suction. 3. To pronounce a vowel or a word with release of breath, as in pronouncing the letter *h*. 4. A fluid or foreign body that is sucked into the airway, *e.g.*, vomitus.

aspiration (as-pi-rā′-shun): 1. The act of drawing in breath; inspiration. 2. The withdrawal of fluids from a body cavity by means of a suction or siphonage apparatus. 3. The sucking of fluid into the airway. **A. BIOPSY,** needle biopsy (*q.v.*). **A. PNEUMONIA,** inflammation of the lung from inhalation of a foreign body, usually fluid or food particles. **NEEDLE A.,** removal of fluid with a long slender needle. **PATHOLOGICAL A.,** the drawing into the respiratory tract of food particles or mucus during unconsciousness or anesthesia. **SUPRAPUBIC A.,** a needle is inserted above the symphysis pubis into the bladder to collect an uncontaminated urine specimen. **TRANSLARYNGEAL A.,** is accomplished by a percutaneous puncture through the cricothyroid membrane. **TRANSTRACHEAL A.,** accomplished by puncture of the wall of the trachea below the larynx; done to obtain a sputum specimen needed for diagnosis of primary pneumonias when a normal cough does not produce enough.

aspirator (as′-pi-rā-tor): A negative-pressure apparatus for collecting material by suction, specifically for withdrawing fluid or gas from a cavity for diagnostic or therapeutic purposes.

asplenia (a-splē′-ni-a): 1. Absence of the spleen. 2. Impaired splenic function.

asporogenic (as-pō-rō-jen′-ik): Not spore-producing, or not produced by spores.

assay (as′-sā): The use of physical, chemical, or biological methods to analyze, test, or examine a substance to determine its purity or the relative proportion of its constituents, or the potency of a drug,—assay, v.

Assembly of Hospital Schools of Nursing: Founded in 1967. Membership: hospital schools of nursing. Functions: to provide support and promote advancement of hospital schools of nursing through educational programs and other activities. Publishes a bimonthly newsletter. Address: American Hospital Association, 840 Lake Shore Drive, Chicago, IL 60611

assertiveness (as-ser′-tiv-nes): A communication technique utilizing statements and actions to forcefully and positively compel recognition of one's position, rights, and status. **A. TRAINING,** a technique that teaches one to make appropriate responses to others, and to openly and honestly express one's feelings in a manner that is both satisfying and respectful while taking into consideration the rights of others as well as one's own.

assessment (a-ses′-ment): 1. A judgment made after evaluating or examining a situation or condition. 2. Any method of measuring the degree of competence of another person's ability to perform physical and/or intellectual skills. **NURSING A.,** involves gathering information from and about a patient, identifying his health care problem and needs, and stating these in terms that relate to the particular problem or condition.

assimilation (as-sim-i-lā′-shun): The process whereby the already digested foodstuffs are absorbed and utilized by the tissues. The constructive phase of metabolism. Syn., anabolism. In psychology, the integration of new experiences into one's consciousness.—assimilable, adj., assimilate, v.

assisted ventilation: Intermittent positive pressure breathing; see under intermittent.

Associate Degree programs in nursing education: See under nursing education.

association (a-sō-si-ā′-shun): A union or close relationship of ideas, things, or persons. **A. AREAS** or **CORTEX,** areas in the cortex of the brain that serve to integrate motor and sensory input. **A. OF IDEAS,** in psychology, the connection between ideas in the cortex so that one idea calls up another that was previously linked with it. **A. TEST,** the subject responds immediately with another word when the examiner speaks a word; the nature of the response and the time it takes for the response are used in diagnosis. **FREE A.,** ideas arising spontaneously when censorship is removed.

astasia (as-tāz′-i-a): Inability to stand erect due to muscle incoordination which is not of physical origin. **A.-ABASIA,** hysterical inability to stand, walk, or perform movements while erect; there is no paralysis or organic pathology; considered a sign of neurosis or of disease of the frontal lobe.

asteatosis (a-stē-a-tō′-sis): Lack or deficiency of secretion by the sebaceous glands. **A. CUTIS,** a skin condition characterized by dryness, scaliness and sometimes fissures; causes include nervous system disorders, senility, contact with irritants such as chemicals, detergents.

astereognosis (a-ster′-e-og-nō′-sis): Loss of the power to recognize the shape and consistency of objects by touching them.

asterixis (a-stēr-ik′-sis): Intermittent, involuntary jerking contractions of muscle groups, those of the wrist and fingers in particular; due to any of several pathological conditions; manifested by flapping tremor of the outstretched hand.

asthenia (as-thē′-ni-a): Thinness, weakness, debility, and lack of strength, particularly muscle strength. The term often forms part of combination words, *e.g.*, neurasthenia. **NEUROCIRCULATORY A.,** an anxiety neurosis associated with chest pains, faintness, palpitation, and extreme fatigue.

asteroid (as′-ter-oyd): Star-shaped.

asthenic (as-then′-ik): Pertaining to asthenia. **A. PERSONALITY,** see personality, asthenic.

asthenocoria (as-thē′-nō-kō′-ri-a): Sluggishness of the pupillary reaction to light.

asthenopia (as-the-nō′-pi-a): 1. Poor vision. 2. Eyestrain or speedy tiring of the eyes, usually due to weakness of the visual organ or muscles and attended by headache, sometimes pain in the eyes, dimness of vision.

asthenospermia (as′-the-nō-sper′-mi-a):

Weakness or reduced motility of the spermatozoa in the semen.

asthma (az′-ma): A disease characterized by recurrent paroxysmal attacks of difficulty in breathing which may be associated with wheezing, cough, sense of suffocation or constriction in the chest; due to bronchiolar constriction and inflammation, often allergic in origin. Occurs most often in children or young adults. Often caused by inhalation or ingestion of substances to which the patient is hypersensitive. A family history of asthma is often present. **ALLERGIC A.**, reaction to a specific allergen such as pollen, dust; attacks are of sudden onset and brief duration. **BRONCHIAL A.**, attacks of breathlessness associated with bronchial obstruction or spasm; characterized by expiratory wheeze. **CARDIAC A.**, paroxysmal dyspnea often seen in left ventricular failure. **EXTRINSIC A.**, caused by something in the environment; allergic **A. FOOD A.**, caused by ingestion of certain foods; characterized by diaphoresis, diminished breath sounds, diffuse prolonged expiratory wheezes, respiratory distress. **GRINDERS' A.**, popular name for silicosis that arises from inhalation of metallic dust. **INTRINSIC A.**, due to some particular physiologic disturbance. **OCCUPATIONAL A.**, seen in persons who are exposed in their work environments to grain dust, wood dust, asbestos, enzymatic detergents. See status asthmaticus under status.

asthmatic (az-mat′-ik): 1. Pertaining to asthma. 2. A person suffering from asthma.

astigmatism (a-stig′-ma-tizm): Defective vision caused by inequality of one or more of the refractive surfaces of the eye, usually the corneal, so that the light rays do not converge to a single point on the retina. May be congenital or acquired. Syn., astigmia.—astigmatic, astigmic, adj.

astomia (a-sto′-mi-a): A congential anomaly characterized by absence of the mouth.—astomatous, astomous, adj.

astragalectomy (as-trag′-a-lek′-to-mi): Excision of the astragalus, now generally called the talus.

astragalus (as-trag′-a-lus): The ankle bone or talus upon which the tibia rests.—astragalar, adj.

astraphobia (as-tra-fō′-bi-a): Morbid fear of lightning and thunderstorms.

astringent (as-trin′-jent): An agent that contracts organic tissue, thus lessening secretion, arresting hemorrhage, diarrhea, etc.—astringency, n.; astringent, adj.

astro-: Combining form denoting star or star-shaped.

astroblast (as′ trō-blast): A cell from which an astrocyte develops.

astroblastoma (as′-trō-blas-tō′-ma): A relatively rare rapidly growing brain tumor arising from and composed of astroblasts.

astrocyte (as′-trō-sīt): A star-shaped cell, particularly a neuroglial or brain cell. See neuroglia.

astrocytoma (as-trō-sī-tō′-ma): A relatively common slow growing primary tumor of the brain and spinal cord tissue; formed from astrocytes; characteristically invades surrounding structures. Usually graded I to IV, depending on the degree of potential malignancy of the tumor. Grades I and II occur most often in children; grades III and IV are the most common of all gliomas, occurring most often in middle or old age. See glioma.

astrocytosis (as′-trō-sī-tō′-sis): An increase in both the number and the size of astrocytes.

astroglia (as-trog′-li-a): Neuroglia (*q.v.*) that is composed of astrocytes.

astroid (as′-troyd): Star-shaped.

astrophobia (as-trō-fō′-bi-a): Morbid fear of the stars and celestial space.

Astrup Technique: A technique for measuring the pH of arterial or capillary blood with a microelectrode; allows for calculation of PCO_2 and bicarbonate concentration.

asyllabia (a-sil-lā′-bi-a): A form of aphasia in which one recognizes individual letters of the alphabet but cannot form them into syllables or comprehend them when combined to form syllables.

asylum (a-sī′-lum) 1. An institution for housing aged or debilitated persons who, for some reason, cannot care for themselves. 2. An old term for a mental hospital.

asymbolia (a-sim-bō′-li-a): Inability to recognize such symbols of communication as words, gestures, signs, etc. Asemia (*q.v.*).

asymmetry (a-sim′-e-tri): In anatomy, uneven or unequal in size, shape, or placement of paired organs or parts on opposite sides of the body.—asymmetric, asymmetrical, adj.

asymptomatic (a-simp-tō-mat′-ik): Exhibiting no symptoms.

asynchronous (a-sin′-krō-nus): 1. A disturbance in coordination. 2. Pertains to the occurrence, at different times, of events that normally occur at the same time. **A. PACEMAKER**, see under pacemaker.

asynclitism (a-sin′-kli-tizm): The condition existing when the planes of the presenting parts of the fetal head and the mother's pelvis are not parallel; the skull bones overlap as a result of labor; cesarean section is usually indicated.

asynergy (a-sin′-er-ji): Failure of organs or parts which normally work together to do so; pertains to muscle groups especially. Also asynergia.—asynergic, adj.

asynesia (as-i-nē′-zi-a): Dullness of intellect; stupidity.

asystemic (a-sis-tem′-ik): Not confined to a specific system.

asystole (a-sis′-tō-le): Imperfect, incomplete, or no contractions of the ventricles of the heart during the systolic phase of the cardiac cycle. Cardiac standstill.

at. no.: Abbreviation for atomic number.

at risk: In health care, at risk situations are those involving possible problems that often can be prevented but which will require medical treatment if allowed to occur.

at. wt.: Atomic weight.

atactic (a-tak′-tik): Ataxic. See ataxia.

atactilia (a-tak-til′-i-a): Loss of ability to recognize impressions received through the sense of touch.

ataractic (at-a-rak′-tik): 1. Pertaining to a state of mental calmness or tranquility. 2. An agent that helps to relieve anxiety thus providing emotional equilibrium and tranquility without causing drowsiness. Syn., tranquilizer, neuroleptic.

ataralgesia (at-ar-al-jē′-zi-a): A method of allaying mental distress and pain associated with certain surgical procedures by sedation combined with analgesia which makes it possible for the patient to remain conscious and alert.

ataraxia (at-a-rak′-si-a): A state of tranquility or calmness in which neither consciousness nor mental faculties are interfered with.—ataractic, adj.

atavism (at′-a-vizm): The reappearance of an hereditary trait which has skipped one or more generations.—atavic, atavistic, adj.

ataxia, ataxy (a-taks′-i-a, a-tak′-si): Defective control and coordination of voluntary muscles; due to a lesion in the central nervous system which may be hereditary or caused by infection, the presence of a tumor, trauma, or atrophy of nervous system tissues. **ACUTE CEREBELLAR A.**, usually unilateral, with hypotonia of muscles on the affected side causing a characterisric posture. **FRIEDREICH'S A.**, occurs in children and young adults; affects chiefly the lower extremities; marked by lateral curvature of the spine, swaying movements, and speech difficulties. **HEREDITARY CEREBELLAR A.**, occurs chiefly in young adults; marked by speech defects and nystagmus; also called Marie's **A.** **LOCOMOTOR A.**, see tabes dorsalis.

ataxiaphasia (a-tak′-si-a-fā′-zi-a): A speech disorder in which the person has the ability to utter words but cannot speak in sentences.

ataxia-telangiectasia (a-taks′-i-a tē-lan′-ji-ek-tā′-si-a): An inherited disorder with onset in infancy or early childhood, characterized by progressive cerebellar ataxia, abnormal eye movements, recurring lung and sinus infections. Syn., Louis-Bar syndrome. See ataxia; telangiectasia.

ataxic (a-taks′-ik): Pertaining to or affected by ataxia. **A. GAIT**, an awkward gait, characterized by walking with the legs far apart, lifting the leg high and then bringing it down so that the entire foot strikes the ground at once; indicative of a spinal cord lesion. **A. SPEECH**, see under speech. **A. TREMOR**, intention tremor; see under tremor.

ataxiophemia (a-tak′-si-ō-fē′-mi-a): Lack of coordination of the muscles involved in producing speech.

atel-, atelo-: Combining forms denoting incomplete or imperfect.

atelectasis (at-e-lek′-ta-sis): 1. Imperfect expansion of the lungs at birth. 2. Collapse of a lung or part of it, resulting in a partial or complete airless state of a lung; due to occlusion of a bronchus or bronchiole caused by tumor, aneurysm, mucous plug, certain drugs, inspiration of a foreign object, a disease such as tuberculosis. Also, a complication following abdominal surgery.—atelectatic, adj.

atelencephalia (at-el′-en-se-fā′-li-a): A congenital anomaly consisting of imperfect or incomplete development of the brain.

atelia (a-tē′-li-a): A congenital anomaly consisting of imperfect or incomplete development of the body or any of its parts. Also ateliosis.

atelocardia (at-el-ō-kar′-di-a): A congenital anomaly consisting of underdevelopment or imperfect development of the heart.

atelocheiria (at-el-ō-kī′-ri-a): A congenital anomaly consisting of imperfect development of the hand.

atelognathia (at-e-log-nā′-thi-a): A congenital anomaly consisting of imperfect development of the jaw, especially the lower jaw.

atelomyelia (at′-e-lō-mī-ē′-li-a): A congenital anomaly consisting of imperfect development of the spinal cord.

athelia (a-thē′-li-a): Congenital absence of the nipples.

athermia (a-ther′-mi-a): 1. Lacking warmth. 2. Without fever.

atheroembolization (ath′-er-ō-em-bō-lī-zā′-shun): A condition in which an embolus consisting of atheromatous intima breaks off from an artery and is carried by the bloodstream to a smaller distal branch.

atherogenic (ath-e-rō-jen′-ik): Capable of producing atheroma.—atherogenesis, n.

atheroma (ath-er-ō′-ma): 1. Deposition of hard yellow plaques of lipoid material in the intimal layers of the arteries; the primary lesion in atherosclerosis (*q.v.*). May be related to high level of cholesterol in the blood. Of great importance in the coronary arteries in predisposing to coronary thrombosis. 2. A sebaceous cyst; see under cyst.—atheromata, pl.; atheromatous, adj.

atheromatosis (ath′-er-ō-ma-tō′-sis): The

presence of multiple atheromata in the arteries. Atherosclerosis.

atherosclerosis (ath′-e-rō-sklē-rō′-sis): The most frequently occurring form of arteriosclerosis, coexisting with atheroma; a disease process that causes thickening of arterial walls and loss of their elasticity; affects chiefly the large and medium sized arteries, especially the aorta, coronary arteries, and peripheral vessels. The WHO definition calls **A.** a complex chemical process involving "a combination of changes in the intima and media, including accumulation of lipids, hemorrhage, fibrous tissue and calcium deposits."—atherosclerotic, adj.

atherosis (ath-er-ō′-sis): Atherosclerosis (*q.v.*).

athetosis (ath-e-tō′-sis): A condition marked by slow, purposeless, involuntary, repeated, sinuous, writhing movements of the fingers and hands, toes and feet; sometimes involving most of the body. Generally due to a brain lesion. Seen chiefly in children in whom it is usually congenital; in older patients it is usually associated with cerebrovascular disease.—athetoid, athetotic, adj.

athlete's foot: See tinea pedis under tinea.

athlete's heart: Lay term for a hypertrophic or dilated heart that is thought to be due to repeated overexertion.

athrepsia (a-threp′-si-a): Marasmus. Term used particularly in reference to children who suffer from progressive physical weakness and emaciation resulting from malnutrition.—athreptic, adj.

athrombia (a-throm′-bi-a): Lack of, or defect in, the clotting of blood.

athymia (a-thī′-mi-a): 1. Congenital absence of the thymus gland. 2. Without spirit or feeling. 3. Dementia.

athyreosis (a-thī-rē-ō′-sis): Deficient secretion of thyroid hormone that results in myxedema (*q.v.*) or cretinism (*q.v.*). See hypothyroidism.

athyroidism (a-thī′-royd-izm): Lack of thyroid secretion because of absence or dysfunction of the gland. May be congenital or acquired; when congenital it produces cretinism (*q.v.*); when acquired in maturity it produces myxedema (*q.v.*). Athyreosis.

atlantal (at-lan′-tal): Pertaining to the atlas.

atlantoaxial (at-lan-tō-ak′-si-al): Pertaining to the atlas and the axis.

atlantooccipital (at-lan′-tō-ok-sip′-i-tal): Pertaining to the atlas and the occipital bone.

atlas: The first cervical vertebra which supports the head; so called because the Greek hero, Altas, was supposed to carry the earth on his shoulders. It articulates with the occipital bone above and the second cervical vertebra (axis) below.—atloid, adj.

atmosphere (at′-mos-fēr): See air.

atmospheric (at-mos-fēr′-ik): Pertaining to the atmosphere. **A. PRESSURE,** the pressure exerted by the weight of the atmosphere (in every direction); it is the sum of the pressures of oxygen, nitrogen, carbon dioxide, and other gases in proportion to their fractional concentration in the air; this amounts to approximately 15 pounds per square inch at sea level, and increases below that level and decreases above it; is also affected by humidity, moist air being lighter than dry air; also known as barometric pressure.

atocia (a-tō′-si-a): Sterility in the female.

atom (at′-om): In physics, the smallest particle of an element capable of existing individually and of taking part in a chemical reaction without losing its identity. In combination with one or more atoms of the same or another element, it makes up all the known kinds of matter. Has a dense central nucleus containing postively charged protons, which is surrounded by negatively charged electrons, equal in number to the nuclear protons, and which move in an orbit around the nucleus.—atomic, adj.

atomic (a-tom′-ik): Pertaining to an atom. **A. NUMBER,** the number of protons in the nucleus of an atom; it is the same for every atom of a given element, and each element has a characteristic number. **A. THEORY,** a theory that the basic unit of all types of matter is the atom. **A. WEIGHT,** the average weight of the atoms of an element compared with that of the atoms of carbon.

atomization (at-om-ī-zā′-shun): A mechanical process whereby a liquid is divided into a fine spray.—atomizer, n.

atomizer (at′-o-mīz-er): A device for converting a liquid into a spray and for throwing a jet of the spray.

atonia, atony (a-tō′-ni-a, at′-ō-ni): Lack of normal tone; refers particularly to muscles.

atonic (a-ton′-ic): Without tone; weak.—atonia, atony, atonicity, n.

atopens (at′-ō-pens): Soluble antigens which function as allergens; found as part of the total protein in many foods including milk, eggs, tomatoes, wheat.

atopic (a-top′-ik): 1. Pertaining to atopy (*q.v.*). 2. Out of place; displaced. **A. ALLERGY,** atopy (*q.v.*).

atopy (at′-op-i): Allergy which is hereditary. Term covers diseases such as hay fever, asthma, urticaria, and eczema where there is a clear family history of these conditions.—atopic, adj.

atoxic (a-toks′-ik): 1. Not poisonous. 2. Not caused by a poison.

atoxigenic (a-tok-si-jen′-ik): Not producing toxin(s).

ATP: Abbreviation for adenosine triphosphate.

atrachelous (a-trak′-e-lus): Having an abnormally small neck or no neck.

atraumatic (a-traw-mat′-ik): Not producing or inflicting damage or injury.

atremia (a-trē′-mi-a): 1. Absence of tremor. 2. An hysterical condition in which the patient is unable to walk although the movements of walking can be performed without discomfort while lying down.

atresia (a-trē′-zi-a): Imperforation or closure of a normal body opening or canal; often congenital. **A. ANI,** imperforate anus. **BILIARY A.,** closure of one or more of the bile ducts; results in jaundice, liver damage, splenomegaly. **CONGENITAL CHOANAL A.,** failure of the sides of the nose to communicate with each other. **DUODENAL A.,** congenital closure of the duodenum or absence of part of it; characterized by vomiting, distention of the epigastrium, symptoms of Down's syndrome. **ESOPHAGEAL A.,** congenital failure of the lumen of the esophagus to develop fully; characterized by persistent vomiting, dyspnea, cyanosis; often associated with a fistula between the esophagus and the trachea. **FOLLICULAR A.,** a normal process occurring in the ovarian follicle when the ovum dies and cyclic degeneration and scar formation occur. **INTESTINAL A.,** a congenital obstruction; may occur at any level, but usually in the ileum. **TRICUSPID A.,** a complex congenital anomaly in which the tricuspid valve fails to develop; the right ventricle and the pulmonary artery are underdeveloped, and there is usually an atrial and ventricular septal defect.

atretic (a-tret′-ik): Characterized by or pertaining to atresia.

atrial (ā′-tri-al): Pertaining to an atrium. **A. FIBRILLATION,** chaotic cardiac irregularity without any semblance of order; the fibers of the atria contract rapidly and convulsively, independently of each other and of the contraction of the ventricles; commonly associated with mitral stenosis and nodular toxic goiter, but also with other diseases of the heart; sometimes seen in general toxic conditions. **A. FLUTTER,** rapid regular cardiac rhythm caused by an irritable focus in the atrial muscle; usually associated with organic heart disease; speed of atrial beats may be between 200 and 400. **A. GALLOP,** extra presystolic sounds heard in the atrium just after atrial contraction and during diastole. **A. SEPTAL DEFECT,** continued patency of the foramen ovale (*q.v.*) after birth. **A. SEPTUM,** the muscular wall that separates the right and left upper chambers of the heart. **A. TACHYCARDIA,** the condition when the atrium has spasms of contracting more frequently than the ventricles; usually referred to as paroxysmal atrial tachycardia (PAT).

atrichia (a-trik′-i-a): Lack or loss of hair. Syn., atrichosis.—atrichous, adj.

atrioseptal (ā-tri-ō-sep′-tal): Pertaining to an atrium of the heart and the septum between the two atria.

atrioseptopexy (ā′-tri-ō-sep′-tō-pek-si): A surgical procedure for correction of an interatrial septal defect.

atrioventricular (ā′-tri-ō-ven-trik′-ū-lar): Pertaining to the atria and ventricles of the heart. Syn., auriculoventricular. **A. BLOCK,** the closing or stopping of the transmission of the circulatory impulse from the atrium to the ventricle through the A-V node. **A. BUNDLE,** see bundle of His. **A. DISSOCIATION,** refers to a condition in which the atria and ventricles beat independently, each in response to its own pacemaker. **A. NODE,** see under node. **A. VALVES,** the valves between the atria and ventricles of the heart; they control the flow of blood through the heart; see mitral and bicuspid.

atrium (ā′-tri-um): A chamber. In anatomy, refers to either of the upper two chambers of the heart; the right atrium collects venous blood from the vena cava and forces it into the right ventricle; the left atrium receives arterial blood from the pulmonary veins and forces it into the left ventricle.—atria, pl.; atrial, adj.

atrophy (at′-rō-fi): Wasting, emaciation, diminution in size and function of an organ or part that had previously reached mature size. May result from a pathological condition or a physiological cause such as aging or disuse.—atrophied, atrophic, adj. **ACUTE YELLOW A.,** massive necrosis of the liver associated with severe infection, toxemia of pregnancy, or ingested poisons. **HEMIFACIAL A.,** may be unilateral or bilateral and involve bones and cartilage as well as muscle; may be congenital or caused by a pathological process; see Romberg's disease. **MUSCULAR A.,** affects primarily the skeletal muscles, may result from interruption of nerve supply, disuse, or pathology of muscle tissue. **PROGRESSIVE MUSCULAR A.,** a chronic disease marked by progressive wasting of the muscles, beginning with those of the upper extremities. **SUDEK'S A.,** a syndrome occurring in a limb a few weeks after fracture, usually of the hand; the part becomes painful, the fingers stiff, warm, and shiny as the bones of the hand become rarefied.

atropine (at′-rō-pēn): A drug derived from the belladonna plant or produced synthetically; used in medicine as a smooth muscle relaxant, to increase the heart rate, and as a mydriatic; also used in treating parkinsonism and frequently given before anesthesia to decrease salivary and bronchial secretions.

ATS: Abbreviation for antitetanus serum. Contains tetanus antibodies. Produces artificial passive immunity. A test dose must be given first. Can cause anaphylaxis.

ATT: Abbreviation for antitetanus toxoid. Contains treated tetanus toxins. Produces artificial active immunity. Does not cause anaphylaxis.

attachment (a-tach′-ment): 1. Something that serves to attach one thing to another. 2. In anatomy, the place or the means by which one structure or body part is fixed to another. 3. Affection or fond regard. 4. In psychology, the attitude or feeling that develops in interpersonal relationships in critical periods of life when one individual is in a dependent situation to another, as occurs in bonding between an infant and its mother, an important experience in development of personality and in one's ability to adapt to the environment.

attendant: A nonprofessional person who performs many different kinds of services in assisting the professional nurse to care for the sick.

attention: The focusing of one's listening, seeing, and thinking on a certain person, thing, or idea to the exclusion of any nonpertinent stimuli. **A. SPAN,** the time interval during which one's attention is centered on a single person, object, idea, or situation.

attention deficit disorder: A fairly common childhood disorder; of two types—one with hyperactivity and one without hyperactivity. In the first type the child is inattentive to instruction, impulsive in action, and hyperactive in the schoolroom; at home the child is inattentive to instruction and unable to concentrate on any activity for any length of time. In type two the symptoms are much the same as in type one except that the child is not hyperactive. The symptoms of either type usually appear at about age 3 and may be associated with mild or moderate mental retardation, epilepsy, cerebral palsy, or other neurological disorders. A third type of attention disorder, the residual type, is usually seen in persons who earlier in life were classified as having an attention disorder with hyperactivity which they may no longer have; however, the symptoms of inattention, impulsivity of action, inability to organize work, and easy distractibility remain. Has also been referred to by several other names including minimal brain damage, minimal brain dysfunction syndrome, hyperkinetic child syndrome, and minimal cerebral dysfunction.

attenuate (a-ten′-ū-āt): To modify, change, or cause to lose virulence.

attenuation (a-ten-ū-ā′-shun): A bacteriological process by which organisms are rendered less virulent by exposure to an unfavorable environment such as drying, heating, or being passed through another organism. They can then be used in the preparation of vaccines.—attenuant, attenuated, adj.; attenuate. v.

attic (at′-ik): The upper part of the cavity of the middle ear.

atticotomy (at-i-kot′-o-mi): A surgical opening into the attic of the middle ear cavity.

attitude: 1. A settled mode of thinking. 2. Posture; position of the body or limbs, particularly a position assumed in illness or abnormal mental states such as catatonia (*q.v.*).

attraction: The force or influence existing mutually between particles or masses which causes them to be drawn toward each other. **CAPILLARY A.**, the force which causes a fluid to be drawn into and to rise in a tube of fine caliber.

attrition (a-trish′-un): 1. The process of eroding or abrading the skin or other body surface. 2. The normal wearing away of tissue or a structure by use.

atypical (ā-tip′-i-k'l): Not typical; unusual, irregular; not conforming to type, *e.g.*, **A.** pneumonia.

A.U.: Abbreviation for *aures unitas* [L.], meaning both ears, or for *auris uterque* [L.], meaning each ear.

Au, au: Chemical symbol for aurum [L.], meaning gold.

audile (aw′-dil): 1. Relating to hearing. 2. Denoting a person with a type of mental imagery which recalls auditory impressions more readily than visual or motor.

audio-, audito-: Combining forms denoting 1) sound; 2) hearing.

audioanalgesia (aw′-di-ō-an-al-jē′-zi-a): The abolition or control of pain by listening to specially recorded music.

audiofrequency (aw′-di-ō-frē′-kwen-si): Any frequency within the normal range of human hearing.

audiogenic (aw-di-ō-jen′-ik): Caused or produced by sound.

audiogram (aw′-di-ō-gram): A graph showing the variations in acuteness of hearing: utilizes a standardized test that determines the individual's hearing threshold at various frequencies and an audiometer.

audiologist (aw-di-ol′-ō-jist): One skilled in audiology and who specializes in treating persons with impaired hearing.

audiology (aw-di-ol′-o-ji): The science dealing with the evaluation and treatment of hearing impairment.—audiological, adj., audiologically, adv.

audiometer (aw-di-om′-e-ter): A delicate electrical instrument for measuring the sharpness and range of hearing for pure tones, speech, and bone and air conduction.

audiometry (aw-di-om′-e-tri): The testing and measuring of hearing acuity by use of an audiometer.

audiosurgery (aw′-di-ō-sur′-jer-i): Surgery on the ear.

audiovisual (aw′-di-ō-viz′-ū-al): Pertaining to both sight and sound; usually refers to communication or teaching techniques.

audit (aw′-dit): An examination of records or

accounts. In health care, a procedure for measuring the outcomes of care and the level of performance of care-giving personnel. See nursing audit.

audition (aw-dish'-un): 1. The act of hearing. 2. Perception of sound.

auditory (aw'-di-tō-ri): Pertaining to the sense or the organs of hearing. **A. AREA,** that portion of the temporal lobe cortex which interprets sound. **A. CANAL,** or **MEATUS,** the canal between the pinna and the ear drum; about 3 cm long, the outer part is made up of cartilage; the inner one-third has a bony wall and contains wax-secreting glands. **A. FATIGUE,** a temporary shift of one's sensitivity threshold for a certain sound following exposure to the sound for a period of time. **A. NERVES,** the eighth pair of cranial nerves; they relay information from the ear to the brain. **A. OSSICLES,** three tiny bones (malleus, incus, and stapes) stretching from the tympanum across the cavity of the middle ear to a membrane that separates the middle from the inner ear. **A. TUBE,** the canal that connects the pharynx with the tympanic cavity; it is partly bony, partly cartilaginous, and lined with mucous membrane. The eustachian tube.

Auerbach's plexus (ow'-er-bakh): A plexus of autonomic nerve fibers situated between the longitudinal and circular fibers of the muscular coat of the stomach and intestines; the myenteric plexus. [Leopold Auerbach, German neuropatholgist. 1828–1897.]

aur-, auri-: Combining forms denoting the ear.

aura (aw'-ra): A premonition; a peculiar sensation or warning, recognized by the patient, of an impending convulsion or seizure such as occurs in migraine and epilepsy. May be auditory, optic, kinesthetic, epigastric, etc. in nature.

aural (aw'-ral): 1. Pertaining to the ear. 2. Pertaining to an aura.

auricle (aw-ri-k'l): 1. The pinna or flap of the external ear. 2. An ear-shaped appendage to either cardiac atrium. 3. Formerly used to refer to the cardiac atrium.—auricular, adj.

auricular (aw-rik'-ū-lar): 1. Pertaining to the ear. 2. Pertaining to an auricle. **A. FIBRILLATION,** see atrial fibrillation, atrial flutter.

auriculectomy (aw-rik-ū-lek'-tō-mi): Amputation of the external structures of the ear; often the result of a knife fight.

auriculotemporal (aw-rik'-ū-lō-tem'-por-al): Pertaining to the ear and the temporal bone.

auriculoventricular: See atrioventricular.

auriculoventriculostomy (aw-rik'-ū-lō-ven-trik'-ū-los'-to-mi): A surgical procedure utilized in treatment of certain forms of hydrocephalus; consists of a polyethylene tube inserted into the lateral ventricle of the brain through a burr hole in the skull and which leads to the right atrium or the superior vena cava; the purpose is to drain excessive cerebrospinal fluid from the ventricle into the general circulation.

auripuncture (aw-ri-pungk'-tur): Puncture of the tympanic membrane (*q.v.*).

auris (aw'-ris): The ear.

auriscope: An instrument for examining the ear; a type of otoscope.

aurotherapy (aw-rō-ther'-a-pi): The use of gold salts in treatment of disease.

aurum (aw'-rum): Gold [L.].

auscultation (aws-kul-tā'-shun): A method of examining internal organs by listening to the sounds they produce; a diagnostic procedure used particularly in examining the heart, lung, pleura, and intestine, and the fetal circulation. It may be 1) immediate, by placing the ear directly against the body; or 2) mediate, by use of the stethoscope.—auscultatory, adj.; auscult, auscultate, v.

auscultatory (aws-kul'-ta-tō-ri): Of, or pertaining to, auscultation. **A. GAP,** a zone of silence sometimes noted when measuring blood pressure by the auscultatory method; occurs chiefly in patients with hypertension or in cases of aortic stenosis.

Austin-Flint murmur: A murmur heard at the apex of the heart in patients with aortic regurgitation into the left ventricle.

Australia antigen: Hepatitis B surface antigen; found in the serum of individuals with acute or chronic serum hepatitis, or in carriers of that disease; is easily transmitted by blood, needles, or other instruments; blood for transfusion is screened for this antigen.

autacoid (aw'-ta-koyd): See autocoid.

autemesia (aw-te-mē'-zi-a): Idiopathic or self-induced vomiting.

autism (aw'-tizm): 1. Schizophrenic syndrome in childhood; thought to be caused by a physical disorder of the brain; usually appears during first three years of life; marked by poor development of language and social skills and abnormal relationships to persons and the environment. 2. A state of morbid self-absorption in which one is dominated by self-centered thoughts that are wishful, symbolic, delusional, hallucinatory, or irrational; and by daydreaming, fantasizing, and detachment from reality, with excessive concentration on oneself.

autistic (aw-tis'-tik): Morbidly self-centered thinking, governed by the wishes of the individual; wishful thinking (phantasy), in contrast to reality thinking. Occurs in schizophrenia (*q.v.*). **A. BEHAVIOR,** self-absorption, refusal to use language or to speak, isolation of self from others, repetitive actions; inability to relate realistically with people in one's environment. **A. LANGUAGE,** sounds invented by a person to express meanings but which are unintelligible to others.

auto-: Combining form denoting relationship to self.

autoagglutination (aw′-tō-a-gloo-ti-nā′-shun): Agglutination of an individual's red blood corpuscles by a factor in his own serum, in the absence of a specific antibody.

autoagglutinin (aw′-tō-a-gloo′-ti-nin): A factor in the blood serum that causes a clumping together of an individual's own cells.

autoamputation (aw′-tō-am-pū-tā′-shun): 1. The spontaneous loss from the body of a finger or appendage, or of an abnormal growth such as a polyp. 2. The resorption or shortening that occurs in fingers in long-standing scleroderma.

autoanalysis (aw′-tō-a-nal′-a-sis): A psychotherapeutic method wherein the individual analyzes his own mental disorder.

autoantibody (aw′-tō-an′-ti-bod-i): An antibody formed in an individual and which reacts against other antigenic substances in the same individual.

autoantigen (aw′-tō-an′-ti-jen): A normal tissue constituent within the body that is capable of stimulating the production of antibody in the tissues of the individual in which it occurs.

autoantitoxin (aw′-tō-an-tī-tok′-sin): An antitoxin produced by the body itself.

autochthonous (aw-tok′-thō-nus): Being present in the place in which it was formed; refers usually to the graft of an individual's own tissue to another part of his body.

autocide (aw′-tō-sīd): A purposely caused death, as occurs when one kills oneself by intentionally causing a lethal accident, typically in a vehicle.

autoclasis (aw-tok′-la-sis): Destruction of a part due to influences within itself.

autoclave (aw′-tō-klāv): 1. An apparatus for sterilizing articles by steam under high pressure. 2. To sterilize articles in an autoclave.

autocoid (aw′-tō-koyd): In biochemistry, any organic substance such as a hormone that is secreted into the blood stream directly and carried by the blood or lymph to the part of the body where its primary action takes place.

autodigestion (aw′-tō-di-jest′-chun): Self-digestion of body tissues by their own secretions. Autolysis (*q.v.*).

autoecholalia (aw′-tō-ek-ō-lā′-li-a): Constant repetition of one's own words or phrases; seen in certain neuropathologic states.

autoechopraxia (aw′-tō-ek-ō-prak′-shi-a): The continual repetition of some action the individual has previously performed.

autoepilation (aw′-tō-ep-i-lā′-shun): The spontaneous loss of hair.

autoeroticism (aw′-tō-e-rot′-i-sizm): Sensual arousal and self-gratification of sexual desire obtained by manipulation of or looking at or touching one's genitalia or other erotic zones, masturbation, or fantasy. Often a characteristic of the period of early emotional development of the child but not limited to this age group.

autogenesis (aw′-tō-jen′-e-sis): Originating within the organism; spontaneous generation.

autogenous (aw-toj′-e-nus): Self-generated; endogenous; originating within the body and not acquired from any outside source. Applied to bone graft, skin graft, etc. **A. VACCINE,** one prepared from the bacteria from the patient's own infection. Also autogenetic, autogenic.

autograft (aw′-tō-graft): A graft in which the tissue is taken from another part of the body which is to receive it.

autohemolysis (aw-tō-hē-mol′-i-sis): Destruction of an individual's red blood cells by a factor in the person's own serum.

autohemotherapy (aw′-tō-hē-mō-ther′-a-pi): The treatment of a person with his own blood which is withdrawn from a vein and reinjected intramuscularly; may be used in cases of recurring urticaria.

autohypnosis (aw-tō-hip-nō′-sis): A state of hypnosis that is self-induced.

autoimmune (aw-tō-im-mūn′): Refers to a disease condition in which the body produces an immunological reaction to its own cells or tissues; includes such diseases as rheumatoid arthritis, myasthenia gravis, lupus erythematosus, hemolytic anemia.

autoimmunity (aw′-tō-im-mū′-ni-ti): The condition of being allergic to one's own tissues.

autoimmunization (aw′tō-im-mū-nī-zā′-shun): Immunization obtained by having an attack of a disease or by processes occuring naturally in the body.

autoinfection (aw-tō-in-fek′-shun): Infection arising from an organism already present within the body or transferred from one part of the body to another by fingers, etc.; self-infection.

autoinoculation (aw′-tō-i-nok-ū-lā′-shun): 1. Inoculation with an organism present in another site in the body; the spread of an infection in the body. 2. Inoculation of an individual with a vaccine prepared from microorganisms from his own body.

autointoxication (aw′-tō-in-tok-si-kā′-shun): Poisoning from faulty metabolic products elaborated within the body, or from some uneliminated toxin generated within the body.

autokinesis (aw-tō-kī-nē′-sis): Voluntary movement.—autokinetic, adj.

autolesion (aw-tō-lē′-zhun): A lesion resulting from an injury or wound that is self-inflicted.

autologous (aw-tol′-ō-gus): 1. Belonging to or part of the same organism; related to self. 2. Derived from the subject itself.

autolysin (aw-tol′-i-sin): A lysin that originates within an organism and is capable of destroying its own tissues and parts.

autolysis (aw-tol′-i-sis): The destruction of tissues or cells by the action of their own digestive enzymes.—autolytic, adj.

automatic (aw-tō-mat′-ik): That which is performed independently of the will; self-regulating; involuntary; spontaneous. **A. BLADDER,** see autonomous bladder.

automaticity (aw-tom-a-tis′-i-ti): The state or condition of being automatic.

automatism (aw-tom′-a-tizm): The involuntary performance of actions that are normally voluntary, without purpose or intention on the part of the individual, and often without the knowledge that they are taking place. May occur in somnambulism, hysteria, and post-epileptic states.

automaton (aw-tom′-a-ton): 1. An apparatus that automatically follows programmed instructions; a robot. 2. Anything that moves or acts of itself. 3. A person who acts or reacts in a predictable or mechanical manner.

automysophobia (aw′-tō-mis-ō-fō′-bi-a): A manic dread of personal uncleanliness.

autonomic (aw-to-nom′-ik): Independent; involuntary; automatic. **A. NERVOUS SYSTEM,** see under nervous system. **A. SPEECH,** see under speech.

autonomous (aw-ton′-o-mus): Independent; self-governing; developing and functioning independently. **A. BLADDER,** see under bladder.

autonomy (aw-ton′-o-mi): Having the ability to function without control by others. In nursing, refers to the amount of discretionary control the nurse has over her performance of nursing actions in the course of professional practice.

autopathy (aw-top′-a-thi): A disease that has no observable external causation; an idiopathic condition.

autopepsia (aw-tō-pep′-si-a): The destruction of the stomach wall by the action of the gastric secretion; autodigestion.

autophagia (aw-tō-fā′-ji-a): The biting of one's own flesh; occurs sometimes in persons with dementia.

autophilia (aw-tō-fil′-i-a): Narcissism; self-love to a pathological degree.

autophobia (aw-tō-fō′-bi-a): Morbid fear of one's self or of being alone.

autoplasty (aw′tō-plas-ti): Replacement or repair of injured or diseased tissues by a graft of healthy tissues from another area of the same body.—autoplastic, adj.; autoplast, n.

autopsy (aw′-top-si): The examination of the organs of a dead body for the purpose of determining the cause of death or of studying the pathological conditions of the organs—Syn., postmortem examination; necropsy. **PSYCHOLOGICAL A.;** in suicidology, a retrospective study of a patient's life after his death.

autoregulation (aw′-tō-reg-ū-lā′-shun): 1. The action of inherent factors and inhibitory feedback systems to largely or completely counteract internal or external changes and stresses; said especially of the circulatory physiology. 2. The tendency of blood flow to an organ or part to remain at or return to the same level regardless of changes in the artery conveying blood to it.

autorrhaphy (aw-tor′-a-fi): The closure of a wound by utilizing the tissues from the area of the wound.

autosensitization (aw′-tō-sen-si-ti-za′-shun): Sensitization to one's own serum or body tissues.—autosensitize, v.

autosepticemia (aw′-tō-sep-ti-sē′-mi-a): Septicemia from a poison that develops within the body and not introduced from the outside.

autoserous (aw-tō-sē′-rus): Pertaining to autoserum. **A. TREATMENT,** treatment by inoculation of an individual with serum obtained from his own blood.

autoserum (aw-tō-sē′-rum): Serum to be administered to the individual from whose blood it was derived.

autosomal (aw-tō-sō′-mal): Pertaining to an autosome. **A. DOMINANT INHERITANCE** (or disease), an inherited disease which affects only one of the parents of the person having it; affects either sex; less serious than recessive inherited disease. **A. RECESSIVE INHERITANCE,** affected individuals tend to be in the same generation; normal parents are the carriers; rare but more severe than dominantly inherited conditions.

autosome (aw′-tō-sōm): One of the ordinary chromosomes, that is, any chromosome other than the X or Y; autosomes are equally distributed among the germ cells.—autosomal, adj.

autosplenectomy (aw′-tō-splē-nek′-tō-mi): A pathologic condition in which the tissues of the spleen shrink and are replaced by fibrous tissue; occurs in sickle cell anemia.

autosuggestion (aw′-tō-sug-jest′-yun): 1. Self-suggestion; uncritical acceptance of ideas arising in the individual's own mind. Occurs in hysteria. 2. The technique of trying to improve health or change behavior by constant repetition of certain phrases; *e.g.*, "Every day in every way I am getting better and better."

autotherapy (aw-tō-ther′-a-pi): 1. Treatment by administration of filtrates of the patient's own secretions. 2. Cure of disease without medical supervision; self-cure.

autotopagnosia (aw′-tō-tōp-ag-nō′-si-a): Loss of the ability to identify the various parts of one's own body; a type of agnosia (*q.v.*).

autotoxicosis (aw′-tō-tok-si-kō′-sis): Autointoxication (*q.v.*).

autotransfusion (aw′-tō-trans-fū′-zhun): 1. The infusion into the patient of the actual blood lost by hemorrhage. 2. Binding the lower extremities and, sometimes, the lower abdomen, to force blood from them to the vital organs.

autotransplantation (aw′-tō-trans-plan-ta′-shun): The surgical procedure of transplanting a graft of tissue from one part of the body to another site on the same person.

autovaccine (aw-tō-vak′-sēn): Autogenous vaccine. See under autogenous.

aux-, auxe-, auxo-: Combining forms denoting 1) growth, enlargement; 2) accelerating, stimulating.

auxesis (awk-sē′-sis): An increase in size or bulk due to growth or expansion of the cells rather than an increase in their numbers.

auxotherapy (awk-sō-ther′-a-pi): Substitution therapy; *e.g.*, organotherapy or hormonotherapy (*q.v.*).

A-V: Abbreviation for atrioventricular or atriovenous. **A-V BLOCK,** a type of heart block in which the impulse between the atria and the ventricles of the heart is either slowed down or blocked.

A-V dissociation: Independent action of the atria and ventricles; a form of heart block.

avascular (a-vas′-kū-lar): Bloodless; not vascular; *i.e.*, without blood vessels. May be normal, as in cartilaginous tissue, or pathological. **A. NECROSIS,** death of tissue from deficient blood supply following injury or disease. It is often a precursor of osteoarthritis.

avascularization (a-vas′-kū-lar-ī-zā′-shun): The act of expelling blood from a part as by application of elastic bandage, by posture, or by ligation.

aversion (a-ver′-zhun): A method of treatment by deconditioning. Effective in some forms of addiction or other abnormal behavior. **A. THERAPY,** involves the use of punishment or unpleasant stimuli to weaken and ultimately eliminate the particular behavior or habit that is unacceptable; also called negative reinforcement and aversive conditioning.

Avery's syndrome: Transient tachypnea of the newborn, with grunting; sometimes seen in full-term infants; usually resolves within two days; may represent a mild form of respiratory distress syndrome.

avian (ā′-vi-an): Pertaining to birds. **A. TUBERCLE BACILLUS,** resembles other types of tubercle bacilli but attacks primarily birds including chickens and ducks; occasionally causes disease in man.

aviation medicine: The branch of medicine that is concerned chiefly with physiological, pathological, and emotional conditions or disturbances resulting from travel in an airplane. Also deals with the problems of transporting the sick and wounded by air.

aviation physiology: That branch of physiology that is concerned with physiological changes that occur during various activities at high altitudes; *e.g.*, flying in an airplane or space vehicle, or mountain climbing.

aviator's disease: A condition marked by headache, drowsiness, vasomotor and other disturbances sometimes seen in aviators.

aviator's ear: Aero-otitis media (*q.v.*).

avidin (av′-i-din): An antivitamin; a specific protein found in raw egg-white. It interferes with the absorption of biotin (*q.v.*), thus producing biotin deficiency.

avirulent (a-vir′-ū-lent): Without virulence (*q.v.*).

avitaminosis (a-vī′-ta-min-ō′-sis): Any disease resulting from a deficiency of one or more essential vitamins in the diet; includes such disease conditions as scurvy, beri-beri, and rickets.

Avogadro's law: Under the same conditions equal volumes of gases contain the same number of molecules.

avoirdupois (av′-er-dū-poy′): The English system of weights and measures.

avulsion (a-vul′-shun): A forcible wrenching or tearing away of a body part or structure; surgical repair is often possible and, if the avulsion is complete, certain body parts may be successfully rejoined.

A & W: Abbreviation for alive and well.

awareness (a-war′-nes): Consciousness. Being awake, conscious, and cognizant of one's self and one's surroundings.

axial (ak′-si-al): In anatomy, pertaining to the axis of a body part or structure. **A. TOMOGRAPHY,** a type of radiology in which a series of cross-sectional images along an axis are combined to make a three-dimentional scan. See computerized axial tomography.

axilla (ak-sil′-a): The armpit.—axillae, pl.; axillary, adj.

axillary (aks′-i-lar-i): Pertaining to the axilla. Term is applied to nerves, blood vessels, lymphatics, nodes.

axion (ak′-sē-on): The brain and spinal cord.

axis (ak′-sis): 1. The second cervical vertebra. 2. An imaginary line passing through the center of a structure, *e.g.*, the median line of the body. **A. CYLINDER,** the axon of a cell.—axes, pl.; axial, adj.

axodendritic (ak′-sō-den-drit′-ik): Pertaining to an axon and to dendrites. **A. SYNAPSE,** a synapse between two neurons wherein the fibers of the axon of one neuron are in direct contact with the dendrites of another neuron.

axon (ak′-son): That process of a nerve cell conveying impulses away from the cell body and toward the next nerve; the essential part of the nerve fiber and a direct prolongation of the nerve cell. Also called axis-cylinder, axis-cylinder process, neuraxon, neurite.—axonal, adj.

axoneuron (ak-sō-nū′-ron): A nerve cell of the central nervous system.

axonotmesis (ak-son-ot-mē′-sis): Peripheral degeneration as a result of damage to the axon of a nerve. The internal architecture is preserved and recovery depends upon regeneration of the axon, and may take many months (about an inch a month is the usual speed of regeneration). Such a lesion may result from pinching, crushing, or prolonged pressure on a nerve without severing it.

axoplasm (aks′-ō-plazm): The cytoplasm of an axon.—axoplasmic, adj.

azo-: Prefix indicating the presence of nitrogen in a substance.

azoospermia (a-zō-ō-sperm′-i-a): Sterility in the male through absence of motile spermatozoa in the semen.

azotemia (az-ō-tē′-mi-a): The presence of pathological amounts of nitrogenous products, principally urea, in the blood. Seen in such conditions as circulatory or renal failure, gastrointestinal hemorrhage, dehydration. Often used synonymously with uremia.—azotemic, adj.

azotenesis (az-ō-te-nē′-sis): Disease or disorder due to an excess of nitrogen products in the blood.

azotometer (az-ō-tom′-e-ter): An instrument used to measure the amount of nitrogen compounds in a solution, particularly the amount of urea in urine.

azotorrhea (az-ō-tō-rē′-a): A condition in which large amounts of nitrogen are eliminated in the stools.

azoturia (az-ō-tū′-ri-a): The presence of excessive amounts of urea or other nitrogenous products in the urine.—azoturic, adj.

azygos, azygous (az′-i-gus): Occurring singly; unpaired, as the **A.** vein.

azymia (a-zim′-i-a): Absence of an enzyme(s).

B

B: 1. Chemical symbol for boron. 2. Abbreviation for a) bacillus; b) base.

B cell: A lymphocyte that originates in the bone marrow; a precursor of the plasma cell, and one of two types of lymphocytes that have important roles in the body's immunologic response.

B lymphocyte (limf′-ō-sīt): A lymphocyte (*q.v.*) that originates in the bone marrow; has antigenic properties; when stimulated by an antigen it differentiates into a plasma cell and produces circulating antibody.

β: beta. For words beginning thus, see under the specific term.

Ba: The chemical symbol for barium.

Babcock sentence test: A test for dementia in which the patient is asked to repeat a complicated sentence.

Babesia (ba-bē′-zē-a): A genus of Sporozoa found in the red blood cells of various animals; may be transmitted to man by ticks.

babesiasis (ba-bē-sī′-a-sis): A malaria-like disease caused by the protozoan parasite *Babesia* which is widely distributed in nature, and is transmitted to man by the bite of an infected wood tick; rodents and other animals harbor the parasite in their red blood cells. Symptoms include nausea and vomiting, fever, sweating, chills, myalgia, arthralgia, hemolytic anemia. Most cases in the U.S. have occurred in Martha's Vineyard and Nantucket, off the Massachusetts coast, and Shelter Island, off the New York coast. There is no known cure; the disease is apparently self-limited. Also called babesiosis.

Babinski (ba-bin′-ski): **B'S. REFLEX**, see under reflex. **B'S. SIGN**, a diminishment or loss of the Achilles tendon reflex, as occurs in sciatica. [Joseph Francois Felix Babinski, French neurologist. 1857–1932.]

baby: An infant from birth to about two years of age or until the child is able to walk and talk. **BABY BATTERING**, term sometimes used to describe child abuse when the victim is under two years of age; includes such abuses as throwing, banging, or violently shaking the infant which may cause bleeding in and around the brain and lead to mental retardation. **BABY BLUES**, colloquial term for transient mild depression occurring after childbirth.

baccalaureate degree nurse (bak-a-law′-rē-at): A nurse who holds a bachelor's degree in nursing from an accredited college or university.

baccalaureate programs in nursing: Beginning in 1909, baccalaureate programs, which are college or university based and grant a bachelor's degree in nursing, have grown steadily. Usually four years in length, these programs offer courses in the liberal arts during the first two years particularly. They prepare students for professional nursing.

baccate (bak′-āt): Resembling a berry in form or structure.

Bacillaceae (bas-i-lā′-sē-ē): A large family of spore-forming organisms commonly found in soil. Most are harmless to man but a few cause serious infections, *e.g., Bacillus anthracis* (anthrax), *Clostridium tetani* (tetanus), *Clostridium welchii* (gas gangrene).

bacillary (bas′-i-lar-i): 1. Pertaining to bacilli. 2. Having a rod-like structure. **B. DYSENTERY**, a severe form of enteritis marked by abdominal pain, fever, severe diarrhea, sometimes bloody stools. Caused by a bacteria of the *Shigella* genus. Especially prevalent in tropical climates. Also called shigellosis.

bacillemia (bas-i-lē′-mi-a): The presence of bacilli in the blood.—basillemic, adj.

bacillicide (ba-sil′-i-sīd): An agent that destroys bacilli.

bacilliform (ba-sil′-i-form): Shaped like a bacillus; rod-shaped.

bacillosis (bas-i-lō′-sis): A general infection caused by bacilli.

bacilluria (bas-i-lū′-ri-a): The presence of bacilli in the urine.—bacilluric, adj.

Bacillus (ba-sil′-us): A term now restricted to a genus of rod-shaped microorganisms of the family *Bacillaceae* (*q.v.*), consisting of aerobic, gram-positive, spore-producing organisms; the majority are saprophytic and nonpathogenic; their spores are commonly only found in soil and dust. **B. ANTHRACIS**, the cause of anthrax in man and animals. **B. CEREUS**, an aerobic bacillus, often causes food poisoning. **B. SUBTILIS**, a common organism in soil and water; occurs frequently as a laboratory contaminant and occasionally it causes disease in man.

bacillus (ba-sil′-us): 1. An organism of the class Schizomycetes. 2. A general term loosely employed to designate any rod-shaped microorganism.—bacilli, pl.; bacillary, adj.

bacillus Calmette-Guérin: A vaccine prepared from bovine tubercle bacilli; intended for use in producing active immunity to tuberculosis in children and young adults. Originally given by mouth, now subcutaneously. Abbreviated BCG.

back: In anatomy, refers to the posterior part of the body from the neck to the pelvis. **FLAT B.**, a **B.** that appears flat because of a reduction in the normal thoracic and lumbar curves. **HOLLOW BACK,** lordosis (*q.v.*) that extends to part or all of the lumbar spine. **HUMP BACK,** kyphosis (*q.v.*); also called hunchback. **POKER BACK,** rigidity of the spine caused by ankylosis commonly associated with rheumatoid arthritis; also called poker spine and bamboo spine. **SWAY BACK,** lordosis (*q.v.*), that extends to all or part of the spine.

back blows: Descriptive of a maneuver used as one of the first steps in relieving airway obstruction in an unconscious patient; several sharp blows in an upward motion are administered with the palm of the hand to the spinal area between the shoulders; if the patient is supine he is rolled to his side toward the nurse and the arm toward the nurse is elevated. An infant may be held face down on the nurse's lap for administration of the back blows.

back rest: A device used to support a bed patient in a semi-reclining or sitting position.

backache (bak′-āk): Any pain in the back, especially the lower back.

backbone: The spinal or vertebral column.

backflow: The flowing of a current or substance in a direction opposite to that it usually takes, *e.g.,* regurgitation.

bacteremia (bak-ter-ē′-mi-a): The presence of bacteria in the bloodstream. May be primary, or secondary when it is associated with the use of an intravascular device or when it develops as a nosocomial infection in a hospitalized patient.—bacteremic, adj.

bacteri-, bacterio-: Combining forms denoting bacteria.

bacteria (bac-tēr′-i-a): One-celled, plant-like microorganisms, visible only under the microscope. A great many varieties are found in man's environment; the majority are not disease producing. **B.** are recognized according to shape, growth needs, staining reactions, and loci of infection in the body. Structurally, there is a protoplast containing cytoplasmic and nuclear material (not seen by ordinary methods of microscopy) within a limiting cytoplasmic membrane, and a supporting cell wall. Other structures such as flagella, fimbriae and capsules may also be present. Individual cells may be spherical (cocci), straight or curved rods (bacilli), or spiral (spirilla); they may form chains or masses, and some show branching with mycelium (*q.v.*) formation. They may produce various pigments including chlorophyll. Reproduction is chiefly by simple binary (*q.v.*) fission. Some live on dead organic matter and so are saprophytes; others live in living tissue and so are parasites. Each variety has its own requirements as to nourishment, light, moisture, pH, etc. Some are pathogenic to man and animals; some cause plant diseases.—bacterium, sing.; bacterial, adj.

bacterial (bak-tēr′-i-al): Pertaining to or caused by bacteria. **B. ENDOCARDITIS,** see endocarditis. **B. RESISTANCE,** the resistance which some organisms, particularly pathogenic organisms, develop for a drug to which they were originally susceptible.

bactericide (bak-tēr′-i-sīd): Any agent that destroys bacteria.—bactericidal, adj.; bactericidally, adv.

bacterid (bac′-ter-id): A skin condition characterized by a recurring or persistent eruption of lesions, particularly on the palms and soles; thought to be due to sensitivity to the bacterial products from an infection elsewhere in the body.

bacteriofluorescein (bak-tē′-ri-ō-floo-ō-res′-ē-in): A fluorescent material produced by certain bacteria.

bacteriogenic (bak-tēr′-i-ō-jen′-ik): 1. Caused by bacteria. 2. Relating to bacteria.

bacterioid (bak-tēr′-i-oyd): Resembling bacteria.

bacteriologist (bak-tēr-i-ol′-ō-jist): One who studies and is expert in the science of bacteriology.

bacteriology (bak-tēr-i-ol′-ō-ji): The science and study of bacteria.—bacteriologically, adv.

bacteriolysin (bak-tēr-i-ol′-i-sin): A specific antibody (*q.v.*) produced in the blood after an infection with an organism and which is capable of destroying the invading organism by lysis.—bacteriolytic, adj.

bacteriolysis (bak-tēr-i-ol′-i-sis): The disintegration and dissolution of bacteria.—bacteriolytic, adj.

bacteriopathology (bak-tēr′-i-ō-path-ol′-o-ji): The study of the bacterial cause of disease.

bacteriophage (bak-tēr′-i-ō-fāj): A filterable virus that destroys bacteria; usually each of several varieties acts against only one specific type of bacteria.

bacteriophagia (bak-ter′-i-ō-fā′-ji-a): The destruction of bacteria by a bacteriophage.

bacteriophobia (bak-tēr′-i-ō-fō′-bi-a): Morbid fear of bacteria or disease-producing organisms.

bacterioprotein (bak-tēr′-i-ō-prō′-tē-in): Any of several protein substances contained in bacteria.

bacteriosis (bak-tēr-i-ō′-sis): Any disease caused by bacteria.

bacteriostasis (bak-tēr′-i-ō-stā′-sis): The prevention or hindrance of bacterial growth and/or multiplication.

bacteriostat (bak-tēr′-i-ō-stat): An agent that prevents or inhibits the growth of bacteria.—bacteriostatic, adj.

bacteriotherapy (bak-tēr′-i-ō-ther′-a-pi): Treatment of disease by introduction of disease into the bloodstream.

bacteriotoxemia (bak-tēr′-i-ō-tok-sē′-mi-a): The presence of bacterial toxins in the circulating blood.

bacteriotoxin (bak-tēr′-i-ō-tok′-sin): A toxin that is produced by bacteria or one that is toxic to bacteria.

bacterium (bak-tēr′-i-um): Singular of bacteria (*q.v.*).

bacteriuria (bak-tēr-i-ū′-ri-a): The presence of bacteria in the urine. Also bacteruria.—bacteriuric, adj.

Bacteroides (bak′-ter-oy′-dēz): A genus of non-sporeforming anaerobic bacteria normally present in the mouth and large intestine. **B. FRAGILIS,** the most common and most virulent **B.**, found in septicemia, appendicitis, and metastatic abscesses of the lung, liver, and pelvis; also called Bacillus fragilis. **B. MELANINOGENESIS,** found in abdominal wounds, kidney infections, puerperal sepsis.

bactometer (bak-tom′-e-ter): A laboratory device for detecting the density and growth of bacteria in urine specimens.

bag: A pouch or sac. **B. OF WATERS,** the membranous sac that contains the amniotic fluid and the fetus. **COLOSTOMY B.**, one worn over the stoma after a colostomy. In obstetrics, a silk or rubber **B.** that is inserted into the uterine cavity and then inflated to induce labor or dilate the cervix; common types are Barnes and Voorhees. See also Ambu bag, Barnes' bag, and Politzer bag.

bag of waters: The amnion and amniotic fluid. See amnion.

bagassosis (bag-a-sō′-sis): A respiratory disorder caused by inhalation of bagasse, the residue that remains after the extraction of sugar from sugar cane and which is used in the manufacture of paper, wallboard and similar products. Symptoms include fever, malaise, anorexia, chills, sweating, dyspnea, and features of bronchopneumonia.

bagging: A relatively easy method of providing positive pressure during suctioning and intermittent sighing; apparatus consists of a Huested valve and an attached bag which is squeezed to deliver air to the lungs.

bahnungstherapie (bah-nungs-ther′-a-pi): A German term for a type of therapy involving repetitive movements which may be passive in the beginning, until a muscle or muscles that have been affected by hemiplegia have regained at least part of their ability to respond to volitional control.

Baker's cyst: A cyst in the popliteal space; formed of synovial fluid that has escaped from the bursa; usually secondary to some other disease; symptoms include pain, swelling, limitation of movement.

baker's itch: Contact dermatitis (*q.v.*) resulting from handling sugar or flour; probably an allergic reaction.

baking soda: Sodium bicarbonate; see under sodium.

BAL: British anti-lewisite. A heavy metal antagonist used in treatment of certain metal poisonings, *e.g.*, arsenic, gold, or mercury poisoning. Also called dimercaprol.

balance (bal′-ans): In physiology, the harmonious relation between the parts and organs of the body and their functions, or between substances in the body. **ACID-BASE B.**, a normal equilibrium or ratio between the acid and base elements of the blood and body fluids, expressed as pH. **ELECTROLYTE B.**, is associated with water **B.**, since the electrolytes are the ions present in body water; term refers to the concentration of ions of electrolytes in the interstitial fluid and the blood plasma which are normally essentially the same. **FLUID B.**, term commonly used to express the concept of both water balance and electrolyte balance in the body. **NITROGEN B.**, balance between the intake and output of nitrogen; *negative nitrogen balance* occurs when more nitrogen is lost than is taken into the body; may happen in such conditions as burns, starvation, fevers, malnutrition. *Positive nitrogen b.* occurs when more nitrogen is taken into than is lost from the body; happens in pregnancy, repair of tissues, and during growth of infants and children. **WATER B.**, 1) the condition in which water intake equals water excreted; or 2) the proper distribution of water between the intercellular and extracellular compartments of the body.

balani-, balano-: Combining forms denoting relationship to the glans penis or glans clitoridis. See glans.

balanic (bal-an′-ik): Pertaining to the glans penis or glans clitoridis.

balanitis (bal-a-nī′-tis): Inflammation of the glans penis, often associated with phimosis. **B. GANGRENOSA,** destruction of part or all of the male external genitalia by infection thought to be due to a spirochete. **B. XEROTICA OBLITERANS,** inflammation of the glans penis with scarring and white induration; the meatus may be stenosed; often occurs in men with diabetes.—balanitic, adj.

balanoblennorrhea (bal′-a-nō-blen-ō-rē′-a): Gonorrheal inflammation of the external surface of the glans penis.

balanoplasty (bal′-a-nō-plas-ti): Plastic surgery of the glans penis.

balanoposthitis (bal′-an-ō-pos-thī′-tis): Inflammation of the glans penis and prepuce.

balanorrhea (bal-a-nō-rē′-a): Purulent or gonorrheal balanitis with copious discharge of pus.

balantidiasis (bal′-an-ti-dī′-a-sis): A disease caused by infection by the *Balantidium coli* organism; symptoms vary from those of mild colitis to acute dysentery and include nausea, vomiting, diarrhea, headache, fever, weakness, abdominal pain, weight loss and, sometimes, ulceration of the colon.

Balantidium (bal-an-tid′-i-um): A genus of ciliated protozoa including species found in the intestine of some animals and man. **B. COLI,** commonly found in hogs and transmittable to man causing a condition characterized by diarrhea and sometimes ulceration of the intestine.

balanus (bal′-an-us): The glans of the penis or clitoris.

baldness: Partial or complete lack of hair on the scalp. See alopecia.

Balkan frame: A frame, usually made of wood or iron pipes, fitted over a bed and to which weights and pulleys are attached; used to suspend immobilized fractured limbs and provide for continuous traction.

ball squeezing: An exercise for strengthening hand and arm muscles; a rubber ball or wad of crumpled newspaper is held in the hand and squeezed at a regular rate several times a day.

Ballance's sign: The presence of a dull sound heard on percussing the right flank when the patient lies on the left side; said to indicate a ruptured spleen.

ball-and-socket joint: A joint in which the round head of one bone fits into a cup-like cavity of another bone permitting full freedom of movement or circumduction (*q.v.*), *e.g.*, the shoulder or hip joint.

ballismus (ba-liz′-mus): The occurrence of violent, quick, jerking, or twisting movements, caused by contraction of arm or leg muscles and seen in Sydenham's chorea. May be bilateral; when it occurs in only one side it is called hemiballism. Also ballism.

ballistocardiograph (ba-lis′-tō-kar′-di-ō-graf): An apparatus for estimating the volume of cardiac output by recording the movement of the body resulting from the contraction of the ventricles and ejection of blood into the aorta. The record of this movement is called a ballistocardiogram.

ballistophobia (ba-lis-tō-fō′-bi-a): Morbid fear of missiles.

balloon or balloon-tip catheter: See Foley catheter under catheter.

ballooning (ba-loon′-ing): Distending a body cavity by the introduction of air or other agent to facilitate its examination or for therapeutic purposes.

ballottement (ba-lot′-ment): 1. Palpation to detect a floating enlarged organ when abdominal ascites is present. 2. Testing for a floating object, especially used to diagnose pregnancy after the sixteenth week and before the twenty-eighth week. A finger is inserted into the vagina and the uterus is pushed forward; if a fetus is present it will fall back, bouncing in its bath of fluid. **RENAL B.,** palpation of the kidney by pushing it suddenly and firmly forward from the back with one hand while the other hand is pressed firmly into the abdominal wall.—ballottable, adj.

balm (bahm): A healing or soothing medication, usually an ointment. Syn., balsam (*q.v.*).

balneary (bal′nē-a-ri): A place where therapeutic baths are given.

balneology (bal-nē-ol′ō-ji): The science of therapeutic baths and bathing.

balneotherapy (bal′-nē-ō-ther′-ap-i): The treatment of disease by the use of baths, *e.g.*, hot, cold, or salt water baths. Also balneotherapeutics.

balneum (bal′nē-um): A bath. See bath.

balsam (bawl′-sam): A pharmaceutical preparation containing resinous substances; used topically for its healing and soothing qualities. **B. OF PERU,** a dark brown viscid substance containing benzoin; used topically in ointment form as a skin protectant and rubefacient. Also called peruvian balsam. **B. OF TOLU,** a yellowish to brown substance obtained from the seeds and fruit of certain legumes; used in pharmaceutical preparations as a stimulant or expectorant; it is an ingredient of tincture of benzoin.

band cells: See under cell.

band keratopathy (ker-a-top′-a-thi): The deposition of calcium salts in the cornea and conjunctiva forming grayish opacities in crescent shapes; they cause itching, irritation, and "red eye."

bandage (ban′-dij): A piece of cloth or other material, of varying size and shape, applied to some part of the body to hold a dressing or splint in place; to support, compress or immobilize a part; prevent or correct a deformity; or to aid in the arrest of hemorrhage. Depending on its purpose and the part to which it is applied, **B.'S** are made of gauze, muslin, flannel, elastic webbing, rubber, adhesive plaster or moleskin, paper, cohesive material which adheres to itself but not to any other substance, and wide-mesh material impregnated with such substances as plaster of Paris, waterglass, chalk, dextrin, starch, etc., which harden or solidify after application. Shapes of bandages are: **ROLLER,** a continuous strip of material of varying length and width, which has been tightly wound; **TRIANGULAR,** half of a piece of material 36 to 40 inches square; **CRAVAT,** a triangular **B.** folded upon itself several times until the desired width is obtained; **TAILED,** made of several strips of material which are joined to each other only in the middle third; **HANDKERCHIEF,** a large square of material, sometimes with ties to hold it in place. Bandages are also classified according to the way they are applied: **CIRCULAR,** applied in several circular turns about a part; **OBLIQUE,** several slanting turns about a part, but the turns do not overlap; **SPIRAL,** several turns about a part, each one higher on the part than the previous one and overlapping it by about two-thirds; **SPIRAL REVERSE,** a spiral **B.** in which the roll of material is given a half-twist at each turn so that the inside of the roll becomes the outside, thus the **B.** is made to fit a part that is not uniform in size throughout; **FIGURE-OF-EIGHT,** a series of turns, each one crossing the previous one at midpoint and then encircling a part above or below the crossing so that the finished **B.** describes a figure eight; **SPICA,** a type of spiral **B.** in which the turns are folded regularly upon themselves in the form of the letter V, a maneuver which helps make the **B.** fit such parts as the shoulder, groin, foot; **RECURRENT,** a series of turns starting in the middle of the area to be covered and then proceeding to either side with each turn overlapping and coming back to the starting point, used for such areas as the tip of a finger, the head, or an amputation stump. **ACE B.,** trade mark for a roller bandage made of elastic material and frequently used to make firm, continuous pressure on a part. **BARTON'S B.,** a figure-of-eight **B.** used to support a fractured lower jaw. **CAPELINE B.,** a spica **B.** applied in the form of a cap or hood to cover the head, shoulder, amputation stump. **COMPRESSION B.,** one applied firmly enough to compress a part but not shut off the blood supply. **DEMIGAUNTLET B.,** covers the hand but not the fingers. **DESAULT'S B.,** binds the elbow to the side, used for fractured clavicle. **ESMARCH'S B.,** a rubber **B.** applied to a limb from the distal end upward, used to expel blood from a part to be operated upon. **KLING B.,** a narrow elastic gauze **B.,** used to produce compression. **SCULTETUS B.,** a many-tailed **B.** for chest or abdomen. **SUSPENSORY B.,** one applied like a sling to support a part, *e.g.*, the scrotum. **VELPEAU'S B.,** one which binds the arm to the chest with the hand resting on the opposite shoulder, used for fractured clavicle. **T-B.,** two strips of material joined like the letter T, used for holding perineal dressings in place.

Band-Aid surgery: Popular term for laparoscopy (*q.v.*).

Bandl's ring (band'-lz): Name given to the ridge that develops when the fibrous tissue that divides the upper muscular segment from the lower fibrous segment of the uterus pulls over the presenting part in prolonged labor and interferes with expulsion of the fetus.

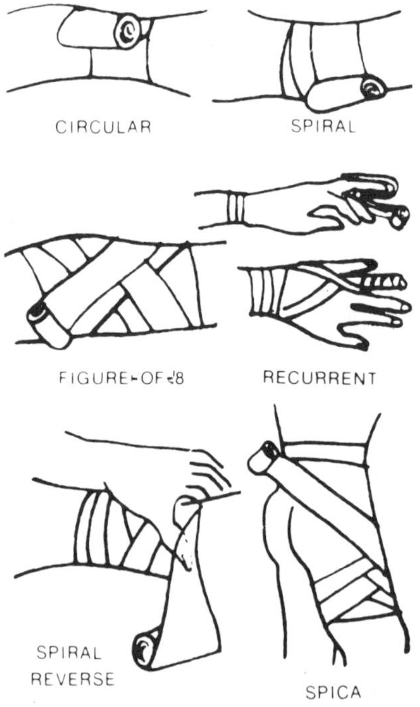

Bandage terminology

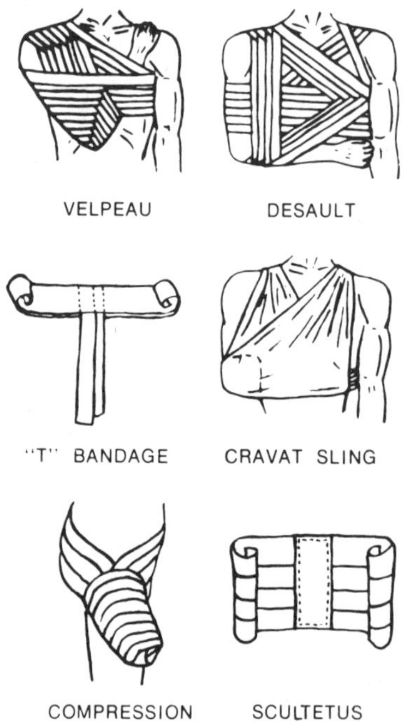

Types of bandages

bandy leg: Bowleg (genu varum).

bank: 1. In medicine, a place for storage of such materials as whole blood, plasma, bone, skin, cornea, or other human tissue, to be used therapeutically, often in reparative surgery. 2. A reserve supply of certain human tissue or blood to be used therapeutically in another person, *e.g.*, eye **B.**, blood **B.**

Banting: Sir Frederick Grant Banting, Canadian scientist 1891–1941; with Charles Herbert Best, American-born physiologist in Canada, and John J. R. Macleod, discoverers of insulin (1922).

Banti's disease or **syndrome:** A disorder of the spleen characterized by gastrointestinal bleeding, anemia, thrombocytopenia, leukopenia, splenomegaly, portal hypertension, weakness and fatigue; progresses usually to cirrhosis of the liver.

baragnosis (bar-ag-nō′-sis): The inability to estimate weight of objects held in the hand; may be a sign of lesion in the parietal lobe. Opp. of barognosis. Syn., abarognosis.

barba (bar′-ba): The beard.

Barbados leg (bar-bā′-dōz): See elephantiasis.

barber's itch: Folliculitis of the beard in which inflammation of the hair follicles of the beard, usually caused by a staphylococcal organism, results in pustules and scab formation. Also called sycosis barbae. See sycosis.

barbituism (bar-bit′-ū-izm): Acute or chronic poisoning caused by excessive use of any of the barbiturates; symptoms include fever, chills, headache, skin eruptions, psychological changes. Also spelled barbiturism.

barbiturates (bar-bit′-ū-rātz): A large group of synthetic compounds derived from barbituric acid and widely used for their hypnotic or sedative effects through depressing the central nervous system. Small changes in the basic structure result in the formation of rapid-, medium-, or long-acting drugs, and a wide range is available. Continued use may lead to tolerance and dependence, hence addiction. Action is potentiated in the presence of alcohol. Overdosage may lead to profound narcosis, respiratory depression, and death. Allergic skin conditions may develop in some patients.

barbotage (bar-bo-tazh′): A method of spinal anesthesia; a small amount of solution from a syringe is injected into the subarachnoid space and the plunger partially withdrawn, allowing the cerebrospinal fluid to mix with the remaining fluid in the syringe. Part of this mixture is then injected and the plunger partially withdrawn again. This process may be repeated several times before all of the medication in the syringe has been injected.

baresthesia (bar-es-thē′-zi-a): The pressure sense.

baresthesiometer (bar′-es-thē-zi-om′-e-ter): An instrument used for estimating an individual's sensitivity to pressure stimuli.

bargaining: A technique sometimes used by very ill patients who try to trade off their present unfavorable condition for a situation that is less serious.

bariatrics (bar-i-at′-riks): The branch of medicine that deals with obesity.

barium (bar′-i-um): A metallic element with several uses in medicine. **B. SULFATE,** a bulky, fine white powder that is tasteless and odorless; used in solution as a radiopaque substance to outline internal structures on x ray. **B. ENEMA,** injection of barium sulfate into the rectum; allows for x-ray visualization of the large intestine. **B. MEAL,** a large amount of barium sulfate is swallowed; allows for x-ray visualization of the action of the esophagus and stomach. **B. SWALLOW,** a small amount of barium sulfate is swallowed to allow for x-ray visualization of the action of the esophagus.

Barlow: **B.'S DISEASE,** infantile scurvy, a deficiency of vitamin C. **B.'S SYNDROME,** a condition characterized by an apical systolic murmur and a click, resulting from mitral regurgitation due to prolapse of the mitral valve. **B.'S TEST** or **SIGN,** the newborn child is placed in supine position, the hips and knees are flexed to 90°, and the hips abducted; if a jerk is felt and a click is heard, the test is a positive sign of congenital dislocation of the hips. [Thomas Barlow, English physician, 1845–1945.]

Barnes' bag: A rubber bag filled with water; used to dilate the cervix and induce premature labor.

barognosis (bar-og-nō′-sis): 1. The ability to estimate weight. 2. The recognition and perception of weight. Opp. of baragnosis (*q.v.*).

baromacrometer (bar′-ō-ma-krom′-e-ter): An instrument for measuring the length and weight of the newborn.

barometer (ba-rom′-e-ter): An instrument used to measure atmospheric pressure.

barometric (bar-ō-met′-rik): Pertaining to or indicated by a barometer. **B. PRESSURE,** the pressure of the atmosphere as indicated by a barometer.

baroreceptor (bar′-ō-re-sep′-tor): A sensory nerve receptor that is sensitive to changes in pressure; chiefly those receptors in the ascending aorta and at the bifurcation of the external and internal carotid arteries which, when stimulated, cause vasodilatation, decreased blood pressure, bradycardia, and decrease in cardiac output.

barosinusitis (bar′-ō-sī-nus-ī′-tis): Inflammation of the frontal sinuses accompanied by edema and hemorrhage; caused by rapid changes in atmospheric pressure, as occur in flying, and deep sea diving. Also called aerosinusitis.

barospirator (bar-ō-spī′-rā-tor): A machine for producing artificial respiration, *e.g.*, the Drinker respirator (*q.v.*).

barotalgia (bar-ō-tal′-ji-a): Pain in the middle ear caused by a difference in the air pressure in it and in the surrounding atmosphere.

barotitis (bar-ō-tī′-tis): Inflammation of the ear caused by rapid changes in atmospheric pressure. **B. MEDIA**, inflammation of the middle ear caused by a difference between the air pressure in the middle ear and that in the environment.

barotrauma (bar-ō-traw′-ma): Injury to the middle ear, ear drum, eustachian tube, or the paranasal sinuses; often caused by blunt chest injury when the glottis is closed and pressure in the airways is increased causing an imbalance between the atmospheric pressure and that within the affected cavity. Trauma to lung tissue may result from the high pressure employed in ventilating patients with PEEP (*q.v.*).

Barr body: Sex chromatin; a small mass of chromatin in the nucleus of all nondividing cells of females. The sex of a fetus can be determined by examination of the amniotic fluid for the presence or absence of this body.

barrel chest: An enlarged thorax which appears rounded and with a widened anterior-posterior measurement; may be normal in some persons as in those living in high altitudes, or pathological as seen in persons with chronic pulmonary emphysema or some other chronic obstructive pulmonary disease; may also be seen in those with kyphosis or asthma.

barren (bar′-en): Sterile, particularly in reference to the female.

Barr-Epstein virus: Herpes-like virus particles thought to be the causative agent in Burkitt's tumor, other tumors, and possibly related to infectious mononucleosis. Also called Epstein-Barr virus.

Barrett's syndrome: A peptic ulcer at the lower end of the esophagus where the lining is similar to that of the stomach. Also called Barrett's esophagus.

Barré-Guillain syndrome: Guillain-Barré syndrome (*q.v.*).

barrier (bar′-ē-er): An obstruction, obstacle, blocking agent. **BLOOD-BRAIN B.**, the mechanism which prevents certain substances such as bacteria or their toxins, or drugs, from passing from the blood to the cerebrospinal fluid or brain. **PLACENTAL B.**, the tissue in the placenta which prevents certain substances from passing from the mother's blood to that of the fetus. **B. NURSING**, a method of preventing the spread of infection from an infected patient to others in the area by the use of isolation technique; see under nursing.

bartholinitis (bar-tō-lin-ī′-tis): Inflammation of a vulvovaginal gland (Bartholin's gland).

Bartholin's duct: 1. The major duct draining the sublingual gland. 2. The ducts that lead from Bartholin's gland to the vulva.

Bartholin's gland: Two small bean-shaped mucus-secreting glands situated at either side of the vagina at the base of the labia minora. [Caspar Bartholin Jr., Danish anatomist 1655–1738.]

Barton, Clara: American teacher who helped care for the wounded during the Civil War by collecting and distributing supplies; influenced the establishment of the American Red Cross in 1882 and was its first president. [1821–1930.]

Bartonella fever: Non-protozoal hemolytic anemia. Occurs in several forms; endemic in Peru. Syn., Oroya fever, Carrion's disease. Probably transmitted by sandflies. Also called bartonelliasis and bartonellosis.

Bartter's syndrome: A hereditary condition of unknown cause, characterized by juxtaglomerular cell hyperplasia, occurring in children with dwarfism, aldosteronism, hypokalemic acidosis, and elevated renin or angiotensin levels.

baruria (ba-rū′-ri-a): The condition in which the urine has an abnormally high specific gravity.

basad (bā′-sad): Toward the base of an object or structure.

basal (bā′-sal): 1. Pertaining to a base. 2. Fundamental.

basal body temperature: The lowest temperature reached by the body during one's waking hours; usually occurs immediately upon wakening in the morning.

basal cell: A cell of the deepest layer of stratified epithelium; see epithelium. **B.C. CARCINOMA**, see under carcinoma. **B. C. EPITHELIOMA**, see under epithelioma.

basal ganglia (bā′-sal gan′-gli-a): Four small islands of grey matter located in the white matter at the base of the cerebrum. The lentiform nucleus, comprising globus pallidus and putamen, together with the caudate nucleus, make up the corpus striatum, which along with the claustrum make up the four **B.G.** Concerned with modifying and coordinating voluntary muscle movement. Site of degeneration in Parkinson's disease. See paralysis.

basal metabolic rate: The rate at which energy is expended by an individual during digestive, physical, and emotional rest, as estimated by measuring the amount of O_2 intake and CO_2 output during a specified time period. Abbreviated BMR.

basal metabolism: The amount of energy used by the body at complete rest, being the minimum necessary for sustaining life.

basal metabolism test: A test for measuring the basal metabolic rate (*q.v.*), which utilizes an apparatus that measures and records the amount of oxygen used per unit of time. The test is performed in the morning before breakfast and preferably after a good night's sleep and 18 hours after taking food. The normal rate is −10 to +10, and is elevated in hyperthyroidism and lowered in hypothyroidism.

basal narcosis (nar-kō′-sis): The preanesthetic administration of narcotic drugs which reduce fear and anxiety, induce sleep and thereby minimize postoperative shock.

base (bās): 1. The lowest part. 2. The wide or broad end of an organ. 3. The main part of a compound. In chemistry, a substance which combines with an acid to form a salt.—basal, basic, basilar, adj.

"baseball" finger: A tearing away of the extensor tendon of the distal phalanx of the finger; caused by a sudden blow on its tip as when catching a baseball. Also called "mallet" finger.

Basedow's disease: Exophthalmic goiter. See thyrotoxicosis.

basement membrane: A thin, delicate, transparent layer of connective tissue underlying the epithelium of mucous membranes and glands.

basi-, basio-: Combining forms denoting base, basic, basis, basilar.

basic: 1. Fundamental. 2. Having properties of a base; alkaline.

basicity (bā-sis′-i-ti): 1. The quality of being basic. 2. The ability to unite with negative ions of an acid.

basicranial (bā′-si-krā′-ni-al): Pertaining to the base of the skull.

basilar (bas′-i-lar): Situated at or pertaining to a base. **B. ARTERY**, artery at the base of the skull, formed by the junction of the right and left vertebral arteries. **B. MEMBRANE**, the structure that forms the floor of the cochlear duct and supports the spiral organ of Corti.

basilar artery insufficiency syndrome: Occurs in patients with sclerosis of the basilar artery but no occlusion. There is insufficient flow of blood through the artery with slow pulse rate, low blood pressure, and symptoms of cardiovascular accident including diplopia, vertigo, numbness, dysarthria, weakness of one side of the body, depressed consciousness.

basilic (ba-sil′-ik): Prominent. **B. VEIN**, a large vein on the inner side of the arm. The **MEDIAN B. VEIN**, at the bend of the elbow, is generally chosen for venipuncture.

basiloma (bas-i-lō′-ma): A basal cell carcinoma.

basioccipital (bā-si-ok-sip′-i-tal): Pertaining to the basilar part of the occipital bone.

basis (bā′sis): A base or foundation. Opp. of apex.

basocyte (bā′-sō-sīt): A basophil or leukocyte cell.

basocytopenia (bā′-sō-sī-tō-pē′-ni-a): Basophilic leukopenia or a decrease in the proportion of basophils in the blood.

basocytosis (bā-sō-sī-tō′-sis): Basophilic leukocytosis or an abnormal increase in the proportion of basophilic leukocytes in the blood.

basoerythrocyte (bā-sō-ē-rith′-rō-sīt): An erythrocyte that contains basophil granules.

basopenia (bās-ō-pē′-ni-a): An absolute or relative decrease in the number of basophils in the bloodstream.

basophil (bā′-sō-fil): 1. A substance, cell, or tissue that stains well with basic dyes. 2. A polymorphonuclear leukocyte distinguished by the presence of large granules which stain intensely with basic dyes and have a relatively lightly staining nucleus; they make up approximately 0.5 to 1.0 percent of the polymorphonuclear leukocytes in the circulating blood; they contain heparin and histamine and are increased in numbers in such pathologic conditions as Hodgkin's disease, smallpox, chickenpox, myelotic leukemia.

basophilia (bā-sō-fil′-i-a): 1. Increase of basophils in the circulating blood. 2. A condition in which red blood cells develop basophilic-staining granules; seen in leukemia, advanced anemia, malaria, lead poisoning and some other toxic states.

basophilic (bās-ō-fil′-ik): Pertaining to an organism that stains readily with basic dyes.

basophobia (bā-sō-fō′-bi-a): Morbid fear of walking.

basoplasm (bā′-sō-plazm): That part of the cytoplasm of a cell that takes an alkaline dye stain readily.

Bassini's operation: A surgical procedure for reconstruction of the inguinal canal in repair of an inguinal hernia.

Batchelor plaster: A plaster of Paris splint used for correcting dislocation of the hip; consists of casts for both legs from ankles to the groins with legs in full abduction and medial rotation, and with the feet attached to a pole. Similar to a frog plaster (*q.v.*).

Bateman's needle: A special needle that has two cannulae; used for giving intravenous injections to infants.

bath: 1. The immersion of all or any part of the body into water or other substance, or the application of a spray, jet, or vapor from a fluid, for cleansing purposes or therapy. 2. The apparatus or place used for bathing. 3. The substance used for bathing. The term is modified according to *a*) temperature, *e.g.*, cold

(18°C), hot (40°C), warm (38°C), tepid (29°C); *b*) medium used, *e.g.*, milk, mud, brine (water rich in salt), starch, wax, water; *c*) medicament added, *e.g.*, sodium chloride, sulfur, potassium permanganate; *d*) function of the medicament, *e.g.*, astringence; *e*) part bathed, *e.g.*, arm; *f*) environment, *e.g.*, bed. **AIR B.**, the therapeutic exposure of the unclothed body to flowing warm moist air. **CHARCOT'S B.**, bathing the body with cold water while standing in hot water. **CONTRAST B.**, immersion of an extremity in hot and cold water alternately. **FINNISH B.**, a sauna **B.**; see sauna. **FOOT B.**, a **B.** for one or both feet. **HALF B., B.** of the hips and lower part of the body. **HIP B.**, the body is immersed in water from the waist down for therapeutic purposes. **LIGHT B.**, exposure of the body or part of it to heat from an electric light bulb in a box or cabinet or under a cradle. **NAUHEIM B.**, one in which the patient is immersed in warm carbonated water. **NEEDLE B.**, one in which water is projected onto the body in fine streams under pressure. **PARAFFIN B.**, the application of heated liquid paraffin. **SAND B.**, a physical therapy procedure wherein the entire body is immersed in either dry or moist warm sand. **SITZ B.**, a hip bath in which the body is immersed in water only up to and including the hips and buttocks. **SPONGE B.**, the body is washed with a wet cloth but is not immersed in water. **SWEAT B.**, warm bath to promote sweating. **TURKISH B.**, a steam **B.** in a cabinet where the temperature becomes increasingly hotter, followed by a rub and massage and then a cold shower. **WAX B.**, paraffin **B.** **WHIRLPOOL B.**, a **B.** in which the water is whirled by a powered device.

bathophobia (bath-ō-fō′-bi-a): An exaggerated fear of deep places or of looking down into deep places.

bathy-: Combining form denoting deep.

bathyanesthesia (bath′-i-an-es-thē′-zi-a): Loss of sensibility in the deeper parts of the body.

bathycardia (bath-i-kar′-di-a): The condition in which the heart is fixed in a lower position than normal.

bathyesthesia (bath′-i-es-thē′-zi-a): Sensibility in the parts of the body below the surface, *e.g.*, the muscle sense.

bathyhyperesthesia (bath-i-hī′-per-es-thē-zi-a): Exaggerated sensitivity of the muscular tissues and other deep body structures.

bathypnea (bath-ip′-ni-a): Deep breathing.

battered baby syndrome: A baby with swollen and bruised portions of body. Radiographically there is subperiosteal new bone at ends of long bones and fracture separation of cartilaginous epiphyses.

battered child syndrome: The result of deliberate trauma inflicted on a young child by custodians; includes any or all of the following conditions: bruises of the skin, burns, multiple fractures, hematomata, malnutrition, retarded growth and development, bone deformities.

battered wife: Any woman who is beaten by her mate regardless of whether he is her husband.

battery: 1. The touching or beating of one person by another without permission, either directly or by use of an object. 2. A series of tests given for a specific purpose. 3. A group of two or more cells grouped together to furnish a source of electric current.

battledore (bat′-el-dōr): **B. PLACENTA**, a placenta in which the umbilical cord is attached to its margin rather than the center.

Battle's sign: An oval-shaped ecchymotic spot at the tip of the mastoid process; usually indicates a basal skull fracture.

batwing ears: Ears shaped like the wings of a bat.

baunscheidtism (bawn′-shīt-izm): A method of producing counterirritation by acupuncture (*q.v.*) using an instrument with several needles; the skin may be rubbed with an irritant such as croton oil or oil of mustard before the treatment, or the needles dipped into an irritant before use. Named for its inventor, Karl Baunscheidt.

Baxter's formula: Used for calculating fluid replacement, particularly in burn victims; based on percent of burned area; 4 ml of Ringer's lactate per kilogram of body weight per percent of body surface burned.

bayonet (bā-ō-net′): **B. FORCEPS**, a forceps that has the blades offset from the handle. **B. LEG**, refers to a backward dislocation of the knee joint.

Bazin's disease: Erythema induratum. A chronic, recurrent disorder, involving the skin of the legs of women. There are deep-seated nodules which later ulcerate. [Antoine Pierre Ernest Bazin, French dermatologist. 1807–1878.]

BBB: 1. Bundle branch block; delay or block of conduction in the left or right branch of the Bundle of His. 2. Blood-brain barrier, see under barrier.

BBT: Abbreviation for basal body temperature.

BCG: Abbreviation for *bacille Calmette-Guérin* (*q.v.*).

b.d.: Abbreviation for *bis die* [L.] meaning twice a day. Also written b.i.d. (*bis in die,* [L.]).

BE: Abbreviation for barium enema. See under barium.

bead (bēd): A small, usually spherical projection. **RACHITIC BEADS**, a series of small, rounded prominences at the points where the ribs join their cartilages; sometimes seen in rickets; also rachitic rosary.

BEAM: *B* rain *e* lectrical *a* ctivity *m* apping. An electroencephalographic procedure used in diagnosing dyslexia and also to study schizophrenia.

bearing down: 1. A pseudonym for the expulsive pains in the second stage of labor. 2. A feeling of weight and descent in the pelvis associated with uterine prolapse or pelvic tumor.

beat: A throb or pulsation as of the heart or an artery. APEX B., in a heart of normal size the apex beat can be seen or felt in the fifth left intercostal space in the midclavicular line; it is the lowest and most lateral point at which an impulse can be detected and provides a rough indication of the size of the heart. DROPPED B., refers to the loss of an occasional ventricular beat. ECTOPIC B., one that does not originate in the sinus node. PREMATURE B., an early beat not in the normal sequence of cardiac impulses.

beating: A massage maneuver consisting of percussion with the ulnar border of the hand and little finger.

Beau's lines: Transverse furrows in the fingernails; indicate a growth disturbance; may be due to infection, trauma, hypercalcemia, systemic disease, coronary occlusion, certain skin diseases.

bechic (bek′-ik): 1. A cough remedy. 2. Acting to control coughing. 3. Pertaining to cough.

Beckwith-Wiedemann syndrome: A hereditary disorder characterized by several congenital anomalies including exophthalmos, macroglossia, and gigantism as well as microcephaly, polycythemia, omphalocele, and port-wine birthmark. Also called Beckwith's syndrome and EMG syndrome.

Beck's triad: Three signs that are characteristic of cardiac tamponade (compression): 1) increased venous pressure, 2) decreased arterial pressure, and 3) diminished heart sounds.

bed: 1. CAPILLARY B., the total mass of capillaries in the body. 2. NAIL B., the modified epidermis lying underneath the fingernails and toenails. 3. A couch or other article of furniture to sleep or rest in or on; the term generally is used to include the frame, springs, mattress, and bed linen. AIR B., one with an inflatable mattress, usually rubber. ANESTHETIC B., one that is prepared to receive a patient who has had a general anesthetic. CIRCOLECTRIC B., a hospital B. that permits vertical turning of the patient; an electric motor turns the entire bed frame which is suspended between hoop-like supports; can be operated by the patient or nurse and permits different positions. CLINTON B., a B. designed to relieve skin pressure; consists of a mattress filled with tiny glass beads through which air is pumped causing the beads to be in constant motion. CLOSED B., a B. that is unoccupied but is prepared to receive a new patient. ETHER B., an anesthetic B. FLOTATION B., one that has a mattress filled with water or some other substance through which air can be circulated; see Clinton B. FRACTURE B., one with an overhead frame for the attachment of fracture appliances. GATCH B., one with a crank attachment to permit raising and lowering of the head and knees. OPEN B., a B. assigned to a patient but not occupied all of the time. OSCILLATING B., a B. that oscillates around its transverse axis as a rocking B., or around its longitudinal axis. ROCKING B., one with a motor attachment which causes it to rock at a regular rate; used as a means of performing artificial respiration. WATER B., one with a rubber mattress partly filled with water; used to prevent bedsores.

bed board: A board placed beneath the mattress to give support to certain areas of the body; often used in cases of low back pain.

bedbug: A blood-sucking insect of the genus *Cimex lectularis;* small, wingless, reddish-brown in color, hard and smooth in appearance, and with a distinctive odor. They live and lay eggs in cracks and crevices of furniture and walls, and can survive long periods without food. They are nocturnal in habit, and an irritating substance in their saliva causes their bites to produce wheals with a central hemorrhagic point. They apparently are not vectors of disease but their bites leave a route for secondary infection. See Cimex.

bedfast: Bedridden. Refers to one who is unwilling or unable to get out of bed.

bedpan: A special, appropriately shaped receptacle used to receive fecal and urinary waste from patients who are bedfast.

bedrail: A device which is fastened to the side of the bed to prevent the patient from falling or getting out of bed.

bedrest: 1. A device used for propping a patient up in bed. 2. Continuous confinement to bed for the purpose of rest.

bedridden (bed′-rid-den): Confined to bed for a prolonged period.

bedsore (bed′-sōr): Decubitus ulcer (*q.v.*).

bedwetting: See enuresis.

bee: An insect of the genus *Apis;* the honeybee. BEESTING, causes redness, pain, local swelling; hypersensitive individuals may have severe anaphylactic reactions and must be treated immediately (usually with epinephrine).

beef tapeworm: *Taenia saginata;* see under Taenia.

Beer's knife: Delicate instrument with triangular blade used in cataract operations for incision of cornea preparatory to removal of lens. [Georg Joseph Beer, Austrian ophthalmologist. 1763–1821.]

beeswax (bēz′-waks): Wax derived from honeycomb; used in preparation of ointments.

behavior (bē-hāv′-yor): In the general sense, conduct, *i.e.*, any observable action or response of an individual. In psychology, the meaningful response of an organism to its environment. **ANTISOCIAL B.**, **B.** that ignores or violates the customs and laws of society. **AUTONOMIC B.**, see under autonomic. **B. DISORDER**, **B.** that 1) deviates noticeably from one's normal **B.**, or 2) is marked by abnormal conduct or mode of action. **B. MODIFICATION**, the bringing about of changes in unacceptable behaviors. **B. REFLEX**, one acquired through training or repetition. **B. THERAPY**, any treatment that attempts to modify one's behavior by any of several techniques, *e.g.*, aversion therapy (*q.v.*) or flooding (*q.v.*). **INCONGRUOUS B.**, **B.** that is inconsistent with the individual's usual behavior. **INVARIABLE B.**, **B.** that is determined by nature, *e.g.*, reflex actions. **OPERANT B.**, 1) **B.** that involves specific responses to stimuli that previously did not provoke a response; or 2) **B.** that seeks to change the environment to produce a desired effect. **PASSIVE-AGGRESSIVE B.**, marked by aggression expressed passively as in pouting, procrastinating, or obstructing. **REGRESSIVE B.**, immature **B.** patterns characterized by partial or complete return to infantile **B.** **RITUALISTIC B.**, a pattern of behavior marked by the performance of certain motor activities in a routinized, consistent manner to relieve anxiety; sometimes used by children to provide security. **SOCIOPATHIC B.**, **B.** characterized by a disregard for the usual social rules and constraints.

behavioral (bē-hāv′-yor-al): Pertaining to behavior. **B. CONTRACTING**, a clinical management tool consisting of a written contract, prepared jointly by the patient and the therapist or health care team, which commits the patient to specific behaviors, states the input expected from the worker or team, and outlines the consequences of behavioral outcomes at various stages during the term of the contract. **B. DISORDERS**, see behavior disorder under behavior. **B. SCIENCES**, those areas of study that are devoted to the development of man's interpersonal relationships and activities, as well as his beliefs and values; includes such widely diverse fields as cultural anthropology, political science, sociology, psychology and psychiatry.

behaviorism (bē-hāv′-yor-ism): A psychological term that denotes an approach to psychology through the study of measurable responses and reactions, *i.e.*, objective, observable behavior, rather than through such subjective phenomena as ideas or emotions. Developed by Watson who insisted that human behavior is predictable, controllable, influenced primarily by the environment, and accessible to understanding through observation chiefly. [John B. Watson, American psychiatrist, 1878–1958.]

behaviorist (bē-hāv′-yor-ist): One who is concerned with the description, prediction, and, sometimes, the control of behavior.

Behçet's syndrome (bā′-sets): A rare condition of unknown cause involving many body systems; symptoms include extensive vasculitis including that of the retina, uveitis, lesions of the mouth and genitalia, pyodermia, arthralgia, neurologic abnormalities; affects primarily young males.

bejel (bej′-el): An endemic, non-venereal, infectious disease found in Arabs of the Near and Middle East, mostly in children; the causative organism is indistinguishable from that which causes syphilis.

bel: A term used to express the relative intensity of a sound. See decibel.

belch: 1. An eructation (*q.v.*). 2. To eructate, or allow gas from the stomach to escape noisily through the mouth.

Bell: **BELL'S MANIA**, an obsolete name for acute delirium. **BELL'S PALSY**, unilateral or bilateral pain and paralysis of the muscles of facial expression, due to a lesion of the seventh cranial nerve; of unknown origin; results in distortion of the face. **B'S. PHENOMENON**, under normal circumstances, the eyes turn sharply upward when the eyelids are closed intentionally, but in individuals with facial palsy the eye on the affected side will turn upward but the lid that should close remains widely open.

belladonna (bel-a-don′-a): A substance obtained from the dried leaves and flowers of a common poisonous plant, the deadly nightshade; the source of atropine, used in medicine for its powerful antispasmodic effect, as a cardiac and respiratory stimulant, for treatment of parkinsonism, as an adjunct to general anesthesia, and to check certain secretions. **B.** is also the source of hyoacyamine, an anticholinergic substance used in the treatment of certain gastrointestinal disorders.

belle indifference: The incongruous unconcern and lack of emotion or anxiety despite incapacitating symptoms, commonly shown by patients with hysteria. First noted by Janet (1893). [Pierre Marie Felix Janet, French psychiatrist, 1859–1947.]

Bellevue bridge: A device used to keep the scrotum elevated when the patient is in the supine position; useful in treatment of epididymitis.

Bellocq's sound or cannula (bel′-oks, kan-ū-la): A curved tube used for plugging the posterior nares in epistaxis.

belly: 1. The abdomen. 2. The fleshy, prominent part of a muscle. **B. ACHE**, colic. **B. BUTTON**, the navel or umbilicus.

Bence Jones protein: Protein bodies appearing in the urine of persons suffering from disease of the bone marrow, *e.g.*, myelomatosis (*q.v.*). Their characteristic quality is that on heating the urine, they are precipitated out of solution at 50° to 60°C; they redissolve on further heating to boiling point and reprecipitate on cooling. [Henry Bence Jones, London physician. 1814–1873.]

Bender gestalt test: A psychological test useful in diagnosing visual-motor defects; the subject is asked to reproduce a series of nine simple designs; his variations from the originals are interpreted in terms of perception and organization, according to gestalt theory.

bends: Decompression sickness. Severe pains in the bones, joints, and muscles and in the abdomen, and general weakness often experienced by a person who goes too quickly from a place of abnormal atmospheric pressure to one of normal pressure; observed in aviators and divers. See caisson disease.

beneceptor (ben′-e-sep-tor): A nerve organ or receptor that receives and transmits stimuli of a beneficial nature. *Cf.* nociceptor.

Benedict's solution (ben′-ē-dikts sol-ū′-shun): A solution of copper sulphate which is easily reduced, producing color changes. Used to detect the presence of sugar.

benign (bē-nīn′): Innocent; mild; nonrecurring; favorable for recovery; the opposite of malignant. **B. POSITIONAL VERTIGO**, see under vertigo. **B. PROSTATIC HYPERTROPHY**, enlargement of the prostate gland; a fairly common condition which may interfere with the flow of urine. **B. TUMOR**, a neoplasm that does not metastasize or invade other tissues but which may, nevertheless, require removal because it presses on an organ and interferes with its function or occupies space needed by other structures.

Benjamin's operation: Osteotomy (*q.v.*) of the femur and tibia, or double osteotomy of these bones, to alter the weight-bearing surfaces; sometimes performed in treatment of osteoarthritis of the knee.

Benzedrene (ben′-ze-drēn): Proprietary name for one of the amphetamines popularly used to stave off sleepiness in people who work long hours; a nervous stimulant that may lead to hyperactivity, paranoid thinking, and other psychotic symptoms; there is a tendency to escalate the dosage and to become addicted.

benzene (ben′zēn): A colorless, inflammable liquid obtained from coal tar. Extensively used as a solvent. Its chief importance in medicine is in industrial toxicology. Continued exposure to it results in leukopenia, anemia, and purpura.

benzidine (ben′-zi-dēn): A chemical compound used for detecting traces of blood and in testing for sulfates in water.

benzocaine (ben′-zō-kān): A chemical substance consisting of white crystals or powder; used in solution as a non-toxic local anesthetic; also used as a dusting powder or in ointment form for pruritus.

benzodiazepines (ben-zō-dī-az′-e-pēns): A group of drugs used as major tranquilizers, *e.g.*, Librium, Valium; administered orally; used in treatment of anxiety states without depression; habit-forming and widely abused.

benzoin (ben′-zoyn): A balsamic resin; has several uses in medicine including use as a stimulating expectorant with administration by inhalation to patients suffering from bronchitis or laryngitis; also used as a topical protectant.

benzyl benzoate (ben′-zil ben′zō-āt): A clear, odorless, aromatic liquid; often used as an active ingredient of a lotion for treatment of scabies (*q.v.*).

bereavement (bē-rēv′-ment): The state of having suffered the loss of a loved one by death. Increasing interest in the topic for nurses has developed with the growth of the hospice movement and sociological interest in death and dying along with the expansion of the nursing role to include comprehensive care of both the dying patient and his or her family.

beriberi (ber′ē-ber′-ē): A deficiency disease caused by lack of thiamine (vitamin B_1). Occurs mainly in the Orient where the staple diet is polished rice; also occurs in areas where there is famine for any length of time and in such places as crowded prisons when the diet is inadequate; rare in the U.S. The symptoms are pain from neuritis, paralysis, muscular wasting, chronic constipation, progressive edema, mental deterioration and, finally, heart failure.

Berkow's method: A method of determining the size of a burn injury in children; more accurate than the rule of nines (*q.v.*). It takes into account the difference in body proportions of children according to their ages; *e.g.*, in infants the head is considered to account for 18 percent of total body surface and the legs for 14 percent. These proportions change until the age of 15; from then on the rule of nines applies.

berylliosis (ber-il-i-ō′-sis): An occupational disease due to inhalation of dust or fumes of beryllium, a metallic element, but may also result from dust particles that enter the body through a lesion in the skin or mucous membrane; symptoms may not appear for several years after exposure and consist chiefly of interstitial fibrosis of lung tissue which impairs lung function, but the liver, skin, and lymph nodes may also be involved.

bestiality (bēs′-ti-al-i-ti): 1. Any animal-like behavior. 2. Sexual intercourse between a human and an animal.

Best's disease: Vitilliform macular dystrophy; see under dystrophy.

beta (bā′ta): The second letter of the Greek alphabet; in chemistry and other types of series, often used to designate the chemical position of a substance in certain compounds. **B. CELLS,** see under cell. **B. RAYS,** see under ray. **B. RECEPTOR,** see under receptor. **B. RHYTHM,** see under rhythm. **B. WAVE,** see under wave.

beta-adrenergic receptor: Any of the adrenergic parts of a receptor of a stimulus that react to norepinephrine and certain other blocking agents by causing relaxation of bronchial muscles, elevated blood pressure and heart rate, and strengthened contraction of cardiac muscle. The opposite of alpha-adrenergic receptor.

beta-blocking agent: An agent that blocks the action of a beta-adrenergic receptor; relieves symptoms of anxiety, diminishes heart rate and cardiac output; may be used in treatment of withdrawal symptoms in alcoholism and drug addiction; some are used in treatment of hypertension and angina pectoris.

betacism (bā′-ta-sizm): A speech defect characterized by using the *b* sound to express other consonants, or by overuse of the sound in speaking.

beta-endorphin (bā′-ta en-dor′-fin): An amino acid peptide involved in many body processes, especially the relief of pain; has a morphine-like activity.

beta-hemolytic streptococcic pharyngitis: Inflammation of the pharynx caused by *Streptococcus pyogenes*.

betel (bē′-tel): A climbing plant of southern Asia; the seed of the fruit, or nut, is wrapped in a leaf of the plant, along with lime, and chewed to produce both stimulating and narcotic effects; continued use causes black discoloration of the teeth; formerly used in Asiatic medicine as a stimulant, astringent, tonic, and counterirritant.

Betz cells: Giant cells of the cerebral cortex in the area anterior to fissure of Roland.

bezoar (be′-zōr): A ball or concretion found in the alimentary tract of certain animals and sometimes in the stomach of man, particularly in psychiatric patients; usually made up of ingested hair and vegetable fibers. In the past thought to have magical therapeutic value, and still used in some parts of the world as a medicament with mystical properties.

bhang (bang): Cannabis sativa. See under cannabis.

Bi: The chemical symbol for bismuth.

bi-: Prefix denoting 1) two, twice; 2) between; 3) affecting two similar parts. In chemistry, double.

biarticular (bī-ar-tik′-ū-lar): Pertaining to or affecting two joints.

biauricular (bī-aw-rik′-ū-lar): Pertaining to or affecting the auricles of both ears.

bibliokleptomania (bib′-li-ō-klep-tō-mā′-ni-a): A morbid desire to steal books.

bibliotherapy (bib-li-ō-ther′-a-pi): The therapeutic use of reading.

bibulous (bib′-ū-lus): Absorbent; spongy.

bicameral (bī-kam′-er-al): Consisting of two chambers or hollows; term often used to describe an abscess which is divided into two cavities by a septum.

bicarbonate (bī-kar′-bō-nāt): A salt of carbonic acid; formed by the combination of water and carbon dioxide under the influence of carbonic anhydrase. **BLOOD B.,** that in the blood, indicating the alkaline reserve; also called plasma **B. SODIUM B.,** a white crystalline powder, used in medicine chiefly as a gastric antacid; also used in solution as a dressing for wounds, for cleansing the mouth, nose, and vagina, as an enema, or as an emollient in bath-water.

biceps (bi′-seps): A muscle possessing two heads or points of origin. **B. BRACHII,** the flexor muscle at the front of the humerus. **B. FEMORIS,** the flexor muscle at the back of the thigh. **B. REFLEX,** contraction of the biceps muscle when its tendon is tapped; this is normal but when greatly increased indicates some pathology.

bichloride (bī-klō′-rīd): A compound, particularly a salt, in which the molecules contain two equivalents of chlorine to one of another element. **B. OF MERCURY,** a corrosive antiseptic, formerly much used both as a germicide and as an antisyphilitic; highly toxic.

bicipital (bī-sip′-i-tal): 1. Two-headed. 2. Pertaining to a biceps muscle. **B. TENDINITIS,** see under tendinitis.

biconcave (bī-kon′-kāv): Being concave or hollow on two surfaces; said of lenses.

biconvex (bī-kon′-veks): Being convex or curving outwardly on two surfaces; said of lenses.

bicornuate (bī-kor′-nū-āt): Having two horns, generally referring to a double uterus or a single uterus possessing two horns. Also bicornate.

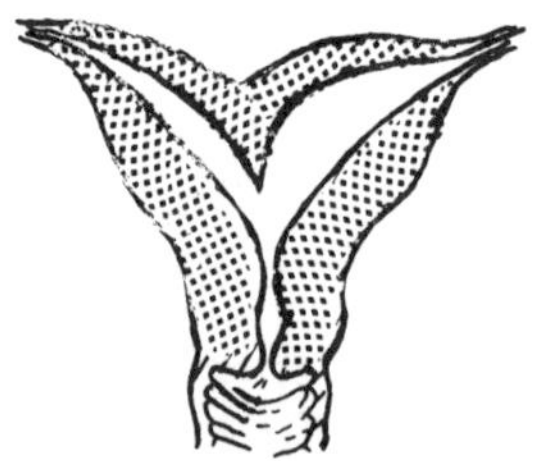

Bicornuate uterus

bicuspid (bī-kus′-pid): Having two cusps or points. **B. TEETH,** the premolars. **B. VALVE,** the mitral valve between the left atrium and ventricle of the heart; it allows blood to flow freely from the left atrium into the left ventricle and prevents backflow from the ventricle to the atrium during ventricular contraction.

b.i.d.: Abbreviation for *bis in dei* [L.], meaning twice a day. Also written b.d.

bidactyly (bī-dak′-ti-li): Absence of all fingers or toes except the first and fifth. See **lobster-claw hand.**

bidet (bē-dā′): A low-set, trough-like basin or sitz bath in which the perineum can be immersed while the legs are outside and the feet on the floor. Can have attachments for douching the vagina or rectum.

biduous (bid′-ū-us): Lasting or remaining for two days.

Bielchowsky's disease: Amaurotic familial idiocy (*q.v.*). Also called Bielchowsky-Jansky disease.

bifid (bī′-fid): Divided into two parts. Cleft. Forked.

bifocal (bī-fō′-kal): Having two foci; term used especially in reference to eyeglasses that have a lens that corrects for near vision set into a lens that corrects for distant vision.

biforate (bī-fō′-rāt): Having two perforations or openings.

bifurcation (bī-fur-kā′-shun): A division or forking into two branches, or the site where such division occurs, *e.g.*, the **B.** of a blood vessel.—bifurcate, adj., and v.

bigeminal (bī-jem′-i-nal): Paired; double. **B. PREGNANCY**, twin pregnancy. **B. PULSE**, two heartbeats followed by a pause before the next two beats; also called pulsus bigeminus; may originate in the atria, the A-V node, or the ventricles.

bigeminy (bī-jem′-i-ni): 1. The condition of occurring doubly or in pairs. 2. A type of heart beat in which two beats occur close together, with the third beat being skipped; a regularly occurring irregularity. Also called bigeminus.

biguanides (bī-gwan′-īds): A group of synthetic drugs given orally in treatment of noninsulin dependent diabetics, particularly the obese; thought to stimulate the uptake of glucose in the absence of insulin.

bilateral (bī-lat′-er-al): 1. Having two sides. 2. Pertaining to both sides of a structure or the body. 3. Occurring on both sides of the body or on right and left structures, as bilateral cataracts.—bilaterally, adv.

bile (bīl): A bitter, alkaline, viscid, greenish-yellow to golden brown, slightly antiseptic fluid secreted by the liver and stored in the gallbladder from which it is released into the duodenum via the common bile duct and where it aids digestion by emulsifying fats, stimulating peristalsis, and preventing putrefaction. It contains water, mucin, lecithin, cholesterol, **B.** salts and the pigments bilirubin and biliverdin. **B. DUCTS**, the hepatic and cystic, which join to form the common **B.** duct.—biliary, bilious, adj.

Bilharzia (bil-har′-zi-a): Syn., *Schistosoma* (*q.v.*).

bilharziasis (bil-hăr-zī′-a-sis): Syn., Schistosomiasis (*q.v.*).

biliary (bil′i-ar-i): Pertaining to bile, the bile ducts, or the gallbladder. **B. CALCULUS**, a gallstone. **B. COLIC**, excruciating, paroxysmal painin the upper right quadrant of the abdomen and referred to the shoulder, due to smooth muscle spasm arising in the bile passages; often caused by pressure of a stone in the gallbladder or its passage through the ducts. **B. DUCTS**, passages in the liver which join the duct from the gallbladder to form the common bile duct. **B. FISTULA**, an abnormal tract conveying bile to the surface or to some internal organ. **B. SYSTEM**, the hepatic (biliary) ducts, gallbladder, cystic duct, and common bile duct; also called the biliary tract or tree.

bilification (bil-i-fi-kā′-shun): The formation and secretion of bile.

biligenesis (bil-i-jen′-e-sis): The production of bile.

bilihumin (bil-i-hū′-min): The insoluble fraction of gallstones.

bilin (bī′-lin): The chief ingredient of bile, consisting mostly of sodium salts of normal bile acids.

bilious (bil′-yus): 1. Pertaining to bile. 2. Pertaining to excess of bile. 3. A popular nonmedical word signifying a digestive upset, often with headache and constipation, and attributed to excess secretion of bile.

bilirubin (bil-i-roo′-bin): A reddish-yellow crystalline pigment that gives bile its orange color; it is a waste product from the normal breakdown of old red blood cells which passes through the liver where it is changed chemically and is excreted chiefly in the feces.

bilirubinemia (bil-i-roo-bi-nē′-mi-a): The presence of more bilirubin in the blood than the slight amount normally found there.

bilirubinuria (bil-i-roo-bi-nū′-ri-a): The presence of more bilirubin in the urine than the slight amount normally found there.

bilitherapy (bil-i-ther′-a-pi): Treatment with bile or bile salts.

biliuria (bil-i-ū′-ri-a): The presence of bile or bile salts in the urine.—biliuric, adj.

biliverdin (bil-i-ver′-din): The green pigment occurring in bile, an oxidation product of bilirubin.

biliverdinuria (bil′-i-ver-di-nū′-ri-a): The presence of biliverdin in the urine.

Billing's ovulation method: A birth control method based on observations by the woman and her interpretation of the symptoms that accompany hormonal changes throughout the menstrual cycle, particularly those which occur around the time of ovulation, and the avoidance of sexual contact from the time she recognizes the approach of ovulation until three days following ovulation.

bills of rights: See Patients' Bill of Rights.

bilobate (bī-lō'-bāt): Having two lobes.

bilobular (bī-lob'-ū-lar): Having two little lobes or lobules.

bimanual (bī-man'-ū-al): 1. Pertaining to both hands. 2. Performed with both hands, *e.g.*, in gynecology, the method of examining internal female genitalia with one hand on the abdomen and the finger or fingers of the other hand in the vagina.—bimanually, adj.

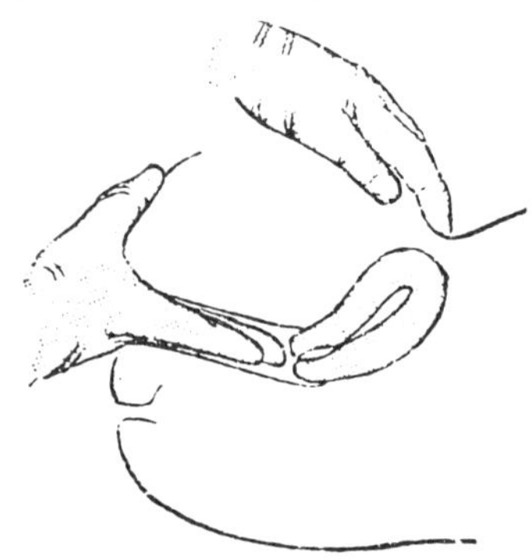

Bimanual examination

bimastoid (bi-mas'-toyd): Pertaining to both mastoid processes.

bimaxillary (bī-mak'-si-ler-i): 1. Pertaining to both jaws. 2. Affecting both jaws.

binary (bī'-na-ri): Made up or consisting of two things; characterized by two. In chemistry, a compound made up of two elements. In anatomy, dividing or separating into two. **B. FISSION**, reproduction of cells by division into two approximately equal parts.

binaural (bī-naw'-ral): Pertaining to, or having, two ears. Applied to a type of stethoscope (*q.v.*).

binauricular (bī-naw-rik'-ū-lar): Pertaining to the auricle of each ear.

binder (bīn'-der): A broad bandage, applied about the abdomen or breasts; often used following surgery or childbirth. **T-BINDER**, a **B.** patterned after the letter T; used to hold perineal or rectal dressings in place.

Binet's test (bē'-nāz): A series of graded intelligence tests in which a child's intelligence level (mental age) is used to measure mental development between the ages of 3 and 12; this is expressed as intelligence quotient, which is arrived at by dividing the mental age by the chronological age. [Alfred Binet, French psychologist. 1857–1911.]

binocular (bin-ok'-ū-lar): 1. The use of both eyes in vision. 2. Pertaining to both eyes. 3. Describing an optical instrument requiring both eyes for its use.

binotic (bin-ō'-tik): 1. Having two ears. 2. Pertaining to both ears.

binovular (bin-ov'-ū-lar): Derived from two separate ova. **B.** twins may be of different sexes. See uniovular.

binuclear (bī-nū'-klē-ar): Having two nuclei.

bio-: Combining form denoting 1) life; 2) living organism or tissue.

bioanalyst (bī-ō-an'-a-list): A person who is specially trained in several clinical laboratory disciplines and in administration, and who has responsibility for the administration and supervision of a clinical laboratory.

bioassay (bī-ō-as'-sā): Assessing the potency or strength of a substance by comparison of the effects it has on living organisms, *e.g.*, animals, with the effects of a standardized preparation. Syn., biological assay.

bioastronautics (bī'-ō-as'-trō-naw'-tiks): The science of the effects of space and interplanetary travel on living organisms, particularly the means of keeping astronauts alive and able to function in outer space under conditions that are hostile to human life.

bioavailability (bī'-ō-ā-vāl-a-bil'-i-ti): The degree to which a drug, other medication, or other substance becomes available for use by the body after administration.

biocatalyst (bī-ō-kat'-a-list): An enzyme.

biochemistry (bī-ō-kem'-is-tri): The branch of chemistry that deals with the changes of organic compounds as they occur in living organisms.—biochemical, adj.

biocidal (bī-ō-sī'-dal): Active against life; causing death, particularly of living microorganisms.

bioclimatology (bī'-ō-klī-ma-tol'-ō-ji): The study of the effects of climate or the natural environment on life.

bioelectricity (bī'-ō-ē-lek-tris'-i-ti): 1. Electric phenomena that occur in living tissues. 2. Effects of electric current on living tissue. **B. TESTS**, tests that detect and record electric currents generated within the body.

bioenergetics (bī'-ō-en-er-jet'-iks): A science that deals with the molecular mechanisms involved in the transformation of energy in the biologic functions of living tissue.

bioengineering (bī'-ō-en-jin-eer'-ing): The application of engineering principles to the biological sciences, especially to medicine and surgery, in the designing of sophisticated mechanical or microelectric devices that are safe for patient use; *e.g.* renal dialysis machines, cardiac pacemakers, electronic monitors.

bioequivalent (bī-ō-ē-kwiv'-a-lent): In pharmacology, refers to the relative equivalency of effect of different forms of a drug; for example, generic and brand-name preparations.

bioethics (bī-ō-eth′-iks): The principles that govern the uses of medical and biological technology, particularly when they have a bearing on human life. Is concerned with the social, ethical, legal, and even theological ramifications of the effects of biomedical research and technology. The term is often used synonymously with medical ethics.

biofeedback (bī-ō-fēd′-bak): A combination of meditation and technology (including monitoring devices) utilized for controlling states of mind to help the person identify, monitor, and even control certain body functions; used in treating stress, neurologic disorders, certain physiologic disturbances such as tension headache. **B. TRAINING**, learning to control body processes such as breathing, heartbeat, and other involuntary body functions including muscle contraction; consists of learning a series of deep relaxation exercises.

bioflavonoids (bī-ō-flā′-vō-noyds): Any of a group of compounds obtained from the rinds of citrus fruits and from many plants; their action in the body is to maintain a normal state of the walls of small blood vessels.

biogenesis (bī-ō-jen′-e-sis): 1. The origin of living organisms. 2. Term used to describe the theory that living organisms can be produced only by organisms already living; opp. to the theory of spontaneous generation.—biogenetic, adj.

biogenics (bī-ō-jen′-iks): A system of self-education achieved by practicing exercises in relaxation and focusing the attention, along with concentration, on spiritual matters; utilizes techniques developed by Coué, Jung, the gestaltists, and others.

biologic (bī-ō-loj′-ik): Pertaining to biology. **B. RHYTHMS**, see under rhythm.

biological (bī-ō-loj′-i-kal): 1. Pertaining to biology. 2. In pharmacy, a preparation made from living organisms or their products and used in the diagnosis, treatment, or prevention of disease; includes the serums, vaccines, antitoxins, and antigens. **B. AGE**, see under age. **B. CLOCK**, the mechanism of a learned 24-hour pattern of sleep and wakefulness; see circadian rhythm. **B. CLOCK THEORY**, holds that aging is due to the running down of an inherent biological clock located in the nucleus of cells that determines the number of divisions a normal cell can undergo before it dies. **B. HALF-LIFE**, the time it takes the body to excrete or eliminate one half of a dose of an administered substance; it is the same for all isotopes of a given element; see half-life.

biological warfare: The use of disease-causing agents such as bacteria, viruses, etc., against both military forces and civilians during the conduct of war.

biologicals (bī-ō-loj′-i-kalz): Complex substances obtained from living organisms and their products, including antigens, antitoxins, serums, and vaccines.

biologist (bī-ol′-ō-jist): A person who is an expert in, or who specializes in, biology.

biology (bī-ol′-ō-ji): The science of life, dealing with the structure, function, and organization of all living things including plants and animals.—biologic, biological, adj.; biologically, adv.

biolysis (bī-ōl′-i-sis): The breaking down of organic matter by the chemical action of such living organisms as bacteria.—biolytic, adj.

biomechanics (bī-ō-me-kan′-iks): The science that deals with the mechanics of the human body, based on the application of principles of physics and engineering to the action of biological systems; includes the study of the environment required by astronauts when in space.

biomedical (bī-ō-med′-i-kal): Pertaining to both biology and medicine.

biomedicine (bī-ō-med′-i-sin): Clinical medicine that utilizes in practice the principles of such natural sciences as biology and biochemistry.

biometer (bī-om′-e-ter): An instrument for measuring the amount of carbon dioxide given off by living tissue.

biometry (bī-om′-e-tri): The application of statistical methods in the study of biology. Biostatistics.

biomicroscope (bī-ō-mī′-krō-skōp): A special microscope with a thin beam of light which permits the examiner to observe minute details within living tissue or organs, the eye, for example. See slitlamp.

biomicroscopy (bī-ō-mī-kros′-ko-pi): 1. The microscopic study of the structure of living cells. 2. The microscopic examination of living tissue in the body. 3. Examination of the cornea, lens, vitreous body, and retina with a slitlamp (*q.v.*).

bion (bī′-on): An individual living thing.

bionics (bī-on′-iks): The science of developing models that parallel the human vertebrate nervous system; may be mathematical, electronic, or physical; applied in cybernetic engineering. See cybernetics.

bionosis (bī-ō-nō′-sis): Any disease caused by a living agent such as a bacterium or a virus.

biophage (bī′-ō-fāj): A parasite. Any living organism that derives its nourishment from another living organism.

biophilia (bī-ō-fil′-i-a): The instinct of self-preservation.

biophysics (bī-ō-fiz′-iks): The branch of knowledge that deals with 1) the physics of living organisms; 2) the applications of the principles and methods of physics to the problems of living organisms.

bioplasm (bī'-ō-plazm): The essential or vital part of the protoplasm of living cells. Protoplasm.

biopsy (bī'-op-si): 1. Observation or examination of a living subject or of tissue taken from a living body, as opposed to a postmortem observation. 2. Term used to describe the removal of a small piece of tissue from a living body for histologic examination needed to establish an accurate diagnosis. **ASPIRATION** or **NEEDLE B.**, examination of tissue removed by a hollow needle. **BIOCHEMICAL B.**, a combination of histological and chemical examination of tissue for diagnostic purposes. **CONE B.**, examination of a cone-shaped piece of tissue; in a cervical **CONE BIOPSY** a circular tapering piece of tissue is excised from the external os of the uterus, for pathological examination. **ENDOSCOPIC B.**, **B.** in which the specimen is obtained by a surgical instrument inserted through an endoscope. **NEEDLE B.**, aspiration **B.** **OPEN B.**, examination of a specimen taken following a surgical incision, to be examined immediately. **PUNCH B.**, **B.** in which the specimen is removed by a punch. **SPONGE B.**, **B.** in which the specimen is obtained by placing a sponge over a lesion or membrane. **STERNAL B.**, examination of bone marrow that is removed from the sternum by puncture or aspiration. **SURFACE B.**, examination of tissue removed from a surface by scraping; used especially to diagnose cancer of the uterine cervix. **TOTAL B.**, examination of an entire organ or part that is removed from the body. **WEDGE B.**, examination of a pie-shaped portion of tissue.

biopsychology (bī'-ō-sī-kol'-o-ji): See psychobiology.

biopsychosocial (bī'-ō-sī-kō-sō'-shul): Pertains to the "whole person" approach to health care which involves the biological, psychological, and social factors involved in an illness.

biorbital (bī-or'-bit-al): Pertaining to or involving the orbits of both eyes.

biorhythm (bī'-ō-rithm): A biologically regulated rhythmic pattern of change in physiologic behavior such as occurs in the menstrual cycle, or the regular variations in body temperature, blood pressure, or mood.

biosocial (bī-ō-sō'-shul): 1. Relating to the biological and social aspects of life. 2. Relating to the human aspects of social life as they are affected by the principles of biology.

biospectroscopy (bī'-ō-spek-tros'-ko-pi): The spectroscopic examination of living tissue and/or of body fluids; clinical spectroscopy. See spectroscopy.

biosphere (bī'-ō-sfēr): All areas of the known universe where life can exist.

biostatistics (bī-ō-sta-tis'-tiks): The science of statistics applied to collected numerical data concerning human populations. Vital statistics.

biostereometrics (bī'-ō-ster-ē-ō-met'-riks): A photographic technique that utilizes two cameras that produce pictures called bodygrams; can detect deformities and serve as the basis for designing prostheses.

biosynthesis (bī-ō-sin'-the-sis): The forming of chemical compounds by synthesis within the living organism.

biotherapy (bī-ō-ther'-a-pi): The treatment of disease with a living microorganism or the product of a living microorganism.

biotic (bī-ot'-ik): Pertaining to life or living organisms.

-biotic: Combining form denoting life, or having life.

biotics (bī-ot'-iks): The study of living organisms and their qualities, functions, and activities.

biotin (bı'-o-tin): One if the water-soluble members of the vitamin B complex which acts as a coenzyme, and is presumed essential to man. Found in varying amounts in many plant and animal foods but chiefly in liver, kidney, egg yolk, milk, yeast, peanuts, unpolished rice; also synthesized from ingested foods in the intestine. Raw egg white in quantities interferes with its absorption. Formerly called vitamin H.

biotomy (bī-ot'-ō-mi): Vivisection.

biotoxicology (bī'-ō-toks-i-kol'-o-ji): The study of toxins and toxic conditions produced by living organisms.

biotransformation (bī'-ō-trans-for-mā'-shun): The chemical and metabolic changes that substances undergo in the body, particularly drugs.

biotripsis (bī-ō-trip'-sis): Wearing away or eroding of the skin, seen mostly in the elderly.

Biot's respiration: See Biot's breathing under breathing.

biotype (bī'-ō-tīp): A group of organisms having the same genotype. See genotype.

biovular (bī-ov'-ū-lar): See binovular.

bipara (bip'-a-ra): A woman who has given birth to two children in two different labors.

biparental (bi'-pa-ren'-tal): 1. Having two parents, one male and one female. 2. Derived from two parents.

biparietal (bī'-pa-ri'-et-al): Pertaining to both parietal bones or both parietal lobes.

biparous (bip'-a-rus): 1. Producing two ova or two offspring at one time. 2. Having borne twins.

bipartite (bī-par'-tīt): 1. Divided into two parts. 2. Consisting of two parts or divisions.

biped (bī'-ped): 1. Any animal with two feet, as man. 2. Two-footed.

bipolar (bī'-pō-lar): Having two poles. **B. NERVE CELL**, a nerve cell with two processes, *i.e.*, an afferent and an efferent process.

bipolar disorders: Major affective neurotic disorders occurring as: **BIPOLAR DISORDER,**

MIXED, in which alternating manic and depressive episodes occur, or have recently occurred, with the two phases being intermixed or alternating. **BIPOLAR DISORDER, MANIC,** in which a manic episode occurs or has occurred recently. **BIPOLAR DISORDER, DEPRESSED,** in which a major depressive episode occurs or has occurred recently. See major depression under depression.

biramous (bī-rā′-mus): Having two rami or branches.

bird fanciers' lung: A condition caused by exposure to avian antigens in dust, feathers, or excreta of birds; extrinsic allergic alveolitis. Also called bird breeder's lung and pigeon breeder's lung.

birefringence (bī-rē-frin′-jens): The quality of splitting a ray of light in two, or of transmitting light unequally in different directions. Also called double refraction.—birefringent, adj.

Birnberg bow: An intrauterine contraceptive device.

birth: The act of expelling the young from the mother's body; delivery; being born. **B. CANAL,** the cavity or canal of the pelvis through which the baby passes during labor. **B. CERTIFICATE,** a legal document given on registration, within a specified period after birth, listing date and place of birth, name and sex of child, names of parents, other pertinent information. **B. CONTROL,** the prevention or regulation of conception by any means; contraception. **B. DEFECT,** congenital defect; see congenital. **B. INJURY,** any injury occurring during parturition, *e.g.*, fracture of a bone, subluxation of a joint, injury to a peripheral nerve, intracranial hemorrhage. **B. PALSY** or **PARALYSIS,** paralysis caused by injury received at or during birth. **B. TRAUMA,** 1) an injury sustained in the process of being born; 2) in psychiatry a hypothesis that relates the shock of being born with the later development of anxiety or neurosis. **PREMATURE B.,** one occurring after the seventh month of pregnancy but before term. **B. RATE,** the number of live births per 1000 population per year.

birth center: A licensed nonhospital alternative delivery service for healthy women with normal uncomplicated deliveries and low risk for complications. Offers minimal medical intervention and allows family and friends to be present. Also offers prenatal and postnatal care. Services are provided chiefly by certified nurse-midwives. May be free standing or run by a hospital in a separate building on hospital grounds.

birth control pill: A contraceptive agent in the form of a pill, taken orally. See contraception, contraceptive.

birthing: Giving birth. **B. CHAIR,** a chair used by women in labor; may have a complicated design or be a simple chair with a large central hole in the seat; allows for the upright position and thought by some to facilitate labor, particularly in the second stage. **BIRTHING BED,** a special bed equipped with levers that control the head, seat, and foot positions; the foot section can be adjusted to provide for Trendelenburg position; the advantage is that the patient does not have to change beds for labor, delivery, and recovery. **BIRTHING ROOMS,** special rooms in hospitals or clinics for family-centered childbirth; husbands and children can take part in the event.

birthmark: A hemangioma or other blemish present on the skin at birth; nevus (*q.v.*).

bis-: Prefix denoting two or twice.

bis in die: Twice a day [L.]. Abbreviated b.d. or b.i.d.

bisalbuminemia (bis′-al-bū-mi-nē′-mi-a): A congenital blood disorder in which the individual's blood contains two serum albumins that differ in their physical responses to electrophoresis.

bisaxillary (bis-ak′-si-lar-i): Pertaining to both axillae.

bisect (bī′-sekt): To divide into two equal parts.—bisection, n.

bisection (bī-sek′-shun): The process of cutting into two parts.

bisexual (bī-seks′-ū-al): 1. Having the interest and characteristics of both sexes. 2. Having gonads of both sexes; hermaphrodite. 3. Relating to both sexes. 4. Consisting of both sexes. 5. In psychiatry, responsive to both sexes.

bisexuality (bī′-seks-ū-al′-i-ti): 1. The condition of being attracted to both males and females in the same degree. 2. The Freudian concept that each individual has components of both sexes in his makeup.

bisferiens (bis-fē′-ri-ens): Refers to a pulse that has two palpable beats during one systole.

bisferious (bis-fē′-ri-us): Striking twice; having two beats, as a pulse; dicrotic.

bisiliac (bis-il′-i-ak): Pertaining to the two ilia or to two iliac parts or structures.

bismuth (biz′-muth): A greyish metal. Various preparations formerly much used internally for their antisyphilitic, antidiarrheal, antiacid, antiseptic and astringent actions; and externally for their protective actions.

bismuthosis (biz-mū-thō′sis): Bismuth poisoning.

bistoury (bis′-tū-ri): A surgical knife, long, narrow, and sometimes curved, for cutting from within outward as in opening an abscess, hernial sac, etc.

bisulfate (bī-sul′-fāt): An acid sulfate derived from sulfuric acid; contains twice the proportion of acid as an ordinary sulfate.

bitartrate (bī-tar′-trāt): A salt resulting from

the neutralization of a tartaric acid. Also called acid tartrate.

bite: Puncture, laceration, or penetration of the skin by human teeth or by an animal or insect. In dentistry, the occlusion of the teeth.

bitemporal (bī-tem'-por-al): 1. Pertaining to both temporal areas of the skull. 2. Pertaining to both temporal lobes of the brain.

Bitot's spots or patches (bē'-toz): Shiny, gray, triangular spots, seen at the sides of the cornea, and associated with vitamin A deficiency. Also called xerosis conjunctiva.

bitrochanteric (bī-trō-kan-ter'-ik): Pertaining to 1) the greater trochanter of both femurs or 2) the greater and lesser trochanter of a femur.

bitters: Bitter tasting medicinal substances that are used as tonics or stomachics (*q.v.*).

bituminosis (bī-too-mi-nō'-sis): A form of pneumoconiosis caused by inhalation of soft-coal dust.

biuret test (bī-ū-ret'): A laboratory test for 1) protein; 2) urea.

bivalent (bī-vā'-lent): 1. In chemistry, refers to a substance that has a valence of two, or one that has two valences; see valence. 2. Double or paired, as two joined chromosomes.

bivalve (bī'-valv): 1. Having two blades, as in a vaginal speculum. 2. To divide a plaster of Paris cast into two portions, an anterior and a posterior half. 3. Having two valves, as mollusks or clams.

biventricular (bī-ven-trik'-ū-lar): Involving or pertaining to both ventricles of the heart.

black damp: See under damp.

Black Death: An extremely virulent form of the plague that ravaged Europe and Asia in the 14th century. Named for the hemorrhagic, blackening spots which formed on the skin. Bubonic plague.

black lung, black lung disease: Pneumoconiosis (*q.v.*). So called by coal miners because the inhalation of coal dust blackens the lungs and slowly destroys the lung tissues.

black widow spider: See Latrodectus mactans.

blackhead: See comedo.

blackout: 1. A condition characterized by failure of vision and unconsciousness of short duration, caused by sudden reduction in the amount of blood reaching the brain and retina. 2. A period of time during alcoholic or other drug intoxication that the individual cannot remember afterward.

blackwater fever: A malignant form of malaria (*q.v.*) occurring in the tropics, especially Africa. There is great destruction of red blood cells, and this causes a very dark colored urine. Other symptoms include high fever, vomiting, jaundice, enlarged liver and spleen, acute renal failure, tachycardia. The prognosis is poor.

Blackwell, Elizabeth: First woman to graduate from a medical school in the U.S. Promoted and assisted in the establishment of the first schools of nursing in this country. [1821–1910.]

bladder: A membranous sac that serves as a receptacle or reservoir for a fluid or gas. **ATONIC B.**, a condition in which there is no sensation in the urinary bladder, with overdistention, incomplete emptying; may or may not be of neurogenic origin; seen in tabes dorsalis and pernicious anemia. **AUTONOMOUS B.**, a condition of the bladder in which the individual has lost control of the function of micturition due to injury of the spinal cord in the lumbosacral region. **GALL B.**, see gallbladder. **HYPOTONIC B.**, a condition of greatly decreased or absent tonus of the detrusser urinae muscle; see detrusser. **ILEAL B.**, see ileoureterostomy. **IRRITABLE B.**, a condition in which extreme sensitivity of the bladder is accompanied by constant desire to urinate. **NERVOUS B.**, a term describing the condition in which one has a constant desire to urinate but cannot empty the bladder. **NEUROGENIC B.**, a term designating any dysfunction of the urinary bladder caused by a lesion in the spinal cord or peripheral nervous system. **PSYCHOGENIC B.**, a term descriptive of a condition in which the patient empties the bladder at increasingly shorter intervals until eventually the bladder fails to fill to any degree before the need to void is felt; caused by one or more nervous and emotional factors. **RECTAL B.**, a term used to describe the results of surgery in which the ureters are transplanted to the rectum. **REFLEX B.**, a condition in which the sensation of bladder distension and ability to control micturition are lost; results from a lesion in the spinal cord; seen in paraplegic patients. **SPASTIC B.**, autonomous **B. STAMMERING B.**, a term describing a condition in which the stream of urine is interrupted several times

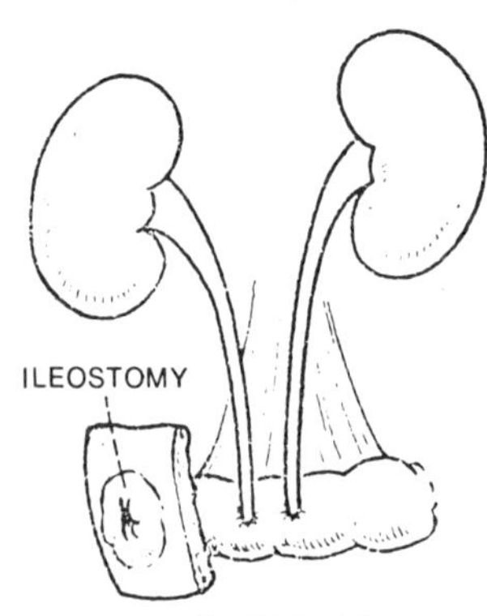

Ileal bladder

during voiding. **UNINHIBITED B.**, a **B.** that has retained the sensation of distention but lost the ability to inhibit voiding; due to a lesion in the cerebral cortex; frequently seen in persons with cardiovascular disease. **UNSTABLE B.**, a **B.** condition to be differentiated from stress incontinence by the fact that a cough, sneeze, or posture change may cause an uninhibited bladder contraction resulting in complete emptying of the bladder whereas in stress incontinence only part of the bladder content leaks out. **URINARY B.**, the muscular bag in the pelvis that serves as a reservoir for urine.

Blalock-Hanlon operation: An operation in which an intra-atrial septum is created to compensate for congenital transposition of the great vessels.

Blalock-Taussig operation: An anastomosis between the subclavian artery and the pulmonary artery; most often performed on a child affected with tetralogy of Fallot; helps increase the blood flow through the lungs and reduces cyanosis by supplying more oxygen to the tissues. [Alfred Blalock, American surgeon, 1899–1964. Helen Taussig, American pediatrician. 1898–1986.]

blanch: 1. To become ashen or pale. 2. To take the color out of.

bland: Mild, nonirritating, soothing. **B. DIET**, see under diet.

blas-, blasto-: Combining forms denoting bud, budding; used particularly in relation to a primitive cell or element in the early stage of development of the embryo.

blast: An immature stage in cell development before the distinctive characteristics of the particular cell appear. Also often used as a word termination to describe a particular kind of cell, *e.g.*, neuroblast.

-blast: Combining form denoting an embryonic or formative unit, especially of living matter.

blastema (blas-tē′-ma): The primitive material from which cells and tissues of the embryo develop.

blastocele (blas′-tō-sēl): The central cavity of the blastula of a developing embryo.

blastocyst (blas′-tō-sist): The modified blastula, consisting of an outer part—the trophoblast, an inner cell mass, and the blastocele; it represents the stage in embryonic development that follows the morula (*q.v.*).

blastocyte (blas′-tō-sīt): An embryonic cell that has not yet become differentiated into its specific type.

blastocytoma (blas-tō-sī-tō′-ma): A neoplasm made up chiefly of immature undifferentiated embryonic tissue. Blastoma.

blastoderm (blas′-tō-derm): A delicate, membranous lining of the zona pellucida of the fertilized ovum. The rudimentary structure from which the embryo is formed.

blastogenesis (blas-tō-jen′-e-sis): 1. Multiplication of an organism by asexual reproduction or budding. 2. Transmission of parental characteristics to offspring by the germ cells.

blastolysis (blas-tol′-i-sis): Dissolution and destruction of the blastocyst (*q.v.*).

blastoma (blas-tō′-ma): A true tumor. A tumor originating from the blastema of tissue or an organ. Syn., blastocytoma.—blastomatous, adj.

blastomere (blas′-tō-mēr): One of the cells resulting from the division of the fertilized ovum.

Blastomyces (blas-tō-mī′-sēz): A genus of fungi pathogenic to man. **B. DERMATITIDIS**, a species of North American fungus that causes blastomycosis (*q.v.*).

blastomycosis (blas′-tō-mī-kō′-sis): Granulomatous and suppurative inflammation characterized by formation of multiple abscesses in skin and subcutaneous tissues, sometimes also affecting the viscera and bones. Caused by infection with an organism of the genus Blastomyces. **NORTH AMERICAN B.**, a pulmonary infection caused by *Blastomyces dermatitidis;* often disseminates to the skin, bones, lungs and other organs; also called Gilchrist's disease.

blastula (blas′-tū-la): The stage of development at which an embryo consists of one or several layers of cells around a central fluid-filled cavity.

BLB mask: Boothby-Lovelace-Bulbulian breathing mask; has an inspiratory and expiratory valve; for use in high altitudes, but also used for clinical administration of oxygen.

bleb: A large blister. See blister, bulla, vesicle.

bleed: 1. To lose blood from a vein or artery. 2. To cause blood to be lost from a vein or artery.

bleeder: 1. A blood vessel that is severed, sometimes during surgery, and from which blood continues to escape. 2. An individual who is subject to frequent loss of blood, as one suffering from hemophilia (*q.v.*).

bleeding: Losing blood as a result of a severed or ruptured blood vessel. **ANOVULATORY B.**, **B.** not associated with ovulation. **B. TIME**, the time required for the spontaneous arrest of bleeding from a skin puncture; under controlled conditions this forms a clinical test and is not to be confused with clotting time. **DYSFUNCTIONAL B.**, uterine **B.** usually due to an endocrine imbalance rather than a tumor or organic disease. **OCCULT B.**, hidden or concealed **B.**, the blood being so changed that it is not easily identifiable.

blennemesis (blen-em′-e-sis): The vomiting of mucus.

blennogenic (blen-ō-jen′-ik): Forming or producing mucus.

blennophthalmia (blen-of-thal′-mi-a): Catarrhal conjunctivitis.—blennophthalmic, adj.

blennoptysis (blen-op′-ti-sis): The expectoration of mucous secretion from the bronchi.

blennorrhagia (blen-ō-rā′-ji-a): A copious mucous discharge.

blennorrhea (blen-ō-rē′-a): Syn., blenorrhagia (*q.v.*). **INCLUSION B.**, acute, purulent conjunctivitis; in infants, this is due to infection from the mother's genital tract during birth; affects both eyes; marked by red swollen lids and purulent discharge. In adults, it is less severe; often acquired venereally or in swimming pools; the discharge is less purulent; usually affects only one eye; also called inclusion conjunctivitis.

blennostasis (blen-nos′-ta-sis): Diminution of an abnormal or excessive mucous secretion.

blennothorax (blen-ō-thō′-raks): An accumulation of mucus in the bronchi.

blennuria (blen-nū′-ri-a): The presence of mucus in the urine.

bleph-, blephar-, blepharo-: Combining forms denoting eyelid.

blepharadenitis (blef′-ar-ad-e-nī′-tis): Inflammation of the Meibomian glands. Also blepharoadenitis.

blepharal (blef′-a-ral): Pertaining to the eyelids.

blepharedema (blef-ar-ē-dē′-ma): Edema of the eyelids.

blepharism (blef′-a-rizm): Spasm of the eyelids.

blepharitis (blef-a-rī′-tis): Inflammation of the eyelids, particularly the edges. **B. MARGINALIS**, chronic inflammation of the eyelid margins, the hair follicles, and the sebaceous glands;) marginal **B. NONULCERATIVE B., B.** marked by hyperemia, thickening, and scaling of the eyelid edges; may be associated with seborrhea of the scalp or psoriasis. **ULCERATIVE B., B.** resulting from bacterial infection of the sebaceous glands of the eyelids; marked by redness, swelling, ulceration with crust formation, photophobia, conjunctivitis.

blepharoatheroma (blef′-a-rō-ath-er-ō′-ma): A tumor of the eyelid.

blepharoblennorrhea (blef′-a-rō-blen-ō-re′-a): Conjunctivitis accompanied by a purulent discharge.

blepharochalasis (blef′-a-rō-kal′-a-sis): Relaxation of the tissues of the eyelid; a horizontal fold of excess tissue develops; may be excessive enough to drop over the pupillary axis.

blepharoconjunctivitis (blef′-a-rō-kon-junk-ti-vī′-tis): Inflammation of the eyelids and the conjunctiva.

blepharodiastasis (blef′-a-rō-dī-as′-ta-sis): Abnormally wide separation of the eyelids or inability to close them completely.

blepharokeratoconjunctivitis (blef′-a-rō-ker′-a-tō-con-junk-ti-vī′-tis): Inflammation involving the edges of the eyelids, the cornea, and the conjunctiva; may be due to infection, irritation, or an allergy.

blepharon (blef′-a-ron): The eyelid; palpebra.—blephara, pl.

blepharoncus (blef-a-rong′-kus): A tumor of the eyelid.

blepharopachynsis (blef′-a-rō-pa-kin′-sis): Abnormal thickening of an eyelid.

blepharophimosis (blef′-a-rō-fī-mō′-sis): Abnormal narrowing of the slit between the eyelids. Also called blepharostenosis.

blepharoplasty (blef′-a-rō-plas-ti): Plastic repair of an eyelid. Sometimes done for cosmetic purposes to remove wrinkles and bulges caused by hereditary factors or aging.

blepharoplegia (blef-ar-ō-plē′-ji-a): Paralysis of an eyelid.

blepharoptosis (blef-a-rō-tō′-sis): Drooping of an upper eyelid. See ptosis.—blepharoptotic, adj.

blepharospasm (blef′-a-rō-spazm): 1. Excessive winking. 2. Spasm of the obicularis oculi muscle producing partial or complete closure of the eyelid for seconds or minutes at a time.—blepharospastic, adj.

blepharosynechia (blef′-a-rō-si-nek′-i-a): Temporary or permanent adhesion of the eyelids to each other.

blind: 1. Unable to see. 2. Closed at one end, as a pouch.

blind spot: The spot at which the optic nerve leaves the retina. It is insensitive to light.

blindness: Loss or lack of ability to see; may be due to disorder of the organ of sight or to a lesion in the central nervous system. **COLOR B.**, a term loosely applied to any deviation from the normal ability to distinguish hues accurately. **CONCUSSION B.**, that caused by violent explosion, gunfire, etc. **DAY B.**, hemeralopia (*q.v.*). **ECLIPSE B.**, may occur while watching an eclipse of the sun without proper eye protection. **FUNCTIONAL B.**, occurs without any disorder of the organ of sight. **LEGAL B.**, less than 20/200 vision in the better of the two eyes, or when visual acuity is restricted to 20 degrees or less. **NIGHT B.**, nyctalopia (*q.v.*). **PSYCHIC B.**, inability to recognize known objects; due to a lesion in the central nervous system. **TOTAL B.**, no light perception whatever.

blink: To close the eyelids and then open them quickly several times in succession. **B. REFLEX**, the reflex action of closing the eyes when the cornea is touched. Also called corneal reflex.

blister: Separation of the epidermis from the dermis by a collection of fluid, usually serum or blood. See vesicle. **FEVER B.**, herpes simplex (*q.v.*) of the lip.

bloat (blōt): To become swollen, puffy, or edematous. Usually refers to abdominal distention; may be caused by air swallowing or by intestinal gas from fermentation of intestinal contents.

block: 1. An obstruction or blockage of a passage. 2. Regional anesthesia. 3. An obstruction in the path of a nerve or muscle impulse. See heart block, nerve block, saddle block.

blood: The red, viscid fluid filling and circulating through the heart and blood vessels; supplies nutritive material to, and carries waste away from, the body tissues. Consists of plasma, a clear straw-colored fluid with particles or corpuscles immersed in it. Corpuscles (blood cells) are of two varieties: 1) red (also called erythrocytes) are nonnucleated, biconcave disks, present in normal blood in amounts ranging from 4,000,000 to 6,000,000 per cu mm; they transport oxygen from the lungs to the tissues and carry carbon dioxide away from the tissues; 2) white cells, or leukocytes, are nucleated, granular, motile cells; the range in normal blood is from 5,000 to 10,000 per cu mm with definite percentages of each of several types; they protect the body by destroying invading organisms. Also present are minute cell fragments called platelets or thrombocytes which are important in the clotting mechanism; the normal range is 200,000 to 500,000 per cu mm. ARTERIAL B., aerated blood which carries oxygen to tissues. DEFIBRINATED B., that in which the fibrin has been removed by agitation and which therefore does not clot. LAKED B., that in which the red cells are hemolyzed. OCCULT B., that which is not visible; its presence is determined by chemical tests. VENOUS B., that which has transported oxygen to the tissues and has picked up carbon dioxide which is being carried back to the lungs. WHOLE B., that from which none of its elements has been removed.

blood agar: A solid culture medium for certain microorganisms; consists of nutrient agar to which blood has been added.

blood bank: A special laboratory where whole blood or its components are collected, typed, and stored until needed for transfusion; may be a unit of a hospital or a separate facility. Currently, whole blood is treated with a preparation of citrate-phosphate-dextrose-adenine to increase the maximal storage time.

blood buffers: A group of substances consisting chiefly of dissolved carbon dioxide and bicarbonate ions which function in the blood to maintain the proper pH of the blood.

blood casts: Casts that contain red blood corpuscles, formed in the renal tubules and found in the urine in certain kidney diseases.

blood clotting: See mechanism of clotting, under clot.

blood corpuscles: Blood cells. See blood, erythrocyte, leukocyte, platelet.

blood count: Calculation of the number of red or white cells per cubic millimeter of whole blood, using a hemocytometer. COMPLETE B.C., includes, in addition to numerical and differential count of white cells, a count of red cells and estimates of hemoglobin, hematocrit, and platelets in a blood sample. Abbreviated CBC. DIFFERENTIAL B.C., an estimate of the relative number of each of the various types of white cells in a cubic millimeter of blood. DIRECT PLATELET COUNT, utilizes a counting chamber and microscope to determine the number of platelets in a cu mm of blood.

blood crossmatching: A technique used for determining the compatibility of bloods, done before transfusion. See blood groups.

blood culture: After withdrawal of blood from a vein, it is incubated in a suitable medium, at an optimum temperature, so that any contained organisms can multiply and so be isolated and identified under the microscope. See bacteremia and septicemia.

blood donor (dō′-nor): An individual who donates some of his blood for use by another, either directly to that person or to a blood bank.

blood dyscrasia: See under dyscrasia.

blood gas: Refers to gases normally present in the blood serum; includes oxygen, carbon dioxide, and nitrogen; Determination of the amounts of gases present is an important procedure in evaluating for treatment patients with serious cardiac, respiratory, or kidney failure and other conditions of stress or shock.

blood groups: All human blood has been classified (by Landsteiner) as belonging to one of four groups (also called types or systems), A, B, AB, and O, the divisions being based on the presence or absence of specific, genetically determined antigens (agglutinogens) located on the surface of the red cells, and of specific antibodies (agglutinins) in the serum. The cells of groups A, B, and AB contain the corresponding agglutinogens (antigens) A, B, and AB; O contains none. The serum of A blood contains anti-B agglutinins; B blood serum contains anti-A agglutinins; O blood serum contains both, and AB contains neither. If incompatible bloods are mixed, *e.g.,* A and B, the agglutinins in the serum of one type will cause agglutination (clumping) of the red cells of the other type, and this may lead to severe, sometimes fatal reaction in the patient. Since O blood cells contain no agglutinogens, it can safely be given to persons with any type of blood and thus is known as the universal donor. Since AB blood contains no agglutinins, persons with such blood can safely receive A, B, and O blood and thus are known as the universal recipients. In addition to the four groups,

Landsteiner and Wiener discovered the Rh (Rhesus) system, which is based on the presence or absence of an hereditary factor known as the Rh factor; blood that contains this factor is called Rh positive and that which does not is called Rh negative. See rhesus. Several other systems more recently identified on the basis of the reaction of cells with antibodies include Auberger, Diego, Duffy, Kell, Kidd, Lewis, Lutheran, MNSs, P, Sutter, Xg.

	AB	A	B	O
AB	O	X	X	X
A	O	O	X	X
B	O	X	O	X
O	O	O	O	O

Compatibility of blood types

O = compatible
X = incompatible
AB = incompatible with all other types
O = compatible with all other types (universal donor)

blood plasma: The liquid portion of whole blood. Composed of over 90 percent water, 6 to 8 percent protein substances; mineral salts; nutrients; gases; waste products; clotting agents; antibodies; and hormones.

blood platelets: Small, circular or oval colorless disks found in the circulating blood, averaging about 250,000 in 1 cu mm of blood. Important in the clotting of blood because they release thrombokinase which, in the presence of calcium, reacts with prothrombin to form thrombin. Syn., thrombocyte.

blood poisoning: Septicemia (*q.v.*).

blood pressure: The lateral pressure of the blood against the blood vessel walls as the column of blood is pumped through them; may be measured indirectly by a sphygmomanometer (*q.v.*) or directly by use of a transducer-monitor system. ARTERIAL B.P., that in the arteries. CENTRAL VENOUS P., the blood pressure in the right atrium, obtained through a procedure in which a soft pliable indwelling catheter is introduced into a suitable vein (usually the internal jugular or the subclavian) and threaded into the right atrium, with the distal end attached to a water manometer and an intravenous setup; the readings on the manometer are measures of cardiac competence, atrial pressure, and ventricular functioning, as well as a guide for fluid replacement. DIASTOLIC B.P., the lowest pressure registered on the apparatus when the left ventricle is in a state of relaxation; the normal adult range is likely to be between 60 and 80 mm. HIGH B.P., see hypertension. SYSTOLIC B.P., the highest point registered on the apparatus when the heart muscle is at the maximum contraction; the normal adult range is likely to be between 110 and 145 mm. VENOUS B.P., that in the veins.

blood sedimentation rate: See erythrocyte sedimentation rate.

blood serum: The clear fluid which exudes when blood clots; it is plasma minus the clotting agents.

blood smear: A drop of blood, placed on a glass slide and then spread and stained for microscopic examination.

blood stream, bloodstream: The flowing blood as it is in the body as opposed to blood that has been withdrawn from the body.

blood substitute: A substance such as human plasma, serum albumin, dextran, gum acacia, or gelatin, given by transfusion in cases of hemorrhage or shock.

blood sugar: The amount of carbohydrate, chiefly glucose, in the circulating blood; expressed in milligrams per 100 milliliters; varies from 80 to 120 mg per 100 ml of blood serum, or 70 to 105 mg per 100 ml of whole blood. This level is controlled by various enzymes and hormones, the most important single factor being insulin (*q.v.*). See hyperglycemia and hypoglycemia.

blood transfusion: The intravenous replacement of lost or destroyed blood by compatible citrated human blood. Also used for severe anemia with deficient blood production and for treatment of shock or severe infections. Fresh blood from a donor or stored blood from a blood bank may be used. It can be given whole, or with some plasma removed (packed-cell transfusion). If incompatible blood is given, severe reaction follows. See blood groups.

blood types: See blood groups.

blood typing: The determination of an individual's blood group by laboratory tests. See blood groups; crossmatching.

blood urea: The amount of urea (*q.v.*) in the blood; varies within the normal range of 20 to 40 mg per 100 ml of blood. The level is virtually unaffected by the amount of protein in the diet when the kidneys, which are the main organs of excretion of urea, are normal. When they are diseased, the blood urea quickly rises. See uremia.

blood urea nitrogen: Nitrogen in the form of urea, found in whole blood and serum; the normal range of 8 to 20 mg per 100 ml of blood or plasma, is altered in disorders of kidney function. Abbreviated BUN.

blood vessels: The tubes which transport the blood throughout the body; arteries, veins, capillaries.

blood volume: The total amount of circulating blood in the body.

blood-brain barrier: See barrier.

bloodletting: The removal of blood from a vein for therapeutic purposes, formerly a popular form of treatment.

bloodshot: Congestion of blood in the small vessels of a localized area, as occurs, *e.g.*, in the conjunctiva when the small vessels dilate and become visible.

Bloom's syndrome: An inherited condition seen primarily in Jewish children; characterized by short stature and underdeveloped facial bones, erythematous facial rash, sensitivity to sunlight; many of these children develop leukemia.

blotch: A spot or blemish, or an abnormally pigmented or reddened area on the skin or a membrane.

blow bottles: A pair of bottles containing water which is blown from one to the other by means of a connecting rubber tube; this forces the patient to exhale against resistance.

blue baby: The appearance produced by insufficient oxygen in the blood; may be due to a congenital defect that allows the arterial and venous blood to become mixed. The appearance, by contrast, of a newborn child suffering from temporary anoxia is described as "blue asphyxia." **BLUE BABY OPERATION,** a procedure designed to ameliorate the lack of adequate oxygenation of an infant's blood caused by the tetralogy of Fallot (*q.v.*).

blue bloater: A patient suffering from chronic bronchitis, polycythemia, alveolar hyperventilation, hypercapnia, or cor pulmonale; is often heavy set, breathless, and has distended neck veins, ankle edema, and a blue or reddish-blue face color. Colloquial.

Blue Cross/Blue Shield: One of the largest voluntary group health agencies in the U.S.; a nonprofit third-party payment organization that functions under state enabling acts in the 50 states; offers health care insurance to individuals and groups in a community at a single set rate and pays the same benefits to all subscribers in the same community. Blue Cross pays all or part of a subscriber's hospital expenses and Blue Shield pays all or part of the subscribers' in-hospital doctor bills and a certain amount of office-based care. For persons over 65, the "Blues" offer policies that cover the gaps in Medicare payments; they also play a large part in the administration of Medicare and Medicaid programs. Some employers include Blue Cross/Blue Shield insurance as part of a fringe benefits program.

blue diaper syndrome: Blue staining of an infant's diaper due to an inborn error of metabolism of tryptophan, which is converted by intestinal flora to indican causing blue discoloration of the urine.—see tryptophan.

blue spot: See Mongolian spot.

blues: Depression; despondency. A colloquialism.

Blumberg's sign: Pain which is produced when the examiner suddenly withdraws pressure on the abdomen; it is indicative of inflammation of the peritoneum.

BMR: Abbreviation for basal metabolic rate.

body: 1. The trunk or frame of a person and the structures it contains as differentiated from the head and extremities. 2. The largest or principal part of an organ, *e.g.*, the body of the uterus. 3. Any mass of material. **B. IMAGE,** the image in an individual's mind of his own body. Distortions of this occur as a result of affective disorders, parietal lobe tumors, or trauma. **B. MECHANICS,** the application of the principles of kinesiology (*q.v.*) to body activities so as to correlate actions of the various parts and thus prevent injuries and problems related to posture. **B. TEMPERATURE,** that of the healthy body; 98.6°F when taken by mouth, usually one degree higher by rectum. **CAROTID B.,** see under carotid. **CAVERNOUS B.,** one of the two erectile columns in the dorsum of the penis and in the clitoris. **CILIARY B.,** see under ciliary. **PERINEAL B.,** see under perineal. **VERTEBRAL B.,** see under vertebral. For other specific bodies, see under the adjectives.

body language: The intentional and unintentional messages transmitted wittingly or unwittingly by facial expression, eye contact, posture, clothing, touching, and body movements; kinesic behavior; varies with race and culture.

Boerhaave's glands (boor′-hav-ez): The sweat glands, first described by Boerhaave. [Hermann Boerhaave, Dutch physician. 1668–1738.]

Bohn's nodules: Small white nodules on the center of the palate of the newborn; of no known significance.

Bohr effect: The influence of carbon dioxide on the oxygen dissociation curve (*q.v.*), causing a shift to the right and indicating a reduction in the affinity of hemoglobin for oxygen. [Neils Bohr, Danish physicist. 1885–1962.]

boil: An acute inflammatory condition surrounding a hair follicle; a furuncle.

bolometer (bō-lom′-e-ter): 1. An instrument for measuring small differences in the amount of heat radiated from a specific body area or part. 2. An instrument formerly used for measuring the force of the heart beat as distinguished from the force of the blood in the blood vessels.

boloscope (bō′-lo-skōp): An instrument for locating metallic foreign bodies in tissues.

Bolton Act: Federal legislation enacted in

1943; established the Nurse Cadet Corps and, for the first time, provided for allocation of federal funds in support of nursing education by paying the tuition of students in the Cadet Corps and giving them a monthly stipend on condition that they remain in nursing for the duration of World War II. Sponsored by Senator Frances P. Bolton, this act had several other effects on nursing education in general including the reduction of the requirement of 36 months to 30 months duration, and the forbidding of discrimination on the basis of race, color or marital state.

bolus (bō′ -lus): 1. A large pill. 2. A soft, pulpy mass of masticated food ready to swallow.

bombé of the iris: Forward displacement of the iris, caused by a blockage in the pupil which prevents forward flow of the aqueous.

bonding: The unique attachment and unity of two people, most often that between an infant and parent, especially the mother, which endures as a warm, secure relationship throughout life; it is brought about by touching, fondling, speaking, and having eye-to-eye contact.

bone: 1. The hard, connective tissue forming the skeleton. 2. Any distinct piece of the skeleton. **B. TISSUE** may be either compact or cancellous. About one third of the total weight is accounted for by the organic matter of the fibrous tissue and the remaining two thirds by the inorganic mineral matter deposited in it. There are 206 named bones in the body; they make up about one-seventh of the body weight. In children the proportion of organic matter is greater, giving a tendency to bend rather than break; in elderly people the mineral content is in greater proportion, causing the bones to become brittle. Bones are classified according to shape as long, short, flat, irregular, and sesamoid. **B. CONDUCTION,** usually refers to conduction of sound waves through the skull to the hearing receptors in the ear by means of a hearing device applied to the exterior of the skull. **B. GRAFT,** transplantation of a piece of healthy bone from one part of the body to another, or from one person to another. Used to repair bone defects, afford support, or to supply osteogenic tissue. See cancellous, compact, marrow.—bony, adj.

bone marrow: The highly vascular, soft, pulpy, network of reticular tissue that fills the cavities of most bones. **RED MARROW,** found in the articular ends of long bones and in the cancellous parts of flat and short bones, bodies of the vertebrae, the cranial diploë, and the sternum and ribs. The main function of red marrow is the development of erythrocytes and granular leukocytes (eosinophils, basophils, and neutrophils). Blood platelets are also formed in the red marrow by fragmentation of large cells known as megakaryocytes. **YELLOW MARROW** consists mostly of fatty connective tissue; it is found in the medullary cavities of the long bones, the femur and humerus in particular.

bone marrow aspiration: The withdrawal, by special needle, of a specimen of bone marrow for diagnostic purposes; usually utilizes the sternum.

bone marrow depression: Decreased or diminished production and maturation of erythrocytes and granulocytes.

bone marrow transplant: The transplantation of bone marrow from a healthy donor into the bloodstream of the another; if successful it starts producing healthy blood cells; may be used in treatment of aplastic anemia.

Bonnevie-Ullrich syndrome: Gonadal dysgenesis. A chromosomal disorder resulting in short stature, webbed neck, facial and other bodily deformities, cardiac anomalies, lymphedema of the hands and feet, sexual infantilism. Also called Turner's syndrome.

booster dose: A later dose given to enhance the effect of an initial or previous dose; usually applied to antigens given for the purpose of producing specific antibodies.

boot: 1. A covering for the foot. 2. A boot-shaped appliance. **UNNA'S PASTE BOOT,** see Unna's boot.

boot therapy: Refers to the application of a plastic boot which is inflated intermittently; used to prevent postoperative thrombophlebitis.

bootling: Refers to a breech presentation of a fetus when one or both feet present first.

borate (bō′ -rāt): A salt or ester of boric acid.

borax (bor′ -aks): A compound of boron, found in certain arid areas; chief use is as a water softener and detergent; it has mild antiseptic properties.

borborygmus (bor-bo-rig′ -mus): Rumbling or gurgling noises caused by the movement of flatus in the intestines.—borborygmi, pl.

Bordetella pertussis (bor-de-tel′ -la pertus′ -is): The organism that causes whooping cough. See pertussis.

boric acid: A common mild antiseptic, used in the form of a solution, ointment, or powder for surface application to skin and mucous membranes of the eye, ear, nose, bladder, etc. Serious and fatal accidents have occurred from internal use or accidental poisoning. Also boracic acid.

Bornholm disease: Epidemic pleurodynia (*q.v.*); probably caused by Coxsacki B virus through contact infection. Symptoms include severe diaphragmatic pain, fever. Also called epidemic myalgia. See fibrositis.

boron (bō′ -ron): A nonmetallic element found

only in combination with other substances; the active principle in boric acid and borax.

Borrelia (bor-rē′-li-a): A genus of spirochetes; among the many species are the organisms that cause various types of relapsing fever.

boss: 1. A rounded projection or eminence as on a bone or tumor; also called bossing. 2. The projection of the spine in kyphosis (*q.v.*).

bosselated (bos′-sel-ā-ted): Having knob-like protrusions.

botany (bot′-a-ni): The branch of biology that deals with plants.

botryoid (bot′-rē-oid): Like a bunch of grapes in appearance.

bottle-mouth syndrome: The development of caries in the deciduous teeth of children who go to sleep with a bottle of milk or juice propped against their teeth.

botulin (bot′-ū-lin): A very active neurotoxin that affects the nervous system; sometimes found in imperfectly preserved or canned nonacid vegetables or meat such as sausage; causes botulism (*q.v.*); is produced by an anaerobic organism *Clostridium botulinum,* widely distributed in soil and the intestines of domestic animals.

botulism (bot′-ū-lizm): A severe type of food poisoning caused by botulin (*q.v.*). Characterized by sudden onset, vomiting, abdominal pain, malaise, dry mouth, dizziness, muscular weakness, cyanosis, and ocular and pharyngeal paralysis, within 24 to 72 hours after eating improperly canned or smoked food that has been contaminated by the *Clostridium botulinum*. Often fatal due to respiratory failure.

bouba (boo′-ba): Yaws (*q.v.*).

Bouchard's nodes: Nodules that appear on the second joints of the fingers; have been associated with gastrectasis.

bougie (boo′-zhē): A flexible, slender cylindrical instrument of varying sizes, shapes and materials; used to explore or dilate a canal such as the anus, urethra, or esophagus, to dilate a stricture of a canal or structure such as the cardiac sphincter, to induce labor, or as a guide for the passage of other instruments.

bougienage (boo-zhē-nazh′): The introduction of a bougie or a cannula into an orifice or a tubular structure of the body for purposes of examination or treatment.

bouillon (boo′-yan): A broth prepared from animal flesh. Used as a food and as a culture medium for bacteria.

Bourneville's disease: Epiloia (*q.v.*).

bouton (boo-ton′): A button; pustule; knob-like swelling or nodule.

boutonniere deformity (boo-ton-yair′): A finger deformity in which the proximal interphalangeal joint is flexed and the distal joint is hyperextended. Also called buttonhole deformity.

bovine (bō-vēn′; bo-vīn′): Pertaining to the cow or ox. The bovine type of the tubercle bacillus (*Mycobacterium tuberculosis*) may infect the bones, glands, and joints in human beings.

bowel (bow′-el): The intestine; the gut. SMALL B., the first 23 ft. of the intestine, the first 10 or 11 in. of which is the duodenum; the next two-fifths is the jejunum and the following three-fifths the ileum. LARGE B. measures 6 ft. in length but is larger in diameter than the small intestine and has other distinguishing features such as the structure of its lining membrane. See colon.

bowel sounds: Heard on auscultation over the abdomen; caused by air mixing with fluid during peristalsis; those heard in the small intestine are high pitched and gurgling while those in the large intestine are lower in pitch and rumbling; their intensity is an indication of peristaltic activity and strength.

Bowen's disease: Intraepithelial squamous cell carcinoma of the skin; the formation of small, red, scaling patches with an irregular surface is characteristic.

bowleg: The outward curving or arching of the leg, or both legs, at and/or below the knee; genu varum.

Bowman's capsule: The expanded beginning of a renal tubule in the kidney. It and the tuft of capillaries that it surrounds make up a malpighian corpuscle.

Boyle's law: At any stated temperature, a given mass of gas varies in volume inversely in proportion to the pressure exerted upon it. [Robert Boyle, English physicist. 1627–1691.]

BP: Abbreviation for 1. Blood pressure 2. British Pharmacopoeia.

BPM: Abbreviation for beats per minute (heartbeats).

brace: An orthopedic appliance used to support a part of the body or to keep it in proper position for functioning.

brachi-, brachio-: Combining forms denoting the arm.

brachial (brā′-ki-al): Pertaining to the arm. Applied to vessels in this region and to a nerve plexus at the root of the neck; see brachial plexus under plexus. B. BIRTH PALSY, paralysis of the arm due to injury to the brachial plexus during delivery.

brachialgia (brā-ki-al′-ji-a): Pain in the arm.

brachialis (brā-ki-al′-is): A muscle of the anterior part of the upper arm; it lies immediately under the biceps brachii; acts to flex the forearm.

brachiocephalic (brāk′-i-ō-se-fal′-ik): Pertaining to the arm and the head.

brachiocrural (brăk′-i-ō-kroo′-ral): Pertaining to both the arm and the leg.

brachiocubital (brăk′-i-ō-kū′-bit-al): Pertaining to both the arm and the forearm.

brachium (brā′-ki-um): 1. The arm, especially from the shoulder to the elbow. 2. Any armlike appendage.—brachia, pl.; brachial, adj.

brachy-: Combining form denoting short, shortness.

brachybasia (brak-i-bā′-zi-a): A shuffling, slow-stepped gait.

brachycardia (brak-i-kar′-di-a): See bradycardia.

brachycephalic (brak-ē-se-fal′-ik): Having a short wide head.—bradycephalia, n.

brachycheilia (brak-i-kī′-li-a): Abnormally short lips. Also brachychilia.

brachydactylia (brak-i-dak-til′-i-a): Abnormal shortness of the fingers and toes, a congenital anomaly. Also brachydactyly.

brachygnathia (brak-i-nā′-thi-a): A congenital anomaly consisting of abnormal shortness of the mandible; a receding lower jaw.

brachymetropia (brak-i-mē-trō′-pi-a): Myopia (*q.v.*).

brachytherapy (brak-i-ther′-a-pi): Radiation therapy with the source of radiation being close to or on the surface of the area being treated.

Bradford frame: A canvas and metal device used for immobilizing the spine or pelvis, resting the trunk or back muscles, or preventing deformity in patients with certain fractures, dislocations or diseases of the spinal or pelvic bones. Consists of a tubular steel frame with two canvas slings allowing a 4- to 6-inch gap to facilitate use of the bedpan. [Edward H. Bradford, American orthopedic surgeon. 1848–1926.]

Bradley method: A method of childbirth preparation consisting of prenatal education in physiological changes and of breathing exercises to promote relaxation during labor; involves both prospective parents.

bradyacusia (brad-i-a-kū′-zi-a): Diminished perception of sound; dullness of hearing.

bradyarrhythmia (brad′-i-ar-rith′-mi-a): Bradycardia (*q.v.*).

bradyarthria (brad-i-ar′-thri-a): Abnormally slow enunciation of words.

bradycardia (brad-i-kar′-di-a): Abnormally slow rate of heart contraction, resulting in a pulse rate of less than 60 beats per minute in an adult, 70 in a child, or 120 in a fetus. In febrile states the expected increase in pulse rate is 10 beats per minute for each degree of rise in body temperature; when the pulse rate does not increase, the condition is called **RELATIVE B. SINUS B.**, a slow heartbeat which originates in the normal sinus pacemaker; often occurs after a myocardial infarction with reduction of the oxygen needs of the myocardium.

bradycardia-tachycardia syndrome: Arrhythmic heart action in which episodes of sinus bradycardia alternate with tachycardia; usually due to pathology of the sinus node. Also called sick sinus syndrome and brady-tachy syndrome.

bradyesthesia (brad-i-es-thē′-zi-a): Abnormal slowness of transmission of sensory impulses or dullness of perception of sensory input.

bradykinesia (brad-i-kī-nē′-si-a): Excessive slowness of voluntary movement and speech; a characteristic of parkinsonism and certain other nervous system disorders.

bradykinin (brad-i-kī′ nin): A polypeptide formed in the blood plasma; it has vasomotor action, increases the permeability of capillary walls, and contributes to the formation of edema.

bradykininogen (brad′-i-kī-nin′ ō-gen): A globulin found in the blood plasma; a necessary precursor to the formation of bradykinin (*q.v.*).

bradylalia (brad-i-lā′-li-a): Abnormal slowness of speech, due to a lesion in the central nervous system such as occurs in Sydenham's chorea.

bradylexia (brad-i-lek′-si-a): Abnormal slowness of reading, usually due to a lesion in the central nervous system.

bradylogia (brad-i-lō′-ji-a): Slowness of speech, resulting from sluggish thinking, as occurs in some mental disorders.

bradypepsia (brad-i-pep′-si-a): Slowness of digestion.

bradyphagia (brad-i-fā′-ji-a): Slowness in eating.

bradyphasia (brad-i-fā′-zi-a): A form of aphasia characterized by slow utterance of speech; bradylalia.

bradypnea (brad-ip-nē′-a): Abnormal slowness of breathing; often the result of central nervous system depression.

bradysphygmia (brad-i-sfig′-mi-a): Abnormal slowness of the pulse; bradycardia.

bradystalsis (brad-i-stal′-sis): Abnormal slowness of peristaltic movement.

bradytocia (brad-i-tō′-si-a): Abnormally slow labor and/or delivery.

brady–: Combining form denoting; 1) slow; 2) dull.

Braille (brāl): A kind of writing and printing used for the blind; the letters are made up of raised points or dots that the blind person can feel.

brain: The encephalon; that part of the central nervous system contained in the cranial cavity. It consists of the cerebrum, cerebellum, pons varolii, midbrain, and medulla oblongata. **B.**

CENTER, a group of nerve cells in a circumscribed area that are concerned with the regulation of a certain function, *e.g.*, sight, hearing, speech, etc. B. SCAN, a diagnostic procedure utilizing a radioactive isotope and a scanner or camera, and a detection instrument that counts the gamma rays being emitted by the particular area being scanned; see scanner. B. STEM, all of the brain except the cerebrum and the cerebellum, *i.e.*, the midbrain, pons, and medulla oblongata; contains afferent and efferent tracks between the brain and spinal cord; functions in control of subconscious and reflex activities. B. TUMOR, see glioblastoma multiforme; meningioma. B. WAVES, see under wave.

brain case: The part of the skull that encloses the brain.

brain concussion: Injury to the tissues of the brain due to trauma such as a violent blow. See concussion.

brain death: Occurs when all brain function is completely and irreversibly destroyed as demonstrated by a "flat" electroencephalogram and lack of brain stem and other reflexes; may result from prolonged anoxia, intracranial hemorrhage, severe head injury. See also under death, and Harvard Criteria for Death.

brain scan: A painless diagnostic procedure in which radioisotopes administered intravenously circulate through the brain where they can be traced and photographed by a scanner (*q.v.*); a useful technique for locating and identifying tumors or other brain lesions.

brain stem: All of the brain except the cerebrum and the cerebellum *i.e.*, the midbrain, the pons varolli, and the medulla oblongata. It extends from the cerebral hemispheres through the foramen magnum and continues as the spinal cord; contains nuclei that affect respiration, blood pressure, the heart race, coughing, swallowing, vomiting and wakefulness.

brain waves: See under wave.

brainstorming (brān′-stor-ming): The spontaneous expression of ideas or thoughts by people meeting in a group without having previously considered the advantages, disadvantages, consequences, or practicality of the ideas or thoughts.

brainwashing: A kind of mental conditioning in which stress and mental torture are used to force a captive person to accept a set of beliefs that are contrary to his former beliefs but in accord with those of his captor.

bran: The husk of grain. The coarse outer part of cereals, especially wheat; high in roughage and the vitamin B complex.

branchial (brang′-ki-al): 1. Pertaining to gills. 2. Pertaining to the fissures or clefts which occur on each side of the neck of the human embryo, and which enter into the development of the nose, ears, and mouth; B. CYST, a swelling in the neck arising from the embryonic remnants of a branchial cleft.

brandy: An alcoholic liquid distilled from wine. Contains about 50% alcohol.

brash: 1. A burning sensation in the stomach caused by excessive acidity and often accompanied by belching of sour, burning fluid. Syn., heartburn, pyrosis; water brash. 2. An attack of illness. 3. The appearance of a rash or eruption.

BRAT diet: Bananas, rice, apples, and tea. A diet formerly often used in treating infants and young children with vomiting and diarrhea, to reestablish electrolyte balance and control dehydration.

Braun-Bohler frame: Traction using a weight and pulley system in treating an oblique fracture that is unstable.

Braxton-Hicks contractions: Intermittent contractions of the uterus during pregnancy; painless but can be felt after about the 16th week; they occur about every 15 or 20 minutes, and are not labor pains. Also called Braxton-Hicks sign, Hicks sign.

Brazelton Neonatal Assessment Scale: A scale used in evaluating the behavioral responses of newborns.

breach of duty: A legal term denoting behavior that is not considered "reasonable." In nursing it usually means that a patient was injured or harmed in some way by something

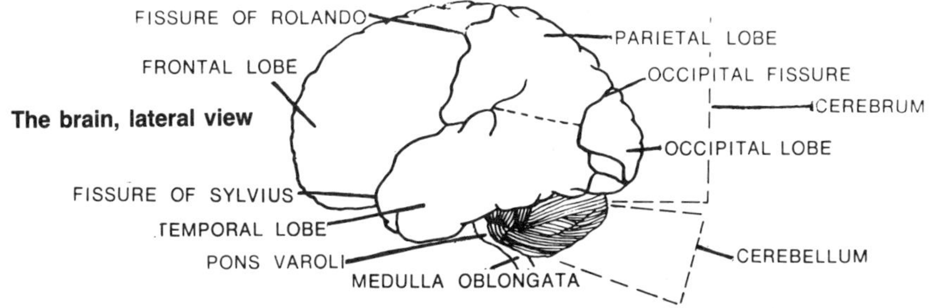

The brain, lateral view

that the nurse did, *e.g.*, causing someone to be burned by a too hot water bag.

break-bone fever: See dengue.

breast: The anterior part of the thorax; the mammary gland. **B. AMPUTATION,** mastectomy (*q.v.*). **B. BONE,** the sternum. **CHICKEN B.,** pigeon **B. FUNNEL B.,** deformity caused by abnormal depression of the sternum. **PIGEON B.,** deformity resulting from prominent sternum, often caused by rickets. **B. PROSTHESIS,** utilized following mastectomy; may be made of foam or filled with air, liquid, or silicone. **B. PUMP,** a hand-operated or electric device for withdrawing milk from the female breast. **B. RECONSTRUCTION,** possible following some operations for breast removal; done to remove scar, replace the nipple and areola, or to introduce a Silastic implant to replace removed breast tissue.

breath: The air inhaled and exhaled during respiration. **B. HOLDING,** a phenomenon seen in young children, usually precipitated by anger, fear, or frustration; the child becomes cyanotic and sometimes loses consciousness briefly and breathing is resumed automatically.

breath sounds: Sounds of air going in and out of the lungs that can be heard with a stethoscope during respiration. **ASTHMATIC B.S.,** characterized by short gasping inspirations and prolonged expirations; high-pitched and wheezing due to narrowing of the airway. **AMPHORIC B.S.,** harsh, high pitched sounds heard in open pneumothorax. **BRONCHIAL B.S.,** high pitched, loud hollow sounds heard over the trachea in the presence of atelectasis and pleural effusion. **BRONCHOVESICULAR B.S.,** blowing sounds of moderate pitch and loudness heard over the scapulae in the back. **CAVERNOUS B.S.,** resemble amphoric **B.S.,** but the sounds are low pitched and hollow. **VESICULAR B.S.,** originate in the alveoli and can be heard over the normal lung.

breath test: A test performed on a person's breath to determine whether he is alcoholically intoxicated. See Breathalyzer.

Breathalyzer (breth′-a-lī-zer): An instrument used for analyzing a person's breath to determine whether the person has imbibed alcohol within a certain period of time, and how much. **B. TEST,** measures expired air to determine the blood alcohol level in percent by weight.

breathe: The act of alternately inhaling air into and exhaling air from the lungs.

breathing (brēth′ ing): The alternate inhalation and exhalation of air to and from the lungs. **APNEUISTIC B., B.** characterized by long inspirations; occurs in severe hypoxia, hypoglycemia, meningitis. **ASTHMATIC B.,** a harsh breathing accompanied by a wheezing sound, expecially on expiration. **BIOT'S B., B.** in a random pattern of deep and shallow respirations occurring irregularly. **CLUSTER B., B.** characterized by clusters of breaths occurring in a disorderly fashion with pauses between the clusters. **COGWHEEL B.,** jerky **B. CONTINUOUS POSITIVE PRESSURE BREATHING, B.** that is assisted by a ventilator that administers air or a mixture of gases under continuous positive pressure which fluctuates to permit air to flow into and out of the lungs; also called continuous positive pressure ventilation; abbreviated CPPB. **DIAPHRAGMATIC B.,** that accomplished chiefly by movements of the diaphragm; also called abdominal **B. EUPNIC B.,** free easy breathing; the type observed in normal persons at rest. **GLOSSOPHARYNGEAL B., B.** accomplished by gulping air rapidly and using the tongue and muscles of the pharynx to force the air into the respiratory tract; neither the main muscles of respiration nor the accessory muscles are involved; also called frog **B., INTERMITTENT POSITIVE PRESSURE B., B.** with the assistance of a respirator that administers air or a mixture of gases under positive pressure during inspiration until a preset pressure is reached; also called intermittent positive pressure ventilation; abbreviated IPPB. **PARADOXICAL B.,** seen after severe chest injury; the injured part bulges during exhalation and is sucked in during inspiration; see flail chest. **PERIODIC B.,** see Cheyne-Stokes respiration under respiration. **POSITIVE PRESSURE B.,** the breathing of air or oxygen that is under a constant pressure relative to the ambient pressure. **PURSED-LIP B.,** exhaling slowly through the mouth with the lips "pursed" as for whistling; it prolongs the exhalation, increases the pressure in the airway, less air is trapped in the alveoli, and more carbon dioxide is eliminated. **STERTOROUS B.,** characterized by a snoring sound on expiration.

breathlessness (breth′-les-nes): 1. Not breathing. 2. Panting or gasping for one's breath. 3. Holding one's breath when deeply disturbed emotionally. **PSYCHOGENIC B.,** abnormal or bizarre breathing patterns; seen in the elderly or the demented.

breech (brēch): The buttocks (*q.v.*). **B. PRESENTATION,** the position of the fetus during labor in which the buttocks instead of the head presents at the uterine orifice.

bregma (breg′-ma): The point on the skull at the junction of the coronal and sagittal sutures; the anterior fontanel.—bregmata, pl.; bregmatic, adj.

Brenner tumor: A tumor of the ovary; may be solid or cystic and contain groups of epithelial cells and connective tissue stroma; usually benign.

Brennerman's ulcers: Ulceration of the urinary meatus in the male. Seen primarily in boys in whom the foreskin has been removed by circumcision leaving the area open to infection.

brephotrophic (bref-ō-trōf′-ik): Pertaining to nutrition of the embryo and newborn.

brevicollis (brev-i-kol′-is): Shortness of the neck.

brewer's yeast: A rich source of vitamin B complex; the dried pulverized cells of a yeast (*Saccharomyces cerevisiae*); so called because it is used in the brewing process.

bridge: A structure that joins two parts or organs. **B. OF NOSE,** the upper part of the external nose, formed by union of the nasal bones. In dentistry, a device bearing one or more artificial teeth which is anchored to the natural teeth.

bridging: Providing relief from pressure by suspending the affected area while supporting the surrounding areas.

Bright's disease: Inflammation of the kidney; nephritis. Term formerly often used to describe glomerulonephritis and other kidney diseases marked by proteinuria. [Richard Bright, English physician. 1798–1858.]

Brill's disease: A mild form of typhus fever that may recur many years after the original infection; rare in the U.S. Also called recrudescent typhus, sporadic typhus, and Brill-Sinsser disease. [Nathan Edwards Brill, American physician. 1860–1925.]

brilliant green: An analine dye that is used as 1) a topical antiseptic and bacteriostatic, or 2) an indicator dye that changes from yellow to green when the pH of the substance is at pH 0.0 to pH 2.6.

brim: The edge or margin of a part. **B. OF THE PELVIS,** the bony ring that divides the true from the false pelvis.

Briquet's syndrome: Hysterical paralysis of the diaphragm with shortness of breath and loss of voice.

brisement (brēz′-mon): A crushing; refers particularly to the breaking up by force of the adhesions in ankylosis.

brittle bones: See osteogenesis imperfecta.

broad ligament: Lateral ligament; double fold of parietal peritoneum which hangs over the uterus and outstretched fallopian tubes, forming a lateral partition across the pelvic cavity.

Broadbent's sign: Visible retraction of the left side and back, in the region of the eleventh and twelfth ribs, synchronous with each heart beat and due to adhesions between the pericardium and diaphragm. See pericarditis. [William Broadbent, English physician. 1835–1907.]

broad-spectrum: A term used to describe an agent, particularly an antibiotic, that is effective against a wide variety of microorganisms.

Broca's area (brok′-a): The motor center for speech; situated at the commencement of the sylvian fissure in the left hemisphere of the cerebrum. Injury to this center results in inability to speak. [Pierre Paul Broca, French surgeon. 1824–1880.]

Brock's operation: An operation for the relief of pulmonary valve stenosis.

Brodie-Trendelenburg test: A test to evaluate the competency of the venous valves in patients with varicose veins of the lower legs.

Brodie's abscess: See under abscess.

Brodmann's areas: Specific numbered areas of the cerebral cortex in the occipital and preoccipital areas that have been identified as the seat of specific functions of the brain.

bromhidrosis (brom-hī-drō′-sis): A profuse fetid perspiration, especially associated with the feet, groin, axillae. Syn., body odor, fetid perspiration, osmidrosis.—bromhidrotic, adj. Also bromidrosis.

bromides (brō′-mīdz): A small group of drugs, compounds of bromine and another element, that have a mild depressant action on the central nervous system; elimination is slow and the drug accumulates in the body causing a toxic condition marked by skin eruptions and mental disturbances; once used extensively as a sedative and in treatment of certain forms of epilepsy but now replaced by agents with less objectionable side effects.

bromine (brō′-mēn): A nonmetallic volatile reddish liquid element; unites with hydrogen to form hydrobromic acid which combines with many metals to form bromides.

bromism (brō′-mizm): Chronic poisoning due to continued or excessive use of bromides; characterized by lethargy, headache, dysarthria, acne-like skin lesions, sometimes mania or psychotic behavior. Also brominism.

bromoderma (brō-mō-der′-ma): Skin eruption resembling acne caused by use of bromine or its compounds. Often a symptom of brominism (*q.v.*). **NODOSE B.,** the occurrence of nodular lesions on the legs in association with bromoderma.

bromohyperhydrosis (brō′-mō-hī′-per-hī-drō′-sis): Excessive secretion of sweat having a fetid odor.

bromomania (brō′-mō-mā′-ni-a): Psychosis or delirium caused by overuse of bromides.

bromomenorrhea (brō′-mō-men-ō-rē′-a): Profuse offensive-smelling menses.

bromopnea (brō-mop-nē′-a): Abnormally foul or fetid breath.

Brompton's cocktail: An .analgesic mixture given on a regular basis to patients with advanced cancer to relieve pain that cannot be controlled by ordinary analgesics without clouding the sensorium. The original recipe called for heroin, cocaine, chloroform water, and ethanol; today it is usually simply an elixer of morphine.

Bromsulphalein (brōm-sul′-fa-lē-in): A preparation of sulfobromophthalein, a dye used in liver function tests; it is injected intravenously. Normally 80% of the dye is removed by the liver and the rest by other organs; in pathological conditions, when the liver is not functioning properly, it removes less of the dye which then remains in the blood. Abbreviated BSP.

bronch-, bronchi-, bronchio-, broncho-: Combining forms denoting: 1) bronchus; 2) bronchiole.

bronchadenitis (brong-kad-e-nī′-tis): Inflammation of the bronchial glands. Also broncho-adenitis.

bronchial (brong′-ki-al): Pertaining to or affecting the bronchi. **B. ASTHMA,** see under asthma; **B. BREATH SOUNDS,** see under breath sounds. **B. HYGIENE,** the maintenance of a clear airway and removal of secretions from the tracheobronchial tree. **B. PNEUMONIA,** see bronchopneumonia. **B. TREE,** the bronchi and all their branching structures. **B. TUBES,** subdivisions of the bronchi after they enter the lungs.

bronchiarctia (brong-ki-ark′-shi-a): Bronchiostenosis (*q.v.*).

bronchiectasis (brong-ki-ek′-ta-sis): Chronic dilatation of the bronchioles; the alveolar sacs become dilated and filled with large quantities of offensive pus. Characterized by productive cough, expectoration of mucopurulent material, fetid breath, and enlargement of the air passages. Usually follows such infection as bronchopneumonia with lobular collapse, which may have occurred in infancy. May lead to greatly limited ventilatory capacity and recurrent infection of the lungs, lung abscess, or amyloid disease. Also bronchiectasia.—bronchiectatic, adj.

bronchiocele (brong′-ki-ō-sēl): A circumscribed area of dilatation in a bronchiole. Bronchocele.

bronchiole (brong′-ki-ōl): One of the minute subdivisions of the bronchi which terminate in the alveoli or air sacs of the lungs.—bronchiolar, adj.

bronchiolectasis (brong-ki-ō-lek′-ta-sis): Dilatation of the bronchioles.

bronchiolitis (brong-ki-ō-lī′-tis): An acute infection of the lower respiratory tract, usually caused by a parainfluenza virus or respiratory syncytial virus (RSV); may be extremely serious in children under three, but in older children the symptoms are usually those of a simple cold. It is spread by contact and by air-borne particles. **B. OBLITERANS,** a complication of inhalation of smoke or other irritating fumes; exudate that forms in the bronchioles obliterates the lumen, resulting in chest pain, unproductive cough, shortness of breath; may be fatal due to respiratory insufficiency. Also called capillary bronchitis and bronchopneumonia.—bronchiolitic, adj.

bronchiolus (brong-ki-ō′-lus): One of the smaller subdivisions of the bronchus.—bronchioli, pl. Syn., bronchiole.

bronchitis (brong-kī′-tis): Inflammation of the bronchial mucous membrane; may be primary or secondary, acute or chronic. **ACUTE B.,** occurs chiefly in young children or elderly persons; usually an extension of infection following a common cold, upper respiratory infection, measles, or influenza. **ACUTE LARYNGEAL B.,** a form of winter croup that resembles diphtheria except that no membrane forms; occurs chiefly in infants under one year of age. **ASTHMATIC B.,** symptoms of asthma associated with an apparent bronchial infection. **CHRONIC B.,** occurs chiefly in older persons; may follow acute **B.,** develop gradually, or be secondary to another condition such as sinusitis, or to cigarette smoking; tends to recur and to be worse in cold, foggy weather; can cause right-sided heart failure, especially when associated with gross emphysema. See cor pulmonale.—bronchitic, adj.

bronchoblennorrhea (brong′-kō-blen-ō-rē′-a): Expectoration of copious mucopurulent sputum, often seen in chronic bronchitis.

bronchocele (brong′-kō-sēl): 1. A circumscribed swelling or dilatation of a bronchus. 2. A goiter.

bronchocephalitis (brong′-kō-sef-a-lī′-tis): Whooping cough. See pertussis.

bronchoconstriction (brong′-kō-kon-strik′-shun): Bronchostenosis (*q.v.*).

bronchoconstrictor (brong′-kō-kon-strik′-tor): Any agent that causes constriction of the bronchi thus decreasing the caliber of the pulmonary air passages.

bronchodilatation (brong′-kō-dil-a-tā′-shun): Widening of the caliber of the bronchi by the use of drugs or by surgical procedure.

bronchodilator (brong-kō-dī′-lā-tor): Any agent or surgical instrument that is used to dilate the bronchi thus increasing the caliber of the pulmonary air passages.

bronchoesophagology (brong′-kō-ē-sof-a-gol′-o-ji): The medical specialty that deals with the diseases and disorders of the tracheobronchial tree and the esophagus.

bronchoesophagoscopy (brong′-kō-ē-sof-a-gos′-kō-pi): Examination of the tracheobronchial tree and the esophagus with special endoscopes.

bronchofiberscope (brong-kō-fī′-ber-scōp): A specially designed fiberscope for visualization of the trachea and bronchi.

bronchogenic (brong-kō-jen′-ik): Arising from a bronchus. **B. CARCINOMA,** any of several types of carcinoma that arise in the bronchi.

bronchogram (brong′-kō-gram): Radiological picture of the bronchial tree after the introduction of a radiopaque material.

bronchography (brong-kog′-raf-i): Preparation of x-ray film after introduction of radiopaque substance into the bronchial tree.—bronchographic, adj.; bronchographically, adv.

broncholith (brong′-kō-lith): A stone or concretion in a bronchus or bronchial tube.

broncholithiasis (brong′-kō-li-thī′-a-sis): The formation and presence of concretions in the tracheobronchial tree.

bronchomalacia (brong′-kō-ma-lā′-shi-a): Softening and degeneration of the elastic and connective tissues of the trachea and bronchi; the condition may be congenital or acquired, and may result eventually in obstructive emphysema or atelectasis.

bronchomycosis (brong-kō-mī-kō′-sis): General term used to cover a variety of fungus infections of the bronchi and lungs, *e.g.*, pulmonary moniliasis, aspergillosis (*q.v.*).—bronchomycotic, adj.

broncopathy (brong-kop′-a-thi): Any disease or abnormality of the bronchi and/or bronchioles.

bronchophony (brong-kof′-o-ni): Abnormal voice sounds as heard through the stethoscope when applied over consolidated lung tissue. See also pectoriloquy.

bronchopleural fistula (brong-kō-ploo′-ral fis′-tūl-a): Pathological communication between the pleural cavity and a bronchus.

bronchopneumonia (brong′-kō-nū-mō′-ni-a): Inflammation of the bronchi and lungs; small areas of the lungs are consolidated and coalesce but do not have a lobular distribution; usually begins at the termini of bronchioles and alveoli and spreads throughout the lungs. Caused by a number of microorganisms including *Streptococcus pneumoniae, Staphylococcus pyogenes,* and *Mycoplasma pneumoniae*; may occur as a primary infection in infants and the aged, in whom it is relatively common, but may also be secondary to measles, whooping cough, upper respiratory infections, and debilitating diseases; may also result from inhalation of noxious gases or dusts or from aspiration of infected material from the respiratory or gastrointestinal tract; in young children the cause is often tthe respiratory syncytical virus (*q.v.*). Symptoms include chest pain, cough with purulent (sometimes bloody) sputum, chills, fever; high pulse and respiration rates; weakness. Complications include pulmonary abscess, empyema, peripheral thrombosis, jaundice, congestive heart failure. Also called lobular pneumonia, bronchial pneumonia, bronchiolitis, and bronchioalveolitis.

bronchopneumonitis (brong′-kō-nū-mō-nī′-tis): Bronchopneumonia (*q.v.*).

bronchopulmonary (brong-kō-pul′-mō-nar-i): Pertaining to the bronchi and the lungs. **B. DYSPLASIA**, a condition that exists throughout life in persons who received oxygen therapy as infants; lungs are overinflated, areas of the lobes are emphysemic, and there is damage to bronchioles and alveoli.

bronchorrhagia (brong-kō-rā′-ji-a): Hemorrhage from the bronchi; see hemoptysis.

bronchorrhea (brong-kō-rē′-a): An excessive discharge from the bronchial mucous membrane.—bronchorrheal, adj.

bronchoscope (brong′-kō-skōp): A curved, lighted, flexible endoscope (*q.v.*) used for examining the interior of the bronchi, removing a foreign body, or taking a specimen for biopsy, etc.—bronchoscopy, n.; bronchoscopic, adj.; bronchoscopically, adv.

bronchoscopy (brong-kos′-kō-pi): Direct visualization of the bronchi with a bronchoscope. Most often done for patients with persistent cough, wheezing, hemoptysis, or with signs of tumor; for viewing or removing an obstruction; to create an airway; or to obtain material for biopsy. **FIBEROPTIC B.**, can be done at the bedside using a local anesthetic. **RIGID B.**, utilizes a rigid scope; is done in the operating room under general anesthesia.

bronchospasm (brong′-kō-spazm): Sudden, temporary constriction of the bronchial tubes due to contraction of involuntary plain muscle in their walls; the chief characteristic of asthma and bronchitis.

bronchospirometer (brong′-kō-spī-rom′-e-ter): An instrument used to measure the oxygen intake and carbon dioxide output of a lung, or of each lung separately.—bronchospirometric, adj.; bronchospirometry, n.

bronchospirometry (brong′-kō-spi-rom′-e-tri): Determination of the functional capacity of either or both lungs or a segment of a lung.

bronchostenosis (brong-kō-ste-nō′-sis): Narrowing of a bronchus.—bronchostenotic, adj.

bronchostomy (brong-kos′-tō-mi): The surgical procedure of creating an opening through the chest wall into a bronchus.

bronchotomy (brong-kot′-ō-mi): A surgical incision into the larynx, trachea, or a bronchus.

bronchotracheal (brong-kō-trā′-kē-al): Pertaining to the bronchi and the trachea.

bronchovasoconstrictor (brong′-kō-vā′-sō-kon-strik′-tor): An agent that causes constriction of the blood vessels in the bronchi.

bronchus (brong′-kus): One of the two tubes into which the trachea divides; each tube enters a lung, where it divides and subdivides. The bronchi serve as passageways for air going into and out of the lungs; they are made up of three coats—an outer fibrous coat, a middle coat of smooth muscle, and an inner coat of ciliated mucous membrane.—bronchi, pl.; bronchial, adj.

brontophobia (bron-tō-fō′-bi-a): Abnormal fear of thunder.

bronze diabetes: See under **diabetes.**

Brooke Formula: A widely used formula for estimating the amount of fluid to be replaced during the first 24 hours of therapy for patients with burns of up to 50 percent of body surface area. It calls for: 1) lactated Ringer's solution, 1.5 ml per kg of body weight per percent of body area burned; 2) colloid (blood, dextran, plasma), 0.5 ml per kg of body weight per percent of area burned; and 3) water (glucose in water), the amount dependent on weight and size of the patient (2000 ml for an adult). One-half of the patient's estimated requirement for the first 24 hours is given during the first eight hours and one-quarter during each of the two following eight-hour periods.

brossage (brō-sazh′): Brushing with a stiff brush to remove granulations, especially from the everted eyelids in cases of trachoma.

Brothers Hospitallers of St. John of God: A religious order founded in Spain in 1538 and spread throughout the world; members were chiefly interested in caring for the mentally ill, but cared for other patients as well; established and maintained hospitals wherever they worked.

brow: The forehead; the region of the supraorbital ridge. **B. PRESENTATION,** the position of the fetus during labor in which the brow presents at the uterine orifice making normal delivery almost impossible.

brown atrophy: Descriptive of changes in the myocardium of aging patients; there is loss of heart weight and infiltration of the muscle cells by lipofuscin (*q.v.*); may or may not be significant.

brown fat: A mass of tissue in the neck and scapular region of the newborn; its function is thought to be the storage of fat and formation of blood. Also interscapular gland.

brown lung disease: Byssinosis (*q.v.*).

brown recluse spider: Loxsosceles reclusa. For effects of bite, see **loxsoscelism.**

brownian movement or motion: The peculiar, random, dancing movements exhibited by finely divided particles in solution; often seen in microscopic viewing of bacteria in suspension.

Brown-Sequard's syndrome: Hemiplegia caused by damage to a lateral half of the spinal cord; associated with ipsilateral motor paralysis, loss of joint and tendon sensation, decreased tactile determination, contralateral anesthesia, and loss of temperature sense.

Bruce treadmill test: An exercise to assess the patient's tolerance for increased exercise or physical activity after myocardial infarction; consists of walking on a slowly moving slightly tilted treadmill which gradually goes faster; the patient is attached to an electrocardiograph machine that measures and records blood pressure at the various speeds.

Brucella (broo-sel′-la): A genus of bacteria causing brucellosis (undulant fever in man; contagious abortion in cattle). **B. ABORTIS** is the bovine strain, **B. MELITENSIS,** the goat strain; both transmissible to man via infected milk. **B. SUIS,** a species of **B.** found in swine; capable of producing severe infection in humans. **B. TEST,** a test for undulant fever.

Brucellaceae (broo-sel-lā′-sē-ē): A large family of rodshaped, gram-negative bacteria that are pathogenic to animals and man; includes *Brucella, Bordetella, Francisella, Hemophilus,* and *Pasteurella.*

brucelliasis (broo-sel-lī′-a-sis): Infection with the *Brucella* group of organisms; brucellosis.

brucellosis (broo-sel-lō′-sis): A generalized acute or chronic infection of animals and man; caused by one of the species of Brucella; rarely transmitted from man to man but spreads from animal to animal and from animal to man. In man, characterized by recurrent attacks of fever and mental depression, headache, malaise, anorexia, anemia, weight loss, weakness, sweating, constipation, muscle and joint pain, splenomegaly. Complications include pnuemonia, arthritis, endocarditis, peripheral neuritis, cirrhosis of the liver, cystitis.

Bruch's membrane: The basal layer of the choroid which is in contact with the pigmented layer of the retina. Also called Henle's membrane.

Brudzinski's sign: Either of two reflexes seen in patients with meningitis. 1. Neck sign; immediate flexion of knees and hips on raising head from pillow. 2. Leg sign; when one leg is flexed onto the abdomen, the other knee and leg tend to flex also. [Josef von Brudzinski, Polish physician. 1874–1917.]

Brugia (broo′-ji-a): A genus of nematode parasites transmitted to man and other mammals by mosquitoes. **B. MALAYI,** a species found in Malaya and other areas in the far East; infestation characterized by lymphangiitis and lymphadenitis.

bruise (brooz): A discoloration of the skin due to an extravasation of blood into the underlying tissues; caused by an impact injury; there is no abrasion of the skin. A contusion.

bruit (broo′-ē): An extracardiac diagnostically important whooshing sound heard on auscultation over a blood vessel, gland, or organ. When heard over an artery it is produced by the passage of blood over an irregular surface or through a narrowed portion of the vessel; when heard over the aorta it may indicate the presence of an aneurysm; when heard over the abdomen it may indicate a constricted or dilated vessel. **DIASTOLIC B.,** a **B.** heard after the second heart sound; usually indicates abnormal valve function. **SYSTOLIC B.**, a **B.** heard between the first and second sounds during the systolic phase of the cardiac cycle.

Brunner's glands: Compound glands in the submucous layer of the duodenal wall.

Bruns' frame: A special frame used for a child or infant with congenital hip dislocation; provides bilateral leg traction and maximum abduction of the leg.

Brun's syndrome: Paroxysmal headache, with visual symptoms, vertigo, vomiting, and sometimes syncope, when the position of the head is suddenly changed; one cause is thought to be a lesion in the 3rd or 4th ventricle of the brain which interferes with the flow of cerebrospinal fluid.

Brushfield's spots: White or pale yellow pinpoint spots seen in the periphery of the iris in children with Down's syndrome; they disappear if the eye color changes to brown; considered diagnostic.

bruxism (bruks'-izm): Grinding of the teeth, especially during sleep.

bruxomania (bruks-ō-mā'-ni-a): Grinding of the teeth during waking hours; a neurotic habit.

BSA: Abbreviation for body surface area.

BSE: Abbreviation for breast self-examination.

BSN: Abbreviation for Bachelor of Science in Nursing.

BSR: Abbreviation for blood sedimentation rate. See erythrocyte sedimentation rate.

BTU: Abbreviation for British thermal unit; the amount of heat required to raise the temperature of one pound of water one degree Fahrenheit.

bubo (bū'-bō): An inflammatory swelling of a lymph node, especially in the groin or axilla, due to absorption of infective material, often proceeding to suppuration. A feature of soft sore (chancroid), lymphogranuloma, inguinale, and plague.—bubonic, adj.

bubonalgia (bū-bō-nal'-ji-a): Pain in the groin or inguinal region.

bubonic plague (bū-bon'-ik plāg): An acute, infectious, frequently fatal disease caused by *yersinia pestis* which is carried in infected rats and transmitted to man by the bite of rat fleas; characterized by chills, fever, and formation of buboes. This was the Black Death of the Middle Ages. See plague.

bubonocele (bū-bon'-o-sēl): An inguinal hernia, particularly one in which the knuckle of intestine has not yet pushed through the external abdominal ring.

bucardia (bū-kar'-di-a): Extreme enlargement of the heart.

bucca (buk'-a): The cheek.

buccal (buk'-al): Pertaining to the cheek or mouth. **B. ADMINISTRATION**, administration of a medication by placing it in the cheek and allowing absorption of it through the oral mucosa. **B. CAVITY**, the part of the oral cavity between the inner surface of the cheek and the teeth. **B. SMEAR**, see under smear.

buccinator (buk'-si-nā-tor): The chief muscle of the cheek.

buccocervical (buk-ō-ser'-vi-kal): Pertaining to the cheek and the neck.

buccogingival (buk-ō-jin'-ji-val): Pertaining to the cheek and the gum.

buccolabial (buk-ō-lā'-bi-al): Pertaining to the cheek and the lips.

buccolingual (buk-ō-ling'-wal): Pertaining to the cheek and the tongue.

buccopharyngeal (buk-ō-fa-rin'-jē-al): Pertaining to the cheek and the pharynx.

buccula (buk'-ū-la): Double chin.

bucking: An informal term referring to gagging on an endotracheal tube.

Buck's extension: See under traction.

bud: In anatomy, a small protuberance on a part resembling the bud of a plant. **TASTE B.**, one of the many end organs for the sense of taste; minute flask-shaped structures located on the tongue, the surface of the soft palate, and posterior part of the epiglottis; contain specialized epithelial cells and fibrils of the nerves of taste.

Budd-Chiari syndrome: Obstruction of the hepatic veins; may be acute or chronic, and either form may be fatal. Cause may be a neoplasm; hepatic disease, stricture or trauma; or systemic infection.

budding (bud'-ing): Asexual reproduction by division into two unequal parts.

Buerger-Allen exercise: Buerger exercise (*q.v.*) plus active exercise of the feet.

Buerger's disease: Thromboangiitis obliterans; obliterative vascular disease of peripheral blood vessels. Occurs more often in men than in women and in smokers than non-smokers.

Buerger's exercise: Designed to treat arterial insufficiency of the lower limbs; consists of alternate elevation and dependence of the legs; a rest period, and then repetition of the exercise. [Leo Buerger, American physician. 1879–1943.]

"buffalo hump": A deposit of fatty tissue in the interscapular area; seen in persons with Cushing's syndrome. Informal.

buffer: 1. A chemical substance which, when present in a solution, causes resistance to pH change (*q.v.*) when acids or alkalis are added. Sodium bicarbonate is one of the chief buffers of the blood and tissue fluids. 2. A substance which tends to offset the reaction of another agent when given in conjunction with it. **BUFFER SYSTEM** in the blood, keeps the pH of the blood serum at normal levels, chiefly by the actions of bicarbonate ions and dissolved carbon dioxide on each other.

bulb: 1. A rounded, globular part of a vessel or tube. 2. Old name for the medulla oblongata. **OLFACTORY B.**, The bulbous end of each olfactory tract; situated on the underside of the anterior lobe of the cerebrum, one on each side of the longitudinal fissure. **VESTIBULAR B.**, the paired masses of erectile tissue at each side of the vaginal opening, joined by a thin strand below the clitoris.

bulbar (bul-bar): 1. Pertaining to a bulbous structure. 2. Pertaining to the medulla oblongata.

bulbitis (bul-bi′-tis): Inflammation of the bulbous part of the urethra.

bulbocavernosis (bul′-bō-kav-er-nō′-sis): One of the muscles of the female pelvic floor; extends from the perineum to the clitoris, one on each side.

bulbonuclear (bul-bō-nū′-klē-ar): Pertaining to the medulla oblongata and the nuclei situated within it.

bulbospinal (bul-bō-spī′-nal): Pertaining to the medulla oblongata and the spinal cord, particularly to the nerve fibers which connect them.

bulbourethal (bul-bō-ū-rē′-thral): Applied to two racemose glands (Cowper's) which open into the bulb of the male urethra.

bulbous (bul′-bus): Resembling a bulb.

bulimia (bū-lim′-i-a): Insatiable appetite or hunger, usually experienced soon after a meal; seen in some cerebral lesions, diabetes mellitus and psychotic states. **B. NERVOSA**, refers to the uncontrollable urge to overeat followed by induced vomiting or purging.

bulkage (bulk′-ij): A material such as agar which increases the volume of the intestinal content, thereby stimulating peristalsis.

bulla (bul′-la): A large watery vesicle; a bleb. In dermatology, bulla formation is characteristic of the pemphigus group of dermatoses, but it also occurs in contact dermatides such as those caused by burns, sunburn, poison oak and poison ivy; in bullous impetigo and dermatitis herpetiformis; and on the palms and soles in scarlet fever and congenital syphilis.—bullae, pl.; bullate, bullous, adj.

bullous pemphigoid (bul′-us pem′-fi-goyd): A chronic skin condition in which large bullae occur over a wide area, especially on the lower abdomen, groin, and inner aspect of the thigh; the tendency to occur increases with age.

BUN: Abbreviation for blood urea nitrogen.

bundle branch block: See under **heart block**.

bundle of His (hiss): Consists of neuromuscular fibers that arise at the atrioventricular node, pass along the interventricular septum, and finally divide into right and left branches that are distributed throughout the ventricular walls. They transmit the impulse for ventricular contraction; failure to do so produces heart block (*q.v.*). [William His, German physician. 1863–1934.]

bundle of Kent: A bundle of modified cardiac muscle tissue which begins at the atrioventricular node, extends into the intraventricular septum, with its branches terminating in the subendocardium of the right and left ventricles.

bunion (bun′-yun): Syn., hallux valgus. A deformity of the head of the metatarsal bone at its junction with the great toe. Friction and pressure of shoes at this point cause the bursa to become inflamed and enlarged thus causing enlargement of the joint and lateral displacement of the great toe. The prominent bone with its bursa is called a bunion. **TAILOR'S B.**, inflammation and enlargement of the head of the fifth metatarsal bone.

bunionectomy (bun-yun-ek′-tō-mi): The surgical removal of a bunion.

buphthalmos (boof-thal′-mos): A condition of infants in which there is an increase in intraocular fluid with consequent increase in the size of the eyeball. Also called congenital glaucoma.

buret, burette (bū-ret′): A graduated glass tube fitted with a stopcock, used for measuring liquids and for delivering an accurately measured amount of a liquid.

Burkitt's tumor: Primary malignant lymphoma occurring chiefly in male children between two and 14 years of age and living in a geographical area of Africa where malaria and other mosquito-borne diseases are endemic; thought to be caused by the Barr-Epstein virus. The rapidly growing tumor occurs most often in the jaw bone and orbit of the eye, but may also occur in abdominal and other organs. [Denis Burkitt, 20th century surgeon in Uganda.]

burn: 1. A lesion of the tissues due to chemicals, dry heat, electricity, flame, friction, or radiation; usually classified in three degrees: a) first degree, erythema; b) second degree, vesiculation; and c) third degree, destruction of epidermis and dermis, and damage to underlying tissues. A fourth degree is recognized when the burn is deep enough to involve fascia, muscle, and bone. 2. In chemistry, to oxidize. 3. To feel the sensation of heat. **CHEMICAL B.**, one due to a caustic chemical. **FLASH B.**, one due to a sudden brief exposure to radiant heat, as that caused by an atomic explosion. **FRICTION B.**, one caused by friction or rapid movement of skin over an abrasive substance or of an abrasive substance over skin; also called brush burn. **RADIATION B.**, overexposure to x rays, ultraviolet rays, radium, or atomic energy. See **rule of nines**.

burn center: A special health care facility designed, staffed, and maintained for the care of severely burned patients; may or may not be an adjunct to another health care facility.

burning foot syndrome: The sensation of burning and other abnormal sensations in the feet and sometimes in the hands; occurs in the elderly, persons with various neurological disturbances, alcoholics, and diabetics.

burnout (burn′-owt): A psychological and physical state characterized by listlessness, pessimism, apathy, and lack of motivation, interest, and energy, particularly in relation to one's work; often appears to be a result of career-related stress such as excessive demands on a person's strength, energy, and resources, disappointment in lack of advancement, or conflict between the job and family responsibilities.

Burow's solution: Aluminum acetate solution; used topically as an astringent and antiseptic in a variety of skin disorders.

burping (burp′-ing): Belching.

burr: 1. **B. CELLS**, red blood cells with blunt cytoplasmic projections like those of acanthocytes; may be seen in the cells of persons with various disorders of the blood, cancer of the stomach, and gastric ulcers, or extensive burns. 2. A rotary cutting instrument used: a) in operations on bones, or b) in dentistry, to open and prepare tooth cavities. **B. HOLES**, holes made in the skull with a burr; for diagnostic purposes, for removing a clot, to aspirate an abscess or cerebrospinal fluid, to permit removal of a brain tumor, or to relieve intracranial pressure. Cranial trephination.

bursa (bur′-sa): A fibrous sac lined with synovial membrane and containing a small quantity of synovial fluid. Bursae are found between 1) tendon and bone; 2) skin and bone; 3) muscle and muscle. Their function is to facilitate movement without friction between these surfaces.—bursae, pl.

bursectomy (bur-sek′-to-mi): The surgical removal of a bursa (*q.v.*).

bursitis (bur-sī′-tis): Inflammation of a bursa; may be acute or may develop slowly after repeated injuries or strain. Characterized by pain, swelling, and tenderness. Prominent locations are the deltoid bursa of the shoulder; the radiohumeral bursa of the elbow, as in miner's, student's, or tennis elbow; and the metatarsophalangeal bursa of the great toe where it becomes the cause of a bunion. **ACHILLES B.**, involves the bursa between the A. tendon and the posterior surface of the calcaneus; characterized by heel pain; frequently occurs in the elderly and often due to ill fitting shoes; also called Haglund's disease. **ISCHIAL B.**, inflammation of the bursa over the tuberosity of the ischium, caused by prolonged sitting; also called weaver's bottom. **OLECRANON B.**, epicondylitis (*q.v.*). **PREPATELLAR B.**, inflammation of the large bursa in front of the patella; also called housemaid's knee.

bursolith (bur′-sō-lith): A concretion within a bursa.

bursopathy (bur-sop′-a-thi): Any disease or disorder of a bursa.

Burton tongs: See under tongs.

butterfly: B. TAPING, a technique utilizing a butterfly-shaped piece of adhesive material to hold the edges of a wound together instead of stitching them, or to hold a tracheostomy tube in place. **B. RASH**, a rash in the shape of a butterfly extending over the nose and cheeks; seen in lupus erythematosus and certain skin disorders.

buttock (but′-ok): One of the two fleshy projections posterior to the hip joints. Formed mainly of the gluteal muscles.

button: A small round plastic device used to plug an opening such as a tracheostomy opening.

butyric (bū-tir′-ik): Relating to butter. **B. ACID**, occurs naturally in butter, cod liver oil, sweat, feces, urine, and other substances; has an unpleasant odor; is a product of the putrefaction of protein.

butyroid (bū′-ti-royd): Resembling butter.

bypass: An auxillary flow, or shunt (*q.v.*). Often applies to a temporary or permanent surgical grafting of blood vessels to detour blood around occluded segments of arteries or veins. **CARDIOPULMONARY B.**, exclusion of the heart and lungs from the circulation; blood is diverted from the right atrium via a pump-oxygenator, and returned to the aorta. **CORONARY B.**, surgical construction of a detour, usually consisting of a graft utilizing a strip from the saphenous vein, through which blood can bypass narrowed or occluded portions of a coronary artery. See also shunt.

byssinosis (bis-in-ō-sis): A chronic industrial disease of the lungs occurring in cotton workers especially, due to inhalation of cotton dust. Also occurs in those working with hemp or flax. Characterized by tightness in the chest, dyspnea, coughing, wheezing; may lead to bronchitis, emphysema, respiratory failure.

C

C: 1. Abbreviation for: a) calorie (large); b) centigrade or Celsius; c) contraction. 2. Chemical symbol for carbon.

c: Abbreviation for: 1) *cum* [L.] meaning with; usually written c̄, or 2) calorie (small).

CA: Abbreviation for chronological age.

Ca: 1. Abbreviation for: a) carcinoma; b) cathode. 2. Chemical symbol for calcium.

cabinet bath: A bath utilizing hot air or steam, and in which only the patient's head is exposed, the rest of the body being in an enclosed box that is heated by electricity.

Cabot's ring bodies: Bluish lines in the form of figures of eight or loops, seen in the stained red blood cells of individuals with severe anemia, especially the anemia that occurs in lead poisoning.

cac-, caco-: Combining form denoting bad, abnormal, defective, deformed, diseased.

cacao (ka-kā'-ō): The seeds from a South American tree, *Theobroma cacao,* from which cocoa, chocolate, and cocoa butter are prepared.

cacesthesia (kak-es-thē'-zi-a): 1. Any disorder of sensibility or of the sense organs. 2. Malaise; unresponsiveness.

cachectic (ka-kek'-tik): Pertaining to or characterized by cachexia.

cachet (ka-shā'): 1. A lens-shaped absorbable capsule for enclosing a dose of medicine to be taken orally. 2. A flat capsule made of circles of rice paper sealed together and enclosing a dose of any bitter powdered drug to be taken orally. 3. A cone-shaped piece of equipment made of lead, used in application of a radioactive substance.

cachexia (ka-kek'-si-a): A term denoting a state of constitutional disorder, malnutrition, general ill health, and wasting away of body tissue. The chief signs are pale mucous membranes, anemia, emaciation, sallow unhealthy skin, and heavy lusterless eyes.—cachectic, adj.

cachinnation (kak-i-nā'-shun): Hysteric or immoderate laughter without any apparent cause; often seen in certain psychoses including schizophrenia.

cacodemonomania (cak-ō-dē'-mon-ō-mā'-ni-a): A mental condition in which the patient believes himself to be possessed by an evil spirit.

cacogenesis (kak-ō-jen'-e-sis): 1. Abnormal growth or development. 2. Congenital malformation. 3. Racial deterioration.

cacoguesia (kak-ō-gū'-si-a): Term usually applies to a bad taste not necessarily due to anything ingested; often occurs with the aura that precedes some epileptic seizures.

cacomelia (kak-ō-mē'-li-a): Congenital deformity of a limb or limbs.

cacoplastic (kak-ō-plas'-tik): 1. Defective growth or development. 2. Lacking ability to grow or develop normally.

cacorhythmia (kak-ō-rith'-mi-a): Abnormal cardiac rhythm.

cacosmia (kak-oz'-mi-a): 1. A foul odor. 2. A hallucination of an odor, particularly of putrefaction.

cacumen (kak-ū'-men): The top or apex of a body part or structure.

cadaver (ka-dav'-er): A corpse or dead body.—cadaveric, cadaverous, adj.

Cadet Nurse Corps: Created in 1943 by Federal legislation to assist in overcoming the nurse shortage during World War II; applicants had to agree to remain in nursing for the duration of the war, were given an allowance that covered their expenses including tuition. Schools of nursing were required to shorten the course to 30 months; discrimination among applicants on the basis of color or marital status was not allowed.

cadmium (kad'-mi-um): A metallic element formerly used in medications but now used chiefly in industry; of importance because of its potential for causing poisoning due to inhalation of cadmium fumes by workers in such industries as electroplating, or from eating foods stored in cadmium-lined containers. Symptoms include nausea, vomiting, dyspnea, prostration, headache, pulmonary edema.

caduceus (ka-dū'-sē-us): Insignia of the medical corps of the U.S. Army. Consists of the wand of Hermes or Mercury entwined with two serpents. The insignia of the medical profession is the staff of Aesculapius which has one serpent twined about it. See also Aesculapius.

caelotherapy (sē-lō-ther'-a-pi): The use of religion in therapeutics.

caesarean: See cesarean.

café au lait spots (ka-fā-ō-lāy'): Flat light brown spots on the skin as seen in neurofibromatosis; may also occur normally in the aging.

caffeine (kaf'-ēn): An odorless, white, bitter powder obtained from the leaves and beans of tea, coffee, maté, and guarana; used medically as a central nervous system stimulant, a cardiac stimulant, a diuretic, and in headache remedies.

caffeinism (kaf'-ēn-izm): A condition induced by excessive use of coffee or other caffeine-containing preparations. Symptoms include insomnia, irritability, palpitation and dyspepsia.

Caffey's disease: A type of hyperostosis (*q.v.*) of infants in which there is swelling of the tissues over the affected bone, fever, irritability, and periods of exacerbation and remission. Also called infantile cortical hyperostosis.

cage: **THORACIC C.**, the bony structure that encloses the organs of the thorax (*q.v.*); is made up of the sternum, ribs, and part of the vertebral column.

caisson disease (kā′-son): A condition variously called decompression illness, the bends, vascular necrosis of bone, divers' disease. Results from sudden reduction in atmospheric pressure as occurs, *e.g.*, in divers on returning to surface, or airmen ascending to great heights. Due to bubbles of nitrogen which are released from solution in the blood; symptoms vary according to the site of these. The condition is largely preventable by proper and gradual decompression technique.

Cal: Abbreviation for large calorie.

calabar (kal′-a-bar): A disease seen chiefly in Africa; caused by a parasitic falarial worm that enters through the skin and causes the development of lumps in the subcutaneous tissue; may also enter the anterior chamber of the eye. Loa loa is one type of this disease.

calamine (kal′-a-mīn): **1.** Zinc carbonate. **2.** A preparation of zinc oxide and ferric oxide, a pink powder used in treatment of certain skin diseases; also used in ointments and lotions as a protective and astringent in treating a variety of skin conditions.

calcaneal (kal-kā′-nē-al): Pertaining to the calcaneus or the heel. **C. SPUR,** a bony outgrowth on the lower surface of the calcaneus; caused by repeated traumatic pressure on the heel. **C. TENDON REFLEX,** Achilles reflex; see under reflex.

calcaneoapophysitis (kal-kā′-nē-ō-a-pof-i-sī′-tis): Pain, swelling, and inflammation of the posterior part of the calcaneus at the insertion of the tendon of Achilles.

calcaneocuboid (kal-kā′-nē-ō-kū′-boyd): Pertaining to the calcaneus and cuboid bones.

calcaneodynia (kal-kā′-nē-ō-din′-i-a): Pain in the heel, especially when standing or walking.

calcaneofibular (kal-kā′ nē-ō-fib′ ū-lar): Pertaining to the calcaneus and the fibula.

calcaneonavicular (kal-kā′-nē-ō-na-vik′-ū-lar): Pertaining to the calcaneus and navicular bones.

calcaneus (kal-kā′-nē-us): The heel bone, os calcis; the largest and strongest of the tarsal bones.

calcar (kal′-kar): A spur or spurlike projection. In biology, a pointed, projecting outgrowth of a part, often calciferous.

calcareous (kal-kā′-rē-us): Pertaining to or containing lime or calcium; of a chalky nature.

calcarine (kal′-kar-in): Pertaining to or resembling a calcar (*q.v.*); spur-shaped.

calcariuria (kal-kā-ri-ū′-ri-a): The presence of calcium salts in the urine.

calcemia (kal-sē′-mi-a): The presence of an excessive amount of calcium in the blood.

calcibilia (kal-si-bil′-i-a): The presence of calcium in the bile.

calcicosis (kal-si-kō′-sis): A lung disease, often occupational, due to inhalation of marble dust (calcium carbonate).

calcifames (kal-sif′ a-mēz): A form of pica in which the individual has an abnormal craving to eat calcium-containing substances.

calciferol (kal-sif′-e-rol): Vitamin D_2. Produced synthetically by ultraviolet radiation of ergosterol; has the most vitamin D activity of any substance produced in this way; occurs also in milk and fish liver oils. Used in treatment of rickets, parathyroid deficiency, lupus vulgaris, and osteomalacia; also used prophylactically.

calciferous (kal-sif′-er-us): Containing calcium, lime, or chalk.

calcification (kal-sif-i-kā′-shun): The hardening of an organic substance by a deposit of calcium salts within it. May be normal as in bone or pathological as when it occurs in arteries or other tissues.

calcify (kal′-si-fī): To deposit mineral salts in the body organs or tissues.

calcinosis (kal-si-nō′-sis): Deposition of calcium in various tissues and parts of the body.

calcipenia (kal-si-pē′-ni-a): Deficiency of calcium in the body.

calciprivia (kal-si-priv′-i-a): Deprivation or loss of calcium from the body.

calcitonin (kal-si-tō′-nin): See thyrocalcitonin.

calcium (kal′-si-um): A soft, white metallic element, essential for the formation and maintenance of bone; 2 percent of body weight is calcium, of which 97 percent is in the bones and teeth. Its deposition in the bones is controlled by the parathyroid gland and its utilization by bone is dependent on vitamin D (*q.v.*). It is a vital electrolyte in the blood, especially in relation to clotting, and to neuromuscular activity. Several of its salts are used in medicine. **C. CARBONATE,** a **C.** compound occurring naturally in bone; also prepared artificially for use in therapy as a source of **C.** and as an antacid. **C. CHLORIDE,** an odorless, white granular compound used in medicine as a diuretic and urine acidifier, and as an antiallergenic; in solution it is used to correct electrolyte imbalance. **C. GLUCONATE,** an odorless tasteless salt of calcium; used in tablet and liquid form as a source of C. **C. LACTATE,** a white powder soluble in water; used as a source of **C.** and as a blood coagulant. **C. TEST,** see Sulkowitch's test.

calciuria (kal-si-ū′-ri-a): The presence of calcium in the urine.

calculogenesis (kal-kū-lō-jen′-e-sis): The origin or development of calculi.

calculosis (kal-kū-lō′-sis): The presence of a calculus or of calculi.

calculus (kal′-kū-lus): An abnormal concretion composed chiefly of mineral substances and formed usually in the passages that transmit secretions, or in the cavities that act as reservoirs for them. Commonly called stones. **ARTHRITIC C.,** A deposit of urates in or around a joint. **BILIARY C.,** one formed in a bile duct or gallbladder; a gallstone. **RENAL C.,** one formed in the kidney. **URINARY C.,** one formed in any part of the urinary tract.—calculi, pl.; calculous, calculary, adj.

Caldwell-Luc operation: The surgical procedure of creating an opening through the canine fossa into the maxillary sinus to facilitate drainage of the sinus.

calefacient (kal-e-fā′-shent): An agent that produces a feeling of warmth in the part to which it is applied.

calf (kaf): The muscular portion at the back of the leg below the knee, formed principally by the bellies of the soleus and gastrocnemius muscles. **C. BONE,** the fibula.—calves. pl.

caliber (kal′-i-ber): The diameter of a round structure such as a tube or canal.

calibrate (kal′-i-brāt): To determine, by measurement or by comparison to a standard, the correct value of each unit of measurement on the scale of an instrument or apparatus.—calibrated, adj.; calibration, n.

caligo (ka-lī′-gō): Dimness or obscurity of vision.

caliper (kal′-i-per): 1. A measuring instrument with two adjustable legs for determining thickness, diameter, or distance. 2. In orthopedics, a splint or brace. **SKIN C.,** a **C.** for measuring the thickness of a skinfold. **WALKING C.,** a splint for the lower extremity; two metal legs extend from the posterior of the thigh to a metal plate attached to the sole of the shoe.

calisthenics (kal-is-then′-iks): Systematic light exercises to preserve health, develop muscles and gracefulness.

callomania (kal-ō-mā′-ni-a): A type of mania in which the person has delusions of personal beauty.

callosity (kal-os′-i-ti): A local hardening of the skin caused by pressure or friction. The epidermis becomes hypertrophied. Most commonly seen on the feet and palms of the hands.

callous (kal′-us): Resembling callus. Hard.

callus (kal′-us): 1. A localized area of thickened skin, the stratum corneum of the palms and soles in particular, resulting from trauma caused by continual friction or pressure. 2. The fibrous tissue that forms at the end of bone in a fracture and which eventually becomes bone.

calor (kā′-lor): Heat; one of the four classic signs of inflammation; see also rubror, tumor, dolor. In physiology, the heat generated by metabolic processes.

caloric (kal-or′-ik): Pertaining to: 1) heat; 2) calories.

caloric test: A test for assessing vestibular function. When a normal ear is irrigated with hot water, there is rotary nystagmus toward that ear; if irrigated with cold water, there is rotary nystagmus toward the opposite ear. In vestibular disease, there is no nystagmus with either hot or cold water irrigation of an affected ear.

calorie (kal′-ō-ri): The unit of measure of heat energy; usually designates the small calorie which is the amount of heat required to raise the temperature of one gram of water 1°C. Usually written with a small *c* and may be abbreviated to cal.; sometimes called gram calorie. The large calorie is the amount of heat required to raise the temperature of 1 kilogram of water 1°C, thus it is 1000 times as large as the small calorie; usually written with a capital C, and may be abbreviated to Cal.; sometimes called kilogram calorie; is used in the study of metabolism. Also calory.

calorific (kal-ō-rif′-ik): Heat-producing. **C. VALUE,** the number of calories produced by a given amount of food, *e.g.*, 1 gram of protein and carbohydrate each liberate 4 calories, 1 gram of fat liberates 9 calories.

calorigenic (ka-lor-i-jen′-ik): 1. Heat-producing. 2. Energy-producing.

calorimeter (kal-ō-rim′-e-ter): An apparatus for measuring heat production. The respiration **C.** is used for determining the body's basal metabolic rate by measuring the heat produced by gaseous exchange in the lungs.

calorimetry (kal-ō-rim′-e-tri): The measurement of the amount of heat given off in a chemical reaction.

calvaria (kal-vā′-ri-a): The vault of the skull; the skullcap. Also calvarium.

Calvé's disease: Osteochondrosis of the vertebrae or of the femur. See osteochondrosis.

calvities (kal-vish′-i-ēz): Baldness.

calycectomy (kal-i-sek′-tō-mi): The surgical removal of a calyx of the kidney.

calyx (kā′-liks): In anatomy, one of the cuplike structures in the renal pelvis into which the pyramids of the renal medulla project.—calices, pl.; caliceal, adj.

camera (kam′-er-a): In anatomy, a cavity, chamber, or ventricle.

camisole (kam′-i-sōl): A canvas shirt with long sleeves, used to restrain violent or irrational patients; a straightjacket.

camp fever: Common name for typhus or typhoid fever.

camphor (kam′-for): A colorless white compound occurring as crystals, granules, or a gum; has a characteristic penetrating odor; obtained from an Asian shrub or tree; used locally as an antipruritic, antiseptic, analgesic, rubefacient, and as a carminative and toothache remedy.

camphorated oil: Cottonseed oil with camphor added; used externally as a counterirritant.

camphorated tincture of opium: A solution of alcohol and water containing opium, anise oil, camphor, benzoic acid, and glycerin; used chiefly as an antidiarrhetic. Syn., paregoric.

camptodactylia (kamp′-tō-dak-til′-i-a): The permanent flexion of one or both interphalangeal joints of one or more fingers; usually the little finger is affected.

Campylobacter (kam-pi-lō-bak′-ter): A genus of gram-negative bacteria; spirally curved rods with a flagella at one or both ends and which move with a corkscrew-like motion. Various species affect man as well as domestic animals. In humans symptoms include fever, night sweats, enteritis, headache, and bloody stools. May be transmitted by drinking water.

campylognathia (kam-pi-lō-nath′-i-a): Harelip (*q.v.*).

canal (ka-nal′): In anatomy, a relatively straight narrow tube, channel, or duct in bone or tissue. For particular canals see under alimentary, auditory, birth, haversian, inguinal, Nuck, Schlemm, semicircular, vaginal, vertebral.

canaliculus (kan-a-lik′-ū-lus): 1. A minute capillary passage. 2. Any small canal, such as the passage leading from the edge of the eyelid to the lacrimal sac, or one of the numerous small canals that lead from the Haversian canals and terminate in the lacunae of bone.—canaliculi, pl.; canalicular, adj.; canaliculization, n.

canalization (kan-a-lī-zā′-shun): 1. Formation of a new channel in tissue. 2. A surgical procedure that provides for drainage of wounds without the use of tubes.

cancellate, cancellated (kan′-sel-āt, -ed): Having a structure that resembles latticework.

cancellous (kan′-sel-us): Resembling latticework; light and spongy, like a honeycomb. Refers particularly to bony tissue that underlies or lies between layers of compact bone in epiphyses, sternum, ribs, vertebrae, and diploë of the skull; the interstices are filled with red bone marrow.

cancer (kan′-ser): A general term for a variety of malignant growths in many parts of the body; often used synonymously with tumor, neoplasm, or malignancy. The growth is purposeless, parasitic, invasive, and flourishes at the expense of the human host. Although the basic etiology is not known, cancer is considered curable if discovered early and if all cancer cells are removed by surgery or destroyed by radiation. Characteristics are the tendency to cause local destruction, to spread by metastasis, to recur, and to cause toxemia. Cancer is broadly classified as either carcinoma, which includes malignant tumors of the skin or mucous membranes, or as sarcoma, which includes tumors of connective tissue.—cancerous, adj.

cancer in situ: Carcinoma in situ; see under carcinoma.

canceremia (kan-ser-ē′-mi-a): The presence of cancer cells in the blood.

cancericidal (kan-ser-i-sī′-dal): Destructive to the cells of cancer.

cancerigenic (kan-ser-i-jen′-ik): Giving rise to a malignant neoplasm. See carcinogen.

cancerophobia (kan-ser-ō-fō′-bi-a): Extreme fear of cancer. Also cancerphobia.

cancerous (kan′-ser-us): Pertaining to, of, or resembling a cancer.

cancroid (kang′-kroid): 1. Squamous cell carcinoma. 2. Pertaining to squamous cell carcinoma. 3. Resembling cancer. 4. Cancer of moderate degree; may be said of skin cancer in particular.

cancrum oris (kan′-krum-or′-is): Gangrenous stomatitis (*q.v.*), occurring in malnourished children; also seen in such debilitating conditions as leukemia, Hodgkin's disease, and severe cases of measles, tuberculosis, malaria or kala-azar. Also noma.

Candida (kan′-di-da): A genus of yeast-like fungi; widespread in nature. *Candida* (*Monilia* or *Oidium*) *albicans* is a commensal of the mouth, throat, vagina, intestinal tract, and skin. Becomes pathogenic in some physiologic and pathologic states. May produce such infections as thrush, vulvovaginitis, balanoposthitis and pulmonary disease. **C. VAGINITIS**, inflammation of the vagina, often recurrent, caused by any of the several species of the Candida genus; characterized by pruritus, swelling of the vulva, and a thick, whitish discharge that adheres to the vaginal walls and is difficult to remove. Treatment includes the topical administration of medicated creams or suppositories; preventive measures include avoidance of tight undergarments and treatment of such underlying conditions as diabetes.

candidiasis (kan-di-dī′-a-sis): Infection with a fungus of the genus *Candida.*, syn., moniliasis, thrush. Characterized by formation of pseudomembranes on mucous surfaces of the respiratory and intestinal tracts and the vagina, skin lesions that resemble eczema, sometimes granulomata. Skin and local infections are usually benign; systemic infections, which may involve the kidney, may be fatal. **ORAL C.**, thrush (*q.v.*).

candy-stripers: Young hospital volunteers; named for the pink and white striped uniforms they wear.

canicola fever (kan-i-kō′-la): Infection of humans by the *Leptospira canicola* from rats, dogs, pigs, foxes, mice, voles and possibly cats. There is high fever, headache, conjunctival congestion, jaundice, severe muscular pains, rigors and vomiting. As the fever abates in about one week, the jaundice disappears. See Weil's disease.

canine (kā′nīn): 1. Resembling a dog. 2. Pertaining to certain teeth, four in all, two in each jaw, situated between the incisors and the premolars, and called cuspids. Those in the upper jaw are commonly known as eye teeth; those in the lower jaw as stomach teeth. **C. SPASM**, see risus sardonicus. **C. FOSSA**, a depression in the maxilla above the canine teeth.

canities (ka-nish′-i-ēz): Grayness or whiteness of the scalp hair.

canker sore: Small white ulcerative sores occurring chiefly on the lips, mouth, and inside of the cheek. See apthae, noma, thrush, and apthous stomatitis.

cannabis (kan′-a-bis): The flowering tops of hemp plants. Seldom used in modern medicine. **C. SATIVA**, a psychotropic agent, popularly known as bhang, hashish, or marijuana, is used illegally as snuff, in cigarettes, and in intoxicating drinks for its euphoric effects which resemble those of opium. **C. INDICA**, Indian hemp, once widely used as a sedative in nervous disorders.

cannabism (kan′-a-biz-em): Poisoning caused by overuse or habitual use of cannabis.

cannon wave: In electrocardiography, a large positive wave that occurs when the right atrium contracts but for some anatomic or pathologic reason, cannot empty its contents.

cannula (kan′-ū-la): A hollow tube contained in a trocar that is introduced into a body cavity after which the trocar is withdrawn and the tube remains in place, where it is used to introduce or withdraw fluid from a cavity, to irrigate a cavity, or to instill medication into a cavity. **BELLOCQ'S C.**, a hollow sound used to pass a thread through the nose and mouth to pull in a plug in treatment of epistaxis. **NASAL C.**, a double pronged device that is placed in the nostrils; has an extension that goes behind the ears and is secured under the chin; a common method of administering oxygen.—cannulas, cannulae, pl.

cannulate (kan′-ū-lāt): To introduce a cannula into a body cavity or tube-like organ.—cannulation, n.

cantharides (kan-thar′-i-dēz): A substance formerly much used externally as a rubefacient or vesicant and internally as an aphrodisiac and diuretic; made from the dried insect, *Cantharis vesicatoria*, a kind of beetle. See Spanish fly.

canthectomy (kan-thek′-to-mi): The excision of a canthus.

canthitis (kan-thī′-tis): Inflammation of the tissues at a canthus or canthi.

canthoplasty (kan-thō-plas′-ti): Plastic surgery on the external canthus of the eye to enlarge the palpebral fissure.

canthorrhaphy (kan-thor′-a-fi): Suturing at either the outer or inner canthus of the palpebral fissure; done to shorten the fissure.

canthus (kan′-thus): The angle formed by the junction of the eyelids. The inner one is known as the nasal **C.** or the medial palpebral commissure, and the outer one as the temporal **C.** or the lateral palpebral commissure.—canthal, adj.; canthi, pl.

Cantor tube: A long slender single-lumen intestinal tube used for long-time intubation; has a sealed rubber balloon at the tip into which mercury is instilled using a syringe and needle.

cap: In anatomy, a cap-shaped protective cover-like structure. **CERVICAL C.**, a thimble-shaped cap that fits over the cervix; a birth control device.

capacity (ka-pac′-i-ti): The ability to hold, receive, or store something. **INSPIRATORY C.**, the volume of air that can be inspired following a normal exhalation. **RESIDUAL C.**, the amount of air that remains in the lung after a maximal respiratory effort. **FUNCTIONAL RESIDUAL C.**, the amount of air that remains in the lung after a normal expiration. **TOTAL LUNG C.**, the sum of the functional residual capacity and the inspiratory capacity, normally 5000–6000 cc for an adult. **VITAL C.**, the greatest volume of air that can be expired after a maximum inspiration.

capeline (kap′-e-lin): See under bandage.

capillarectasia (kap′-i-lar-ek-tā′-zi-a): Dilatation of the capillaries.

capillaritis (kap-i-lar-ī′-tis): 1. Inflammation of the capillaries. 2. A skin disorder characterized by rupture of superficial capillaries and the consequent development of pigmented spots on the skin; cause unknown.

capillary (kap′-i-lar-i): 1. Hair-like. 2. A tiny thin-walled vessel, forming part of the network which facilitates rapid exchange of substances between the contained fluid and the surrounding tissues. **ARTERIAL C.**, a minute vessel distal to an arteriole; carries arterial blood. **BILE C.**, begins in a space in the liver and joins others to form a bile duct. **BLOOD C.**, unites an arteriole and a venule. **C. FRAGILITY**, refers to a high potential for rupture of the blood capillaries. **LYMPH C.**, begins in the tissue spaces throughout the body and joins others, eventually forming a lymphatic vessel. **C. MEMBRANE**, the basement membrane (*q.v.*) which allows diffusion of oxygen and nutrients and osmosis of water. **VENOUS C.**, a tiny vessel proximal to a venule; carries venous blood.

capillary fragility test: A test to evaluate the ability of the capillaries to resist conditions of increased pressure or anoxia.

capillus (ka-pil′-lus): A hair, specifically of the head.—capilli, pl.

capistration (kap-i-strā′-shun): Phimosis (*q.v.*).

Capital Commentary: A news column that appears monthly in *The American Nurse (q.v.)* during the time that the U.S. Congress is in session. Its purpose is to keep nurses informed about legislative matters that concern nurses and the nursing profession.

capitate (kap′-i-tāt): 1. Head-shaped; having a rounded extremity. 2. The largest of the eight carpal bones, so called because it has a head-shaped process.

capitation (kap-i-tā′-shun): Any uniform payment or fee payable per capita. In medical practice, the term is applied to an arrangement whereby the physician receives an annual set amount for his services to a patient, regardless of how much actual medical care the patient needs and receives. **CAPITATION GRANT**, in nursing education, refers to grants of federal funds to schools of nursing according to the number of students they enroll and graduate.

capitulum (ka-pit′-ū-lum): A small, rounded head or prominence on a bone by which it articulates with another bone.

Caplan's syndrome: A form of pneumoconiosis associated with rheumatoid arthritis; characterized by the formation of numerous nodular lesions throughout the lungs.

-capnia: A combining form denoting the presence of carbon dioxide.

capotement (ka-pōt′-mōn): A splashing sound heard in dilatation of the stomach.

capsid (kap′-sid): The protective protein coat that surrounds the nucleic acid component of viruses.

capsitis (kap-sī′-tis): Inflammation of the capsule that encloses the crystalline lens.

capsulated (kap′-sū-lā-ted): Enclosed within a capsule.

capsulation (kap-sū-lā′-shun): To surround a part with a capsule. Encapsulation.

capsule (kap′-sul): 1. The ligaments that surround a joint. 2. An absorbable gelatinous or rice paper container for a dose of oral medicine. 3. The outer membranous covering of certain organs, such as the kidney, liver, spleen, adrenals.—capsular, adj.

capsulectomy (kap-sū-lek′-to-mi): Surgical excision of a capsule. Usually refers to a joint or lens; less often to the kidney.

capsulitis (kap-sū-lī′-tis): Inflammation of a capsule of an organ or joint. **ADHESIVE C.**, inflammation of a joint that results in limited motion; when it occurs in the shoulder is often referred to as frozen shoulder.

capsulolenticular (kap′-sū-lō-len-tik′-yū-lar): Pertaining to the lens of the eye and its capsule.

capsuloplasty (kap′-sū-lō-plas-ti): Plastic surgery for repair of a joint capsule.

capsulorrhaphy (kap-sū-lor′-a-fi): Suture of a capsule; usually refers to the surgical repair of a torn joint capsule.

capsulotomy (kap-sū-lot′-o-mi): Incision of a capsule, usually referring to that surrounding the crystalline lens of the eye.

caput (kap′-ut): 1. A general term applied to the superior extremity of an organ or other body part. 2. The superior extremity of the body; the head. **C. MEDUSAE**, dilated veins in the area immediately surrounding the umbilicus, with blood flowing away from the umbilicus; seen in the newborn and in patients with cirrhosis of the liver; so called because the pattern of the veins resembles the snake-haired Medusa; also called caput medusae syndrome. **C. SUCCEDANEUM**, a serous effusion or edema overlying the scalp periosteum on an infant's head; the result of pressure during labor; disappears quickly.

car sickness: A form of motion sickness (*q.v.*).

carbamide (kar′-bam-īd): A product of protein metabolism; urea (*q.v.*); produces diuresis when used intravenously with dextrose solution.

carbaminohemoglobin (kar-bam′-i-nō-hē-mō-glō′-bin): Hemoglobin united with carbon dioxide; one of the forms in which carbon dioxide exists in the blood.

carbohemia (kar-bō-hē′-mi-a): An excessive amount of carbon dioxide in the blood. Also carbonemia.

carbohydrase (kar-bō-hī′-drās): Any of several enzymes that act as a catalyst in the hydrolysis of carbohydrates to simple sugars.

carbohydrate (kar-bō-hī′-drāt): An organic compound containing carbon, hydrogen, and oxygen, the latter two usually present in the same proportion as in water. Formed in nature by photosynthesis in plants. Carbohydrates are heat producing; they include starches, sugars, and cellulose and are classified as monosaccharides, disaccharides, polysaccharides, and heterosaccharides. They make up about half of our food intake and include such foods as cereals, rice, breads, most vegetables, especially the legumes and potatoes, and most fruits. A deficiency of C. in the diet leads to fatigue and electrolyte imbalance; excessive consumption may lead to obesity, dental decay, and, possibly, hypertension, diabetes, or kidney disorders.

carbohydraturia (kar′-bō-hī-dra-tū′-ri-a): The presence of an excess of carbohydrates in the urine; glycosuria.

carbol-fucsin (kar′-bol-fook′-sin): A dark purple solution containing phenol, resorcinol, acetone, alcohol, and distilled water; used externally as an antifungal preparation. **C. STAIN,** a solution used for staining certain acid-fast bacteria including the tubercle bacillus; contains phenol and basic fucsin in distilled water.

carbolic acid (kar-bol′-ik as′-id): Phenol (*q.v.*). Formerly much used as an antiseptic and germicide. Irritating to the skin and highly poisonous.

carbolism (kar′-bōl-izm): Poisoning with phenol (carbolic acid).

carboluria (kar-bō-lū′-ri-a): Green or dark colored urine due to excretion of carbolic acid, as occurs in carbolic acid poisoning.

carbometer (kar-bom′-e-ter): An instrument for determining the amount of carbon dioxide that is given off with the breath. Also carbonometer.

carbon: A non-metallic element present in all organic compounds. **C. DIOXIDE,** a tasteless, colorless gas; a waste product of many forms of combustion and metabolism, excreted by the lungs. When dissolved in a fluid, carbonic acid is formed; a specific amount of this in the blood produces inspiration; in cases of insufficiency, inhalations of **C.D.** act as a respiratory stimulant. It is also mixed with O_2 in anesthetic gases to stimulate respiration. In its solid form—**C.D.** snow—it is used as an escharotic and refrigerant. **C. MONOXIDE,** an insidious, colorless, odorless gas, present in illuminating gas, the exhaust of combustion motors and the products of incomplete combustion of wood and coal. It forms a stable compound with hemoglobin, thus robbing the body of its oxygen-carrying mechanism; signs of hypoxia ensue. **C. TETRACHLORIDE,** a colorless liquid with an odor similar to chloroform. Used chiefly as a solvent and detergent. No longer used in medicine.

carbon dioxide: See under carbon.

carbon dioxide "snow": Dry ice; solid carbon dioxide with a temperature of −79° Centigrade; in medicine, used to destroy certain skin lesions.

carbon monoxide: See under carbon.

carbonaceous (kar-bō-nā′-shē-us): Pertaining to or containing carbon.

carbonate (kar′-bon-āt): 1. To charge with carbon dioxide. 2. Any salt of carbonic acid.—carbonated, adj.

carbonemia (kar-bō-nē′-mi-a): An excessive amount of carbon dioxide in the blood.

carbonic acid: A solution of carbon dioxide in water; often called carbonated water.

carbonic anhydrase (kar-bon′-ik an-hī′-drās): An enzyme that acts as a catalyst in the synthesis and decomposition of carbonic acid from and to carbon dioxide and water, a step in the removal of carbon dioxide from the tissues and into the blood and alveolar air.

carbonuria (kar-bo-nū′-ri-a): An excess of carbon dioxide or other carbon compounds in the urine.

carbonyl chloride (kar′-bō-nil klō′-rid): Phosgene; a poisonous gas, developed for use in warfare.

carboxyhemoglobin (kar-bok′-si-hē-mō-glō′-bin): A stable compound formed by the union of carbon monoxide and hemoglobin; the red blood cells thus lose their respiratory function, as occurs in carbon monoxide poisoning.

carboxyhemoglobinemia (kar-boks′-i-hēm-ō-glō-bin-ē′-mi-a): The presence of carboxyhemoglobin in the blood.

carbuncle (kar′-bung-k′l): An acute, circumscribed, painful, suppurative inflammation (usually caused by a staphylococcic organism) involving several hair follicles and surrounding subcutaneous tissue, forming an extensive slough with several discharging sinuses. Frequently occurs on the back of the neck and most often in men; diabetics are particularly susceptible.—carbuncular, adj.

carbunculosis (kar-bung-kū-lō′-sis): The formation of several carbuncles simultaneously or in rapid succession.

carcin-, carcino-: Combining forms denoting cancer.

carcinoembryonic antigen (kar′-sin-ō-em-brē-on′-ik an′-ti-jen): An antigen normally present in the fetus and, in very small amounts, in the adult; tests for its presence are of use in determining the existence of a malignancy, or of metastasis of a malignant tumor, and whether surgical removal of a malignant tumor is advisable.

carcinogen (kar′-sin-ō-jen): Any cancer-producing substance or agent, *e.g.*, friction, injury, pressure, coal tar and its products, prolonged exposure to heat, sun, or radiation.—carcinogenic, adj.; carcinogenicity, n.

carcinogenesis (kar′-si-nō-jen′-e-sis): 1. The production or origin of cancer. 2. The process by which normal cells are transformed into cancer cells.—carcinogenic, adj.; carcinogenicity, n.

carcinogenicity (kar′-sin-ō-jen-is′-i-ti): Pertaining to the ability to cause cancer.

carcinoid (kar′-sin-oyd): Refers to a circumscribed tumor, usually benign and occurring in the gastrointestinal tract. **C. SYNDROME,** a condition thought to be due to secretion of serotonin from **C.** tumors that have metastasized to the liver; characterized by intense flushing of the face, angiomas of the skin, watery diarrhea, edema, ascites, bronchial spasm, sudden drop in blood pressure, stenosis of the tricuspid and pulmonary valves, and right heart failure.

carcinolytic (kar′-si-nō-lit′-ik): Destructive of carcinoma cells or pertaining to such destruction.

carcinoma (kar-si-nō′-ma): A malignant new growth derived from epithelial and glandular tissues, which tends to infiltrate into surrounding tissues and to spread by metastasis; the cells resemble those of the tissue where the growth is found. **ADENOSQUAMOUS C.,** a type of adenocarcinoma composed of both glandular and squamous malignant elements; occurs as an endometrial **C.,** most often seen in older women. **BASAL CELL C.,** a slow-growing, usually painless ulcer, usually occurring on the upper part of the face of older persons; may start as only a scaly patch or as a pearly raised papule with small capillaries; seldom metastasizes; highly curable. Occasionally seen also on the vulva of women over 60, where it begins as a small nodule, grows steadily and slowly, and eventually ulcerates. **BRONCHOGENIC C., C.** of the lungs; arises in the epithelium of the bronchial tubes. **C. IN SITU,** an asymptomatic condition; cells resembling cancer cells grow from the basal epithelial layer and finally involve the whole epithelium so that its layers can no longer be recognized; the term is often applied to **C.** of the cervix; also called preinvasive **C. CHORIONIC C., C.** composed of cells that are characteristic of the chorion of the embryo; occurs in the testes and ovaries and sometimes in other parts of the body; see choriocarcinoma. **EPIDERMOID C.,** squamous cell **C. MEDULLARY C.,** a poorly differentiated malignant neoplasm composed mostly of epithelial cells with little or no stroma; often occurs in the breast. **MELANOTIC C.,** malignant melanoma; see under melanoma. **SCIRRHOUS C., C.** with a hard structure owing to the formation of dense connective tissue. **SQUAMOUS CELL C.,** an invasive **C.** containing anaplastic squamous cells, arising in the squamous epithelium; often occurs on the lower lip; limited metastasis and curability; also called epidermoid cyst.

carcinomatophobia (kar′-si-nō-ma-tō-fō′-bi-a): Morbid fear of carcinoma.

carcinomatosis (kar-si-nō-ma-tō′-sis): A condition in which carcinoma is widespread throughout the body. Also carcinosis.

carcinomatous (kar-si-nō′-ma-tus): 1. Pertaining to carcinoma or cancer. 2. The condition of being malignant.

carcinosarcoma (kar′-si-nō-sar-kō′-ma): A tumor which has the cells and characteristics of both carcinoma and sarcoma; occurs most often in the uterus, esophagus, or thyroid gland.

carcinosis (kar-si-nō′-sis): The presence of cancer throughout the body; carcinomatosis.

card-, cardia-, cardio-: Combining forms denoting: 1) the heart, or 2) heart action.

cardia (kar′-di-a): The esophageal opening into the stomach.

-cardia: Combining form denoting a heart condition.

cardiac (kar′-di-ak): 1. Pertaining to the heart. 2. Pertaining to the cardia. 3. A person who has heart disease. 4. An agent or drug which acts especially on the heart. **C. ARREST,** complete cessation of the heart's activity. **C. ARRHYTHMIA,** abnormal rhythm of the heartbeat. **C. ASTHMA,** see asthma. **C. ATROPHY,** fatty degeneration of the heart muscle. **C. BED,** one which can be manipulated so that the patient is supported in a sitting position. **C. BODY SURFACE MAPPING,** an electrocardiographic technique utilizing many electrodes producing signals that are fed into a computer which filters out the important readings; gives more information than the ordinary ECG about possible abnormalities. **C. CATHETERIZATION,** see under catheterization. **C. COMPENSATION,** the maintenance of effective circulation in cases of cardiac disease or disorder, by some mechanism such as hypertrophy of the muscle. **C. COMPRESSION,** 1) constriction of the heart which renders it unable to fill completely; may be due to pericardial fibrosis, or the accumulation of blood in the pericardial sac; 2) a procedure used in cardiopulmonary resuscitation; see cardiac massage. **C. CYCLE,** the period from the beginning of one heart beat to the beginning of the next; includes systole, diastole, and rest period. **C. DECOMPENSATION,** inability of the heart to maintain normal circulation; symptoms are dyspnea, cyanosis, and edema. **C. EDEMA,** gravitational dropsy. **C. FAILURE,** sudden fatal stoppage of the heart. **C. INDEX,** the volume per minute of cardiac output per square meter of body surface; in the normal adult person the average output is approximately 2.2 liters per minute. **C. INSUFFICIENCY,** inability of the heart to function normally. **C. MASSAGE,** external or closed-chest massage consists of rhythmic compression of the lower end of the sternum every one and a half to two seconds; internal or open-chest massage consists of rhythmic compression of the heart after the chest has been opened surgically. **C. MONITORING,** involves recording the activity of the heart; three methods are 1) hardware **C.M.,** continuous monitoring of a patient on bed rest; 2) telemetry **C.M.,** monitoring the heart of an ambulatory patient; and 3) Holter **C.M.,** the use of a Holter monitor (*q.v.*) for 24 hours for a patient undergoing cardiac rehabilitation. **C. MURMURS,** see **MURMUR. C. NEUROSIS,** a form of anxiety neurosis characterized by chest pains, palpitation, dyspnea, faintness; also called neurocirculatory asthenia. **C. ORIFICE,** the opening between the esophagus and the stomach. **C. OUTPUT,** the volume of blood expelled by either ventricle of the heart per unit of time, usually per minute; computed by multiplying the heart rate by the stroke volume. **C. PACING,** regulating the rate of contraction of the heart muscle by means of an artificial cardiac pacemaker. **C. RESERVE,** 1) the ability of the heart to increase its output to meet increased biological requirements; 2) the difference between **C.** output at rest and during maximum physical effort. **C. STANDSTILL,** the sudden cessation of contraction of the myocardium. **C. TAMPONADE,** compression of the heart; can occur in surgery or result from penetrating wounds of the heart which cause hemorrhage into the pericardium; may also result from rapid production of effusion with the patient becoming pale with clammy extremities, engorgement of the neck veins, faint heart sounds, dependent edema, and hepatomegaly.

cardiac care unit: A critical care unit for patients with myocardial infarction: monitors are used to assess immediately changes in the status and functioning of the cardiac system. Abbreviated CCU.

cardial (kar′-di-al): Pertaining to the cardia (*q.v.*).

cardialgia (kar-di-al′-ji-a): 1. Literally, pain in the heart. 2. A painful sensation in the "pit of the stomach;" often called heartburn.

cardianeuria (kar′-di-a-nū′-ri-a): Lack of tone in the heart muscle.

cardiataxia (kar′-di-a-tak′-si-a): Irregularity of heart action due to incoordination of the contractions.

cardiectasis (kar-di-ek′-ta-sis): Dilatation of the heart.

cardiectomy (kar-di-ek′-to-mi): Surgical removal of the cardiac end of the stomach.

cardinal (kar′-di-nal): Primary or fundamental, as cardinal signs—temperature, pulse, respiration.

cardioaccelerator (kar′-di-ō-ak-sel′-e-rā-tor): An agent that speeds up the action of the heart.

cardioaortic (kar′-di-ō-ā-or′-tik): Pertaining to the heart and the aorta.

cardiocatheterization (kar′-di-ō-kath-e-ter-ī-zā′-shun): cardiac catheterization; see under catheterization.

cardiocele (kar′-di-ō-sēl): The protrusion of the heart from its cavity through an opening in the diaphragm or a wound.

cardiocentesis (kar′-di-ō-sen-tē′-sis): Surgical puncture of the heart.

cardiochalasia (kar′-di-ō-ka-lā′-zi-a): Weakening or incompetence of the cardiac orifice of the stomach.

cardiocirrhosis (kar′-di-ō-sir-rō′-sis): Cirrhosis of the liver accompanied by heart disease.

cardioclasis (kar-di-ok′-la-sis): Rupture of the heart.

cardiodiaphragmatic (kar′-di-ō-dī-a-frag-mat′-ik): Pertaining to the heart and the diaphragm.

cardiodiosis (kar′-di-ō-di-ō′-sis): Dilatation of the esophageal opening into the stomach by means of an instrument introduced through the esophagus.

cardiodynamics (kar′-di-ō-dī-nam′-iks): The study of the forces involved in the functions and actions of the heart.

cardiodynia (kar′-di-ō-din′-i-a): Pain in the heart.

cardioesophageal (kar′-di-ō-ē-sof-a-jē′-al): Pertaining to the stomach and the esophagus, particularly to their junction.

cardiogenesis (kar′-di-ō-jen′-e-sis): The development of the heart in the embryonic stage of life.

cardiogenic (kar′-di-ō-jen′-ik): 1. Pertaining to the development of the heart. 2. Developing or having its origin in the heart, *e.g.*, the shock in coronary thrombosis. **C. SHOCK,** occurs when the cardiac output of blood is inadequate to meet body requirements.

cardiogram (kar′-di-ō-gram): A tracing, on special paper, showing the activity of the heart muscle; obtained by cardiography. Electrocardiogram.

cardiograph (kar′-di-ō-graf): An instrument for recording graphically the force and form of the heart beat.—cardiographic, adj.; cardiographically, adv.

cardiohepatic (kar′-di-ō-hē-pat′-ik): Pertaining to the heart and the liver.

cardioinhibitor (kar′-di-ō-in-hib′-i-tor): An agent that slows or restrains the action of the heart.—cardioinhibitory, adj.

cardiokinetic (kar′-di-ō-kī-net′-ik): 1. Stimulating heart action. 2. An agent that influences heart action.

cardiolith (kar′-di-ō-lith): A stone or concretion in the heart tissue.

cardiologist (kar-di-ol′-ō-jist): One who specializes in the study and treatment of heart diseases.

cardiology (kar-di-ol′-o-ji): That branch of medicine that deals with the heart, its functions and diseases.

cardiomalacia (kar′-di-ō-mā-lā′-shi-a): Softening of the heart muscle, due to a pathologic condition.

cardiomegaly (kar′-di-ō-meg′-a-li): Enlargement of the heart.

cardiometry (kar-di-om′-e-tri): The procedure of measuring the size of the heart or the force exerted by its contractions.

cardiomyoliposis (kar′-di-ō-mī-ō-lī-pō′-sis): Fatty degeneration of the heart muscle.

cardiomyopathy (kar′-di-ō-mī-op′-a-thi): A disorder of heart muscle; acute, sub-acute, or chronic; cause may be obscure; may be associated with endocardial or pericardial pathology.—cardiomyopathic, adj.

cardiomyotomy (kar′-di-ō-mī-ot′-o-mi): The operation of incising constricting muscle at the junction of the esophagus and the stomach to relieve dysphagia in cardiospasm (*q.v.*).

cardionephric (kar′-di-ō-nef′-rik): Pertaining to the heart and the kidneys.

cardioneurosis (kar′-di-ō-nū-rō′-sis): 1. Functional neurosis associated with cardiac symptoms. 2. Neurosis characterized by intense concern with one's heart in the absence of any pathology.

cardiopathy (kar-di-op′-a-thi): Any heart disorder or disease.—cardiopathic, adj.

cardiopericarditis (kar′-di-ō-per-i-kar-dī′-tis): Inflammation of the heart muscle and pericardium.

cardioplasty (kar′-di-ō-plas-ti): Plastic surgery on the esophageal opening into the stomach.

cardioplegia (kar′-di-ō-plē′-ji-a): Cardiac arrest as may result from a direct blow or injury. May also be an elective procedure, utilizing drugs, during cardiac surgery.

cardiopneumatic (kar′-di-ō-nū-mat′-ik): Pertaining to the heart and respiration.

cardioptosis (kar-di-op′-to-sis): Downward displacement of the heart.

cardiopulmonary (kar′-di-ō-pul′-mō-ner-i): Pertaining to the heart and lungs. **C. ARREST,** the absence of effective circulation or respiration, or both. **C. BYPASS,** see bypass. **C. RESUSCITATION,** see resuscitation.

cardiopyloric (kar′-di-ō-pī-lor′-ik): Pertaining to the cardia and the pylorus (*q.v.*).

cardiorenal (kar′-di-ō-rē′-nal): Pertaining to the heart and kidneys.

cardiorespiratory (kar′-di-ō-res-pī′-ra-to-ri): Pertaining to the heart and the respiratory system.

cardiorrhaphy (kar-di-or′-a-fi): The procedure of suturing the heart muscle.

cardiorrhexis (kar-di-ō-rek′-sis): Rupture of the heart wall.

cardiosclerosis (kar-di-ō-skle-rō′-sis): Hardening of the heart muscle.

cardioscope (kar′-di-ō-scōp): An instrument fitted with a lens and illumination, for examining the inside of the living heart.—cardioscopic, adj.; cardioscopically, adv.

cardiospasm (kar′-di-ō-spazm): Persistent spasm of the cardiac sphincter between the esophagus and the stomach, causing secondary dilation of the upper part of the esophagus and thus giving rise to substernal pain and sometimes regurgitation. Usually no pathological change is found but the pain is easily mistaken for cardiac pain.

cardiosphygmograph (kar′-di-ō-sfig′-mō-graf): An instrument for recording the heart movement and the pulse.

cardiotachometer (kar′-di-ō-ta-kom′-e-ter): An instrument for recording the heart rate continuously over days or longer.

cardiotherapy (kar′-di-ō-ther′-a-pi): Treatment of heart diseases and disorders.

cardiothoracic (kar′-di-ō-thō-ras′-ic): 1. Pertaining to the heart and thoracic cavity. 2. Pertaining to a specialized branch of surgery. **C. RATIO,** the size of the heart as compared to the size of the thoracic cage.

cardiothyrotoxicosis (kar′-di-ō-thī-rō-tok-si-kō′-sis): Toxic hyperthyroidism accompanied by cardiac involvement.

cardiotocography (kar′-di-ō-tō-kog′-ra-fi): A combination of electrocardiography and tocography (*q.v.*). The fetal heart rate is obtained by a microphone placed on the mother's abdomen or by an electrode to the fetal scalp. At the same time the uterine contractions are measured by tocography. Both measurements are recorded on a monitoring device.

cardiotomy (kar-di-ot′-o-mi): 1. Surgical incision of the heart. 2. An operation in which the cardiac sphincter is cut in order to reduce stricture of the esophagus.

cardiotonic (kar′-di-ō-ton′-ik): Increasing the contractility of the heart muscle and slowing its rate, thus increasing efficiency of the cardiac pumping. Usually refers to agents which have this effect, especially drugs.

cardiotoxic (kar′-di-ō-tok′-sik): Having a toxic or harmful effect upon the heart.—cardiotoxicity, adj.

cardiovalvulitis (kar′-di-ō-val-vū-lī′-tis): Inflammation of the heart valves.

cardiovalvulotomy (kar′-di-ō-val-vū-lot′-o-mi): A surgical procedure for correction of valvular stenosis, consisting of excision or cutting of a heart valve; usually refers to the mitral valve.

cardiovascular (kar′-di-ō-vas′-kū-lar): Pertaining to the heart and blood vessels. **C. SYSTEM,** the heart and blood vessels by which the blood is pumped and circulated throughout the body; it transports the oxygen from the lungs to the tissues and returns carbon dioxide to the lungs to be removed.

cardioversion (kar′-di-ō-ver′-zhun): Restoration of the heart's normal rhythm by applying brief discharges of direct-current electricity across the intact chest and into the heart muscle to stop an arrhythmia or control fibrillation, and allow the normal heart to take over; usually an emergency measure. It is called defibrillation when used to correct ventricular fibrillation.

cardioverter (kar′-di-ō-ver-ter): An instrument used to deliver a brief direct-current electric shock to the heart to terminate certain arrhythmias.

carditis (kar-dī′-tis): Inflammation of the heart. A word seldom used without a descriptive prefix, *e.g.*, endo-, myo-, pan-, peri-. **RHEUMATIC C.**, associated with rheumatic fever; may be severe, causing congestive heart failure, pericarditis, and enlargement of the heart. **STREPTOCOCCAL C.**, occurs as a result of a streptococcal infection.

CARE: An international voluntary organization concerned with nutrition and health for the less fortunate people of the world.

care: See under the adjectives: acute, closed, coronary, cooperative, coordinated home care, long-term, self.

care contracting: A procedure whereby the care giver and the patient commit themselves to a precisely defined course of action and activities, usually in writing, stating specifically certain behaviors that are to occur and the conditions under which they are to occur, and establishing rewards and punishments appropriate to the outcomes.

care plan: An individual plan for the care of a particular patient. For a nursing care plan, data regarding the patient's needs are obtained from the nursing assessment report, the specific nursing activities to be carried out are outlined, the desired goals are stated, and priorities are set. The purpose of care plans is to improve patient care, minimize duplication or omission of care activities, and to assure that special problems are taken care of.

career ladder: In nursing, refers to a system whereby health care agencies promote individuals in recognition and reward for advanced educational activities, experience, or performance in nursing practice. Also descriptive of the progress of the nurse who advances from the lowest level required for registration to attainment of the doctoral degree.

caregiver: Any person who is involved in identifying, preventing, or treating patients, or in rehabilitating them; includes professionals, nonprofessionals, and community health workers.

caries (kā′-ri-ez): Inflammatory decay of bone or teeth, usually associated with pus formation. **SPINAL C.**, Pott's disease (*q.v.*).—carious, adj.

carina (ka-rī′-na): Any keel-like structure. Usually refers to the **C. TRACHAE**, a ridge at the base of the trachea where it separates to form the right and left bronchi.—carinal, adj.

cariogenic (kar-i-ō-jen′-ik): Conducive to the development of caries.

Carlen's tube: An endotracheal tube for older children.

carminative (kar-min′-a-tiv): 1. Having the power to relieve flatulence and associated colic. 2. An agent that helps to prevent the formation of gas and is capable of causing gas to be expelled from the gastrointestinal tract.

carneous (kar′-nē-us): Fleshy. **C. MOLE**, see mole.

carnivorous (kar-niv′-o-rus): Subsisting entirely or chiefly on meat.

carnophobia (kar-nō-fō′-bi-a): Morbid aversion to meat as food.

carotenase (kar′-ō-tē-nās): An enzyme that converts carotene into vitamin A.

carotene (kar′-ō-tēn): A yellow pigment, found in carrots, sweet potatoes and other yellow vegetables, leafy vegetables, milk fat and other fats, and egg yolk; is converted into vitamin A in the liver. A provitamin.

carotenemia (kar-o-te-nē′-mi-a): The presence of an excessive amount of carotene in the blood; in large quantities it produces yellowing of the skin.

carotid (kar-ot′-id): The principal arteries on each side of the neck, which supply blood to the head and neck. They arise from the aortic arch on the left and the innominate artery on the right. At the bifurcation of each common carotid artery into the internal and external carotid arteries there are: 1) the **C. BODIES**, a collection of chemoreceptors which, being sensitive to chemical changes in the blood, protect the body against lack of oxygen and aid in the reflex control of the blood pressure, heart rate, and respiration; and 2) the **C. SINUS**, a slight dilatation of the common carotid artery at its bifurcation; it contains baroreceptors in its walls which are sensitive to pressure changes; pressure on the sinus causes vasodilation, slowing of the heart, and a drop in blood pressure.

carotid sinus syndrome: A condition characterized by bradycardia, severe hypotension, dizziness, faintness; caused by overactivity of the carotid sinus reflex.

carotidynia (ka-rot′-i-din′-i-a): A syndrome consisting of throbbing neck pain and tenderness over the course of the carotid artery and temporomandibular joint, and headache; relatively rare. Also spelled carotodynia.

carpal (kar′-p'l): Pertaining to the wrist.

carpal tunnel (kar′-pal): A deep cavity on the palm side of the carpus with a fibrous band across it forming a tunnel which accommodates the median nerve and some of the tendons of the hand. **C.T. SYNDROME,** a fairly common symptom complex due to compression on the median nerve in the carpal tunnel; characterized by pain, paresthesia, atrophy of the thenar muscles, edema of the fingers, numbness, and tingling in the area of the hand innervated by the median nerve, with weakness, sometimes extending to the elbow; most severe at night. The compression may be caused by swelling of the structures in the tunnel and compression of the nerve as it passes through the fascial band. Most common in middle-aged women. Also called carpotunnel syndrome.

carpectomy (kar-pek′-to-mi): Excision of a carpal bone.

carphology (kar-fol′-o-ji): Involuntary picking at the bedclothes; an extremely grave symptom seen in great exhaustion, high fevers, delirium. Syn., floccillation.

carpometacarpal (kar′-pō-met-a-kar′-pal): Pertaining to the carpal and metacarpal bones, the joints between them, and the ligaments joining them.

carpopedal (kar′-pō-ped′-al): Pertaining to the wrist and foot or to the hands and feet. **C. SPASM,** spasm of the hands and feet, or of the thumbs and great toes, as sometimes seen in tetany.

carpophalangeal (kar′-pō-fa-lan′-jē-al): Pertaining to the wrist and the fingers.

carpoptosis (kar-pop-tō′-sis): Wristdrop.

carpus (kar′-pus): The wrist. The eight small bones and surrounding structures between the hand and the forearm. The bones, arranged in two rows, are the navicular, lunate, triangular, pisiform, trapezium, greater multangular, lesser multangular, capitate, and hamate.—carpal, adj.

carrier (kar′-i-er): 1. A healthy animal or human host who harbors a pathogenic or potentially pathogenic microorganism in the absence of discernible disease and serves as a possible source of infection. **ACTIVE C.,** one who becomes a **C.** after recovering from the disease. 2. An insect vector that transmits an infection. 3. A heterozygote (*q.v.*) that carries a recessive gene together with its normal allele.

cartilage (kar′-til-ij): Gristle; a tough connective tissue, characterized by firmness and having no neurovascular supply. There are three main varieties: 1) **HYALINE C.,** a semitransparent substance of a pearly bluish color possessing considerable elasticity; 2) **YELLOW ELASTIC C.,** possesses a network of yellow elastic fibers, branching and anastomosing in all directions; it is a true cartilage found, *e.g.*, in the external ear; and 3) white fibrocartilage, consists of dense white fibrous tissue of great strength and rigidity; it forms the intervertebral disks. **ARTICULAR C.,** the **C,** at the joint surfaces of bones; provides smooth surfaces for movement without friction. **ARYTENOID C.,** one on either side forming the posterior wall of the upper rim of the larynx; their function is to regulate the opening and closing of the space between the vocal cords. **COSTAL C.,** one of several cartilages that attach the first seven ribs to the sternum. **CRICOID C.,** lies below the thyroid **C.**; shaped like a signet ring with the broad part at the back; forms the lateral and posterior walls of the larynx; lined with ciliated epithelium. **ENSIFORM C.,** the xiphoid process of the sternum. **EPIPHYSEAL C.,** that present at the ends and shafts of the long bones in children; it allows for growth in length. **THYROID C.,** the large cartilage of the larynx, in the front of the neck; "Adam's apple."

cartilaginous (kar-ti-laj′-i-nus): Composed of or pertaining to cartilage.

caruncle (kar′-ung-k'l): A red, fleshy projection. **LACRIMAL C.,** a small reddish projection near the inner canthus of the eye; caruncula lacrimalis. **HYMENAL C.,** the tabs of skin that remain around the oriface of the vagina after rupture of the hymen. Also called caruncula myrtiformes.

carus (kār′-rus): Stupor; coma.

cary-, caryo: Combining forms denoting relationship to a nucleus; same as kary-, karyo-.

case: **C. HISTORY,** a biography of a patient's physical and pathological experiences, collected for scientific purposes; sometimes obtained by interview, sometimes collected over the years; includes the history of the present condition for which he is being treated. **C. RECORD,** all of the data that accumulated about a patient's history, disease, treatment, etc. during his hospital stay; it is placed in the permanent files of the hospital and is admissible as evidence in court. **C. STUDY,** a method of learning about various diseases and their treatment; includes gathering, organizing, and recording all relevant data concerning a specific condition or status of an individual patient.

caseation (kā-zē-ā′-shun): The precipitation of casein in milk to form cheese. **C. NECROSIS,** necrosis of tissue whereby it is changed to a dry, crumbly consistency resembling cheese; characteristically associated with pulmonary tuberculosis.

casein (kā′-sē-in): A protein formed when milk enters the stomach. Coagulation occurs, due to the action of rennin on the caseinogen in the milk, splitting it into two proteins, one being casein. The casein combines with calcium and a clot is formed.

caseinogen (kā-sē-in′-ō-jen): The precursor of casein; a substance present in milk that is converted into casein by the action of rennin in the stomach.

caseous (kā′-zē-us): Resembling cheese or having the nature and consistency of cheese; often refers to a certain type of necrosis of tissue.

cast: 1. Fibrous material and exudate that has been molded to the form of the cavity or tube in which it has collected, *e.g.*, **RENAL C.** or **URINARY C.**; it can be identified under the microscope and classified according to its constitution as bloody, epithelial, fatty, etc. 2. A commonly used term for any abnormal turning of the eye. 3. A stiff bandage or dressing made of crinoline or like material impregnated with plaster of Paris or other hardening material; used to immobilize a part in cases of fracture or dislocation and in various orthopedic conditions. **AIRPLANE C.**, a spica cast that covers the upper torso as well as the affected arm and holds it in an abducted position. **BANJO C.**, one with a large ring extension that holds the fingers in extension by the use of rubber bands; used mostly for finger fractures. **BODY C.**, a **C.** that encloses the trunk; may extend from the neck to the groin; used for treating diseases and injuries of the vertebrae. **CYLINDER C.**, a semirigid **C**, applied to the lower leg; extends from the thigh to the ankle; used for treating ankle and knee injuries. **GAUNTLET C.**, encloses the wrist and extends to the palm; used for treating fractures of the metacarpus and phalanges. **MINERVA JACKET**, a **C.** used in treatment of fractures of the cervical vertebrae; encloses the forehead, chin, occiput, and neck and extends down over the shoulders and trunk. **SPICA C.**, used to immobilize an extremity by incorporating part of the body along with the injured extremity; the **SHOULDER SPICA** is used for treating fractures of the proximal humerus; the **THUMB SPICA** is used in fractures of the navicular bone in the wrist; the **HIP SPICA** is used in fractures of the femur, and in some hip, pelvic, and tibial fractures; the **TOE SPICA** is used after surgery for bunions and incorporates all or part of the foot. **TURNBUCKLE JACKET**, a spica jacket **C.** which may include the head and arm; the side of the jacket is split and a turnbuckle inserted to allow for gradual opening of the two halves as correction progresses; used in treatment of scoliosis. **WALKING C.**, a rubber walker is attached to a leg and foot cast to permit the patient to ambulate. See also Unna's boot.

cast brace: A device used with a walking cast to permit early ambulation following fracture of the tibia.

Castellani's paint (kas-tel-an′-ēz): A preparation containing carbol-fuchsin used as a skin disinfectant and in the treatment of certain fungal infections of the skin.

Castle's factor: A substance secreted by the stomach; necessary for the absorption of vitamin B_{12} (cyanocobalamin); deficiency or lack of this factor results in pernicious anemia. Also called Castle's intrinsic factor.

castor oil: Obtained from the seed of the castor bean; used in medicine as a purgative; oleum ricini.

castration (kas-trā′-shun): The removal of testes or ovaries. **C. ANXIETY**, the unfounded fear of loss of one's genital organs; may be precipitated by some humiliating or worrisome life event or by feelings of guilt over forbidden sexual desires; in children it usually arises from guilt over oedipal feelings. Also called castration complex. See also Oedipus.

casualty (kaz′-ū-al-ti): An accidental or other type of injury, or a person who has suffered such an injury.

CAT: 1. **CAT SCAN**, see computerized axial tomography. 2. Childrens Apperception Test.

cat scratch fever: A minor local inflammatory lesion with redness, swelling, slight ulceration or papule formation at the site of a scratch wound; chills, malaise, rash, and fever of an undulating type may develop; probably caused by a virus. Regional lymph nodes may become involved and eventually suppurate. Symptoms usually disappear in 2 to 3 weeks. Apparently worldwide, not seasonal and shows no preference for age or sex.

cata-: Prefix denoting down, under, lower, away, against, through, concealed, along with.

catabasis (ka-tab′-a-sis): The stage during which a disease declines in severity.

catabiosis (kat′-a-bī-ō′-sis): Normal physiologic aging of a cell or group of cells.

catabolism, katabolism (ka-tab′-ō-lizm): The series of chemical reactions in the living body in which complex substances, taken in as food, are broken down into simpler ones, accompanied by the release of energy. This energy is needed for anabolism and the other activities of the body.—catabolic, adj.

catabolite (ka-tab′-ō-līt): Any product of catabolism (*q.v.*).

catagen (kat′-a-jen): The brief period in the hair growth cycle after the hair is formed and before the resting period that precedes shedding. See telogen.

catagenesis (kat-a-jen′-e-sis): 1. Involution. 2. Retrogression.

catalase (kat′-a-lās): An enzyme found in many plant and animal tissues, and especially in anaerobic bacteria; catalyzes the decomposition of hydrogen peroxide into water and oxygen. **C. TEST**, a screening test for urinary tract infection or other inflammatory kidney disease.

catalepsy (kat′-a-lep-si): A conscious but trance-like state in which the muscles are rigid so that the subject remains in a fixed position over an indefinite period of time.—cataleptic; cataleptoid, adj.

catalysis (ka-tal′-i-sis): A change in the rate at which a chemical action proceeds, produced by an agent which is not itself affected by the reaction. May be positive or negative.—catalytic, adj.

catalyst (kat′-a-list): An agent that produces catalysis (*q.v.*). It does not undergo any change during the process. Syn., catalyzer, enzyme, ferment.

catalyze (kat′-a-līz): To act as a catalyst or to influence a chemical reaction without taking part in it.

catamenia (kat-a-mē′-ni-a): Menstruation.—catamenial, adj.

catamnesis (kat-am-nē′-sis): Term used to describe the medical history of a patient: 1) after an initial examination or illness, or 2) in the interim between a patient's discharge from hospital and a follow-up examination.

cataphasia (kat-a-fā′-zi-a): A disorder of speech characterized by the constant repetition of certain words or phrases.

cataphoresis (kat′-a-fō-rē′-sis): Electrophoresis (*q.v.*).

cataphrenia (kat-a-frē′-ni-a): A mental state that resembles dementia and which tends to be temporary.

cataphylaxis (kat-a-fi-lak′-sis): The migration of leukocytes and antibodies to the site in the body that has been invaded by an infective organism.

cataplasia (kat-a-plā′-zi-a): Atrophy or degeneration of tissues in which they revert to an earlier, or embryonic state.

cataplasm (kat′-a-plaz'm): 1. A powder applied to the skin. 2. A poultice.

cataplexy (kat′-a-plek-si): A condition of sudden powerlessness due to muscular rigidity caused by intense emotional upheaval such as fear or shock, or hypnotic suggestion. The patient remains conscious; recovery is usually complete.—cataplectic, adj.

cataract (kat′-a-rakt): A progressive clouding of the crystalline lens of the eye or its capsule, or both, causing blurring of vision; may be due to senility, trauma, or diabetes mellitus; may also be congenital in infants who have a viral infection in utero. **CONGENITAL C.**, may be due to the mother's having rubella during early pregnancy. **HARD C.**, contains a hard nucleus, tends to be dark in color, and occurs in older individuals. **SENILE C.**, a hard **C.** that occurs as a result of the aging process. **SOFT C.**, one without a hard nucleus; occurs at any age but particularly in the young. Cataract usually develops slowly and when mature is called "ripe."—cataractous, adj.

catarrh (ka-tarh′): An old term for inflammation of mucous membrane with a constant flow of mucus; applied especially to the upper respiratory tract. **AUTUMNAL C.**, hay fever (*q.v.*). **POSTNASAL C.**, Chronic rhinopharyngitis. **VERNAL C.**, allergic rhinitis and conjunctivitis, caused by spring pollens.

catastrophic (kat-a-strof′-ik): Sudden; disastrous; violent; life-threatening. **C. CARE**, care involving use of life-support techniques and devices provided for severely traumatized or seriously acutely ill patients. **C. HEALTH INSURANCE**, a type of insurance covering medical and other care for seriously ill or injured individuals.

catastrophism (ka-tas′-trō-fizm): The theory or assumption that senescence begins late in life and follows a rapid course to death, as opposed to the belief that senescence occurs at a rather uniform rate throughout the life span.

catatonia (kat-a-tō′-ni-a): A type of behavior that may occur in schizophrenia; the patient may assume certain odd postures for indefinite periods, have muscular spasms, refuse to speak, become negative, stuporous or indifferent to the environment.—catatonic, adj.

catch syndrome: A benign condition marked by transient pain in the chest which is relieved by taking a deep breath in small graduated steps; may or may not be indicative of a pathological condition.

catchment area: A term used to describe the geographic area from which a mental health facility or other health care facility draws its clientele.

catecholamine (kat-e-kōl′-a-mēn): Any one of a group of compounds that are secreted largely but not exclusively by the adrenal gland and which have the power to cause physiological changes resembling those caused by the action of the sympathetic nerves. Includes dopamine, norepinephrine, and epinephrine. Also produced synthetically as drugs for use as sympathomimetics; see sympathomimetic.

catgut (kat′-gut): A form of ligature and suture of varying thickness, strength and absorbability, prepared from sheep's intestines. After sterilization it is hermetically sealed in glass tubes according to size. The plain variety is usually absorbed in 5 to 10 days. Chromicized **C.** and iodized **C.** will hold for 20 to 40 days.

catharsis (ka-thar′-sis): 1. A cleansing or purging, said particularly of the intestine. 2. A method used in Freudian psychiatry; the analyst urges the patient to talk freely about things that come to mind during a train of thought and thus purge his mind of the memories of painful or unpleasant experiences that may be causing his psychological disturbance; syn., abreaction (*q.v.*).

cathartic (ka-thar′-tik): 1. Producing catharsis (*q.v.*). 2. An agent that promotes evacuation of the intestine. Cathartics are classed as laxatives or purgatives, according to the type and degree of evacuation they produce.

catheter (kath′-e-ter): A slender, hollow, flexible tube of varying lengths, bores and shapes, that is inserted into a structure (*e.g.*, a vein or hollow organ); used to distend a hollow tube or passage, to distend or maintain an opening, or for injecting, instilling, or withdrawing fluid from a body cavity. Catheters are made of soft and hard rubber, gum elastic, glass, rubberized silk; silver and other metals; some are radiopaque. Catheters are often designated as French; sizes 16–18 French are usually used for adults. To convert from French scale to millimeters divide by 3; see French scale. ARGYLE CHEST CATHETER, a size 32 to 36 French catheter that is inserted in the 4th or 5th intercostal space at the midaxillary line of the affected side and connected to underwater seal and suction, to reestablish negative pressure in the pleural space for a patient with pneumothorax; in cases of hemothorax, the 36 French catheter is inserted in the second intercostal space. BALLOON C., see Foley c. BROVIAC C., a C. designed for use in administering hyperalimentation. CARDIAC C., a long, slender C., designed for passage through a blood vessel into the heart. DEPEZZAR C., Malecot C. FEMALE C., a short C. for catheterizing the urinary bladder of female patients. FOLEY C., a common type of indwelling C. held in place by an attached inflated balloon. HICKMAN C., used for administering hyperalimentation; it is designed to also allow for withdrawal of blood and administration of medications. INDWELLING C., one fastened in place for continuous drainage of the urinary bladder. INLYING C., one inserted for infusion after doing a cutdown. INTRACATHETER, a C., inserted through a needle; used for intravenous infusions; the venipuncture is made with the needle and the C. is then inserted into the vein through the needle. JACQUES C., has a rounded end and an opening at the side. MALE C., a long catheter for use in catheterizing the male bladder. MALECOT C., has a protuberance at the distal end; used to drain the bladder through a suprapubic opening. NASAL C., used to pass food into the stomach or to administer oxygen through the nose. NONRETENTION C., one used to empty the urinary bladder or to collect a clean urine specimen; is removed after use. RETENTION C., indwelling C. or self-retaining C., one fitted with a device to hold it in position when prolonged drainage of the urinary bladder is required. SUCTIONING C., one used to suction the upper respiratory tract; introduced through the nasotracheal route. SWAN-GANZ C., a balloon-tipped, flow-directed, multilumen C. used for hemodynamic monitoring; has a transistorized thermistor that detects changes in blood temperatures which are used to compute cardiac output; it also measures right and left ventricular pressures and pulmonary capillary wedge pressure in the smallest pulmonary vessels accessible to the catheter. A transducer attached to the external end of the catheter translates pressure waves into electrical impulses; thus waves appear on an oscilloscope and the digital values are displayed on the monitor. Used in diagnosing and managing patients with heart failure from myocardial infarction or cardiogenic shock, those with pulmonary edema or pulmonary embolus, those who haave undergone cardiac bypass surgery. WHISTLE-TIPPED C., one with an opening on the end as well as the side.

catheterization (kath-e-ter-ī-zā′-shun): Insertion of a catheter into a body cavity or channel, often the urinary bladder. CARDIAC C., an invasive procedure consisting of the insertion of a fine, polyethylene or radiopaque nylon tubing via the basilic, median cubital, basilar, or femoral vein into the heart to: 1) record pressures; 2) introduce an opaque substance prior to x ray; 3) withdraw blood samples; and 4) determine blood flow in the heart. Either the right or left heart and one or more chambers may be catheterized. CONTINUOUS C., provides for continuous drainage of the bladder through an indwelling catheter. INTERMITTENT C., C. that is performed at intervals to remove accumulated urine from the bladder. SUPRAPUBIC C., is accomplished by surgically inserting an indwelling catheter through an opening just above the pubis.

catheterize (kath′-e-ter-iz): To introduce a catheter into a body cavity; often refers to the urinary bladder. See also cardiac catheterization under catheterization.

cathexis (ka-thek′-sis): In psychiatry, the conscious or unconscious fixing of one's psychic energy on some particular thing, person, or concept.—cathetic, adj.

cathode (kath′-ōd): The negatively charged terminal of an electrode or an electrolytic cell, as in a storage battery.

cation (kat′-ī-on): A positively charged ion; the opposite of anion (*q.v.*).

catopric (ka-top′-rik): Pertaining to the branch of physics that deals with the principles of reflected light. C. TEST, a test for cataract utilizing the reflection of images from the capsules of the lens and cornea.

catoptrophobia (kat-op-trō-fō′-bi-a): Morbid fear of mirrors or of breaking them.

catylase test (kat′-i-lās): A screening test for urinary tract infections.

cat's eye: CAT'S-EYE AMAUROSIS, blindness in one eye characterized by bright reflection from the pupil. CAT'S-EYE PUPIL, an elongated, slit-like pupil.

cauda (kaw′-da): A tail or tail-like appendage. In anatomy, refers to a structure resembling such an appendage. C. EQUINA, the lower end of the spinal cord; it is a bundle of roots of all the spinal nerves below the first lumbar; resembles a horse's tail.

cauda equina syndrome: A condition characterized by a dull, aching, radiating pain in the sacrum, bladder, and perineal area; caused by compression of the spinal nerve roots.

caudad (kaw′-dad): Toward the posterior, lower, or distal end.

caudal (kaw′-dal): 1. Pertaining to a cauda. 2. In anatomy, refers to an inferior or lower position. C. BLOCK, caudal anesthesia; induced by intermittent or continuous injection of an anesthetic into the caudal portion of the spinal canal.

caudal regression syndrome: A congenital anomaly in which the lumbar, sacral, and coccygeal vertebrae fail to develop normally; often associated with neurologic defects.

caul: A part or all of the amnion which sometimes covers or envelopes the head of the fetus at birth. "Angel's veil," in olden days thought to be a good omen.

cauliflower ear: A partially deformed auricle, usually due to injury; frequently seen in professional boxers.

cauloplegia (kaw-lō-plē′-ji-a): Paralysis of the penis.

causal (kaw′sal): Pertaining to a cause, as the agent causing a disease.

causalgia (kaw-sal′ji-a): Excruciating burning neuralgic pain, resulting from physical trauma to cutaneous nerve fibers.

causa mortis (kaw′-za mor′-tis): By reason of impending death. Specifically, the term refers to a gift made by one who is about to die.

caustic (kaw′-stik): 1. Corrosive or destructive to living tissue, or agents that produce this effect. Used therapeutically to destroy granulation tissue, warts, polypi. Carbolic acid, nitric acid, carbon dioxide snow, silver nitrate, and potassium hydroxide are most commonly employed. 2. Able to burn, corrode, or otherwise destroy by chemical action.

caustic soda: Sodium hydroxide; see under sodium.

cauterize (kaw′-ter-īz): 1. To apply a cautery. 2. To destroy tissue by heat, chemical action, or electricity.—cauterization, n.

cautery (kaw′-ter-i): A caustic agent or device such as a chemical, hot iron, electricity, or extreme cold to destroy living tissue. ACTUAL C., a hot iron used to apply direct heat. CHEMICAL C., a chemical substance used to burn or sear tissue. ELECTRIC C., a platinum wire maintained at red heat by an electric current. PAQUELIN'S C., a form of C. in which the hollow platinum point is kept at the required heat by a current of benzene which is constantly pumped into it.—cauterization, n.; cauterize, v.

cava (kā′-va): Plural of cavum. A vena cava.

caval (kā′-val): Pertaining to the vena cava.

cavamesenteric shunt (kā′-va-mes-en-ter′-ik): The upper end of the inferior vena cava is anastomosed to the superior mesenteric vein; used in children when the portal vein is blocked. See shunt.

Cavell, Edith L.: British nurse, matron of a Red Cross Hospital in Belgium during World War I; worked with the underground and helped about 200 imprisoned English, French, and Belgian soldiers to escape; was arrested by the Germans, tried, and convicted, and was executed October 12, 1915. [1865–1915]

cavernous (kav′-er-nus): Pertaining to a cavity or hollow. C. BODY, see under body. C. RESPIRATIONS, see under respiration. C. SINUS, see under sinus.

caviar spots (kav′-i-ar): Varicosities of small vessels under the tongue producing small, smooth red to brown papules; seen mostly in the elderly.

cavitary (kav′-i-ter-i): Pertaining or referring to a cavity or to the presence of many cavities.

cavitation (kav-i-tā′-shun): The formation of a cavity as in pulmonary tuberculosis.

cavitis (kā-vī′-tis): Inflammation of a vena cava.

cavity (kav′-i-ti): A hollow; an enclosed area within the body. ABDOMINAL C., that area below the diaphragm and above the pelvis; the abdomen. BUCCAL C., the mouth. CEREBRAL C., the ventricles of the brain. CRANIAL C., the brain box formed by the bones of the cranium. DENTAL C., a hollow formed in a tooth as a result of decay of the organic matter following decalcification of the inorganic outer part of the tooth; syn., caries (pl.). DORSAL C., the cavity enclosed by the vertebrae and the bones of the cranium. GLENOID C., see under glenoid. MEDULLARY C., the hollow center of a long bone, containing yellow bone marrow or medulla. NASAL C., that in the nose, separated into right and left halves by the nasal septum. ORAL C., the buccal cavity. PELVIC C., that formed by the pelvic bones, more particularly the part below the iliopectineal line and containing primarily the rectum and reproductive organs. PERITONEAL C., a potential space between the parietal and visceral layers of the peritoneum. Similarly, the PLEURAL C. is the potential space between the pulmonary and parietal pleurae which, in health, are in contact in all phases of respiration. SPINAL C., contains the spinal cord. SYNOVIAL C., the potential space in a synovial joint. THORACIC C., the part of the trunk lying above the diaphragm. TYMPANIC C., the cavity of the middle ear; see under ear. UTERINE C., that of the uterus, in the form of a small triangle, the base extending between the orifices of the uterine tubes. VENTRAL C., the body **C.**, in front of the spinal column; encloses the mouth, throat, thorax, abdomen and pelvis.

cavography (ka-vog′-ra-fi): Radiography of the inferior or superior vena cava.

cavum (kā′-vum): A cavity or space.—cava, pl.; caval, adj.

cavus (kā′-vus): Concave; hollow. **PES C.**, a foot deformity in which there is a high longitudinal arch and a depressed metatarsal arch. Syn., nondeforming clubfoot.

CBC: Abbreviation for complete blood count. See blood count.

CBS: Abbreviation for chronic brain syndrome.

CC: Abbreviation for: 1) chief complaint; 2) current complaint.

cc: Abbreviation for cubic centimeter.

CCU: Abbreviation for: 1) coronary care unit; 2) cardiac care unit.

CDC: Abbreviation for Centers for Disease Control.

CDH: Abbreviation for congenital dislocation of the hip.

cecal (sē′-kal): Pertaining to the cecum.

cecectomy (sē-sek′-to-mi): Operation for removal of the cecum or part of it, or an incision into it.

cecitis (sē-sī′-tis): Inflammation of the cecum.

cecocolic (sē-kō-kol′-ik): Pertaining to the cecum and the colon.

cecocolostomy (sē′-kō-kō-los′-to-mi): A surgically created anastomosis between the cecum and the colon.

cecoileostomy (sē′-kō-il-ē-os′-to-mi): A surgically created anastomosis between the cecum and the ileum.

cecoptosis (sē-kop-tō′-sis): Downward displacement of the cecum.

cecorectostomy (sē′-kō-rek-tos′-to-mi): A surgically created anastomosis between the cecum and the rectum.

cecosigmoidostomy (sē′-kō-sig-moid-os′-to-mi): A surgically created anastomosis between the cecum and the sigmoid flexure of the colon.

cecostomy (sē-kos′-to-mi): A surgically established fistula between the cecum and the anterior abdominal wall, done to bypass an area of the cecum that is diseased, obstructed, or congenitally absent; the bowel content is voided into a collection bag attached to the skin.

cecotomy (sē-kot′-ō-mi): The operation of making an incision into the cecum.

cecum (sē′-kum): The blind, pouch-like commencement of the colon in the right iliac fossa; it is separated from the ileum by the ileocecal valve. The vermiform appendix is attached to it.—cecal, adj.

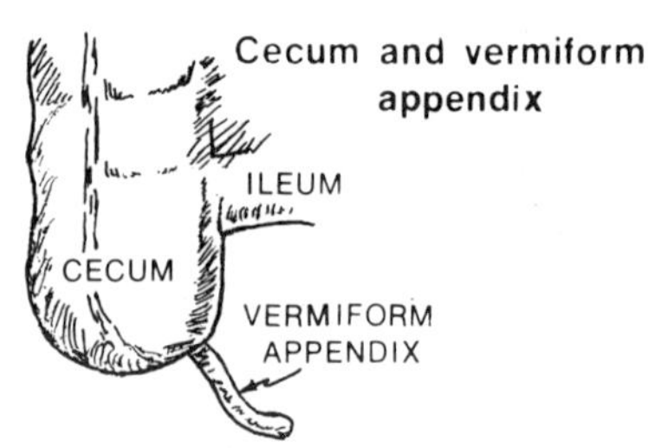

ceiling limit: The level of a toxic substance in the work environment that should not be exceeded.

-cele: Combining form denoting: 1. Tumor. 2. Hernia.

celiac (sē′-li-ak): Pertaining to or relating to the abdomen. **C. DISEASE**, nontropical sprue; occurs primarily in young children but also in adults; characterized by malabsorption of fats and inability to digest certain gluten grains, pain, vomiting, diarrhea, distention, malnutrition, bulky foul-smelling stools; cause unknown; may be hereditary. **C. CRISIS**, an acute attack of diarrhea and vomiting resulting in dehydration and acidosis.

celialgia (sē-li-al′-ji-a): Pain in the abdomen.

celiectasia (sē′-li-ek-tā′-zi-a): Abnormal distention of the abdomen.

celiectomy (sē-li-ek′-to-mi): The surgical removal of any abdominal organ.

celiocentesis (sē′-li-ō-sen-tē′-sis): Surgical puncture of the abdominal cavity. Also celioparacentesis.

celiocolpotomy (sē′-li-ō-kol-pot′-o-mi): Surgical incision into the abdominal cavity by way of the vagina.

celiohysterectomy (sē′-li-ō-his-ter-ek′-to-mi): Surgical removal of the uterus via an abdominal incision; abdominal hysterectomy.

celioma (sē-li-ō′-ma): A tumor of the peritoneum, particularly a mesothelioma (*q.v.*).

celiomyositis (sē′-li-ō-mī-ō-sī′-tis): Inflammation of the abdominal muscles.

celiopathy (sē-li-op′-a-thi): Any abdominal disease.

celiopyosis (sē′-li-ō-pī-ō′-sis): Suppuration within the abdominal cavity, especially of the peritoneum.

celioscopy (sē-li-os′-ko-pi): Syn., laparoscopy, peritoneoscopy (*q.v.*).

celiotomy (sē-li-ot′-o-mi): The making of an incision into the abdominal cavity; usually refers to one through the loin or flank, but may also be made through the abdominal wall or the vagina.

cell: A mass of protoplasm containing a nucleus. The basic physiologic and structural unit of all living things. Consists of a central core, the nucleus, which is made up of nucleoplasm, enclosed in a membrane, and surrounded by cytoplasm, the whole being enclosed in a membrane which separates it from other cells. Certain cells are non-nucleated, *e.g.*, erythrocytes, and others are multinucleated, *e.g.*, the leukocytes. **ARGYROPHILIC C.,** cells that are capable of being stained by silver salts. **BAND C.,** a neutrophil with a nucleus in the form of a continuous band which may be coiled, twisted, or in the shape of a horseshoe; see neutrophil. **B CELLS,** beta lymphatic cells that migrate directly into tissues without passing through the thymus; they mature into plasma cells and are responsible for the production of immunoglobulins. **BETA CELLS,** cells that make up most of the bulk of the Islands of Langerhans in the pancreas; they secrete insulin. **C. MEMBRANE,** the semipermeable membrane that bounds all animal cells; the cell wall. **T-CELL,** a lymphocyte derived from the thymus and which participates in the body's immune defenses; in the gate control theory T-cells are assumed to respond to both excitatory and inhibitory impulses to cause or inhibit a response by the body to certain stimuli.

cell-mediated immunity: A specific type of immune reaction thought to be initiated by T-lymphocytes. See T-cell.

cellophane (sel′-ō-fān): A derivative of cellulose, made into a thin, transparent, highly impermeable sheet or tube; used in face masks and as a protective covering for wound and surgical dressings.

cellular (sel′-ū-lar): Pertaining to or composed of cells.

cellulicidal (sel′-ū-li-sī′-dal): Destructive to cells.

cellulitis (sel-ū-lī′-tis): A diffuse inflammation of connective tissue, especially the loose subcutaneous tissue. When it involves the pelvic tissues in the female it is called parametritis. When it occurs in the floor of the mouth it is called Ludwig's angina.

celluloneuritis (sel′-ū-lō-nū-rī′-tis): Inflammation of nerve cells.

cellulose (sel′-ū-lōs): A carbohydrate forming the outer walls of plant and vegetable cells. A polysaccharide which cannot be digested by man but supplies roughage for stimulation of peristalsis.

celom (sē′-lom): The body cavity of the fetus; from it the principal cavities of the trunk arise. Also coelom.

celoscope (sē′-lō-skōp): A lighted instrument for viewing the abdominal cavity.

Celsius (sel′-si-us): Swedish astronomer [1701–1744] who invented a thermometric scale in which the boiling point of water at sea level is 100 degrees and the melting point of ice is zero degrees (centigrade thermometer).

cement (sē-ment′): 1. Any plastic material used to bind contiguous objects or materials together. 2. Any material used for filling teeth or making other dental repairs. 3. The hard, white, bone-like substance covering the roots of the teeth; cementum.

censor (sen′-sor): Term employed by Freud to define the resistance which prevents repressed material from readily reentering the conscious mind from the subconscious (unconscious) mind unless they are disguised in some way.

center: 1. A group of neurons concerned with the control of a particular activity or function; usually named for the function they control, *e.g.*, respiratory center, auditory center, etc. 2. The midpoint of a body.

Centers for Disease Control: A federal agency in the Public Health Service, established to protect the health of the nation by providing leadership and direction in the investigation, identification, prevention, control, and eradication of preventable and other diseases. The major components are the Center for Infectious Diseases, Center for Environmental Health, Center for Health Promotion and Education, Center for Prevention Services, Center for Professional Development and Training, and Center for Occupational Safety and Health. Address, 1600 Clifton Rd., N.E., Atlanta, Ga 30333

centesis (sen-tē′-sis): A puncture of a body cavity with a trocar, needle, or aspirator. Often used with other word elements to indicate the part of the body involved, *e.g.*, abdominocentesis.

centi-: Prefix used in the metric system to indicate one one-hundredth.

centigrade (sen′-ti-grād): Having one hundred divisions or degrees. Usually applied to the Celcius thermometric scale in which the freezing point of water is fixed at 0 and the boiling point at 100 degrees.

centigram (sen′-ti-gram): A metric unit of weight; one one-hundredth part of a gram. Abbreviated cg or cgm.

centiliter (sen′-ti-lē-ter): One one-hundredth of a liter. Approximately 10 cc. Abbreviated cl.

centimeter (sen′-ti-mē-ter): In metric linear measurement, one one-hundredth of a meter. 0.3937 of an inch. Abbreviated cm.

centrad (sen′-trad): Toward a center, or toward the median line of the body.

central core disease: An inherited, progressive disorder characterized by slow weakening of skeletal muscles; so called because on biopsy the central core of muscles stains abnormally.

central nervous system: That part of the nervous system consisting of the brain, spinal cord, spinal nerves and their end organs.

central venous pressure: See under blood pressure.

centrifugal (sen-trif′-ū-gal): Efferent. Having a tendency to move away or outward from a center or from the cerebral cortex.

centrifuge (sen′-tri-fūj): An apparatus that rotates at high speed, thereby increasing the force of gravity so that substances of different densities are separated; usually used to separate particulate material from a suspending liquid.—centrifuge, v.t.

centrilobular (sen′-tri-lob′-ū-lar): In the central part of a lobule; usually refers to a lobule of the liver.

centriole (sen′-tri-ōl): Either of two cylindrical granules in the cytoplasm of cells which migrate to opposite poles during cell division and determine the arrangement of the spindles in the dividing cell.

centripetal (sen-trip′-et-al): Afferent. Having a tendency to move toward a center or toward the cerebral cortex.

centromere (sen′-trō-mēr): The part of the chromosome to which the spindle fiber is attached during mitosis (*q.v.*).

centrosome (sen′-trō-sōm): A minute spot in the cytoplasm of animal cells supposedly concerned with the division of the nucleus and which, in mitosis, draws the divided chromosomes to opposite sides of the dividing cell. See mitosis.

centrosphere (sen′-trō-sfēr): A small body near the nucleus of an animal cell which contains the centrosome.

centrum (sen′-trum): A center.

cephal-, cephalo-: Combining forms denoting head.

cephalad (sef′-a-lad): Toward, or in the direction of, the head.

cephalalgia (sef′-al-al′-ji-a): Pain in the head; headache. Also spelled cephalgia.

cephalhydrocele (sef-al-hī′-drō-sēl): A serous cyst under the scalp.

cephalic (sef-al′-ik): Pertaining to the head; near the head. C. INDEX, the ratio of the width to the length of the head. C. VERSION, an obstetric maneuver to change the fetal lie to a head presentation to facilitate delivery.

-cephalic, -cephalism, -cephaly: Combining forms denoting 1) the head; 2) headed or having a head.

cephalin (sef′-a-lin): A fraction of a phospholipid that exists in the brain from which it is extracted and used as a clotting agent in blood coagulation work. C. FLOCCULATION TEST, a laboratory test for diagnosing liver disease; it detects the presence of jaundice before it is observable in the patient.

cephalitis (sef-a-lī′-tis): Encephalitis (*q.v.*).

cephalocaudal (sef′-a-lō-kaw′-dal): 1. Refers to the long axis of the body, *i.e.*, from head to foot. 2. Refers to something going in both a cephalic and caudal direction, or going in a direction from the head to the lower part of the body.

cephalocele (sef′-a-lō-sēl): Hernia of the brain; protrusion of part of the cranial contents through the skull. ORBITAL C., protrusion of some of the cranial contents into the orbit of the eye; a birth defect usually accompanied by other eye defects.

cephalocentesis (sef′-a-lō-sen-tē′-sis): Surgical puncture of the head; usually refers to the insertion of a trocar or cannula into the brain to drain off the fluid of a hydrocephalus or of an abscess.

cephalodynia (sef-a-lō-din′-i-a): Pain in the head; headache.

cephalogyric (sef-a-lō-jī′-rik): Pertaining to turning or to rotary motions of the head.

cephalohematoma (sef-a′-lō-hē-ma-tō′-ma): A collection of blood beneath the fibrous covering of the skull. Also spelled cephalhematoma.

cephaloid (sef′-a-loyd): Resembling the head.

cephalomeningitis (sef′-a-lō-men-in-jī′-tis): Inflammation of the meninges of the brain.

cephalometer (sef-a-lom′-e-ter): An instrument for measuring the head dimensions.

cephalometry (sef-a-lom′-e-tri): Measurement of the living human head.

cephalomotor (sef-a-lō-mō′-tor): Pertaining to movements of the head.

cephalo-orbital (sef′-a-lō-or′-bi-tal): Pertaining to the skull and the orbits.

cephalopelvic (sef′-a-lō-pel′-vik): Term used in referring to the size of the head of the fetus in utero in relation to the size of the mother's bony pelvis. C. DISPROPORTION, a disparity between the size of an infant's head and that of the maternal pelvis or of the opening of the pelvis.

cephaloplegia (sef′-a-lō-plē′-ji-a): Paralysis of the muscles of the head and face.

cephalosporins (sef-a-lō-spōr′-ins): A group of broad-spectrum penicillinase-resistant antibiotics derived from *Cephalosporium,* a genus of fungi found in soil. Effective against gram-negative and gram-positive organisms including E. coli, Klebsiella, Hemophilius influenzae, Aerobacter, and Proteus. Used in treatment of certain severe infections of the respiratory and genitourinary tracts, bloodstream, bones and joints, and in staphylococcal and streptococcal infections of skin and soft tissues.

cephalothoracopagus (sef′-a-lō-thor-a-kop′-a-gus): Conjoined twins united at their heads, necks, and thoraces.

cephalotomy (sef-a-lot′-o-mi): An operation to reduce the circumference of the fetal head in order to assist its delivery.

cephalotripsy (sef-a-lō-trip′-si): In obstetrics, the instrumental crushing of the fetal head when delivery is impossible.

cephalotrypesis (sef′-a-lō-trī-pē′-sis): Trephining of the skull.

cerat-, cerato-: Combining forms denoting: 1. The sclera. 2. Horny tissue.

cerate (sē′-rāt): A preparation for external use; has a wax or fat base; consistency is between that of an ointment and a plaster; does not melt at ordinary temperatures.

cerato-: For words beginning thus see also words beginning kerato-.

cerclage (ser-klazh′): 1. A technique used in reducing a fracture; a wire or other nonabsorbable material is placed around the bone to hold it in the reduced position until the permanent fixation is accomplished. 2. The technique of stitching edges of an incompetent uterine cervix together with nonabsorbable sutures to prevent spontaneous abortion; the sutures are removed at term.

cerea flexibilitas (sēr′-e-a fleks-i-bil′-i-tas): The "waxy" flexibility often seen in patients with catatonic schizophrenia in which an arm or leg remains in any position in which is it placed.

cerebellar (ser′-e-bel′-ar): Pertaining to or involving the cerebellum. C. ATAXIA, a condition marked by muscular incoordination, due to a lesion or disease of the cerebellum; see also ataxia. C. GAIT, a characteristic wide-based, unsteady, staggering, lurching gait; due to a lesion or disease of the cerebellum.

cerebellitis (ser-e-bel-lī′-tis): Inflammation of the cerebellum.

cerebellospinal (ser′-e-bel-ō-spī′-nal): 1. Pertaining to the cerebellum and the spinal cord. 2. Proceeding from the cerebellum to the spinal cord, as a descending cerebellospinal tract; see under tract.

cerebellum (ser-e-bel′-um): That part of the brain which lies behind and below the cerebrum and above the pons and medulla oblongata; consists of two lateral hemispheres with a narrow central portion; its chief functions are the coordination of fine voluntary movements and the maintenance of equilibrium.—cerebellar, adj.

cerebral (ser-ē′-bral, ser′-e-bral): Pertaining to or affecting the cerebrum. C. ACCIDENT or CEREBROVASCULAR ACCIDENT, a common occurrence, caused by reduced blood supply to cerebral neurons; may result from hemorrhage, stenosis of cerebral arteries, embolism, or thrombosis. C. CORTEX, the outermost cellular layer of gray matter covering the cerebrum; is responsible for higher mental activities during consciousness. CEREBRAL DEATH, see brain death. C. CRY, the high-pitched cry of an infant; may be indicative of meningitis. C. DIPLEGIA, results from a birth injury to both hemispheres causing double hemiplegia and lack of development of limbs. C. HEMORRHAGE, hemorrhage into the cerebrum from a ruptured artery; may result from hypertension or arteriosclerosis. C. HERNIA, a hernia in which some of the brain substance protrudes through an opening in one of the bones of the skull as may occur after surgery or injury. C. LOCALIZATION, the specification of a certain area in the brain that controls a particular function such as speech, vision, etc. C. MENINGITIS, inflammation of the meninges of the brain. See meningitis. C. PALSY, a nonprogressive, persistent disorder of motor power resulting from an impairment in the development of the nervous system, due to a birth injury of cerebral motor nerves; covers a large group of disabilities, the most common of which is lack of muscular control; symptoms appear in infancy or early childhood. Several types are recognized: 1) ataxic, in which many muscles are involved; 2) spastic, the most common form, in which attempts to use affected muscles results in incoordinated movements; 3) athetoid, in which severe muscular incoordination is uncontrolled and uncontrollable; and 4) flaccid, in which muscular incoordination is very severe. C. THROMBOSIS, thrombosis occurring in a cerebral blood vessel.

cerebralgia (ser-e-bral′-ji-a): Headache.

cerebrate (ser′-e-brāt): To use the mind; to think.

cerebration (ser-e-brā′-shun): Functional or mental activity of the cerebrum; thinking.

cerebritis (ser-e-brī′ tis): Inflammation of the cerebrum.

cerebrology (ser-e-brol′-o-ji): The scientific study of the brain and its functions.

cerebromalacia (ser′-e-brō-ma-lā′ shi-a): Softening of the substance of the cerebrum.

cerebromedullary (ser′-e-brō-med′-ū-la-ri): Pertaining to the cerebrum and the spinal cord.

cerebromeningitis (ser′-e-brō-men-in-jī′ tis): Inflammation of the brain and its meninges.

cerebropathy (ser′-e-brop′-a-thi): Any disease or disorder of the brain.

cerebroretinal (ser′-e-brō-ret′-i-nal): Pertaining to or involving both the brain and the retina. C. ANGIOMATOSIS, see von Hippel-Landau disease. C. DEGENERATION, a condition characteristic of a group of hereditary degenerative diseases, *e.g.*, amaurotic familial idiocy, Niemann-Pick disease, and infantile Gaucher's disease; marked by retinal changes and progressive dementia.

cerebrosclerosis (ser′-ē-brō-sklē-rō′-sis): Hardening of the substance of the cerebrum.

cerebroside (ser′-e-brō-sīd): A lipid substance found in body tissues, particularly brain and nerve tissue.

cerebrospinal (ser′-e-brō-spī′-nal): Pertaining to the brain and spinal cord. **C. FEVER,** an epidemic form of cerebrospinal meningitis (*q.v.*). **C. FLUID,** the fluid filling the ventricles of the brain and the central canal of the spinal cord; also found in the cranial and subarachnoid spaces; it is colorless, odorless, and clear, with a specific gravity of 1.007; contains protein and a few white cells but no red cells; has a fluctuating glucose level; and a normal pressure of 80–180 millimeters of water when the patient is lying down. **C. GANGLIA,** ganglia located on the dorsal root of each spinal nerve; see ganglion. **C. MENINGITIS,** inflammation of the meninges of the spinal cord. **C. NERVE,** one that runs from or to the brain or spinal cord, *i.e.*, a central nervous system nerve. **C. PUNCTURE,** usually refers to a lumbar puncture, *i.e.*, a puncture into the subarachnoid space between the third and fourth lumbar vertebrae. **C. SYSTEM,** consists of the brain, spinal cord, and the nerves emanating from or running to them.

cerebrotonia (ser′-e-brō-tō′-ni-a): A temperamental trait manifested by restraint, inhibition in regard to physical enjoyment, apprehensiveness, and a tendency toward concealment.

cerebrovascular (ser′-ē-brō-vas′-kū-lar): Pertaining to the blood vessels of the brain, especially to pathological conditions or changes in these vessels. **C. ACCIDENT,** the rupture of a blood vessel within or near the brain, as occurs in cerebral hemorrhage, a stroke, a transient ischemic attack, or a change in the blood supply in the brain as a result of embolism or thrombosis that causes neurological dysfunction.

cerebrum (ser′-e-brum, se-rē′-brum): The largest and uppermost part of the brain; it does not include the cerebellum, pons and medulla. The longitudinal fissure divides it into two hemispheres, each containing a lateral ventricle. The internal substance is white, the outer convoluted cortex is gray.—cerebral, adj.

certifiable (ser-ti-fī′-a-b'l): Term used in reference to: 1. Infectious or industrial diseases which, by law, are reportable to health authorities. 2. A person who behaves in such a way that he is considered to have a psychosis severe enough to require his placement in a psychiatric institution.

Certificate of Need: Popular term for a law requiring a review of facilities already available to institutions applying to qualify for federal funds for use in various health care programs, the main objective being containment of hospital costs.

certification (ser-ti-fi-kā′-shun): The process whereby a nongovernmental agency or association recognizes that an individual or an agency has met predetermined standards set for it by the certifying agency. For health care agencies, certification is granted by the American Hospital Association's Joint Commission on Accreditation for Hospitals. For nurses, the American Nurses' Association conducts programs for certification. The ANA certification, designed in 1973, identifies members of the profession who practice at a higher level than that required for state licensure. Candidates must hold a current license to practice as an R.N., have had experience in the area of certification, and pass a written examination to demonstrate currency in practice. The ANA conducts certification programs for the following, all of whom may be designated by the initials R.N.,C.: Community Health Nurse; Adult Nurse Practitioner; Family Nurse Practitioner; School Nurse Practitioner; Gerontological Nurse; Gerontological Nurse Practitioner; Maternal and Child Health Nurse; High-Risk Perinatal Nurse; Pediatric Nurse Practitioner; Medical-Surgical Nurse; Clinical Specialist in Medical-Surgical Nursing; Psychiatric and Mental Health Nurse. The American Nurses' Association also conducts programs for certification of administrators who have had experience in nursing administration or consultation; these nurses may be certified in Nursing Administration (R.N.,C.N.A.) or Nursing Administration, Advanced (R.N.,C.N.A.A.). The various health care specialties have their own specialty boards some of which are responsible for certification of their members. Certification by the ANA is for five years, after which the nurse may apply for recertification, and is not to be confused with registration or licensing.

Certified Laboratory Technician: A clinical laboratory worker specially trained to perform routine laboratory tests.

Certified Nurse-Midwife: A nurse-midwife who has had training in both nursing and midwifery, and has met the certification requirements of the American College of Nurse-midwives.

ceruloplasmin (sē-roo-lō-plaz′-min): A protein found in plasma; contains most of the copper normally present in plasma; is markedly decreased in hepatolenticular degeneration.

cerumen (se-roo′-men): Earwax. The soft, yellowish-brown, wax-like secretion of the ceruminous glands in the external auditory canal.—ceruminous, ceruminal, adj.

cervical (ser′-vi-kal): Pertaining to the neck, or to the neck of an organ. **C. ADENITIS,** inflammation of the lymph glands or nodes of the neck. **C. CANAL,** the lumen of the cervix uteri which leads from the body of the uterus to the vagina. **C. CAP,** a rubber contraceptive cap that fits over the end of the uterine cervix. **C. COLLAR,** an appliance used to keep the head in neutral or slightly fixed position. **C. HALTER,** a device used to increase vertebral separation and thus relieve pressure on cervical nerves; see c. traction halter under traction. **C. INCOMPETENCE,** painless dilatation of the cervix of the pregnant uterus; usually causes termination of the pregnancy. **C. RIB,** a riblike process that sometimes appears on a cervical vertebra; may present no problems or it may press on the brachial plexus when it causes **C.** rib syndrome. **C. NERVES,** the first eight pairs of spinal nerves. **C. VERTEBRAE,** the first (upper) seven bones of the spinal column.

cervical disc syndrome: A condition characterized by pain radiating to the shoulder and arm; due to compression of the cervical nerve roots.

cervical rib syndrome: A group of symptoms caused by pressure on the brachial plexus and the cervical subclavian artery by a supernumerary cervical rib and/or the large scalene muscles. Symptoms include pain over the shoulder and back of the neck, but particularly in the forearm and ulnar area of the hand where it is accompanied by tingling, numbness, coldness, cyanosis, anesthesia, weakness, and muscular atrophy.

cervicectomy (ser-vi-sek′-to-mi): Amputation of the cervix of the uterus.

cervicitis (ser-vi-sī′-tis): Acute or chronic inflammation of the uterine cervix.

cervicoauricular (ser′-vi-kō-aw-rik′-ū-lar): Pertaining to the neck and the ear.

cervicobrachial (ser′-vi-kō-brā′-ki-al): Pertaining to the neck and upper arm.

cervicocolpitis (ser′-vi-kō-kol-pī′-tis): Inflammation of the uterine cervix and the vagina.

cervicodynia (ser-vi-kō-din′-i-a): A cramp or pain in the neck.

cervicofacial (ser′-vi-kō-fā′-shi-al): Pertaining to the face and neck.

cervicorectal (ser′-vi-kō-rek′-tal): Pertaining to the cervix of the uterus and the rectum.

cervicovaginitis (ser′-vi-kō-vaj-i-nī′-tis): Inflammation of the uterine cervix and the vagina.

cervicovesical (ser′-vi-kō-ves′-i-kal): Pertaining to both the uterine cervix and the urinary bladder.

cervix (ser′-viks): A neck or constricted part of an organ. **C. UTERI,** the neck of the uterus. **INCOMPETENT C.,** occurs usually at about the 16th to 20th week of pregnancy when the cervix dilates painlessly; a suturing procedure is sometimes utilized to avoid abortion; see cerclage.

cesarean section (se-sar′-ē-an): Delivery of a fetus via an incision through the abdominal and uterine walls. So called because Caesar was supposed to have been born that way. Also caesarean.

cesium (sē′-zi-um): A rare metallic element in the alkali group. Several of its salts have actions similar to those of potassium and have been used experimentally in medicine. **C. BROMIDE,** used in infrared spectrometry. **C-137,** has a half-life of 30 years; encapsulated, it is used as a source of radiation for therapeutic purposes. Also caeseum. Chemical symbol, Cs.

cesticidal (ses-ti-sī′-dal): Destructive to tapeworms of the subclass *Cestoda.*

cestode (ses′-tōd): Tapeworm. See Taenia.—cestoid, adj.

cestodiasis (ses-tō-dī′-a-sis): Infestation with cestodes (*q.v.*).

cevitamic acid (sev-i-tam′-ik as′-id): Ascorbic acid (*q.v.*).

cf.: Abbreviation for compare.

CFT: Abbreviation for complement fixation test. See complement.

Chadwick's sign: See Jacquemier's sign.

chafing (chāf′-ing): Irritation of the skin due to: 1) irritants; or 2) two skin surfaces rubbing together.

Chagas' disease: An acute or chronic condition occurring chiefly in South and Central America; caused by infestation with the parasite *Trepanosoma cruzi,* transmitted to man by the bite of various bugs; characterized by fever, lymph gland involvement, splenomegaly, megacolon, sometimes encephalitis, arrhythmia, and chronic heart disease often resulting in death from heart failure. [Carlos Chagas, Brazilian physician. 1879–1934.]

chain reaction: A series of events each of which initiates or influences a following reaction.

chalasia (ka-lā′-zi-a): The relaxation of a body opening, particularly one that is normally guarded by a sphincter muscle. May be a cause of regurgitation or vomiting by infants when there is no other sign of distress.

chalazion (ka-lā′-zi-on): A cyst on the edge of the eyelid from retained secretion of the meibomian glands. Similar to a stye, but painless. May disappear or may need to be surgically evacuated.—chalazia, pl.

chalicosis (kal-i-kō′-sis): A lung disease caused by inhalation of stone dust. Found chiefly among stonecutters. Pneumoconiosis (*q.v.*).

chalkitis (kal-kī′-tis): An occupational disorder marked by inflammation of the eyes; caused by workers rubbing their eyes after handling brass.

chalone (kā′-lon): Any one of several inhibitors of mitosis that is active within the tissue in which it is elaborated; inhibits proliferation of cells and is thought to be reversible in action.

chalybeate (kal-ib′-ē-āt): 1. Containing iron, as occurs in the waters of various spas. 2. A pharmaceutical preparation containing iron.

chamber: In anatomy, an enclosed space or cavity, *e.g.*, the **C.'S** of the heart, or the anterior and posterior **C.'S** of the eye. See also hyperbaric oxygen chamber under hyperbaric.

Chamberlen forceps: The original obstetric forceps, invented by Dr. Peter Chamberlen [English obstetrician 1560–1631] but first described in the literature in 1773.

chamecephaly (kam-e-sef′-a-li): The condition of having a flat head with a low cephalic index (*q.v.*).—chamecephalic, adj.

CHAMPUS: Abbreviation for *C*ivilian *H*ealth and *M*edical *P*rograms for *U*niformed *S*ervices (*q.v.*).

chancre (shang′-ker): A primary lesion, usually of syphilis or chancroid; formed at the site of infection two to three weeks after infection; usually on the lips, genitals, or fingers; consists of an ordinary round or oval red spot that may go unnoticed as it is usually painless; may develop into a papule, ulcer or erosion that is highly infectious. Associated with swelling of local lymph glands. Also called hard chancre and hunterian chancre.

chancroid (shang′-kroyd): A type of nonsyphilitic venereal infection caused by *Hemophilus ducreyi;* prevalent in warmer climates; associated with uncleanliness; transmitted by sexual contact; characterized by regional lymph node involvement, and multiple painful, ragged ulcers on the penis or vulva that have a purulent exudate.

Chandelier's sign: Tenderness of the cervix on digital examination and a feeling of fullness or masses at the sides of the pelvis; an indication of pelvic inflammatory disease.

change of life: The menopause (*q.v.*).

character (kar′-ak-ter): The sum total of the known and predictable mental characteristics of an individual, particularly his conduct. **C. CHANGE,** denotes change in the form of conduct to one foreign to the patient's natural disposition, *e.g.* indecent behavior in a hitherto respectable person. Common in the psychoses. **C. DISORDER,** term given to a pattern of behavior that is disapproved or unacceptable in the person's social environment.

characteristic (kar′-ak-ter-is′-tik): 1. A specific, distinguishing attribute or trait. 2. A structural or functional feature of an organism.

characterology (kar′-ak-ter-ol′-o-ji): The study of character and personality and their development.

charcoal (char′-kōl): The residue after burning organic substances at a high temperature in an enclosed vessel. Used in medicine for its adsorptive and deodorant properties. **ACTIVATED C., C.** that has been treated to increase its adsorptive power; used in treating diarrhea and as an antidote in some poisonings.

Charcot-Marie-Tooth disease: Progressive neuropathic muscular dystrophy. See muscular dystrophy.

Charcot's joint (shar′-kōs): Complete disorganization of a joint associated with syringomyelia or advanced cases of tabes dorsalis (locomotor ataxia). Condition is painless. Also called neurogenic joint disease and Charcot's arthropathy. **C. TRIAD,** late manifestations of disseminated sclerosis—nystagmus, intention tremor and staccato speech. [Jean Martin Charcot, French neurologist and clinician. 1825–1893.]

charge nurse: The title usually given to the nurse who is in charge of a particular unit of a hospital when the head nurse is off duty.

charlatan (shar′-la-tan): One who pretends to have knowledge or skills which he does not possess; a quack.

Charles' law: States that, at constant pressure, the volume of a given mass of gas is directly proportional to the absolute temperature. Also called Gay-Lussac's law.

charley horse: Soreness, stiffness and pain in a muscle or tendon following injury or excessive athletic activity. Term usually restricted to the quadriceps muscle. Slang.

chart: A record of data; may be in tabular or graph form. **GENEALOGICAL C.,** a design showing all descendents of a common ancestor; may be used to determine whether a disease is due to presence of a particular gene. **PATIENT'S CHART,** an individual record that is kept for each hospital patient. Common usage refers to a collection of forms for recording various types of information, *e.g.*, laboratory and x-ray examination reports; patient's temperature, pulse and respirations; nurses' notes, including their observations of the patient's condition, food intake, etc. The chart becomes part of the hospital's permanent records; it is a legal document. **SNELLEN'S C.,** a chart of block letters used in testing vision.

charting: The recording on a patient's chart of the important data about a patient and his illness, his medical and nursing care, and the progress and outcome of his disorder.

Chassaignac's tubercle (shas-ān-yahks′): A landmark structure; located at the level of the thyroid on the 6th cervical vertebra; the most prominent of the cervical vertebrae.

chaulmoogra oil: A substance formerly much used in the treatment of leprosy; now largely replaced by the sulfones and sulfonamides.

CHB: Abbreviation for complete heart block.

CHD: Abbreviation for coronary heart disease.

Chediak-Higashi syndrome: A progressive congenital disorder characterized by albinism, pancytopenia, photophobia, enlarged liver and spleen, and a tendency to develop malignant lymphoma; usually fatal.

cheek: The side wall of the oral cavity.

cheil-, cheilo-: Combining forms denoting relationship to the lips.

cheilalgia (kī-lal′-ji-a): Pain in the lips.

cheilectomy (kī-lek′-to-mi): Surgical excision of part of the lip.

cheilectropion (kī-lek-trō′-pi-on): An abnormal outward turning of the lips.

cheilitis (kī-lī′-tis): Inflammation of the lip(s).

cheilognathopalatoschisis (kī′-lō-nath′-ō-pal-a-tos′-ki-sis): A cleft of the upper lip, upper jaw, and both hard and soft palates.

cheilophagia (kī-lō-fā′-ji-a): Lip-biting.

cheiloplasty (kī′-lō-plas-ti): Any plastic operation on the lip.

cheilorrhaphy (kī-lor′-a-fī): Suturing of a cut or lacerated lip, or repair of a harelip.

cheiloschisis (kī-lōs′-ki-sis): Harelip.

cheilosis (kī-lō′-sis): Fissuring and scaling of the lips, especially at the angles of the mouth, usually resulting from riboflavin deficiency.

cheilotomy (kī-lot′-o-mi): Incision of the lip.

cheir-, cheiro-: Combining forms denoting relationship to the hand.

cheiralgia (kī-ral′-ji-a): Pain in the hand. Also cheiragra.

cheirarthritis (kī-rar-thrī′-tis): Inflammation of the joints of the fingers and hands.

cheirology (kī-rol′-o-ji): See chirology.

cheiromegaly (kī-rō-meg′-a-li): Abnormal enlargement of the hands.

cheiroplasty (kī′-rō-plas-ti): Plastic surgery on the hand.

cheiropompholyx (kī′-rō-pom′-fo-liks): Symmetrical eczematous eruption of the skin of the hands (especially fingers) characterized by the formation of tiny vesicles and associated with itching or burning. On the feet the condition is called podopompholyx.

cheirospasm (kī′-rō-spazm): Writer's cramp (*q.v.*).

chelating agents (kē′-lā-ting): Soluble organic compounds that can fix certain metallic ions into their molecular structure; the chelates resulting from this action are used therapeutically in treatment of certain metal poisonings and the new compound formed in the body is excreted in the urine.

chelation (kē-lā′-shun): The interaction between a metallic substance and an organic compound having both a carboxyl (OH) group and a hydroxyl (HO) group so as to form a ring type structure.

chemical (kem′-i-kal): 1. Of or pertaining to chemistry. 2. A substance produced by or used in a chemical process. **C. CHANGE,** the transformation of a substance into a different substance through a chemical reaction. **C. FORMULA,** the composition or structure of a substance as represented by chemical symbols. **C. REACTION,** the interaction of two or more substances which results in chemical change. **C. SYMBOL,** a single capital letter or a capital and small letter used as an abbreviation for an atom of an element. **C. WARFARE,** the use in war of toxic gases, incendiary substances, and poisonous chemicals.

cheminosis (kem-i-nō′-sis): Any pathological condition caused by a chemical.

chemistry (kem′-is-tri): The science that deals with the composition, structure, properties, behavior, and reactions of substances and the changes they may undergo.

chemo-: Combining form denoting relationship to: 1) chemistry; 2) a chemical.

chemoceptor (kēm′-ō-sep-tor): Chemoreceptor (*q.v.*).

chemonucleolysis (kē′-mō-nū-klē-ol′-i-sis): A technique for treating lumbar disk disease. Consists of injecting a proteolytic enzyme into the intervertebral disk.

chemopallidectomy (kē′-mō-pal-i-dek′-to-mi): The destruction of a predetermined section of globus pallidus by the injection of chemicals. The operation is performed for the relief of parkinsonism and other similar conditions that are marked by muscle rigidity.

chemoprophylaxis (kē′-mō-prō-fi-lak′-sis): The prevention of a specific disease (or recurrent attack) by administration of chemotherapeutic agents.—chemoprophylactic, adj.

chemopsychiatry (kē′-mō-si-kī′-a-tri): Treatment of mental or emotional disorders by administration of drugs.

chemoreceptor (kē′-mō-rē-sep′-tor): 1. A chemical linkage in a living cell having an affinity for, and capable of combining with, certain other chemical substances. 2. A sensory end organ that responds to a chemical stimulus.

chemoserotherapy (kē′-mō-sēr-ō-ther′-a-pi): Treatment of infection by a combination of drugs and serum.

chemosis (kē-mō′-sis): An edema or swelling of the bulbar conjunctiva.—chemotic, adj.

chemosuppressive (kē′-mō-sup-pres′-iv): Syn., chemoprophylactic. See chemoprophylaxis.

chemosurgery (kē-mō-sur′-jer-i): The destruction of diseased or unwanted tissue by the application of chemical agents.

chemosynthesis (kē-mō-sin′-the-sis): In physiology, the production of carbohydrates by use of energy derived from a chemical reaction rather than from light. See photosynthesis.

chemotaxis (kē-mō-tak′-sis), chemotaxy: Response of organisms to chemical stimuli, attraction towards a chemical being positive **C.**, and repulsion being negative **C.**

chemothalamectomy (kē′ mō-thal-a-mek′-

to-mi): Destruction of part of the thalamus by the injection of a chemical; similar to chemopallidectomy (*q.v.*). Done for the relief of tremor.

chemotherapy (kē-mō-ther′-a-pi): The oral, intramuscular, or intravenous administration of a specific chemical agent to arrest the progress of, or eradicate, a specific pathologic condition in the body without causing irreversible injury to healthy tissue; widely used in the treatment of cancer.

chemtrode (kem′-trōd): A small hollow tube that can be implanted in the brain and used to deliver small amounts of chemicals to specific areas.

chenodeoxycholic acid (kē′-nō-dē-oks-i-kō′-lik as′-id): A normal constituent of bile; has been used in treatment of gallbladder disease since it allows the cholesterol in gallstones to dissolve.

cherry angioma: See under angioma.

cherry-red spot: A bright red spot(s) seen on the macula (*q.v.*) in infants with infantile amaurotic idiocy, Niemann-Pick disease, or Gaucher's disease.

chest: The thorax (*q.v.*). **C. CAVITY,** the upper division of the body cavity, containing the heart, lungs, and related structures. **C. TUBES,** tubes inserted into the second intercostal or fifth intercostal space for the removal of air or fluid from the pleural cavity; usually attached to a water-seal apparatus. **FLAIL CHEST,** an unstable thoracic cage due to fracture in which two or more ribs are detached; the segment is drawn inward on inspiration and pushed outward on exhalation; loss of rigidity of the chest wall may lead to inadequate ventilation and result in respiratory failure. See also barrel chest; funnel breast; pigeon breast.

chestmobile: A vehicle outfitted as a clinic which travels from place to place for the purpose of making chest x rays of the general population.

Cheyne-Stokes respiration: A breathing pattern in which the respirations gradually increase in depth, then decrease in depth, and then stop altogether for a period, after which the pattern is repeated. See under respiration.

CHF: Abbreviation for congestive heart failure.

chi square: A technique used in research to analyze differences among variables, expressed as a ratio; it is obtained by dividing the square of the differences between the variables observed and the expected frequencies divided by the theoretic frequencies of the variables.

Chiari-Frommel syndrome: A postpregnancy condition marked by prolonged lactation, amenorrhea, and atrophy of the uterus; thought to be caused by pituitary dysfunction.

chiasm (kī′-azm): An X-shaped crossing or decussation. **OPTIC C.** or **CHIASMA OPTICUM,** the meeting of the optic nerves; where the fibers from the medial or nasal half of each retina cross the middle line on the ventral surface of the brain to join the optic tract of the opposite side. Also chiasma.

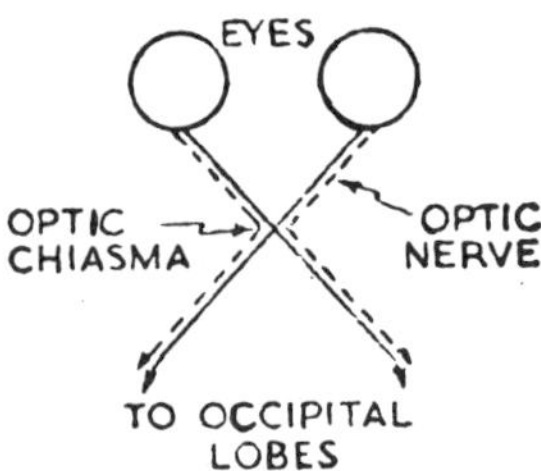

Optic chiasm

chiasma (kī-az′-ma): Chiasm.—chiasmata, pl.

chiasmatic (kī-az-mat′-ik): Pertaining to a chiasm. Also chiasmal.

chicken breast: See pigeon breast.

chickenpox: A mild, specific, highly contagious disease of childhood, caused by a virus. Successive crops of vesicles appear first on the trunk; they scab and heal without causing scars. Syn., varicella.

chigger (chig′-er): A minute larval mite that burrows into the skin of warm-blooded animals. In man its bite produces a wheal (*q.v.*) which itches intensely. Not the same as jigger.

chigoe (chig′-o): The sand flea of South America and southern U.S.; burrows into the skin of the feet and legs causing intense irritation that may progress to ulceration.

chilblain (chil′-blān): Congestion and swelling attended with severe itching and burning sensation in reaction to damp, cold weather; fingers, toes and ears are affected particularly. Erythema pernio.

child abuse: Beating, starving, neglecting, sexually or emotionally abusing, mistreating, or demeaning of a child by parents or other adult, often one who is emotionally disturbed; reportable in most states; often a social or legal agency becomes involved in preventing further abuse and in getting treatment for the abuser. See also battered child syndrome and baby battering under baby.

Child Health Act of 1967: Provides for the establishment of a wide variety of maternal and child health care services, with federal and state funding, and with the objective of providing comprehensive health care for children.

childbearing: Pregnancy and the delivery of a child. **C. PERIOD,** the years of a woman's life during which she can normally bear children, *i.e.,* the years between puberty and menopause.

childbed: The state of a woman being in labor or bringing forth a child. **C. FEVER,** puerperal fever (*q.v.*).

childbirth: Term applied to the normal termination of pregnancy with the birth of an infant. **FAMILY-CENTERED C.,** siblings and other family members are present during the birth process; birth takes place in the home or birthing room, etc.; incorporates the infant into the family unit immediately. **NATURAL C.,** popular term for a form of **C.** that emphasizes reduction or elimination of the use of drugs; patient is prepared by courses in which she learns the anatomy and physiology involved, and practices a regimen of exercises during pregnancy.

childhood: The period of life between infancy and puberty. **C. SCHIZOPHRENIA,** that which occurs before puberty; characterized by autism (*q.v.*) and immaturity.

Childrens' Bureau: A federal government agency established in 1912; provided leadership for many progressive child health and welfare programs until 1969 when its functions were distributed among numerous other federal, state, and local agencies.

chill: A sudden sensation of cold, accompanied by shivering, often followed by rise in body temperature. Sometimes the initial symptom of an acute infection such as pneumonia; a characteristic symptom of malaria.

chilo-: For words beginning thus see words beginning cheilo-.

chimera (ki-mēr′-a): In genetics, refers to an individual whose body contains cells from two different cell lines that are derived from two different zygotes.

chimney sweep's cancer: Scrotal carcinoma. A squamous cell carcinoma due to chronic exposure to coal soot.

chin: The mentum; the lower anterior prominence of the mandible.

chionablepsia (kī-ō-na-blep′-si-a): Snow-blindness.

chiro-: For words beginning thus see also words beginning cheiro-.

chirology (kī-rol′-ō-ji): A method of communicating with or between deaf-mutes through hand signals. Dactylology.

chiropodist (kī-rop′-o-dist): One qualified in chiropody (*q.v.*). Podiatrist.

chiropody (kī-rop′-o-di): The treatment of corns, callosities, bunions and toenail conditions. Podiatry.

chiropractic (kī-rō-prak′-tik): A system of treatment based on the theory that disease is caused by impingement on the spinal nerves and that relief or cure can be effected through manual manipulation of the spinal column.

chiropractor: One who practices chiropractic (*q.v.*).

chiropsia (kī-rop′-si-a): Friction applied with the hands; massage.

chirospasm (kī′-rō-spazm): Writer's cramp (*q.v.*).

Chlamydia (kla-mid′-i-a): A genus of parasitic gram-negative organisms: two species are 1) **C. PSITTACI** which causes psittacosis and 2) **C. TRACHOMATIS,** a serious sexually transmitted pathogen which causes lymphogranuloma venereum (*q.v.*), inclusion conjunctivitis, blinding trachoma, epididymitis, pelvic inflammation, cervicitis, urethritis, salpingitis, prostatitis, Reiter's syndrome, infant pneumonia.

chloasma (klō-az′-ma): Painless yellowish or dark brown patches on the skin; melasma. **C. GRAVIDARUM,** patches of brown discoloration on the forehead, cheeks, nipples and along the median line of the abdomen, occurring during pregnancy; sometimes called "mask of pregnancy."

chlor-, chloro-: Combining forms denoting a green color.

chloramines (klor′-a-mēns): Chlorine compounds used as topical antiseptics and disinfectants.

chlorate (klō′-rāt): Any salt of chloric acid.

chlordane (klor′-dān): An organic insecticide; may cause poisoning in humans if ingested, inhaled, or absorbed.

chloremia (klō-rē′-mi-a): 1. Decrease in the hemoglobin and red cells; chlorosis (*q.v.*). 2. The presence of more than the normal amount of chlorides in the blood.

chlorhydria (klor-hī′-dri-a): An excess of hydrochloric acid in the gastric juice.

chloride (klō′-rīd): A salt of hydrochloric acid; a compound composed of two substances, one of which is chlorine that carries a negative charge of electricity.

chloride of lime: See under chlorinated.

chloridemia (klō′-ri-dē′-mi-a): The presence of chlorides in the blood.

chloriduria (klō′-ri-dū′-ri-a): More than the normal amount of chlorides in the urine.

chlorinated (klōr′-in-ā-ted): Said of a substance to which chlorine has been added, *e.g.*, water. **C. LIME,** a substance made by passing chlorine over hydrated lime; formerly much used as a disinfectant, fumigant and deodorant; also called chloride of lime.

chlorination (klōr-i-nā′-shun): The procedure of adding chlorine to a substance to disinfect it, *e.g.*, water, sewage.

chlorine (klor′-ēn): A yellowish-green gaseous element with an irritating, suffocating odor. Represented by the symbol Cl.

chloroanemia (klor-ō-a-nē′-mi-a): See chlorosis.

chloroform (klor′-ō-form): A clear, colorless,

volatile, heavy liquid with a sweetish taste, once much used as a general anesthetic.

chloroleukemia (klō′-rō-lū-kē′-mi-a): A type of leukemia in which no perceptible tumor masses occur, but the organs and body fluids have a definite green color on autopsy.

chloroma (klō-rō′-ma): A condition in which multiple malignant greenish-yellow growths develop, especially on the periosteum of the facial and cranial bones and the vertebrae. Observed most frequently in children and young adults.

chlorophenothane (klō′-rō-fēn′nō-thān): The insecticide, dichloro-diphenyl-trichloroethane; called DDT. See DDT and dicophane.

chlorophyll (klō′-rō-fil): The coloring matter of green plants; essential for photosynthesis (*q.v.*). Now prepared synthetically for use in medicine and as a deodorant.

chloropicrin (klō-rō-pik′-rin): A poisonous oily liquid used as a disinfectant and fungicide.

chloropsia (klō-rop′-si-a): A visual defect that causes objects to appear green.

chloroquine (klor′-ō-kwin): A chemical used as an antimalarial and antiamebic.

chlorosarcoma (klō-rō-sar-kō′-ma): See chloroma.

chlorosis (klō-rō′-sis): An old name for simple iron deficiency anemia occurring especially in young women.

chloruresis (klōr-ūr-ē′-sis): Excretion of chlorides in the urine.

chloruretic (klor-ū-ret′-ik): 1. Promoting urinary excretion of chlorides. 2. An agent that promotes urinary excretion of chlorides.

CHN: Abbreviation for Community Health Nurse; see under nurse.

choana (kō′-a-na): Funnel-shaped opening. The posterior nasal orifices or nares (*q.v.*).—choanae, pl.; choanal, adj.

choanal (kō′-a-nal): Pertaining to a choana. C. ATRESIA, obstruction occurring in a choana; refers often to obstruction in the airway of the newborn.

chocolate cyst: See under cyst.

choke: To strangle or suffocate due to obstruction or compression of the trachea or larynx.

choke damp: Dangerous atmosphere sometimes formed in coal mines due to gradual absorption of oxygen from the air and the giving off of carbon dioxide from the coal. Black damp.

choked disk: Swelling and protrusion of the optic disk (*q.v.*); occurs in several disease conditions including brain tumor.

chol-, chole-, cholo-: Combining forms denoting bile, gall.

cholagogue (kō′-la-gog): A drug that causes an increased flow of bile into the intestine.

cholalic acid (kō-lal′-ik as′-id): Cholic acid (*q.v.*).

cholangiocarcinoma (kō-lan′-ji-ō-kar-si-nō′-ma): An adenocarcinoma occurring usually within an intrahepatic bile duct.

cholangiogram (kō-lan′-ji-ō-gram): An x-ray film demonstrating the bile ducts. TRANSHEPATIC PERCUTANEOUS C., a roentgenologic procedure whereby a radiopaque dye is injected by needle through the abdominal wall into the biliary tree and the movement of the dye into the liver is observed on a fluoroscopic screen; used to differentiate between intrahepatic and extrahepatic jaundice.

cholangiography (kō-lan-ji-og′-ra-fi): Radiographic examination of hepatic, cystic, and bile ducts.

cholangiohepatitis (kō-lan′-ji-ō-hep-a-tī′-tis): Severe inflammation of the liver and small bile ducts in the liver; often associated with fluke infestation which causes obstructions in the ducts.

cholangiolitis (kō-lan′-ji-ō-lī′-tis): Inflammation of the bile ducts within the liver.

cholangioma (kō-lan′-ji-ō′-ma): A tumor in a bile duct, especially a duct within the liver.

cholangiopancreatography (ko-lan′-ji-ō-pan-krē-a-tog′-ra-fi): Radiographic demonstration of the bile ducts and the pancreatic ducts following administration of a radiopaque dye; utilizes a fiberscope.

cholangiotomy (kō-lan-ji-ot′-o-mi): Surgical incision into a bile duct.

cholangitis (kōl-an-jī′-tis): Inflammation of a bile duct; symptoms include pain in the upper right abdominal quadrant, fever, nausea, vomiting, jaundice.

cholecalciferol (kō′-lē-kal-sif′-er-ōl): Vitamin D_3, found in butter, egg yolk, and fish liver oils; also prepared synthetically. An antirachitic vitamin.

cholecyst (kō′-lē-sist): The gallbladder.—cholecystic, adj.

cholecystagogue (kō′-lē-sis′-ta-gog): An agent that stimulates activity of the gallbladder and promotes the flow of bile from it.

cholecystalgia (kō′-lē-sis-tal′-ji-a): Biliary colic; may be due to inflammation of the gallbladder or to the obstruction of a cystic duct by a gallstone.

cholecystangiogram (kō′-lē-sis-tan′-ji-ō-gram): Film demonstrating gallbladder, cystic and common bile ducts after administration of opaque medium.

cholecystectasia (kō′-lē-sis-tek-tā′-zi-a): Dilatation of the gallbladder.

cholecystectomy (kō-lē-sis-tek′-to-mi): Surgical removal of the gallbladder.

cholecystenterostomy (kō′-lē-sis-ten-ter-os′-to-mi): The surgical establishment of an anastomosis between the gallbladder and the small intestine.

cholecystic (kō-lē-sis′-tik): Pertaining to the gallbladder.

cholecystitis (kō-lē-sis-tī′-tis): Inflammation of the gallbladder; may be acute or chronic.

cholecystocholangiogram (kō′-lē-sis-tō-kō-lan′-ji-ō-gram): x ray of the gallbladder and the bile ducts.

cholecystocolonic (kō′-lē-sis-tō-kō-lon′-ic): Pertaining to the gallbladder and the colon or to a communication between them.

cholecystocolostomy (kō′-lē-sis-tō-kō-los′-to-mi): The surgical establishment of an anastomosis between the gallbladder and some portion of the colon, usually the upper part.

cholecystoduodenostomy (kō-lē-sis′-tō-du-ō-dēn-os′-to-mi): The establishment of an anastomosis between the gallbladder and the duodenum. Usually necessary in cases of stricture of common bile duct, which may be congenital or due to previous inflammation or operation.

cholecystogastrostomy (kō-lē-sis′-tō-gas-tros′-to-mi): The surgical establishment of an anastomosis between the gallbladder and the stomach; a palliative operation when the common bile duct is obstructed by an irremovable growth.

cholecystogram (kō-lē-sis′-tō-gram): An x-ray picture of the gallbladder obtained by cholecystography (*q.v.*).

cholecystography (kō-lē-sis-tog′-ra-fi): Radiographic examination of the gallbladder after it has been rendered opaque by the ingestion or intravenous injection of an opaque medium.—cholecystographic, adj.; cholecystographically, adv.; cholecystograph, n.

cholecystojejunostomy (kō-lē-sis′-tō-jē-jū-nos′-to-mi): The surgical establishment of an anastomosis between the gallbladder and the jejunum. Usually performed to relieve obstructive jaundice due to a growth in the head of the pancreas.

cholecystokinase (kō-lē-sis-tō-kīn′-ās): An enzyme that promotes the breakdown of cholecystokinin.

cholecystokinin (ko-lē-sis-tō-kīn′-in): A hormone secreted by the mucous membrane of the upper part of the small intestine; stimulates contraction of the gallbladder and the secretion of pancreatic enzymes. Also called pancreozymin.

cholecystolithiasis (kō-lē-sis′-tō-li-thī′-a-sis): Cholelithiasis (*q.v.*).

cholecystolithotripsy (kō-lē-sis′-tō-lith′-ō-trip-si): The procedure of crushing gallstones within the gallbladder.

cholecystopathy (kō′-lē-sis-top′-a-thi): Any pathology of the gallbladder.

cholecystostomy (ko-le-sis-tos′-to-mi): A surgically established fistula between the gallbladder and the abdominal surface; used to provide drainage in empyema of the gallbladder or after removal of stones.

cholecystotomy (kō-lē-sis-tot′-o-mi): A surgical incision in the abdominal wall for the purpose of removing gallstones or providing for drainage.

choledochal (kō-lē-dōk′-al): Pertaining to or affecting the common bile duct.

choledochectomy (kō-led-ō-kek′-to-mi): Surgical excision of part of the common bile duct.

choledochitis (kō-led-ō-kī′-tis): Inflammation of the common bile duct.

choledochoduodenostomy (kō-led′-ō-kō-dū′-ō-den-os′-to-mi): The formation of a passageway between the common bile duct and the duodenum.

choledochogastrostomy (kō-led′-ō-kō-gas-tros′-to-mi): The surgical establishment of an anastomosis between the common bile duct and the stomach.

choledochojejunal (kō-led′-o-kō-jē-jū′-nal): Pertaining to the common bile duct and the jejunum.

choledochojejunostomy (kō-led′-o-kō-jē-jū-nos′-tō-mi): The surgical establishment of an anastomosis between the common bile duct and the jejunum.

choledocholith (kō-led′-o-kō-lith): A stone in the common bile duct.

choledocholithiasis (kō-led′-ō-kō-lith-ī′-a-sis): The presence of a stone or stones in the common bile duct.

choledocholithotomy (kō-led′-ō-kō-li-thot′-om-i): Surgical removal of a stone through an incision in the common bile duct.

choledocholithotripsy (kō-led′-o-kō-lith′-ō-trip-si): Crushing of a gallstone within the common bile duct.

choledochopancreatography (kō-led′-ō-kō-pan-krē-a-tog′-ra-fi): Visual examination of the common bile duct and the pancreatic duct with a fiberoptic endoscope.

choledochoscope (kō-led′-ō-kō-skōp): An instrument for viewing the interior of the common bile duct.

choledochostomy (ko-led-ō-kos′-to-mi): Drainage of the common bile duct through an incision in the abdominal wall, usually after exploration for a stone.

choledochotomy (ko-led-ō-kot′-o-mi): An incision into the common bile duct.

cholehemia (ko-le-hē′-mi-a): The presence of bile in the blood.

cholelith (kō′-lē-lith): A gallstone.

cholelithiasis (kō′-lē-li-thī′-a-sis): The presence of stones in the gallbladder or bile ducts.

cholelithotomy (kō′-lē-li-thot′-o-mi): Operation for the removal of gallstones through an incision in the gallbladder.

cholemesis (kō-lem′-e-sis): Vomiting of bile.

cholemia (kō-lēm′-i-a): The presence of bile in the blood.—cholemic, adj.

cholepoiesis (kō-lē-poy-ē′-sis): The formation of bile in the liver.

cholera (kol′-er-a): An acute, infectious, enteric disease, endemic and epidemic in Asia; caused by the potent endotoxin produced by the *Vibrio comma* (also called *Vibrio cholerae*); spread mainly by contaminated food and water, overcrowding, and generally unsanitary conditions. Symptoms include copious "rice-water" stools, accompanied by agonizing cramp; severe, persistent vomiting; malaise; headache; muscular weakness; dehydration with depletion of minerals and electrolyte imbalance; rapid respirations; slow pulse rate; and circulatory collapse. The mortality rate is very high. Preventive measures include the use of cholera vaccine; boiling all drinking water; and cooking all foods; in addition, isolating and treating carriers.

choleresis (kol-er-ē′-sis): The elaboration of bile by the liver.

choleric temperament (kol′-er-ik): One of the four classic types of temperament (*q.v.*); hasty and prone to emotional outbursts; easily angered; irascible and hot tempered; all without discernible cause.

cholerrhagia (kol-er-rā′-ji-a): Excessive flow of bile.

cholestasis (kō-les′-ta-sis): Diminution or arrest of the flow of bile.—cholestatic, adj.

cholesteatoma (kō-les-tē-a-tō′-ma): A benign, slow-growing encysted tumor, often containing cholesterol; occurs chiefly in the middle ear and mastoid region as a result of chronic otitis media, but also occurs in the meninges, skull, or brain.

cholesterase (kō-les′-ter-ās): An enzyme that splits up cholesterol.

cholesteremia (kō-les-ter-ē′-mi-a): Excess cholesterol in the blood. Also cholesterolemia.

cholesterol (kō-les′-ter-ol): A pale yellow crystalline substance occurring as granules or particles; of a fatty nature, occurring in foods of animal origin; found in brain, nerves, liver, kidneys, blood cells, and plasma, and is a major normal constituent of bile and bile acids. Not easily soluble and may crystallize in the gallbladder and form gallstones, and along arterial walls in atherosclerosis. When irradiated it forms vitamin D. Important in maintaining the permeability of cell walls, and synthesis of steroid hormones, and in the functioning of certain body systems, *e.g.*, the nervous system. Normal values for human serum, 150–250 mg/ml. Investigators differ as to whether diets high in cholesterol may be responsible for certain circulatory diseases, atherosclerosis in particular.

cholesterolemia (kō-les-ter-ol-ē′-mi-a): Cholesteremia (*q.v.*).

cholesterolopoiesis (kō-les′-ter-ol-ō-poy-ē′-sis): The synthesis of cholesterol by the liver.

cholesteroluria (kō-les′-ter-ol-ū′-ri-a): Cholesterol in the excreted urine.

cholesterosis (kō-les-ter-ō′-sis): Abnormal deposition of cholesterol, especially in the gallbladder; due to faulty metabolism of lipids. Also cholesterolosis.

choletherapy (kō-lē-ther′-a-pi): The use of bile as a medication.

cholic acid (kō′-lik as′-id): One of the principal acids found in human bile, usually in conjunction with glycine and taurine; an important aid to digestion.

choline (kō′-lēn): A chemical found in most animal tissues as a constituent of lecithin and acetylcholine. Part of the vitamin B complex, and known to be a growth factor. Appears to be necessary for fat transportation in the body. Useful in preventing fat deposition in the liver in cirrhosis. Richest sources are dairy products, liver, kidney, brain, wheat germ, brewer's yeast, egg yolk.

choline acetyltransferase (kō′-lēn a-set-il-trans′-fer-ās): An enzyme necessary for the formation of acetylcholine (*q.v.*).

cholinergic (kō-lin-er′-jik): Refers to parasympathetic nerves that liberate acetylcholine at their terminations when a nerve impulse passes. See **adrenergic**. **C. CRISIS**, severe muscular weakness and respiratory depression caused by an excess of acetylcholine in the body; likely to occur in patients with myasthenia gravis as a result of overdose of anticholinesterase drugs. **C. FIBERS**, nerve fibers that liberate acetylcholine at the synapse.

cholinesterase (kō-lin-es′-ter-ās): An enzyme that hydrolyzes acetylcholine into choline and acetic acid, at nerve endings. Present in all body tissues.

cholorrhea (kōl-ō-rē′-a): Excessive secretion of bile.

choluria (kō-lū′-ri-a): The presence of bile in the urine.—choluric, adj.

chondr-, chondri-, chondro-: Combining forms denoting cartilage.

chondral (kon′-dral): Cartilaginous; relating to cartilage.

chondralgia (kon-dral′-ji-a): Pain in a cartilage. Chondrodynia.

chondrectomy (con-drek′-to-mi): The surgical removal of a cartilage.

chondrification (kon-dri-fi-kā′-shun): Conversion into cartilage.—chondrify, v.

chondritis (kon-drī′-tis): Inflammation of cartilage.

chondroadenoma (kon′-drō-ad-e-nō′-ma): An adenoma containing cartilaginous elements. See adenoma.

chondroangioma (kon′-drō-an-ji-ō′-ma): An angioma containing cartilaginous elements. See angioma.

chondroblast (kon′-drō-blast): An embryonic cell that produces cartilage.

chondroblastoma (kon′-drō-blas-tō′-ma): A rare tumor, usually occurs in the epiphyses of long bones; generally benign; most often seen in young males.

chondrocalcinosis (kon′-drō-kal-si-nō′-sis): The deposit of calcium salts in cartilaginous tissue, particularly that of the joints of the hands and feet. See pseudogout.

chondrocostal (kon-drō-kos′-tal): Pertaining to the costal cartilages and ribs.

chondrocyte (kon′-drō-sīt): A cartilage cell.

chondrodynia (kon-drō-din′-i-a): Pain in a cartilage.

chondrodystrophy (kon-drō-dis′-trō-fi): A defect or disorder of cartilage formation. See achondroplasia.

chondroendothelioma (kon′-drō-en-dō-thē-li-ō′-ma): An endothelioma containing cartilaginous elements.

chondrofibroma (kon-drō-fī-brō′-ma): A chondroma that contains fibrous elements.

chondrogenesis (kon-drō-jen′-e-sis): The formation of cartilage.—chondrogenic, adj.

chondroid (kon′-droyd): Resembling cartilage.

chondroitin (kon-drō′-i-tin): A nitrogenous substance which, combined with protein in the form of chondroitin sulfate, is one of the chief constituents of cartilage.

chondrolipoma (kon-drō-li-pō′-ma): A benign tumor containing both cartilaginous and fatty tissue.

chondrolysis (kon-drol′-i-sis): Dissolution of cartilage.—chondrolytic, adj.

chondroma (kon-drō′-ma): A benign, slow-growing, painless tumor of cartilage. Tends to recur after removal. It causes no pain.

chondromalacia (kon-drō-mal-ā′-shi-a): Abnormal softness of cartilage, occurring most often in the knee. May be congenital in which case the bones of the stillborn fetus are soft and pliable.

chondromatosis (kon-drō-ma-tō′-sis): A congenital condition, marked by the presence of many chondromata affecting chiefly the growing ends of long bones and bones of hands and feet; usually unilateral, resulting sometimes in shortening and deformity of the affected limb.

chondromatous (kon-drō′-ma-tus): 1. Of or pertaining to a chomdroma. 2. Of the nature of cartilage.

chondromucoid (kon′-drō-mū′-koyd): A glycoprotein; one of the main constituents of cartilage.

chondromyoma (kon′-drō-mī-ō′-ma): A myoma that contains cartilaginous elements.

chondromyxosarcoma (kon′-drō-mik-sō-sar-kō′-ma): A sarcoma containing both cartilaginous and mucous elements.

chondro-osseous (kon-drō-os′-ē-us): Consisting of cartilage and bone.

chondropathy (kon-drop′-a-thi): Any disease of the cartilaginous tissue.

chondroplasty (kon′-drō-plas-ti): Plastic surgery on cartilage.

chondroprotein (kon-drō-prō′-tē-in): One of several glucoproteins occurring naturally in cartilage.

chondrosarcoma (kon′-dro-sar-kō′-ma): A rapidly growing malignant neoplasm of cartilage occurring most frequently near the ends of long bones.—chondrosarcomatous, adj.; chondrosarcomata, pl.

chondroseptum (kon-drō-sep′-tum): The part of the nasal septum that is composed of cartilage.

chondrosis (kon-drō′-sis): The formation of cartilage.

chondrosteoma (kon′-dros-tē-ō′-ma): An osteoma that contains cartilaginous tissue. Osteochondroma.

chondrosternal (kon-drō-ster′-nal): Pertaining to the rib cartilages and sternum.

chord (kord): Cord.

chorda (kor′-da): A collection of fibers forming a cord; a tendon. **C. TYMPANI,** a branch of the facial nerve which passes through the tympanic cavity and joins the lingual branch of the trigeminal nerve; its fibers are distributed over the anterior two-thirds of the tongue; infection of the middle ear or mastoid may cause temporary or permanent loss of taste sensation for sweet, salt, and sour.

chordae (kor′-dē): Plural of chorda. **C. TENDINAE,** fine, white, glistening cords stretching between the atrioventricular valves and the papillary muscles of the heart. When the muscles contract, the chordae are tightened, thus preventing the cusps of the atrioventricular valves from being swept back into the atria during ventricular contraction.

chordee (kor-dē′): Downward bending of the penile shaft; painful on erection; usually due to urethritis; common in gonorrhea. **CONGENITAL C.,** a cord-like anomaly extending from the scrotum up the penis, pulling it downward in an arc; congenital hypospadias is also present.

chorditis (kor-dī′-tis): Inflammation of a cord; usually refers to the spermatic or vocal cords.

chordoma (kor-dō′-ma): A malignant tumor arising from the remains of the embryonic notochord; may occur anywhere along the vertebral column from the base of the skull downward, often in the sacrococcygeal area.

chordotomy (kor-dot′-o-mi): Surgical division of any cord, particularly the anterolateral nerve pathways in the spinal cord, to give relief from intractable pain. Temporary relief, as for severe burns or shingles, may be obtained by direct electric chordotomy under local anesthesia. Also cordotomy.

chorea (kō-rē′-a): A nervous disorder of the extremities and face, sometimes the entire body; characterized by ceaseless, rapid, spasmodic, jerky, purposeless movements that are beyond the control of the individual. The childhood type is also called rheumatic chorea or St. Vitus' dance. **HUNTINGTON'S CHOREA,** an inherited, degenerative, and ultimately fatal chorea that is not usually evident until the fourth or fifth decade of life; characterized by insidious onset, loss of muscle tone, hand and body tremor, head-nodding, mental deterioration and psychoses. Also called Woody Guthrie disease after the folk singer who died of it in 1967. **SENILE C.,** a benign chorea characterized by late onset and relatively few signs of mental deterioration. **SYDENHAM'S CHOREA,** occurs mainly in children; characterized by moderate convulsive movements; chorea minor.

choreiform (kō-rē′-i-form): Resembling chorea (*q.v.*), particularly the rapid, jerky, purposeless movements of chorea.

choreoathetosis (kō′-rē-ō-ath-e-tō′-sis): A nervous condition characterized by both choreic and athetoid movements. See **athetosis.** **PAROXYSMAL C.,** a syndrome in which sudden movements trigger attacks of choreoathetoid movements or tonic posturing of certain parts of either or both sides of the body; often familial.

choreomania (kō-rē-ō-mā′-ni-a): Dancing mania; term often used to describe a type of epidemic chorea seen in the Middle Ages.

choreophrasia (kō-rē-ō-frā′-zi-a): The constant repetition of meaningless words or phrases.

chorioadenoma (kō′-ri-ō-ad-e-nō′-ma): An adenomatous tumor of the chorion (*q.v.*). **C. DESTRUENS,** a type of hydatidiform mole which may be transported to distant sites, particularly the lungs. Also called metastasizing, malignant, or invasive mole.

chorioamnionitis (kō′-ri-ō-am′-ni-ō-nī′-tis): Inflammation of the fetal membranes, associated with a bacterial infection.

chorioangioma (kō′-ri-ō-an-ji-ō′-ma): A vascular tumor of the chorion arising from placental capillaries.

choriocarcinoma (kō′-ri-ō-kar-si-nō′-ma): An extremely malignant tumor occurring most often in young women, starting in the uterus and less often in the ovary; spreads rapidly to the lungs, liver, brain, vagina, and pelvic organs. May follow abortion, ectopic pregnancy, or normal pregnancy, or may develop from hydatidiform mole (*q.v.*).

choriogenesis (kō-ri-ō-jen′-e-sis): The development of the chorion (*q.v.*).

choriomeningitis (ko′-ri-ō-men-in-jī′-tis): Cerebral meningitis involving the choroid plexuses; see **choroid plexus,** under **plexus.** It is caused by a virus, affects chiefly young adults, and occurs most often during the fall and winter months.

chorion (kō′-ri-on): The outermost of four fetal membranes that form the embryonic sac which surrounds the embryo; it secretes chorionic gonadotropin during the first months of pregnancy and becomes an important part of the placenta. **C. FRONDOSUM,** the part of the **C.** that bears the chorionic villi (*q.v.*).

chorionepithelioma (kō′-ri-on-ep-i-thē-li-ō′-ma): A highly malignant tumor arising from chorionic cells, usually those of the uterus but also those of other female generative organs and the testes; may follow hydatidiform mole (*q.v.*), abortion, or even normal pregnancy; quickly metastasizes, especially to the lungs. Syn., choriocarcinoma. Also chorioepithelioma.

chorionic (kō-ri-on′-ik): Pertaining to the chorion (*q.v.*). **C. GONADOTROPIN,** a hormone normally produced by the chorion of a fertilized ovum. **C. VILLI,** many finger-like projections from the chorion through which the exchange of gases, nutrients, and waste products between the maternal and fetal blood takes place.

chorionitis (kō-ri-on-ī′-tis): Inflammation of the chorion.

choroid (kō′-royd): The middle pigmented vascular coat of the posterior five-sixths of the eyeball, continuous with the iris in front. It lies between the sclera externally and the retina internally, and prevents the passage of light rays. **C. PLEXUS,** see under **plexus.**—choroidal, adj.

choroiditis (kō-royd-ī′-tis): Inflammation of the choroid. **C. GUTTATA,** degenerative change affecting the retina around the macula lutea; believed to be caused by an atheromatous condition of the arteries; seen in older people; also called Tay's choroiditis.

choroidocyclitis (ko′-roy-dō-si-klī′-tis): Inflammation of the choroid and ciliary body.

choroidoretinal (kō-roy′-dō-ret′-in-al): Pertaining to both the choroid and the retina.

choroidoretinitis (kō-roy′-dō-ret-in-ī′-tis): Inflammation of both the choroid and the retina.

Christian Science: A religion founded by Mary Baker Eddy in 1866; it teaches that cause and effect are mental and that sin, illness, and death may be overcome through the practice of spiritual healing that is based on a full understanding of the principles of healing as taught by Jesus.

Christmas disease: Allied to hemophilia (*q.v.*). Caused by a hereditary deficiency of clotting factor IX (plasma thromboplastin component). Named for the patient in whom it was first described.

Christmas factor: Factor IX, a precoagulant factor normally present in plasma but deficient in patients with hemophilia B (Christmas disease, *q.v.*).

chrom-, chromat-, chromato-, chromo-: Combining forms denoting: 1) color; 2) pigment.

chromaffin (krō-maf′-in): Term used in reference to certain cells that take up and stain strongly yellow or brown with chromium salts; said of certain cells seen mostly in the adrenal medulla and less frequently along the sympathetic nerves and the abdominal aorta.

chromaffinoma (krō-maf-i-nō′-ma): 1. Any tumor containing chromaffin cells. 2. Pheochromocytoma (*q.v.*).

chromatelopsia (krō-mat-e-lop′-si-a): Imperfect perception of colors; color blindness.

chromatic (krō-mat′-ik): Pertaining to 1) color; 2) chromatin (*q.v.*).

chromatid (krō′-ma-tid): Either of the two like chromosomes that result from the longitudinal splitting of a chromosome as a step in preparation for mitosis; each chromatid eventually becomes a chromosome.

chromatin (krō′-ma-tin): The part of the cell nucleus that stains most readily with basic dyes; it consists of nucleic acid and proteins, the DNA-containing part of the nucleus; the physical basis of heredity.

chromatism (krō′-ma-tizm): 1. Abnormal pigmentation. 2. An abnormal condition characterized by hallucinatory perceptions of colored light.

chromatodermatosis (krō′ ma-tō-der-ma-tō′-sis): Any disease of the skin accompanied by discoloration. Also chromodermatosis.

chromatodysopia (krō′-ma-tō-dis-ō′-pi-a): Imperfect perception or differentiation of colors. Color blindness.

chromatogenous (krō-ma-toj′-e-nus): Producing color or pigmentation.

chromatogram (krō-mat′-ō-gram): The graphic record produced by chromatography (*q.v.*).

chromatography (krō-ma-tog′-ra-fi): The separating of a substance made up of closely related compounds by allowing a solution or mixture of them to seep through an adsorbent material into a scaled vertical glass; the different solutes move through the material at different speeds resulting in bands of different colors at different levels in the glass. Also called column chromatography.—chromatographic, adj.

chromatoid (krō′-ma-toyd): Pertaining to, resembling, or having the properties of chromatin.

chromatometer (krō-ma-tom′-e-ter): An instrument for measuring the intensity of color or color perception.

chromatophil (krō-mat′-ō-fil): A cell or tissue that stains readily; chromophil.

chromatophore (krō-mat′-ō-for): 1. A pigmented connective tissue cell. 2. A pigmented phagocytic cell found chiefly in the skin, mucous membranes, and the choroid coat of the eye and, sometimes, in melanomas.

chromatopseudopsis (krō′-ma-tō-sū-dop′-sis): Color blindness.

chromatopsia (krō-ma-top′-si-a): A visual defect in which objects that are normally seen as colorless are seen as having color. May be due to optical or psychic disturbances or to the use of certain drugs.

chromatosis (krō-ma-to′-sis): Abnormal pigmentation of the skin, as in Addison's disease (*q.v.*).

chromaturia (krō-ma-tū′-ri-a): The excretion of urine of an abnormal color.

chromesthesia (krō-mes-thē′-zi-a): The association of a perception of color with a sensation of hearing, taste, smell, or touch.

chromhydrosis (krōm-hī-drō′-sis): The secretion of colored sweat.

chromicize (kro′-mi-sīz): To treat or to impregnate with chromic acid or a chromium salt.

chromium (krō′-mi-um): A hard, grayish metallic element. Chemical symbol, Cr.

chromoblastomycosis (krō′-mō-blas-tō-mī-kō′-sis): Any of a group of fungal skin infections characterized by itching and the appearance of nodules and papillomas which frequently progress to warty plaques or ulceration; seen on the feet, legs, and exposed areas.

chromocyte (krō′-mō-sīt): Any colored or pigmented cell.

chromocytometer (krō-mō-sī-tom′-e-ter): An instrument for measuring color, particularly one which measures the hemoglobin in red blood cells.

chromogen (krō′-mō-jen): Any substance that may give color to another substance.

chromogenic (krō-mō-jen′-ik): Producing a pigment.

chromonychia (krō-mō-nik′-i-a): Any abnormal or unusual coloring of the nails.

chromophil (krō′-mō-fil): A cell, tissue, or structure that takes a deep stain easily. **C. GRANULES**, see Nissl(s) bodies. **C. TUMOR**, see pheochromocytoma.—chromophilic, adj.

chromophobe (krō′-mō-fōb): Any cell or tissue that does not stain readily, especially the cells of the anterior hypophysis. **C. ADENOMA**, the most common type of pituitary tumor with symptoms resembling those of a space-occupying lesion due to pressure on nervous system tissues; made up of chromophobe cells.

chromophytosis (krō-mō-fī-tō′-sis): 1. Discoloration of the skin. 2. Tinea versicolor (*q.v.*).

chromopsia (krō-mop′-si-a): Chromatopsia (*q.v.*).

chromoptometer (krō-mop-tom′-e-ter): An instrument for measuring an individual's perception of color.

chromosome (krō′-mo-sōm): Any one of the microscopic, dark-staining, thread-like bodies which develop from the nuclear material of the cell and which split longitudinally during cell division, one half going into the nucleus of each daughter cell. They carry the hereditary factors (genes), the number being constant for each species; they are also responsible for the determination of sex. The sex chromosomes are called X and Y; the female cell always contains two X chromosomes and the male cell contains one X and one Y chromosome.

chromotropic (krō-mō-trōp′-ik): Attracting color or pigment.

chron-, chrono-: Combining forms denoting relationship to time.

chronaxia, chronaxie (krō-nak′-si-a, krō-nak′-sē): The length of time an electric current must flow in order to excite the tissue being tested.—chronaxic, adj; chronaxy, n.

chronic (kron′-ik): Slowly developing, lingering, longlasting Opp. of acute.—chronically, adj.; chronicity, n.

chronic brain syndrome (CBS): An irreversible organic disorder; may be caused by viral or degenerative disease of the nervous system; often associated with brain trauma, encephalitis, meningitis, metabolic disorders, senility, cerebral arteriosclerosis; characterized by disorientation, faulty memory and comprehension.

chronic care: See long-term care.

chronic obstructive pulmonary disease (COPD): Term used in referring to pulmonary diseases of uncertain origin, characterized by persistent interference with air flow during expiration; usually consists of emphysema with destruction of the distal air spaces, bronchitis, and bronchoconstriction, any one of which symptoms may predominate. Also called chronic obstructive lung disease.

chronicity (krō-nis′-i-ti): The quality or state of being chronic.

chronobiology (kron′-ō-bī-ol′-o-ji): The study of the mechanisms underlying predictable time-dependent biological rhythms that occur during human growth, development, and aging, including the menstrual, sleep/wake, and rest/activity cycles, and the heartbeat.

chronogenesis (kron-ō-jen′-e-sis): The history and development of an organism or groups of organisms.—chronogenetic, adj.

chronognosis (kron-og-nō′-sis): Sensitivity to the passage of time.

chronograph (kron′-ō-graf): An instrument for measuring and recording small amounts of time in certain psychophysical experiments.

chronological age (kron-ō-loj′-i-kal): Age from birth; one's calendar age.

chronotropic (kron′-ō-trōp′-ik): Having an effect on the rate of rhythmic movements, *e.g.*, the heartbeat. **C. DRUGS**, may increase or decrease the heart rate, depending on the drug.

Chron's disease: Chronic inflammation of areas in the small intestine, of unknown cause; characterized by pain, flatulence, ulceration, persistent and recurring diarrhea; chief complications are perforation and hemorrhage.

Chrysops (kris′-ops): A genus of flies found world-wide; commonly called deerflies; they are the vectors of several disease organisms.

chrysotherapy (kris-ō-ther′-a-pi): Treatment with compounds of gold.

chthonophagia (thon-ō-fā′-ji-a): The habit of eating dirt. Syn., geophagia. Also chthonophagy.

chukka boot (chuk′-ka): An orthopedic boot or shoe that has a three-quarter upper; it covers the malleolus.

Chvostek's sign (shvos′-teks): Excessive twitching of the facial muscles on tapping the facial nerve. A sign of tetany. [Franz Chvostek, Austrian surgeon. 1835–1884.]

chyle (kīl): Digested fats which, as an alkaline milky fluid, pass from the small intestine via the lymphatics to the blood stream.—chylous, adj.

chylemia (kī-lē′-mi-a): The presence of chyle in the circulating blood.

chylidrosis (kī-li-drō′-sis): Sweat that has a milky appearance.

chylification (kī-lif-i-kā′-shun): The formation of chyle in the intestine and its absorption by the lacteals.—Syn., chylopoiesis.

chylocele (kī′-lō-sēl): A collection of chyle in the tunica vaginalis of the testis.

chylomicron (kī-lō-mī′-kron): A microscopic particle found in the intestinal lymphatics and blood during and after meals; made up chiefly of triglycerides but also contains small amounts of protein, cholesterol, and phospholipids.

chylopericardium (kī′-lō-per-i-kar′-di-um): The presence of a milky fluid in the pericardium; may result from trauma or from obstruction of the thoracic duct.

chylorrhea (kī′-lō-rē′-a): 1. The production of an excessive amount of chyle. 2. Diarrhea with stools that are milky in color, due to rupture of lymphatics of the small intestine.

chylosis (kī-lō′-sis): The conversion of food into chyle in the intestine and its absorption by the tissues.

chylothorax (kī-lō-thō′-raks): The accumulation of chyle (*q.v.*) in the thoracic cavity; may be caused by trauma to the thoracic lymphatic duct, *e.g.*, as may occur in fracture dislocation of thoracic vertebrae or during intrathoracic surgical procedures.

chylous (kī′-lus): Pertaining to or resembling chyle.

chyluria (kī-lū′-ri-a): Chyle in the urine giving it a milky appearance. Can occur in some nematode infestations, when either a fistulous communication is established between a lymphatic vessel and the urinary tract, or the distension of the urinary lymphatics causes them to rupture.—chyluric, adj.

chymase (kī′-mās): An enzyme found in the gastric juice; it acts to hasten the action of pancreatic juice.

chyme (kīm): Partially digested food which as an acidic, creamy-yellow, thick fluid, passes from the stomach to the duodenum. Its acidity controls the pylorus so that **C.** is ejected at frequent intervals.—chymous, adj.

chymotripsinogen (kī-mō-trip-sin′-o-jen): A precursor of chymotripsin; part of the pancreatic secretion.

chymotrypsin (kī-mō-trip′-sin): Proteolytic enzyme of the pancreatic secretion; also prepared synthetically. Along with trypsin, **C.** acts to stimulate catabolism of proteins.

Ci: Abbreviation for Curie.

cibophobia (sī-bō-fō′-bi-a): 1. An intense dislike of food. 2. A morbid fear of eating.

cicatrectomy (sik-a-trek′-tō-mi): The surgical excision of a scar.

cicatricial (sik-a-trish′-al): Pertaining to or resembling a scar.

cicatrix (sik′-a-triks): A scar; formed from connective tissue in the healing of a wound. See keloid .—cicatricial, adj.; cicatrization, n; cicatrize, v.

cicatrization (sik′-a-trī-zā′-shun): Scarring.

-cide: Combining form denoting kill, killing, or to kill.

ciguatera (sēg-wah-ter′-a): A serious, sometimes fatal, toxicity caused by the ingestion of certain large, tropical fish, especially the barracuda, red snapper, and grouper, which have fed on smaller fish that have ingested a particular blue-green alga; symptoms include diarrhea, myalgia, visual disturbances, vomiting, dysesthesias, paresthesias.

cilia (sil′-i-a): 1. The eyelashes. 2. Microscopic hair-like projections from certain epithelial cells. Membranes containing such cells are known as ciliated membranes, for example, those lining the respiratory tract and fallopian tubes.—cilium, sing.; ciliary, ciliated, cilial, adj.

ciliary (sil′-i-a-ri): Hair-like. **C. APPARATUS,** the nerves, muscles, and other structures of the eye that are concerned with adjusting the lens of the eye for vision at varying distances. **C. BODY,** a specialized structure in the eye connecting the anterior part of the choroid to the circumference of the iris; it is composed of the ciliary muscles and processes. **C. MUSCLES,** fine hair-like muscle fibers arranged in a circular manner to form a grayish-white ring immediately behind the corneoscleral junction. **C. PROCESSES,** 70 to 80 in number, are projections on the under surface of the choroid which are attached to the **C.** muscles. **C. REFLEX,** see under reflex.

ciliospinal (sil′-i-ō-spī′-nal): 1. Pertaining to the ciliary body (see under ciliary) and the spinal cord. 2. Referring to the ciliary center in the lower cervical and upper thoracic section of the spinal cord which governs the dilatation of the pupil. 3. **C. REFLEX,** see under reflex.

cillosis (sil-lō′-sis): Spasmodic twitching of the muscles of the eyelid.

Cimex (sī′-meks): A genus of insects of the family Cimicidae. **C. LECTULARIUS,** the common bedbug, parasitic to man; bloodsucking. See bedbug.

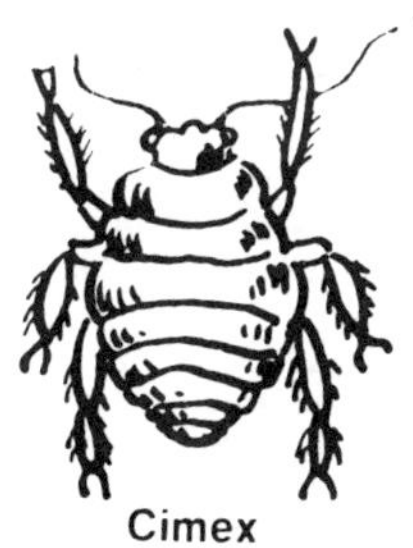
Cimex

cinchona (sin-kō′-na): The dried bark or root of the South American tree, Cincona; the source of quinine, quinidine, and cinchonine; used mainly in treatment of malaria and as cardiac depressants.

cinchonism (sin′-kon-izm): Poisoning from cinchona or one of its alkaloids; quininism (*q.v.*); symptoms include severe tinnitus, deafness, headache, visual disturbances, nausea, vomiting, diarrhea.

cineangiocardiography (sin′-ē-an′-ji-ō-kar-di-og′-ra-fi): Motion picture of the passage of contrast medium through the heart and blood vessels.

cineangiography (sin′-ē-an-ji-og′-ra-fi): Motion picture angiography (*q.v.*).

cinecystourethrography (sin′-ē-sist-ō-ū-rē-throg′-ra-fi): Radiographic demonstration of the lower urinary tract following the introduction of a radiopaque dye into the bladder; the organs are observed on a television monitor before, during, and after voiding.

cinefluorography (sin′-ē-floo-or-og′-ra-fi): Motion picture photography of images on a fluoroscopic screen.

cineradiography (sin′-e-rā-di-og′-ra-fi): Moving picture radiography showing an organ in motion or action.

cingulectomy (sin-gū-lek′-to-mi): The surgical removal of part or all of the singulate gyrus of the cortex; see gyrus.

cingulum (sin′-gū-lum): A collection of association fibers located in the cingulus gyrus of the brain; see gyrus.

cion (sī′-on): The uvula (*q.v.*).

cionectomy (sī-ō-nek′-to-mi): Excision of part or all of the uvula.

cionitis (sī-ō-nī′-tis): Inflammation of the uvula.

circadian (ser′-kā-di-an): Pertaining to a period of 24 hours. **C. RHYTHM,** rhythm within a periodicity of 24 hours, especially in relation to biologic variations.

circinate (ser′-si-nāt): In the form of a circle or segment of a circle, *e.g.*, the skin eruptions of late syphilis, ringworm, etc.

circle of Willis: An anastomosis of arteries at the base of the brain, formed by the union of the branches of the internal carotids with the branches of the basilar artery. [Thomas Willis, physician to James II. 1621–1675].

CircOlectric bed: See under bed.

circotomy (sir-sot′-o-mi): The incision of a varicosity.

circulating nurse: One who works in the operating theatre, usually an R.N., who is free to obtain needed supplies and deliver them to the operating team, to answer anesthesiologists' requests for assistance, and perform other duties that the "scrub" nurse and the operating team are not free to carry out.

circulation (ser-kū-lā′-shun): Passage in a circle. In anatomy, often refers to movement of blood in the body. **C. OF BILE,** the passage of bile from the liver cells where it is formed to the gallbladder, then via the bile ducts to the duodenum and intestine where the bile salts and fats are reabsorbed into the blood. **C. OF CEREBROSPINAL FLUID,** takes place from the ventricles of the brain to the cisterna magna, from whence the fluid bathes the surface of the brain, and cord, including its central canal. It is absorbed into the blood in the cerebral venous sinuses. **COLLATERAL C.,** that established through anastomotic communicating channels, when there is interference with main blood supply. **CORONARY C.,** that of blood through the heart walls. **EXTRACORPOREAL C.,** blood is taken from the body, directed through a machine (heart-lung, artificial kidney) and returned to the general **C. FETAL C.,** that of blood through the fetus, umbilical cord and placenta. **LYMPH C.,** that of lymph collected from the tissue spaces, which passes via capillaries, vessels, glands and ducts back into the blood stream. **PORTAL C.,** that of venous blood (collected from the intestines, pancreas, spleen and stomach) to the liver before return to the heart. **PULMONARY C.,** deoxygenated blood leaves the right ventricle, flows through the lungs where it becomes oxygenated and returns to the left atrium of the heart. **SYSTEMIC C.,** oxygenated blood leaves the left ventricle and after flowing throughout the body, returns deoxygenated to the right atrium.—circulatory, adj.; circulate, v.

circulatory (ser′-kū-la-tor-i): Pertaining to circulation, particularly of the blood. **C. ARREST,** cessation of circulation of the blood through the heart; may be due to hypoxia, pericardial effusion, arrhythmias due to drugs, electric current; often fatal. **C. SYSTEM,** a system of channels through which nutrient fluids and oxygen are carried to the cells of the body; usually refers to vessels that carry blood.

circum-: Prefix denoting around, surrounding, on all sides.

circumanal (ser-kum-ā′-nal): Surrounding the anus.

circumcision (ser-kum-sizh′-un): Excision of the prepuce or foreskin of the penis. **FEMALE C.,** excision of part or all of the prepuce, the clitoris, and the labia. (*q.v.*).

circumcorneal (ser-kum-kor′-nē-al): Surrounding the cornea.

circumduction (ser-kum-duk′-shun): 1. The circular movement of an organ or part around a central axis; *e.g.*, the eye or a limb. 2. The active or passive swinging of a limb in such a manner that it describes a cone-shaped figure with the apex of the cone being fixed at a joint and the distal end being moved to form a complete circle.

circumferential pneumatic compression: Treatment by application of a body garment (or trousers) which can be inflated sufficiently to produce pressure adequate to control internal hemorrhage from major arteries and veins; can also be used as an air splint for fractures of leg bones. Not to be used in the presence of pulmonary edema, head, neck, or chest injuries, or hemorrhage from the upper extremities.

circumflex (ser′-kum-fleks): Winding round, designating particularly an artery or nerve that has a winding course. **C. NERVE,** that supplying the deltoid muscle.

circumlocution (ser-kum-lō-kū′-shun): 1. Evasiveness in speech. 2. Using an unusually large number of words to express an idea; a device used by the aphasic to express a word that he is unable to retrieve.

circumocular (ser-kum-ok′-ū-lar): Surrounding the eye.

circumoral (ser-kum-ō′-ral): Surrounding the mouth **C. PALLOR,** a pale appearance of the skin around the mouth, in contrast to the flushed cheeks. A characteristic of scarlet fever.—circumorally, adv.

circumscribed (ser′-kum-scrībd): Limited; confined to a limited area.

circumstantiality (ser′-kum-stan-shi-al′-i-ti): A condition seen in schizophrenia and senile dementia; the patient is apparently aware of what he wants to express but cannot get beyond utterances that are beside the point.

circumvallate (ser-kum-val′-lāt): Surrounded by a raised ring or by a trench, as the papillae of the tongue.

circumvascular (ser-kum-vas′-kū-lar): Surrounding a blood vessel.

circus movement: In electrocardiography, the term applies to a continuous movement of a wave that arises in an ectopic focus and travels in a circle around a ring of muscle within the atrial wall, with the result that only part of the impulse is conducted to the ventricle.

cirrhosis (sir-ro′sis): 1. Hardening of an organ. 2. Diffuse permanent damage to an organ. Applied almost exclusively to degenerative changes in the liver with resulting fibrosis; associated developments may include ascites (*q.v.*), obstruction of circulation through the portal vein, with hematemesis, jaundice, and enlargement of the spleen. **ALCOHOLIC C.,** Laennec's **C. CRYPTOGENIC C., C.** of unknown cause; often seen in patients with a history of hepatitis or alcoholism. **LAENNEC'S C.,** the **C.** of the liver that develops in alcoholics; hobnail liver.

cirsectomy (ser-sek′-to-mi): The surgical excision of all or part of a varicose vein.

cirsoid (ser′-soyd): Resembling a tortuous dilated vein (varix, *q.v.*). **C. ANEURYSM,** a tangled mass of pulsating blood vessels, usually seen as a subcutaneous tumor on the scalp.

cirsomphalos (sir-som′-fa-los): A varicose condition involving the navel. See **caput medusae** under **caput.**

cisplatin therapy: The use of cisplatin, an antineoplastic agent, in the treatment of metastatic ovarian and testicular cancer.

cissa (sis′-a): Pica (*q.v.*).

cistern (sis′-tern): A reservoir or large enclosed space for the storage of fluid, particularly the areas in the subarachnoid space where cerebrospinal fluid is stored. See also **cisterna.**

cisterna (sis-ter′-na): Any closed space serving as a reservoir for a body fluid. **C. CHYLI,** the dilated part at the beginning of the thoracic duct which receives lymph from several lymph-collecting vessels. **C. MAGNA,** a subarachnoid space in the cleft between the medulla oblongata and the cerebellum.—cisternal, adj.

cisternal puncture: See **puncture.**

cisternogram (sis-ter′-nō-gram): An x-ray photograph of the posterior fossa of the cranium after the injection of a contrast medium.—cisternography, n.

cistoid (sis′-toyd): 1. Like a bladder. 2. Like a cyst. 3. A tumor that resembles a cyst in that it contains fluid or pulpy material but which has no capsule.

citrate (sī′-trāt): A compound of citric acid and a base.

citrated (sī′-trāt-ed): Containing a citrate; refers particularly to blood or milk to which a solution of potassium or sodium citrate, or both, has been added.

citrate-phosphate-dextrose-adenine: A preparation commonly used as an anticoagulant in whole blood (for transfusion) because it increases the maximal storage time. Abbreviated CPDA.

citric acid (sit′-rik): Occurs widely in fruits, especially in lemons and limes. Prevents scurvy; also has a diuretic action.

citrin (sit′-rin): A mixture of bioflavonoids (*q.v.*) that act in the body to reduce permeability of the capillaries; useful in the treatment of certain purpuras. Also thought to enhance the action of vitamin C in prevention of scurvy. Found in rose hips, citrus fruits, and black currants. Also known as vitamin P complex.

citrulline (sit′-rul-līn): An amino acid first found in watermelon; thought to be involved in formation of urea in the liver.

citrullinuria (sit′-rul-li-nū′-ri-a): The presence of large amounts of citrulline in the urine; usually accompanied by increased levels also in the blood and cerebrospinal fluid.

citta (sit′-a), cittosis (sit-tō′-sis): Pica (*q.v.*).

Civilian Health and Medical Programs for Uniformed Services (CHAMPUS): A federally supported insurance program (Department of Defense) that provides for purchasing health care in the private sector for dependents of active duty personnel and of military retirees, and for dependents of military personnel killed in action.

Cl: Chemical symbol for chlorine.

clairvoyance (klar-voy′-ans): The act or power of knowing about events without the use of the senses. Extrasensory perception; insight; divination.

clamp: Usually refers to an instrument used to compress vessels to prevent hemorrhage or to compress organs in order to prevent their contents from spilling into the operative field.

clang association: A way of speaking that is marked by the association of words that are similar in sound; rhyming speech. Seen in schizophrenia and the manic phase of bipolar disorder.

clap: A slang term for gonorrhea.

clapping: A massage maneuver involving a type of percussion; the hands are either held flat or cupped and are brought down rapidly and repeatedly; often used on the chest to dislodge bronchial secretions.

Clark's rule: A formula for calculating the correct dose of medicine for a child:

$$\frac{\text{weight of child in lbs.}}{150} \times \text{adult dose} = \text{child's dose}$$

-clasis: A combining form meaning breaking up.

clasp-knife phenomenon: A reflex in which a muscle or group of muscles that has previously offered resistance to passive movement suddenly yields, causing a movement like the snapping shut of a clasp-knife blade. Occurs chiefly in patients with spastic hemiparesis.

-clast: A combining form denoting something that breaks something else or causes separation of its parts.

clastothrix (klas′-tō-thriks): Brittleness of the hair.

claudicant (claw′-di-kant): 1. Pertaining to claudication (*q.v.*). 2. A person suffering from intermittent claudication.

claudication (klaw-di-kā′-shun): Limping, ataxic gait, or pain due to interference with the blood supply to the legs. The cause may be disease or spasm of the vessels themselves. **INTERMITTENT C., C.** characterized by severe pain in the calves when the person is walking; but after a short rest he is able to continue.

claustrophilia (klaws-trō-fil′-i-a): A morbid fear of being in open spaces and an obsession to remain indoors with all windows and doors locked.

claustrophobia (klaws-trō-fō′-bi-a): Morbid fear of enclosed places, or of being locked in.—claustrophobic, adj.

clavicle (klav′-i-k'l): The collarbone. It articulates with the sternum at one end and the acromion process of the scapula at the other.—clavicular, adj.

clavicular (kla-vik′-ū-lar): Pertaining to the clavicle. **C. NOTCH,** a depression on either side of the upper end of the sternum for articulation of the medial ends of the clavicles.

clavus (klā′-vus): A corn or horny area on the skin. **C. HYSTERICUS,** a pain described as feeling like having a nail driven into one's head.

clawfoot (klaw′-foot): Deformity in which the longitudinal arch of the foot is increased in height, and associated with clawing of the toes. It may be acquired or congenital in origin. Syn., pes cavus.

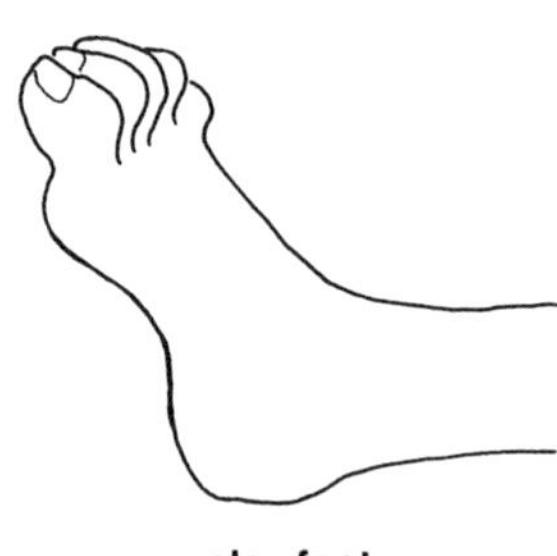

clawfoot

clawhand: A condition in which the hand is clawed and radially deviated due to paralysis of the flexor carpi ulnaris, ulnar half of the flexor digitorum longus, and the small muscles of the hand. Occurs in leprosy, syringomyelia, and in lesions of the ulnar and radial nerves.

clean: Uncontaminated; free of microorganisms. Frequently used to refer to objects that have had no contact with patients in isolation units, or to instruments, etc. that have been sterilized and kept free from contact with microorganisms.

Clean Air Act of 1970: Amended in 1977, legislation aimed at setting standards for protection of the air environment. It directs the Environmental Protection Agency to reduce particulate emissions to a specified percentage of the existing level. It is assumed that the reduced exposure will improve the public health.

clean-catch specimen: A urine specimen used in examination for the presence of bacteria. The periurethral area is thoroughly cleansed and a sterile receptacle for the urine is held so it does not touch the body; the patient voids and discards a small amount of urine before collecting the specimen. Female patients are instructed to hold the labia apart while voiding.

cleavage (klēv′-ij): 1. The segmentation by mitosis of the fertilized ovum, with the resulting cells becoming smaller with each division. 2. The splitting of a molecule into two or more smaller molecules. 3. Linear clefts in the skin, most prominently in the skin of the palms and soles.

cleft: A long, narrow fissure, particularly one

that develops in the embryo. **C. LIP,** harelip (*q.v.*). **C. PALATE,** congenital failure of fusion between the right and left palatal processes. If complete, it extends through both hard and soft palates, thus forming a single cavity for the nose and mouth; often associated with harelip.

cleid-, cleido-: Combining forms denoting the clavicle.

cleidocostal (klī-dō-kos′-tal): Pertaining to the clavicle and the ribs.

cleidocranial (klī-dō-krā′-ni-al): Pertaining to the cranium and the clavicle. **C. DYSOSTOSIS,** a rare hereditary condition in which there is defective ossification of the cranial bones and the clavicles.

cleidohumeral (klī-dō-hū′-mer-al): Pertaining to the clavicle and the humerus.

cleidorrhexis (klī-dō-rek′-sis): The fracturing of a clavicle; usually refers to fracture of a fetus's clavicle during difficult labor.

cleidoscapular (klī-dō-skap′-ū-lar): Pertaining to the clavicle and the scapula.

cleidosternal (klī-dō-ster′-nal): Pertaining to the clavicle and the sternum.

cleidotomy (klī-dot′-o-mi): Cutting of one or both clavicles to reduce the width of the shoulders of a fetus to facilitate delivery through a contracted pelvis or when the fetus is unusually large or dead.

cleptomania (klep-tō-mā′-ni-a): Kleptomania (*q.v.*).

clergyman's knee: Inflammation of the infrapatellar bursa over the tibial tuberosity; often the result of kneeling in the upright position.

click: A sharp brief sound. **EJECTION C.,** a single high-pitched sound usually heard early in systole; arises from one of the great vessels or when the aortic or pulmonary valve opens forcefully; most often associated with septal defects, sometimes with hypertension. **JOINT C.,** a sharp, high-pitched sound heard on joint movement. **ORTOLANI'S C.,** a click that is felt in a congenitally dislocated hip when the thigh is abducted when in flexion and the head of the femur slides over the rim of the acetabulum. **SYSTOLIC C.,** a sharp click heard during systole; often indicates a mitral valve defect—clicking, adj.

client: In nursing, an individual who seeks and/or receives nursing care services, either from a health care facility or from a health care professional.

climacteric (klī-mak′-ter-ik): The symptoms that accompany the cessation of ovarian function. It marks the end of the period of possible reproduction by the female, as evidenced by cessation of the menstrual periods; other bodily and emotional changes may occur. In the male, it marks the beginning of the period of lessening sexual activity, usually between the ages of 40 and 60.

climacterium (klī-mak-tē′-ri-um): Climacteric (*q.v.*). **C. PRAECOX,** premature appearance of the symptoms and physical changes associated with the climacteric.

climatology (klī-ma-tol′-o-ji): The study of climate and its effects on health and disease.

climatotherapy (klī-ma-tō-ther′-a-pi): The treatment of disease by exposure to a climate different from the one in which the patient normally lives.

climax (klī′-maks): 1. The period of greatest intensity of a disease; the crisis of a disease. 2. The sexual orgasm.—climactic, adj.

clinic (klin′-ik): 1. A center for examination, study and treatment of outpatients. 2. Medical instruction, with the examination of patients, before a group of medical students; usually conducted at the bedside. 3. A type of medical practice wherein a group of medical specialists work cooperatively.

clinical (klin′-i-kal): 1. Pertaining to a clinic. 2. Pertaining to the actual observation and treatment of sick persons as distinguished from theoretical or experimental observations. **C. NURSE SPECIALIST,** see under nurse. **C. DIAGNOSIS,** see under diagnosis. **C. NURSING,** see under nursing. **C. THERMOMETER,** a self-registering thermometer used to determine the temperature of the human body; its range is from 94 to 110 degrees Fahrenheit and from 34.4 to 42 degrees Centigrade (Celsius).

clinical (klin′-i-k′l): 1. Pertaining to a clinic. 2. Practical observation and treatment of sick persons as opposed to theoretical study. **C. DIAGNOSIS, D.** that is based on physical signs of disease, physical examination, and the patient's history: does not include laboratory tests.

clinician (kli-nish′-an): 1. A physician who is engaged in clinical practice rather than research. 2. A professional nurse with a Masters degree and experience and who has received certification in a particular field of nursing practice.

clinicopathology (klin′-i-kō-path-ol′-o-ji): The diagnosis of disease by observation of the patient's signs and symptoms, combined with a study of laboratory findings.

Clinitest (klin′-i-test): Trade name for a reagent tablet used in testing urine for sugar, particularly by patients at home; the administration kit contains the reagent tablets, and the equipment needed for conducting the test.

clinodactylism (kli-no-dak′-til-izm): A congenital defect consisting of abnormal bending or deviation of the fingers and/or toes. Clinodactyly.

clinoid (klin′-oyd): Resembling a bed.

clinometer (kli-nom′-e-ter): An instrument for measuring cyclophoria (*q.v.*). Also called clinoscope.—clinometry, n.; clinometric adj.

Clinton bed: See under bed.

clip: A malleable metal staple that is fixed in the skin with a special forceps to hold the edges of a surgical wound together.

clithrophobia (klith-rō-fō′-bi-a): Morbid fear of being locked in.

clitoral (klit′-or-al): Pertaining to the clitoris. **C. STAGE,** the stage in girls' psychosexual development that compares with the phallic stage in boys.

clitoridectomy (klit′-or-i-dek′-to-mi): Surgical removal of the clitoris; female circumcision.

clitoriditis (klit′-ō-ri-dī′-tis): Inflammation of the clitoris. Also clitoritis.

clitoridotomy (klit′-or-i-dot′-o-mi): Incision into or excision of part of the clitoris.

clitoris (klit′-or-is): A small, erectile, highly erotogenic body situated just below the mons veneris at the junction anteriorally of the labia minora; the homologue of the penis in the male.—clitoral, clitoridean, adj.

clitorism (klit′-ō-rizm): Hypertrophy of the clitoris.

cloaca (klō-ā′-ka): 1. The common opening of the intestinal and urogenital tract in fishes and birds and reptiles. 2. In osteomyelitis, the opening in the sheath covering the bone through which pus and necrotic debris escapes.

clofibrate (klō-fī′-brāt): A liquid chemical with a characteristic odor (chlorophenoxyisobutyrate); used in treatment of cholesterolemia; it reduces the plasma levels of cholesterol, triglycerides, and uric acid.

clone (klōn): 1. One of a group of individuals with like genetic makeup; produced by asexual reproduction of a single individual. 2. A group of cells produced by a single cell by the process of mitosis.—clonal, adj.; cloning, v.

clonic (klon′-ik): Of the nature of clonus; pertains particularly to generalized seizures that are characterized by the rapid, alternating contraction and relaxation of muscles.

clonic-tonic: See tonic-clonic.

clonorchiasis (klō-nor-kī′-a-sis): An infection of the liver caused by the presence of the adult worms of the fluke, *Clonorchis sinensis,* in the biliary channels.

Clonorchis sinensis (klō-nor′-kis si-nen′-sis): A tapeworm (Chinese liver fluke) found in the Far East; infects both animals and man. Man becomes infected by eating raw or undercooked fish; attacks primarily the biliary passages producing symptoms of enlarged liver, edema, and diarrhea; often fatal.

clonus (klō′-nus): A series of regular, rapid, intermittent muscular contractions and relaxations following stimulation; usually indicates central nervous system disease and affects mostly the arms and legs.

closed: **C. CARE,** care in an institution or behind closed doors; may be in a medical facility, nursing home, or boarding home which is not connected with other systems of care. **C. CHEST DRAINAGE,** continuous drainage of the pleural cavity by means of an intercostal drainage tube that is attached to an airtight collecting bottle to which suction is applied. **C. DOOR POLICY,** a policy in psychiatric treatment which not only keeps patients behind closed doors, but keeps mentally well patients from associating with the mentally ill, thus preventing any influence these people may have on the attitudes and possible recovery of the mentally ill. **C. HEART MASSAGE,** rhythmic compression of the chest by hand pressure applied over the sternum. **C. HEART SURGERY,** that performed without making an incision into the chest cavity. **C. REDUCTION OF FRACTURE,** reduction by manipulation of the bone without making an incision in the skin. **C. TREATMENT OF BURNS,** the use of an occlusive dressing after cleansing the area and applying a topical medication.

Clostridium (klos-trid′-i-um): A bacterial genus; large gram-positive anaerobic, variously shaped, pathogenic bacilli found as commensals of the gut of animals and man, and as saprophytes in the soil. Produces endospores which are widely distributed. Many species are pathogenic for man because of the endotoxins produced, *e.g.,* **C. BOTULINUM** (botulism); **C. PERFRINGENS** (gas gangrene); **C. SPOROGENES,** a species of **C.** that frequently contaminates deep wounds; considered nonpathogenic, but causes a foul odor in wounds; **C. TETANI** (tetanus); **C. WELCHII** (gas gangrene).

clot: 1. A semisolid mass. Usually refers to

Mechanism of clot formation

Injury to blood vessel causes

↓

Blood platelets to disintegrate
and release

↓

Thromboplastin
which is converted into

↓

Prothrombin
which unites with calcium to form

↓

Thrombin
which causes

↓

Fibrinogen in the blood
to be converted into

↓

Fibrin
which unites with the cellular elements
in the blood to form a

↓

Clot

blood; fibrin forms a network that holds the formed elements in the blood in a mass. 2. To form into a clot; to coagulate.

clotting factor: Any of several substances in the blood that are concerned with the clotting process; principally fibrinogen, fibrin, prothrombin, thrombin, thromboplastin, and calcium ions.

clotting time: The time it takes for shed blood to clot. This is determined by test and differs from bleeding time in that it involves only the ability of the blood to clot, whereas bleeding time also involves the ability of the small capillaries to constrict.

Cloward procedure: A surgical procedure for immobilizing the cervical spine when external measures cannot maintain proper alignment; consists of fusion of the anterior spine of the cervical vertebra involved; utilizes a bone graft from another part of the body.

clubbed fingers: Fingers that are swollen with bulbous enlargement of the terminal phalanges, usually without any osseous change. See clubbing.

clubbing: Refers to the bulbous enlargement of the ends of the phalanges due to proliferation of the soft tissues without the same degree of change in the bones. May be familial and insignificant. Also sometimes seen in children with certain congenital heart defects and in adults with heart, lung, or gastrointestinal diseases.

clubfoot: A congenital malformation in which the foot is twisted out of shape or position; may be either unilateral or bilateral. See talipes.

clubhand: A congenital deformity analogous to clubfoot; type most commonly seen is the result of defective development of the radius.

clumping: See agglutination.

cluneal (kloo′-nē-al): Pertaining to the buttocks.

clunis (kloo′-nis): The buttock.—clunes, pl.

cluster: 1. C. HEADACHE; see under headache. 2. C. WELL BABY CLINIC; clinic care arranged so that mothers meet in groups for viewing films and hearing lectures by a pediatrician and nurse practitioner, followed by individual examination of their infants.

cluttering (klut′-ter-ing): Confused speech which is rapid and indistinct with syllables and letters being dropped.

Clutton's joints: Symmetrical swelling of joints, usually painless, the knees often being involved. Associated with congenital syphilis. [Henry Hugh Clutton, English surgeon. 1850–1909.]

clysis (klī′-sis): 1. The cleansing or washing out of a cavity. 2. Term used when administering fluids by other than the oral route: subcutaneously (hypodermoclysis); intravenously (venoclysis); rectally (proctoclysis).

clyster (klis′-ter): An enema.

cm: Abbreviation for centimeter.

cnemis (nē′-mis): The tibia or shin bone.—cnemic, cnemial, adj.

CNM: Abbreviation for Certified Nurse-Midwife.

CNS: Abbreviation for central nervous system.

Co: Chemical symbol for cobalt.

CO: 1. Chemical formula for carbon monoxide. 2. Abbreviation for cardiac output.

C/O: Abbreviation for complains of.

CO_2: Chemical formula for carbon dioxide.

coagulant (kō-ag′-ū-lant): 1. An agent that causes or speeds clotting of the blood. 2. Having the effect of increasing the tendency of the blood to clot.

coagulase (kō-ag′-ū-lās): A clotting enzyme, *e.g.*, thrombin, rennin. Also produced by some bacteria (*e.g.*, *Staph. aureus*), which clot plasma. Used to type bacteria into C. negative and positive.

coagulate (kō-ag′-ū-lāt): 1. To change from a fluid to a solid jelly-like mass, or to clot. 2. To cause a clot or curdle.—coagulation, coagulability, n.; coagulable, adj.

coagulation (kō-ag-ū-lā′-shun): 1. The process of changing a liquid to a solid or thickened state; the formation of a clot. 2. The process of changing fluid plasma of the blood to a solid gel by the conversion of fibrinogen to fibrin. C. FACTORS, see under factor. COAGULATION TIME, see clotting time.

coagulometer (kō-ag-ū-lom′-e-ter): An instrument for determining the clotting time of blood.

coagulopathy (kō-ag-ū-lop′-a thi): Any disorder of blood coagulation.

coagulum (kō-ag′-ū-lum): Any coagulated mass. Scab.

coal tar: Thick black substance obtained from coal by distillation. Used in a variety of pharmaceutical preparations.

coal workers' pneumoconiosis: See under pneumoconiosis.

coalesce (kō-a-les′): To grow together; to unite into a mass. Often used to describe the development of a skin eruption when discrete areas of affected skin coalesce to form sheets of a similar appearance, *e.g.*, in psoriasis, pityriasis rubra pilaris.—coalescence, n.; coalescent, adj.

coaptation (kō-ap-tā′-shun): The procedure of correctly aligning or placing displaced parts, as the ends of a fractured bone. C. SPLINT, a splint that prevents fragments of a bone from overriding.

coarctation (kō-ark-tā′-shun): Contraction, stricture, narrowing; applied to a vessel or canal. **C. OF THE AORTA,** a pressing together or narrowing of the aorta or part of it; may be a congenital heart defect or may be due to pathological narrowing of the median coat of the artery.

coarctotomy (kō-ark-tot′-a-mi): Surgical division of a stricture.

coating: A covering. **C. OF PILLS,** a covering to conceal an unpleasant taste. **ENTERIC C.,** covering for a medicament which prevents its being absorbed from the stomach; the coating dissolves in the intestine only.

Coat's disease: A condition in which there is chronic, progressive exudation of the retina; seen most often in children and young adults.

cobalamin (kō-bal′-a-min): Part of the Vitamin B_{12} group.

cobalt (kō′-balt): A mineral element considered nutritionally essential in minute traces; thought to be linked with iron and copper in prevention of anemia. Co^{60}, a radioisotope frequently used in radiotherapy for cancer.

coca (kō′-ka): The leaves of several varieties of the South American shrub, *Erythroxylon,* from which cocaine is obtained.

cocaine (kō-kān′): A crystalline alkaloid obtained from coca leaves; used as a narcotic; habituating. **C. HYDROCHLORIDE,** a hydrochloride of cocaine, used as a topical anesthetic.

cocainism (kō′-kān-izm): Mental and physical degeneracy caused by a morbid craving for, and excessive use of, cocaine.

Cocayne syndrome: A rare hereditary disorder characterized by premature aging; degenerative changes occur with great rapidity; other pathological changes include the development of cataracts, hypertension, glaucoma, arthritis, hearing loss, mental deficiency, unsteady gait, and degeneration of retinal pigment.

coccidiodomycosis (kok-sid-i-oy′-dō-mī-kō′-sis): An acute infection caused by inhalation of wind-borne spores of the fungus, *Coccidioides immitis;* endemic in southwestern U.S., Mexico, and South America; symptoms resemble those of influenza—fever, cough, sweats; usually self-limiting; also called valley fever, desert fever, San Joaquin Valley fever. A more serious form is progressive involving several other body systems; symptoms include anorexia, weight loss, severe joint pain, lymphadenopathy, the development of cutaneous nodules; complications include cranial nerve palsies, pulmonary lesions, meningitis; often fatal.

coccobacillus (kok′ō-ba-sil′-us): A short, thick, somewhat ovoid bacterial cell.—coccobacillary, adj.

coccogenous (kok-oj′-e-nus): Produced by cocci.

coccoid (kok′-oyd): Resembling a micrococcus.

coccus (kok′-us): A spherical or nearly spherical bacterium. Often classified according to the way it arranges itself, as can be seen under the microscope: diplococcus, when it occurs in pairs; streptococcus, when it occurs in chains; staphylococcus, when it occurs in bunches resembling bunches of grapes.—cocci, pl.; coccal, coccoid, adj.

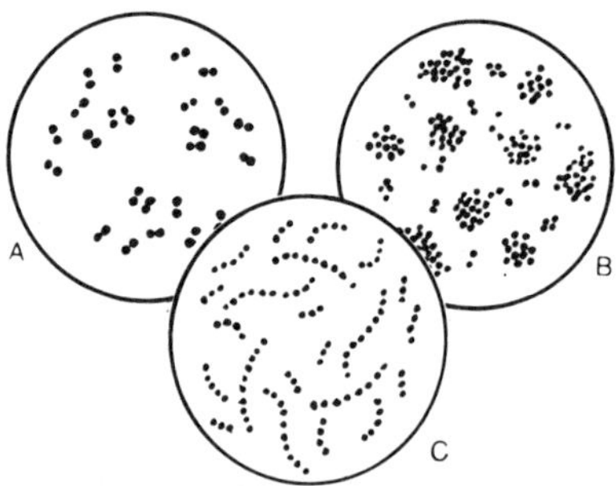

Cocci. A. diplococci. B. staphylococci. C. streptococci.

-coccus: Combining form denoting berry-shaped. Used primarily in forming generic names of microorganisms.

coccy-: A combining form denoting coccyx.

coccydynia (kok-si-din′-i-a): Pain in the coccygeal area. Also coccyalgia.

coccygeal (kok-sij′-ē-al): Pertaining to or located in the region of the coccyx. **C. NERVE,** one of the lowest pair of the spinal nerves.

coccygectomy (kok-si-jek′-to-mi): Surgical removal of the coccyx.

coccygeopubic (kok-sij′-ē-ō-pū′-bik): Pertaining to the coccyx and the pubes.

coccygeus (kok-sij′-ē-us): Pertaining to the coccyx. **C. MUSCLE,** a muscle that extends from the pubis to the sacrum and coccyx; one of the two muscles that make up the pelvic diaphragm, the muscular floor that supports the pelvic organs.

coccygodynia (kok′-si-gō-din′-i-a): Syn., coccydynia (*q.v.*).

coccyx (kok′-siks): The last bone at the base of the vertebral column. It is triangular in shape and curved slightly forward. It is composed of four rudimentary vertebrae, cartilaginous at birth, ossification being completed at about the 30th year.—coccygeal, adj.

cochlea (kok′-lē-a): A tightly coiled, fluid filled, spiral canal resembling a snail shell, in the anterior part of the bony labyrinth of the inner ear; contains the essential organ of hearing, the organ of Corti, where the movement of special hair cells that are the receptors of sound waves stimulate the auditory nerve.—cochlear, adj.

cochleitis (kok-le-ī′-tis): Inflammation of the cochlea. Also cochlitis.

cochleovestibular (kok′-lē-ō-ves-tib′-ū-lar): Pertaining to the cochlea and the vestibule of the ear.

cocoa (kō′-kō): The seeds of *Theobroma cacao*. The powder is made into a nourishing pleasant beverage. Contains theobromine and caffeine. **C. BUTTER,** the fat obtained from the roasted seeds; is used in suppositories, ointments and as an emollient.

cod liver oil: Oleum morrhuae. The oil extracted from the liver of fresh codfish. Contains vitamins A and D and on that account is used as a dietary supplement in cases of mild deficiency. Also used as a preventive of rickets in children. Now often replaced by purer forms or concentrates of vitamins A and D.

Code Blue: Term used for indicating that a person in irreversible coma is not to be resuscitated if it appears that death is imminent. Also called No Code.

Code for Nurses: Included in *Code for Nurses with Interpretive Statements,* published by the American Nurses Association in 1950 and revised in 1976. It delineates the functions and principles of conduct of professional nurses, and presents guidelines adopted by the Association for carrying out responsibilities consistent with ethical obligations of the profession and quality in nursing care. See Appendix XI.

codeine (kō′-dēn): An alkaloid of opium; similar to morphine in action and habituating; used in medicine for its analgesic, sedative, hypnotic, antitussive, antidiarrheal and narcotic effects.

codon (kō′-don): A basic informational unit of the genetic code, being a segment of the DNA molecule that specifies a certain amino acid.

coelom (sē′-lom): A cavity in the embryo; eventually it divides into the pericardial, pleural and peritoneal cavities.

coenzyme (kō-en′-zīm): An enzyme activator, *e.g.,* bile which facilitates the action of lipase in the digestion of fats.

cofactor: 1. Any factor functioning in cooperation with another factor. 2. A coenzyme.

coffee-ground vomitus: Vomitus containing partly digested blood; has the appearance of coffee grounds.

Cogan's syndrome: A non-syphilitic keratitis with progressive bilateral deafness and tinnitus, pain in the eyes, photophobia, impaired vision; probably due to vasculitis; occurs chiefly in young adults.

cognition (kog-ni′-shun): The mental process involved in thinking, perceiving, knowing, comprehending, reasoning, judging, remembering, and being aware of one's thoughts and of objects. **C.** is one of the three aspects of mind, the others being affection (feeling or emotion) and conation (willing or desiring); these aspects of mind work as a whole but any one of them may dominate any mental process. **C. DEVELOPMENT,** refers to the development of the acquisition of conscious thought, intelligence, and problem-solving ability, an orderly process which begins in childhood. **C. THERAPY,** refers to any of several treatment methods that help an individual to alter the mental processes involved in perceiving, thinking, and reasoning that are maladaptive to his environment.

cognitive (kog′-ni-tiv): Related to or involving perception, including the elements of comprehension, judgment, memory, and reasoning. **C. BEHAVIOR THERAPY,** in psychiatry, a method of using intellectual and verbal techniques to help patients identify and modify or overcome inappropriate feelings and behavior; the emphasis is on voluntary control of behavior. **COGNITIVE LEARNING THEORY,** the theory that it is the person's interpretation of the environment that determines which actions are or are not rewarding, which positive reinforcements are viewed as bribes, and which negative reinforcements are viewed as punishment. See also operant learning theory.

cogwheel rigidity: A type of movement in certain neurologic conditions; when a hypertonic muscle is passively stretched it resists and responds with a rhythmic jerkiness of movement. Also called cogwheel resistance, cogwheel phenomenon.

cohabitation (kō-hab-i-tā′-shun): The living together of a man and woman as man and wife; they may or may not be legally married.

cohort (kō′-hort): A group of individuals having some common factor or objective; a colleague, supporter, or associate.

coil: 1. A spiral or winding structure; helix. 2. An intrauterine contraceptive device. **C. GLAND,** a sweat gland.

coitophobia (kō-i-tō-fō′-bi-a): Morbid dread or fear of coitus.

coitus (kō′-i-tus): The act of sexual intercourse with a person of the opposite sex; copulation. **C. INTERRUPTUS,** intercourse in which the penis is withdrawn before ejaculation occurs. **C. RESERVATUS,** intercourse in which ejaculation is avoided, with the penis remaining in the vagina until flaccid.

col-, coli-, colo-: Combining forms denoting colon.

cola: See kola.

colalgia (kō-lal′-ji-a): Pain in the colon.

colchicine (kōl′-chi-sēn): A pale yellow bitter alkaloid powder obtained from a European tree; used in suppression and treatment of gout.

COLD: Abbreviation for chronic obstructive lung disease.

cold: 1. Opp. of heat. 2. A catarrhal inflammation of the upper respiratory tract; may be caused by infection or allergy.

cold abscess: An abscess that does not exhibit the usual signs, *i.e.*, redness, heat, swelling.

cold agglutination test: A test that demonstrates the cold agglutination phenomenon, that is, human erythrocytes of the group O type will agglutinate at 0° to 10°C, but not at normal body temperatures in cases of atypical pneumonia, trypanosomiasis, some viral infections, and several other disorders.

cold sleep: Hypothermia (*q.v.*).

cold sore: A small vesicle or blister that appears, usually around or within the mouth, during a cold or a disease attended by fever. Often multiple. See herpes. Also fever blister.

cold, wet sheet pack: A form of therapy in which the patient is wrapped in cold, wet sheets; as the body heat warms the sheets, the excited or agitated patient becomes calmed.

Cole tube: An endotracheal tube for children; size 8–18 French.

colectomy (kō-lek′-to-mi): Excision of part or all of the colon.

coleitis (kōl-ē-ī′-tis): Vaginitis.

coleocystitis (kol-ē-ō-sis-tī′-tis): Inflammation of the vagina and the urinary bladder.

coleoptosis (kōl-ē-op′-tō-sis): Prolapse of the vaginal wall.

coleotomy (kōl-ē-ot′-ō-mi): Colpotomy (*q.v.*).

colibacillemia (kō′-li-bas-i-lē′-mi-a): The presence of *Escherichia coli* in the blood.

colibacillosis (kō′-li-bas-il-ō′-sis): Infection caused by *Escherichia coli*.

colibacilluria (kō′-li-ba-sil-ū′-ri-a): The presence of colon bacilli in the urine.

colibacillus (kō′-li-ba-sil′-us): The colon bacillus; found in the intestine of man and many animals. *Escherichia coli*.

colic (kol′-ik): 1. Abdominal pain that occurs in waves with relatively painless periods between the spasms of pain. 2. A complex syndrome seen in infants under three months of age; characterized by excessive crying, apparent severe abdominal pain, pulling up of the legs and clenching of the fists. **BILIARY C.**, spasm of smooth muscle in a bile duct, caused by a gallstone. **GALLBLADDER C.**, acute cholecystitis (*q.v.*). **INTESTINAL C.**, abnormal peristaltic movement of an irritated intestine, causing abdominal pain. **PAINTER'S C.**, spasm of the intestine and constriction of mesenteric vessels; associated with lead poisoning as may occur in painters. **RENAL C.**, spasm of a ureter due to the presence of a stone. **UTERINE C.**, dysmenorrhea.—colicky, adj.

colic (kō′-lik): Pertaining to or involving the colon.

colicin (kōl′-i-sin): A protein secreted by certain strains of *Escherichia coli* that act to destroy other strains of the same species.

colicky (kol′-i-ki): 1. Resembling or causing colic. 2. A person suffering from colic.

colicystitis (kō′-li-sis-tī′-tis): Cystitis caused by *Escherichia coli*.

coliform (kō′-li-form): A word used to describe any bacterium of fecal origin which is morphologically similar to *Escherichia coli*.

colipyuria (kō′-li-pī-ū′-ri-a): Pus in the urine associated with infection caused by *Escherichia coli*.

colitis (ko-lī′-tis): Inflammation of the colon; acute or chronic. **ACUTE C.**, occurs suddenly as a result of infection or irritation; accompanied by pain and diarrhea. **AMEBIC C.**, caused by an ameba. **GRANULOMATOUS C.**, inflammation of the colon characterized by formation of granulomas. **MUCOUS C.**, often seen in neurotic individuals; accompanied by colic, diarrhea, and passage of mucus in stools. **PSEUDOMEMBRANOUS C.**, a relatively rare syndrome; may appear in postoperative patients who have received certain antibiotics; symptoms include diarrhea, pain, cardiac collapse, and formation of a pseudomembrane over the mucosa of the bowel with necrosis; often fatal. **SPASTIC C.**, irritable colon; see under colon. **ULCERATIVE C.**, an inflammatory and ulcerative condition of the mucosa of the colon; of unknown cause. Characteristically it affects young and early middle-aged adults, producing periodic bouts of diarrheal stools containing mucus and blood. Often chronic, it may vary in severity from a mild form with little constitutional upset to a severe, dangerous, and prostrating illness.

coliuria (kō-li-ū′-ri-a): See colibacilluria.

collagen (kol′-la-jen): An albuminoid substance, arranged in bundles, insoluble in water. It is the main protein constituent of the white fibers of connective tissue and cartilage and the organic substance of bone. The **COLLAGEN DISEASES** are characterized by an inflammatory lesion of unknown origin with widespread pathology of the connective tissues and affecting the small blood vessels; they include dermatomyositis, lupus erythematosus, polyarteritis (periarteritis) nodosa, and scleroderma, rheumatoid arthritis, and rheumatic fever.—collagenic, collagenous, adj.

collagen sponge (kol′-a-jen): A birth control device consisting of a sponge which absorbs the ejaculate and keeps it away from the cervix while the semen content deteriorates.

collagenase (kol-aj′-in-ās): A proteolytic enzyme that hydrolyzes collagen fibers and gelatin; an endotoxin produced by *Clostridium perfringens* (*q.v.*); attacks primarily subcutaneous and muscular tissues.

collagenolysis (kō-laj′-e-nol′-i-sis): The dissolution of collagen.

collagenosis (ko-laj-e-nō′-sis): Collagen disease; see under collagen.

collapse: 1. Extreme physical or nervous prostration. 2. The falling in of a hollow organ or vessel, *e.g.*, collapse of lung from change of air pressure inside or outside the organ. C. THERAPY, artificial pneumothorax (*q.v.*), induced to collapse and immobilize a lung. Also collapsotherapy.

collarbone: The clavicle (*q.v.*).

collateral (kō-lat′-er-al): Accessory, secondary. C. CIRCULATION, established by blood flowing in nearby anasatomosing small vessels when a main vessel has become blocked.

Colles' fracture: See under fracture.

Collet's syndrome: Glossolaryngoscapulopharyngeal hemiplegia of the muscles innervated by the ninth, tenth, eleventh, and twelfth cranial nerves; may be due to fracture of the posterior part of the skull.

colliquative (kol-lik′-wa-tiv): 1. Profuse; excessive. 2. Characterized by excessive fluid discharge.

collodion (ko-lō′-di-on): A flammable, viscous solution of pyroxylin, ether and alcohol. It forms a flexible film on the skin and is used mainly as a protective dressing. FLEXIBLE C., collodion mixed with camphor and castor oil.

colloid (kol′-loyd): A glue-like noncrystalline substance; diffusible but not soluble in water and unable to pass through an animal membrane. Some drugs can be prepared in their colloidal form. C. GOITER, abnormal enlargement of the thyroid gland, due to the accumulation in it of viscid, iodine-containing colloid.—colloidal, adj.

colloma (ko-lō′-ma): A colloid cancer; a carcinomatous tumor in which the substance has degenerated to a glue-like condition.

collopexia (kol-ō-pek′-si-a): The surgical fixation of the neck of the uterus.

collum (kol′-um): 1. The neck. 2. A neck-like part.

collyrium (kol-lir′-i-um): 1. Eyewash. 2. Eye drops.

coloboma (kō-lō-bō′-ma): A notch-like defect in the eye, characterized by a fissure or absence of tissue; often bilateral; seen most commonly in the iris, ciliary body, or choroid; may be congenital or pathological.

colocecostomy (kō′-lō-sē-kos′-tō-mi): Cecocolostomy (*q.v.*).

colocentesis (kō′-lō-sen-tē′-sis): Surgical puncture of the colon, usually to relieve distention.

coloclysis (kō-lok′-li-sis): Irrigation of the colon.

colocolostomy (kō′-lō-ko-los′-to-mi): An anastomosis between two parts of the colon not formerly contiguous.

colocystoplasty (kōl-ō-sis′-tō-plas-ti): Operation to increase the capacity of the urinary bladder by using part of the colon.—colocystoplastic, adj.

coloileal (kō-lō-il′-ē-al): Pertaining to the colon and the ileum.

colon (kō′-lon): The large bowel extending from the cecum to the rectum. In its various parts it has appropriate names—ascending C., transverse C., descending C., sigmoid C. IRRITABLE C., one in which there is a tendency to hyperperistalsis, colic, and sometimes diarrhea; emotional stress is thought to be a contributing factor.—colonic, adj.

colonic (kō-lon′-ik): Pertaining to the colon. C. LAVAGE, the introduction of a large amount of fluid into the colon to cleanse and flush it out.

colonization (kol′-on-ī-zā′-shun): 1. The formation of compact groups of microorganisms as occurs when bacteria begin to reproduce on the surface of or within a culture medium, or in a location to which they have metastasized. 2. Innidiation (*q.v.*).

colonopathy (kō′-lon-op′-a-thi): Any disease of the colon.

colonorrhagia (kō-lon-ō-rā′-ji-a): Hemorrhage from the colon.

colonorrhea (kō-lon-ō-rē′-a): Discharge of mucus from the colon.

colonoscope (kō-lon′-ō-skōp): An instrument for examining the lower part of the colon.—colonoscopy, n.

colonoscopy (kō-lon-os′-kō-pi): Examination of the colon, usually with a flexible fiberoptic endoscope.

colony (kol′-on-i): A mass of bacteria, growing on a culture, which is the result of multiplication of one or more organisms. A colony may contain many millions of individual organisms and become macroscopic (*q.v.*); its physical features are often characteristic of the species. C. COUNT, bacterial count; a method of estimating the number of bacteria in a unit of sample. C. COUNTER, a device for counting colonies of bacteria growing in culture medium.

coloproctectomy (kō-lō-prok-tek′-to-mi): Surgical removal of the colon and the rectum.

coloproctitis (kō-lō-prok-tī′-tis): Inflammation of the colon and the rectum.

coloproctostomy (kō-lō-prok-tos′-to-mi): An anastomosis between the colon and the rectum.

coloptosis (kō-lop′-tō-sis): The downward displacement of the colon.

color blindness: Achromatopsia. See under blindness.

color index: A term used to indicate the relative amount of hemoglobin in red blood cells of a patient. It is the ratio of the percentage of hemoglobin (100 percent = 14.6 G of hemoglobin per 100 ml) to the percentage of red blood cells (100 percent = 5 million per cu mm). The normal index ranges from 0.85 to 1.1.

color scotoma: Color blindness in only a part of the visual field.

Colorado tick fever: See Rocky Mountain spotted fever.

colorectal (ko-lō-rek′-tal): Pertaining to the colon and the rectum.

colorectitis (kō-lō-rek-tī′-tis): Inflammation of the colon and the rectum.

colorectum (kō-lō-rek′-tum): The lower ten inches of the bowel including the distal part of the colon and the rectum considered together, regarded as an organic entity.

colorimeter (kul-ō-rim′-e-ter): An instrument used in chemical analyses to determine intensity of color in a substance when needed to determine the amount of its presence, *e.g.*, for measuring the amount of hemoglobin in the blood.

colorimetry (kul-ō-rim′-i-tri): Chemical analyses involving the use of a colorimeter.

colorrhagia (kō-lō-rā′-ji-a): An abnormal discharge from the rectum.

colorrhaphy (kō-lor′-a-fi): Suturing of the colon.

colosigmoidostomy (kō′-lō-sig-moy-dos′-tō-mi): An anastomosis between the sigmoid and another part of the colon.

colostomate (kō-los′-to-māt): A person who has a colostomy.

colostomy (kō-los′-to-mi): A surgically established fistula between the colon and the surface of the abdomen; this acts as an artificial anus and may be temporary or permanent. **TRANSVERSE C.**, a surgical anastomosis between the ileum and the transverse colon.

colostrum (kō-los′-trum): The thin pale yellow serous fluid secreted in the breasts during the first few days after parturition, before the formation of true milk is established. It contains white blood cells, protein, water, and carbohydrates, and is immunologically active; rich in lactalbumin; acts as a laxative for the infant. **C. CORPUSCLE** or **BODY**, one of many round bodies containing fat droplets found in colostrum early in lactation and again when milk is dimishing; thought to be modified leukocytes; a galactoblast.

colotomy (kō-lot′-o-mi): Incision into the colon.

colovaginal (kō-lō-vaj′-in-al): Pertaining to the colon and the vagina.

colovesical (kō-lō-ves′-i-kal): Pertaining to the colon and the urinary bladder.

colp-, colpo-: Combining forms denoting: 1. A fold or hollow. 2. The vagina.

colpalgia (kol-pal′-ji-a): Pain in the vagina.

colpatresia (kol-pa-trē′-zi-a): Atresia or closing up of the vagina.

colpectomy (kol-pek′-to-mi): Surgical excision of the vagina, or part of it.

colpeurysis (kōl-pū-ris′-is): Surgical dilatation of the vagina.

colpitis (kol-pī′-tis): Inflammation of the vagina.

colpocele (kol′-pō-sēl): A hernia into the vagina.

colpocystitis (kol′-pō-sis-ti′-tis): Inflammation of the vagina and the urinary bladder.

colpohysterectomy (kol′-pō-his-ter-ek′-to-mi): Surgical removal of the uterus through the vagina.

colpoperineoplasty (kol′-pō-per-i-nē′-ō-plas-ti): Plastic repair of the vagina and perineum.

colpoperineorrhaphy (kol′-pō-per-in-ē-or′-a-fī): The surgical repair of an injured vagina and perineum.

colpoplasty (kol′-pō-plas-ti): Plastic surgery of the vagina.

colpoptosis (kol-pop-tō′-sis): Prolapse of the vagina.

colporrhaphy (kōl-por′-a-fi): 1. Surgical repair of a tear in the vagina. 2. Suturing of the vaginal wall to narrow the vaginal canal.

colporrhexis (kōl-pō-rek′-sis): 1. Rupture or laceration of the vaginal vault. 2. The forcible tearing away of the uterine cervix from the vaginal walls; a rare occurrence during childbirth.

colposcope (kol′-pō-skōp): An endoscope for viewing the vagina and cervix —colposcopic, adj.; colposcopically, adv.; colposcopy, n.

colposcopy (kōl-pos′-kō-pi): Examination of the vagina and cervix by means of a colposcope.

colpostenosis (kol-pō-ste-nō′-sis): Constriction or narrowing of the vaginal canal.

colpotomy (kol-pot′-ō-mi): Incision of the vaginal wall. **POSTERIOR C.**, performed to drain an abscess in the pouch of Douglas through the vagina.

colpoxerosis (kōl-pō-zē-rō′-sis): Abnormal dryness of the vaginal mucous membrane.

columella (kol-ū-mel′-la): In anatomy, a small column or column-like structure. **C. NASI**, the fleshy margin of the nasal septum. **C. COCHLEA**, the central pillar of the cochlea.—columellae, pl.

column (kol′-um): In anatomy, a structure of the body resembling a column or pillar, *e.g.*, the spinal column. **RENAL C.**, one of the structures that lie between the pyramids in the cortex of the kidney; see kidney. **VERTEBRAL C.**, see under vertebral.

coma (kō′-ma): A prolonged state of complete loss of consciousness, from which the patient cannot be awakened; insensibility. Seen in alcoholism and other poisonings, diabetes, epilepsy, encephalitis, brain tumor, hematoma, vascular diseases. **DIABETIC C.**, occurs suddenly in patients with diabetes mellitus; due to excess of insulin in the blood and the resulting severe acidosis. **HEPATIC C.**, **C.** that accompanies hepatic encephalopathy; see under encephalopathy. **HYPERGLYCEMIC C.**, **C.** due to an excess of glucose in the circulating blood. **HYPOGLYCEMIC C.**, **C.** due to an excess of insulin in relation to the glucose content of the circulating blood. **INSULIN C.**, **C.** due to an excess of insulin in the blood; see also insulin shock therapy under therapy.

comatose (kō′-ma-tōs): In a state of coma.

combat fatigue: A state of physical and emotional fatigue experienced by soldiers in military combat. Also called combat neurosis, battle neurosis, and shell shock.

combustion (kum-bust′-shun): In chemistry, rapid oxidation accompanied by heat and sometimes light.

comedo (kom′-ē-dō): Blackhead. A wormlike cast formed of sebum which occupies the outlet of a sebaceous gland in the skin. Comedones have a black color because of oxidation; a feature of acne vulgaris.—comedones, pl.

comedocarcinoma (kō′-mē-dō-kar-sin-ō′-ma): A type of carcinoma of the breast; some of the milk ducts are filled with cells that form casts which resemble those of blackheads when expressed.

comes (kō′-mēz): In anatomy, a blood vessel that accompanies another vessel or a nerve trunk.

comma bacillus (kom′-ma bas-il′-us): **VIBRIO COMMA**, the comma-shaped organism that causes cholera. Also called *Vibrio cholerae*.

commensal (kō-men′-sal): One of two organisms living in a state of commensalism (*q.v.*) without invading tissues or causing infection; however, when transferred to an abnormal site, some commensals are potentially pathogenic.

commensalism (ko-men′-sal-izm): The harmonious living together of two organisms, one of which obtains food, protection or other benefit from the other without either damaging or benefitting the other.

comminuted (kom′-i-nūt-ed): Broken or shattered into a number of small pieces; term often used to denote a shattering fracture of a bone.—comminution, n.

commissure (kom′-mi-shūr): 1. The point or line of union between two parts, *e.g.*, the angle or corner of the eyelids or lips. 2. A band of nerve fibers that cross from one side of the brain or spinal cord to the other.

commissurotomy (kom-is-shūr-ot′-o-mi): Surgical division of a fibrous band or ring. Usually refers to surgery on the band that surrounds the mitral orifice; relieves mitral stenosis.

commitment (ko-mit′-ment): The legal placing of a mentally ill person in an institution that is devoted to the care of such persons and from which he may not leave when he chooses. Justification for commitment is usually based on the belief that the person is dangerous to himself and/or others.

common bile duct: The duct formed by the union of the hepatic and pancreatic ducts; empties into the duodenum.

common cold: See cold.

commotio retinae (kō-mō′-shi-ō ret′-i-nē): Disturbance of retinal function with sudden blindness following a blow on or near the eyeball; there is usually no recognizable lesion and sight is usually regained.

communicable (ko-mū′-ni-ka-b'l): Transmissible from one source to another or from one person to another, either directly or indirectly. **C. DISEASE**, an infectious disease that is transmitted from one person to another, directly or by an animal or insect vector, or a carrier. See also reportable communicable disease.

Communicable Disease Center: See Centers for Disease Control.

communication (kuh-mū′-ni-kā′-shun): The process of exchanging thoughts or information in a reciprocal relationship; may be carried on verbally or nonverbally as, *e.g.*, by writing, gestures, facial expression, or body behavior.

community (ko-mū′-ni-ti): A group of people living in the same geographic area and under the same government. **C. HEALTH**, the discipline concerned with preventing disease and prolonging life through organized effort to control communicable disease, provide services for early diagnosis and treatment of disease, and provide health maintenance education for individuals, families, and the community at large. **C. HEALTH CLINIC**, included in this category are the neighborhood health centers, women's clinics, abortion clinics, family planning centers, and mental health centers. **C. HEALTH NURSE**, see under nurse. **C. HEALTH NURSING**, see under nursing. **C. HEALTH SERVICE**, pertains to any planned health service provided for a population rather than an individual. **C. MEDICINE**, the branch of medicine concerned with the health status of populations rather than individuals, and with conditions that affect health and the purity of food, milk, water, etc. The stress is on prevention but facilities for inpatients, outpatients, and hospital and clinic patients are often included in such a center.

Community College nursing programs: See Associate Degree programs, under nursing education.

compact (kom-pakt', kom'-pakt): Dense or solid in structure. C. BONE, the hard outer layer of bones, especially the long bones.

compartment (kom-part'-ment): 1. A small enclosure within a larger space, *e.g.*, the areas between muscle groups in the leg. 2. One of the two main fluid-containing areas in the body: a) the INTERCELLULAR C., the space occupied by the fluid within the cell walls; makes up about 40 percent of total body weight; and b) THE EXTRACELLULAR C., the space occupied by the plasma and interstitial fluid; makes up about 30 percent of total body weight.

compartmental syndrome (com-part-men'-tal): A condition in which increased pressure within a compartment interferes with the circulation of blood to the contents of that space.

compatibility (kom-pat-i-bil'-i-ti): Suitability; congruity. The property of a substance that enables it to mix with another without ill effects, *e.g.*, two medicines, blood plasma and cells. See blood groups.—compatible, adj.

compensate (kom'-pen-sāt): To counterbalance a lack or defect in a bodily or physiologic function.

compensation (kom-pen-sā'-shun): 1. A form of compromise. 2. A psychic mechanism employed by a person to cover up a weakness by exaggerating a more socially acceptable quality. 3. The state of counterbalancing or making up for a structural or functional defect or deficiency through overgrowth of another organ or increased function of unimpaired parts of the same organ. CARDIAC C., a condition in which adequate circulation is maintained in patients with cardiac disease.

complaint (kom-plānt'): A lay term used to describe a disease, ailment, or group of symptoms which cause the individual to seek medical advice.

complement (kom'-ple-ment): Any of a group of several factors normally present in plasma that are of importance in the mechanism of immunity. Thermolabile and nonspecific, they are absorbed into antigen-antibody complexes and this leads to the completion of reactions such as bacteriolysis and the killing of bacteria. C. FIXATION TEST, a test that measures the amount of complement fixed by any given antigen-antibody complex.

complemental (kom-ple-men'-tal): Complementary. C. AIR, see air.

complementary (kom-ple-men'-ta-ri): Supplying a deficiency.

complete blood count: Includes, in addition to numerical and differential count of white blood cells, a count of red cells and estimates of platelets, hemoglobin, and hematocrit. Abbreviated CBC.

complex (kom'-pleks): A Freudian term for a series of emotionally charged ideas, repressed because they conflict with ideas acceptable to the individual, but which significantly influence attitudes and behaviors. CAIN C., rivalry and destructive impulses between brothers. CASTRATION C., fear of loss or damage of one's sexual organs as punishment for forbidden sexual desires. ELECTRA C., a syndrome attributed to suppressed sexual desire of a daughter for her father; also called father C. INFERIORITY C., an abnormal feeling of being inferior which causes an individual to behave in an overly assertive, aggressive manner; may stem from organic inferiority, low social status, or from an emotional disturbance resulting from not being able to attain one's goals. INVERTED OEDIPUS C., refers to a girl who feels hopeful love for her mother and an ambivalent love-hatred for her father, with whom she identifies and copies in her personality, developing masculine behaviors, the result being that she may become homosexual. LEAR C., lustful desire of a father for his daughter. MOTHER C., Oedipus C. OEDIPUS C., a syndrome attributed to suppressed sexual desire of a son for his mother. PERSECUTION C., paranoia (*q.v.*). SUPERIORITY C., 1) an exaggerated feeling of being superior; 2) intense striving for superiority as compensation for supposed inferiority.

compliance (kom-plī'-ans): 1. The quality or behavior of yielding to pressure, suggestion, or force. 2. In physiology, an expression of the ability of an air- or fluid-filled organ such as the lung or bladder to yield to pressure or force. 3. In respiratory conditions, the elasticity of the lung or the ease with which it is inflated. 4. In health care, the extent to which a patient agrees with and carries out the prescribed activities of a therapeutic regimen in terms of agreeing with and accepting the specific requirements, taking the recommended medications, keeping appointments, and making changes in his lifestyle required by the regimen. See also noncompliance.

complication (kom-pli-kā'-shun): In medicine, a concurrent condition or disease, or an accident or second disease arising in the course of primary disease and adding to its severity.

compos mentis (kom'-pos men'tis): A Latin term meaning of sound mind.

compound (kom'-pownd): A substance composed of two or more elements, chemically combined in a definable proportion to form a new substance with new properties. **C. FRACTURE,** see **fracture.**

comprehension (kom-pre-hen′-shun): The act of grasping, with the mind, meaning and relationships or the knowledge that results from this action.

compress (kom′-pres): A pad or folded piece of cloth applied firmly to a part to cover a wound, exert pressure or control hemorrhage, or to relieve pain, swelling or inflammation. May be dry or wet, hot or cold.

compression (kom-presh′-un): 1. The state of being compressed. 2. The act of pressing or squeezing together. **CEREBRAL C.,** arises from any space-occupying intracranial tumor, hemorrhage, or other lesion. **DIGITAL C.,** pressure applied by the fingers, usually to an artery to stop bleeding. **C. BANDAGE,** see under **bandage.**

compromise (kom′-pro-mīz): A mental mechanism whereby a conflict (*q.v.*) is evaded by disguising the repressed wish to make it acceptable in consciousness.

compulsion (kom-pul′-shun): An irresistible, repetitive urge to engage in some act that the individual knows is irrational, or against his best judgment or his usual standards of behavior. The term is also descriptive of thoughts, fears, and use of words over which the individual has no control.

compulsive (kom-pul′-siv): 1. Having the power of compulsion (*q.v.*). 2. Pertaining to acts performed under compulsion. **C. PERSONALITY,** one characterized by an irresistible impulse to perform, under compulsion, acts that have to do with such qualities as orderliness or cleanliness.

compulsiveness (kom-pul′-siv-ness): An uncontrollable urge to perform certain physical actions or rituals; in psychiatry, considered a defense mechanism.

computerized axial tomography (CAT): Painless diagnostic procedure for examining soft tissues; consists of a radiographic scan in which hundreds of x-ray pictures are taken as a camera revolves through 180 degrees; the pictures are fed into a computer which integrates them and a cross section picture is displayed on a computer screen. The procedure, called CAT scan, allows for visualization of gray matter, necrotic tissue, and tumors, is utilized in determing the location and size of brain tumor and such conditions as cancer of the pancreas, and in injuries of the liver, spleen, pancreas, or kidney.

computerized tomography: Computerized axial tomography (*q.v.*).

CON: Abbreviation for Certificate of Need.

conarium (kō-nā′-ri-um): The pineal gland.

conation (kō-nā′-shun): The act of willing, desiring, striving. The conscious tendency to action. One of the three aspects of mind, the others being cognition (awareness, understanding) and affection (feeling or emotion.)

conative (kon′-a-tiv): Pertains to 1) the act of making an effort or of striving; 2) the exertive power of the mind; the will power.

concatenation (kon-kat′-e-nā′-shun): A series of events or objects occurring in sequence or together.

concave (kon′-kāv′): Having a somewhat depressed or hollowed out surface like the inner surface of a bowl. Opp. to convex.

concavity (kon-kav′-i-ti): A hollowed out space or depression on the surface of an organ or structure.

conceive (kon-sēv′): 1. To become pregnant. 2. To form a conception of.

concentrate (kon′-sen-trāt): 1. To bring together at a common point. 2. To increase the strength or bulk of a substance by condensing it. 3. A pharmaceutical preparation that has been strengthened by evaporation of some of its liquid content.—concentration, adj.

concentration (kon-sen-trā′-shun): 1. Close or fixed attention. 2. Strength or density. 3. The ratio of the solute to the volume of a solution.

concept (kon′-sept): 1. A mental image resulting from abstracting and recombining certain qualities or characteristics of a number of ideas and forming them into a generalization. 2. An idea or thought.

conception (kon-sep′-shun): 1. The union of an ovum and a spermatazoon to begin a new life. 2. The act of becoming pregnant. 3. An abstract mental image or idea, or the act of forming such an image or idea.

conceptus (kon-sep′-tus): That which is conceived; a fetus; an embryo.

concha (kon′-ka): A shell or shell-like structure.—conchae, pl. **AURICULAR C.,** the external ear. **NASAL CONCHAE,** three long thin bony projections from the lateral walls of the nasal cavity; identified according to position as superior, medial, and inferior.

conchotomy (kon-kot′-o-mi): The excision of a concha.

concomitant (kon-kom′-i-tant): Occurring at the same time or together.

concrescence (kon-kres′-ens): A growing together or union of parts that are normally separate.

concretion (kon-krē′-shun): A deposit of hard material in the tissues or in a natural cavity of the body; a calculus.

concurrent (kon-kur′-ent): Occurring at the same time or acting together. **C. INFECTION,** two or more infections occurring in an individual at the same time. **C. DISINFECTION,** the immediate disinfection of discharges from the body of an infected person or of materials that have been contaminated by such discharges or by the patient.

concussion (kon-kush′-un): A violent shaking or jarring of the body or a part of it as may result from a fall, a hard blow, or an explosion, or the condition resulting from such an action. **BRAIN C.**, a morbid condition resulting from a violent impact to the head; characterized by partial or complete transient loss of consciousness, dizziness, pallor, coldness, visual disturbances, unequal pupils, and sometimes an increase in pulse rate and incontinence of urine and feces; recovery is usually swift and complete except when injury is severe, or is repeated, as occurs in boxers, for example.

condensation (kon-den-sā′-shun): 1. The process of becoming thicker, or more dense or compact. 2. The process of changing a gas into a liquid or a liquid into a solid. 3. A psychological process whereby two or more concepts or events are fused into a single symbol; often occurs in dreams.

condition: 1. A state of being, as of health or disease. 2. To produce, through training or repeated application, a particular response to a particular stimulus.—conditioned, adj.

conditioned: 1. **C. REFLEX**, see under reflex. 2. **C. RESPONSE**, a response aroused by some stimulus other than that which naturally produces it. 3. **C. STIMULUS**, one to which a conditioned reflex has been developed.

conditioning: Term sometimes used synonymously with learning. Specifically, a process whereby a person learns to modify or adapt his behavior when certain stimuli are applied. In group therapy, a technique used to help the patient learn to cope with discomfort and to carry on with his daily activities. **NEGATIVE C.**, learning in which a neutral stimulus produces a desired response after repeated application of the stimulus, along with the stimulus that originally produced the desired response. **OPERANT C., C.** that is the result of rewarding (or not punishing) the individual who, having once responded to a stimulus in a desired manner, is likely to respond similarly to the same stimulus in the future.

condom (kon′-dom): A flexible rubber or plastic sheath worn over the penis as a contraceptive or as protection against venereal disease or of AIDS (*q.v.*).

conduction (kon-duk′-shun): 1. The transmission of heat, light, or sound waves through suitable media. 2. The passage of electrical currents and nerve impulses through body tissues. **C. SYSTEM**, in cardiology, consists of the S-A node, the A-V junction, the bundle of His, right and left bundle branches, and the Purkinje fibers; it conducts impulses through the heart to produce the heartbeat. **C. TEST**, an electrical test to determine whether a nerve is capable of transmitting nerve impulses. **C. TIME**, the time it takes for a nerve to react to stimulation, measured by a recording device such as an electromyograph. **C. VELOCITY**, the speed with which a nerve impulse is transmitted; expressed in meters per second.

conductive (kon-duk′-tiv): Pertaining to conduction. **C. HEARING LOSS**, a defect in the external or middle ear causing an impedance to sound-wave conduction, without loss of interpretation of sounds; various appliances that compensate for this loss are available.

conductivity (kon-duk-tiv′-i-ti): In physiology, the ability to transmit an impulse from one point to another in the body; said of nerves and the heart.

conductor (kon-duk′-tor): A substance or medium which transmits heat, light, sound, electric current, etc. **POOR, GOOD,** or **NONCONDUCTOR**, designate degrees of conductivity.

condylar (kon′-di-lar): Pertaining to a condyle.

condylarthrosis (kon′-di-lar-thrō′-sis): A joint in which an ovoid surface or condyle fits into an elliptical articular surface.

condyle (kon′-dil): A rounded, knuckle-like projection at the articular end of a bone, such as occur on the humerus and tibia; they articulate with adjacent bones and provide anchorage for ligaments.

condylectomy (kon-di-lek′-to-mi): Excision of a condyle.

condyloid (kon′-di-loyd): Resembling a condyle.

condyloma (kon-di-lō′-ma): Papilloma. **C. ACUMINATUM**, a pointed dry wart found under the prepuce in the male and on the vulva and vestibule of the female, or on the skin of the perineal area; not necessarily venereal. **C. LATUM**, a flat, highly contagious, moist, venereal wart with a grayish yellow discharge; found on the vulva, penis, anus, and axillae in late secondary syphilis.—condylomata, pl.; condylomatous, adj.

cone: A solid figure that has a circular base and tapers to a point. In anatomy, usually refers to one of the cone-like bodies found along with the rods in one of the layers of neurons in the retina; together the rods and cones are the receptors for light stimuli. **C. BIOPSY**, see under biopsy.

confabulation (kon-fab-ū-lā′-shun): A symptom common in confusional states when there is impairment of memory for recent events. The gaps in the patient's memory are filled in with fabrications of his own invention. Occurs in senile and toxic confusional states, cerebral trauma and Korsakoff's syndrome (*q.v.*).

confection (kon-fek′-shun): In pharmacology,

a preparation in which drugs are mixed with honey, syrup, or sugar.

confidential information: Privileged communication. A statement made to a physician or certain other people in positions of trust which, by law, cannot be revealed, even in court.

confidentiality (kon′-fi-den-shē-al′-i-ti): The ethical principle that a caregiver may not disclose information about a patient without his consent and that such information will be used only in connection with his treatment or in planning for his health care.

confinement (kon-fīn′-ment): Restraint of an individual within a designated area. Specifically, refers to the termination of pregnancy, labor, and the delivery of an infant; lying-in.

conflict (kon′-flikt): A mental struggle caused by the simultaneous presence of two incompatible contrasting impulses, desires, or drives which are of equal or comparable intensity. The conflict is termed intrapsychic when it occurs between urges within the personality, and extrapsychic when it occurs between urges within the self and the environment. When the conflict becomes intolerable, one of the urges may be suppressed and result in some form of neurosis.

confluent (kon′-floo-ent): Becoming merged; flowing together. In medicine, a uniting as of neighboring pustules, *e.g.*, **C. SMALLPOX**, a variety in which the pustules coalesce.—confluence, n.

confusion (kon-fū′-shun): Term used to describe a mental state which is out of touch with reality and associated with clouding of consciousness and impairment of the patient's ability to think clearly, perceive, and respond decisively; often accompanied by disorientation as to time, place, and person. May be due to decreased cerebral blood flow, damage to brain tissue, or mental disturbance; may also be present following epileptic fits, and in cerebral arteriosclerosis, trauma, or severe toxemia.

confusional state (kon-fū′-zhun-al): Mental confusion manifested in either chronic brain syndrome (*q.v.*) or as a symptom of some general disease. **SYMPTOMATIC C.S.**, temporary disruption of cerebral function, often reversible if the underlying disease is recognized and treated.

congener (kon′-je-ner): One of two or more substances or things that are allied or akin. In anatomy, term is applied to muscles that have a common action or function. See synergism.

congenital (kon-jen′-it-al): Referring to mental or physical conditions that are present at birth; they are acquired during development in the uterus and are to be differentiated from conditions that are hereditary (*q.v.*). **C. ANOMALY**, an abnormality present at birth. **C. DISLOCATION OF THE HIP**, an anomaly due to faulty formation of the acetabulum. **C. HEART DISEASE**, developmental anomalies of the heart, resulting postnatally in imperfect oxygenation of the blood, manifested by cyanosis and breathlessness; later there is clubbing of the fingers. See clubbing, blue baby. **C. MEGACOLON**, Hirschprung's disease (*q.v.*). **C. SYPHILIS**, acquired by the fetus from the mother during intrauterine life.

congestion (kon-jes′-chun): Hyperemia; abnormal accumulation of blood in a part or an organ. **ACTIVE C.**, due to increased flow of blood to the part or to dilatation of the vessels. **HYPOSTATIC C.**, occurs in the lowest part of an organ or part; due to gravity and impaired circulation. **PASSIVE C.**, results from slowing down of venous return, as in the lower limbs or the lungs.—congest, v.; congestive, adj.

congestive heart failure: Inability of the heart to maintain an adequate output of blood from one or both ventricles, resulting in manifest congestion and overdistension of certain veins and organs with blood, an inadequate blood supply to the body tissues, and excessive retention of water and salt; usually chronic. Clinical manifestations include arteriosclerotic or hypertensive heart disease, dyspnea, nocturia, tachycardia, gallop rhythm, splenomegaly.

conglutinate (kon-gloo′-ti-nāt): To adhere or stick together as if by a glutinous substance.—conglutination, n.; conglutinant, adj.

conglutination (kon-gloo-ti-nā′-shun): The abnormal joining together of two contiguous bodies or surfaces.

Congo red: A coal tar dye which is injected into the blood stream in a test for free acid in the gastric contents or for the presence of amyloid disease.

coniasis (kō-nī′-a-sis): The presence of dust-like particles in the gallbladder; to be differentiated from gallstones.

coniology (kō-ni-ol′-o-ji): The science of atmospheric dust and its effects on human health.

coniometer (kō-ni-om′-e-ter): A device for measuring the amount of dust in the atmosphere in a particular location.

coniosis (kō-ni-ō′-sis): A pulmonary disease caused by the inhalation of dust. See pneumoconiosis.

conization (kon-i-zā′-shun): Removal of a cone-shaped part of the cervix by the knife or cautery.

conjoint (kon-joynt′): 1. Joined together. 2. Pertaining to two things that are done together.

conjugal (kon′-jū-gal): Pertaining to marriage or to a husband and wife.

conjugate (kon′-jū-gāt): 1. Paired; working together. 2. **OBSTETRIC C.**, the true conjugate diameter, an important diameter of the pelvis. See diameter. **C. OCULAR MOVEMENTS**, close coordination of eye movements to keep them both looking at the same object.

conjugation (kon-jū-ga′-shun): The joining together of two substances to form another substance. In chemistry, the joining together of two compounds, *e.g.*, a toxic substance and a substance from the body, to form a compound that the body can eliminate.—conjugated, adj.

conjunctiva (kon-jungk-tī′-va): The delicate transparent mucous membrane that lines the inner surface of the eyelids and reflects over the exposed anterior surface of the eyeball. **BULBAR C.**, that which covers the anterior third of the eyeball. **PALPEBRAL C.**, that which lines the eyelids.

conjunctival (kon-jungk-tī′ val): Pertaining to or affecting the conjunctiva. **C. REFLEX,** see under reflex. **C. SAC** or **CUL-DE-SAC,** the potential space, lined with conjunctiva, between the eyelids and the eyeball, particularly that between the lower lid and the eyeball.

conjunctivitis (kon-jungk-ti-vī′-tis): Inflammation of the conjunctiva; may be bacterial, viral, or allergic in origin. **CATARRHAL C.**, pinkeye; may be due to Hemophilus or staphylococcus organisms, or to pollutants in the atmosphere; marked by burning of the eyes, photophobia, and mucous or purulent discharge. **FOLLICULAR C.**, dense infiltration of the connective tissue of the conjunctiva; due to irritation or a virus. **GONORRHEAL C.**, an acute, severe form of **C.**; caused by the *Neisseria gonorrhoeae* organism; may progress to panophthalmitis. **INCLUSION C.**, **C** of the newborn; acquired during passage through the birth canal; often caused by *Chlamydia trachomatis*. **PURULENT C.**, characterized by discharge of pus. **"SWIMMING POOL" C.**, **C.** often acquired in swimming pools; acute and purulent; also called inclusion **C.**

conjunctivoma (kon-junk-ti-vō′ ma): A tumor involving the conjunctional tissue.

connective tissue: The binding and supportive tissues of the body, the principal varieties of which are 1) areolar, 2) fibrous and 3) elastic. Adipose and lymphoid tissue, bone, and cartilage belong to the same group of bodily structures.

Conn's syndrome: Primary hyperaldosteronism; may be associated with adrenal tumor. See aldosteronism.

consanguinity (kon-san-gwin′-i-ti): Blood relationship.—consanguineous, adj.

conscious (kon′-shus): 1. Being aware; capable of voluntary perception in response to stimuli and of having subjective experiences. 2. Refers to all mental phenomena of which one is aware. 3. Being awake and in full possession of one's mental faculties.

consciousness (kon′-shus-nes): 1. Being conscious (*q.v.*). 2. Awareness of self and of one's environment at any given time, with each instance of awareness being experienced as a thought, perception, idea, sensation, or emotion. In psychoanalysis, that part of one's psychic or mental life of which one is aware and that is accessible to others through verbal report or by inference from one's behavior. See also drowsiness, stupor, coma.

consensual (kon-sen′-sū-al): 1. Pertaining to involuntary movements that occur simultaneously with voluntary movements. 2. Pertaining to excitation that occurs involuntarily in response to stimulation of another part. 3. A similar reaction of both pupils to a stimulus applied to only one eye.

consent: The voluntary consent of a patient (or of someone authorized to give consent) that is required prior to any surgical, diagnostic, or special therapeutic procedure, except in emergency situations requiring immediate surgery to preserve life. **INFORMED C.**, based on full disclosure of the whole truth before the patient submits to any surgery or invasive tests; the consent form states the diagnosis; treatment planned, drugs or procedures to be employed; prognosis; the risks involved; alternative therapies; and whether the hospital intends to conduct research or experimental studies on the patient. The form must be signed by the patient, unless he is mentally incompetent or a minor (when a surrogate assumes this responsibility), and must be witnessed. It is the responsibility of the physician to obtain informed consent.

conservative (kon-serv′-a-tiv): Descriptive of a treatment aimed at preserving health or restoring diseased or injured parts to normal, as opposed to radical or heroic treatment measures.

consolidation (kon-sol-i-dā′-shun): Becoming solid, as, for instance, the state of the lung due to exudation and organization in lobar pneumonia.

constipation (kon-sti-pā′-shun): An implied chronic condition of infrequent and often difficult evacuation of feces; may be due to lack of normal tone of the intestine, insufficient food or fluid intake, obstruction, the presence of tumor or diverticuli, or to habitual failure to empty the rectum. **ACUTE C.**, signifies obstruction or paralysis of the gut; of sudden onset. **HYPOTONIC C.**, due to lack of motility of the colon; the stool remains soft but becomes impacted in the rectum. **HYPERTONIC C.**, **C.** in which there is increased contraction of the bowel but the stool is not evacuated and becomes hard and dry from reabsorption of water.

constitution (kon-sti-tū′-shun): The physical and mental makeup of a person.

constrict (kon-strikt′): To contract or draw together.

constriction (kon-strik′-shun): 1. A morbid sensation of being tightly squeezed or bound. 2. A narrowing or binding of a tissue or part as occurs in syndactyly (*q.v.*). 3. The narrowing of a blood vessel or of an opening such as the pupil.

consultation (kon-sul-tā′-shun): In medicine a discussion by two or more physicians concerning the specific aspects of a pathological condition in a particular patient.

consumption (kon-sump′-shun): 1. The act of consuming or using up. 2. A wasting of body tissues; in this sense, the term was formerly much used for pulmonary tuberculosis (which "consumed" the body).—consumptive, adj.

contact (kon′-takt): 1. A mutual touching or connection. 2. Direct or indirect exposure to infection. 3. A person who has been so exposed. **C. DERMATITIS**, a type of eczema due to irritants, friction, sensitivity. **C. LENS**, of glass or plastic, worn under the eyelids in direct contact with conjunctiva (in place of spectacles) for therapeutic or cosmetic purposes.

contactant (kon-tak′-tant): A substance that may come into contact with the skin; often refers to an allergen (*q.v.*) or other substance that may cause contact dermatitis.

contagion (kon-tā′-jun): 1. Communication of disease from person to person. 2. A contagious disease. 3. The living organism by which a disease is transferred from person to person.—contagious, adj.; contagiousness, n.

contagious (kon-tā′-jus): 1. Capable of transmission from one person to another, by direct or indirect contact. 2. Highly communicable, referring to a disease that is easily transmitted from one person to another.

contagium (kon-tā′-ji-um): Any infective matter that may spread a disease.

contaminant (kon-tam′-i-nant): A substance or object that contaminates (*q.v.*).

contaminate (kon-tam′-i-nāt): 1. To soil or infect with extraneous matter, particularly pathogenic bacteria. 2. To render unfit for human use by pollution with unhealthful or disease-producing elements, *e.g.*, pollution of drinking water.—contamination, n.

continence (kon′-ti-nens): 1. Self-restraint; refusal to yield to an impulse or desire, *e.g.*, voluntary refrainment from sexual intercourse. 2. The ability to retain a bodily discharge until the conditions are proper for evacuation, *e.g.*, urine or feces.

continent (kon′-ti-nent): In medicine, the state of being able to control such normal bodily functions as defecation or urination until conditions are proper for carrying them out.

continuing education: For nurses, formal planned courses of instruction for practicing professional nurses for the purposes of updating nurses' knowledge and skills, developing professionalism in nursing, and assisting nurses in advancing their careers. Participation in continuing education programs and accumulation of a specific number of C.E. credits is now a requirement for relicensure in many states.

continuous: Extending without interruption or cessation. **C. BATH**, one in which the patient is kept immersed in water at 32 to 37°C; a therapeutic measure for quieting agitated psychiatric patients. **C. POSITIVE AIRWAY PRESSURE**, a technique of respiratory assistance involving the use of a respirator when it is necessary to increase the functional capacity of the lung, expand atelectic areas within the lung, and to diminish the tendency of alveoli to collapse on expiration; especially useful in treating infants with hyaline membrane disease. Abbreviated CPAP. Also called positive pressure breathing.

contra-: Prefix denoting against, opposed.

contraception (kon-tra-sep′-shun): The voluntary and artificial prevention of conception or impregnation.

contraceptive (kon-tra-sep′-tiv): An agent or device used to prevent conception, *e.g.*, condom, spermaticidal vaginal cream, soft diaphragm to cover the mouth of the uterus, intrauterine contraceptive device (IUD), or pills that are taken orally.—contraception, n.

contract (kon-tract′, kon′-tract): 1. To draw together; shorten; decrease in size. 2. To acquire by contagion or infection.

contract (kon′-trakt): 1. An agreement, usually written, between two individuals with differing interests and concerns to describe their future actions; specifies conditions under which behavior is to occur, and usually includes the consequences of not following the conditions as outlined. 2. In clinical psychology, written **CONTINGENCY CONTRACTS** between therapist and patient are utilized as instruments for achieving certain agreed upon behaviors; the contingencies are specified, and the patient agrees to treatment which includes the behaviors agreed upon.

contractile (kon-trak′-til): Possessing the ability to shorten—usually occurs as a response to a stimulus; a particular characteristic of muscle tissue.

contraction (kon-trak′-shun): Shortening, especially applied to muscle fibers. **ISOMETRIC C., C.** of a muscle in which there is no change in its length because there is no movement of a joint; also called static contraction. **ISOTONIC C., C.** of a muscle that results in motion and, consequently, a change in its length.

contracture (kon-trak′-chur): Permanent shortening of a muscle, tendon, or scar tissue, or fibrosis of tissue supporting a joint, producing a deformity and limiting movement of the joint; may result from disuse or improper position. **DUPUYTREN'S C.**, painless, chronic flexion of the fingers, especially the third and fourth, toward the palm; etiology uncertain. [Guillaume Dupuytren, French surgeon. 1777–1835.] **VOLKMANN'S C.**, a rapidly developing flexion deformity of the wrist and fingers, with loss of power, resulting from fixed contracture of the flexor muscles of the forearm. The cause is ischemia of the muscles by injury or obstruction to the brachial artery near the elbow. Sometimes follows improper use of a tourniquet. [Richard von Volkmann, German surgeon. 1830–1889.]

contraindication (kon′-tra-in-di-kā′-shun): A sign, symptom, or condition suggesting that a certain line of treatment (usually used for that disease) should be discontinued or avoided.

contralateral (kon-tra-lat′-er-al): Pertaining to, located on, or occurring in or on the opposite side.—contralaterally, adv.

contrast medium: A substance that is radiopaque and which helps to outline an organ or space on x-ray films; may be swallowed, injected intravenously, or introduced by enema.

contrecoup (kon′-tr-koo): Injury or damage at a point opposite the impact, resulting from transmitted force. More likely to occur in an organ or part containing fluid, as the skull.

control: 1. To maintain influence over the conduct of a situation, function, or activity. 2. A standard against which to measure an experiment or test. 3. A subject chosen to participate in an experiment under the same circumstances as the subjects in a study with the exception of the omission of one variable being investigated.

Controlled Substances Act: Passed in 1970, this Act practically replaced the Harrison Narcotic Act of 1914 and the 1956 Narcotic Control Act which dealt with federal control of narcotics, hallucinogens, stimulants, and depressants. The 1970 Act gives the federal and state governments control of such additional substances as poisons, caustics, corrosives, and amphetamines.

contusion (kon-tū′-zhun): A bruise; slight bleeding into tissues while the skin remains unbroken.—contuse, v.

conus (kō′-nus): **C. ARTERIOSUS**, the cone-shaped eminence of the right ventricle of the heart; the pulmonary artery trunk arises from it. **C. MEDULLARIS**, the cone-shaped lower end of the spinal cord; also called conus terminalis.

convalescence (kon-va-les′-ens): The period of recovery following an illness, operation, or accident.—convalescent, adj. and n.

convalescent (kon-va-les′ent): Pertaining to convalescence. **C. CARRIER**, a person who continues to carry the pathogenic organisms within his body during recovery from a disease. **C. SERUM**, blood serum of a patient recently recovered from a specific disease, sometimes given by injection to another person to prevent the occurrence of the disease.

convection (kon-vek′-shun): Transfer of heat from the hotter to the colder part; the heated substance (air or fluid), being less dense, tends to rise. The colder portion, flowing in to be heated, rises in its turn, thus **C.** currents are set in motion.

converge (kon-verj′): To come to a point, as light rays do when passing through a lens.—convergence, n.; convergent, adj.

convergence (kon-ver′-jens): Moving together toward a common point, as occurs when the two eyes move in coordination toward fixation on the same point or object.

conversion (kon-ver′-zhun): 1. Correction of the position of a fetus, or part of it, during labor. 2. In psychiatry, a freudian term for the defense mechanism whereby intrapsychic conflicts are expressed in a variety of sensory or motor symptoms such as pain, blindness, deafness, paralysis, or other loss of function. **C. DISORDERS**, see hysterical neurosis, conversion type, under neurosis. **C. APHONIA**, see under aphonia.

convex (kon-veks′): Having an evenly rounded external surface that bulges outward. Opp. to concave (*q.v.*).

convoluted (kon′-vō-loo-ted): Folded, curved, contorted, twisted, or winding.

convolutions (kon-vō-loo′-shunz): Folds, twists or coils as found in the intestine, renal tubules and surface of brain.—convoluted, adj.

convulsant (kon-vul′-sant): An agent that causes convulsions.

convulsion (kon-vul′-shun): Violent, uncontrolled, involuntary contractions of groups of muscles, resulting from abnormal stimulation from many causes. Occurs with or without loss of consciousness. **CLONIC C.**, alternating contraction and relaxation of muscle groups. **FEBRILE C.**, usually a generalized **C.** occurring in children with fever. **TONIC C.**, sustained muscular rigidity.—convulsive, adj. Also called fit, seizure.

convulsive (kon-vul′-siv): Related to, producing, or characterized by convulsions. **C. DISORDER**, any condition characterized by convulsions, particularly the various types of epilepsy. **C. THERAPY**, one of the physical methods of treatment for mental disorders, notably depressive states, mania, stupor; before introduction of electroshock therapy, drugs were widely used to produce the convulsions that are basic to this kind of therapy. Also known as electroplexy, electrotherapy, electroconvulsive therapy. See insulin shock.

Cooley's anemia: Thalassemia (*q.v.*). [Thomas Benton Cooley, American pediatrician. 1871–1945.]

Coombs' test: DIRECT C. TEST, used in early diagnosis of erythroblastosis fetalis and in crossmatching blood for high-risk recipients. INDIRECT C. TEST, used to detect various minor blood type factors, including the Rh factor.

cooperative care: A care program in which a family member or close friend lives in the hospital with an adult patient, assists in routine duties and learns how to care for the patient at home. Parents stay with their children, thus reducing the child's fears and loneliness. The system also reduces the cost of hospitalization.

Cooper's droop: Jargon for pendulous breasts; caused by sagging of the suspensory ligaments of the breast; see Cooper's ligaments, 3.

Cooper's ligaments: 1. A band of fascia attached to the iliopectineal spine and the pubic spine. 2. A group of fibers that connect the olecranon with the coronoid process at the elbow joint. 3. The suspensory ligaments of the breast.

coordinated home care: Care given to a patient in his home; a centrally administered program under the direction of a physician; provides for nursing care planning, evaluation of care, and follow-up procedures; includes needed social work and other community health services.

coordination (kō-or'-di-nā'-shun): Moving or functioning in harmony. MUSCULAR C., the harmonious action of muscles, permitting free, smooth and efficient movements under perfect control.

co-ossify (kō-os'-i-fī): To grow or become joined together by ossification (*q.v.*).

cootie (koo'-ti): The body louse (slang).

COPD: Abbreviation for chronic obstructive pulmonary disease.

cope (kōp): The ability to deal with problems and stresses.

coping (kō'-ping): 1. Behavior that protects a person from feelings of anxiety; includes such unconscious mechanisms as denial, rationalization, repression, etc. 2. The problem-solving efforts employed by an individual in making a choice among possible alternatives for adapting to a crisis event. C. STRATEGIES, planned techniques whereby the individual under stress attempts to regain emotional equilibrium and freedom from the stress-inducing situation.

copiopia (kōp-i-ō'-pi-a): Eyestrain; asthenopia (*q.v.*).

copious (kōp'-i-us): Profuse; abundant.

copper: A reddish-brown metallic element; found in small amounts in many vegetable and animal tissues; also present in some enzymes and necessary in small amounts for good health. Copper salts have little use in medicine except the sulfate which is used in astringent lotions and in treating phosphorus poisoning; it is also a constituent of Benedict's solution and Fehling's solution which are used for testing urine for glucose. Copper functions with iron in its transformation into hemoglobin; is excreted in the urine.

copr-, copra-, copro-: Combining forms denoting feces, dung, filth.

copracrasia (kop-ra-krā'-si-a): Lack or loss of ability to control the discharge of feces.

copremesis (kop-rem'-e-sis): The vomiting of material containing feces.

coproctic (kop-rok'-tik): Relating to or resembling feces.

coprolagnia (kop-rō-lag'-ni-a): A sexual perversion in which the individual derives pleasure from thinking about, handling, or seeing feces.

coprolalia (kop-rō-lā'-li-a): The use of filthy speech, especially of words relating to feces; occurs as a symptom in mentally disordered persons, most commonly in those suffering from cerebral deterioration or trauma affecting the frontal lobes of the brain.

coprolalic (kop-rō-lal'-ik): A person who uses filthy or obscene language.

coprolith (kop'-rō-lith): A stony concretion or hard mass of fecal material in the intestine.

coprology (kop-rol'-o-ji): The study of feces.

coprophagy (kop-rof'-a-ji): The eating of dung or feces; in humans, a symptom of severe neurosis.

coprophilia (kop-rō-fil'-i-a): An abnormal interest in filth, especially feces.

coproporphyria (kop-rō-por-fir'-i-a): A hereditary disease in which large amounts of coproporphyrin are excreted, chiefly in the feces.

coproporphyrin (kop-rō-por'-fi-rin): Naturally occurring porphyrin in the feces, formed by bilirubin. Also found in the urine of patients with coproporphyrinuria, a metabolic disorder.

coproporphyrinuria (kop'-rō-por-fir-in-ū'-ri-a): The excretion of an abnormal amount of coproporphyrin in the urine.

copropraxia (kop-rō-prak'-si-a): Vulgar or obscene gestures.

coprostasis (kop-ros'-ta-sis): Fecal impaction in the intestine. Also coprostasia.

coprozoic (kop-rō-zō'-ik): Found in or living in feces.

copulation (kop-u-lā'-shun): Sexual intercourse.

cor (kor): The muscular organ that keeps the blood circulating in the body; the heart.

cor pulmonale (kor pul-mo-nal'-ē): Chronic or acute right ventricular hypertrophy or acute strain of the right heart following disorders of the lungs; sometimes accompanied by heart failure; usually persistent. Signs and symptoms include edema, liver congestion, hepatomegaly, ascites, high venous blood pressure, substernal pain, cough, dyspnea, syncope on exertion.

cor triatrium (kor-trī-ā′-tri-um): A congenital cardiac anomaly which may be of several types; most commonly, the heart has three instead of two atria.

coracobrachialis (kor′-a-kō-brā-ki-al′-is): A muscle on the medial side of the upper arm.

coracoid (kor′-a-koid): 1. Beak-shaped. 2. Denoting a process of the upper part of the scapula.

cord: A long, rounded, flexible, thread-like structure. SPERMATIC C., that which suspends the testes in the scrotum. SPINAL C., a cord-like structure which lies in the spinal column, reaching from the foramen magnum to the first or second lumbar vertebra; consists of an inner core of gray matter surrounded by a layer of white matter that is composed mostly of myelinated nerve fibers. It is a direct continuation of the medulla oblongata and is about 18 in. long in the adult. UMBILICAL C., the navel-string, attaching the fetus to the placenta; gives passage to the umbilical vein and arteries; it is about two feet long and ½ inch in diameter. VOCAL CORDS, membranous bands in the larynx, the vibrations of which are responsible for the production of voice.

cordate (kor′-dāt): Heart-shaped.

cordial (kord′-yal): 1. An invigorating preparation used for its stimulating effect on the heart and circulation. 2. An alcoholic preparation with a pleasant taste, used for its stimulating effect on the digestion.

corditis (kor-dī′-tis): Inflammation of the spermatic cord.

cordotomy (kor-dot′-ō-mi): See chordotomy.

core: Central portion, often applied to the mass of necrotic material in the center of a boil. C. TEMPERATURE, see body temperature under temperature.

corectasis (kō-rek′-ta-sis): Dilatation of the pupil; usually refers to dilatation caused by some pathologic condition.

corectopia (kō-rek-tō′-pi-a): An abnormality of the eye in which the pupil is not in the center of the iris.

corediastasis (kō-rē-dī-as′-ta-sis): Dilatation of the pupil or a state of dilatation of the pupil of the eye.

Cori cycle: An energy cycle occurring in carbohydrate metabolism in which muscle glycogen is broken down in the peripheral tissues producing lactic acid which is carried to the liver where it is converted into liver glycogen that is converted into glucose which is then carried to the muscles where it is reconverted into muscle glycogen.

Cori's disease: Glycogen storage disease, Type III. A rare hereditary condition characterized by hepatomegaly, acidosis, stunted growth, and the deposit of large amounts of glycogen in the heart, liver, and skeletal muscles; thought to be due to an enzyme deficiency.

corium (kō′-ri-um): The internal layer of the skin lying immediately beneath the epidermis, composed of a dense bed of connective tissue with many blood vessels; also contains the hair follicles, the sweat glands and their ducts, and the sebaceous glands and their ducts, as well as smooth muscle tissue. Also called the dermis, true skin, cutis vera.

corn: A cone-shaped overgrowth and hardening of epidermis, with the point of the cone in the deeper layers, as on a toe; produced by friction or pressure. HARD C., usually occurs over a toe joint. SOFT C., occurs between the toes. Lay term for clavus.

cornea (kor′-nē-a): The outwardly convex transparent membrane forming part of the anterior outer coat of the eye. It covers the iris and the pupil and admits light, occupies about one-sixth of the circumference of the eyeball, and merges backwards into the sclera. C. GUTTATA, degeneration of the cornea; may progress to dystrophy of the epithelial cells; see Fuch's dystrophy under dystrophy. C. PLANA, congenital flatness of the cornea.

corneal (kor′-nē-al): Pertaining to the cornea. C. GRAFT, the replacement of opaque corneal tissue with healthy, transparent human cornea from a donor. C. REFLEX, see under reflex. C. TRANSPLANT, see keratoplasty.

corneitis (kor-nē-ī′-tis): Inflammation of the cornea.

Cornelia de Lange's syndrome: 1. A congenital syndrome marked by anomalies of the limbs, hirsutism, bushy eyebrows, micrognathia, low set ears, short stature, and mild to severe mental retardation; sometimes there are defects of the ribs and sternum, less than the normal number of fingers and toes, and a high arched palate. 2. The condition of having congenitally large muscles, often associated with spasticity.

corneoblepharon (kor′-nē-ō-blef′-a-ron): Adhesion of the eyelid to the cornea.

corneo-iritis (kor′-nē-ō-ī-rī′-tis): Inflammation of the cornea and the iris.

corneomandibular (kor′-nē-ō-man-dib′-ū-lar): Pertaining to the cornea and the mandible. C. REFLEX, movement of the lower jaw to one side in response to irritation of the cornea of the opposite eye when the patient's mouth is open.

corneoplasty (kor′-nē-ō-plas-ti): Syn., keratoplasty. See corneal graft.

corneosclera (kor-nē-ō-sklē′-ra): The cornea and the sclera considered together.—corneoscleral, adj.

corneoscleral (kor-nē-o-sklē′-ral): Pertaining

to the cornea and sclera, as the circular junction of these structures. **C. LIMBUS,** the circumference of the cornea where it joins the sclera.

corneous (kor′-nē-us): Horny.

corneum (kor′-nē-um): The horny outer layer of the skin; the stratum corneum.

cornified (kor′-ni-fīd): Pertains to tissue that has been converted into a horny state.—cornification, n.

cornu (kor′-nū): Any horn-shaped structure.—cornua, pl.; cornual, cornuate, adj.

corona (kō-rō′-na): A crown. In anatomy, refers to a crown-like eminence or a surrounding structure. **C. DENTIS,** the crown of a tooth. **C. RADIATA,** 1) a mass of white nerve fibers that pass from the internal capsule to every part of the cerebral cortex; 2) a mass of granulosa cells derived from the graafian follicles that surround the zona pellucida (*q.v.*); persists for some time after ovulation.

coronal (kōr-ō′-nal): 1. Pertaining to any crown-like structure. 2. Pertaining to the crown of the head. **C. SUTURE,** the jagged transverse line of union between the parietal and frontal bones of the cranium.

coronary (kor′-o-nar-i): Crown-like; encircling in the manner of a crown; said of a blood vessel or nerve that encircles a part or organ. **C. ARTERIES,** the right and left arteries that supply blood to the heart itself; the first pair to be given off by the aorta as it leaves the left ventricle. Spasm or narrowing of these vessels produces angina pectoris. **C. OCCLUSION,** stoppage of flow through the coronary arteries by an obstruction. **C. SINUS,** the channel receiving most cardiac veins and opening into the right atrium. **C. THROMBOSIS,** occlusion of a coronary vessel by a clot of blood.

coronary artery bypass: Open-heart surgery, done to improve circulation to the heart muscle. With the patient established on the heart-lung machine, one end of a section of healthy blood vessel (often taken from the saphenous vein of the leg) is affixed to a coronary artery and the other end to the ascending aorta, thus bypassing an obstructed or narrowed coronary artery. The graft may be 15 to 20 cm in length. Double, triple, or quadruple grafts are done to relieve blockage in several areas of the coronary arteries; these areas are predetermined by coronary arteriography before surgery. Bypassing is also sometimes done to relieve the pain of angina pectoris. See coronary artery under coronary, arteriography, heart-lung machine, and bypass.

coronary artery disease: Any of the pathological conditions that affect the arteries of the heart, particularly those that lessen the flow of oxygen and other nutrients to the heart muscle. Atherosclerosis is the most common cause of CAD, and angina is the most common symptom. Causes include cigarette smoking; hypertension; diets high in cholesterol, fats, salt, and coffee, and deficiencies in certain vitamins.

coronary care unit: A specially equipped and staffed area in a hospital that provides concentrated, specialized care for the treatment of patients who have suffered a coronary (*q.v.*) thrombosis and for observation of those with signs and symptoms of impending heart attack. Abbreviated CCU.

coronary heart disease: A condition caused by a deficiency of oxygen in the myocardium; usually due to narrowing of the lumen of the coronary arteries and/or the presence of coronary atheromas; may be temporary or permanent; the outstanding symptom is pain; may be associated with coronary thrombosis and myocardial infarction, and may result in sudden death. Also called ischemic heart disease.

coronavirus (kō-rō-na-vī′-rus): One of a large group of viruses that are capable of causing acute disease of the upper respiratory tract. So called because when viewed with the electron microscope, the virion appears to be surrounded by a crown with projections that are bulbous at the tip. Also written corona virus.

coroner (kor′-o-ner): A public official, often a physician, whose main duty is to investigate, in the presence of a jury, any death not obviously due to natural causes.

coronoid (kor′-ō-noyd): Crown-like, *e.g.*, **C.** process of the ulna and of the ramus of the mandible.

corotomy (kō-rot′-o-mi): Iridotomy (*q.v.*).

corporeal (kor-po-rē′-al): Pertaining to the physical, material body; not spiritual.

corpse (korps): A dead body. Cadaver.

corpulence (kor′-pū-lens): Obesity; fatness. —corpulent, n. Also corpulency.

corpus (kor′-pus): 1. A discrete mass of material, *e.g.*, specialized tissue. 2. The body of an animal or man, especially a dead body. 3. The main part of an organ or structure. **C. ALBICANS,** the degenerated corpus luteum which atrophies and remains on the surface of the ovary as a white scar. **C. CALLOSUM,** a band of white nerve fibers passing beneath the longitudinal fissure and connecting the two cerebral hemispheres. **C. CAVERNOSUM,** two cylinders of erectile tissue that make up the greater part of the penis. **C. LUTEUM,** the yellow, progesterone-secreting body formed in the ovary after rupture of a graafian follicle; if pregnancy supervenes, it persists and enlarges. **FALSE C.L.,** is formed in the non-pregnant state and persists for approximately one month, when it is reabsorbed. **TRUE C.L.,** occurs in pregnancy, persists for six months, and has almost disappeared by the end of the 9th month. **C. SPONGIOSUM PENIS,** the cylinder of erectile tissue surrounding the penile urethra. **C. STRIATIUM,** a stalklike arrangement of gray and white matter at the base of the brain, thought to have a steadying effect on voluntary movement, but no power of initiation of same.—corpora, pl.

corpuscle (kor′-pus′l): A microscopic mass of protoplasm. There are many named varieties but the term generally refers to the red and white blood cells. See erythrocyte and leucocyte.—corpuscular, adj.

corrective (ko-rek′-tiv): 1. Changes, counteracts or modifies something harmful. 2. A drug that modifies the action of another drug.

Corrigan's pulse: See under pulse.

corrosion (ko-rō′-zhun): The slow wearing away or destruction of a part or tissue.

corrosive (ko-rō′-siv): 1. A caustic; a substance that weakens or destroys the surface or substance of a tissue or other material. 2. Having the power to weaken or destroy the surface or substance of tissue or other material.

corset (kor′-set): An orthopedic appliance that encircles the trunk or part of it, or a part of a limb. MILWAUKEE C., see Milwaukee brace.

cortex (kor′-teks): 1. The outer bark or covering of a plant. 2. The outer layer of an organ beneath its capsule or membrane. CEREBELLAR C., the superficial layer of gray matter covering the cerebellum. CEREBRAL C., the thin layer of convoluted gray matter on the surface of the cerebral hemispheres; it controls most of the complex sensory-motor reactions and is the seat of memory, thought, and language. ADRENAL C., the thick outer portion of the adrenal gland which encloses the medulla of the gland. RENAL C., the smooth-textured outer layer of the kidney; it extends in columns between the pyramids of the medulla; is composed chiefly of glomeruli and secretory cells.—cortices, pl.; cortical, adj.

Corti: ORGAN OF C., the elongated spiral structure lying on the basilar membrane of the cochlea and containing the hair cells where the fibers of the auditory nerve begin; the actual receptor for hearing. [Alfonso Corti, Italian anatomist. 1822–1888.]

cortical (kor′-ti-kal): Pertaining to or referring to a cortex.

corticifugal (kor-ti-sif′-ū-gal): Moving or conducting away from the cortex; said particularly of nerve fibers. Also corticofugal.

corticoafferent (kor′-ti-kō-af′-er-ent): Pertaining to nerves that carry impulses toward the cerebral cortex.

corticobulbar (kor′-ti-kō-bul′-bar): Pertaining to the cerebral cortex and the medulla oblongata. C. TRACT, passes from the cerebrum through the medulla; some motor nerve fibers cross over here as they pass downward, others do not.

corticoefferent (kor′-ti-kō-ef′-er-ent): Pertaining to nerves that carry impulses away from the cerebral cortex.

corticoid (kor′-ti-koyd): A name for the several groups of steroid substances produced by the adrenal cortex and for synthetic compounds with similar actions. Examples of the three main groups are: hydrocortisone, cortisone, prednisolone and prednisone in the first; desoxycortone acetate (DCA or DOCA) in the second; and the sex hormones in the third.

corticomedullary (kor′-ti-cō-med′-ū-lar-i): Pertaining to the cortex and the medulla of an organ.

corticospinal (kor′-ti-kō-spī′-nal): Pertaining to the cortex of the brain and the spinal cord. C. TRACTS, tracts of motor nerve fibers that descend from the cerebral cortex, pons, and medulla where they cross to form lateral and anterior tracts of fibers that descend the spinal cord; they are concerned with fine motor movements.

corticosteroid (kor′-ti-kō-stē′-royd): Any of the hormones produced by the adrenal cortex, or any synthetic substitute.

corticosterone (kor-ti-kos′-ter-ōn): A secretion of the adrenal cortex; influences the metabolism of carbohydrates, potassium and sodium.

corticotropin (kor′-ti-kō-trō′-pin): The hormone of the anterior pituitary gland which specifically stimulates the adrenal cortex to produce steroid hormones. Available commercially as a purified extract of animal anterior pituitary glands (ACTH); only active by injection. Also corticotrophin.

corticotropin releasing factor: A factor produced in the hypothalamus which stimulates the release of corticotropin by the anterior pituitary gland.

cortisol (kor′-ti-sōl): A glucocorticoid (*q.v.*); steroid hormone secreted by the adrenal cortex. Hydrocortisone (*q.v.*). Also called 17-hydrocorticosterone.

cortisone (kor′-ti-sōn): A hormone produced in the adrenal cortex; also produced synthetically; important in carbohydrate metabolism and in body response to stress; converted into cortisol before use by the body. An excess of C., occurs in Cushing's syndrome. It has powerful anti-inflammatory properties, and is used in ophthalmic conditions, rheumatoid arthritis, pemphigus and Addison's disease. Side-effects, such as salt and water retention, may limit its therapeutic use.

coruscation (kor-us-kā′-shun): The subjective sensation of light flashes before the eyes.

corymbiform (ko-rim′-bi-form): In a cluster; said of lesions that are grouped around a larger lesion, as seen in tenia versicolor (*q.v.*).

Corynebacterium (kō-rī-nē-bak-tē′-ri-um): A bacterial genus: gram-positive, rodshaped bacteria, averaging 3 microns in length, showing irregular staining in segments (metachromatic granules). Many strains are parasitic; some are pathogenic, *e.g.*, *C. diphtheriae*, which produces a powerful exotoxin and is the cause of diphtheria. **C. VAGINALIS**, see Gardnerella vaginitis under Gardnerella.

coryza (kō-rī′-za): An acute upper respiratory infection of short duration, usually due to a filterable virus; highly contagious; attacks produce only temporary immunity. Also called acute rhinitis.

cosmetic (koz-met′-ik): 1. Relating to that which is done to improve the appearance, *e.g.*, **c.** surgery. 2. A preparation used to improve the appearance.

cost-, costi-, costo-: Combining forms denoting rib(s).

cost effective: Refers to the least costly plan for meeting specific objectives, or to a service that is less costly than one to which it is being compared; often a factor when considering health care plans.

costa (kos′-ta): A rib.—costae, pl.; costal, adj.

costal (kos′-tal): Of or pertaining to a rib or ribs. **C. ANGLE**, the angle formed by the right and left costal cartilages at the xiphoid process. **C. BREATHING**, breathing that involves primarily the chest structures; occurs in patients with gastric or abdominal pain or distention, and in paralytics. See also costal cartilage under cartilage.

costectomy (kos-tek′-to-mi): Surgical removal of one or more ribs or part of one or more ribs.

costicartilage (kos-ti-kar′-ti-lij): The cartilage of a rib.

costive (kos′-tiv): 1. Pertaining to or producing constipation.2. An agent that slows intestinal motility.

costocervical (cos-tō-ser′-vi-kal): Pertaining to the ribs and the neck.

costochondral (kos-tō-kon′-dral): Pertaining to the ribs and the costal cartilages.

costochondritis (kos′-tō-kon-drī′-tis): Inflammation of a costal cartilage; characterized by anterior chest wall pain, swelling, redness, tenderness to touch. See also Tietze's syndrome.

costoclavicular (kos′-tō-kla-vik′-ūl-ar): Pertaining to the ribs and the clavicle. **C. SYNDROME**, syn. for cervical rib syndrome.

costophrenic (kos-tō-fren′-ik): Pertaining to the ribs and the diaphragm. **C. ANGLE**, the angle at the junction of the costal and diaphragmatic pleurae.

costopneumopexy (kos-tō-nū′-mō-pek-si): The surgical fixation of the lung to a rib.

costosternal syndrome (kos-tō-ster′-nal): A condition in which the patient experiences intermittent pain in the entire anterior chest wall that is intensified by deep inspiration; may last for months.

costotomy (kos-tot′-o-mi): Excision of all or part of a rib.

costovertebral (kos-tō-ver′-te-bral): Pertaining to a rib and a vertebra. **C. ANGLE**, the angle formed by the last rib and the lumbar vertebrae, on either side.

cot: FINGER C., a rubber or plastic covering for the finger; used when examining a body passage as the rectum or vagina, or as a protective covering over a bandage. Also called finger stall. **C. DEATH**, sudden infant death syndrome (*q.v.*).

COTA: Abbreviation for Certified Occupational Therapy Assistant.

cotton-mill fever: Byssinosis (*q.v.*).

cotton-wool patches: Fluffy white patches seen on the retina in patients with lupus erythematosus and hypertensive retinopathy. Also called cotton-wool exudate and cotton-wool spots.

cotyledon (kot-i-lē′-don): One of the subdivisions of the uterine surface of the placenta.

cotyloid (kot′-i-loid): Cup-shaped; pertaining to the acetabular cavity.

cough (kawf): 1. A sudden forcible noisy expulsion of air from the lungs in an effort to expel mucus or other extraneous matter from the air passages; may be productive or unproductive. 2. A chronic or transient condition characterized by frequent coughing due to irritation of the respiratory mucosa. 3. To expel air forcefully after a deep inspiration and closure of the glottis. **C. REFLEX**, an involuntary protective nervous response to irritation of the mucosa of the larynx, trachea, or bronchi, which causes coughing. **C. SYNCOPE**, fainting following a severe coughing spell. **WHOOPING C.**, see pertussis.

coulomb (koo′-lom): The amount of electricity transferred by a current of one ampere in one second.

Council of Diploma Schools of Nursing: One of the Councils of the National League for Nursing. Defines the role and competencies expected of graduates of diploma schools of nursing; deals with issues concerning these programs.

Councilman's bodies: Round acidophilic bodies originating in the liver cells in viral hepatitis, yellow fever, and other diseases of the liver.

counter-: A combining form denoting: 1. Contrary, opposite, adverse. 2. Complementary, corresponding, alternate.

counteraction (kown-ter-ak′-shun): The action of a drug or other therapeutic agent which opposes that of some other drug or agent.

counterconditioning (kown′-ter-kon-dish′-un-ing): The application of a stimulus which ordinarily produces a certain emotional response, simultaneously with another stimulus that produces an opposite response, with the purpose of changing the affective value of the first stimulus.

counterextension (kown′-ter-eks-ten′-shun): Traction upon the proximal extremity of a fractured limb, opposing the pull of the extension apparatus on the distal extremity.

counterirritant (kown-ter-ir′-it-ant): An agent that, when applied to the skin, produces an inflammatory reaction (hyperemia), relieving congestion in underlying organs.—counterirritation, n.

counterirritation (kown′-ter-ir-i-tā′-shun): Superficial irritation causing inflammation that relieves congestion in deeper lying organs.

counterphobia (kown′-ter-fō′-bi-a): A reaction in which the individual attempts to overcome a fear by seeking out situations that are consciously feared.

countershock (kown′-ter-shok): Usually refers to an electric shock given via two electrodes placed on the chest to convert atrial or ventricular fibrillation to normal rhythm.

counterstain: A second stain of a different color applied to a smear to make the organisms that are to be viewed microscopically more distinct.

countertraction (kown-ter-trak′-shun): In orthopedics, a traction that effects another type of traction; sometimes used in reducing fractures.

countertransference (kown′-ter-trans-fer′-ens): 1.The psychiatrist's conscious or unconscious emotional reactions to the patient; see transference. 2. An emotional response of the nurse to the patient that is inappropriate to the therapeutic relationship.

coup (koo): Stroke. **COUP DE SOLEIL,** sunstroke.

coup-countrecoup injury (koo-kon′-tre-koo): Injury, usually to the brain, beneath the point of impact and more extensive injury to the opposite side of the brain.

coupling (kup′-ling): In cardiology, a term used to describe a pulse in which two beats occur in rapid succession followed by a slight pause; often a sign of digitalis poisoning.

Courvoisier's law: States that dilatation of the gallbladder does not usually occur as a result of obstruction of the common bile duct by a gallstone, but is due to some pathological condition such as carcinoma of the pancreas.

couvade syndrome (koo′-vād): The psychophysiologic response of a pregnant woman's husband who experiences the same symptons as his wife, including nausea, vomiting, abdominal pains; a custom among certain primitive tribes.

Couvelaire uterus: See under uterus.

coverglass (kuv′-er-glas): A small piece of special optical glass that is placed over a specimen on a slide for microscopic study.

Cowling's rule: A rule for determining the correct dosage of medicines for children:

$$\frac{\text{age (in yrs. at nearest birthday)}}{24} \times \text{adult dose} = \text{child's dose}$$

cowperitis (kow-per-ī′-tis): Inflammation of the bulbourethral glands (Cowper's).

Cowper's glands (kow′-perz): Bulbourethral glands. Two in number, lying lateral to the membranous urethra, below the prostate gland, and deep to the perineal membrane. They open via short ducts into the anterior (penile) urethra. [William Cowper, English surgeon. 1666–1709.]

cowpox: Vaccinia. Virus disease of cows. Lymph is used in vaccination of humans against smallpox (variola).

coxa (kok′-sa): The hip joint. **C. PLANA,** flattening of the femoral head due to osteochondritis of the epiphysis; also called osteochondritis deformans juvenilis (*q.v.*). **C. VALGA,** an increase in the normal angle between the neck and shaft of the femur. **C. VARA,** a decrease in the normal angle between the neck and shaft of the femur.—coxae, pl.

coxalgia (kok-sal′-ji-a): Literally, pain in the hip joint. Often used as syn. for hip joint disease.

coxitis (kok-sī′-tis): Inflammation of the hip joint.

coxodynia (kok-sō-din′-i-a): Coxalgia (*q.v.*).

coxotuberculosis (kok′-sō-tū-ber-cū-lō′-sis): Tuberculosis of the hip joint.

coxsackievirus (kok-sak′-e-vī-′-rus): One of a large group of enteroviruses that produce symptoms resembling those of poliomyelitis but without the paralysis; associated with cardiac conditions, pneumonia, hepatitis, acute hemorrhagic conjunctivitis, aseptic meningitis, encephalitis, and an influenza-like fever. First isolated in Coxsackie, New York. Also written Coxsackie virus.

CPAP: Abbreviation for continuous positive airway pressure.

CPK: Abbreviation for creatine phosphokinase.

CPPB: Abbreviation for continuous positive pressure breathing. See under breathing.

CPR: Abbreviation for cardiopulmonary resuscitation; see under resuscitation.

cps: Abbreviation for cycles per second. See Hertz.

CPT: Abbreviation for Current Procedural Terminology, a listing of standard terminology in common use for describing medical procedures and services.

crab louse (krab lows): Pediculus pubis (*q.v.*).

"crack": A highly concentrated, highly addictive, chemically reconstituted, and relatively inexpensive preparation of cocaine that is sold in the form of small rocks or pebbles and is smoked rather than snorted. Produces more intense "highs" and "lows" than the powdered form of cocaine and leads more quickly to addiction.

crackling (krak′-ling): Fine, moist crepitant-like sound heard on auscultation of the lungs; lower in pitch than crepitant sounds; also called subcrepitant sounds. See **crepitus.**

cradle: A frame, usually of wood or wire, used to keep the bed clothes from contact with an injured or fractured limb; also used when dry heat is being applied to an extremity. **C. CAP,** an accumulation of grayish-yellow crust-like material on the crown of the scalp of an infant with eczema or one who is not shampooed regularly.

cramp: Spasmodic, involuntary, painful contraction of a muscle or group of muscles. Occurs in tetany, food poisoning and cholera. In gynecology, a colloquial term for dysmenorrhea. **HEAT C.,** muscular spasm attended by weak pulse, dilated pupils and prostration, seen in those who work in intense heat and who lose much salt and water through perspiration, *e.g.*, stokers, miners. **MUSCLE C.,** sudden painful involuntary contraction of a skeletal muscle. **WRITERS' C.,** an occupational disease characterized by spasmodic contraction of muscles of fingers, hand and forearm; a similar condition occurs in others whose occupations involve use of fine muscles.

crani-, cranio-: Combining forms denoting skull.

craniad (krā′-ni-ad): Toward the cranium or head.

cranial (krā′-ni-al): Pertaining to the cranium (*q.v.*). **C. CAVITY,** the cavity of the skull which contains the brain. **C. DECOMPRESSION,** reduction of excessive pressure on the brain by means of surgery. **C. FOSSA,** any one of the three shallow depressions on the upper surface of the base of the skull. **C. NERVE,** any one of the twelve pairs of nerves given off by the brain rather than the spinal cord; they are named and numbered in the following order: 1, olfactory; 2, optic; 3, oculomotor; 4, trochlear; 5, trigeminal; 6, abducens; 7, facial; 8, acoustic; 9, glossopharyngeal; 10, vagus; 11, accessory; 12, hypoglossal.

craniectomy (krā-ni-ek′-to-mi): Surgical removal of a portion of skull.

craniocele (krā′-ni-ō-sēl): Protrusion of part of the cranial contents through a defect in the bones of the cranium.

craniocerebral (krā′-ni-ō-ser′-e-bral): Pertaining to the cranium and the cerebrum.

craniocervical (kra′-ni-ō-ser′-vi-kal): Pertaining to the head and neck.

cranioclasis (krā-ni-ok′-la-sis): Crushing of the fetal skull to facilitate delivery in unusually difficult labor.

craniofacial (krā′-ni-ō-fā′-shal): Pertaining to the cranium and the face. **C. DYSTOSIS,** see under **dystosis.**

craniofenestria (krā′-ni-ō-fen-es′-tri-a): A condition in which there is defective development of the bones of the cranium; in some areas no bone whatever is formed.

craniomalacia (krā′-ni-ō-ma-lā′-shi-a): Abnormal softness of the skull bones.

craniomegaly (krā-ni-ō-meg′-a-li): Enlargement of the head.

craniometry (krā-ni-om′-e-tri): The science that deals with the measurement of the skull and face.

craniopagus (kra-ni-op′-a-gus): Conjoined twins that are united at their heads.

craniopharyngioma (krā′-ni-ō-fa-rin-jē-ō′-ma): A solid or cystic benign congenital brain tumor in the area of the pituitary; associated with intracranial pressure on the hypothalamus and optic chiasm; causes visual impairment and hormone disturbances; seen in children and young adults.

cranioplasty (krā′-ni-ō-plas-ti): Surgical repair of a skull defect.—cranioplastic, adj.

craniosacral (krā′-ni-ō-sā′-kral): Pertaining to the skull and sacrum. Applied to the parasympathetic nervous system.

cranioschisis (krā-ni-os′-ki-sis): Congenital fissure of the skull.

craniosclerosis (krā′-ni-ō-sklē-rō′-sis): Abnormal thickening of the cranial bones.

craniospinal (krā′-ni-ō-spī′-nal): Pertaining to the cranium and the spine.

craniostenosis (krā′-ni-ō-stē-nō′-sis): Premature fusion of the cranial sutures with consequent cessation of growth, resulting in deformity and a small skull.

craniosynostosis (krā′-ni-ō-sin-os-tō′-sis): Premature closure of the cranial sutures before or shortly after birth; due to hypercalcemia; the resulting abnormal shape of the head depends on the sutures involved. Brain growth is restricted and mental retardation often follows. Also craniostosis.

craniotabes (krā′-ni-ō-tā′-bēz): A softening and wasting of the cranial bones, and widening of the sutures and fontanels occurring in infancy, due to lack of normal mineralization of the bones.—craniotabetic, adj.

craniotome (krā′-ni-ō-tōm): An instrument used in performing craniotomy (*q.v.*); it is operated by a high-speed drill powered by compressed air. Utilized to speed labor when the fetus is dead.

craniotomy (krā-ni-ot′-o-mi): A surgical opening of the skull in order to remove a growth, relieve pressure, evacuate blood clot, arrest hemorrhage, or to reduce the size of the head of an unborn dead infant to facilitate its delivery.

cranium (krā′-ni-um): The part of the skull enclosing the brain. It is composed of eight bones: the occipital, two parietals, frontal, two temporals, sphenoid and ethmoid.—cranial, adj.

cranium bifidum (krā′-ni-um bif′-i-dum): A fissure of the cranium, usually along the midline. A congenital condition often associated with meningocele.

crash cart: An emergency cart containing supplies, equipment, instruments and drugs needed for cardiopulmonary resuscitation or other life-saving procedures. Items that have been used are immediately replaced and the cart is returned to a designated location where it is readily available. A tag listing the contents is tied to the handle.

crash team: An organized team in a hospital trained to be available in any emergency; includes nurses, physicians, anesthetists, and helpers. A crash cart is kept ready for their use; it is equipped with drugs and equipment needed to handle emergency situations in patients with cardiac, respiratory, circulatory, or central nervous system conditions.

-crasia: A combining form denoting combination, mixing, constitution.

craving (krā′-ving): A persistent hunger or need for a drug or other substance; may be the result of either physical or psychological factors.

C-reactive protein: A globulin found in the serum of persons with inflammation or necrosis; tests for the presence of this protein are used in diagnosing rheumatic fever. Abbreviated CRP.

cream of tartar: Potassium bitartrate; used as a saline cathartic.

creatinase (krē-at′-i-nās): An enzyme that acts as a catalyst in the decomposition of creatine.

creatine (krē′-a-tin): In biochemistry, a crystalline substance synthesized in the body; found chiefly in vertebrate muscle tissue; combines with phosphate to form phosphocreatine, a source of quickly available energy for the muscles; is increased in pregnancy and decreased in hypothyrodism. **C. KINASE,** an enzyme found in cardiac and skeletal muscle; is active in the conversion of phosphocreatine and adenosine diphosphate to creatinine and adenosine triphosphate; used in several diagnostic tests including those for muscle disorders. **C. PHOSPHOKINASE,** **C.** kinase; abbreviated CPK. **C. CLEARENCE TEST,** a test for renal function.

creatinemia (krē-a-ti-nē′-mi-a): The presence of an excess of creatine in the blood.

creatinine (krē-at′-i-nin): A waste substance that is an end product of protein metabolism and is found in muscle, blood, and urine; it is liberated from muscle and secreted in the urine at a constant rate. **C. CLEARANCE TEST,** a test for measuring glomerular filtration, a major function of the kidney that decreases in renal disease. **C. PHOSPHOKINASE,** an enzyme found in cardiac muscle, skeletal muscle, and brain tissue; helps control the amount of energy available for use in the body; is elevated in disorders involving cardiac muscle, cardiac surgery, and cardiac defibrillation; abbreviated CPK.

creatinuria (krē-a-ti-nū′-ri-a): Increased or abnormal amounts of creatinine in the urine. Occurs in metabolic disorders and conditions in which muscle is rapidly broken down, *e.g.*, acute fevers, starvation.—creatinuric, adj.

credentialing (kre-den′-sha-ling): A broad term pertaining to the process that determines whether individuals, institutions or programs are in compliance with established standards. In nursing, the term includes licensure of nurses, certification of practitioners of specialties, and the accreditation of programs in nursing education or agencies offering nursing services.

Credé's method (krē-dāz′): 1. A method of delivering the placenta by gently rubbing the fundus of the uterus until it contracts, and then by squeezing the fundus, expressing the placenta into the vagina whence it is expelled. 2. Periodically pressing on the urinary bladder to expel urine; also called Credé's maneuver. 3. The placing of one drop of 1 percent silver nitrate in each eye of the newborn child to prevent ophthalmia neonatorum (*q.v.*). [Karl Sigmund Franz Credé, German obstetrician. 1819–1892.]

cremaster muscle (krē′-mas-ter): Name given to an extension of the internal oblique muscle over the spermatic cord and testis; the corresponding muscle in the female is underdeveloped.—cremasteric, adj.

cremation (krē-mā′-shun): The burning or incineration of the body of a deceased person.

crenate (krē′-nāt): Scalloped, indented or notched. In physiology, descriptive of the indented edges of red blood cells that have shrunken from exposure to air or to a hypertonic solution. Also crenated.—crenation, n.

crenotherapy (kren-ō-ther′-a-pi): Treatment by mineral spring waters. Also called caunotherapy.

creosote (krē′-ō-sōt): Colorless to yellowish oily liquid obtained from wood tar; used in expectorants and disinfectants.

crepitant (krep′-i-tant): Pertaining to, having, or producing a crackling sound.

crepitation (krep-i-tā′-shun): 1. Grating of bone ends in fracture. Also crepitus. 2. Crackling sound heard via stethoscope in lung infections. 3. Crackling sound elicited by pressure on emphysematous tissue.

crepitus (krep′-i-tus): 1. A dry, crackling sound such as might be produced by the grating ends of a broken bone, or as heard by stethoscope in some pneumonias. 2. The noisy discharge of flatus from the bowel.

cresol (krē′-sol): Colorless to brownish aromatic liquid obtained from wood tar; disinfectant. Lysol is a proprietary name for a compound solution of **C.**

crest: A projection or ridge, especially at the border of a bone.

cretin (krē′-tin): A person affected with cretinism (*q.v.*).

cretinism (krē′-tin-ism): A condition originating in fetal life or early infancy; due to congenital thyroid deficiency; characterized by stunted mental and physical development, dwarfism, large head, thick legs, pug nose, dry skin, scanty hair, swollen eyelids, short neck, protruding abdomen, clumsy uncoordinated gait.—cretin, n.; cretinistic, cretinoid, cretinous, adj.

Creutzfeldt-Jacob syndrome (disease): A rare spongiform encephalopathy of viral origin occurring chiefly in older people; characterized by degeneration of the pyramidal and extrapyramidal systems, progressive dementia, muscular weakness and tremor; usually fatal.

crib death: Death of an infant who has presented no symptoms of illness; occurs usually during first four or five months of life; sometimes thought to result from a sudden overwhelming infection. See sudden infant death syndrome.

cribriform (krib′-ri-form): Perforated, like a sieve. **C. PLATE,** that portion of ethmoid bone that forms the roof of the nasal cavity; has many perforations for the passage of fibers of the olfactory nerve.

cricoid (krī′-koyd): Ring-shaped. Applied to the cartilage forming the inferior posterior part of larynx.

cricoidectomy (krī′-koy-dek′-to-mi): Excision of the cricoid cartilage.

cricopharyngeal (krī′-kō-fa-rin′-jē-al): Pertaining to the cricoid cartilage and the pharynx.

cricothyroid membrane or ligament (krī-kō-thī′-royd): A sheet of fibroelastic connective tissue which is attached at its lower edge to the cricoid cartilage, at its upper edge to the thyroid cartilage, with the lateral parts of its upper margin forming the vocal ligaments.

cricothyrotomy (krī′-kō-thī-rot′-o-mi): An incision through the skin and the cricoid and thyroid cartilages, required in some instances to create and maintain a patent airway; may be preliminary to emergency tracheostomy.

cricotracheotomy (krī′-kō-trā-kē-ot′-o-mi): The procedure of making an incision into the trachea through the cricoid cartilage.

cricovocal (krī-kō-vō′-kal): Pertaining to the cricoid cartilage and the vocal cords.

cri-du-chat (krē-du-shah′): A syndrome consisting of a group of congenital anomalies including brachycephaly, low forehead, wide-spaced eyes, strabismus, micrognathia, and mental retardation; characterized by a catlike cry in infants.

Crigler-Najjar syndrome: A rare congenital condition characterized by nonhemolytic jaundice, the presence of large amounts of bilirubin in the blood, severe central nervous system disorders; due to a deficiency of the hepatic enzyme, glucuronide transferase.

-crine: A suffix denoting secretion, or secreting.

crisis (krī′-sis): 1. The turning point or an abrupt change in the course of a disease, as the point of defervescence in fever. 2. Muscular spasm in tabes dorsalis referred to as visceral crisis (gastric, vesical, rectal, etc.). 3. A period of stress or an episode that interferes with normal functioning activities. **ADDISONIAN C.,** a sudden onset or worsening of the signs and symptoms of Addison's disease. **ANAPLASTIC C.,** a transient condition caused by disappearance of red blood cells from the bone marrow; may develop during serious infections or in certain hemolytic disorders. **ASTHMATIC C.,** status asthmaticus; see under status. **CHOLINERGIC C.,** respiratory failure resulting from overtreatment with anticholinesterase drugs. **DIETL'S C.,** a complication of ptosis of the kidney; the chief symptom is severe sudden pain in the kidney that may follow the intake of large amounts of water but is usually due to kinking of the ureter; other symptoms are nausea, vomiting, hypotension, tachycardia, scanty blood-stained urine; possibly collapse. **MATURATIONAL C.,** one that occurs during life periods marked by social, physical, or psychological change. **MYASTHENIC C.,** sudden deterioration with weakness of respiratory muscles due to an increase of myasthenia. **OCULOGYRIC C.,** see oculogyric. **SITUATIONAL C.,** one that arises as a result of a stressful event. **THYROTOXIC C.,** sudden return of symptoms of thyrotoxicosis, due to a shock, injury, or thyroidectomy.

crisis intervention: A term used to describe a brief type of treatment in which a psychotherapist or a team intervenes in a situation in order to assist the family and the patient to secure help in solving an immediate problem; may include medications, referral to a community agency, changing the patient's environment, etc.

crista galli (kris′-ta gal′-lī): Superior triangular portion of ethmoid bone. Likened to a cock's comb.

criteria (krī-tēr'-i-a): Standards on which a judgment or decision may be based.—criterion, sing.

critical (krit'-i-kal): 1. Arising from or characterized by crisis. 2. Implying serious risk or uncertainty as to outcome. 3. Crucial.

critical care unit: A special unit in a health care facility where patients with critical disorders or diseases of the vital physiological systems (cardiovascular, respiratory, renal, electrolytic, neurologic) are provided with the care required to sustain life. May be combined with an intensive care unit.

CRNA: Abbreviation for Certified Registered Nurse Anesthetist.

crocodile tears syndrome: Excessive flow of tears in some patients with facial paralysis when chewing or ingesting strongly flavored foods.

Croft's splint: A plaster of Paris splint cut in two halves so that it can be removed for massage or other treatment.

Crohn's disease: Regional ileitis; a chronic intestinal disorder in which segments of the intestine become inflamed and swollen; cause unknown. May be acute or chronic; onset usually before age 35; symptoms include nausea, vomiting, diarrhea, abdominal pain, fever, weight loss, malaise. Chief complications are perforation and hemorrhage. Also called regional colitis, regional enteritis, granulatomatous colitis. [Burrill B. Crohn, American gastroenterologist. 1884–1983.]

cross contamination: The introduction of infectious material from one source to another.

cross dependence: A condition in which one drug can prevent withdrawal symptoms in an addict who is withdrawing from use of another drug.

cross infection: A second infection superimposed upon another infectious disease from which the patient is suffering; often the result of direct or indirect contact with another person or patient in the same care facility.

cross section: A cut or slice made through an object at right angles to the long axis.

cross tolerance: A condition in which tolerance to one drug produces a reduced response to another drug in the same general class.

crossed: **C. EXTENSOR RESPONSE,** a normal response in the newborn; when the infant is in the supine position and the sole of one foot is stroked, it responds by flexing the other leg and then adducting and extending it to try to push the stimulus away. **C. LATERALITY,** a combination of right-handedness and left-eyedness, or vice versa.

cross-eye: Convergent strabismus (*q.v.*). A squint in which one or both eyes turn inward toward the nose. Esotropia.—cross-eyed, adj.

crossmatching: A procedure for determining the compatibility of bloods before transfusion. See **blood types, blood crossmatching.**

crotch (krotch): The angle formed by the parting of two leg-like parts or branches. In anatomy, the angle formed by the inner side of the thigh and the trunk.

croton oil (krō'-ton): A drastic purgative derived from the seed of a shrub of the genus *Croton;* considered unfit for human use.

croup (kroop): A condition resulting from acute spasmodic laryngitis, occurring in infants and children, most often at night; characterized by harsh, brassy cough, crowing inspirations, dyspnea, and with or without membrane formation. Croupy breathing in a child is often called stridulous, meaning noisy or harsh-sounding. Narrowing of the airway gives rise to the typical attack with crowing inspiration; may result from edema, allergy, inflammation of the larynx, spasm. **C. KETTLE,** a kettle for producing steam or medicated vapor which is either directed into a **C.** tent or allowed to escape into the air to humidify it; used in croup and bronchial conditions. **C. TENT,** a covering for the head and shoulders into which a stream of steam or medicated vapor is directed; used to relieve croup and some other respiratory conditions.—croupous, croupy, adj.

Croupette (kroo-pet'): Trade mark for a piece of equipment consisting of a small plastic tent with an ice-cooled nebulizer; used in treatment of upper respiratory infections to provide humidity, oxygen, and a cool environment for infants and small children; helps to liquefy secretions and reduce muscular spasms of the larynx; especially useful in tracheobronchitis.

crown: The highest or topmost part of anything. In anatomy, the topmost part of an organ or structure, *e.g.*, the top of the head.

crowning (krown'-ing): The phase in the second stage of labor when part of the fetal scalp can be seen at the vaginal orifice.

crow's feet: Wrinkles emanating from the outer canthus of the eye in a fan-like pattern.

crucial (kroo'-shal): 1. Cross-shaped. 2. Severe; essential, as being decisive.

cruciate (krū'-shi-āt): Shaped like a cross. **C. LIGAMENTS OF THE KNEE,** strong thick ligaments that run from the intercondylar area of the tibia to the femur and cross within the knee joint; they provide stability to the joint and prevent dislocation of the tibia.

crural (kroor'-al): 1. Pertaining to the leg. 2. Leg-like.

crus (kroos): 1. The leg from the knee to the foot. 2. A term applied to various parts of the body which resemble a leg or root.—crural, adj.; crura, pl.

crush injury: An injury in which the physical force caused by crushing, pressure, or by blast is transmitted to the soft tissues, bones or viscera. Often refers to injuries of the chest when there may or may not be fractured ribs; symptoms include severe breathing difficulty immediately after the injury; later the person may develop edema of the lungs, dyspnea, cyanosis; sometimes fatal.

crush syndrome: Traumatic uremia. A condition resulting from damage to the renal tubules because their blood supply has been interfered with. Following an extensive trauma to muscle, there is a period of delay before the effects of renal damage manifest themselves. There is an increase of nonprotein nitrogen of the blood, with oliguria, proteinuria and urinary excretion of myohemoglobin. Loss of blood plasma to damaged area is marked. Symptoms include thirst, nausea, somnolence, hypertension, features of severe shock, pulmonary edema, and cardiac involvement.

crust: A hardened covering formed on a lesion on the surface of the skin from the accumulation of dried exudate and other debris. A scab.

crutch: A staff to support and aid the disabled in walking; it is long enough to reach from the armpit to the ground, has a concave crosspiece to fit the armpit and a crossbar for the hand. **C. PALSY,** paralysis or weakness of one or both of the upper extremities caused by compression of the brachial plexus or of the radial nerve. **CANADIAN C.,** a **C.** that is shorter than one that reaches to the axilla; it has a leather cuff that reaches to the midarm level.

Crutchfield tongs: A type of cranial skeletal calipers used for traction of the cervical spine. See traction, cervical.

crutchwalking: Walking with the aid of crutches when normal weight bearing is not possible. Several gaits are utilized, depending on the particular orthopedic problem involved. In the **TWO-POINT GAIT,** the person advances the right foot and the left crutch together, then the left foot and right crutch together. In the **THREE-POINT GAIT,** the person advances both crutches and the affected leg together, then the unaffected leg. In the **FOUR-POINT GAIT,** the person puts one crutch forward, then the opposite leg, then the other crutch, and then the other leg. In the **SWING-THROUGH GAIT** both crutches are advanced, the legs are swung through to a point past the crutches, then the crutches are brought to the legs. In the **SWING-TO GAIT,** the crutches are advanced and then the legs are brought to the crutches.

crux (cruks): A cross or structure shaped like a cross. **C. OF THE HEART,** the area around the junction of the walls of the four chambers of the heart.

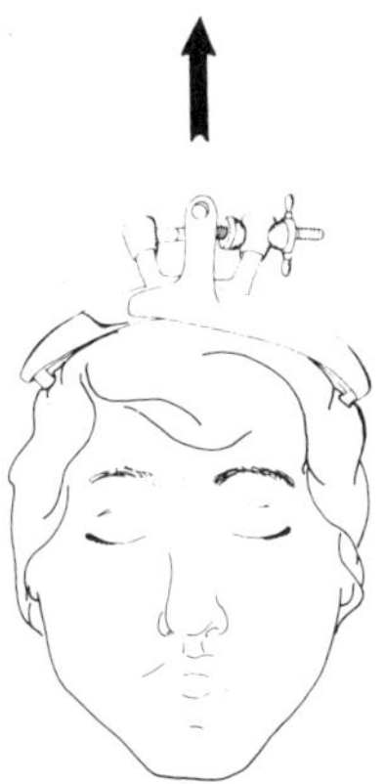

Crutchfield tongs

cry-, cryo-: Combining forms denoting relationship to 1) cold; 2) freezing.

cryalgesia (krī-al-jē′-zi-a): Pain resulting from the application of cold.

cryanesthesia (krī-an-es-thē′-zi-a): Loss of sensation or perception for coldness.

cryesthesia (krī-es-thē′-zi-a): Unusual sensitivity to cold.

crym-; crymo-: Combining forms denoting relationship to 1) cold; 2) frost.

crymodynia (krī-mō-din′-i-a): Rheumatic pain brought on by damp or cold weather.

crymotherapy (krī-mō-ther′-a-pi): Cryotherapy (*q.v.*).

cryobiology (krī′-ō-bî-ol′-o-ji): The branch of biology that deals with the effects of low temperatures, or freezing, on living tissues.

cryocautery (krī′-ō-kaw′-ter-i): The destruction of living tissue by the application of extreme cold, *e.g.*, solid carbon dioxide.

cryoextraction (krī′-ō-ek-strak′-shun): A technique for removing the lens of the eye by use of a cryoprobe.

cryoextractor (krī′-o-ek-strak′-tor): An instrument with a tip that can be cooled to extremely low temperatures (cryoprobe); used in the operation for extraction of a cataractous lens.

cryofibrinogen (krī′-ō-fī-brin′-ō-jen): Fibrinogen that has the unusual quality of precipitating in temperatures of 4°C, and redissolving when the temperature reaches 37°C.

cryofibrinogenemia (krī′-ō-fī′-brin-ō-jen-ē′-mi-a): The presence of cryofibrinogen in the blood.

cryogenic (krī-ō-jen′-ik): 1. Pertaining to or causing very low temperatures. 2. Describing any means or apparatus involved in the production of low temperatures.

cryogenics (krī-ō-jen′-iks): Low temperature physics; concerned with the production of very low temperatures and the phenomena that occur at those temperatures.

cryoglobulin (s) (krī′-ō-glob′-ū-lin): A group of abnormal serum proteins that precipitate on exposure to cold and redissolve when returned to body temperature.

cryoglobulinemia (krī′-ō-glob-ū-lin-ē′-mi-a): A condition in which cryoglobulin is present in the blood; seen in patients with multiple myeloma and some other pathological conditions.

cryohypophysectomy (krī′-ō-hī-pof′-i-sek′-to-mi): The destruction of the pituitary gland by cryotherapy.

cryometer (krī-om′-e-ter): A thermometer for measuring extremely low temperatures.

cryonics (krī-on′-iks): The practice of using intense cold therapeutically for such purposes as producing local anesthesia, or removing superficial skin lesions, and including the freezing of dead bodies and maintaining them at temperatures of -196°C in a sealed capsule suspended in liquid nitrogen.

cryopexy (krī′-ō-pek-si): Surgical fixation with freezing, as in the procedure for replacement of a detached retina.

cryophake (krī′-ō-fāk): A device used to freeze the crystalline lens of the eye to facilitate its removal in cataract surgery.

cryophilic (kri-ō-fil′-ik): Favoring or growing best at low temperatures.

cryoprecipitate (krī′-ō-prē-sip′-i-tāt): A precipitant substance containing Factor VIII; derived by rapidly freezing fresh human plasma from a single donor, then slowly thawing which removes all factors not related to clotting; used to help prevent or control hemorrhage and in treating hemophilia.

cryoprobe (krī′-ō-prōb): An instrument used for freezing tissue. Can be used for biopsy; causes little tissue damage and seeding of malignant cells. Also used in surgical treatment of conditions in various areas of the body, *e.g.*, brain, eye, prostate gland; the cells die and then may be removed surgically or by the body's own waste removal system.

cryosurgery (krī′-ō-sur′-jer-i): The destruction of tissue by the application of extreme cold, *e.g.*, the destruction of an area in the thalamus for treatment of parkinsonism, or the treatment with cold of malignant tumors of the skin. Also chryosurgery, crymosurgery.

cryothalamectomy (krī′-ō-thal-a-mek′-to-mi): The destruction of part of the thalamus by cold, done to relieve the tremor and rigidity of Parkinson's disease and other hyperkinetic conditions.

cryotherapy (krī-ō-ther′-a-pi): Therapeutic use of extreme cold, either local or general.

crypt (kript): In anatomy, a small sac, follicle, or pit-like depression opening on a free surface of an organ or of the body. **ANAL C.**, one of the depressions between the folds of mucous membrane in the anal canal. **CRYPTS OF LIEBERKÜHN**, intestinal glands; simple tubular glands in the mucous membrane of the intestine, thought to be concerned with secretion of intestinal enzymes. **TONSILLAR C.**, one of several crypts in the palatine tonsils.

crypt-, crypto-: Combining forms denoting 1) hidden, covered, invisible; 2) latent.

cryptesthesia (krip-tes-thē′-zi-a): The subconscious perception of an occurrence that is not usually perceptible to the senses.

cryptitis (krip-tī′-tis): Inflammation of the mucous membrane lining the anal crypts.

Cryptococcaceae (krip′-tō-kok-kā′-sē-a): A genus of yeast-like fungi including several that are pathogenic to man, *e.g., Cryptococcus, Candida, Trichosporum,* and *Pityrosporon.*

cryptococcosis (krip′-tō-kok-ō′-sis): A subacute or chronic infection involving the lungs, bones, or skin, but especially the brain and meninges; caused by *Cryptococcus neoformans* (*q.v.*).

Cryptococcus (krip-tō-kok′-us): A genus of fungi. **C. NEOFORMANS** is pathogenic to man; it has a marked predilection for the central nervous system causing symptoms similar to those of tuberculosis, cancer, brain tumor, even insanity; it may also affect the skin, liver, spleen, or joints.

cryptogenic (krip-tō-jen′-ik): Of unknown or obscure cause; often refers to anemia. **C. EPILEPSY**, idiopathic epilepsy. **C. FIBROSING ALVEOLITIS**, an uncommon condition of diffuse interstitial pulmonary fibrosis; symptoms include dyspnea, hypoxia, unproductive cough, cardiac failure; also called Hamman-Rich pulmonary fibrosis.

cryptoinfection (krip-tō-in-fek′-shun): A hidden or latent infection.

cryptolith (krip′-tō-lith): A concretion or stone formed within a gland follicle or a crypt; the tonsil is a frequent site.

cryptomenorrhea (krip′-tō-men-ō-rē′-a): Retention of the menses although other symptoms of menstruation may be present. Due to a congenital obstruction such as an imperforate hymen or atresia of the vagina. Syn., hematocolpos.

cryptomnesia (krip-tom-nē′-zi-a): Subconscious memory; the recall of a forgotten episode or event which seems new to the individual.

cryptorchidectomy (krip′-tor-kid-ek′-to-mi): Surgical removal of an undescended testis.

cryptorchidopexy (krip′-tor-ki-dō-pek′-si): Surgical fixation of an undescended testis in the scrotum.

cryptorchism (krip-tor′-kizm): A developmental defect whereby the testes do not descend into the scrotum; in **TRUE C.**, they remain in the abdominal cavity; in **ECTOPIC C.**, they remain within the inguinal canal. Also cryporchidism.—cryptorchid, n. and adj.

crystallin (kris′-ta-lin): Either of two globulins; the principal constituents of the lens of the eye.

crystalline (kris′-ta-līn): Like a crystal; transparent. Applied to various structures. **C. LENS,** a transparent biconvex body, oval in shape, which is suspended just behind the pupil and the iris of the eye, and separates the aqueous from the vitreous humor. It is slightly less convex on its anterior surface and it refracts the light rays so that they focus directly on the retina.

crystalloid (kris′-ta-loid): 1. Resembling a crystal. 2. A substance that forms a true solution; the opposite of a colloid (*q.v.*).

crystalluria (kris-tal-lū′ri-a): Excretion of crystals in the urine.—crystalluric, adj.

crystalluridrosis (kris′-tal-lū-ri-drō′-sis): Crystallization on the skin of perspiration containing urinary elements.

CS: Abbreviation for clinical specialist.

CSF: Abbreviation for cerebrospinal fluid.

CT: Abbreviation for computerized tomography.

Ctenocephalides (ten-ō-sē-fal′-i-dēz): A common genus of fleas. **C. CANIS,** a species of **C.** found on dogs; can transmit tapeworm to man. **C. FELIS,** a species of **C.** found on cats as well as dogs; may attack humans.

Cu: Chemical symbol for copper.

cu cm: Abbreviation for cubic centimeter.

cu mm: Abbreviation for cubic millimeter.

cubic centimeter (kū′-bik sen′-ti-mē-ter): 1. A mass of material that, in cube form, measures 1 centimeter on each side. Abbreviated cu cm or cc. 2. In liquid capacity it is equal to one one-thousandth of a liter or 0.27 fluidrams; called milliliter and abbreviated ml.

cubital tunnel syndrome: Pain, tenderness, weakness, paresthesia, and atrophy occurring along the ulnar nerve distribution in the hand and forearm; caused by an injury to the ulnar nerve at the elbow.

cubitus (kū′-bi-tus): 1. The forearm. 2. The bend between the arm and forearm. **C. VALGUS,** a greater than normal degree of valgus at the elbow joint; in severe cases the ulnar nerve may be affected. **C. VARUS,** the carrying angle of the elbow is decreased; may be due to previous surgery, injury, or infection.

cuboid (kū′-boid): Shaped like a cube; one of the tarsal bones.

cuboideometatarsal (kū-boy′-dē-ō-met-a-tar′-sal): Pertaining to the cuboid bone and the metatarsals or the articulation between them.

cuboideonavicular (kū-boy′-dē-ō-na-vik′-u-lar): Pertaining to the cuboid and navicular bones or the ligaments connecting them.

cuirass (kwē-ras′): 1. A covering, bandage or cast for the chest. 2. A mechanical apparatus fitted to the chest for artificial respiration.

cul-de-sac (kul′-de-sak): A blind pouch or a cavity closed at one end. **C. OF DOUGLAS,** see Douglas' pouch.

culdocentesis (kul-dō-sen-te′-sis): The aspiration of pus or any other fluid from Douglas' pouch through a retrovaginal puncture or incision.

culdoscope (kul′-dō-skōp): An endoscope used via the vaginal route. See culdoscopy.

culdoscopy (kul-dos′-kō-pi): Passage of a culdoscope through the posterior vaginal fornix, behind the uterus, to enter the peritoneal cavity, for viewing the internal genitalia.—culdoscopic, adj.; culdoscopically, adv. A form of peritoneoscopy, laparoscopy.

culdotomy (kul-dot′-o-mi): An incision into the cul-de-sac called Douglas' pouch (*q.v.*).

-cule: Suffix denoting small.

Culex (kū′-leks): A genus of mosquitoes that act as vectors of certain diseases. *C. fatigans* or *quinquefasciatus* is the most common vector of *Wuchereria bancrofti,* a species of filaria found in warm regions throughout the world.

Culicidae (kū-lis′-i-de): The Diptera family of insects which includes the mosquitoes.

culicide (kū′-li-sīd): An agent that destroys gnats and mosquitoes.—culicidal, adj.

Cullen's sign: A bluish-red discoloration around the umbilicus; may be indicative of intraabdominal hemorrhage, or ruptured ectopic pregnancy; sometimes also seen in acute pancreatitis.

culture (kul′-chur): 1. The development of microorganisms on artificial media under ideal conditions for growth. 2. A growth of microorganisms on a culture medium. 3. The act of cultivating microorganisms on an artificial medium. 4. The total pattern or lifestyle of an individual or group as judged by speech, intellectual and artistic achievement, beliefs, and institutions that are characteristic of a community or population. **C. MEDIUM,** a sterile preparation suitable for the cultivation and growth of microorganisms; may have a meat infusion as a base. **MIXED C.,** growth of two or more organisms in the same culture. **PURE C.,** specific growth of only one species of organism in a culture.

cumulative action (kū'-mū-lā-tiv): Occurs when the dose of a slowly excreted drug is repeated too frequently. This can be dangerous as, if the drug accumulates in the system, toxic symptoms may occur, sometimes quite suddenly. Long acting barbiturates, thyroid extract, strychnine, mercurial salts and digitalis are examples of drugs with a cumulative action.

Cumulative Index to Nursing and Allied Health Literature: A cumulative index to English language nursing and allied health publications, published bi-monthly, with an annual cumulation, by the Glendale Adventist Medical Center, Glendale, California.

cumulus (kū'-mū-lus): A small heap or mound. **C. OOPHORUS,** a small solid mass of follicular cells surrounding the ovum and protruding into the fluid in the cavity of the graafian follicle.

cuneate (kū'-nē-āt): Wedge-shaped.

cuneiform (kū-nē'-i-form): 1. Wedge-shaped. 2. Any one of the three small wedge-shaped bones of the tarsus, or the pyramidal bone of the wrist.

cunnilingus (kun-i-lin'-gus): Oral stimulation of the female genitalia.

cunnus (kun'-us): The female genitalia; the vulva.

cup: In anatomy, a cup-shaped part or structure. **C. ARTHROPLASTY,** a surgical procedure whereby the acetabulum is reshaped and the head of the femur is replaced with a metallic prosthesis.

cupping (kup'-ing): 1. A once popular method of counterirritation. A small, bell-shaped glass (in which the air is expanded by heating, or exhausted by compression of an attached rubber bulb) is applied to the skin, resultant suction producing hyperemia—dry **C.** When the skin is scarified before application of the cup it is termed wet **C.** 2. Rapid, rhythmic tapping over the lungs with the cupped hands; often performed along with vibration produced by placing the fingertips firmly on the area over the lungs and shaking the arms; done to loosen tenacious mucus in the bronchial tree.

cupr-; cupro-: Combining forms meaning copper.

cupruresis (kū-proo-rē'-sis): The presence of copper in the urine.

curare (kū-rar'-ē): A bitter poison, sometimes used as a drug; prepared as an abstract of a variety of South American plants. Inert when given orally but a powerful muscle relaxant when given by intravenous or intramuscular routes. Sometimes used to promote muscle relaxation in convulsions, spasms, shock, and as an adjunct of anesthesia. Has been known to cause death from paralysis of respiratory muscles. Syn., Indian arrow poison.

curarization (kū-rar-i-zā'-shun): The administration of curare until the desired therapeutic effect is achieved.

curative (kūr'-a-tiv): 1. Having a tendency to heal or cure. 2. Related to or useful in curing disease and restoring health.

cure (kūr): 1. To heal or restore to health. 2 A restoration to health. 3. A system or special course of treatment. 4. A medicine or agent used in treating a disease.

curet, curette (kū-ret'): 1. A spoon-shaped instrument or metal loop for scraping the walls of a cavity or other surface (curetting) to remove growths or other abnormal or diseased tissue, or to obtain material for biopsy. 2. To remove growths or other abnormal tissue from a surface such as bone or from the walls of a cavity, as the uterus, by scraping with a spoon-shaped instrument.

curettage (kū-re-tazh'): The scraping of unhealthy or exuberant tissue from a cavity or from a surface such as bone, using a spoon-shaped instrument. **SUCTION C.**, a **C.** using a suction device, often to produce abortion during the first trimester of pregnancy. **VACUUM C.**, suction **C.**—curet, v.

curettings (kū-ret'-ingz): The material obtained by scraping or curetting and usually sent for examination in the pathology laboratory.

Curie, Pierre and **Marie:** French chemist (1859–1919) and his Polish-born scientist wife, Marie Curie (1867–1934); known for their discovery of radium in 1898.

curie (kū'-rē): A unit of measurement of radioactivity; it is that quantity of any radioactive nuclide that has 3.700×10^{10} disintegrations per second.

curietherapy (kū-rē-ther'-a-pi): Treatment by emanations from any radioactive source; originally referred to treatment by radon or radium.

Curling's ulcer: An acute ulcer of the duodenum, usually multiple, most often occurring as a result of stress associated with severe burns.

current (kur'-rent): Something which flows. **ALTERNATING C.**, an electric current that periodically reverses its flow. **DIRECT C.**, an electric current that always flows in the same direction.

Current Procedural Terminology: A publication of the American Medical Association that lists the AMA-approved terminology and coding for use in describing medical procedures and services.

A Curriculum Guide for Schools of Nursing: This book, published in 1937 and sponsored by the National League for Nursing Education, replaced the two earlier publications, *Standard Curriculum for Schools of Nursing* (1917) and *A Curriculum for Schools of Nursing* (1929), all of which were widely used by nurse educators.

curvature of the spine: An abnormal curve in the spinal column; may be to the front (lordosis), to the back (kyphosis) or to the side (scoliosis).

cushingoid (kush′-ing-oyd): 1. Having the appearance of a person with Cushing's disease or syndrome; said of the appearance resulting from the administration of corticosteroid drugs. 2. Having the appearance of one with Cushing's disease or syndrome, but none of the other features of that disorder.

Cushing's disease: A rare disorder, mainly of females, characterized by symptoms of Cushing's syndrome, principally virilism, obesity of trunk and face, hyperglycemia, glycosuria, and hypertension. Due to intrinsic and excessive hormone stimulation of the adrenal cortex by tumor or by hyperplasia of the anterior pituitary gland.

Cushing's syndrome: A disorder similar to Cushing's disease, but commoner, in which excessive hormonal excretion of adrenocorticotropic hormone is caused by intrinsic hyperplasia or, most often, by tumor of the adrenal cortex *per se,* or by prolonged administration of glucocorticoids. Occurring most often in females, the symptoms include fatness of the face ("moon" face), neck and trunk, abnormal distribution of the hair and hypertrichosis, florid complexion, hypertension, kyphosis due to softness of the vertebrae, muscular weakness, polycythemia, atrophy of the genital organs, impotence, and amenorrhea. Also called hyperadrenocorticism; basophilism; pituitary basophilism. [Harvey Williams Cushing, American surgeon. 1869–1939.]

cusp (kusp): A projecting point such as that of the edge of a tooth or a leaflet of a valve such as the heart valves that control the flow of blood between the atria and ventricles; the tricuspid valve in the right heart has three cusps, the mitral (bicuspid) valve in the left heart has two.

cuspid (kus′-pid): A tooth having only one cusp; the third tooth on either side from the midline of the jaws; a canine tooth.

cut-, cuti-: Combining forms denoting skin or cuticle.

cutaneous (kū-tā′-nē-us): Relating to the skin. **C. LEISHMANIASIS,** see under leishmaniasis. **C. TAG,** see acrochordon. **C. URETEROSTOMY,** transplantation of the ureters so that they open on to the skin of the abdominal wall.

cutdown (kut′-down): A small surgical incision to expose a vein into which a needle, cannula, or catheter is inserted for the administration of intravenous fluids or medications.

cuticle (kū′-ti-k'l): The epidermis (*q.v.*); dead epidermis, as that which surrounds a nail. See eponychium.—cuticular, adj.

cutin (kū′-tin): An impermeable waxy substance on or in the pores of cell walls.

cutireaction (kū-ti-rē-ak′-shun): An inflammatory reaction on the skin occurring in certain infectious diseases or upon injection into it of a preparation of the organism causing a specific disease.

cutis (kū′-tis): The corium or deeper layer of the skin; derma; true skin. **C. ANSERINA,** erection of the papillae of the skin due to contraction of the arrectores pilorum; produced by fear, cold, excitement or other stimulus. Often called gooseflesh or goose pimples. **C. MARMORATA,** transient pinkish or purplish mottling of the skin, seen chiefly in children on exposure to cold. **C. RHOMBOIDALIS NUCHAE,** thickening and furrowing of the skin, especially of the neck, from years of exposure to sun and weather. **C. VERA,** the dermis.

cutitis (kū-tī′-tis): Inflammation of the skin; dermatitis.

CV: Abbreviation for cardiovascular.

CVA: Abbreviation for 1. Cerebrovascular accident; a stroke. 2. Costovertebral angle.

CVP: Abbreviation for central venous pressure.

cyan-, cyano-: Combining forms denoting dark blue.

cyanemia (sī-a-nē′-mi-a): Bluishness of the blood, as in cyanosis; due to insufficient oxygen.

cyanide (sī′-a-nīd): Any compound containing cyanogen with the −CN radical; all are deadly poisons.

cyanocobalamin (sī-an-ō-kō-bal′-a-min): Vitamin B_{12}, a member of the vitamin B complex; essential to life. **C.** is a red crystalline, water-soluble, substance containing cobalt; essential for the metabolism of fats, proteins, and carbohydrates, and for normal formation of blood cells; deficiency results in pernicious anemia and brain damage. Found in liver, kidney, eggs, fish, meats, dairy products. Used prophylactically and as a specific in treatment of pernicious anemia; also useful in treatment of several other anemias, sprue, polyneuritis, and herpes zoster. Also called cobalamin, and intrinsic factor.

cyanoderma (sī-a-nō-der′-ma): A bluish discoloration of the skin.

cyanopathy (sī-an-op′-a-thi): Cyanosis.

cyanopia (sī-a-nō′-pi-a): A visual defect in which the individual sees all objects as blue.

cyanosis (sī-a-nō′-sis): A bluish tinge manifested by hypoxic tissue, observed most frequently under the nails, lips and skin. It is always due to lack of oxygen, and the causes of this are legion. **CENTRAL C.,** blueness seen on warm surfaces such as the oral mucosa and tongue, due to impaired gas exchange between the alveoli and the pulmonary capillaries. **PERIPHERAL C.,** blueness of the hands, feet, tip of the nose; disappears on massage of the part; due to low cardiac output; occurs after chilling, smoking, ingestion of certain drugs.—cyanotic, cyanosed, adj.

cyanotic (sī-a-not′-ik): Refers to the bluish purple discoloration of the mucous membranes and skin due to insufficient oxygen in the capillaries.

cyasma (sī-az′-ma): The peculiar freckle-like discoloration of the skin sometimes occurring in pregnant women.

cybernetics (sī-ber-net′-iks): The comparative study of electronic communication systems which combines the disciplines of neurophysiology, mathematics, and electrical engineering; it is concerned with the processes of information flow through which the brain controls the body and through which computers control machines. It supports the hypothesis that the functioning of the human brain is similar to that of electronic control devices.

cyclarthrodial (sik-lar-thrō′-di-al): Pertaining or referring to a cyclarthrosis (*q.v.*).

cyclarthrosis (sik-lar-thrō′-sis): A pivot joint; one which allows for rotation.

cycle (sī-k'l): A regular series of movements or events; a sequence which recurs regularly. CARDIAC C., the series of movements through which the heart passes in performing one heart beat which corresponds to one pulse beat and takes about one second. See diastole and systole. MENSTRUAL C., the periodically recurring series of changes in breasts, ovaries and uterus culminating in menstruation. See also Krebs' cycle.—cyclic, cyclical, adj.

cyclectomy (sī-klek′-to-mi): Excision of part of the ciliary portion of the eyelid or of a piece of the ciliary body (*q.v.*).

cyclical (sī-klik-al): Pertaining to or occurring in a cycle or cycles. C. SYNDROME, term used currently for premenstrual symptom complex, to emphasize that these symptoms are due to normal physiological interaction between several endocrine glands under the cyclical control of the hypothalamus and pituitary. C. VOMITING, periodic attacks of vomiting, associated with ketosis: no demonstrable pathological cause; occurs in nervous persons, children in particular.

cyclitis (sik-lī′-tis): Inflammation of the ciliary body of the eye, often coexistent with inflammation of the iris. See iridocyclitis.

cyclochloroiditis (sī′-klō-kō-roy-dī′-tis): Inflammation of the ciliary body and the choroid.

cyclocryotherapy (sī′-klō-krī-ō-ther′-a-pi): A treatment for glaucoma that utilizes diathermy to freeze the ciliary body.

cyclodialysis (sī-klō-dī-al′-i-sis): Surgical establishment of communication between the anterior chamber of the eye and the suprachoroidal space to relieve intraocular pressure in glaucoma.

cyclodiathermy (sī-klō-dī′-a-ther-mi): Destruction by diathermy of a portion of the ciliary body; done in cases of glaucoma.

cycloid (sī′-kloyd): In psychiatry, descriptive of behavior characterized by alternating periods of well-being and happiness with mild depression.

cyclokeratitis (sī′-klō-ker-a-tī′-tis): Inflammation of the cornea and the ciliary body.

cyclophoria (sī-klō-for′-i-a): Heterophoria that is characterized by a tendency for the eyes to deviate from their anterior-posterior axis and to rotate around their vertical axis; due to lack of equilibrium and weakness of the oblique muscles of the eye. See heterophoria.

cyclophosphamide (sī-klō-fos′-fa-mīd): A preparation of nitrogen mustard with cytotoxic effects; used in medicine as an antineoplastic agent.

cyclopia (sī-klō′-pi-a): A developmental anomaly in which there is a single orbital fossa; associated with severe defects of the brain and facial skeleton, including absence of the nose.

cycloplegia (sī-klō-plē′-ji-a): Paralysis of the ciliary muscle of the eye with consequent loss of the power of accommodation.—cycloplegic, adj.

cycloplegic (sī-klō-plē′-jik): 1. Pertaining to cycloplegia. 2. A drug or agent that causes temporary paralysis of the ciliary muscle.

cyclopropane (sī-klō-prō′-pān): A highly flammable and explosive anesthetic gas; of low toxicity and produces anesthesia rapidly; now largely replaced by nonflammable substances.

cyclops (sī′-klops): A congenital anomaly in which the individual has only one eye or in whom the two eye sockets are fused. See cyclopia.

cyclosporin A (sī-klō-spōr′-in): A substance derived from a fungus; used in helping the body resist infections following organ transplants.

cyclothorax (sī-klō-thō′-raks): The leakage of lymph from the thoracic or other lymphatic duct into the pleural cavity; a rare phenomenon that may result from surgical trauma, malignancy, or chest injury; treatment is surgical.

cyclothymia (sī-klō-thī′-mi-a): An affective disorder characterized by a tendency to alternation between moods of elation and depression that are not caused by external circumstances.—cyclothymic, adj.

cyclotomy (sī-klot′-o-mi): A drainage operation for the relief of glaucoma, consisting of an incision through the ciliary body.

cyclotron (sī′-klō-tron): An apparatus that gives high energy to certain particles by means of an alternating electric field and a powerful magnet; these particles can produce neutrons or can impart artificial radioactivity to various substances.

cyesis (sī-ē′-sis): Pregnancy. See also pseudosyesis.

cylindroid (sil′-in-droyd): 1. Shaped like a cylinder. 2. A variously shaped, twisted, false mucous cast in urine; has the same significance as a cast.

cylindroma (sil-in-drō′-ma): A tumor containing elongated twisted strands of hyaline material; may be benign as certain tumors of the skin that develop from sweat glands or hair follicles, seen chiefly on the scalp or face; or malignant, as certain tumors of the salivary glands, basal cell carcinomas, and epitheliomas.

cylindruria (sil-in-drū′-ri-a): The presence of an increased number of cylindroid casts in urine; they are formed in the nephron and are diagnostic of renal rather than urinary tract disease.

cyllosis (sil-ō′-sis): Clubfoot.

cynanthropy (sin-an′-thrō-pi): A delusion or mania in which the patient believes himself to be a dog and imitates one by barking and growling.

cynophobia (sī-nō-fō′-bi-a): A morbid or unreasonable fear of dogs.

cynorexia (sī-nō-rek′-si-a): Morbidly excessive hunger or appetite. See also bulimia.

cypridophobia (sip-ri-dō-fō′-bi-a): 1. A morbid fear of contracting a venereal disease. 2. Morbid fear of sexual intercourse.

cyrtosis (ser-tō′-sis): Kyphosis (*q.v.*) or other unnatural spinal curvature.

-cyst-: Suffix denoting a bladder.

cyst (sist): 1. The encapsulated stage in the life cycle of certain protozoa. 2. An encapsulated area, filled with fluid or semi-fluid material, in the dermis or subcutaneous tissue. **ADVENTITIOUS C.**, one formed about a foreign body or exudate. **BRANCHIAL C.**, one in the neck region arising from anomalous development of the embryonal branchial cleft(s). **CHOCOLATE C.**, a **C.** filled with degenerated blood; the ovaries are the most usual site. **CHOLEDOCHAL C.**, a congenital dilatation of the common bile duct which is usually manifested early in life; characterized by pain, enlarged liver, jaundice, cirrhosis, tumor; also called choledochous **C.**, and bile **C.** **COLLOID C.**, contains jelly-like material; occurs particularly in the third ventricle. **DERMOID C.**, congenital in origin, usually occurring in the ovary, containing elements of hair, nails, skin, teeth, etc. **EXTERNAL ANGULAR DERMOID C.**, a **C.** usually occurring above the eye on the lateral aspect of the eyebrow; an anomoly occurring in a neonate or infant. **FOLLICULAR C.**, occurs in the ovary when the graafian follicle fails to rupture; menstrual irregularities and menorrhagia may result. **HYDATID C.**, the envelope in which *Taenia echinococcus* (tapeworm) produces its larvae—usually in the liver. **INCLUSION C.**, a **C.** that develops from the implantation of epidermal tissue into another structure of the body; may occur in embryonic development or following trauma. **MEIBOMIAN C.**, see chalazion. **NABOTHIAN C.**, cystlike formations in the Nabothian glands of the cervix; caused by occlusion of the outlets for the secretion of the glands. **OVARIAN C.**, ovarian new growth, usually cystic but may be solid, such as fibroma. To be differeniated from a cystic ovary (*q.v.*); **O. C.** is enucleated from the ovary which is conserved. **PAPILLARY C.**, an ovarian **C.** in which there are nipple-like (papillary) outgrowths from the wall. May be benign or malignant. **PILONIDAL C.**, a sacrococcygeal dermoid **C.** containing hairs. **RETENTION C.**, caused by blocking of a duct, as a ranula (*q.v.*). **SEBACEOUS C.**, retention **C.** of a sebaceous gland (wen). **THYROGLOSSAL C.**, a cystic distension of the thyroglossal duct near the hyoid bone in the neck region.

cyst-, cysti-,cysto-: Combining forms denoting a fluid-filled sac, as the gallbladder or urinary bladder.

cystadenocarcinoma (sis-tad′-e-nō-kar-sin-ō′-ma): A malignant glandular tumor consisting of a solid mass containing cysts; most often seen in the ovary.

cystadenoma (sis′-tad-e-nō′-ma): An innocent cystic new growth of glandular tissue; may contain thick, viscid fluid or clear, thin fluid. **MUCINOUS C.**, a large cyst, usually ovarian, filled with thick fluid resembling mucin; tends to grow rapidly in later life; may become malignant.

cystalgia (sis-tal′-ji-a): Pain in a bladder, especially the urinary bladder.

cystathionine (sis-ta-thī′-ō-nēn): An intermediate product in the conversion of methionine to cysteine, an inherited condition associated with mental deficiency.

cystathioninuria (sis′-ta-thī′-ō-nin-ū′-ri-a): Excessive excretion of thionine, an intermediate product in conversion of methionine (*q.v.*) to cysteine; an inherited condition. Associated with mental subnormality.

cystectomy (sis-tek′-to-mi): 1. Usually refers to the surgical removal of part or the whole of the urinary bladder; this may involve transplantation of one or both ureters cutaneously or into the bowel. 2. Surgical removal of the cystic duct or of the cystic duct and the gallbladder. 3. The excision of a cyst. 4. Removal of part of the capsule of the crystalline lens, a procedure in the operation for removal of a cataract. **OVARIAN C.**, excision of a cyst from an ovary with conservation of the remaining ovarian tissue.

cysteine (sis′-tē-in): A sulfur-containing amino acid found in most proteins.

cystic (sis′-tik): 1. Pertaining to the urinary

bladder or the gallbladder. 2. Pertaining to or resembling a cyst. **C. BREAST DISEASE,** fibrocystic disease of the breast; see under **fibrocystic.** **C. DEGENERATION,** degeneration of tissue with formation of cysts. **C. DUCT,** the duct that leads from the gallbladder and joins the hepatic duct from the liver to form the common bile duct. **CYSTIC FIBROSIS,** an inherited condition characterized by accumulation of thick tenacious mucus which obstructs tubular structures particularly the bronchioles; symptoms include a high level of electrolytes in the sweat, deficient pancreatic functioning, dyspnea, productive cough, voracious appetite, abdominal cramps, bulky malodorous stools, impaired growth; affects about one in every 2500 children; occurs most often in Caucasian children; prognosis beyond adolescence is poor; survival depends on avoidance of pulmonary infections; see **mucoviscidosis; fibrocystic.** **C. MASTITIS,** cystic breast disease.

cysticercoid (sis-ti-ser′-koyd): A larval tapeworm.

cysticercosis (sis-ti-ser-kō′-sis): Infestation of man with Cysticercus (*q.v.*). Symptoms include loss of weight, nervousness, muscular pains; in severe cases the brain may be invaded and convulsions, paralysis, or mental retardation occur. Most cases are contracted in the Far East.

Cysticercus (sis-ti-ser′-kus): The larval form of various tapeworms. After ingestion, the ova do not develop beyond this form in man.

cystiform (sis′-ti-form): Resembling a cyst.

cystine (sis′-tēn): A sulphur-containing amino acid, produced by the breaking down of proteins during the digestive process. **C. STONES,** sometimes occur as a deposit in urine or forming stones in the bladder.

cystinemia (sis-ti-nē′-mi-a): The presence of cystine in the blood.

cystinosis (sis-tin-ō′-sis): Metabolic disorder in which crystalline cystine is deposited in the body, especially in the kidneys. Cystine and other amino acids are excreted in the urine. Renal insufficiency, renal rickets or dwarfism may result. Fanconi's syndrome. See **aminoaciduria.**

cystinuria (sis-ti-nū′-ri-a): A hereditary disorder in which cystine appears in the urine; often associated with liver disease or jaundice. A cause of renal stones.—cystinuric, adj.

cystitis (sis-tī′-tis): Inflammation of a bladder, the urinary bladder in particular. May be acute or chronic, primary or secondary to stones, etc., but the exciting cause is usually bacterial; may be associated with pathologic conditions of the kidney, prostate, or ureters; more common in women than men because the urethra is short. Symptoms include pain on urination, frequency, hematuria. **CYSTIC C., C.** characterized by formation of multiple cysts in the bladder wall. **INTERSTITIAL C.,** chronic **C.** which extends into the deeper tissues of the bladder, often accompanied by ulcer formation. See also **trigonitis.**

cystocarcinoma (sis′-tō-kar-si-nō′-ma): Cystadenocarcinoma (*q.v.*).

cystocele (sis′-tō-sēl): Prolapse or pouching of the posterior wall of the urinary bladder into the anterior vaginal wall. See **colporrhaphy.**

cystodiathermy (sis-tō-dī′-a-therm-i): The application of a cauterizing electrical current to the walls of the urinary bladder; usually done through a cystoscope.

cystodynia (sis-tō-din′-i-a): Pain in the urinary bladder.

cystoelytroplasty (sis-tō-ē-lit′-rō-plas-i): Surgical repair of a vesicovaginal fistula.

cystoepithelioma (sis′-tō-ep-i-thē-li-ō′-ma): An epithelioma that is undergoing cystic degeneration.

cystofibroma (sis-tō-fī-brō′-ma): A fibrous tumor containing cysts.

cystogenesis (sis-tō-jen′-e-sis): The formation of cysts.

cystogram (sis′-tō-gram): An x-ray film demonstrating the urinary bladder. **MICTURATING C.,** taken during the act of passing urine.

cystography (sis-tog′-ra-fi): Radiography of the urinary bladder after it has been rendered radiopaque.—cystographic, adj.; cystographically, adv.

cystoid (sis′-toyd): 1. Like a bladder. 2. Like a cyst. 3. A tumor that resembles a cyst in that it contains fluid or pulpy material but which has no capsule.

cystolith (sis′-tō-lith): A stone in the urinary bladder.

cystolithectomy (sis′-tō-li-thek′-to-mi): Removal of a stone or stones from the urinary bladder by cutting into the bladder.

cystolithiasis (sis-tō-lith-ī′-as-is): The presence of a stone in the urinary bladder.

cystoma (sis-tō′-ma): A tumor containing cysts, especially one in or near an ovary.

cystometer (sis-tom′-e-ter): An instrument used to measure the pressure within the urinary bladder in relation to its capacity; used in studies of bladder function.

cystometrogram (sis-tō-met′-rō-gram): A graphic record, made with a cystometer (*q.v.*), of the changes in pressure within the urinary bladder under various conditions; used in the study of certain disorders of bladder function.

cystomorphous (sis-tō-mor′-fus): Resembling a cyst or a bladder in structure.

cystomyxoma (sis′-tō-mik-sō′-ma): A myxoma (*q.v.*) in which cysts have developed.

cystopexy (sis′-tō-pek-sē): The surgical fixation of the bladder in a new position.

cystoplasty (sis′-tō-plas-ti): Surgical repair of the bladder.—cystoplastic, adj.

cystoplegia (sis-tō-plē′-ji-a): Paralysis of the urinary bladder.

cystoprostatectomy (sis′-tō-pros-ta-tek′-to-mi): Surgical removal of the urinary bladder and the prostate gland.

cystopyelitis (sis-tō-pī-e-lī′-tis): Inflammation of the urinary bladder and the pelvis of the kidney.

cystopyelonephritis (sis-tō-pī′-e-lo-ne-frī′-tis): Inflammation of the urinary bladder associated with pyelonephritis.

cystorectocele (sis-tō-rek′-tō-sēl): Herniation of the urinary bladder and the rectum into the vagina.

cystorrhagia (sis-tō-rā′-ji-a): Hemorrhage from the urinary bladder.

cystorrhaphy (sis-tor′-a-fi): Suturing of the urinary bladder.

cystorrhea (sis-tō-rē′-a): Mucous discharge from the urinary bladder.

cystosarcoma (sis′tō-sar-kō′-ma): A sarcoma in which cysts have developed. **C. PHYLLOIDES**, a large fibroadenoma of the breast; aggressive, tends to metastasize.

cystoscope (sis′-tō-skōp): An endoscope equipped with a light and viewing lenses for examining the urinary tract.—cystoscopic, adj.

cystoscopy (sis-tos′-kō-pi): Observation of the bladder by means of a fiberoptic cystoscope (*q.v.*), for diagnostic purposes.

cystostomy (sis-tos′-to-mi): The operation whereby a fistulous opening is made into the bladder via the abdominal wall.

cystotome (sis′-tō-tōm): 1. A knife used in cataract surgery. 2. A knife used for incising the gallbladder or urinary bladder. Also cistotome.

cystotomy (sis-tot′-o-mi): 1. Incision into the urinary bladder or gallbladder; may be done to remove calculi or a tumor. **PERINEAL C.**, one in which the opening into the urinary bladder is made through the perineum. **SUPRAPUBIC C.**, one in which the opening into the urinary bladder is made just above the symphysis pubis. 2. Incision into the capsule of the crystalline lens.

cystoureteritis (sis′-tō-ū-rē-ter-ī′-tis): Inflammation of the urinary bladder and either or both ureters.

cystoureterogram (sis′-tō-ū-rē′-ter-ō-gram): An x-ray of the urinary bladder and ureters.

cystourethritis (sis′-tō-ū-rē-thrī′-tis): Inflammation of the urinary bladder and urethra.

cystourethrogram (sis-tō-ū-rē′-thrō-gram): An x-ray film demonstrating the urinary bladder and the urethra.

cystourethrography (sis′-tō-ū-rē-throg′-ra-fi): Radiographic examination of the urinary bladder and the urethra after they have been rendered radiopaque.—cystourethrographic, adj.; cystourethrographically, adv.

cystourethropexy (sis′-tō-ū-rē′-thrō-pek-si): Forward fixation of the bladder and upper urethra in an attempt to combat incontinence of urine.

cystourethroscope (sis-tō-ū-rē′-thrō-skōp): An instrument for examining the urinary bladder and the urethra.

cystourethroscopy (sis′-tō-ū-rē-thros′-ko-pi): A procedure utilizing the cystourethroscope to examine the bladder, urethra and urethral orifices for diagnostic purposes or to perform urethral catheterization.

cyte-, cyto-: Combining forms denoting 1) cells; 2) cytoplasm.

cythemolysis (sī-thēm-ol′-i-sis): Dissolution of blood cells, erythrocytes and leukocytes.

cytoarchitecture (sī′-tō-ar′-ki-tek-chur): The structural arrangement of cells.

cytobiology (sī-tō-bī-ol′-o-ji): The study of cell biology.

cytoblast (sī′-tō-blast): The nucleus of a cell.

cytochemistry (sī′-tō-kem′-is-tri): The study of the different chemical compounds within living cells.

cytocide (sī′-tō-sid): An agent that destroys cells.

cytoclasis (sī-tok′-la-sis): The destruction or necrosis of cells.

cytodendrite (sī-tō-den′-drīt): Dendrite.

cytodiagnosis (sī′-tō-dī-ag-nō′-sis): Diagnosis by microscopic study of cells. **EXFOLIATIVE C.**, diagnosis by the examination of cells from the external or internal surfaces of the body. See cytology.

cytogenesis (sī-tō-jen′-i-sis): The genesis and development of cells.—cytogenic, adj.

cytogenetic (sī-tō-jen-et′-ik): Pertaining to cytogenetics. **C. DISORDERS**, congenital malformations.

cytogenetics (sī-tō-je-net′-iks): That branch of biology concerned with the origin, development, structure, functions, etc. of cells, particularly of the chromosomes and genes.

cytogerontology (sī′-tō-jer-on-tol′-o-ji): The study of cellular changes due to the aging process.

Cytoglomerator (sī-tō-glom′-e-rā-tor): A machine that is used for freezing donated blood for long-time storage after the plasma has been extracted and the red cells coated with glycerol; the freezing temperature is −85°C; this process has increased the storage life of blood.

cytoglycopenia (sī′-tō-glī-kō-pē′-ni-a): A deficiency of glucose content in the body cells or the blood cells.

cytoid (sī′-toyd): Resembling a cell.

cytokalipenia (sī′-tō-kal-i-pē′-ni-a): A deficiency of potassium in the body cells or the blood cells.

cytokinesis (sī-tō-kin-ē'-sis): The changes that take place in the cytoplasm of a cell during mitosis and fertilization.

cytology (sī-tol'-ō-ji): Subdivision of biology, consisting of the study of the structure, function and pathology of the body cells. **EXFOLIATIVE C.**, microscopic study of cells from the surface of an organ or lesion after suitable staining.—cytologic, adj.

cytolysin (sī-tol'-i-sin): A substance or antibody that is capable of causing cells to dissolve. When a **C.** acts upon a specific type of cell, it is named accordingly, *e.g.*, hemolysin.

cytolysis (sī-tol'-i-sis): The degeneration, destruction, disintegration or dissolution of living cells.—cytolytic, adj.

cytomegalic inclusion disease: A disease of the newborn especially; due to infection with a cytomegalovirus (*q.v.*) which often occurs before birth; in the neonate is characterized by enlarged spleen and liver, small head, diarrhea, hematemesis, hematuria, cerebral hemorrhage, anemia, mental and motor retardation. Diagnostic cells that contain large acidophil intranuclear inclusions are found in the ducts or acini of the salivary glands, also sometimes in other organs, *e.g.*, liver, kidney. Congenital form is the most severe; formerly thought to be rare in adults; but it has been reported in that age group as an illness resembling infectious mononucleosis.

cytomegalovirus (sī-tō-meg'-a-lō-vī'-rus): One of a group of several DNA viruses, closely related to the herpes viruses, that infect monkeys and rodents as well as man, causing mononucleosis, cytomegalic inclusion disease, and various pulmonary disorders. Although it is not highly contagious, studies show that by age 35 most adults have been infected with it. When it is acquired in utero it sometimes causes deafness or hearing loss, and mental retardation. It causes serious illness in the newborn and in those on immunosuppressive therapy, especially those who have had a transplant. The virus is spread by saliva, breast milk, blood, and semen.

cytomegaly (sī-tō-meg'-a-li): Marked enlargement of cells.—cytomegalic, adj.

cytometer (sī-tom'-e-ter): A standardized device for measuring and counting cells, especially blood cells.

cytomorphology (sī'-tō-mor-fol'-o-ji): The morphology of body cells.

cytomorphosis (sī-tō-mor-fō'-sis): The changes occurring in cells in the course of their development.

cytomycosis (sī-tō-mī-kō'-sis): A fungal infection characterized by enlargement of the spleen, leukopenia, fever; attacks the phagocytes of the blood; often fatal. Also called histoplasmosis.

cyton (sī'-ton): The cell body of a neuron.

cytopathic (sī-tō-path'-ik): Pertaining to pathologic changes in cells.

cytopathology (sī-tō-pa-thol'-o-ji): The branch of pathology that deals with alterations within cells.

cytopenia (sī-tō-pē'-ni-a): A deficiency of blood cells or in the cellular elements in blood.

cytophagy (sī-tof'-a-ji): The engulfing of cells by other cells. See phagocytosis.

cytopheresis (sī-tō-fer-ē'-sis): The removal of cells, especially white blood cells, from whole blood and returning the remaining blood to the donor.

cytophysiology (sī'-tō-fiz-ē-ol'-o-ji): The physiology of cells.

cytoplasm (sī'-tō-plazm): The living material (protoplasm) of the cell other than that of the nucleus.

cytoscopy (sī-tos'-ko-pi): The microscopic examination of cells.

cytosome (sī'-tō-sōm): The cell body exclusive of the nucleus.

cytotechnologist (sī'-tō-tek-nol'-ō-jist): A person who specializes in 1) preparing cells for examination, and 2) examining them.

cytotoxic (sī'-tō-tok'-sik): 1. Pertaining to any substance that is toxic to cells. 2. An agent that damages or deranges cellular organization. Applied to a group of drugs used for treatment of carcinomas and reticuloses.

cytotoxin (sī'-tō-tok'sin): A toxin or antibody that is destructive to specific cells of certain organs, or which inhibits their functioning. See antibodies, cytotoxic.

cytotrophoblast (sī-tō-trof'-ō-blast): The inner (cellular) layer of the trophoblast (*q.v.*).

cytozoic (sī-tō-zō'-ik): Living on or within cells; parasitic.

cytozyme (sī'-tō-zīm): Thromboplastin (*q.v.*).

cyturia (sī-tū'-ri-a): An abnormal number of cells, of any kind, in the urine.

Czerny's sign: Retraction rather than bulging of the abdomen on inspiration; a sign of a central nervous system disorder such as chorea.

D

D: Abbreviation for: 1. Diopter. 2. Dexter, meaning right, *e.g.*, OD, oculus dexter (right eye). 3. Distal. 4. Dorsal. 5. Dose. 6. Died.

D and C: Abbreviation for dilatation of the cervix and curettage (*q.v.*) of the uterus.

DA: Abbreviation for developmental age. See developmental.

Da Costa's syndrome: Neurocirculatory asthenia; see under asthenia.

Dacron (dak′-ron): Trade name for a synthetic textile fiber; resistant to stretching and wrinkling. Sometimes used in replacement surgery.

dacry-, dacryo-: Combining forms denoting 1) lacrimal, or 2) tears.

dacryadenalgia (dak′-ri-ad-e-nal′-ji-a): Pain in or around a lacrimal gland. Also dacryoadenalgia.

dacryadenoscirrhus (dak′-ri-ad-e-nō-skir′-us): A scirrous tumor of a lacrimal gland.

dacryagogatresia (dak′-ri-a-gog-a-trē′-zi-a): Obstruction of a lacrimal duct.

dacryagogue (dak′-ri-a-gog): An agent that promotes the flow of tears.—dacryagogic, adj.

dacryoadenectomy (dak′-ri-ō-ad-e-nek′-to-mi): Surgical incision of a lacrimal gland.

dacryoadenitis (dak′-ri-ō-ad-e-nī′-tis): Inflammation of a lacrimal gland. It is a rare condition which may be acute or chronic. Also dacryadenitis.

dacryoblennorrhea (dak′-ri-ō-blen-ō-rē′-a): Mucous discharge from the lacrimal gland through the lacrimal duct; often chronic.

dacryocyst (dak′-ri-ō-sist): Old term for the tear sac (lacrimal sac).

dacryocystectasia (dak′-ri-ō-sis-tek-tā′-zi-a): Dilatation of a lacrimal duct.

dacryocystectomy (dak′-ri-ō-sis-tek′-to-mi): Excision of any part or all of the lacrimal sac.

dacryocystitis (dak′-ri-ō-sis-tī′-tis): Inflammation of the tear sac, which usually results in abscess formation and obliteration of the tear duct, giving rise to epiphora (*q.v.*); usually bilateral.

dacryocystography (dak′-ri-ō-sis-tog′-ra-fi): Radiographic examination of the tear drainage apparatus after it has been rendered radiopaque.—dacryocystographic, adj.; dacryocystogram, n.

dacryocystorhinostomy (dak′-ri-ō-sis′-tō-rī-nos′-to-mi): An operation to establish drainage from the lacrimal sac into the nose when there is an obstruction in the nasolacrimal duct.

dacryocystotomy (dak′-ri-ō-sis-tot′-o-mi): Surgical incision of the lacrimal duct; usually done to facilitate drainage.

dacryolith (dak′-ri-ō-lith): A concretion that develops in the lacrimal sac and may obstruct the lacrimal duct.

dacryolithiasis (dak′-ri-ō-li-thī′-a-sis): The presence of concretions in the lacrimal sac and/or duct.

dacryoma (dak-ri-ō′-ma): A tumor or swelling causing an obstruction of the lacrimal puncta or duct.

dacryorrhea (dak-ri-ō-rē′-a): Excessive secretion and flow of tears.

dacryostenosis (dak′-ri-ō-ste-nō′-sis): Stenosis or narrowing of the lacrimal flow system.

dactyl (dak′-*): A digit, finger, or toe.—dactyli, pl.; dactylar, dactylate, adj.

dactyl-, dactylo-: Combining forms denoting relationship to a digit, finger, or toe.

-dactylia, dactyl-: Combining forms denoting digit, finger, or toe.

dactylion (dak-til′-i-on): Webbing or adhesion of the fingers. See syndactyly.

dactylitis (dak-ti-lī′-tis): Inflammation of a finger or toe.

dactylogram (dak-til′-ō-gram): A fingerprint.

dactylography (dak-ti-log′-ra-fi): The scientific study of fingerprints.

dactylology (dak-til-ol′-o-ji): The finger sign method of communication used by deaf and dumb people. Fingerspelling.

dactylolysis (dak-ti-lol′-i-sis): 1. The loss of a finger or toe by accident or by surgery. 2. The surgical correction of syndactyly. **D. SPONTANEA**, the disappearance of a digit, as may occur in leprosy.

dactylomegaly (dak-ti-lō-meg′-a-li): Abnormal enlargement of one or more of the fingers or toes.

dactylus (dak′-til-us): A finger or toe.

Dakin's solution: A neutral antiseptic solution formerly much used for cleansing wounds; contains 0.5 percent solution of sodium hypochlorite. [Henry D. Dakin, English chemist in America. 1880–1952.]

Daltonism (dawl′-ton-izm): 1. Color blindness; named after John Dalton, English chemist and physicist [1766–1844], who was afflicted with it. 2. Red-green color blindness.

Dalton's law: States that the pressure exerted by a mixture of gases is equal to the sum of the partial pressures of the gases in the mixture. So long as there is no interaction between the gases, each gas in a mixture is absorbed by a given amount of solvent in proportion to its own partial pressure.

dam: A thin sheet of latex rubber, or a piece of it, that may be used 1) to separate tissues or organs from each other during surgery; 2) to isolate a tooth from mouth fluids during dental surgery; 3) to serve as a drain.

damp: 1. Humid or moist. 2. Pertaining to noxious or foul gases found in mines and caves. **BLACK D.**, noxious atmosphere that collects in a mine from the absorption of oxygen and the giving off of carbon dioxide by coal.

dance: **DANCE THERAPY**, see under therapy. **D. REFLEX**, see under reflex. **ST. VITUS' DANCE**, see under chorea.

dance therapy: Consists of guiding clients toward self-expression through dance movements or other rhythmic movements of the body; usually conducted with groups.

dancing eye-dancing feet syndrome: Opsoclonus (*q.v.*), along with muscle twitching and jerking; usually occurs in children; cause not known.

dander: In medicine, minute scales of skin, hair, fur, or feathers of animals which may cause allergic reactions in persons sensitive to them.

dandruff (dan′-druf): 1. The dried scaly material normally shed by the scalp. 2. Seborrheic dermatitis of the scalp; see under dermatitis.

dandy fever: Dengue (*q.v.*).

Dandy-Walker syndrome: A condition characterized by hydrocephalus due to distention of the fourth ventricle of the brain; thought to be caused by constriction of the foramina of Luschka and Magendi.

dark adaptation: The adjustment of the retina and iris for seeing in a dim light or in darkness.

Darrow's solution: A solution used in fluid therapy; contains the electrolytes normally found in plasma plus an added amount of potassium.

dartos (dar′-tos): A thin layer of smooth muscle tissue that makes up part of the superficial fascia of the scrotum; it envelops the testes. Cold causes it to contract, thus bringing the testes closer to the abdomen for warmth; warmth causes it to relax, thus the testes are kept at a fairly even temperature. Also tunica dartos.

Darwinian tubercle: A blunt pointed tubercle that projects from the upper part of the helix of the external ear; when it is abnormally enlarged it is referred to as Darwinian ear.

Darwinism (dar′-wi-nizm): The theory proposed by Darwin that higher organisms have evolved from lower forms in response to natural and environmental influences. [Charles Darwin, English naturalist. 1809–1882.]

DASE: Denver Articulation Screening Examination; an examination to discriminate between normal development in the acquisition of speech sounds and developmental delay; used for children 2½ to 6 years of age.

Datura stramonium (dā-tū′-ra stra-mō′-ni-um): A plant of the genus *Datura;* yields several alkaloids used in medicine, including scopolamine, hyoscyamine, and atropine.

daughter cell: A cell resulting from subdivision of a mature mother cell.

Dawson's encephalitis: Subacute sclerosing panencephalitis; see under panencephalitis.

day blindness: Inability to see well in bright daylight; hemeralopia.

day care center: A facility that sponsors a program of child care away from home for part of the 24-hour day; may be operated as a business or as a community social agency.

day hospital: A center where non-hospitalized patients, particularly older persons who do not require surgical intervention or 24-hour nursing care, spend a substantial amount of their waking time and are provided with needed diagnostic, medical, nursing, and rehabilitative services. The center may or may not be attached to a general or rehabilitation hospital, and operates on the professional level of a hospital.

day treatment: Treatment given in a care facility during the day only, sometimes in a hospital, as a substitute for inpatient care. Patients spend the day at the facility receiving psychotherapy, occupational therapy, pharmacotherapy, and certain nursing care. Utilized for rehabilitative therapy, for maintaining long-term patients, or as a means of giving intermediate care between hospital and home care until the patient is capable of independent living.

daydream: A pleasant reverie indulged in while awake; an imagining usually involving pleasant visions or wishful thinking.—daydream, v.

db, DB: Abbreviations for decibel(s).

DC: Abbreviation for direct current, a current that flows in one direction only. See AC. **DC CARDIOVERSION**, the use of direct current in cardioversion (*q.v.*).

DD: Abbreviation for differential diagnosis.

DDST: Denver Developmental Screening Test: Used for assessing children's developmental disorders.

DDT: Dichloro-diphenyl-trichloroethane. A powerful insecticide, effective on contact, formerly used worldwide against lice, flies, mosquitoes, and many other insects, especially in agriculture and in mass community programs designed to eliminate certain diseases. Recent governmental restrictions have curtailed its use since the chemical is toxic to humans.

de novo (de-nō′-vō): A Latin term meaning over again or anew.

deacidification (dē′-a-sid-i-fi-kā′-shun): The neutralization of an acid or correction of a condition of acidity.

dead space: 1. In the respiratory tract, the **ANATOMICAL D.S.** consists of those parts of the nose, mouth, and terminal bronchioles that do not take part in the exchange of oxygen and carbon dioxide; the **PHYSIOLOGICAL D.S.** consists of the anatomical **D.S.** plus that in the alveoli which does not take part in exchange of gases. 2. In a hypodermic syringe, the space at the tip of the syringe and in the hub of the needle after an injection.

deaf (def): Partially or completely unable to hear. May be due to anatomic defect, dysfunction or disease of the ear or part of it, brain disorder, or dysfunction of the vestibulocochlear nerve.—deafened, adj.; deafness, n.

Deaf Olympics: Quadrennial world games for the deaf.

deafferentation (dē′-af-fer-en-tā′-shun): Eliminating or interrupting afferent impulses, usually by destroying the afferent nerve pathway.

deafmute (def′-mūt): A person who lacks both the sense of hearing and the ability to speak. Also spelled deaf mute.—deafmutism, adj.

deafness (def′-nes): Lack, loss, or impairment of usable hearing; may be acute or chronic; congenital or acquired. **ACOUSTIC, BOILERMAKER'S** or **OCCUPATIONAL D., D.** that occurs in individuals who work in extremely noisy places. **AVIATORS' D.**, an occupational disease of aviators; may be temporary or permanent; caused by prolonged exposure to loud noise. **CENTRAL D., D.** caused by alterations in the auditory pathways and/or the auditory center of the brain. **CONDUCTION D., D.** that results from interference with conduction of sound waves within the ear; due possibly to the presence of hardened wax or to infection of the outer or middle ear. **HYSTERICAL D., D.** that appears and disappears in hysterical people without discernible physical cause. **NERVE D., D.** that results from damage to the auditory nerve. **ORGANIC D., D.** due to a defect in the ear or auditory apparatus. **PRESBYCUSIC D.**, see presbycusia. **PSYCHIC D.**, a condition in which the person hears sounds but does not comprehend them. **SENSORIMOTOR D.**, the **D.** that occurs in old age; usually due to presbycusia; may also be due to a lesion in the cochlear division of the 8th cranial nerve; also called perceptive **D. SENSORINEURAL D., D.** due to a lesion in the acoustic nerve or the central neural pathways, or both. **SIMULATED D.**, feigned **D. TONE D.**, inability to distinguish musical sounds. **TOXIC D., D.** due to the effect of toxins on the auditory nerve. **WORD D., D.** in which sounds are heard, but interpretation of words is impossible.

deaminase (dē-am′-i-nās): An enzyme that catalyzes the splitting off of an amino group from an organic compound.

deamination (dē-am-in-ā′-shun): 1. The removal of an amino from an organic compound. 2. A process occurring in the liver whereby amino acids are broken down and urea formed. Also deaminization.

dearticulation (dē′-ar-tik-ū-lā′-shun): The dislocation of a joint.

death: The permanent cessation or end of life. In the past death was said to occur when the heart ceased to beat and respiration stopped. **CLINICAL DEATH** occurs at the time of cardiac or respiratory arrest, and **BIOLOGICAL DEATH**, which is irreversible, 3 to 8 minutes later when the body cells have become anoxic. The tendency today is to include **BRAIN DEATH**, the irreversible cessation of brain function, in determining the time of death. Criteria for determining brain death were established in 1968 by the Ad Hoc Committee of the Harvard Medical School to Examine the Definition of Brain Death. These criteria include: 1) unreceptivity and unresponsivity to external stimuli; 2) no movement or breathing for at least one hour; 3) no reflexes can be elicited; and 4) a "flat" electroencephalogram, run for at least 10 minutes and repeated after 24 hours with no change. **D. CERTIFICATE**, a document that the physician is required to fill out and file after the death of a patient; it contains vital information about the person and the cause of the death. **D. INSTINCT**, an unconscious tendency toward self-destruction which may be expressed in a variety of aggressive acts usually aimed at one's self; thought by Freud to co-exist with the "life" instinct. **D. MASK**, a mold, usually of the face of a person, made after death. **D. RATE**, the ratio of deaths over a certain period of time among 1000 of the population in a certain area. **D. RATTLE**, sound sometimes heard in dying patients; caused by the loss of the cough reflex and the breathing of air through mucus that has collected in the trachea. **D. STRUGGLE, AGONY, THROE**, a final twitching or convulsion sometimes seen in a dying person.

debilitant (dē-bil′-i-tant): 1. An agent that weakens or enfeebles. 2. Causing debility.

debilitate (dē-bil′-i-tāt): To make weak or to enfeeble.—debilitating, adj.

debility (dē-bil′-i-ti): A state of weakness, feebleness or infirmity. See also asthenia.

débridement (dā-brēd′-mon): In surgery, thorough cleansing of a wound with removal of all foreign matter and devitalized, injured or infected tissue.—debride, v.

debris (de-brē′): Accumulated devitalized tissue or foreign matter.

dec-; deca-: Prefixes denoting 1) ten; 2) multiplied by ten.

decacurie (dec-a-kū′-rē): A unit of radioactivity; ten curies.

decadence (dek′-a-dens): A process or condition of deterioration, decline, or decay.

decagram (dek′-a-gram): In the metric system, ten grams.

decalcification (dē′-kal-si-fik-ā′-shun): Removal of calcium or calcium salts, as from teeth in dental caries, bone in disorders of metabolism.

decalcify (dē-kal′-si-fī): To deprive of calcium, as in decalcification of bones.

decaliter (dek′-a-lē-ter): In the metric system, liquid volume equal to ten liters.

decameter (dek′-a-mē-ter): In the metric system, a measure of length equal to ten meters.

decancellation (dē-kan-se-lā′-shun): The surgical removal of cancellous bone.

decannulation (dē-kan-ū-lā′-shun): The removal of a cannula (*q.v.*), especially a tracheostomy cannula.

decant (dē-kant′): To pour off a liquid without disturbing the sediment or precipitate in it.

decapeptide (dek-a-pep′-tīd): A polypeptide that contains ten amino acid groups.

decapitation (dē-kap-i-tā′-shun): 1. The removal of the head from the body. 2. The removal of the head of a bone from its shaft.

decapsulation (dē-kap-sū-lā′-shun): Surgical removal of a capsule, *e.g.*, the capsule of the kidney.

decay rate: In radiobiology, the rate at which a radioactive substance decays; radioactive disintegration.

decedent (dē-sē′-dent): A dead person.

decentration (dē-sen-trā′-shun): An ophthalmologic term applied to the condition in which the visual axis does not coincide with the axis of the lens.

decerebellation (dē-ser-e-bel-ā′-shun): Removal of the cerebellum; usually refers to experimental removal for study.

decerebrate (dē-ser′-e-brāt): 1. To remove the cerebrum. 2. To eliminate cerebral function by transecting the brain stem. 3. Without cerebral function; a state of deep unconsciousness. **D. POSTURE** or **POSITION,** a condition of the unconscious patient in which all four limbs are spastic; the legs are hyperextended at the hip and knee, the shoulders are rotated inward, and the arms are flexed at the elbow; indicates severe damage to the cerebrum. **D. RIGIDITY,** flexion of the arms, wrists, and fingers, and extension of the legs; indicates interruption in the corticospinal tracts in the cerebral hemisphere.—decerebrate, n.; adj.

deci-: Combining form denoting one-tenth (in the metric system).

decibel (des′-i-bel): A standard unit that has been adopted for measuring the amount of sound perceptible to the normal ear; it is the smallest change in sound intensity that the normal ear can detect; one tenth of a bel (*q.v.*). Abbreviated DB or db.

decidua (dē-sid′-ū-a): The endometrial lining of the uterus thickened and altered for reception of the fertilized ovum, and which is shed when pregnancy terminates and during menstruation. **D. BASALIS,** the part of the **D.** that lies under the embedded ovum and forms the maternal part of the placenta. **D. CAPSULARIS,** that part of the **D.** that lies over the developing fetus; it surrounds the chorionic sac. **D. MENSTRUALIS,** that part of the outer layer of the endometrium that is shed during menstruation. **D. VERA,** the part of the decidua lining the rest of the uterus; also called the **D. PARIETALIS.**—decidual, deciduate, adj.

deciduation (dē-sid-ū-ā′-shun): The shedding of the decidua (*q.v.*).

deciduoma malignum (dē-sid-ū-ō′-ma ma-lig′-num): A malignant tumor which forms at the site of the placenta during or following a pregnancy; develops from retained decidua; usually develops after a hydatidiform mole, but may follow an abortion, a tubal pregnancy or a normal pregnancy; metastasizes quickly, especially to the lung. Also called choriocarcinoma and chorionepithelioma.

deciduous (dē-sid′-ū-us): Not permanent; said of something that is shed or falls out, at maturity. Term often applied to the teeth of the primary dentition; see under **dentition.**

decigram (des′-i-gram): One-tenth of a gram.

deciliter (des′-i-lē-ter): One-tenth of a liter.

decimeter (des′-i-mē-ter): One-tenth of a meter.

decipara (de-sip′-ar-a): A woman who has given birth to ten viable offspring.

decoagulant (dē-kō-ag′-ū-lant): An agent or substance that reduces the coagulability of the blood by reducing the amount of coagulants or procoagulants in it.

decoction (dē-kok′-shun): In pharmacology, a liquid medicinal susbstance prepared by boiling the ingredients, usually vegetable substances.

decompensation (dē′-kom-pen-sā′-shun): 1. A failure of compensation, particularly in heart disease; inability of the heart to maintain adequate circulation. 2. In psychiatry, the deterioration of existing defenses, resulting in exacerbation of pathologic behavior.

decompose (dē′-kom-pōz′): To decay or rot.

decomposition (dē′-kom-pō-zish′-un): 1. The separation of a substance into simpler compounds or its constituent elements. 2. The chemical breakdown of a substance. 3. Rot; decay; putrefaction.

decompression (dē′kom-presh′-un): Removal of pressure or of a compressing force. **ABDOMINAL D.,** removal of pressure from the abdomen during the first stage of labor; improves blood supply and results in shorter and less painful labor. **D. OF THE BRAIN,** achieved by trephining the skull. **D. OF THE BLADDER,** achieved in cases of chronic urinary retention by continuous or intermittent drainage via catheter inserted into the urethra. **D. CHAMBER,** a compressed air chamber for gradual reduction of barometric pressure; used when returning deep-sea divers and caisson workers to the surface, to avoid decompression sickness. **CARDIAC D.**, removal of fluid from the pericardial sac by means of an incision into the sac. **D. SICKNESS**, caisson disease (*q.v.*).

deconditioning (dē-kon-dish′-un-ing): A type of therapy used in patients with neurotic phobias; after discussing with the patient his/her particular fear, the therapist gradually exposes the patient to the fear itself with further discussion following each exposure.

decongestant (dē-kon-jes′-tant): An agent that reduces congestion.

decongestion (dē-kon-jest′-yun): Relief or reduction of congestion (*q.v.*).—decongestive, adj.

decontamination (dē′-kon-tam-in-ā′-shun): The process of destroying, removing, or neutralizing potentially harmful agents, *e.g.*, bacteria, war gas, or radioactive materials, from persons, objects, or an area.—decontaminate. v.

decorticate (dē-kor′-ti-kāt): To remove the cortex or outer covering of any organ or structure. **D. POSTURE**, that assumed by a person with a lesion at or above the brain stem; spontaneous spasms of rigidity occur, with the arms flexed and adducted, the hands clenched, the legs rotated inwardly and extended, and the feet in plantar flexion.—decortication, n.

decortication (dē-kor-ti-kā′-shun): Surgical removal of cortex or outer covering of an organ such as the brain, kidney, or lung. **D. OF LUNG**, carried out when thickening of the visceral pleura prevents re-expansion of the lung as may occur in chronic empyema. The visceral pleura is peeled off the lung, which is then re-expanded by positive pressure through an anesthetic apparatus.

decrudescence (dē′-kroo-des′-ens): The lessening of intensity of symptoms of a disease.

decubation (dē-kū-ba′-shun): The period in the course of an infectious disease after the symptoms have subsided and lasting until complete recovery.

decubitus (dē-kū′-bi-tus): The recumbent position; lying down. **D. ULCER**, an ulceration or pressure sore, usually occurring in a patient long confined to bed, arising from continual pressure of the flesh over a bony prominence or from friction, obesity, emaciation, impaired circulation to the part, paralysis, old age, lowered vitality, lack of cleanliness, failure to keep the bed dry, smooth and free of irritating particles. The usual sites are the buttock, hip, shoulder, heel, elbow. The first warning is redness of the area, which becomes hot and tender, later smarting. Discoloration ensues and is followed by breaking of the skin, thus producing an open sore which may or may not become infected and which sloughs before healing takes place by granulation. Skin grafting may be necessary. See **pressure areas.**—decubiti, pl.; decubital, adj.

decussation (dē-kus-ā′-shun): Intersection; the crossing of symmetrical structures in the form of an X at a point beyond their origin, as in the optic and pyramidal tracts. Chiasm.—decussate, v.

dedentition (dē-den-tish′-un): The loss or shedding of teeth.

deductive reasoning: The logical thinking process that proceeds from general to specific.

deer fly: A biting fly commonly found in western U.S.; the vector of tularemia (*q.v.*).

deer-fly fever: Tularemia (*q.v.*).

defecation (def-e-kā′-shun): Discharge of fecal matter from the rectum; evacuation of the bowels.—defecate, v.

defect (dē′-fekt): 1. An imperfection or flaw. 2. The malformation or absence of a body part or organ.

defeminization (dē′-fem-i-nī-zā′-shun): The loss or diminishment of feminine sexual characteristics, *e.g.*, increased muscle mass and decreased breast size; often the result of dysfunction or removal of the ovaries. **VOLUNTARY D.**, the voluntary giving up of feminine characteristics and assumption of those of males.

defense mechanism: In psychiatry, an unconscious maneuver that helps to prevent, and to obtain relief from, anxiety or emotional distress. Among the many mechanisms employed are conversion, denial, disassociation, identification, rationalization, repression, substitution, and sublimation.

defensive medicine: Medical practice characterized by the reliance of the physician on objective tests rather than on personal judgment alone in making decisions as to diagnosis and treatment; usually the purpose is to provide protection against possible lawsuits being brought by patients.

deferens (def′-er-ens): Vas deferens (*q.v.*).

defervescence (def-er-ves′-ens): The time during which a fever is declining. If the body temperature falls rapidly it is spoken of as crisis; if it falls slowly the term lysis is used—defervescent, adj.

defibrillation (dē-fib-ri-lā′-shun): The arrest of fibrillation of the cardiac muscle (atrial or ventricular), and restoration of normal rhythm. Usually refers to treatment by application of electric shock (cardioversion).—defibrillate, v.

defibrillator (dē-fib′-ri-lā-tor): 1. Any agent (*e.g.*, an electric shock) that interrupts ventricular fibrillation and restores normal rhythm. 2. An apparatus that administers electric shock used for defibrillation.

defibrinate (dē-fī′-brin-āt): To remove fibrin, particularly from blood or serum.—defibrinated, adj.; defibrination, n.

deficiency disease: Any disease resulting from a deficiency of essential nutrients, vitamins, or minerals in the diet, or an inability of the body to utilize any of these substances. Dehydration; diabetes mellitus, specific vitamin deficiencies, and deficiencies in potassium, calcium, magnesium, and iron intake are the most common of these disorders.

deflection (dē-flek′-shun): A turning aside or a state of being turned aside. **D. OF THE NASAL SEPTUM,** displacement to one side of the bone separating the two nasal cavities, leading to discomfort; often corrected by surgery.

defloration (def-lō-rā′-shun): The rupturing of the hymen, however it is brought about.

deflorescence (def-lō-res′-ens): The disappearance of a skin eruption; usually refers to that of an exanthematous disease.

defluvium (dē-floo′-vi-um): 1. Falling out of the hair. 2. Falling out of the nails.

deformity (dē-fōrm′-i-ti): Congenital or acquired malformation, disfigurement or distortion of the body or a part of it when the deviation from normal is apparent. **GUNSTOCK D.,** deformity of the elbow caused by fracture of either condyle of the humerus; the forearm is displaced to one side. **LOBSTER-CLAW D.,** congenital absence of all fingers except the first and fifth; bidactyly. **MADELUNG'S D.,** congenital, accidental, or pathological dislocation of the lower end of the ulna with radial deviation of the hand. **SPRENGEL'S D.,** a **D.** consisting of a congenitally high scapula and permanent elevation of the shoulder; often associated with other deformities. [Otto G. K. Sprengel, German surgeon. 1852–1915.]

degeneracy (dē-jen′-er-a-si): A state of deterioration of physical and mental functioning, or of social behavior, sexual behavior in particular.

degeneration (dē-jen-er-ā′-shun): 1. Deterioration in quality or function. 2. Regression from more to less specialized type of tissue. **AFFERENT D.,** degeneration spreading upward along sensory nerves. **AMYLOID D.,** a wax-like change in tissues. **CASEOUS D.,** cheese-like tissue resulting from atrophy in a tuberculoma or gumma. **COLLOID D.,** mucoid degeneration of tumors. **CYSTOID D. OF THE RETINA,** a condition characterized by the formation of cystic spaces in the retina. **FATTY D.,** characterized by the presence of droplets of fat in atrophic tissue, as in the myocardium. **HYALINE D.,** said of connective tissue, especially of blood vessels, in which the tissue takes on a homogeneous or formless appearance. **MACULAR D.,** pathological changes in the macula lutea that results in loss of central but not peripheral vision; may be hereditary or be caused by atherosclerosis, trauma, or senility; a leading cause of blindness in people over 60 years of age. **SENILE D.,** the clinical picture of old age in which acuity of thought is blunted. **SUBACUTE COMBINED D.,** a complication of untreated pernicious anemia, starting with paresthesia. **WALLERIAN D., D.** of a motor or sensory nerve fiber that has been cut off from its source of nutrition and is ultimately destroyed.—degenerative, adj.; degenerate, v.

degenerative (dē-jen′-er-a-tiv): Referring to progressive deterioration of cells, tissue, or a body part. **D. DISEASE,** one in which loss of efficiency or function of an organ, structure, or tissue is gradual and progressive and usually nonreversible, *e.g.*, arteriosclerosis. **D. JOINT DISEASE,** a chronic disorder of the joint cartilage, enlargement of the bone, and pain on activity; affects primarily the weightbearing joints and the distal interphalangeal joints of the fingers; occurs chiefly in older people.

degerm (dē-jerm′): To disinfect, by mechanical cleansing or use of an antiseptic.

deglutition (deg-loo-tish′-un): The process of swallowing, partly voluntary, partly involuntary.

degradation (deg-ra-dā′-shun): The reduction of a chemical compound to a simpler one that has fewer carbon atoms.

degustation (dē-gus-tā′-shun): The act of tasting.

dehiscence (dē-his′-ens): The process of splitting or bursting open, as of a wound.—dehisce, v.; dehiscent, adj.

dehumanize (dē-hū′-man-īz): To deprive one of individuality, human qualities, and attributes.

dehydrant (dē-hī′-drant): An agent that reduces the amount of water in the body by dehydration (*q.v.*).

dehydrate (dē-hī′-drāt): To remove water from any substance or source, including the body.

dehydration (dē-hī-drā′-shun): Loss or removal of fluid. In the body, this condition arises when the fluid intake fails to replace fluid loss. This is liable to occur when there is bleeding, diarrhea, excessive sweating, fever, polyuria, or vomiting, and usually upsets the body's electrolyte balance; may also cause tachycardia, impaired sensorium, and decreased intraocular pressure. If suitable fluid replacement cannot be achieved orally, parenteral administration is usually prescribed. **HYPOTONIC D., D.** in which, proportionally, the loss of electrolytes exceeds the loss of water. **ISOTONIC D., D.** in which there is a proportionate loss of water and electrolytes.

7-dehydrocholesterol (dē-hī′-drō-kō-les′-ter-ōl): A sterol found in the skin which forms vitamin D_3 when properly irradiated.

dehydrocorticosterone (dē-hī′-drō-kor-ti-kos′-ter-ōn): 11-dehydrocorticosterone, the chemical name for a steroid from the adrenal cortex; it has some effect on protein and carbohydrate metabolism.

dehydroepiandrosterone (dē-hī′-drō-ep-i-an-dros′-ter-ōn): An androgen (*q.v.*) occurring in normal urine; may also be synthesized from cholesterol.

dehydrogenase (dē-hī-droj′-en-ās): Any of a class of enzymes that activates or mobilizes a substance so that it gives up its hydrogen and transfers it to an acceptor other than oxygen.

dehydrogenate (dē-hī-droj′-en-āt): To remove hydrogen from a compound.

dehypnotize (dē′-hip′-nō-tīz): To arouse a person from hypnosis.

deinstitutionalization (dē′-in-sti-tū′-shi-nal-ī-zā′-shun): Refers to the movement to place institutionalized persons in the community and provide the necessary supportive services; the goal is rehabilitation; the persons are usually disabled in some way.

deionize (dē-ī′-ō-nīz): The removal of ions from a fluid to produce a mineral-free substance.

déjà vu phenomenon (dā-zha voo′ fe-nom′-e-non): Intense feeling of familiarity as if something had been seen, or had happened, before.

dejecta (dē-jek′-ta): Excrement.

dejection (dē-jek′-shun): 1. Mental depression. 2. Defecation (*q.v.*).

Dejerine-Sottas disease (de-zher-ēn′ sō′-tas): Progressive hypertrophic interstitial neuropathy; a rare inherited disease characterized by polyneuritis and greatly thickened peripheral nerves, atrophy of the muscles of the distal parts of the legs.

delactation (dē-lak-tā′-shun): 1. Weaning. 2. Cessation of the secretion of milk.

deLange's syndrome: See Amsterdam dwarfism under dwarfism.

deleterious (del-e-tē′-ri-us): Hurtful, injurious, destructive, noxious, pernicious.

Delhi boil: See oriental sore.

delimitation (dē-lim-i-tā′-shun): 1. Setting limits or bounds. 2. Preventing the spread of disease in an individual or in the community.

delinquency (dē-lin′-kwen-si): Unacceptable, antisocial behavior which is sometimes in violation of law, including such offenses as theft, vandalism, and truancy. Used especially with reference to children or adolescents.

delinquent (dē-lin′-qwent): 1. Failing or neglecting to do what the law and society require, committing misdemeanors and offenses, and behaving in an unacceptable manner; often refers to an adolescent. 2. A person who behaves in an unacceptable antisocial, and, sometimes, illegal manner.

delipidation (dē-lip-i-dā′-shun): The removal of lipid by the use of fat solvents.

deliquescent (del′-i-kwes′-ent): Capable of absorbing moisture from the atmosphere thus becoming liquid.—deliquescence, n.

deliriant (dē-lir′-i-ant): 1. Capable of producing delirium. 2. A drug that may induce delirium. A person who exhibits symptoms of delirium.

delirium (dē-lir′-i-um): A state of frenzy or uncontrollable excitement, characterized by disorientation, mental confusion, impulsive behavior, incoherent speech; often accompanied by delusions and hallucinations. May be present in various forms of mental disease but more frequently seen in patients with high fever, a toxic condition, or injury; usually of short duration. **D. TREMENS,** a violent form of delirium resulting from prolonged use of alcohol; the patient is confused, terrified, and restless; has a marked tremor and hallucinates; also called mania à potu. In psychiatry, a condition occurring in primary degenerative dementia of senile onset; see Appendix VI.—delirious, adj.

delouse (dē-lowz′): To remove lice from or to destroy lice.

delta: The fourth of a series. **D. WAVE,** see under wave.

deltoid (del′-toyd): Triangular. **D. MUSCLE,** large shoulder muscle, the apex of which is inserted into the midshaft of the humerous. **D. LIGAMENT,** the large ligament on the medial side of the ankle.

delusion (dē-lū′-zhun): A false fixed belief held only by the affected person, which cannot be altered by argument or appeal to reason; found as a psychotic symptom in several types of psychopathy, notably schizophrenia, paranoia, senile psychosis, mania, and the depressive states, including involutional melancholia. **D. OF GUILT, D.** occurring in psychotic depressed persons. **D. OF GRANDEUR,** megalomania (*q.v.*). **HYPOCHONDRIACAL D., D.** of bodily disease in spite of no evidence; occurs in schizophrenic persons. **NIHILISTIC D., D.** pertaining to nothingness; the person believes the world and everything in it, including himself, has ceased to exist. **PARANOID D.,** the person wrongfully believes that some one or some thing wishes to do him harm. **D. OF PERSECUTION,** the false notion that one is being willfully persecuted by a particular person or group of persons; the patient is hostile, aggressive, suspicious. **RELIGIOUS D.,** the patient thinks he hears voices that give direct commands from God. **SOMATIC D.,** the fixed belief that one has an imaginary lesion or supposedly abnormally functioning organ. **SYSTEMATIZED D.,** a **D.** in which the patient distorts the truth to justify his actions or reasoning.

delusional (dē-lū′-zhun-al): Pertaining to or characteristic of delusions. **D. SPEECH,** excessive verbalization of delusions of grandeur or of persecution.

demarcation (dē-mar-kā′-shun): 1. A separation or distinction. 2. An outlining of the junction of diseased and healthy tissue; often refers to the line formed at the edge of a gangrenous area.

demasculinization (dē-mas′-kū-lin-ī-zā′-shun): The loss or diminishment of normal masculine characteristics.

demedicalization (dē-med′-i-kal-ī-zā′-shun): 1. The tendency in health care programs and activities to lessen the autonomy of the physician-patient relationship by emphasizing the importance of healthful behavior, elaborating codes of patients' rights, utilizing nurse practitioners, and de-emphasizing the sick role by referring to patients as clients or consumers. 2. A trend in rehabilitation to remove a disabled person from medical supervision after he has been stabilized and is able to be personally responsible for managing his life.

demented (dē-ment′-ed): Insane; deprived of reason.

dementia (dē-men′-shi-a): An organic mental disorder severe enough to prevent normal social and occupational functioning and deterioration of one's intellectual abilities along with alterations in one's memory, judgment, and personality. **PRIMARY DEGENERATIVE DEMENTIA, SENILE ONSET** (after age 65 and at or before age 65), formerly referred to as senile or presenile dementia; mental deterioration marked by loss of memory, disturbed sleep patterns, disorientation, delusions, preoccupation with death, and false notions of persecution; progresses to total lack of ability to deal with the environment. **TOXIC D., D.** due to use of some toxic substance; see Substance-induced Organic Mental Disorders in Appendix VI. **ARTERIOSCLEROTIC D., D.** characterized by headache, dizziness, and confusion; runs a fluctuating course with steady intellectual decline. **ATHEROSCLEROTIC D., D.** resulting from changes in the blood supply to the brain cells; often accompanied by physical and neurologic disorders, impairment of the intellect, memory, and personality. **D. PARALYTICA,** general paresis; see paresis. **D. PRAECOX,** obsolete term for schizophrenia that develops during adolescence or early adult life. **DEGENERATIVE D.,** see under Dementias Arising in the Senium and Presenium, in Appendix VI. **D. PUGILISTICA,** cerebral concussion resulting from repeated blows to the head as happens to professional boxers. **MULTI-INFARCT D.,** a common form of **D.,** resulting from a series of small strokes in the brain that destroy brain tissue. **D.** occuring in persons with substance-induced organic mental disorders, see under Organic Mental Disorders, in Appendix VI.

demi-: Prefix denoting half, one-half.

demineralization (dē-min′-er-al-ī-zā′-shun): The loss of mineral salts from the body, the bones in particular. See decalcification.

demise (dē-mıs′): Death.

Demodex folliculorum: A mite found in the hair follicles and sebaceous glands of the nose and face; causes enlargement of the hair follicles.

demography (dē-mog′-ra-fi): The study of mankind or of human populations, especially their size, density, geographic distribution, physical environments, and vital statistics, including birth and mortality rates, and sometimes morbidity rates.—demographic, adj.

demoniac (dē-mō′-ni-ak): 1. Suggestive of a demon. 2. Influenced by a demon. 3. One regarded as possessed by a demon.

demonomania (dē′-mon-ō-mā′-ni-a): The psychotic belief that one is possessed by devils.

demonophobia (dē′-mon-ō-fō′-bi-a): Abnormal fear of demons and devils.

demulcent (dē-mul′-sent): 1. Soothing; softening. 2. A slippery mucilaginous fluid that allays and soothes inflammation, especially of the mucous membranes.

demyelinate (dē-mī′-e-lin-āt): To remove or destroy the myelin sheath of a nerve or nerves.—demyelination, n., demyelinize, v.

denarcotize (de-nar′-kō-tīz): 1. To deprive one of a narcotic drug that one has been taking or has become addicted to. 2. To remove the narcotic qualities from a drug, especially an opiate.

denaturant (dē-nā′-tūr-ant): A substance that, when added to another, will make the latter unfit for its usual use.

denatured (dē-nā′ churd): 1. Having its natural characteristics modified so as to make it unfit for human consumption, *e.g.*, alcohol. 2. Adulterated.

dendriform (den′-dri-form): Tree-shaped or branch-like.

dendrite or dendron (den′-drīt, den′-dron): One of the branched filaments that are given off from the body of a nerve cell; it is the part of the neuron that transmits impulses from the terminations of other neurons to the nerve cell body.—dendritic, adj.

dendritic (den-drit′-ik): Pertaining to or resembling a dendrite. **D. ULCER,** a linear corneal ulcer that sends out tree-like branches; usually caused by herpes simplex.

denervation (dē-ner-vā′-shun): The act of depriving an area of its nerve supply. Usually refers to incision, excision, or blocking of a nerve.—denervate, v.

dengue (den′-gā): An acute, epidemic, febrile disease that occurs sporadically in the tropical and subtropical parts of the world. The cause is an arbovirus transmitted by the Aedes mosquito. Characterized by headache, fever, rheumatic pains, sore throat, a spotty skin eruption. **HEMORRHAGIC D.**, a serious form of **D.** which affects primarily children; symptoms include prostration, respiratory distress, hemorrhage, circulatory collapse, and shock.

denial: 1. In psychology, a defense mechanism, usually unconscious, whereby a person does not admit that certain facts exist, or he avoids disagreeable realities in order to avoid pain, anxiety, or guilt feelings. 2. Refusal to perceive; often part of a normal phenomenon such as occurs in the fantasies of children at play.

denidation (den-i-dā′-shun): The expulsion of the degenerated uterine mucous membrane during menstruation.

Denis Browne splint: See under splint.

denitrogenation (dē-nī′-trō-je-nā′-shun): The removal of dissolved nitrogen from the body, by breathing nitrogen-free gas, a treatment to prevent the development of caisson disease or aeroembolism.

dens: 1. A tooth. 2. The odontoid process of the axis that provides a pivot on which the atlas can rotate, thereby allowing for rotary movements of the head.—dentes, pl.

densimeter (den-sim′-e-ter): A device for determining the density of a liquid.

density (den′-si-ti): 1. The closeness of the particles in a substance. 2. The mass of a given substance per unit volume. 3. The number of inhabitants per unit of a given area.

dent-; denta-; dento-: Combining forms denoting relationship to a tooth or teeth.

dental (den′-tal): Pertaining to the teeth. **D. ANESTHESIA**, anesthesia for dental operations. **D. CARIES**, disintegration of the substance of teeth; **D.** cavities. **D. CALCULUS**, the deposit of mineral matter on the teeth; tartar. **D. PLAQUE**, a thin deposit of mucoid material on the teeth. **D. PROSTHESIS**, a substitute for natural teeth. **D. PULP**, the vascular tissue in the pulp cavity and root canals of the teeth.

dental hygienist: A person educated and specially trained to provide such dental services as cleaning teeth, taking x rays, and giving assistance to dentists in other ways that are permitted under their license which is issued by the National Board of Dental Examiners after the individual has taken a written and practical examination.

dental technician: A person who has had special training in the making of such dental appliances as bridges, dentures, crowns, etc.; may have taken an educational course or learned on the job.

dentalgia (den-tal′-ji-a): Toothache.

dentate (den′-tāt): Having teeth or pointed, teeth-like projections.

dentia (den′-shi-a): 1. A condition relating to teeth and their development. 2. A word element relating to teeth. **D. PRAECOX**, the presence of erupted teeth at birth, or the premature eruption of teeth. **D. TARDA**, delay in eruption of teeth beyond the normal time for their appearance.

dentifrice (den′-ti-fris): A powder, paste, or liquid for cleansing the teeth.

dentigerous (den-tij′-er-us): Having teeth.

dentin (e) (den′-tēn): The hard material, similar to bone, that makes up the chief substance of the teeth. It encloses the pulp cavity, is covered with enamel on the crown and cementum on the root of a tooth.

dentinogenesis (den′-ti-nō-jen′-e-sis): The formation of dentin. **D. IMPERFECTA**, a hereditary condition in which teeth are small, the pulp cavity is lacking, and early wearing away of the crown and enamel destroys the teeth.

dentinoma (den′-ti-nō-ma): A benign tumor of dentin.

dentist (den′-tist): A person trained for the practice of dentistry.

dentistry (den′-tis-tri): The branch of medicine that is concerned with the prevention, diagnosis, and treatment of diseases of the teeth and surrounding tissues, and with restoring missing natural dental structures.

dentition (den-tish′-un): 1. The process of teething. 2. The character and arrangement of an individual's teeth. **PRIMARY D.**, eruption of the deciduous, milk or temporary teeth. **SECONDARY D.**, eruption of the adult or permanent teeth.

dentoalveolar (den′-tō-al-vē′-ō-lar): Pertaining to the alveolus of a tooth or alveoli of the teeth. **D. ABSCESS**, the formulation of an abscess around the root of a tooth.

dentoalveolitis (den′-tō-al-vē-ō-lī′-tis): A purulent inflammation in the alveoli of the teeth; periodontal disease. See pyorrhea.

dentoid (den′-toid): Toothlike.

dentulus (den′-tū-lus): The state of having one's natural teeth.

denture (den′-chur): A set of teeth. Term usually designates an artificial replacement of one, several or all of the natural teeth.

denude (dē-nūd′): To remove a covering or to lay bare.—denudation, n.

Denver Developmental Screening Test: A popular, reliable test for evaluating a child's development and for identifying delayed development in such areas as social adaptation, fine motor activities, and use of language; most useful in children between ages of one month and six years. Abbreviated DDST.

deodorant (de-ō′-dōr-ant): Any substance that destroys or masks an (unpleasant) odor.—deodorize, v.

deodorizer (de-ō′-dor-ī-zer): An agent that absorbs or neutralizes an odor.—deodorize, v.

deorsumversion (dē-or′-sum-ver′-zhun): The act of turning downward; usually refers to the simultaneous turning downward of both eyes.

deossification (dē-os-i-fi-kā′-shun): Removal or reduction in the amount of mineral content of a bone or bones.

deoxidation (dē-ok-si-dā′-shun): The removal of all or part of the oxygen from a compound.—deoxidize, v.

deoxy-; desoxy-: Prefixes denoting 1) loss or removal of oxygen from a compound, or 2) replacement of the OH group by a hydrogen atom.

deoxycorticosterone (dē-ok′-si-kor-ti-kos′-ter-ōn): A steroid substance produced in the adrenal cortex, concerned chiefly with metabolism and retention of salt and water, and with excretion of potassium; used in the treatment of adrenal insufficiency; also desoxycorticosterone and deoxycortone.

deoxygenate (dē-ok′-si-jen-āt): To deprive an organism of oxygen. To remove all or part of the oxygen from a compound.—deoxygenation, n.

deoxyhemoglobin (dē-ok′-si-hēm-ō-glō′-bin): Hemoglobin that is not associated with oxygen.

deoxyribonuclease (dē-ok′-si-rī-bō-nū′-klē-ās): An enzyme that serves as a catalyst for the hydrolysis of deoxyribonucleic acid (DNA).

deoxyribonucleic acid (DNA) (dē-ok′-si-rī-bō-nū-klē′-ik as′-id): A derivative of nucleic acid, DNA is found in the nuclei and protoplasm of animal cells, many plant cells, most bacterial cells, and many viruses; is the carrier of genetic information in living cells and considered to be the autoreproducing component of chromosomes; is required for the replication of proteins and for cell reproduction. Genes are segments of the DNA molecules which consist of two long chains of alternate sugar and phosphate groups twisted into a double helix; see Watson-Crick helix under helix. Also spelled desoxyribonucleic.

Department of Health, Education and Welfare (DHEW): A federal government department, established in 1953; administered more than 200 programs, over half of which were health related. Reorganized in 1979 when Education became a separate department and the title for the other services was changed to Health and Human Services.

Department of Health and Human Services (DHHS): A major federal department having responsibility for most of the national health programs. Created in 1979 by a regrouping of the units within the Department of Health, Education, and Welfare. Now includes the Office of Human Development Services; the Public Health Service; the Health Care Financing Administration; the Social Security Administration; the National Institutes of Health; Centers for Disease Control; the Veterans Administration; and the Alcohol, Drug Abuse, and Mental Health Administration.

depend: 1. To hang or hang down. 2. To rely, as for support. 3. To be contingent to.—dependence, n.; dependent, adj.

dependence: CHEMICAL D., the need of body tissues for the continued use of any abused chemical substance, including drugs and alcohol; if not satisfied regularly, withdrawal symptoms occur. CROSS D., a condition in which one drug causes dependence but its use can prevent the development of withdrawal symptoms from another, possibly more harmful drug. PHYSICAL D., chemical D. PSYCHOLOGICAL D., a condition marked by intense desire for the pleasurable effects of a drug which invariably leads to use of that drug.

dependency (dē-pen′-den-si): The condition of being dependent on someone or something. D. NEEDS, in psychiatry, the needs for love, mothering, affection, food, shelter, protection, and so on. D. RATIO, refers to the number of persons in the nonworking years (under 20 and over 65) of each 100 persons in the working years (20–64); in the U.S., this ratio was 86 to 100 in 1975, but is gradually increasing as more people are living longer.

depersonalization (dē-per′-sun-al-ī-zā′-shun): A subjective state in which the person loses his sense of reality and of his own personality, and may feel that he no longer exists; caused by partial or total disruption of the ego and self-concept; occurs in schizophrenia and sometimes in depressive states.

depigmentation (dē-pig-men-tā′-shun): Partial or complete loss of pigment.—depigmented, adj.

depilate (dep′-i-lāt): To remove hair from.—depilatory, adj., depilation, n.

depilatories (dē-pil′-a-tor-ēz): Substances usually made in pastes (*e.g.*, barium sulphide) which remove excess hair temporarily; they do not act on the papillae, consequently the hair grows again. See epilation.

deplete (dē-plēt′): 1. To empty or deprive of a principal substance. 2. To reduce the strength of a person or substance.

depletion (dē-plē′-shun): 1. Withdrawal or removal of a body constituent, especially blood. 2. An exhausted state, often referring to results of loss of blood. **D. SYNDROME,** a condition resulting from loss of essential body constituents or from inadequate intake of protein and calories.

deplumation (dē′-ploo-ma′-shun): Loss of the eyelashes.

depolarization (dē-pō′-lar-ī-zā′-shun): The removal, destruction, or neutralization of the electrical polarity of a substance. In neurophysiology, the tendency of the cell to become positive in relation to the potential in the substances surrounding the cell.—depolarize, adj.

deposit (dē-poz′-it): 1. Sediment; dregs; a precipitate. 2. Morbid particles of matter that have collected in a body tissue or cavity.

depot (dē′pō): A place in the body where a substance, *e.g.*, fat or drugs, can be stored and from which it can be released and distributed.

depravation (dep-ra-vā′-shun): 1. Deterioration or degeneration. 2. Perversion.

depraved (dē-prāvd′): 1. Deteriorated. 2. Abnormal.—depravity, n.

depressant (dē-pres′-ant): An agent that reduces or slows the functional activity of an organ or system of the body; often refers to certain drugs.

depressed (dē-prest′): 1. Below the normal level. 2. Refers to the condition of depression; see depression. 3. **D. FRACTURE,** a skull fracture in which the fractured part of the bone is depressed below the level of the other cranial bones.

depression (dē-presh′-un): 1. A hollow place or an indentation, *e.g.*, a fossa in a bone. 2. Diminution of power or activity, either mental or physical. 3. A mood or feeling state characterized by sadness, discouragement, and self-doubt that may occur when one has lost, or thinks he will lose, a loved one or something valued; may be brought about by the actions or critisisms of others or failure to meet self-set goals. 4. In psychiatry, depression states are now classified as neurotic disorders and categorized as major affective disorders, and further categorized as bipolar disorders that are identified as mixed, manic, or depressed, and as major depression, single episode or recurrent (see Appendix VI). Depression is considered neurotic when the condition follows an event or situation that the individual can identify, and psychotic when it is due to a traumatic situation that the individual can identify and is accompanied by severe functional impairment, including insomnia, anorexia, weight loss, impotence, and often delusions. **ANACLITIC D.** occurs in young children often due to neglect; characterized by apathy, anorexia, frequent stools, progressive marasmus; sometimes fatal. **INVOLUTIONAL D., D.** occurring during menopause. **ORGANIC D., D.** associated with a physical disorder, usually one of the nervous system. **RETARDED D., D.** characterized by reduced motility and speech; may be associated with schizophrenia.

depressive (dē-pres′-iv): 1. Pertaining to depression. 2. Causing depression. **D. NEUROSIS,** a disorder in which the individual seeks relief, or partial relief, through depression and self-depreciation. **D. PERSONALITY,** a type of personality characterized by low spirits, subservience, and vulnerability to disappointment. **D. PSEUDO-DEMENTIA,** see Ganser syndrome. **D. STATE,** a mental disorder characterized by severe depression. **D. STUPOR,** a condition characterized by muteness, unresponsiveness, retention of both urine and feces for long periods, and possibly death from starvation.

depressor (dē-pres′-or): Anything that depresses a bodily activity or function. Applies to muscles, drugs, nerves, as well as instruments. **TONGUE D.,** a spatula-like blade, usually of wood, used to hold the tongue down during examination of mouth and throat.

deprivation (dep-ri-vā′-shun): The loss, absence, removal or withholding of powers, or things that are needed. **D. SYNDROME,** usually the result of parental rejection of offspring; may include malnutrition, dwarfism, pot-belly, gluttonous appetite, superficial attachment to any adult.

depulization (dep-ū′-lī-zā′-shun): The removal or eradication of fleas from an area or an animal.

depurant (dep′-ū-rant): 1. Having a cleansing or purifying action. 2. An agent that cleanses or purifies.

depurate (dep′-ū-rāt): To purify, cleanse, or refine.—depuration, n.

DeQuervain: [F. DeQuervain, Swiss surgeon. 1868–1940.] **DEQ'S. DISEASE,** tenosynovitis at the styloid process of the radius, with pain on using the hand or thumb; caused by trauma or over-use which causes a thickening of the synovial lining of the tendon sheath of the abductor pollicis longus and extensor pollicis longus muscles. **DEQ'S. FRACTURE;** fracture of the navicular bone with displacement of the lunar bone. **DEQ'S. THYROIDITIS,** a condition characterized by sudden pain and enlargement of the thyroid gland, accompanied by fever, malaise, sweating; self-limited; cause not known, but thought to be due to a viral infection.

der-: A combining form denoting relationship to the neck.

deradenitis (der-ad-e-nī′-tis): Inflammation of the lymph glands of the neck.

derangement (dē-rānj′-ment): 1. Mental disorder. 2. A disturbance in the normal order or arrangement of a part or an organ.

derealization (dē-rē′-al-ī-zā′-shun): Feelings of unreality and detachment from one's surroundings; may occur simultaneously with depersonalization; a symptom often found in schizophrenic and depressive states.

dereism (dē′-rē-izm): Mental activity characterized by fantasizing that continues uninterrupted by logic or events occurring in the environment; autism; daydreaming.—dereistic, adj.

derivative (dē-riv′-a-tiv): In chemistry, a chemical substance that is not original or fundamental, but which is derived from another substance.

derived (dē-rīvd′): Developed or formed from something else.

-derm: Combining form denoting 1) skin; 2) cutaneous.

derm-, derma-, dermat-, dermato-, dermo-: Combining forms denoting skin.

derma: The skin; specifically, the corium (*q.v.*).—dermic, dermal, adj.

-derma: Combining form denoting: 1. Skin; integument. 2. An abnormal or pathologic condition of the skin.

dermabrasion (der-ma-brā′-zhun): A surgical procedure for the removal of acne scars, tattoos, or nevi. Wire brushes, sandpaper or other abrasives are used.

Dermacentor (der-ma-sen′-tor): A genus of ticks. **D. ANDERSONI,** the vector of the western type of Rocky Mountain spotted fever. **D. VARIABILIS,** the dog tick, vector of the eastern type of Rocky Mountain spotted fever and one of the vectors of tularemia.

dermafat (der′-ma-fat): The adipose content of the skin.

dermal (der′-mal): Relating to the skin, especially the true skin. **D. GRAFT,** a skin graft utilizing a split or full thickness of dermis. **D. SENSE,** recognition of the sensations of heat, cold, pain, or pressure through stimulation of receptors in the skin.

dermatalgia (der-ma-tal′-ji-a): Localized pain in the skin with no lesion at the site of the pain; sometimes due to a nervous disorder. Syn., dermatodynia, dermalgia.

dermatitis (der-ma-tī′-tis): Inflammation of the skin, acute or chronic, and by custom limited to conditions that present with one or more of the following symptoms at some stage: itching, redness, blisters, crusting, scaling, oozing, fissuring, thickening, hardening, or abnormal pigmentation. **ACTINIC D.,** caused by sunlight; not a sunburn. **ATOPIC D.,** chronic eczematous **D.,** usually affecting the face, antecubital, and popliteal areas. **CONTACT D.,** caused by touching a substance to which the person is sensitive, *e.g.*, a chemical, cosmetic, or plant such as poison ivy, oak, or sumac; syn., ivy poisoning, atopic **D.,** irritant **D. D. ARTEFACTA,** self-induced **D.,** produced by heat, chemicals, or other means. **D. DYSMENORRHOEICA, D.** that occurs during the menstrual period, usually on the face. **EXFOLIATIVE D., D.** characterized by pink to deep red skin color, intense itching, branny desquamation. **EXFOLIATIVE D. OF INFANCY,** a type of pemphigus; starts with a red patch or blister. **D. HEIMALIS,** a recurrent eczema occurring in cold weather; winter itch. **D. HERPETIFORMIS,** an intensely itchy skin eruption of unknown cause, most commonly characterized by vesicles, bullae, and pustules on urticarial plaques, which remit and relapse; when occurring in pregnancy it is known as hydros gravida. **D. MEDICAMENTOSA,** skin eruption due to drugs taken internally. **NUMMULAR D.,** a vesicular **D.** with coin-shaped patches, usually seen on the forearms and legs. **OCCUPATIONAL D.,** occurs as a result of handling some sensitizing agent while at work. **SEBORRHEIC D., D.** occurring in areas where oil glands abound, *e.g.*, the face, scalp, pubis, around the anus; characterized by yellowish-gray oily scales. **SECONDARY EXFOLIATIVE D., D.** that may arise during treatment with certain drugs, *e.g.*, arsenic, gold, etc. **STASIS D.,** chronic inflammation of the skin of the legs; associated with vascular statis in the lower extremities. **TRAUMATIC D.,** due to exposure to irritating substances or physical agents. **VARICOSE D.,** usually seen in the lower part of the leg; due to varicosities of the smaller veins. **D. VENENATA,** contact **D. WEEPING D.,** an oozing **D.** that results from scratching to relieve itching. **X-RAY D.,** due to exposure to x rays.—dermatitides, pl.

dermato-autoplasty (der′-ma-tō-aw′-tō-plas-ti): The grafting to a denuded area of skin taken from some other part of the patient's own body.

dermatocellulitis (der′-ma-tō-sel -ū-li′-tis): Inflammation of the skin and subcutaneous tissue.

dermatochalasis (der′-ma-tō-ka-lā′-sis): Relaxation and abnormal looseness of the skin; when it occurs around the eyes the skin hangs over the lid margin, giving the eyes a hooded or baggy appearance.

dermatoconiosis (der′-ma-tō-kō-ni-ō′-sis): Any skin disorder caused by dust.

dermatocyst (der′-ma-tō-sist): Any cyst of the skin.

dermatofibroma (der′-ma-tō-fī-brō′-ma): A fibrous, tumor-like nodule that develops on the skin; benign and often multiple; seen mostly on the extremities of adults; tends to recur after removal.

dermatofibrosarcoma (der′-ma-tō-fī′-brō-sar-kō′-ma): A fibrosarcoma of the skin; see fibrosarcoma.

dermatoglyphics (der-ma-tō-glif′-iks): The skin patterns or surface markings, especially those found on the palms of the hands and soles of the feet. They have been classified and are used as identification since they are unique to each individual and never change.

dermatographia (der-mat-ō-graf′-i-a): See dermographia.

dermatoheteroplasty (der′-ma-tō-het′-er-ō-plas-ti): The grafting of skin taken from the body of another.

dermatologist (der-ma-tol′-o-jist): A physician who studies skin diseases and is skilled in their treatment. A skin specialist.

dermatology (der-ma-tol′-o-ji): The medical specialty which deals with the skin, its structure, functions, diseases and their treatment.—dermatological, adj.; dermatologically, adv.

dermatolysis (der-ma-tol′-i-sis): Abnormal looseness of the skin, usually congenital, causing it and the subcutaneous tissues to hang in folds. Also called dermatomegaly.

dermatome (der′-ma-tōm): 1. An instrument used in cutting a thin slice of skin, particularly for use in skin grafting. 2. An area of skin that is enervated by sensory fibers from a single spinal nerve. There is considerable overlapping of the contiguous dermatomes.

dermatomycosis (der′-ma-tō-mī-kō′-sis): Any fungal infection of the skin.—dermatomyocotic, adj.

dermatomyoma (der′-ma-tō-mī-ō′-ma): A leiomyoma of the skin.

dermatomyositis (der′-ma-tō-mī-ō-sī′-tis): An acute or chronic non-suppurative inflammation of the skin and muscles that presents with edema and muscle weakness; abrupt or sudden

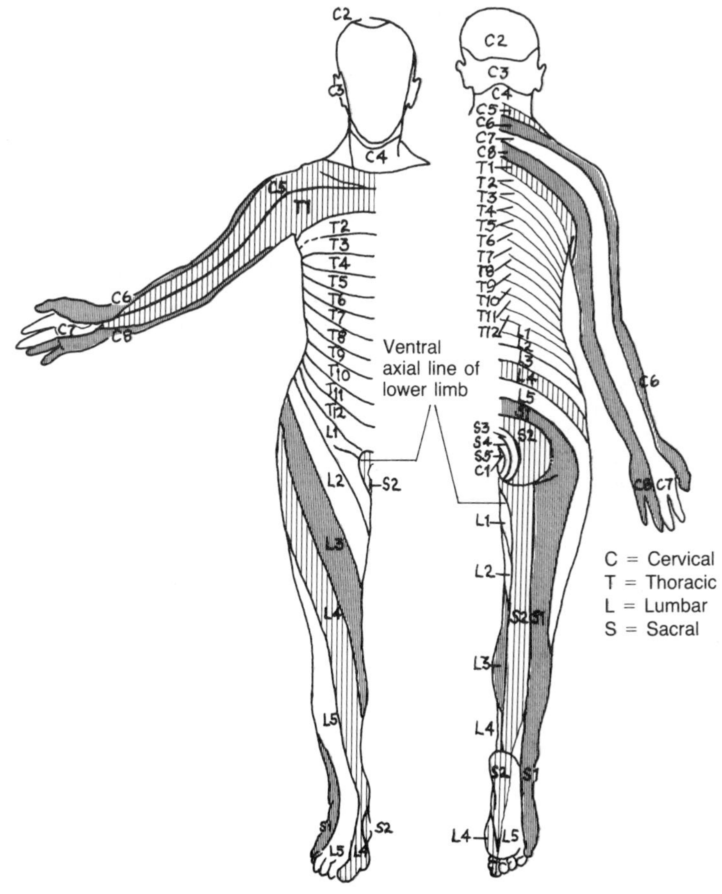

Dermatomes

in onset. Similar to polymyositis except that it is accompanied by a rash which usually appears over the knuckles, elbows, and knees. Often occurs in association with visceral cancer.

dermatoneurosis (der′-ma-tō-nū-rō′-sis): An inflammation of the skin that is due to some nerve abnormality or is a symptom of some form of neurosis.

dermatopathology (der′-mat-ō-pa-thol′-o-ji): A subspecialty of pathology that is concerned with diseases of the skin.—dermatopathologic, adj.

dermatopathophobia (der′-ma-tō-path-ō-fō′-bi-a): Abnormal dread of contracting a skin disease. Also dermatophobia.

dermatopathy (der-ma-top′-a-thi): Any disease or disorder of the skin.

Dermatophagoides farinae: The common household dust mite, which causes allergic reactions in sensitive individuals.

dermatophylaxis (der′-ma-tō-fī-lak′-sis): Protection of the skin against infection.

dermatophyte (der′-ma-tō-fīt): One of a group of fungi that invade the superficial skin causing such skin diseases as tinea pedis, eczema, and ringworm.

dermatophytosis (der′-ma-tō-fī-tō′-sis): An eruption caused by one of the dermatophytes (*q.v.*). Most commonly seen on the feet (athlete's foot). Characterized by itching, small vesicles, fissures and scaling. See **tinea pedis.**

dermatoplasty (der′-ma-tō-plas′-ti): Plastic repair of the skin; skin grafting.

dermatorrhagia (der′-ma-tō-rā′-ji-a): Hemorrhage into or from the skin.

dermatosclerosis (der′-ma-tō-sklē-rō′-sis): Scleroderma (*q.v.*).

dermatosis (der-ma-tō′-sis): Generic term for skin disease.—dermatoses, pl.

dermatotherapy (der′-ma-tō-ther′-a-pi): The treatment of skin disorders.

dermatothlasia (der′-ma-tō-thlā′-zi-a): An abnormal uncontrollable tendency to pinch or bruise one's skin.

dermatoxerasia (der′-ma-tō-ze-rā′-si-a): Roughening or drying of the skin. Syn., xeroderma (*q.v.*).

dermatozoon (der-ma-tō-zō′-on): Any animal parasite of the skin.

dermatozoonosis (der′-mat-ō-zō-ō-nō′-sis): Infestation of the skin with a dermatozoon.

dermatrophia (der-ma-trō′-fi-a): Atrophy of the skin.

-dermia: Combining form denoting a skin condition.

dermis (der′-mis): The true skin; the cutis vera; the layer below the epidermis.—Syn., corium.

dermitis (der-mī′-tis): Dermatitis (*q.v.*).

dermographia (der-mō-graf′-i-a): A condition in which wheals occur on the skin after a blunt instrument or fingernail has been lightly drawn over it. Seen in vasomotor instability and urticaria. Also dermatographia.

dermoid (der′-moyd): Pertaining to or resembling skin and/or its related tissues. **D. CYST,** a benign teratoma (*q.v.*); when it occurs in the ovary it may contain sebaceous fluid, hair, and sometimes, teeth and bone; is usually unilateral and seen mostly in women between 20 and 35 years of age.

dermoidectomy (der-moy-dek′-tō-mi): Surgical removal of a dermoid cyst.

dermometer (der-mom′-e-ter): An instrument for measuring, in ohms, the electric resistance of the skin.

dermometry (der-mom′-e-tri): Measurement of the electrical resistance of the skin.

dermonecrosis (der′-mō-nē-krō′-sis): Necrosis of the skin.—dermonecrotic, adj.

dermopathy (der-mop′-a-thi): Any skin disease.

dermosynovitis (der′-mō-sin-ō-vī′-tis): Inflammation of the skin that overlies an inflamed tendon sheath or bursa.

dermotropic (der-mō-trop′-ik): Having an affinity for the skin.

DES: Abbreviation for diethylstilbestrol (*q.v.*).

desalination (dē′-sal-i-nā′-shun): The process of removing salt from a substance.

desaturation (dē-sat′-ū-rā′-shun): The process of converting a saturated substance into an unsaturated one by the removal of hydrogen.

Descemet's membrane (des-e-māz′): The fine, elastic membrane that lines the posterior surface of the cornea.

descending (dē-sen′-ding): Directed or extending downward. **D. AORTA,** the part of the aorta between the distal end of the arch and the bifurcation into the iliac arteries. **D. COLON,** the part of the colon between the splenic flexure and the sigmoid colon. **D. NEURITIS,** weakness or paralysis of muscles, beginning at the shoulder and spreading downward toward the hands and feet. **D. TRACT,** a collection of nerve fibers that conduct impulses down the spinal cord.

desensitization (dē-sen′-si-tī-zā′-shun): The neutralization or lessening of acquired hypersensitiveness to some agent acting on the skin or internally. Used in asthma and for treatment of people who have become allergic to drugs such as penicillin and streptomycin. The process usually consists of giving small, repeated doses of the protein to which the person is sensitive. **SYSTEMATIC DESENSITIZATION,** in psychiatry, a procedure in behavioral therapy whereby the patient is repeatedly exposed to scenes depicting an anxiety-causing situation while relaxing the deep muscles, with the expectation that the real-life situation will no longer produce an anxiety reaction.

desensitize (dē-sen′-si-tīz): 1. To render a

person insensitive to an antigen by the administration of a series of small, steadily increasing doses of a particular allergen. 2. To deprive a person of sensation by nerve block with an anesthetic drug or by sectioning a particular nerve. 3. In psychiatry, to relieve or remove a person's phobia by frequent exposure to the stressful situation or by repeated discussions of it.—desensitization, n.

desexualize (dē-seks′-ū-a-līz): To castrate (*q.v.*).

DESI ratings: A system of rating *d*rugs as to their *e*ffectiveness for *s*pecific *i*ndications, promulgated by the Food and Drug Administration in 1972.

desiccant (des′-i-kant): Promoting dryness of a substance by absorbing or expelling water from it, or an agent that does this.

desiccate (des′-i-kāt): To dry out thoroughly.—desiccation, n.

-desis: Combining form denoting binding or fusing.

desmalgia (dez-mal′-ji-a): Pain in a ligament.

desmectasis (dez-mek′-ta-sis): The stretching of a ligament.

desmitis (dez-mī′-tis): Inflammation of a ligament.

desmodynia (dez-mō-din′-i-a): Pain in a ligament.

desmoid (dez′-moid): 1. Resembling a tendon or fibroid. 2. A tough, firm, circumscribed mass or tumor in skeletal muscle and fascia, produced by over-proliferation of fibroblasts in striated muscle and sometimes in periosteum, and, possibly, by trauma; most apt to occur in muscles of the head, neck, upper arm, and lower extremity.

desmology (dez-mol′-o-ji): 1. The art of bandaging. 2. The study of ligaments.

desmotomy (dez-mot′-o-mi): The incision of a ligament.

desoxycorticosterone (des-ok′-si-kor-ti-kos′-ter-ōn): deoxycorticosterone (*q.v.*).

desoxyribonucleic acid: Deoxyribonucleic acid (*q.v.*).

desquamation (des-kwa-mā′-shun): Shedding or flaking off, usually referring to the normal shedding of the superficial layer of the skin. Commonly increased after diseases attended by a rash, *e.g.*, scarlet fever, measles.—desquamate, v.; desquamative, adj.

DEST: Denver Eye Screening Test; used for testing visual acuity in children 3 years of age and older.

dest.: Abbreviation for destilla [L.] meaning distilled.

detachment (dē-tach′-ment): **D. OF THE RETINA,** the separation of the inner, neural layer of the retina from the pigment layer. Retinal detachment.

detelectasis (det-e-lek′-ta-sis): Collapse of an organ due to loss of normal inflation.

detergent (dē-ter′-jent): A purifying or cleansing agent resembling soaps in the ability to emulsify oils and hold them in suspension, but differing in chemical composition.

deterioration (dē-tēr-i-ō-rā′-shun): The state of being worse or becoming worse.—deteriorate, v.

determinism (dē-ter′-min-izm): In psychiatry, the concept that all emotional and mental life is determined by preexisting conditions or forces outside of one's control, that one has no freedom of choice, and that the individual is incapable of purposeful, self-generated action.

detoxication (dē-tok-si-kā′-shun): The process of removing the poisonous property of a substance.—detoxicant, adj., n.; detoxicate, v.

detoxification (dē-toks′-i-fi-kā′-shun) A major mode of medical treatment by which the effects of a drug are lessened in victims of overdosage or in addicts. **D. UNIT,** a unit in a health care facility that provides for medically supervised withdrawal from addiction to alcohol or other drugs.—detoxify, v.

detrition (dē-trish′-un): A wearing off or away by friction, rubbing, or use.

detritus (dē-trī′-tus): Organic or nonorganic matter produced by detrition, or waste matter resulting from disintegration or wearing away of tissues.

detrusor (dē-troo′-ser): Term applied to any part of the body that pushes downward. **D. URINAE,** the external longitudinal layer of muscle of the urinary bladder that contracts to empty the bladder.

detubation (dē-tū-bā′-shun): The withdrawal of a tube.—detubate, v.

detumescence (dē-tū-mes′-ens): Diminution or subsidence of: 1) swelling; 2) erectile genital organs.

deuteranopia (dū′-ter-a-nō′-pi-a): Colorblindness in which red and green are incorrectly perceived, green in particular.—deuteranopic, adj.

deutero-: Combining form denoting second.

deuteropathy (dū-ter-op′-a-thi): A pathological condition that is secondary to another disease.

devascularize (dē-vas′-kū-lar-īz): To remove the blood supply to an area by destroying, obstructing, or removing the blood vessel(s).—devascularization, n.

development: In human biology, the gradual growth and maturation of the body systems, of adaptability to the environment, and of creative expression.—developmental, adj.

developmental: Pertaining to development. **D. AGE,** an individual's age as estimated from the degree of his anatomical development. **D.**

AGRAPHIA, delayed development in learning to write. **D. ALEXIA**, delayed development in learning to read. **D. APHASIA**, delayed development in learning to speak. **D. DYSLEXIA**, greater than normal difficulty of the school-age child in learning to read. **D. QUOTIENT**, the score derived by dividing the child's mental age (as measured by the Gesell Development Schedules) by his chronological age, and multiplying by 100; abbreviated DQ. **D. TASKS**, the knowledge and skills that an individual needs to learn at different stages throughout the aging process.

deviancy (dēv' i-an-si): Variation from the norm in quality, state, or behavior.

deviant (dē' -vi-ant): 1. Varying from an accepted normal standard. 2. Something that differs from what is considered normal, especially a person whose behavior or characteristics vary from what is acceptable in the group to which he belongs.

deviate (dē' -vi-āt): 1. To vary from the norm or from the accepted standard. 2. A person whose attitude and behavior differ from the norm or from the accepted social and moral standard. 3. A sexual pervert.

deviation (dē-vi-ā' -shun): 1. A departure from normal. 2. Failure to conform to normal standards. In optics, strabismus (*q.v.*).

device (dē-vīs'): Something contrived or constructed for a particular purpose or use. **CONTRACEPTIVE D.**, one used to prevent conception. **INTRAUTERINE D.**, a **D.** that is inserted into the uterus to prevent conception by preventing implantation of a fertilized ovum; abbreviated IUD.

Devic's disease: Neuromyelitis optica (*q.v.*).

devitalize (de-vı' -tal-īz): To destroy or deprive of life, vitality, force, effectiveness. In dentistry, to destroy the pulp and nerve supply of a tooth.—devitalization, n.

devolution (dev' -ō-lū' -shun): Catabolism; degeneration. The opposite of evolution.

dexamethasone (dek-sa-meth' -a-sōn): A synthetic substance resembling cortisol in biological action; used in medicine as an anti-inflammatory agent.

dexter (deks' -ter): Related to or situated on the right. In anatomy, on the right-hand side.

dextr-, dextro-: Combining forms denoting the right, or toward the right side.

dextrad (deks' -trad): Toward the right.

dextrality (deks-tral' -i-ti): The voluntary preferential use of the right one of the paired organs of the body, as the eye or hand.

dextran (deks' -tran): A blood plasma substitute or expander obtained from the action of a specific bacterium (*Le conostoc mesenteroides*) on sucrose; available in several preparations. Used in treatment of shock, severe burns, hemorrhage, hypovolemia, hydration, and certain kidney diseases.

dextrimaltose (deks' -tri-mal' -tōs): A sugar preparation used in infant formulas; contains maltose and dextrin.

dextrin (deks' -trin): A soluble polysaccharide formed during the hydrolysis of starch.

dextrinuria (deks-tri-nū' -ri-a): The presence of dextrin in the urine.

dextrocardia (deks' -trō-kar' -di-a): Refers to either of two types of congenital phenomena: 1) the heart is slightly rotated and transposed almost entirely to the right side of the chest; or 2) the left chambers of the heart are on the right side and the right chambers are on the left side.

dextrocular (deks-trok' -ū-lar): 1. Right-eyed. 2. Having greater visual power in the right eye.

dextroduction (deks' -trō-duk' -shun): The movement of either eye to the right.

dextrogastria (deks' -trō-gas' -tri-a): Displacement of the stomach to the right.

dextromanual (deks-trō-man' -ū-al): Right-handed.

dextropedal (deks-trop' -e-dal): Preferential use of the right leg and foot.

dextroposition (deks' -trō-pō-zish' -un): Displacement to the right. **D. OF THE HEART**, displacement of the heart into the right half of the thorax.

dextrose (deks' -trōs): 1. Glucose (*q.v.*); a soluble, readily absorbed and utilized carbohydrate (monosaccharide); may be given by almost any route; widely used by intravenous infusion in dehydration, shock, and postoperatively. Also given orally as a readily absorbed sugar in acidosis and other nutritional disturbances. 2. The end product of carbohydrate digestion.

dextrosinistral (deks' -trō-sin' -is-tral): Extending from right to left. Also descriptive of a person who is left-handed but has trained himself to use the right hand for certain performances, *e.g.*, writing.

dextrosuria (deks-trō-sū' -ri-a): The presence of dextrose in the urine.

dextroversion (deks' -trō-ver' -zhun): A moving or turning to the right, as of the eyes.

DHHS: Abbreviation for Department of Health and Human Services (*q.v.*).

dhobie itch : Tinea cruris; a fungal infection of the skin of the groin and inner thigh, seen most often in the obese and in warm climates; a type found in the laundrymen of India is thought to be caused by a laundry-marking ink made from the cashew nut. See tinea.

di-: A prefix denoting two; twice; double.

dia-: A prefix denoting between, apart, across, through, completely.

diabetes (dī-a-bē' -tēz): Any of a group of metabolic disorders marked by the excessive secretion and excretion of urine and excessive thirst; when used without qualification it means

D. MELLITUS. BRITTLE D., D. that is difficult to control because of alternating episodes of hyperglycemia and hypoglycemia; also called unstable **D.** or labile **D. BRONZE D., D.** that also involves the liver; the skin is deeply pigmented; see hemochromatosis. **DRUG-INDUCED D., D.** caused by certain chemicals that may have a cytotoxic effect on the beta cells of the pancreas or may antagonize insulin and thus increase hyperglycemia. **GESTATIONAL D., D.** that occurs during pregnancy. **D. INNOCENS,** a condition marked by glycosuria that is not associated with pancreatic disease. **D. INSIPIDUS,** a disease caused by inadequate secretion of antidiuretic hormone by the pituitary gland; may be congenital or follow injury or infection; characterized by dehydration, polydipsia, and polyuria. **INSULIN-DEPENDENT, KETOSIS-PRONE D., D.** that develops before the age of 16 (formerly called juvenile-onset **D.**); symptoms are more severe than in noninsulin-dependent, ketosis-resistant **D. LIPOTROPHIC D., D.** characterized by deficient storage of fat in the body. **D. MELLITUS,** a chronic disorder characterized by faulty carbohydrate metabolism, due mainly to a relative or absolute lack of effective insulin, which results in alterations in the metabolism of fats and proteins; the urine is pale and of high specific gravity because of its sugar content. Other features include dehydration, polydipsia, polyuria, weight loss, lassitude, retinopathy, neuropathy, nephropathy, lowered resistance to infection, decreased ability of wounds to heal and vascular abnormalities; in more advanced cases there is coma and ketosis. Sometimes leads to accelerated atherosclerosis affecting particularly the blood vessels of the eye, kidneys, and nerves. **NEUROGENOUS D., D.** that occurs in association with certain brain lesions. **NONINSULIN-DEPENDENT, KETONE RESISTANT D., D.** that usually occurs in obese individuals over 40 years of age; they have a variable but less than normal amount of plasma insulin, and their **D.** can often be controlled by diet alone or by an oral hypoglycemic drug; formerly called adult onset **D. SECONDARY D., D.** that is secondary to disease of the pancreas, liver, or any of several other organs. **STARVATION D.,** glycosuria following ingestion of glucose after prolonged fasting; attributed to a reduced ability to form glycogen. **SUBCLINICAL D., D.** in which the glucose tolerance test is abnormal but the patient has no other clinical signs of diabetes.

diabetic (dī-a-bet′-ik): 1. Pertaining to diabetes. 2. An individual suffering from diabetes. **D. ACIDOSIS,** caused by an excess of ketone bodies in the blood; signs include thirst, air hunger, weakness, headache, coma. **D. CATARACT,** see cataract. **D. COMA,** see coma. **D. DIET,** a diet that consists of calculated amounts of protein, carbohydrates, and fats, with sugar restricted. **D. GANGRENE,** that occurring in diabetic patients, often following an injury. See gangrene. **D. IDENTIFICATION CARD,** one carried by diabetics; lists patient's and doctor's names, addresses, and telephone numbers, states the kind and amount of insulin the patient is receiving, and directions for treatment should the person become ill when in a public place. **D. KETOACIDOSIS,** see ketoacidosis. **D. RETINOPATHY,** see retinopathy.

diabetogenic (dī-a-bet′-ō-jen′-ik): Causing diabetes.

diabetogenous (dī-a-be-toj′-e-nus): Caused by diabetes.

diabetologist (dī-a-be-tol′-o-jist): A physician who specializes in the care of people with diabetes.

diaceturia (dī-as-e-tū′-ri-a): The presence of diacetic (acetoacetic) acid in the urine.

diacetylmorphine (dī-a-sē′-til-mor′-fēn): Heroin.

diachorema (dī-a-kō-rē-′-ma): Feces.

diachoresis (dī-a-kō-rē′-sis): Defecation.

diadochokinesia (dī-ad′-ō-kō-kī-nē′-zi-a): The normal function of being able to terminate one motor activity and rapidly substitute another, opposite action, *e.g.*, rapidly changing from the prone to the supine position.

Diagnex Blue test: A test utilizing a dye, Azuresin, which is taken by mouth; determines the presence of hydrochloric acid in the stomach; is positive if the patient's urine has a blue color; not used as much as formerly.

diagnose (dī′-ag-nōs): To recognize the distinctive signs and symptoms of a disease or disorder.

diagnosis (dī-ag-nō′-sis): The name of a disease or condition that distinguishes it from other diseases or conditions. **CLINICAL D., D.** based on physical examination, and the patient's history; does not include laboratory tests. **DIFFERENTIAL D., D.** made after comparing the symptoms of two or more diseases. **LABORATORY D., D.** arrived at after laboratory study of specimens taken from the patient. **POSTMORTEM D., D.** based on findings at autopsy. **SEROLOGICAL D., D.** based on laboratory study of the patient's blood serum. **TENTATIVE D.,** one judged by apparent symptoms and facts pending further study and examination. diagnoses, pl.; diagnose, v.; diagnostic, adj.

Diagnosis Related Groups (DRG): A cost control system in which patients are categorized as to age and diagnosis or surgical procedure, according to 467 different groupings; used in estimating how much each patient in a DRG may be expected to cost the hospital in service by anticipating the amount of service the patient may require and the length of hospital stay. It allows hospitals that are reimbursed by Medicare to collect in advance for services and improves their cash flow. If the length of hospital stay is shorter than the DRG estimate, the hospital makes a profit; if the stay is longer than the DRG estimate, the hospital suffers a loss.

diagnostic (dī-ag-nos′-tik): 1. Pertaining to diagnosis. 2. Serving as evidence in diagnosis.—diagnostician, n.

Diagnostic and Statistical Manual of Mental Disorders: A publication of the American Psychiatric Association, revised periodically. Lists the official classification of diagnoses of mental disorders and provides data helpful in planning treatment programs. Commonly referred to by acronym and number of latest edition (the revised version of the third edition published in 1987 is referred to as DSM-III-R). Health care workers are required to use the nomenclature in DSM-III-R when reporting psychiatric disorders or when filling in insurance forms for patients.

diagnostician (dī-ag-nos-tish′-un): A physician whose chief field of interest and practice is in making diagnoses.

dialysance (dī-al′-i-sans): A measure of the rate of exchange that takes place between the blood and the bath fluid in hemodialysis or peritoneal dialysis, in a certain time period, usually one minute.

dialysate (dī-al′-i-sāt): 1. The fluid used in dialysis. 2. The part of the liquid that passes through a dialyzing membrane in dialysis. **D. BATH,** the isotonic solution used in dialysis; contains almost all of the ions found in the blood and that diffuse across a semipermeable membrane and are needed to establish normal blood levels.

dialysis (dī-al′-i-sis): 1. A process that occurs naturally in the body during digestion, respiration, and urine formation. 2. The separation of certain substances in solution by taking advantage of their differing diffusibility through a porous membrane to remove metabolic waste products, poisons, toxins, drugs taken in overdose, or to correct electrolyte imbalance. **EXTRACORPOREAL D., D.** that utilizes the artificial kidney; see hemodialysis. **PERITONEAL D.,** a method of irrigating the peritoneum by continuously or intermittently infusing dialyzing fluid into the peritoneal cavity by a soft peritoneal catheter where it remains for a preset period of time during which an exchange takes place between the dialyzing fluid and the body fluids containing waste products of metabolism, and then the fluid is withdrawn into a collecting bag.

dialysis disequilibrium syndrome: A condition occurring usually one to two hours after the start of dialysis; characterized by nausea, vomiting, mental confusion including hallucinations, and sometimes convulsions.

dialyzer (dī′a-līz-er): The apparatus used in performing dialysis, or the membrane in the apparatus.

diameter (dī-am′-e-ter): In anatomy, a straight line between two opposite points of a structure that is more or less spherical or cylindrical in shape, *e.g.*, the cranium and the bony pelvis.

diapedesis (dī′-a-pe-dē′-sis): The passage of blood cells through the unbroken vessel walls into the tissues, usually refers to passage of white cells through capillary walls in response to infection or injury.—diapedetic, adj.

diaper rash: An eruption in the diaper area of infants caused by friction, infection, feces, urine, moisture, heat; macropapular in nature but may become excoriated; a monilial infection is sometimes involved.

diaper test: A test for early detection of phenylketonuria (*q.v.*). A drop of 5 to 10% ferric chloride solution is dropped onto a recently wet diaper; if phenylketone bodies are present, the spot will turn green; if the urine is normal, the spot will remain yellow. Test is repeated at intervals because it does not always give positive results even though the infant is suffering from phenylketonuria.

diaphoresis (dī′-a-fō-rē′-sis): Perspiration, particularly that which is excessive; may be associated with muscular activity, stress, use of certain drugs, exposure to heat, fever.

diaphoretic (dī′-a-fō-ret′-ik): 1. An agent that induces diaphoresis; a sudorific. 2. Pertaining to diaphoresis.

diaphragm (dī′-a-fram): 1. The dome-shaped musculomembranous partition between the thorax above and the abdomen below; the chief muscle of respiration. 2. Any partitioning membrane, such as that used in dialysis. 3. A saucer-like contraceptive rubber cap with a spring that fits over and occludes the cervix.

diaphragmalgia (dī′-a-frag-mal′-ji-a): Pain in the diaphragm.

diaphragmatic (dī′-a-frag-mat′-ik): Pertaining to the diaphragm. **D. BREATHING,** see under breathing. **D. FLUTTER,** rapid rhythmic contractions of the diaphragm which may simulate cardiac pain. **D. HERNIA,** see under hernia.

diaphragmatocele (dī′-a-frag-mat′-ō-sēl): Hernia through the diaphragm.

diaphragmitis (dī′-a-frag-mī′-tis): Inflammation of the diaphragm.

diaphyseal (dī-a-fiz′-ē-al): Pertaining to or involving a diaphysis.

diaphysectomy (dī′-a-fī-sek′-to-mi): Excision of part of the shaft of a long bone.

diaphysis (dī-af′-i-sis): The shaft of a long bone.—diaphyses, pl.; diaphyseal, adj.

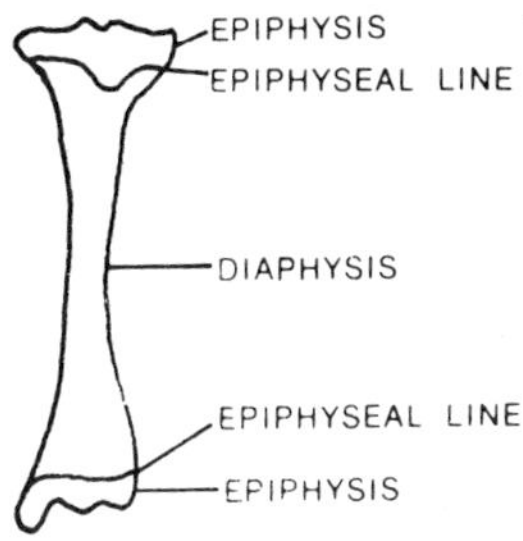

diaphysis

diaphysitis (dī-af-i-sī′-tis): Inflammation of a diaphysis. **TUBERCULOUS D., D.** caused by the tubercle bacillus.

diarrhea (dī-a-rē′-a): Loose or watery and frequent evacuation of stools, with or without discomfort. **BACTERIAL D.**, caused by contaminated food. **CHRONIC D.**, often associated with diverticulosis, colitis, and cancer of the colon. **DIETETIC D.**, due to overindulgence in laxative foods. **EPIDEMIC D., D.** of the newborn, a highly contagious infection seen in maternity hospitals. **FOOD POISONING D.**, a serious condition caused by food contaminated with bacterial toxins, especially those of the *Salmonella* group. **SUMMER D.**, occurs chiefly in children in exceptionally hot weather. **TRAVELERS' D.**, occurs commonly in travelers in tropical or subtropical areas particularly; often thought to be due to imperfect sanitation and caused by the Escherichia coli organism.

diarrheogenic (dī′-a-rē-ō-jen′-]-ik): Producing diarrhea.

diarthric (dī-ar′-thrik): Pertaining to two joints or affecting two joints at the same time.

diarthrosis (dī-ar-thrō′-sis): A synovial, freely movable joint, such as the hip joint.—diarthrodial, adj.; diarthroses, pl.

diastalsis (dī-a-stal′-sis): The downward moving wave of contraction in the small intestine during digestion.—diastaltic, adj.

diastase (dī′-a-stās): A specific enzyme in certain plant cells and in the digestive juice; it converts starch into sugar. **PANCREATIC D.** is excreted in the urine (and saliva) and therefore estimation of urinary **D.** may be used as a test of pancreatic function.

diastasis (dī-as′-ta-sis): 1. A separation of bones without fracture; dislocation. 2. The separation of the epiphysis from the body of a bone. **D. RECTI ABDOMINIS**, separation of the rectus abdominalis at the midline; results from weakening of the supporting tissues, usually as a result of pregnancy or surgery.

diastema (dī-a-stē′-ma): 1. An abnormally wide space between teeth. 2. A cleft or space, particularly one that is congenital.

diastematomyelia (dī-a-stē′-ma-tō-mī-ē′-li-a): A congenital condition in which the spinal cord is spilt into halves separated by a fibrous band; each half has its own dural sac; occurs most often in spina bifida.

diastole (dī-as′-tō-li): The normal relaxation period of the cardiac cycle, when the heart rests, the muscle fibers lengthen, and the respective chambers fill with blood. Alternates with systole (*q.v.*).

diastolic (dī-a-stol′-ik): Pertaining to the diastole. **D. MURMUR**, an abnormal sound heard during diastole; occurs in valvular diseases of the heart. **D. PRESSURE**, the blood pressure during the relaxation phase of the cardiac cycle; it is the lowest pressure reached during any ventricular cycle.

diataxia (dī-a-tak′-si-a): Ataxia affecting both sides of the body.

diathermy (dī′-a-ther-mi): The passage of a high frequency electric current through the tissues whereby heat is produced. When both electrodes are large, the heat is diffused over a wide area according to the electrical resistance of the tissues. In this form it is widely used in the treatment of inflammation, especially when deeply seated (*e.g.*, sinusitis, pelvic cellulitis). When one electrode is very small the heat is concentrated in this area and becomes great enough to destroy tissue. In this form (surgical diathermy) it is used to stop bleeding during surgery by coagulation of blood, or to cut through tissue in operations for malignant disease.

diathesis (dī-ath′-e-sis): An inherited predisposition or combination of attributes that makes a person susceptible to certain diseases or classes of diseases. **HEMORRHAGIC D.**, bleeding **D.**; a predisposition to spontaneous hemorrhage.

DIC: Abbreviation for disseminated intravascular clotting.

dicephalous (dī-sef′-a-lus): Two-headed.

dichorionic (dī′-kō-ri-on′-ik): Having two chorions. **D. TWINS**, twins having separate chorions.

dichotomy (dī-kot′-o-mi): A division into two parts, classes, or groups that are normally mutually contradictory or exclusive.—dichotomization, n.; dichotomous, adj.

dichromatopsia (dī′-krō-ma-top′-si-a): Color blindness in which the individual is able to recognize and distinguish only two of the three primary colors red, blue, and green; either the red-green or the blue-yellow system is lacking, the first type being relatively common and the second being the rarest of all types of color blindness.

dichromophil (di-krō′-mō-fil): Pertaining to a cell or tissue that takes both a basic and acidic stain.

Dick test: A skin test for susceptibility or immunity to scarlet fever whereby a small amount of scarlet fever toxin (erythrogenic toxin of *Streptococcus pyogenes*) is injected subcutaneously; the appearance of a small area of reddened skin at the injection site within 24 hours indicates susceptibility. [George F. Dick, 1881–1967; Gladys R.H. Dick, 1881–1963. Chicago physicians.]

dicophane (dī′-kō-fān): Chlorophenothane, a well-known highly toxic insecticide formerly sometimes used against pediculosis capitis and other body parasites as a lotion or dusting powder. See DDT.

dicrotic (dī-krot′-ik): Pertaining to, or having a double beat, as indicated by a second expansion of the artery during diastole. **D. PULSE,** a small wave of distension of the blood vessel after the normal beat. **D. WAVE,** the second rise in the tracing of a dicrotic pulse.

didactylism (dī-dak′-til-izm): The congenital condition of having only two fingers on one hand or two toes on one foot; bidactyly.

didelphia (dī-del′-fi-a): The congenital condition of having a double uterus.—didelphic, adj.

DIDMOAD: Abbreviation for a rare inherited syndrome that appears in diabetics; stands for *d*iabetes *i*nsipidus, *d*iabetes *m*ellitus, *o*ptic *a*trophy, and *d*eafness.

didymitis (did-i-mī′-tis): Inflammation of a testis; orchitis.

didymous (did′-i-mus): Growing or arranged in a pair or pairs.

-didymus (did′-i-mus): A combining form meaning 1) a testis, or 2) a conjoined pair of twins with the first element of the word designating the part of the bodies that is not fused.

diencephalic syndrome (dī-en-se-fal′-ik): Emaciation; failure to thrive. Seen in infants and children; due to a diencephalic tumor. Also called Russell's syndrome.

diencephalon (dī-en-sef′-a-lon): That part of the forebrain or cerebrum lying between the telencephalon and the mesencephalon; contains the thalamus, hypothalamus, and the greater part of the third ventricle.

diesterase (dī-es′-ter-ās): An enzyme such as nuclease which acts to split the bonds binding the nucleotides in nucleic acid.

diet: 1. The food normally consumed in the course of living. 2. A prescription of food that is required by a patient or permitted to him. 3. To eat only simple, easily digested food in limited quantities. **ACID-ASH D.,** a **D.** that yields an acidic residue; may be prescribed to help prevent the formation of urinary calculi; consists of cereals, fish, eggs, and meat, with restrictions on fruits and vegetables and the elimination of milk and cheese. **ANDRESON D.,** an acid neutralizing **D.** consisting of a mixture of milk, cream, gelatin, and glucose; prescribed for bleeding ulcer and after surgery. **BALANCED D.,** one that contains all the elements in the correct quantities needed for growth and repair of body tissues. **BLAND D.,** one that contains no stimulating or irritating foods. **DIABETIC D.,** one adapted to the needs of a diabetic patient; contains weighed amounts of fats, carbohydrates, and proteins. **FULL LIQUID DIET,** consists of only liquids, but includes ice cream and cream soups. **HIGH CALORIC D.,** one that provides 4000 or more calories per day. **KETOGENIC D.,** one high in fat, low in protein and carbohydrate. **LIGHT D.,** one suitable for a person taking little exercise, *e.g.*, a bed patient or convalescent; includes foods from the Basic Four group, but excludes foods that are difficult to digest and those that are fried, highly seasoned, or spicy. **LOW CALORIE D.,** one that provides 1000 calories or less per day. **LOW FAT DIET,** one low in fat; antiketogenic **D. LOW PROTEIN D.,** one containing the minimum amount of protein. **LOW RESIDUE D.,** one low in cellulose and fiber; prescribed in certain bowel disorders. **LOW SALT D.,** one low in sodium, often used in treatment of edema, hypertension, congestive heart disease. **MACROBIOTIC D.,** see under macrobiotic. **NEPHRITIC D.,** one low in nitrogen content and eliminating spices, alcohol, and condiments. **RICE D.,** a low fat, low salt, low cholesterol **D.** consisting of rice and fruit supplemented with vitamins and iron; used in treatment of arterial hypertension and chronic kidney disease. **SIPPY D.,** a dietary regimen for treatment of peptic ulcer. The objective is to neutralize the hydrochloric acid in the stomach by frequent feedings; starting with milk and cream only and gradually adding bland foods as the symptoms subside until finally the patient is able to take a normal diet. **SOFT DIET,** one consisting of milk, eggs, custard, mashed potatoes, ice cream, or other nonirritating easily digested foods. **VEGETARIAN D.,** one in which all flesh foods are eliminated in favor of vegetables, cereals and dairy products.—dietary, dietetic, adj.

dietetics (dīe-tet′-iks): The interpretation and application of the scientific principles of nutrition to feeding in health and disease.

diethylstilbestrol (DES) (dī-eth′-il-stil-bes′-trōl): A synthetic estrogenic substance used therapeutically as a substitute for natural estrogenic hormones. Should not be used during pregnancy since there have been instances of daughters of women who took DES during pregnancy developing cancer of the cervix.

dietitian (dī-e-tish′-un): One who applies the principles of nutrition to the feeding of an individual, or a group of individuals in various settings, *e.g.*, hospitals, institutions, schools, restaurants, hotels, etc. **THERAPEUTIC D.,** one involved in treatment of patients through modification of their diet.

dietotherapy (dī-et-ō-ther′-a-pi): Scientific management of the diet in the treatment of disease.

differential (dif-fer-en′-shul): Related to or constituting a difference. **D. BLOOD COUNT,** the estimation of the relative proportions of the different leukocyte cells in the blood, with the normal differential count being 1) granular leukocytes; eosinophils, 1–4%, basophils, 1-4%, and neutrophils, 51–67%; and 2) non-granular leukocytes; lymphocytes, 25–33%, monocytes, 2–6%. **D. DIAGNOSIS,** diagnosis based on comparison of the symptoms of diseases that have similar manifestations, and evaluating the signs and symptoms that are dissimilar. **D. FORGETTING,** selective forgetting, especially the faster forgetting of erroneous responses than of correct ones. **D. STAIN,** a stain used to differentiate bacteria; see Gram's stain under stain.

diffusate (di-fū′-zāt): Material that passes through or has passed through a membrane; dialysate.

diffuse (di-fūz′, di-fūs′): 1. To pour out, extend, or scatter. 2. Scattered or spread throughout a substance or an area; not localized or limited. 3. To spread out or disperse.

diffusion (di-fū′-zhun): The process of homogenization whereby liquids, solutions, gases and some solids intermingle when brought into contact, with the molecules from an area of higher concentration moving to an area of lower concentration until the two substances are of equal density.—diffuse, v. See dialysis.

digastric (dī-gas′-trik): Having two bellies; said of muscles, especially those that have two fleshy parts separated by tendinous tissues, *e.g.,* the gastrocnemius muscle.

digest (dī-jest′): In physiology, to change food by mechanical and chemical processes, in the mouth, stomach and intestines, so tnat it can be absorbed by the body.

digesta (dī-jes′-ta): The contents of the stomach and intestine in the process of being digested.

digestant (dī-jest′-ant): An agent that aids in digestion of food.

digestion (dī-jest′-yun): The mechanical and chemical process by which food is broken down in the gastrointestinal tract and rendered absorbable.—digestible, digestive, adj.; digestibility, n.; digest, v.

digestive (dī-jes′-tiv): Pertaining to digestion **D. SYSTEM,** the organs associated with the ingestion and digestion of food; includes the mouth and associated structures, pharynx, esophagus, stomach, small and large intestine, and associ-

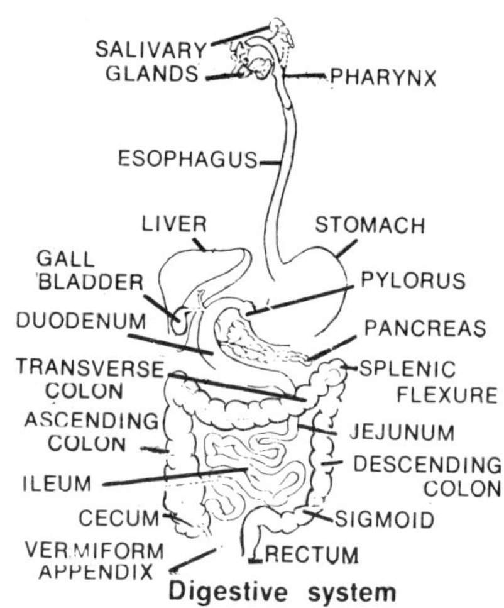

Digestive system

ated glands; also called alimentary system; digestive canal, or tract. **D. TUBE,** alimentary **T.,** see under alimentary.

digit (dij′-it): In anatomy, a finger or toe.—digital, adj.

digital (dij′-i-tal): Relating to, resembling, or performed by a digit, particularly a finger.

digitalgia (dij-i-tal′-ji-a): Pain in a finger or toe.

digitalis (dij-i-tal′-is): A drug prepared from the leaf of the common foxglove plant, which is the source of a large group of drugs used exclusively in cardiac conditions to strengthen and slow the heartbeat. Especially useful in auricular fibrillation and congestive heart failure. The purple foxglove furnishes the glycosides digitalin and digitoxin while the white foxglove furnishes digoxin. These drugs have a cumulative effect.

digitalism (dij′-i-tal-izm): 1. The effect of digitalis in the body. 2. Symptoms caused by overdosage or poisoning by digitalis.

digitalization (dij-i-tal-ī-zā′-shun): Physiological saturation with digitalis, to obtain optimum therapeutic effect.—digitalize, v.

digitate (dij′-i-tāt): Having digits or finger-like processes.

digitoplantar (dij-i-tō-plan′-tar): Pertaining to the toes and the sole of the foot.

digitoxin (dij-i-toks′-in): A cardiotonic glucoside that comes from several species of *Digitalis;* has an action similar to that of digitalis; useful in treatment of congestive heart failure.

digitus (dij′-i-tus): Digit; a finger or toe. **D. FLEXUS,** hammertoe (*q.v.*).—digiti, pl.

diglossia (dī-glos′-i-a): A congenital anomaly in which the two halves of the tongue fail to unite; a bifid tongue.

dihydrotheelin (dī-hī-drō-thē′-e-lin): Estradiol (*q.v.*).

dihydroxyphenylalanine (dī-hī-drok′-si-fen-il-al′-a-nēn): Dopa (*q.v.*).

dihysteria (dī-his-ter′-i-a): The presence of a double uterus.

dil.: Abbreviation for dilue [L.], meaning dilute or dissolve.

dilatation (dil-a-tā′-shun): The condition of being stretched or enlarged. May occur physiologically, pathologically, or be induced artificially.—dilate, v.; dilation, n.

dilatation and curettage: Dilatation of the cervix and scraping of the lining of the uterus. Done to remove any remaining contents of the uterus after abortion, to obtain material for histological examination or diagnosis, for treatment, or when radon or radium seeds are to be implanted. Abbreviated D&C.

dilatation and evacuation: An operation to remove the products of conception; the cervix is dilated and the uterus curetted by suction or other method of curettage.

dilate (dī′-lāt): To expand or enlarge.

dilation (dī-lā′-shun): The act of dilating or stretching of an orifice or cavity of the body.

dilator (dī′-lā-tor): Anything that dilates or stretches an opening or canal or a part of the body, *e.g.*, a muscle, drug, instrument, or other device.

diluent (dil-u′-ent): A diluting or dissolving agent.

dilute (dī-lūt′): 1. To make weaker or thinner by the addition of liquid. 2. Descriptive of a solution that has been weakened or thinned, thereby lessening its potency.

dilution (dī-lū′-shun): 1. The state of being diluted. 2. A solution that has been made weaker or thinner.

dimorphism (dī-mor′-fizm): The condition of having, or of existing in, two different forms. **SEXUAL D.**, the condition of having some of the characteristics of both sexes.

dimorphous (dī-morf′-us): Having the quality of existing in two distinct forms.

dimple (dim′-p'l): A slight depression in bone or other body tissue.—dimpling, n.

dimpling (dim′-pling): A depression in the skin caused by retraction; occurs in subcutaneous tumors, especially in those of the breast. May also occur at sites of repeated insulin injection.

Diogenes syndrome: A condition characterized by a grossly abnormal life style; the person lives in filthy surroundings, sometimes with many animals as pets, but is intellectually normal, often very bright, and resists any attempts to change his or her way of life.

diopsimeter (dī-op-sim′-e-ter): An instrument used to measure the field of vision.

diopter, dioptre (dī-op′-ter): A unit of measurement in refraction. A lens of one diopter has a focal length of 1 meter.

dioptometer (dī-op-tom′-e-ter): An instrument used for measuring the refractive ability of the eye.

dioptric (dī-op′-trik): Pertaining to refraction and refracted light.

diorthosis (dī-or-thō′-sis): The surgical correction or straightening of a deformed or injured extremity.

diotic (dī-ō′-tik): Pertaining to or affecting both ears.

diovulation (dī-ov-ū-lā′-shun): The discharge of two ova during one ovulatory cycle.

dioxide (dī-ok′-sīd): An oxide in which the molecules contain two oxygen atoms.

dipeptidase (dī-pep′-ti-dās): An enzyme that catalyzes the splitting of dipeptides into amino acids.

dipeptide (dī-pep′-tīd): A peptide that yields two amino acids on hydrolysis.

diphallus (dī-fal′-us): A congenital condition in which there is a complete or incomplete second penis or clitoris.

diphasic (dī-fā′-zik): Occurring in two stages or phases.

diphenylhydantoin (dī′-fen-il-hī-dan′-tō-in): A white odorless, powdery substance, soluble in water; used for its anticonvulsant action in the treatment of grand mal epilepsy. Also called phenytoin.

diphtheria (dif-thē′-ri-a): An acute, specific, highly infectious, epidemic and endemic disease caused by the *Corynebacterium diphtheriae* [Klebs-Loeffler bacillus]; transmitted by direct and indirect contact and carriers. Primarily a disease of children, occurring in the fall and winter months; protection is obtained by immunization, usually combined with immunization for pertussis and tetanus. Characterized by the formation of a grayish, leathery, adherent membrane growing on an epithelial surface which bleeds on removal, and the development of a potent systemic toxin that may attack the heart muscle and nerves. **CUTANEOUS D.**, a form that affects the skin, characterized by deep ulcerating lesions; associated with poor hygiene. **LARYNGEAL D.**, membranous croup; a serious condition seen primarily in infants. **NASAL D.**, **D.** confined to the nose; usually mild; but may spread to surrounding structures and tissues. **PHARYNGEAL D.**, that which affects primarily the pharynx. **WOUND D.**, name given to a false membrane that forms on the surface of a wound. **D. ANTITOXIN**, a serum containing antibodies that neutralize the **D.** toxin; obtained from horses that have been immunized to the toxin produced by *Corynebacterium diphtheriae*. **D. TOXIN**, a protein exotoxin produced by the *Corynebacterium diphtheriae;* is responsible for the development of symptoms of diphtheria. **D. TOXIN-ANTITOXIN,** a mixture used to produce active immunity against the disease; now largely replaced by diphtheria toxoid. **D. TOXOID, D.** toxin that has been detoxified; used to produce active immunity to diphtheria.

diphtheritic (dif-thē-rit′-ik): Resembling, caused by, pertaining to, or affected with diphtheria.

diphtheroid (dif′-ther-oyd): 1. Any bacterium resembling the *Corynebacterium diphtheriae*. 2. A disease that resembles diphtheria but is not caused by the *Corynebacterium diphtheriae*.

diphyllobothriasis (dī-fil′-ō-both - rī′-a-sis): Infection with the fish tapeworm of the genus *Diphyllobothrium*.

Diphyllobothrium (dī-fil-o-both′-ri-um): A genus of tapeworms. **D. LATUM,** a family of broad tapeworms, including the common fish tapeworm, which occurs in man as a result of eating raw or improperly cooked fish.

diplacusis (dip-la-kū′-sis): A pathological condition of the cochlea that results in the same sound being heard differently in each ear.

diplegia (dī-plē′-ji-a): Symmetrical paralysis of the same parts on both sides of the body. **CONGENITAL** or **INFANTILE D.,** birth palsy. **FACIAL D., D.** affecting both sides of the face. **SPASTIC D.,** see Little's disease. Cf. paraplegia.—diplegic, adj.

diplo-: A combining form denoting double, twice, two-fold.

diplobacillus (dip′-lō-ba-sil′-us): A pair of short rod-shaped organisms joined end to end as a result of incomplete fission.

diplocardia (dip-lō-kar′-di-a): A condition in which the right and left sides of the heart are partially separated by a deep fissure.

diplocephalus (dip′-lō-sef′-a-lus): See dicephalus.

diplococcus (dip′-lō-kok-′-us): A coccal bacterium characteristically occurring in pairs, *e.g.*, the pneumococcus.

diplocoria (dip′-lō-kō′-ri-a): A double pupil.

diploë (dip′-lō-ē): The cancellous tissue between the outer and inner layers of compact bone, *e.g.*, the flat bones of the skull.—diploetic, adj.

diploic (dip-lō′-ik): 1. Diploetic. 2. Double. 3. Pertaining to the diploë. **D. VEINS,** the large, thin-walled veins situated in the diploe of the cranial bones.

diploid (dip′-loyd): 1. Having two sets of chromosomes; a normal occurrence in the somatic cells of humans. 2. An individual having two full sets of chromosomes that are homologous.—diploidy, n.

diploma programs in nursing: At one time most professional nurses were graduates of diploma programs which were hospital-based and usually three years in length. Entrance requirements included graduation from a college preparatory program in high school. With the advent of the associate degree and baccalaureate degree programs, the diploma programs have steadily declined in number.

diploneural (dip-lō-nū′-ral): Being supplied with two nerves; said of certain muscles.

diplopia (dip-lō′-pi-a): Double vision; the perception of two images of only one object.

diplopiometer (dip-lō-pi-om′-e-ter): A device for measuring diplopia.

diplosomatia (dip-lō-sō-mā′-shi-a): The condition of being completely formed twins that are joined at some part of their bodies.

dipodia (dī-pō′-di-a): A congenital anomaly characterized by the presence of an extra foot.

dipsesis (dip-sē′-sis): Thirst.—dipsetic, adj.

dipsogen (dip′-sō-jen): An agent that induces thirst and intake of fluids.

dipsomania (dip-sō-mā′-ni-a): Alcoholism in which uncontrollable drinking occurs in bouts, often with long periods of sobriety between.—dipsomaniac, adj., n.

dipsophobia (dip-sō-fō′-bi-a): Abnormal fear of drinking, particularly of alcoholic beverages.

dipsosis (dip-sō′-sis): Abnormal thirst, or a craving for unusual drinks.

dipsotherapy (dip-sō-ther′-a-pi): Treatment by withholding or limiting the amount of fluid allowed the patient.

dipstick (dip′-stik): A strip of cellulose impregnated with chemicals that will react with certain substances in the urine and discolor the strip.

dipus (dī′-pus): Having two feet; usually refers to a conjoined twin monster that has only two feet.

direct (di-rekt′): 1. Straight. 2. Without anything between or intervening. **D. CONTACT,** referring to the passing of a disease directly from one person to another. **D. CURRENT,** an electric current that flows continuously; opp. to alternating current. **D. TRANSFUSION,** tranfusion of blood directly from one person to another.

director (di-rek′-tor): 1. A grooved instrument used for guiding the knife in surgical operations. 2. A person in a position involving guiding or directing.

Director of Nursing: A professional nurse who is responsible for the care of patients in a health care facility, for administering the nursing department, for the development and evaluation of nursing staff members, and for determining the standards of nursing care and the policies for the nursing department.

dirt-eating: Geophagia or chthonophagia (*q.v.*).

dis-: Prefix denoting: 1. To do the opposite of; reverse; deprive of; exclude. 2. Absence of; opposite of. 3. Not. 4. Same as dys-.

disability: As a medical term, refers to any lasting impairment of physiological, anatomical, or psychological functioning caused by an injury, illness, or birth defect, with resultant loss of learning power, or limitation of one's capacity to perform some key life functions or activities.

disaccharidase (dī-sak′-a-ri-dās): An enzyme that acts to hydrolyze disaccharide into two monosaccharides.

disaccharide (dī-sak′-a-rīd): Any one of a class of carbohydrates ($C_{12}H_2O_{11}$) that yields two molecules of monosaccharide on hydrolysis, *e.g.*, lactose, maltose, sucrose.

disacchariduria (dī-sak′-a-rī-dū′-ri-a): The presence of a disaccharide in the urine; usually refers to either lactose or sucrose.

disarticulation (dis-ar-tik-ū-lā′-shun): A disjointing, or separation at a joint.

disc (disk): Disk (*q.v.*).

discharge (dis-charj′): 1. To liberate or set free. 2. Material that is expelled, evacuated, or flows away from a body cavity or wound, *e.g.*, feces, urine, pus. 3. The flowing away of a secretion or excretion. 4. To release a patient from a health care facility.

dischronation (dis-krō-nā′-shun): A disturbance in one's consciousness of time.

discission (di-sizh′-un): A cutting into or division; specifically, the rupturing of the lens capsule in surgery for soft cataract.

discitis, diskitis (dis-kī′-tis): Inflammation of a disc, particularly an intervertebral or articular disk.

discoid (dis′-koyd): Having the shape of a disk.

discrete (dis-krēt′): Separate; not continuous. Often said of skin lesions that do not blend or join others. Opp. to confluent (*q.v.*).

discrimination (dis-krim-i-nā′-shun): The ability to perceive distinctions. **D. IN HEARING**, the ability to discriminate between words having the same or very similar sounds.

discus (dis′-kus): A disk.

disease (di-zēz′): Sickness, illness. A departure from a state of health caused by an interruption or modification of any of the vital functions, and characterized by a definite train of symptoms. **ACUTE D.**, an abnormal condition of the body characterized by sudden onset of symptoms of a violent nature, and by a short course terminating in either recovery or death. **CHRONIC D.**, an abnormal condition of the body; of long continuance; marked by lack of violent symptoms, sometimes ending in recovery. **COMMUNICABLE D.**, one that is transferable from one person to another by means of the causative organism. **CONGENITAL D.**, one that is present at birth; may or may not be due to hereditary factors. **DEGENERATIVE D., D.** that is the result of cellular and tissue changes that occur naturally in old age. **FUNCTIONAL D.**, dysfunction of some part of the body with no obvious pathology to account for it. **HEREDITARY D., D.** that is transferred from parent to offspring genetically. **IATROGENIC D., D.** induced by a physician or by a treatment being utilized for some other condition. **IDIOPATHIC D., D.** for which the cause is not known. **INFECTIOUS D., D.** that may be transmitted. **PSYCHOSOMATIC D., D.** that originates in the person's mind or emotions. **SUBCLINICAL D., D.** in which the symptoms have not yet appeared. **TERMINAL D., D.** from which the person cannot be expected to recover.

disengagement (dis-en-gāj′-ment): 1. The emergence from a confined space, in particular the emergence of the infant's head from the vagina during childbirth. 2. A process in which the individual withdraws from society, disregards personal obligations and ties, and is in turn disregarded by society; happens chiefly in the elderly. **D. THEORY**, implies that both society and the aged prepare for death by withdrawal and by gradually reducing their life contacts, a process that leads to poor relationships, egocentricity, and, sometimes, depression; often the result of physiological deficits such as deafness.

disequilibrium (dis-ē′-qwi-lib′-ri-um): Lack or loss of balance; may be physical or mental. **D. SYNDROME**, a condition seen in persons who are severely catabolic; marked by restlessness, twitching, jerking, mental confusion.

disimpact (dis-im-pakt′): To remove an impaction, as of feces in the rectum.—disimpaction, n.

disinfect (dis-in-fekt′): To kill pathogenic organisms by physical or chemical means or to cause them to become inert; refers particularly to cleansing of inanimate objects.—disinfection, n.

disinfectant (dis-in-fek′-tant): An agent that is used to destroy pathogenic organisms or to cause them to be inert.—disinfectant, adj.

disinfection (dis-in-fek′-shun): A vague term, implying the destruction of pathogenic microorganisms, except spores, by physical or chemical means; can refer to the action of antiseptics as well as disinfectants.

disinfestation (dis′-in-fes-tā′-shun): Extermination of such infesting agents as insects, parasites, or rodents, especially lice. Delousing.

disinhibition (dis′-in-hi-bish′-un): The abolition or removal of an inhibition.

disintegrate (dis-in′-te-grāt): To decompose or break up.—disintegration, n.

disintoxication (dis′-in-tok-si-kā′-shun): 1.

Detoxication (*q.v.*). 2. Treatment to assist an addict to overcome his drug habit.

disjoint (dis-joynt′): To separate at a joint or to disarticulate; said of separating bones from their natural relationships at joints.

disk: A circular or rounded, flattened organ or structure. ARTICULAR D., a fibrocartilage or fibrous tissue pad found in some synovial joints. INTERVERTEBRAL D., a layer of fibrocartilage between the bodies of the vertebrae; consists of a fibrous ring with a pulpy center. OPTIC D., the intraocular portion of the optic nerve formed by the fibers converging from the retina and appearing as a white disk. SLIPPED D., herniated D., see under herniated. Also disc, discus.

diskectomy (dis-kek′-to-mi): The surgical removal of an intervertebral disk. Also discectomy.

diskitis (dis-kī′-tis): Inflammation of a disc; usually refers to an intervertebral disk. Also discitis.

diskogram (disk′-ō-gram): Roentgenogram of an intervertebral disk(s) following injection of a radiopaque medium. Also discogram.

diskography (dis-kog′-ra-fi): X ray of an intervertebral disk after it has been rendered radiopaque.—diskographic, adj.; diskographically, adv.; diskograph, n. Also discography.

diskopathy (dis-kop′-a-thi): Any disease or disorder involving an intervertebral disk. Also discopathy.

dislocation (dis-lō-kā′-shun): A displacement of organs or articular surfaces, more especially of a bone at a joint; accompanied by pain and deformity. Syn., luxation.—dislocated, adj.; dislocate, v.

dismemberment (dis-mem′-ber-ment): Amputation of an extremity or part of it.—dismember, v.

disobliteration (dis-ob-lit-er-ā′-shun): Removal of that which blocks a vessel, most often intimal plaques in an artery, when it is called endarterectomy (*q.v.*).

disorder (dis-or′-der): A disturbance or abnormality of physical or mental health or function.

disorientation (dis′-ō-ri-en-tā′-shun): Permanent or temporary loss of orientation or of the ability to identify one's self in relation to time, place, and person. May occur as a result of trauma, severe illness, the use of alcohol or certain drugs, or psychiatric disturbance. When it is a result of organic brain disease, D. for time and place occurs before D. for person.

disparate (dis′-pa-rāt): Unequal; not alike; unmatched.

dispensary (dis-pen′-sa-ri): 1. Once an important health care facility in urban United States; usually connected with a large hospital or medical center; provided clinic or outpatient care, usually to the indigent, at little or no cost. 2. A pharmacy in a hospital or clinic where medications are dispensed.

dispense (dis-pens′): In pharmaceutical practice, to prepare and deliver medicines.

dispersion (dis-per′-zhun): 1. The act of separating or scattering. 2. The incorporation of particles of one substance into another, as occurs in solutions and suspensions.—disperse, v.

displacement (dis-plās′-ment): 1. Removal from the normal position; dislocation. 2. In psychiatry, a defense mechanism whereby an emotion provoked by one person or situation is transferred to another less threatening person or situation. 3. In chemistry, the action whereby one substance in a compound is displaced by another, either by volume or by weight.—displaceability, adj.

disposition (dis-pō-zish′un): A prevailing tendency, mood, attitude.

disproportion (dis-prō-por′-shun): In anatomy, lack of normal relationship between two body areas or parts. CEPHALO-PELVIC D., in obstetrics, the head of the fetus is too large or the pelvis too small to allow the head to engage. See engagement.

dissect (dis-sekt′): 1. To cut apart or separate; applied particularly to tissues of a cadaver for anatomical study. 2. In surgery, to separate a structure by cutting or tearing along the natural lines rather than by making a wide incision.

dissection (di-sek′-shun): 1. The act or process of dissecting. 2. An anatomical specimen obtained by dissection. BLUNT D., a method of separating tissues along natural lines by using a finger or blunt instrument instead of cutting. SHARP DISSECTION, the separation of tissues by cutting with a scalpel, scissors, or other sharp instrument.

disseminated (dis-sem′-i-nā-ted): Widely extended, scattered, or distributed. D. INTRAVASCULAR COAGULATION, an acute or chronic disorder of clotting in which platelets and clotting factors are depleted by hemorrhage or some other circumstance; sometimes occurs as a secondary condition in trauma or following the administration of large amounts of thromboplastic substances. Abbreviated DIC.

dissimilate (dis-sim′-i-lāt): To break a substance down into its component parts; to produce energy or to separate out materials to be eliminated. The reverse of assimilate.—dissimilation, n.

dissociation (dis-sō′-shi-ā′-shun): 1. The separation or breakdown of a complex substance into simpler parts. 2. The release of ions in solution by electrovalent compounds; also called ionization. 3. In psychiatry, a defense mechanism in which the mind achieves non-recognition and isolation of certain unpalatable facts. This involves the actual splitting off from consciousness of all the unpalatable ideas so that the individual is no longer aware of them. D. is commonly observed in such involuntary states as hysteria, schizophrenia, fugue, somnambulism, and dual personality, but is seen in its most exaggerated form in delusional psychosis.

dissociation curve: A graphic curve showing the amount of oxygen that combines with hemoglobin in the blood; it shifts to the right when less than the normal amount of oxygen is taken up and to the left when the normal amount is taken up.

dissociative disorders: See under dissociation, 3.

dissolution (dis-sō-lū′-shun): 1. The chemical separation of a compound into its component elements. 2. The liquefaction of a solid substance. 3. Death.

dissolve (di-zolv′): 1. To cause a substance to pass into solution by placing it in a solvent. 2. To melt or liquefy a substance.

dissonance (dis′-sō-nans): A combination of tones that produce harsh or disagreeable sounds.

dist: Abbreviation for distilled or distil.

distal (dis′-tal): Farthest from the head, center, or any point of reference. Located away from the center of the body and toward the extremities.—distally, adv.; distad, adj. Cf. proximal.

distensible (dis-ten′-si-b'l): Capable of being distended.

distention (dis-ten′-shun): The state of being enlarged or distended. ABDOMINAL D., that which occurs after some operations when there is an abnormal accumulation of gas in the intestines.

distichia (dis-tik′-i-a): The presence of an extra row of eyelashes at the inner border of the eyelid, which turn in and rub on the cornea; a congenital anomaly.

distil, distill (dis-til′): To change a liquid to vapor by the application of heat and then, by cooling, to change the vapor to a liquid.

distillation (dis-til-ā′-shun): The process of driving off gas or vapor by heating solids or liquids, and then condensing the resulting product(s).—distil, distill, v.

distoclusion (dis′-tō-kloo′-zhun): Malocclusion of the teeth in which the teeth and lower jaw are in a distal or recessive position in relation to the upper jaw and teeth.

distomiasis (dis-tō-mī′-a-sis): Infestation with trematodes or flukes; most often the liver, gallbladder and bile ducts, lungs, or blood vessels.

distortion (dis-tor′-shun): The state of being twisted out of the natural position or shape. In psychiatry, a mechanism through which the individual disguises or denies material that he cannot accept and substitutes material that is less offensive to his self-concept.

distractibility (dis-trak′-ti-bil′-i-ti): Inability to focus or keep the attention on any one subject; susceptibility to distraction.

distraction (dis-trak′-shun): 1. The dislocation of joint surfaces caused by extension but without injury to the parts involved. 2. Anything that diverts the attention. 3. Great mental or emotional distress, confusion, or disturbance.

distress (dis-tres′): Anguish or suffering, physical or mental.

disulfide (dī-sul′-fīd): A chemical compound consisting of molecules in which there are two atoms of sulfur to one of the reference substance.

disulfiram (dī-sulf′-ir-am): An anti-intoxicant; a chemical substance that interferes with the metabolism of alcohol in the body; used in treatment of alcoholism. Trade name, Antabuse.

disuse phenomenon: A condition that results from a person's inability to benefit from rehabilitation therapy following an illness that prevented normal ambulation; therapy is directed to both physical and psychological causes.

diurese (dī-ū-rēs′): The act of causing or producing diuresis.

diuresis (dī-ū-rē′-sis): Increased secretion and excretion of urine.

diuretic (dī-ū-ret′-ik): 1. Having the effect of increasing the flow of urine. 2. An agent that increases the flow of urine.

diuria (dī-ū′-ri-a): Frequency of urination during the waking hours.

diurnal (dī-er′-nal): 1. Occurring or recurring during the daytime. 2. Recurring every day.

divalent (dī-vā′-lent): Having a valence of 2.

divergence (dī-ver′-jens): A spreading out or drawing apart from a common point. In ophthalmology, the abduction of one eye or of both eyes at the same time.—divergent, adj.

diversion (dī-ver′-zhun): A turning aside or the act of diverting from a course. URINARY D., the surgical procedure of creating an alternate route for the elimination of urine; following removal or all or part of the urinary bladder, the ureters are severed from the bladder and attached to the ileum or sigmoid, or they may be brought out to the surface of the abdominal wall. See ileal conduit under ileum.

diversional (dī-ver′-shun-al): Tending to produce relaxation or diversion. D. THERAPY, a pastime that causes a person to turn his thoughts away from himself and his problems.

divers' ear: Middle ear inflammation caused by sudden changes in atmospheric pressure; often a symptom in decompression sickness.

diverticulectomy (dī′-ver-tik-ū-lek′-to-mi): Surgical excision of a diverticulum (*q.v.*).

diverticulitis (dī′-ver-tik-ū-lī′-tis): Inflammation of one or more diverticula.

diverticulosis (dī′-ver-tik-ū-lō′-sis): A condition in which there are many diverticula, especially in the sigmoid colon.

diverticulum (dī′-ver-tik′-ū-lum): A circumscribed pouch or sac of variable size protruding from the wall of a tube or hollow organ; occurs chiefly in the intestine, but also in the rest of the alimentary tract, including the esophagus, and in the urinary tract; may be congenital or acquired. **MECKEL'S D.**, a blind tube that arises from the ileum at some distance from the ileocecal valve; it represents a persistent end of the embryonic yolk stalk. **ZENKER'S D.**, a pharyngoesophageal **D.**—diverticula, pl.; diverticular, adj.

divulse (di-vuls′): To separate or pull apart forcibly.—divulsion, n.

Dix, Dorothea, Lynde: Prominent American philanthropist and reformer, known for her influence in securing reforms in the treatment of the insane, prisoners, and the sick poor. As Superintendent of the U.S. Army nurses during the Civil War, she organized and directed volunteer women caretakers of the sick and wounded soldiers. [1802–1887].

dizygotic (dī′-zī-got′-ik): Referring to twins that develop from two fertilized ova; termed fraternal twins.

dizziness (diz′-i-nes): A disturbed, unpleasant sense of one's relationship to space, in which objects seem to whirl about; giddiness. May be due to disturbance in any of the body systems that normally keep one aware of his or her position in space.

DJD: Abbreviation for degenerative joint disease.

DNA: Abbreviation for deoxyribonucleic acid (*q.v.*).

DNA viruses: A group of viruses that includes the herpesviruses, adenoviruses, papoviruses, poxviruses, and the bacteriophages, all of which have a core of deoxyribonucleic acid.

DNR: Abbreviation for do not resuscitate.

D.O.: Abbreviation for Doctor of Osteopathy.

DOA: Abbreviation for dead on arrival.

Dobell's solution: An antiseptic solution formerly much used as a gargle, mouth wash; composed of sodium borate, sodium bicarbonate, phenol, glycerine, and water.

Dobhoff tube: A special long feeding tube that is inserted through the mouth into the duodenum; used for duodenal feedings.

doctor: 1. A person licensed to practice medicine, dentistry, or veterinary medicine. 2. To treat the sick or injured. 3. To dilute, tamper with, or falsify.

Döderlein's bacillus: A large, gram-positive, nonpathogenic rod bacterium commonly found in the vagina; also found in the intestine when the diet is rich in milk or milk products; said to be identical with *Lactobacillus acidophilus*. [Albert Döderlein, German obstetrician and gynecologist. 1860–1941.]

DOE: Abbreviation for dyspnea on exertion.

dolich-, dolicho-: Combining forms denoting long and/or narrow.

dolichocephaly (dol-i-kō-sef′-a-li): A condition in which the head is longer than it is broad.—dolichocephalus, n.; dolichocephalous, dolichocephalic, adj.

dolichocolon (dōl-i-kō-kō′-lon): An abnormally long and dilated colon.

dolichoderus (dol-i-kō-dēr′-us): Having an abnormally long neck.

dolichofacial (dol-i-kō-fā′-shal): Having an abnormally long face.

doll's-eye sign: A phenomenon that occurs when the eyeballs fail to turn to the right when the head is turned to the left, and vice versa; or that fail to turn downward when the head is turned up and back, and vice versa. This deviation from the normal reflex (failure to occur) indicates pressure on the midbrain and pons where the nuclei for the third, fourth, and sixth cranial nerves are located.

dolor (dō′-lor): Pain.

dolorific (dō-lor-if′-ik): Causing pain.

dolorology (dō-lor-ol′-ō-ji): The study of pain and its management.

domatophobia (dō-ma-tō-fō′-bi-a): Abnormal fear of being in a house or other closed structure; a type of claustrophobia.

domicillary care (dom′-i-sil-a-ri): Care provided in homes for the aged, supervised boarding homes, or other facilities for people who are not quite able to manage living independently.

dominance (dom′-in-ans): 1. In genetics, the ability of one of a pair of genes to suppress the other (recessive) gene. 2. In neurology, the tendency of one side of the brain to be more important than the other in controlling certain functions, *e.g.*, speech, handedness. 3. In psychiatry, a predisposition to play an important or controlling role in interpersonal relationships.

dominant (dom′-in-ant): In genetics, refers to a character possessed by one parent, which in the offspring masks the corresponding alternative character derived from the other parent. Opp. to recessive. See Mendel's law. **D. HAND**, the hand of greater skill, *e.g.*, in writing. **D. HEMISPHERE**, the cerebral hemisphere that appears to be more important in the control of body movements; it is contralateral to the **D.** hand.

donee (dō-nē′): One who receives something from another, as blood in a transfusion.

donor (dō′-nor): One who supplies living tissue or material to be used by another. **UNIVERSAL D.**, a person who has group O blood which, in an emergency, can safely be given to patients with blood of any type.

dopa (dō′-pa): An amino acid produced by the oxidation of tyrosine; a precursor of dopamine and an intermediate product in the synthesis of norepinephrine, epinephrine, and melanin. The naturally occurring form, L-dopa, and the synthetic form, levodopa, are used in the treatment of Parkinson's disease.

dopamine (dō′-pa-mēn): A neurotransmitter found in the brain; an intermediate product in the synthesis of epinephrine and norepinephrine, which increases cardiac output and renal blood flow but does not produce peripheral vasoconstriction. In Parkinson's disease there is a depletion of dopamine in the caudate nucleus of the brain.

dope (dōp): 1. Any drug taken habitually for other than medical purposes. 2. To administer or take a habit-forming drug. **D. ADDICT**, a person who is physically and psychologically dependent on a drug, due to habitual use.

Doppler: 1. **D. DEVICE**, a highly sensitive ultrasonic device for measuring the blood pressure of infants and children. 2. **D. EFFECT**, the observable change in the frequency of an acoustic or electromagnetic wave; due to the relative movement of the source of the wave and the observer away from or toward each other. **D. FLOWMETER**, an ultrasonic device for measuring the circulation of blood in the extremities. **D. PHENOMENON** or **PRINCIPLE**, see D. effect. **D. SHIFT**, the amount of change in the frequency of light, sound, or frequency waves that occurs as the wave source and the observer move toward or away from each other. **D. ULTRASONIC TEST**, a test that utilizes an ultrasonic probe and transducer for detecting shifts in sound that are reflected from a blood vessel and augmented by an audio speaker. [Christian Johann Doppler, Austrian physicist and mathematician. 1803–1853].

doraphobia (dor-a-fō′-bi-a): Abnormal fear of touching the skin or fur of animals.

dorsad (dor′-sad): Toward the back.

dorsal (dor′-sal): Pertaining to the back, or the posterior part of an organ. Opp. to ventral. **D.** surface of the foot refers to the top of the foot; **D.** surface of the hand refers to the back of the hand. **D. RECUMBENT POSITION**, see under position.

dorsalgia (dor-sal′-ji-a): Pain in the back.

dorsi-, dorso-: Combining forms denoting relationship to the back or back part of the body.

dorsiduct (dor′-si-dukt): To draw toward the dorsum or the back.

dorsiflexion (dor-si-flek′-shun): Bending backwards, as of the hand or foot. In the case of the great toe—upwards. See Babinski's reflex.

dorsocentral (dor-sō-sen′-tral): At the back and in the center.

dorsolateral (dor-sō-lat′-er-al): Toward or pertaining to the back and the side of the body.

dorsolumbar (dor-sō-lum′-bar): Pertaining to the back in the region of the lower thoracic and upper lumbar vertebrae.

dorsomedial (dor-sō-mē′-di-al): Pertaining to or toward the midline of the back of the body.

dorsonasal (dor-sō-nā′-zal): Pertaining to the bridge of the nose.

dorsonuchal (dor-sō-nū′-kal): Pertaining to the back of the neck.

dorsosacral (dor-sō-sā′-kral): Pertaining to the dorsal and sacral regions. **D. POSITION**, lithotomy position; see under position.

dorsum (dor′-sum): The back or the surface that corresponds to the back.—dorsa, pl.

dosage (dō′-sij): 1. The determination of the proper amount of a medicinal agent to be given. 2. The giving of prescribed amounts of a medicinal agent. 3. The amount of a medication to be given at one time.

dose (dōs): A quantity of any therapeutic agent to be given at any one time, or at stated intervals, as an amount of medicine or a quantity of radiation. **BOOSTER D.**, one given some time after a primary immunization to maintain protection of the individual. **DIVIDED D.**, one given in fractional amounts at specific intervals. **ERYTHEMA D.**, the smallest amount of radiation that will produce reddening of the skin within ten days to two weeks after application. **LETHAL D. (LD)**, one likely to cause death. **MAINTENANCE D.**, one given in protracted illness to keep the patient under an influence achieved by an initial dose of a drug. **MAXIMUM D.**, the largest amount of a drug that can be given with safety. **MINIMUM D.**, the smallest amount of a drug that will produce the desired effect. **MINIMAL LETHAL DOSE (MLD)**, the smallest amount of toxin that will kill a laboratory animal. **OPTIMAL D.**, the amount of an agent that will produce the desired effect without any undesirable effects. **SENSITIZING D.**, the initial **D.** of an allergen; the patient has no antibodies to it.

dosimeter (dō-sim′-e-ter): A device that measures the amount of exposure to x rays or other radioactive emanations; worn by health care personnel who are in frequent contact with radioactive substances or emanations.

dosimetry (dō-sim′-e-tri): The determination of dosages. In radiography, the measurement of doses of x-ray or of radioactive emanations.

dossier (dōs′-ē-ā): The file that contains the accumulated case history of a patient.

dotage (dō′-tij): Senility; mental weakness or foolishness in the aged.

dotard (dō′-tard): A person who is his dotage.

double: **D. DECOMPOSITION,** a chemical reaction in which the ions of two compounds exchange places and two new compounds are formed. **D. PNEUMONIA,** pneumonia in both lungs. **D. VISION,** diplopia (*q.v.*).

double-blind: Refers to a manner of conducting experiments with neither experimenter nor subjects knowing the controlling elements; the objective is to secure statistically reliable results.

douche (doosh): A stream of water, gas or vapor directed against the body or into a body cavity for cleansing or therapeutic purposes.

"doughnut": A simple doughnut-shaped device made of cotton wrapped with gauze bandage; used to protect heels, elbows, and other pressure points where decubitus ulcers are likely to develop.

Douglas' pouch: Rectouterine pouch; see under pouch.

dowager's hump: Kyphosis of the upper back resulting from osteoporosis, particularly of the thoracic spine.

downer or downs: Slang for a drug or drugs having a depressive action.

Downey cells: Atypical lymphocytes, which may be seen on a peripheral blood smear from a patient with infectious mononucleosis and certain other viral infections.

Down's syndrome: A congenital anomaly caused by one of two types of abnormality of chromosome 21: 1) failure of the chromosome to divide; infants with this anomaly are usually born of older mothers; 2) an abnormality within the chromosome itself with the total number of chromosomes being normal; infants with this anomaly are usually born of younger mothers, and there is high risk of recurrence in subsequent pregnancies. This syndrome is characterized by mental subnormality and such physical features as oval tilted eyes, short flat-bridged nose, thickened tongue, flattened occiput, pallor, smaller than normal brain, broad hands and feet with widened space between first and second digits, stubby fingers, hyperflexibility of joints, and generally retarded growth. Also called mongolism and Trisomy 21.

doxogenic (dok-sō-jen′-ic): Caused by or resulting from one's own mental processes and conceptions, said of certain diseases.

D.P.: Abbreviation for: 1. Doctor of Pharmacy; 2. Doctor of Podiatry.

D.P.H.: Abbreviation for Diploma in Public Health.

DPT: Abbreviation for diphtheria-pertussis-tetanus (vaccine).

DQ: Abbreviation for developmental quotient.

dr: Abbreviation for dram.

drachm: See dram.

dracunculiasis (drā-kung′-kū-lī′-a-sis): Infestation with the guinea worm, *Dracunculus medinensis;* symptoms include ulcerative lesions on the lower extremities, pruritus, nausea, vomiting, dyspnea; seen chiefly in the Near East, Central Africa, China.

Dracunculus medinensis (dra-kung′-cū-lus med-i-nen′-sis): The guinea worm (*q.v.*); a parasitic worm that inhabits the subcutaneous and intermuscular tissues of certain animals and in man in whom it causes ulcers of the feet and legs; seen particularly in Africa, Arabia, and India; the embryos of the organism are discharged into raw water through a break in the skin and taken up by small custraceans, which serve as the intermediate host.

draft, draught (draft): 1. A current of air circulating in a limited space. 2. A large dose of liquid medicine to be taken at a single swallow.

dragee (dra-zhā′): A large sugar-coated capsule or pill.

drain (drān): 1. To draw off by degrees an accumulation of such material as pus, lymph, or secretion. 2. A device or substance that provides a channel or means of exit for the discharge from a wound or cavity.

drainage (drān′-ij): The withdrawal, or flow, of fluid from a wound or cavity. **POSTURAL D.,** that achieved by putting the patient in a position in which gravity aids the process. **TIDAL D.,** drainage of a paralyzed urinary bladder utilizing an apparatus that allows for filling the bladder to a certain level and then emptying it either by siphonage or gravity. **UNDERWATER SEAL D.,** a chest drainage system that prevents air from reentering the chest; involves the use of a bottle containing normal saline solution, with two tubes going through openings in the bottle cap, one of which is submerged in the solution and the other attached to the patient's chest catheter. As the patient breathes, air bubbles up in the solution and escapes through the second tube. More complicated systems utilize two or three bottles and allow for suctioning. **D. TUBE,** a hollow tube of glass, rubber, or other material, inserted into a cavity or a wound to allow fluids to escape.

dram: One-eighth of an ounce, in the Apothecaries' System; 60 grains by weight; 60 minims by fluid measurement; one teaspoonful by household measurement.

drape (drāp): A sheet of fabric or other material used to cover parts of the body that do not need to be exposed for examiniation or carrying out a procedure.—drape, v.

drastic (dras′-tik): Term applied to a treatment or medication that has a powerful or thorough effect.

draw sheet: A narrow sheet placed crosswise on the bed to protect the lower sheet. It can be removed when soiled by pulling to the side.

drawer sign: A sign considered diagnostic of rupture of the cruciate ligament of the knee; the patient sits with the knee flexed at 90°; if the tibia glides anteriorally, the anterior cruciate ligament is ruptured; if the tibia glides posteriorally, the posterior cruciate ligament is ruptured.

drepanocyte (drep′-a-nō-sīt): A sickle cell (*q.v.*).

drepanocytemia (drep′-nō-sī-tē′-mi-a): Sickle cell anemia; see under anemia.

dressing (dres′-ing): 1. Any material or substance applied to a wound or lesion to cover it, to prevent infection, to aid in healing, or to absorb drainage. 2. The application of any one of various materials to protect or cover a wound or lesion. **DRY D.**, a **D.** consisting of dry material such as absorbent gauze. **WET D.**, a **D.** that has been moistened with plain water or a fluid containing a medication.—dressings, pl.

Dressler beat: A fusion beat heard in digitalis toxicity; indicates that an ectopic impulse is originating in the ventricle.

Dressler's syndrome: Post-myocardial infarction syndrome (*q.v.*).

DRG: Abbreviation for Diagnosis Related Groups (*q.v.*).

dribble (drib′-'l): 1. To drool. 2. To fall in drops, as urine from the bladder of patients with distended or paralyzed bladder.

drift: 1. A condition caused by muscle weakness following mild hemiparesis; the hand pronates when the patient stands with arms outstretched and the palms facing each other; the foot becomes everted when the patient sits with legs extended, feet together, and eyes closed. 2. Movement of teeth from their normal position, due to loss of other teeth.

Drinker respirator: An alternating pressure machine for administering artificial respiration; consists of a metal tank that encloses the entire body except the head; often called an iron lung.

drip: 1. To instill a medication drop by drop, *e.g.*, eye drops. 2. The slow continuous drop-by-drop administration of a solution into a body cavity. **INTRAVENOUS D.**, continuous drop-by-drop instillation of a solution into a vein; nutrients or drugs may be added to the solution. **MURPHY D.**, continuous drop-by-drop instillation of fluid into the rectum. **POSTNASAL D.**, dripping of irritating material from the posterior nares into the pharynx, often a feature of sinusitis.

drive: 1. An urgent, instinctive need that causes one to press for its satisfaction, *e.g.*, the sex drive. 2. A powerful concern or interest that motivates one to consistent and continual effort.

dromomania (drō-mō-mā′-ni-a): An uncontrollable impulse to wander away from one's home.

dromophobia (drō-mō-fō′-bi-a): Morbid fear of walking about or roaming away from home.

dromotropic (drō-mō-trō′-pik): Having an effect on the conductivity of nerves. **D. DRUGS**, drugs that may speed up or slow conductivity of nerve impulses, depending on the drug.

drool: 1. To let saliva or other liquid run from the mouth. 2. To flow from the mouth, as saliva.

drooling (droo′-ling): Uncontrolled salivation.

drop: **D. ATTACK**, loss of equilibrium and falling, without vertigo or loss of consciousness, followed by rapid recovery. **D. FOOT.** an abnormal downward position of the foot due to paralysis of the flexors of the foot; often due to pressure of bedclothes on the foot or to poorly fitted casts or splints. Also called footdrop. **EAR D.**, medication to be dropped into the ear. **EYE D.**, medication to be dropped into the conjunctival sac. **NOSE D.**, medication to be dropped into the nose. **WRIST D.**, flaccid paralysis of the wrist as a result of injury to a nerve by fracture or trauma.

droplet (drop′-let): A very small drop. **D. INFECTION**, one transmitted by small droplets expelled when talking, sneezing or coughing. **D. NUCLEI**, microscopic particles that, when surrounded by moisture, become airborne.

dropsy (drop′-si): A common term used to describe an abnormal accumulation of fluid in cellular tissue or a cavity. See anasarca, ascites, hydrocephalus, hydrops, hydrothorax.—dropsical, adj.

drowsiness (drowz′-i-nes): A state of semi-wakefulness characterized by lethargy, sleepiness, lessened sensibility, sometimes confusion.

Dr.P.H.: Abbreviation for Doctor of Public Health.

drug: 1. A substance used in the diagnosis, prevention, or treatment of disease; often of vegetable or chemical origin. 2. A medicine or substance that is capable of modifying one or more functions of the body or mind. **D. ABUSE**, use of any drug for other than medical treatment. **D. ADDICTION**, a state in which habitual use of a drug has 1) created a strong physical and/or psychological dependence that cannot be controlled; 2) causes the individual to concentrate his activities on securing the required drug to the exclusion of other forms of socially acceptable activity; and 3) has resulted in a condition wherein withdrawal of the substance causes severe distress symptoms. **D. DEPENDENCE**, the physical need or psychological desire for continuous use of a drug over a period of time and the compulsion to take it continuously to experience its pleasurable effects and to prevent withdrawal symptoms; pertains to both drug abuse and drug addiction, including dependence on alcohol, the hallucinogens, narcotics, analgesics, tranquilizers, or marijuana. **D. REACTION,** an unexpected or undesirable effect produced by a drug and which may or may not be harmful, ranging from nausea, skin rash, nervousness, and gastrointestinal upset to anaphylactic shock; see anaphylactic. **D. RESISTANCE,** the ability to develop resistance to the bacteriostatic action of certain drugs. **D. TOLERANCE,** the decreasing effect of a drug with continued administration so that larger and larger doses are required to produce the same effect.

drug fever: Fever, with chills, urticaria, myalgia, angioedema, arthralgia; usually due to a hypersensitivity to certain drugs; may occur in a few days or up to two weeks after starting certain drug therapies.

drug-fast: A term used to describe resistance of bacteria to the bacteriostatic action of drugs.

drum: In anatomy, the ear drum or tympanic membrane. Also called drumhead.

drunkard's arm: See Saturday night palsy under palsy.

drunkenness: Intoxication, particularly that produced by alcoholic beverages.

drusen (droo′-sen): Small colloid or hyaline bodies seen in the retinal pigment cells in degeneration of Bruch's membrane (*q.v.*).

dry: Not wet; free from and not associated with moisture. **D. COUGH,** one not productive of mucus or phlegm. **D. GANGRENE,** death of tissue due to interference with the blood supply to the part. **DRY ICE,** solid carbon dioxide. **D. LABOR,** labor following premature rupture of the amniotic sac. **D. SOCKET,** alveolitis following extraction of a tooth.

dry eye syndrome: Lack of adequate secretion of tears; a common condition that may be due to irritation from any cause; is increased in persons taking diuretics and following cataract surgery. Symptoms include dryness of the conjunctiva, burning, sensation of a foreign body in the eye. Symptoms are increased in persons taking antihistamines or following cataract surgery. Treatment includes use of artificial tears or of a humidifier or vaporizer.

DTP: Diphtheria and tetanus toxoids combined with pertussis vaccine, used for active immunization of normal infants and children.

DTs: Abbreviation for delirium tremens. See delirium.

dual (doo′-al): Consisting of two parts. **D. PERSONALITY,** see under personality.

Dubin-Johnson syndrome: An inherited error in metabolism resulting in reduced capacity to excrete bilirubin; signs and symptoms include nonhemolytic jaundice and the presence of coarse brown granules in the cells of the liver.

Duchenne: [G.B.A. Duchenne, French neurologist. 1807–1875.] **DUCHENNE'S DISEASE,** tabes dorsalis; see under tabes. **DUCHENNE'S MUSCULAR DYSTROPHY,** pseudohypertrophic infantile muscular dystrophy; see under dystrophy. **DUCHENNE'S PARLYSIS,** progressive bulbar paralysis; see under paralysis.

Duchenne-Griesinger disease: An inherited disorder, marked by wasting and weakness of calf and shoulder muscles, waddling gait, scoliosis. Symptoms appear in childhood and increase until the individual is unable to walk; death usually occurs in early teens from respiratory infection. Also called pseudohypertrophic muscular dystrophy.

"duckbill" prosthesis: A device for laryngectomees; consists of a narrow tube with a valve at the end which allows lung air to be directed from the trachea to the esophagus. The Blom-Singer prosthesis.

Ducrey's bacillus (*Haemophilus ducreyi*) (dū-krāz′): Small gram-negative rod. The causative organism of soft chancre (chancroid), a venereal disease. [Augosto Ducrey, Italian dermatologist. 1860–1940.]

duct (dukt): A passageway or tube, especially one for the passage of secretions or excretions. **EJACULATORY DUCTS,** two fine tubes, one on either side, commencing at the union of the seminal vesicle with the vas deferens, and terminating at their union with the prostatic urethra.

duction (duk′-shun): 1. The act of leading, conducting, or bringing. 2. Movements of the eyes into positions upward, downward, toward the nose, and toward the temples.

ductless (dukt′-les): Having no duct, as the ductless glands. See endocrine gland.

ductule (dukt′-ūl): A small duct.

ductus (duk′-tus): Duct. **D. ARTERIOSUS,** a fetal blood vessel connecting the left pulmonary artery to the aorta, to bypass the lungs in the fetal circulation; it normally closes at birth. **D. VENOSUS,** a fetal blood vessel connecting the umbilical vein to the inferior vena cava, thus the venous blood bypasses the liver; it ceases to function at birth but remains in the liver as a ligament. See also common bile duct (ductus choledochus); ejaculatory ducts (ductus ejaculatorius); lactiferous ducts (ductus lactiferi); nasolacrimal duct (ductus nasolacrimalis); parotid duct (ductus parotideus), also called Stensen's duct; suderiferus duct (ductus suderiferus); thoracic duct (ductus thoracacius); vas deferens (ductus deferens).

Duhamel's operation: An operation to correct a congenital abnormality in the lower intestinal tract of infants with Hirschprung's disease (*q.v.*). See also megacolon.

duipara (dū-ip′-a-ra): A woman who has given birth to two viable children.

dull: 1. Lacking mental alertness. 2. Not sharp. 3. Not resonant, said of sounds heard on examination by percussion.

dumb (dum): 1. Mute; unable to speak. 2. Stupid (slang).

dum-dum fever: Kala-azar (*q.v.*).

dummy: Term sometimes used synonymously with placebo (*q.v.*).

dumping syndrome: The name given to the symptoms which often follow a partial gastrectomy—bilious vomiting, nausea, sweating, palpitation, and a feeling of faintness and weakness after meals.

Dunant, Henri: Swiss philanthropist whose work with the wounded at the battle of Solferino during the Napoleonic Wars inspired him to work for an organization to aid wounded soldiers and eventually led to the establishment of the International Red Cross in 1864. [1828–1920].

duodenal (dū-ō-dē′-nal, dū-od′-e-nal): Pertaining to or affecting the duodenum.

duodenectasis (dū-ō-de-nek′-ta-sis): Chronic dilatation of the duodenum.

duodenectomy (dū-ō-de-nek′-tō-mi): Surgical excision of all or part of the duodenum.

duodenitis (dū-od-e-nī′-tis): Inflammation of the duodenum.

duodenocholangeitis (dū-ō-dē′-nō-kōl-an-jē-ī′-tis): Inflammation of the duodenum and the common bile duct.

duodenocholecystostomy (dū-ō-dē′-nō-kō-lē-sis-tos′-tō-mi): Surgical creation of a passage between the gallbladder and the duodenum.

duodenoduodenostomy (dū-ō-dē′ nō-dū-ō-dē-nos′ tō-mi): An anastomosis of two sections of the duodenum, done to correct an abnormality that prevents duodenal contents from passing through the lumen.

duodenoenterostomy (dū-ō-dē′-nō-en-ter-os′-tō-mi): The formation of an anastomosis between the duodenum and another part of the intestine.

duodenoileostomy (dū-ō-dē′ nō-il-ē-os′-tō-mi): The surgical creation of an anastomosis between the duodenum and the ileum.

duodenojejunal (dū-ō-dē′-nō-je-joo′-nal): Pertaining to the duodenum and the jejunum.

duodenojejunostomy (dū-ō-dē′-je-joo-nos′-to-mi): Surgical formation of an anastomosis between the duodenum and the jejunum.

duodenopancreatectomy (dū-ō-dē′-nō-pan-krē-a-tek′-tō-mi): Surgical removal of part of the duodenum that encircles the head of the pancreas along with the head of the pancreas.

duodenorrhaphy (dū-ō-de-nor′-a-fi): Suturing of the duodenum following reparative surgery or injury.

duodenoscopy (dū-od-e-nos′-kō-pi): Examination of the interior of the duodenum by means of an endoscope.

duodenostomy (dū-od-e-nos′-tō-mi): Surgical creation of an opening into the duodenum with the establishment of a fistula between it and another cavity or the outside.

duodenotomy (dū-od-e-not′-ō-mi): Incision into the duodenum.

duodenum (dū-ō-dē′-num du-od′-e-num): The fixed, curved, first portion of the small intestine, eight to ten inches long, connecting the stomach above to the jejunum below.—duodenal, adj.

dupp (dup): A syllable used to describe the second sound heard at the apex of the heart in auscultation. It is higher pitched and shorter than the first sound, lupp.

Dupuytren's contracture: See under contracture.

dura mater (dū′-ra mā′-ter): The outermost, fibrous, and toughest of the three meninges that surround the brain and spinal cord.—dural, adj.

duritis (dū-rī′-tis): Inflammation of the dura; also called pachymeningitis.

duroarachnitis (dū′-rō-ar-ak-nī′-tis): Inflammation of the dura mater and the arachnoid membrane.

Dutch cap: A contraceptive device that covers the cervix.

dwarf (dwarf): 1. An abnormally short or undersized person, especially one whose body proportions are abnormal. 2. To prevent, or preventing normal growth and development.

dwarfism (dwarf′-izm): Abnormal smallness or development of the body. **AMSTERDAM D.,** a congenital syndrome in which severe mental retardation is associated with many anatomical abnormalities including short stature with short tapering fingers, short wide head, low-set ears, bushy eyebrows, fish-like mouth, excessive hairiness; 10 percent of the afflicted have epilepsy; also called deLange's syndrome. **PITUITARY D., D.** due usually to hypofunction of the hypophyseal or anterior lobe of the pituitary gland; but may also result from pituitary lesions or trauma, or from deficiency of thyrotrophic and adrenocorticotrophic hormones; in young persons characterized by stunted growth and development, childish appearance, and delayed sexual maturation; in older persons the outstanding characteristic is premature senility. **THANATOPHORIC D.,** severe congenital dwarfism with very small limbs, narrow chest, long head, flattened vertebral bodies; death occurs early due to pulmonary difficulties.

Dx: Abbreviation for diagnosis.

dyad (dī′-ad): A pair. A couple, *e.g.*, mother and father, mother and baby. In cytology, either of two spiral filaments that are joined by the centrosome and constitute a chromosome; they separate during cell division and each becomes a chromosome in the daughter cells.—dyadic, adj.

dynamic (dī-nam′-ik): Pertinent to or having physical energy or force. **D. PSYCHOLOGY**, a psychological approach that stresses the element of energy in mental processes.

dynamics (dī-nam′-iks): 1. The branch of mechanics that deals with forces and the laws governing them. 2. The various forces operating in a field. 3. The implementation of the mechanics of a situation or procedure. 4. In psychiatry, the determination of how individuals develop emotional reactions and patterns of behavior.

dynamogenesis (dī′-na-mō-jen′-e-sis): The generation of force or energy, especially as occurs in muscles and nerves in response to stimulation.

dynamometer (dī-na-mom′-et-er): An apparatus that measures the strength of a muscular contraction. **SQUEEZE D.**, a **D.** that measures the strength of the grip.

dynamoscope (dī-nam′-ō-scōpe): An instrument resembling a stethoscope for auscultating muscle contraction.

dyne (dīn): A unit of force; the amount of force that, when applied to a one-gram mass for one second, will accelerate the mass by one centimeter per second.

dys-: Prefix denoting painful, difficult, abnormal, diseased, impaired, faulty, poorly.

dysacousia (dis-a-koo͞′-zi-a): 1. An impairment of hearing in which the individual may be able to perceive sound but cannot discriminate certain syllables or words in terms of understanding them. 2. An impairment of hearing in which certain ordinary sounds produce pain or discomfort. Also disacousia, disacusis.

dysadrenalism (dis-ad-rē′-nal-izm): Any disorder of the adrenal gland or of adrenal function.

dysadrenocorticism (dis′-ad-rē-nō-kor′-ti-sism): Any disorder resulting from deranged function of the adrenal cortex and the cortical hormones.

dysaphia (dis-ā′-fi-a): Impairment in the sense of touch (pressure).

dysarthria (dis-ar′-thri-a): Difficulty in articulating words; may be due to a cerebellar disturbance, spasticity of the tongue or muscles of speech, or emotional stress.—dysarthric, adj.

dysarthrosis (dis-ar-thrō′-sis): Any joint deformity, disease or other condition limiting movement.

dysautonomia (dis-aw-tō-nō′-mi-a): Any dysfunction of the autonomic nervous systsm. **FAMILIAL DYSAUTONOMIA**, a hereditary condition characterized by motor incoordination, hyporeflexia, emotional instability, defective lacrimation; appears to occur most often in persons of Jewish descent; also called familial autonomic dysfunction.

dysbasia (dis-bā′-zi-a): Difficulty in walking, particularly when it is due to a nervous system lesion.

dysbulia (dis-bū′-li-a): Weakness of the will; uncertainty and indecisiveness.

dyscalculia (dis-kal-kū′-li-a): A decrease in one's ability to work mathematical problems; due to an injury to, or disease of, the brain.

dyscheiria (dis-kī′-ri-a): A disturbance of sensibility in which the person is unable to tell which side of the body has been touched. Also spelled dyschiria.

dyschesia (dis-kē′-zi-a): Constipation with accumulation of feces in the rectum and difficult or painful defecation. Also dyschezia.

dyschondroplasia (dis-kon-drō-plā′-zi-a): A disease affecting the growth of long bones, metacarpals and phalanges; the cartilage develops regularly but ossifies very slowly, thus arresting the growth of the long bones while the head and trunk develop normally. This produces a condition of stocky dwarfism.

dyschromatopsia (dis-krō-ma-top′-si-a): Disorder, impairment, or loss of color vision.

dyschromia (dis-krō′-mi-a): Any discoloration of the skin or hair.

dyscoria (dis-kō′-ri-a): Abnormal shape, form, or reaction of the pupil.

dyscrasia (dis-krā′-zi-a): An old term referring to the humors (*q.v.*) of the body; see **humeralism**. **BLOOD D.**, a general term for blood disease; often refers to a pathological condition marked by the presence of abnormal components in the blood.

dysdiadochokinesia (dis-dī-ad′-ō-kō-kī-nē′-si-a): Inability to perform alternating movements rapidly, *e.g.*, rotation or supination of the arm; usually indicates a cerebellar disorder; also sometimes seen in minimally brain-damaged children.

dysdipsia (dis-dip′-si-a): Difficulty in swallowing liquids.

dysendocriniasis (dis′-en-dō-krin-ī′-a-sis): Any functional disorder of the hormone-secreting glands.

dysentery (dis′-en-ter-i): A term for a variety of disorders that may be epidemic or endemic and that are characterized by inflammation and sometimes ulceration of the intestines accompanied by evacuation of watery stools containing blood and mucus and attended by colic and tenesmus. Causative agent is usually a bacterium, protozoon or parasitic worm that is spread chiefly through contaminated food or water. **AMEBIC D., D.** caused by the *Entamoeba histolytica*. **BACILLARY D., D.** caused by a bacillus of the genus *Shigella*. See **amebiasis**.—dysenteric, adj.

dysesthesia (dis-es-thē′-zi-a): Impairment of the sense of touch.

dysfunction (dis-funk′-shun): Abnormal functioning of any body organ or part. **COLONIC D.**, sluggish muscular action of the colon resulting in distention and constipation. **MINIMAL BRAIN D.**, that which may be caused by an inherited metabolic defect or damage or destruction of brain cells before birth; or it may follow infection with high fever, trauma, or lack of oxygen. Affected children may be hyperactive, have a short attention span, and be poor learners. **UTERINE D.**, the slowing down or cessation of uterine contractions during labor; inertia uteri.

dysgammaglobulinemia (dis-gam′-ma-glob′-ū-li-nē′-mi-a): Imperfect production or abnormality of the gamma globulins in the blood serum; often associated with poor resistance to infection.

dysgenesis (dis-jen′-e-sis): Malformation during embryonic development. **ALAR D.**, abnormal development of the sacroiliac joint. **GONADAL D.**, term applied to a variety of developmental anomalies involving the gonads; see pseudohermaphroditism, hermaphroditism, Turner's syndrome.

dysgerminoma (dis-jer-mi-nō′-ma): A solid ovarian or testicular tumor of low grade malignancy. It is not hormone-secreting, as it is developed from cells that date back to the undifferentiated state of gonadal development, *i.e.*, before the cells have either male or female attributes.

dysgeusia (dis-gū′-si-a): Impairment in the sense of taste, or perversion of taste; those affected often say that all foods have a vile taste.

dysgnosia (dis-nō′-si-a): Any disorder of intellectual function.

dysgraphia (dis-graf′-i-a): Impairment of the physical power to write; often the result of a brain lesion.

dyshematopoiesia (dis-hē′-ma-tō-poy-ē′-si-a): Imperfect blood formation.

dyshidrosis (dis-hid-rō′-sis): 1. Any abnormality in the production of sweat. 2. A vesicular skin eruption, occurring chiefly on the hands and feet; thought to be caused by a blockage of the sweat glands at their orifices; pompholyx (*q.v.*).

dyskeratosis (dis-ker-a-tō′-sis): Abnormal keratinization of epidermal tissue.

dyskinesia (dis-kī-nē′-si-a): Impairment of the ability to perform voluntary movements. **TARDIVE D.**, etiology not always known; may occur as a side effect of certain psychotropic drugs; characterized by facial tics and grimaces; blinking, chewing, sucking, and lip-smacking movements; choreoathetotic movements of the trunk may occur as well as torticollis, pelvic thrusting, foot-tapping; resembles parkinsonism in many ways.

dyslalia (dis-lā′-li-a): Difficulty in talking due to structural defect of speech organs.—dyslalic, adj.

dyslexia (dis-lek′-si-a): Impairment of the ability to read with comprehension; the child usually has difficulty with groups of letters, but the intelligence is unimpaired; often associated with poor instruction in reading, impaired hearing, or emotional stress.

dyslogia (dis-lō′-ji-a): 1. Delay or interference in the development of the power of speech; often due to a central nervous system lesion. 2. Inability to think logically or to reason.

dysmasesis (dis-ma-sē′-sis): Difficulty in mastication.

dysmaturity (dis-ma-tūr′-i-ti): Signs of incomplete or retarded growth at birth; "small for dates" (*q.v.*). To be distinguished from prematurity.

dysmelia (dis-mē′-li-a): A congenital malformation characterized by shortening or complete absence of one or more limbs.

dysmenorrhea (dis-men-ō-rē′-a): Painful or difficult menstruation. **CONGESTIVE D.**, that which occurs during the premenstrual period; may be due to ischemia and water retention; characterized by dull aching pain in the lower abdomen accompanied by feelings of depression and irritability. **PRIMARY D.**, seen mostly in girls in their mid- and late teens; arises 24 hours before menstruation starts and is worst during the first 12 hours; causes are muscle incoordination, changes in hormonal secretion; may be accompanied by nausea and diarrhea. **SECONDARY D.**, seen mostly in women in their late 20s; pain starts before menstruation begins and continues through the flow; may be due to retroversion of the uterus, to pelvic inflammation, or endometritis; may be accompanied by anxiety and depression. **SPASMODIC D.**, pain limited to the lower abdomen and back, accompanied by nausea and faintness; starts on the first day of the menses; due to muscle contractions.

dysmetria (dis-mē′-tri-a): Impairment of the sense of distance in controlling muscular action, *e.g.*, hand movements that overshoot the mark, as in the finger-nose test; seen in persons with cerebellar lesions.

dysmnesia (dis-nē′-si-a): A naturally poor or impaired memory.

dysmorphia (dis-mor′-fi-a): Deformity; abnormality in shape.

dysmorphogenesis (dis-mor-fō-jen′-e-sis): The process of abnormal tissue formation, particularly that which occurs in the developing fetus resulting in a malformed infant.

dysopia (dis-ō′-pi-a): Impaired vision.

dysorexia (dis-o-rek′-si-a): A diminished or unnatural appetite.

dysosmia (dis-oz′-mi-a): Impairment of the sense of smell.

dysosteogenesis (dis-os-tē-ō-jen′-e-sis): Defective bone formation. Also dysostosis.

dysostosis (dis-os-tō′-sis): Defective formation of a bone or bones. **CLEIDOCRANIAL D.**, defective ossification of cranial bones and of the clavicle. **CRANIOFACIAL D.**, a rare birth defect consisting of a premature closure of the skull sutures, underdevelopment of the maxillae, exophthalmos, strabismus, nystagmus. **MANDIBULOFACIAL D.**, Treacher-Collins syndrome (*q.v.*). **METAPHYSEAL D.**, a form of **D.** in which the metaphases of long bones are spottily calcified and remain largely cartilaginous.

dysoxia (dis-ok′-si-a): Abnormal utilization of oxygen by the tissues either because of diminished supply or because of impairment of the cells' ability to utilize oxygen.

dyspareunia (dis-pa-roo′-ni-a): Painful or difficult coitus in women.

dyspepsia (dis-pep′-si-a): Disturbed digestion, characterized by heartburn, gas, nausea and a sense of over-fullness; indigestion. May be due to morbid condition of some organ or part of the digestive system or to the psychic effects of emotional tension, anxiety, fits of temper, etc. dyspeptic, adj.

dysphagia (dis-fā′-ji-a): Painful or difficult swallowing; may result from local mouth or throat disorders, anxiety, or certain central nervous system disorders.

dysphasia (dis-fā′-zi-a): Loss or impairment of power to use or understand language due to injury or damage to the brain.—dysphasic, adj.

dysphemia (dis-fē′-mi-a): Stammering.

dysphonia (dis-fō′-ni-a): Unnatural sound of the voice, as hoarseness, or difficulty in pronouncing sounds; due to organic, functional, or psychic causes.

dysphoria (dis-fō′-ri-a): Unpleasant mood; malaise; restlessness. Opp. of euphoria.

dyspigmentation (dis′-pig-men-tā′-shun): A disorder of pigmentation; either the skin or the hair may be affected.

dysplasia (dis-plā′-zi-a): Abnormal development of organs, tissues, or cells. **CERVICAL D.**, a progressive **D.** of the cervix; seen most often in young women; may lead to carcinoma. **FIBROMUSCULAR D.**, idiopathic **D.** leading to stenosis of the arteries, especially the renal artery, causing hypertension; usually seen in young women. **MONOSTOTIC D., D.** in which only one bone becomes deformed due to displacement by fibrous tissue. **POLYOSTOTIC D.**, same as monostotic **D.** except that more than one bone is involved, usually on only one side of the body.

dyspnea (disp′-nē-a): Difficult or painful breathing. **EXERTIONAL D.**, that which occurs during even moderate exercise and is relieved when the exercise is discontinued. **EXPIRATORY D., D.** in which the expiratory time is prolonged; caused by obstruction in the bronchioles or small bronchi; may be associated with asthma, bronchitis, or obstructive emphysema. **INSPIRATORY D., D.** caused by some hindrance to the intake of air; may be due to presence of a foreign body, laryngitis, tumor, or compression of the trachea; often stridulous. **NOCTURNAL D., D.** that increases steadily during the day until by night it is very distressing. **ORTHOSTATIC D., D.** that occurs when one is in the erect position. **PAROXYSMAL D., D.** that occurs when one is lying down, particularly at night; associated with congestive heart failure.

dyspraxia (dis-prak′-si-a): Difficulty in performing, or partial loss of ability to perform, coordinated movements.

dysproteinemia (dis-prō′-tē-in-ē′-mi-a): Any disorder or derangement of the protein content of the blood. **FAMILIAL IDIOPATHIC D., D.** due to a genetic defect that results in an increase in the production of globulin in relation to the albumin content.

dysraphism (dis′-ra-fizm): Failure of fusion between parts that normally unite.

dysreflexia (dis-rē-flek′-si-a): Abnormal or faulty physiological reflexes; may occur in patients with spinal cord injury; triggered by a distended bladder or rectum, or by hyperirritability of skin. **AUTONOMIC D.**, due to spinal cord injury at or above the T-6 level; occurs as a crisis in response to some noxious stimulus such as distended bladder or bowel, urinary stones, or decubitus ulcer; symptoms include pounding headache, facial flush, diaphoresis, and paroxysmal hypertension, the last resulting in retinal hemorrhage, seizures, and sometimes stroke, which may be fatal.

dysrhythmia (dis-rith′-mi-a): Disordered or abnormal rhythm. **CEREBRAL D.**, disturbance or irregularity of brain waves as recorded by electroencephalography.

dyssocial (dis-sō′-shul): Pertaining to the behavior of an individual who disregards the social and moral codes of the community and engages in predatory, illegal, sometimes criminal, activities.

dysstasia (dis-stā′-si-a): Difficulty in standing.

dyssynergia (dis-sin-er′-ji-a): A disturbance in muscular coordination; due to lack of cooperation between agonist and antagonist muscles that usually act in unison. Ataxia.

dystaxia (dis-tak′-si-a): Difficulty in controlling voluntary movements. Mild ataxia (*q.v.*).

dysthanasia (dis-tha-nā′-zi-a): Slow, painful death.

dysthesia (dis-thē′-zi-a): Impatience, ill temper, fretfulness.

dysthymia (dis-thī′-mi-a): 1. Any condition that is attributed to a malfunctioning thymus during childhood. 2. In psychiatry, mental depression or despondency; may be associated with hypochondriasis.

dystocia (dis-tō′-si-a): Difficult, slow, or abnormal labor or delivery.

dystonia (dis-tō′-ni-a): Disordered or defective muscle tone. **D. MUSCULORUM DEFORMANS,** a relatively rare hereditary disease characterized by involuntary contractions of muscles, particularly those of the trunk, arms, and legs, which occur chiefly when walking.—dystonic, adj.

dystopia (dis-tō′-pi-a): Displacement or malposition of an organ.—dystopic, adj.

dystrophia (dis-trō′-fi-a): Dystrophy. **D. ADIPOSO-GENITALIS,** Fröhlich's syndrome (*q.v.*).

dystrophy (dis′-trō-fi): Term applied to many disorders, musculoskeletal disorders in particular, that arise from faulty nutrition. **FUCH'S D., D.** characterized by erosion of the epithelium of the cornea. **LANDOUZY-DÉJERINE D.**, a form of muscular **D.** in which there is atrophy of the face, shoulder girdle and arm; characterized by inexpressive face, drooping shoulders, contractures, absent tendon reflexes, inability to raise the arms; also called facioscapulohumeral D. **LIMB-GIRDLE D.**, a hereditary, slowly progressive type of muscular **D.**; begins in childhood; may involve either the shoulder or pelvic girdle. **MUSCULAR D.**, a group of familial, progressive, primary degenerative muscle disorders characterized by atrophy and wasting away of muscles, affecting primarily children and young adults; of unknown cause. Several types are recognized with the **DUCHENNE TYPE** being the most severe; onset begins before five years of age; characterized by pseudohypertrophy of muscles followed by atrophy, skeletal deformities, lordosis, protruding abdomen, congestive heart failure, and frequent respiratory infections. **MYOTONIC D., D.** characterized by progressive weakness and atrophy of muscles of the face and limbs especially, early baldness, cataracts, often mental deficiency. **SYMPATHETIC REFLEX D., D.** characterized by superficial or deep pain in an upper or lower extremity, with throbbing, burning, aching, local edema and erythema; occurs after some physical disturbance in that extremity. **VITELLIFORM D.**, congenital degeneration of the macula; occurs in childhood; characterized by yellow or reddish lesions that eventually form pigmented areas on the macula, causing loss of central vision; syn., Best's disease.

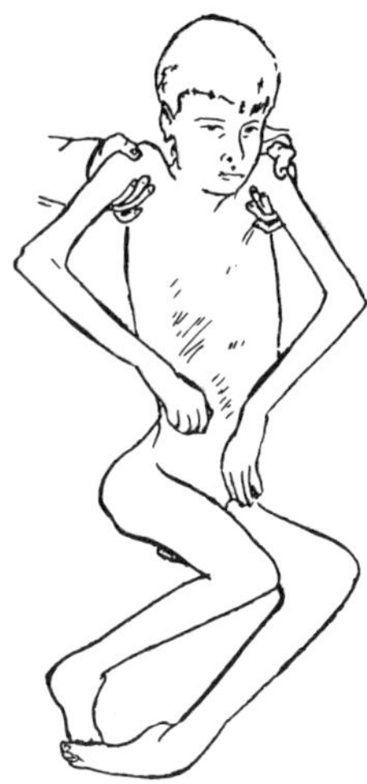

Muscular dystrophy

dysuria (dis-ū′-ri-a): Difficult or painful urination.

E

E. coli (kō′-li): See Escherichia coli, under Escherichia.

E trisomy: See under trisomy.

Eagle test: A precipitation test for syphilis.

ear: The organ of hearing. **EXTERNAL E.**, consists of the semicircular flap on the side of the head called the auricle or pinna and the external auditory meatus or canal that extends to the middle ear from which it is separated by the tympanum or ear drum. **MIDDLE E.**, consists of an air-containing cavity, bounded laterally by the tympanum; anteriorly it communicates with the eustachian tube and thus with the throat. Stretched across this cavity are the tiny bones, the malleus, incus and stapes; these bones are in contact with the tympanic membrane and with one of the openings into the inner ear; their function is to transmit sound waves from the tympanum to the inner ear. **INTERNAL** or **INNER E.**, the deepest part of the ear; consists of a bony labyrinth in which a similar membranous labyrinth is suspended in a fluid called perilymph. It is divided into the vestibule, cochlea and three semicircular canals and contains a fluid called endolymph. Its walls hold the endings of the nerve of hearing. **E. DRUM**, the membrane that separates the external from the middle ear; also called tympanic membrane, tympanum. **E. LOBE**, the lower, usually fleshy part of the pinna. **E. PLUG**, a small device of wax, rubber, or plastic worn in the external auditory canal to keep out noise, water when swimming, etc. E. wax, cerumen (*q.v.*).

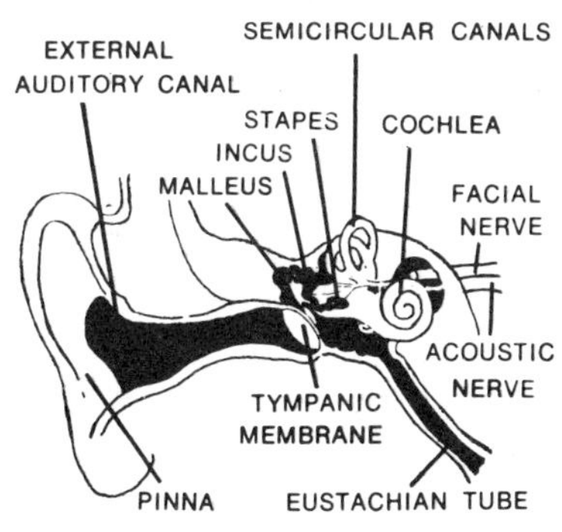

The ear

ear drops: Liquid medication to be instilled into the external canal of the ear, drop by drop.

earache (ēr′-āk): Pain in the ear. Syn., otalgia, otodynia.

Early Periodic Screening Diagnosis and Treatment: A requirement of the Medicaid program that all states maintain a program for determining the physical and mental defects of children in the program and provide both short- and long-term care. Abbreviated EPSDT.

Eastern equine encephalitis: See under encephalomyelitis.

Eaton agent: A species of *Mycoplasma pneumoniae,* the causative agent in primary atypical pneumonia, an acute systemic disease involving the lungs and characterized by high fever, cough, debility.

Eaton-Lambert syndrome; a condition of myasthenia most often seen in patients with oat-cell carcinoma of the lung; the muscles of the trunk, pelvis, and shoulder girdle are most affected. Also called Lambert-Eaton syndrome.

EB virus: Epstein-Barr virus (*q.v.*).

Eberthella: Former name for *Salmonella typhi,* the causative agent in typhoid fever. [Karl J. Eberth, German physician. 1835–1926.]

Ebola virus disease: First recorded in the U.S. in 1976. Involves cutaneous lymph nodes; symptoms include headache, muscle and abdominal pain, diarrhea, intravascular clotting; often fatal.

ebonation (ē-bō-nā′-shun): Removal of bone fragments from a wound after an injury.

ebriety (ē-brī′-e-ti): Habitual drunkenness. Also inebriety, ebrietas.

Ebstein's anomaly: Malformation of the leaflets of the tricuspid valve, usually associated with a septal defect. The valve is displaced downward into the right ventricle causing dilatation of the right atrium and cardiomegaly.

ebullition (eb-ū-lish′-un): 1. The state or process of boiling; effervescence. 2. A sudden, violent emotional outburst.

eburnation (ē-bur-nā′-shun): A disease condition in which bone becomes dense and hard like ivory.

ecbolic (ek-bol′-ik): Any agent that stimulates contraction of the gravid uterus and hastens expulsion of its contents.

eccentric (ek-sen′-trik): 1. Abnormal or peculiar in manner, speech, or ideas. 2. Proceeding outward from a center.

ecchondroma (ek-kon-drō′-ma): A benign tumor composed of cartilage that protrudes from the surface of the bone in which it arises. Also ecchondrosis.

ecchymoma (ek-i-mō′-ma): A slight hematoma or swelling due to a bruise and resulting from subcutaneous extravasation of blood.

ecchymosis (ek-i-mō′-sis): An extravasation of blood under the skin; marked by purple discoloration gradually changing to brown, green, yellow. Syn., bruise.—ecchymoses, pl.; ecchymosed, ecchymotic, adj.

eccoprotic (ek-ō-prot′-ik): Purgative; laxative.

eccrine (ek′-rin): Of or pertaining to secretions, particularly that of the sweat glands.

eccrinology (ek-ri-nol′-o-ji): The branch of anatomy and physiology that deals with the secretions and excretions of the exocrine glands. See **exocrine**.

eccrisis (ek′-ri-sis): 1. The excretion of waste products from the body. 2. Any bodily waste; excrement.

eccyesis (ek-sī-ē′-sis): Ectopic pregnancy; See under **ectopic**.

ecdemic (ek-dem′-ik): Neither epidemic nor endemic, ecdemic refers to a disease that is carried to an area from a distant source.

ECF: Abbreviation for extracellular fluid.

ECG: Abbreviation for electrocardiogram. Also EKG.

echinococcosis (ek′-i-nō-kok′-ō-sis): Infestation with the larval form of a tapeworm of the genus *Echinococcus;* characterized by the formation of hydatid cysts, especially in the liver.

Echinococcus (ek-i-nō-kok′-us): A genus of small tapeworms that infest primarily carnivores; occasionally man becomes infested with the larvae which cause development of hydatid cysts, especially in the liver.

echoacousia (ek′-ō-a-koo′-si-a): A disturbance of hearing in which a sound is heard after the stimulus that produced it has ceased.

echocardiography (ek′-kō-kar-di-og′-ra-fi): A painless procedure for recording the echo produced by directing ultrasound waves through the chest wall; shows the position and motion of the heart walls and great vessels; particularly useful in evaluating certain heart structures and abnormalities and in diagnosing and treating valvular heart disease.

echoencephalography (ek′-ō-en-sef-a-log′-ra-fi): A noninvasive technique in which ultrasonic waves are beamed at both sides of the head; the echos from the central part of the brain, which are recorded on a graphic tracing, may indicate the presence of a central mass in the brain; useful in detecting abscesses, blood clots, injury, or tumor within the brain.—echoencephalogram, n.

echogram (ek′-ō-gram): The pictorial representation of body structures and activity obtained by recording the echo produced by a technique utilizing ultrasound.

echolalia (ek-ō-lā′-li-a): Pathologic, meaningless repetition of words or phrases one has just heard. Occurs most commonly in schizophrenia and dementia; sometimes in toxic delirious states. A characteristic of all infants' speech.—echolalic, adj.

echomimia (ek′-ō-mim′-i-a): Echopathy. A neurosis in which the individual purposelessly repeats the actions or words of another.

echo-ophthalmolography (ek′-ō-of-thal-mō-log′-ra-fi): The use of ecogram (*q.v.*) to examine the eye and its orbit for possible pathology or disorder.

echopony (ek-of′-o-ni): The echo of a vocal sound heard during auscultation of the chest.

echopraxia (ek′-ō-prak′-si-a): Pathologic, involuntary repetition of acts one has seen performed by others; often performed without any expression or emotion.—echopractic, adj.

echovirus (ek-ō-vī′-rus): Enteric Cytopathic Human Orphan, name given to a group of viruses originally found in stools of diseaseless children; most them appear to be harmless but several have been known to cause various respiratory infections, enteritis, and non-bacterial meningitis.

eclabium (ek-lā′-bi-um): Eversion of a lip or lips.

eclampsia (ek-lamp′-si-a): 1. A severe manifestation of toxemia of pregnancy, often accompanied by convulsions and sometimes coma; associated with hypertension, edema, proteinuria, oliguria; other symptoms include headache, blurred vision, gastric pain; complications include cerebral hemorrhage, retinal hemorrhage, sometimes with blindness, pulmonary edema, renal failure, premature detachment of the placenta. May also occur during the puerperium. 2. A sudden convulsive attack.—eclamptic, adj.

eclamptogenic (ek-lamp-tō-jen′-ik): 1. Convulsant; causing convulsions. 2. Causing eclampsia.

eclectic (ek-lek′-tik): Refers to the practice of selecting what seems to be the best from diverse systems, sources, etc. In medicine, refers to the use of biologic, psychologic, sociologic, and cultural factors by physicians in constructing the framework within which they practice.—eclecticism, n.

ecmnesia (ek-nē′-zia): Impaired memory for recent events with normal memory of remote ones. Common in old age and in early cerebral deterioration.

ecography (ē-kog′-ra-fi): The use of ultrasound as a diagnostic aid in differentiating between solid and cystic structures within the body. The technique involves measuring the variations in echoes reflected by ultrasonic vibration of bodies of varying density. Ultrasonography.

ecology (ē-kol′-o-ji): The branch of biology that deals with the interactions of organisms with their environments and with each other.

ecosystem (ē′kō-sis-tem): A community and its environment functioning as a unit in nature; ecological system.

ecphorize (ek-fō′-rīz): To revive a memory or an engram (*q. v.*).

ecphyadectomy (ek-fī-a-dek′-tō-mi): Appendectomy (*q. v.*)

ecphyaditis (ek-fī-a-dī′-tis): Appendicitis.

ECS: Abbreviation for: 1. Electroconvulsive shock. 2. Electrocerebral silence.

ecstasy (ek′-sta-sē): A state of exaltation, exhilaration or delight; a trance.—ecstatic, adj.

ecstrophy (ek′-strō-fī): Exstrophy (*q.v.*).

ECT: Abbreviation for electroconvulsive therapy. See electrotherapy.

ectad (ek′-tad): Outward; without.

ectasia (ek-tā′-zi-a): An overstretching or dilatation of a tubular organ or vessel. **MAMMARY DUCT E.**, inflammation of the collecting ducts of the mammary gland with a sticky multicolored discharge from the nipple, accompanied by pain, itching, and redness around the nipple. **SENILE E.**, dilated tufts of capillaries appearing as red or purplish spots on the skin of the upper chest and trunk of older persons.

-ectasia, -ectasis: Combining forms denoting dilatation, stretching.

ecthyma (ek-thī′-ma): A pyogenic skin infection occuring chiefly on the thighs and legs, most often seen in tramps, filthy persons, and neglected children and characterized by large flat papules, with hardened bases and thick brownish crusts, that ulcerate and heal with pigmented scars. A similar condition may occur in syphilis.

ecto-: Combining form denoting external, outer, outside, situated on, out of place.

ectoblast (ek′-tō-blast): The ectoderm (*q.v.*).

ectocardia (ek-tō-kar′-di-a): A congenital condition in which the heart is misplaced, either within or outside the thoracic cavity.

ectocinerea (ek-tō-si-nē′-rē-a): The cortical part of the gray matter of the brain.

ectocolostomy (ek-tō-kō-los′-to-mi): The surgical formation of a communication between the colon and the abdominal wall.

ectoderm (ek′-tō-derm): The external primitive germ layer of the embryo. From it are developed the skin structures, the nervous system, organs of special sense, mucous membrane of the mouth and anus, pineal gland and part of the pituitary and adrenal glands.—ectodermal, adj.

ectodermosis (ek′-tō-der-mō′-sis): Any disease or disorder due to congenital maldevelopment of an organ or tissue derived from the ectoderm, *e.g.*, skin, eyeball, retina, nervous system.

ectogenous (ek-toj′-e-nus) 1. Introduced from or originating outside the body. 2. Capable of developing apart from the host; said of bacteria, particularly the pathogens.—ectogenic, adj.

ectomorph (ek′-tō-morf): An individual whose body build tends to be lean and fragile, with thin muscles and slightly underdeveloped digestive organs. Compare with endomorph and mesomorph.—endomorphic, adj.

-ectomy: Combining form denoting a cutting out; surgical removal.

ectoparasite (ek-tō-par′-a-sīt): A parasite that lives on the exterior surface of its host.—ectoparasitic, adj.

ectopia (ek-tō′-pi-a): Displacement of an organ or structure, especially if congenital. **E. CORDIS**, displacement of the heart; may be in the abdomen or outside the chest wall. **E. LENTIS**, displacement of the crystalline lens of the eye. **E. VESICAE**, a congenital anomaly in which the urinary bladder protrudes through or opens onto the abdominal wall.—ectopic, adj.

-ectopia: Combining form denoting a condition in which an organ or part is out of place.

ectopic (ek-top′-ik): 1. Occurring at an abnormal time, in an abnormal place, or in an abnormal position. 2. Situated outside a normal position, said of an organ or part; may be congenital or acquired. **E. BEAT**, a heartbeat caused by an impulse that originates in an area other than the sinoatrial node. **E. FOCUS**, a group of cells in the heart which may or may not be able to control the heartbeat when the natural pacemaker fails to function normally. **E. GESTATION, E.** pregnancy. **E. PREGNANCY**, extrauterine pregnancy; the fertilized ovum fails to reach the uterus but becomes implanted elsewhere; in most cases the site is the fallopian tube but sometimes it is the peritoneal cavity. At about the 6th week of pregnancy, the tube ruptures, causing a surgical emergency. This is a serious condition and may be accompanied by severe pain, shock and intra-abdominal hemorrhage. Prognosis is good if diagnosis and treatment are early, poor if treatment is omitted or unduly delayed.

ectoplasm (ek′-tō-plazm): The outer layer of protoplasm of a cell.

ectopy (ek′-to-pi): Displacement or malposition.

ectozoa (ek-tō-zō′-a): Animal parasites living on the outside of the body of the host.—ectozoon, sing.

ectrodactylia (ek-trō-dak-til′-i-a): Congenital absence of one or more fingers or toes or parts of them.

ectrogeny (ek-troj′-e-ni): The congenital absence of any organ or part of the body.

ectromelia (ek-trō-mē′-li-a): Congenital absence of one or more of the long limb bones. Also, congenital absence of one or more of the limbs. See amelia.

ectropion (ek-trō′-pi-on): An abnormal turning out of a part, as of an eyelid when it is due to laxity of the structures that support it; this causes eversion with resulting exposure of the lid conjunctiva. **CERVICAL E.**, outward turning of the edges of the endocervix; usually results from chronic cervicitis or laceration of the external os. **SENILE E., E.** due to atrophy of the eyelid or flaccidity of the lid muscles.

ectrosyndactyly (ek-trō-sin-dak′-ti-li): A congenital anomaly in which some of the digits are partly or entirely missing and the others are webbed.

ECV: Abbreviation for extracellular volume.

eczema (ek′-ze-ma): An all-inclusive term used to describe a non-contagious condition of the skin; may be chronic. Characterized by redness, inflammation, itching, formation of vesicles, papules or pustules that discharge and later become scaly and crusted. Cause is unknown but the condition is usually associated with allergies, drug sensitivity, fungus infection, nutritional deficiency, uncleanliness. **CRAQUELÉ E., E.** characterized by round erythematous lesions. **INFANTILE E.**, an allergic **E.** of infants from about two months to two years. often limited to forehead and cheeks; very irritating; due to an allergy to foods, baby oil, or powder, etc. **NUMMULAR E.**, eczema characterized by coin-shaped scaly lesions. **STASIS E.**, stasis dermatitis (*q.v.*). **E. VACCINATUM**, generalized vaccinia resulting from inoculation with vaccinia virus when there is an existing topical eczema; symptoms include crops of vesicles over the entire body, high fever, malaise, enlargement of lymph nodes; has a high mortality.—eczematous, adj.

EDD: Abbreviation for expected date of delivery.

edema (ē-dē′-ma): Localized or general swelling due to the accumulation of fluids in the cells, intercellular spaces, and serous cavities. **ANGIONEUROTIC E.**, acute, localized, transitory swelling of the subcutaneous and submucosal tissues; may be a hereditary condition or due to a food or drug allergy, or may be of nervous origin; marked by sudden onset, sometimes fever and arthralgia; involves chiefly the face and lips, larynx, viscera, and extremities. **CARDIAC E.**, often results from congestive heart failure, reduced cardiac output, hypertension or hypotension; most marked in the extremities. **DEPENDENT E., E.** occurring in the extremities and lower part of the body. **NUTRITIONAL E.**, occurs in starvation or prolonged malnutrition; results from protein deprivation along with excessive intake of water and salt. **ORTHOSTATIC E., E.** of the legs which may develop in psychiatric patients who exhibit catatonia and stand in one position for a long period of time. **PERIORBITAL E.**, fluid which collects in the tissues around the eye. **PITTING E., E.** in which pressure on the tissues produces long-lasting depressions. **PULMONARY E.**, a form of waterlogging of the lungs resulting from left ventricular failure or mitral stenosis; also sometimes due to overloading of intravenous solutions. **RENAL E.**, results from disturbed kidney function in nephritis.

edematogenic (e-dem-a-tō-jen′-ik): Producing or resulting in edema.

edentulous (ē-den′-tū-lus): Without teeth.

EDNA: Abbreviation for Emergency Department Nurses Association.

EDTA: Abbreviation for ethylenediaminetetraacetic acid, a substance that is mixed with blood specimens to prevent them from clotting.

Edwards procedure: A surgical procedure for correcting congenital transposition of the aorta and pulmonary arteries.

Edwards syndrome: Trisomy 18 Syndrome (see under Trisomy).

EEG: Abbreviation for electroencephalogram.

EENT: Abbreviation for eye, ear, nose, and throat.

effacement (ē-fās′-ment): 1. A change or obliteration of form or features. 2. The shortening of the cervical canal during labor until it becomes a circular orifice continuous with the lower part of the uterus.

effect (ē-fekt′): A condition or result produced by some agent, force, or action.

effector (ē-fek′-tor): 1. A motor or secretory nerve ending in a muscle, gland, or organ. 2. A muscle that contracts or gland that secretes in response to a nerve impulse.

effemination (ē-fem-i-nā′-shun): The development of feminine attributes in a male.

efferent (ef′-er-ent): Carrying, conveying, or conducting away from a center. Opp. to afferent. **E. NERVE**, one that conveys impulses away from the central nervous system to a part of the body such as a muscle or gland.

effervescent (ef-er-ves′-ent): Bubbling, foaming, giving off gas bubbles.

effleurage (ef-loo-razh′): A long, deep or superficial stroking movement used in massage.

efflorescence (ef-lō-res′-ens): In medicine, a rash or skin eruption in which the lesions are numerous and conspicuous.

efflorescent (ef-lō-res′-ent): Descriptive of a crystalline substance that has become dry and powdery due to loss of water content.

effluvium (ef-floo′-vi-um): 1. An exhalation or emanation, expecially one that is foul smelling. 2. A shedding, especially of hair.

effort syndrome: A form of anxiety neurosis, manifesting itself in a variety of cardiac symptoms such as palpitation, precordial pain, shortness of breath for which there is no pathological explanation, and fatigue. Usually appears in persons with inadequate personality when confronted with hard or dangerous tasks. Syn., soldier's heart; neurocirculatory asthenia.

effusion (ē-fū′-zhun): Extravasation or escape of fluid into a tissue or cavity; may be serous, bloody, or purulent. **ENCYSTED E.**, the effused fluid is enclosed in a cyst, sac, or bladder. **PERICARDIAL E.**, the accumulation of fluid exudate in the pericardial sac following pericarditis, most commonly associated with pyogenic infections, acute fibrinous pericarditis, rheumatic fever, or tuberculosis. **PLEURAL E.**, effused fluid in the space between the lungs and pleura; may be bloody, purulent, or chylous; see chylothorax, empyema, hemothorax. **PULMONARY E.**, the presence of fluid in the air sacs and interstitial tissue of the lungs.

EFM: Abbreviation for electronic fetal monitoring.

egest (ē-jest′): To discharge unabsorbed food residue from the digestive tract.—egestion, n.

egesta (ē-jes′-ta): Material that has been egested; excreta.

ego (ē′-gō): 1. Self-esteem. 2. In psychoanalytic theory, the unconscious self, the "I", that part of personality that deals with reality and is influenced by social forces. It modifies behavior by unconscious compromise between the primitive instinctual urges (the id), internalized parental and social prohibitions (the superego), and reality.

egocentric (ē-go-sen′-trik): Self-centered; selfish; limited in outlook to one's own wishes and desires. Syn., egotropism.—egocentrism, n.

egomania (ē-gō-mā′-ni-a): Morbid preoccupation with self and self-esteem.

egophony (ē-gof′-o-ni): A peculiar voice sound resembling the bleating of a goat, heard over the upper chest cavity of persons suffering from pleurisy with effusion.

egotism (ē′-gō-tizm): Overvaluation of one's self; self-conceit.—egotistic, adj.

Ehlers-Danlos syndrome: A hereditary condition characterized by hyperelasticity of the skin, fragility of the skin capillaries, a tendency to bruise easily with the development of soft subcutaneous tumors, hyperextension of the joints, and various visceral anomalies.

Ehrlich [Paul Ehrlich, German bacteriologist. 1854-1915.]: **EHRLICH'S SIDE-CHAIN THEORY**, postulated that body cells consist of a stable nucleus and unstable side chains or chemoreceptors which, under certain conditions, are overproduced and released into body fluids; these free receptor groups become antibodies and are capable of combining specifically with certain antigen molecules. **EHRLICH'S 606**, arsphenamine (Salvarsan), discovered in 1909 as a result of his 606th experiment; the first specific treatment known for syphilis, yaws, and related infections.

Einthoven's triangle: In electrocardiography, an equilateral triangle with apices at the right and left shoulder and left hip, with each apex being equally distant from the center of the triangle, which is the heart. Used in electrocardiology for locating the standard limb leads.

Eisenmenger (ī′-sen-meng-er) [Victor Eisenmenger, German physician. 1864-1932.]: **EISENMENGER'S SYNDROME**, a condition in which a congenital septal defect allows for shunting of blood from the right side of the heart to the left side, with the result that some oxygen-poor blood gets pumped into the circulation and some oxygen-rich blood gets pumped into the lungs; symptoms include pulmonary hypertension and cyanosis. **EISENMENGER'S TETRALOGY**, a congenital anomaly consisting of ventricular septal defect, dextroposition of the aorta, dilatation of the pulmonary artery, and right ventricular hypertrophy.

eiweissmilch (ī′-vīs-milch): A preparation for infant feeding; consists of milk with added casein and calcium oxide and a reduced amount of lactose. Used in nutritional disturbances.

ejaculation (ē-jak-u-lā′-shun): A sudden emission or expulsion, said particularly of semen. **PREMATURE E.**, **E.** at the beginning of or prior to coitus. **RETARDED E.**, occurs when the individual cannot effect **E.** when desired. **RETROGRADE E.**, occurs when semen is ejaculated into the bladder; may occur in diabetic males.

ejaculatory (ē-jak′-ū-la-tor-i): Pertaining to ejaculation. **E. DUCTS**, see under duct.

ejection click: A sound produced by the heart; caused by the sudden dilatation of the pulmonic artery and the aorta or to the forceful opening of the aortic valve; may indicate some pathologic condition but also heard in many normal, healthy persons.

EKG: Abbreviation for electrocardiogram. Also ECG.

elastance (ē-las′-tans): A measure of the ability of an organ or structure to return to its original form when its contents are removed; refers often to an air-filled lung or fluid-filled urinary bladder.

elastic (ē-las′-tik): Capable of being stretched, twisted, or distorted and then resuming its natural shape. **E. BANDAGE**, a bandage of rubber or woven elastic material used to exert continuous pressure on edematous or swollen limbs, broken ribs, or varicose veins. **E. STOCKING**, a stocking made of woven elastic material; used to exert pressure on veins in the lower limbs. **E. TISSUE**, connective tissue made up of yellow elastic fibers.

elasticity (ē-las-tis′-i-ti): The ability of a material to undergo distortion and return to its original size, shape, and condition.

elastin (ē-las′-tin): The protein substance that forms the base of yellow elastic tissue.

elastinase (ē-las′-tin-ās): An enzyme that acts to dissolve elastic tissue by its action on elastin. Also elastase.

elastofibroma (ē-las′-tō-fī-brō′-ma): A tumor consisting of both elastic and fibrous tissue; usually occurs in the subscapular area, particularly of the elderly.

Elastoplast: Trademark for a type of elastic bandage made of cotton cloth without rubber, has porous, adhesive, non-fray edges.

elastosis (ē-las-tō′-sis): Degeneration of elastic tissue. **SENILE E.**, a dermatosis of old age, marked by degeneration of the elastic and collagen fibers in sun-exposed skin.

elation (ē-lā′-shun): Joyfulness; excitement that is marked by increased physical and mental activity. It becomes pathological when not consistent with the patient's circumstances.

elbow: The joint between the arm and forearm. **E. JERK**, involuntary bending of the elbow when the triceps muscle is struck suddenly. **MINER'S E.**, inflammation and enlargement of the bursa over the tip of the elbow caused by leaning on the elbow while digging. When seen in students it is called **STUDENT'S E. NURSEMAID'S ELBOW**, subluxation of the head of the humerus. **TENNIS E.**, radiohumeral bursitis; inflammation of the epicondyle of the humerus; occurs in those who engage in certain sports including tennis, but also occurs as a result of some unusual strain; due to repeated, sudden, jerky, vigorous movement of the extended forearm.

eldering: The aspect of the aging process that is influenced by the social group and culture in which one grows up and ages.

elderly (el′-der-li): Pertaining to individuals who are beyond middle age but not yet considered old. See old.

elective (ē-lek′-tiv): Term applied to procedures, usually surgical, that may be advantageous to the patient but not necessary to save his life; either the physician or the patient may make the choice as to whether to perform the procedure at all or to schedule it for some convenient future date.

Electra complex (e-lek′-tra kom′-plex): Term derived from Greek mythology. Refers to excessive fondness of a daughter for her father. The female counterpart of the Oedipus complex (*q.v.*)

electric shock therapy: See electroconvulsive.

electrical silence: Absence of electrical activity of the brain as shown on the electroencephalogram; brain death.

electricity (ē-lek-tris′-i-ti): A fundamental physical entity of nature, now believed to be caused by the motion of positively and negatively charged particles; is observable in its attraction and repulsion of electrified bodies and the phenomena of luminescence and heating effects.

electrocardiogram (ēlek-trō-kar′-di-ō-gram): A graphic recording of the electrical changes in the heart muscle during the cardiac cycle; obtained with an electrocardiograph (*q.v.*). Abbreviated EKG, ECG.

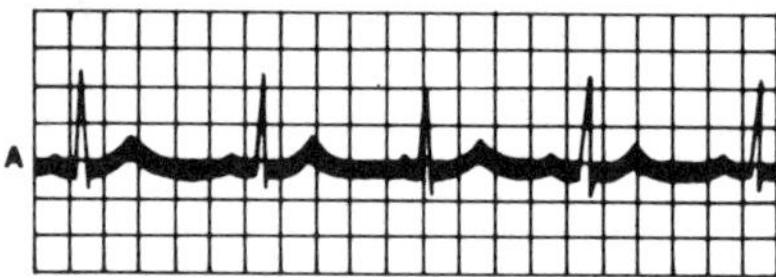

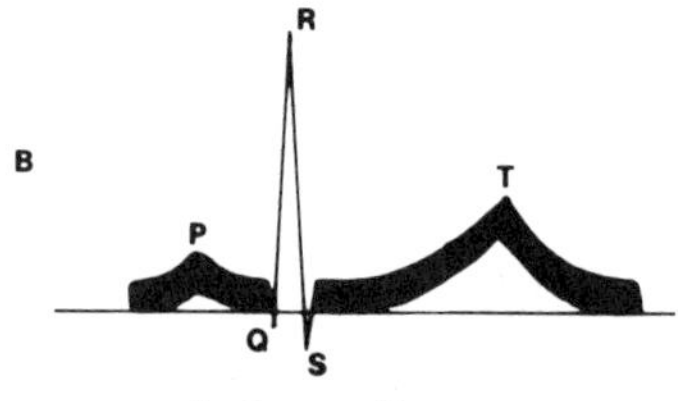

electrocardiogram

electrocardiograph (ē-lek-trō-kar′-di-ō-graf): An instrument containing a string galvanometer through which passes the electrical current produced by the heart's contraction. The electric impulses arising in the heart are picked up by several electrodes placed on the patient's body and amplified, and a permanent record (electrocardiogram) of these oscillations is made on a moving drum of graph paper.

electrocardiography (ē-lek′-trō-lar-di-og′-ra-fi): The process and technique of recording and interpreting the electrical activity of the heart.

electrocardiophonograph (ē-lek′-trō-kar′-di-ō-fō′-nō-graf): An instrument that records electrical potentials simultaneously with heart sounds produced during contraction of the heart muscle.

electrocardioscope (ē-lek-trō-kar′-di-ō-skōp): An instrument for visualizing the interior of the chambers of the heart.

electrocauterization (ē-lek′-trō-kaw-ter-ī-zā′-shun): Cauterization by means of a wire heated by direct or alternating current of electricity.

electrocoagulation (ē-lek′-trō-kō-ag-ū-lā′-shun): A technique of surgical diathermy. Coagulation of bleeding points, or hardening of tumors or diseased tissue by the application of electricity.

electroconvulsive (ē-lek′-trō-kon-vul′-siv): Usually refers to therapy for some mental disorder; consists of passing an electric current through the patient's brain, producing a convulsion and coma.

electrocorticography (ē-lek′-trō-kor-ti-kog′-ra-fi): An electroencephalogram in which the electrodes are attached directly to the cortex of the brain.—electrocorticographic, adj.; electrocorticographically, adv.

electrode (ē-lek′-trōd): In electrotherapy, a conductor in the form of a pad or plate whereby electricity enters or leaves the body.

electrodesiccation (ē-lek′-trō-des-i-kā′-shun): A technique of surgical diathermy in which a high-frequency current is applied to tissue with a needle electrode; there is drying and subsequent removal of the tissue.

electrodiagnosis (ē-lek′-trō-dī-ag-nō′-sis): The use of graphic recordings of electrical irritability of tissues in diagnosis.—electrodiagnostic, adj.

electroencephalogram (ē-lek′-trō-en-sef′-a-lō-gram): A graphic record made with the electroencephalograph (*q.v.*). Abbreviated EEG.

electroencephalograph (ē-lek′-trō-en-sef′-a-lō-graf): An instrument for obtaining a recording of the electric currents developed in the brain by means of electrodes that may be attached to the scalp or the surface of the brain, or placed within the substance of the brain. The electrodes pick up electric changes produced by activity in the brain and amplify them for recording. The record is an electroencephalogram (EEG), useful in localizing brain lesions or tumors and in studying some forms of mental disorder and brain function.—electroencephalographic, adj., electroencephalographically, adv.

electroencephalography (ē-lek′-trō-en-sef-a-log′-ra-fi): The recording of electric currents developed in the brain. See electroencephalograph.

electroexcision (ē-lek′-trō-ek-siz′-zhun): The excision of tissue or a body part by electrosurgical means. See electrosurgery.

electrogastrogram (ē-lek-trō-gas′-trō-gram): The graphic record made by electrogastrography (*q.v.*). Abbreviated EGG.

electrogastrography (ē-lek′-trō-gas-trog′-ra-fi): The measuring of the electrical activity of the stomach by means of swallowed gastric electrodes.

electrogoniometer (ē-lek′-trō-gō-ni-om′-e-ter): An instrument for measuring angular positions and the amplitude of movement at a joint.

electrogram (ē-lek′-tro-gram): A recording, on paper or film, of an electrical event, as occurs, *e.g.*, in an electrocardiogram.

electrohemostasis (ē-lek′-trō-hē-mos′-ta-sis): The arrest of hemorrhage by the use of electrocautery.

electrokymograph (ē-lek-trō-kī′-mō-graf): An apparatus for photographing and showing the motion of the heart and other organs on a fluoroscopic screen.

electrokymography (ē-lek′-trō-kī-mog′-ra-fi): The technique of recording the motion of the heart and other organs by x-ray photography.

electrolarynx (ē-lek-trō-lar′-inks): Any of several types of electronic devices that enable laryngectomees who can use esophageal speech (*q.v.*) to communicate. See esophageal speech under esophageal.

electrologist (ē-lek-trol′-o-jist): A person who uses an electric current by means of a needle electrode, to remove hair, warts, moles, birthmarks, etc.

electrolysis (ē-lek-trol′-i-sis): 1. Chemical decomposition of a substance by passage of an electric current through it. 2. Destruction and permanent removal of hairs (epilation), moles, spider nevi, etc. by means of electricity.

electrolyte (e-lek′-trō-līt): 1. A liquid or solution of a substance that is capable of conducting electricity and is decomposed by the passage of it; see electrolysis. 2. In physical chemistry, any substance that dissociates into positive and negative ions when in solution; in physiology, refers to body anions and cations. **E. BALANCE,** 1) the normal state when there is the correct balance between positive and negative ions in body fluids, tissues, and blood; 2) the state of the body in relation to intake and output of electrolytes.

electrolyte and fluid balance: See fluid and electrolyte balance.

electromassage (ē-lek′-trō-ma-sazh′): The application of a current of electricity to the body combined with massage.

electrometrogram (e-lek-trō-met′-rō-gram): A device for recording the changes in electric potential that occur with contraction of the muscles of the uterus.

electromyogram (ē-lek-trō-mī′-ō-gram): 1. An electrophysiological recording of the electric activity of a muscle, either that which occurs spontaneously or that which is produced by an electric current. 2. A graphic recording of movements of the eye during reading. Abbreviated EMG.

electromyograph (ē-lek-trō-mī′-ō-graf): An instrument used for measuring the electrical currents generated in muscle tissue activity.

electromyography (ē-lek′-trō-mī-og′-ra-fi): 1. A graphic recording of electrical currents generated when a muscle contracts as a result of the application of an electric stimulus. 2. The science and study of the recordings made by an electromyograph.

electromyoneurography (ē-lek′-trō-mī-ō-nū-rog′-ra-fi): A procedure used in studying neuromuscular action; involves the measuring and recording of the action potentials and conduction velocities of sensory and motor nerves by means of an electric current applied directly to skeletal muscle; useful in locating nerve lesions.

electron (ē-lek′-tron): The unit of negative electricity that, revolving around a nucleus of positive electricity, constitutes the atom. Thought to be the ultimate constituent of all matter. **E. MICROSCOPE,** a modern **M.** that differs from the ordinary **M.** in several ways; in particular, instead of using ordinary light it utilizes electron beams that have a much shorter wave length than ordinary visible light and this allows for much greater magnification. **E. THEORY,** the theory that all bodies are complex structures made up of atoms together with still smaller particles—electrons, protons, and neutrons.

electronarcosis (ē-lek′-trō-nar-kō′-sis): Narcosis or unconsciousness produced by passing an electric current through the brain. Used in treating certain mental disorders.

electroneurolysis (ē-lek′-trō-nū-rol′-i-sis): Destruction of a nerve by the application of electricity.

electroneuromyography (ē-lek′-trō-nū′-rō-mī-og′-ra-fi): A method of recording the electrical changes and the velocity with which they are conducted along the peripheral nerves; used in studying neuromuscular conduction and various nerve lesions.

electroneurostimulation (ē-lek′-trō-nū′-rō-stim-ū-lā′-shun): Electric stimulation with electrodes; used in treatment of a weak muscle or muscles, pain of unknown origin, or involuntary muscular action.

electronic (e-lek-tron′-ik): 1. Relating to or carrying electrons (*q.v.*). 2. Pertaining to devices that operate on the principles of electronics (*q.v.*).

electronics (ē-lek-tron′-iks): A special branch of physics that deals with the behavior of electrons in gases or vacuums, and with the operation and functioning of electronic devices.

electronystagmography (ē-lek′-trō-nī-stag-mog′-ra-fi): The electroencephalographic recording of eye movements for use in assessing nystagmus.

electro-oculogram (ē-lek′-trō-ok′-ū-lō-gram): A graphic record of the changes in electric potential that occur with movements of the muscles that control the eye. Abbreviated EOG.

electrophoresis (ē-lek-trō-fō-rē′-sis): Migration of charged collodial particles in solution to the positive or negative pole when an electric current is passed through the solution.

electrophysiology (ē-lek′-trō-fiz-e-ol′-o-ji): The science or study of physiology in its relation to electric phenomena produced in the normal body.

electroplexy (ē-lek′-trō-plek-si): Electric shock; may be intentional as in electroshock therapy or accidental by lightning or electrocution.

electropuncture (e-lek-trō-punk′-chur): The use of needles as electrodes for applying electric current to a nerve or muscle.

electropyrexia (ē-lek′-trō-pī-rek′-si-a): High body temperature produced by a special electrical apparatus. Used in fever therapy.

electroradiology (ē-lek′-trō-rā-di-ol′-ō-ji): The branch of medicine that deals with the use of electricity and x-ray in the treatment of disease.

electroretinogram (ē-lek′-trō-ret′-i-nō-gram): Graphic record of electrical response of the retina after stimulation by light. Abbreviated ERG.

electroretinograph (ē-lek′-trō-ret′-i-nō-graf): An instrument for measuring the electrical response of the retina to stimulation by light; utilized in the diagnosis and study of various eye disorders.—electroretinographic, adj.; electroretinography, n.

electroscission (ē-lek′-trō-sizh-un): The division of tissues using an electrocautery knife.

electroshock (ē-lek′-trō-shok): Shock produced by applying an electric current to the brain. **E. THERAPY,** see electroconvulsive.

electrospectography (ē-lek′-trō-spek-tog′-ra-fi): A recording of electroencephalographic wave patterns, and their study and interpretation. See electroencephalograph.

electrostimulation (ē-lek′-trō-stim-ū-lā′-shun): The therapeutic or experimental use of electricity to stimulate tissue.

electrosurgery (ē-lek-trō-ser′-jer-i): The use of electricity in surgery, *e.g.*, the electric knife, electric needle, or hot electric wire.

electrosynthesis (ē-lek-trō-sin′-the-sis): The formation of a compound by means of electricity.

electrotaxis (ē-lek-trō-tak′-sis): The movement of plant or animal cells or organisms to either a positive or negative pole in response to an electric stimulus.

electrothanasia (ē-lek′-trō-tha-nā′-zi-a): Electrocution; death caused by application of an electric current.

electrotherapy (ē-lek-trō-ther′-a-pi): Treatment of disease by means of electricity, *e.g.*, diathermy, electroshock therapy. Also electrotherapeutics, electroshock, electroplexy.

electrotonus (ē-lek-trō-tō′-nus): The changes that occur in the irritability of a muscle or nerve by the passage of an electric current through it.

electuary (ē-lek′-tū-a-ri): A medication in paste form, consisting of a powdered drug mixed with honey or a sweet syrup, to be allowed to dissolve in the mouth before swallowing.

element (el′-e-ment): One of the constituents of a compound. The elements are primary substances which alone or combined with other elements in compounds, constitute all matter. The basic unit of an element is the atom.—elementary, adj.

-eleo: Combining form denoting oil.

eleoma (ēl -ē-ō′-ma): A mass or swelling, sometimes granulomatous; usually caused by injection of an oil or an oily substance into subcutaneous or muscle tissue.

eleopathy (ē-lē-op′-a-thi): A diffuse boggy, fatty swelling, usually of the joints of the lower extremities, following contusion or other injury and attributed to the formation of an oily substance that has an irritating effect on the subcutaneous cellular tissue.

eleotherapy (ē-lē-ō-ther′-a-pi): The use of oil in therapeutics. Also oleotherapy.

elephantiasis (el-e-fan-tī′-a-sis): A chronic disease, usually of the tropics, caused by an obstruction in the lymphatics. Often due to filaria (*q.v.*) but in non-tropical areas may occur as a result of syphilis or recurrent streptococcal infections. Characterized by thickening and hardening of the skin and subcutaneous tissues and hypertrophy of the affected areas; legs and external genitalia most often affected. Also Barbados leg, pachydermia.—elephantiod, elephantiasic, adj.

elevator (el′-e-vā-tor): 1. An instrument for lifting or separating parts, *e.g.*, periosteum from bone. 2. An instrument for extracting roots of teeth. 3. One of the extraocular muscles.

eliminant (ē-lim′-in-ant): An agent that increases excretion of waste materials.

elimination (ē-lim-i-nā′-shun): The removal of wastes from the body.

elinguation (ē-ling-gwā′-shun): Surgical removal of the tongue. Glossectomy.

Elisa test: A test used to detect the presence of antibodies to the AIDS virus in samples of blood from transfusion; first used in 1985. May give false negatives or false positives, so a follow-up test is given after a positive result.

elixir (ē-lik′-ser): A clear, sweetened, flavored, often alcoholic, solution containing a medicinal agent; administered by mouth.

elliptocyte (ē-lip′-tō-sīt): An elliptically shaped erythrocyte.

elliptocytosis (e-lip′-tō-sī-tō′ sis): A rare hereditary type of anemia in which many of the red blood cells are oval in shape; seen in certain blood dyscrasias, thalassemia, and in pernicious, sickle cell, and iron deficiency anemias.

elute (ē-lūt′): In chemistry, to separate material from an adsorbent by washing in a suitable solvent.

Ely's sign: A sign indicating the presence of hip-joint disease or irritation of the psoas muscle; the patient lies on the table with his feet hanging over the edge, the heel is brought up to the buttock and if the movement cannot be completed, the sign is said to be positive.

emaciation (e-mā-shi- ā′-shun): Excessive leanness, or wasting of body tissue.—emaciate, v.

emaculation (ē-mak′-ū-lā′-shun): The removal of spots or other blemishes or lesions from the skin.

emanation (em-a-nā′-shun): 1. Exhalation. 2. That which is given off, such as the gaseous disintegration products of radioactive substances.

emanatorium (em-a-na-tor′-i-um): A special facility for treatment with a radioactive element by use of radioactive water or by inhalation.

emanotherapy (em-a-nō-ther′-a-pi): Treatment by inhalation of air charged with a natural radioactive element, usually radon.

emasculation (e-mas-kū-lā′-shun): Castration.

embalm (em-balm′): To treat a dead body with preservatives to prevent its decay.

embolalia (em-bō-lā′-li-a): The insertion of meaningless words in a sentence.

embolectomy (em-bō-lek′-to-mi): Surgical removal of an embolus.

embolemia (em-bō-lē′-mi-a): The presence of an embolus or emboli in the bloodstream.

embolic (em-bol′-ik): Pertaining to an embolus or an embolism.

embolism (em′-bō-lizm): The sudden obstruction of a blood vessel by a bit of foreign matter, *e.g.*, a clot, air bubble, fat particle, or clump of bacteria that is brought to the site by the blood current. **AIR E., E.** caused by a bubble of air; usually occurs following surgery or injury to a blood vessel, but may also be a serious complication of intravenous therapy. **ARTERIAL E., E.** that is usually characterized by sudden onset of pain, ischemia, coldness of the part supplied by the artery, absent or diminished pulses. **FAT E., E.** caused by a tiny drop of fat in the bloodstream; most commonly occurring in association with diabetes, pancreatitis, fatty liver disease, skeletal trauma. **PULMONARY E., E.** that occurs when a bubble of air or fat, but most often a free flowing clot in the circulation, becomes lodged in the pulmonary artery or a branch of it causing an impedance of pulmonary circulation characterized by sudden respiratory distress, pleural pain, restlessness; may be a serious complication of intravenous therapy.

embolization (em-bō-lī-zā′-shun): The therapeutic occlusion of a blood vessel, usually by introducing into the circulation any of several substances that will occlude the vessel.

embolus (em′-bō-lus): A body such as a clot or an air bubble transported in the blood until it causes obstruction by blocking a blood vessel. Besides clots and air bubbles, emboli may consist of masses of bacteria, tumor cells, parasites, tissue fragments, or fat globules.—emboli, pl.

embrocation (em-brō-kā′-shun): The application of a liquid to the body, especially by rubbing.

embryectomy (em-brē-ek′-tō-mi): The surgical removal of the products of conception; particularly in ectopic pregnancy.

embryo (em′-brē-ō): The early stage in the development of an organism, particularly one that is produced by the fertilization of an egg following fusion of the gametes (*q.v.*) resulting in a zygote which undergoes progressive cell division producing an embryo. In human anatomy, the term is applied to the conceptus from the time of generation until all of the internal and external organs are present and undergoing further development, which occurs at approximately the end of the seventh week of pregnancy, after which it is called a fetus.

embryoctomy (em-bri-ok′-to-mi): Feticide; the intentional destruction of the embryo or the fetus in utero for abortion or when delivery is impossible.

embryogenesis (em′-brē-ō-jen′-e-sis): 1. The period in prenatal development when the characteristics of the embryonic body are established; usually considered to extend from the second through the eighth week, after which the conceptus is called a fetus. 2. The development of a new individual by the process of sexual reproduction.

embryologist (em-brē-ol′-o-jist): A physician who specializes in embryology.

embryology (em-brē-ol′-o-ji): Study of the development of an organism from fertilization to etrauterine life.—embryological, adj., embryologically, adv.

embryoma (em-brē-ō′-ma): A tumor that develops from embryonic cells.

embryonic (em-brē-on′-ik): 1. Pertaining to an embryo. 2. Rudimentary.

embryopathia (em-brē-ō-path′-i-a): Embryopathy. **E. RUBEOLARIS**, the developmental anomalies occurring in children born of mothers who had German measles (rubella) during early pregnancy.

embryopathy (em-brē-op′-a-thi): A disease of abnormal condition resulting from interference with the normal development of the embryo or fetus. More serious if it occurs during the first three months. Includes the rubella syndrome, anomalies that occur in the fetus as a result of the mother's having had German measles (rubella) early in pregnancy.

embryotocia (em-brē-ō-tō′-si-a): Abortion.

embryotomy (em-brē-ot′-o-mi): Mutilation of the fetus to facilitate removal from uterus when natural birth is impossible. May consist of craniotomy, decapitation, cleidotomy, or evisceration.

embryotoxon (em-brē-ō-tok′-son): An opaque ring around the cornea; resembles arcus senilis (*q.v.*). May be congenital, in which case it is called arcus juvenilis.

emergency (ē-mer′-jen-si): 1. A pathological condition which develops suddenly and requires immediate medical therapy or surgical intervention. 2. A suddenly occurring threat to life or health, such as an epidemic or a disaster, that calls for immediate attention to seriously ill or injured victims.

emergency cart: See crash cart.

Emergency Department Nurses Association (EDNA): The national professional organization for nurses working in emergency departments; sponsors continuing education programs and several publications including the bimonthly *Journal of Emergency Nursing*. Address, 666 North Shore Drive, Suite 1729, Chicago IL 60611.

Emergency Medical Systems Act of 1973: Provides for allocation of federal funds for community-based life support systems, training of emergency medical technicians, and facilities for transporting patients to hospital or other care facility.

Emergency Medical Technician: A paraprofessional person who has had special training in emergency care, the standards for training being set by the U.S. Department of Transportation. The 81-hour course includes instructions in the transportation of seriously ill persons, cardiopulmonary resuscitation, control of bleeding, splinting and bandaging, administration of oxygen, and delivery of babies. Some states require that every emergency vehicle carry at least one emergency medical technician who must qualify for reaccreditation every two years. Abbreviation EMT.

emergent (e-mer′-jent): In emergency care, refers to the patient whose acute or life-threatening condition requires quick judgment and immediate attention.

Emergicenter: Name given to emergency care centers that provide services to patients with non-life-threatening conditions; located in shopping malls, industrial areas, and other places where people congregate. A type of freestanding ambulatory surgical center (*q.v.*).

emesis (em′-e-sis): Vomiting.

-emesis: Combining form denoting vomiting.

emetic (ē-met′-ik): 1. Causing the act of

vomiting. 2. Any agent used to produce vomiting.

EMG: Abbreviation for electromyogram.

EMI: The American Medical Association's emergency symbol; consists of a star and the staff of Aesculapius. Adopted by the World Medical Association in 1964. A wallet-size identification card is available from the American Medical Association, EMI, Department of Health Education, 525 N. Dearborn St., Chicago, IL 60610.

EMI scanner: Name given to the first computerized axial tomograph (manufactured in England by Electrical and Musical Instruments). The machine permits safe, painless serial viewing of organs or parts of the body that do not show up on x-ray photographs; used especially for viewing the brain.

-emia: Combining form denoting 1) blood, 2) a condition of blood.

eminence (em′-i-nens): A prominence or projection, especially on the surface of a bone.

emiocytosis (ē′-mi-ō-sī-tō′-sis): The passage of granular cell material through the cell membrane; said particularly of the insulin granules in the cells of the Islands of Langerhans, which migrate to the cell membrane where they fuse, the membrane ruptures, and the insulin passes out of the cell into the circulation.

emission (ē-mish′-un): An ejacultion or sending forth, specifically an involuntary ejaculation of semen. **NOCTURNAL E.,** involuntary emission of semen during sleep, occurring in normal males beginning with puberty.

emmenagogue (ē-men′-a-gog): An agent or measure used to regulate or induce menstruation.

emmenia (ē-mē′-ni-a): The menses (*q.v.*).

emmenology (em-e-nol′-o-ji): The sum of knowledge about the physiology and pathology of menstruation.

emmetropia (em-e-trō′-pi-a): Normal or perfect vision.—emmetropic, adj.

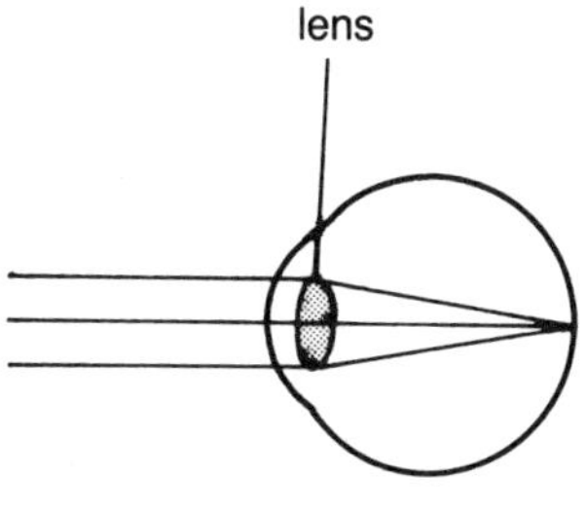

Emmetropia

emollient (ē-mol′-i-ent): An agent that softens and soothes skin or mucous membrane.

emotion (ē-mō′-shun): A strong feeling such as fear, anger, grief, joy, or love, or an aroused mental state recognized in ourselves by certain bodily changes, and in others by certain characteristic behavior.

emotional (ē-mō′-shun-al): Characteristic of or caused by emotion. **E. BIAS,** tendency to allow one's **E.** attitude to affect logical judgment. **E. ILLNESS,** a mental disorder. **E. INSTABILITY,** a condition characterized by hysterical behavior. **E. LABILITY,** fluctuations in emotional expression that are beyond the person's control; may shift from crying to laughing, from anger to fear, and so on; often due to a frontal lobe lesion. **E. MATURITY,** the state of having achieved maximum emotional control. **E. REACTION,** reaction based on emotion rather than logic. **E. STATE,** effect of emotions on normal mood, *e.g.*, agitation.—emotionality, n.

empathy (em′-pa-thi): The ability to perceive and share the feelings of another through insightful awareness of that person's feelings and emotions and what they mean. To be distinguished from sympathy.—empathic, adj.; emphathize, v.

emphlysis (em′-fli-sis): An exanthematous disease characterized by vesicular eruption, with the lesions becoming scabby.

emphraxis (em-frak′-sis): 1. Clogging or obstruction; often refers to the pores of the sweat glands. 2. An impaction.

emphysema (em-fi-sē′-ma): A nonreversible chronic pulmonary disorder, often secondary to smoking or the hazards of certain occupations; characterized by the breakdown of the septal walls between the alveoli, destruction of the connective tissue that is responsible for the elastic recoil of the lung, and the resulting gaseous distention of the tissues or organs with air. **CENTRIACINAR E.,** affects chiefly the bronchioles rather than the alveoli; there is focal dilatation of air spaces which are scattered throughout normal tissue of the entire lung; also called centrilobular **E. INTERSTITIAL E.,** a condition in which air is trapped in the lung tissue instead of moving into the alveoli; occurs in respiratory distress syndrome of infants. **OBSTRUCTIVE E.,** overdistention of the lung resulting from partial obstruction of the air passages, which allows air to enter the alveoli but interferes with expiration. **PANACINAR E.,** panlobular **E.,** affects all lung segments; the alveoli atrophy and the vascular bed is destroyed. **PULMONARY E.,** alveolar distention, which may be 1) generalized; often accompanying chronic bronchitis, or 2) localized, occurring distally to partial obstruction of a bronchus or in alveoli adjacent to a segment of collapsed lung. **SUBCUTANEOUS E.,** air or gas in subcutaneous tissues; when it occurs in the connective tissue under the skin it is called **CUTANEOUS E. SURGICAL E.,** air or gas in subcutaneous tissues following surgery or trauma.—emphysematous, adj.

empirical (em-pir′-i-kal): Refers to a theory or mode of treatment based on observation and experience rather than reasoning or speculation.—empiricism, n.

emporiatrics (em-pō-ri-at′-riks): The branch of medicine that deals with the health of travelers throughout the world.

emprosthotonos (em-pros-thot′-o-nos): A tetanic spasm in which the body becomes tense and the feet and head are brought forward; when face downward, the body is incurving with only the forehead and feet touching the bed. The position is opposite to that seen in opisthotonos (*q.v.*).

"empty nest" syndrome: Usually refers to a phenomenon experienced by couples when the youngest of their children reaches maturity and leaves the home.

emptysis (emp′-ti-sis): Hemoptysis (*q.v.*).

empyema (em-pī-ē′-ma): A collection of pus in a cavity, hollow organ, or space; if unspecified, refers to pus in the pleural cavity.—empyemic, adj.

empyesis (em-pī-ē′-sis): 1. Suppuration. 2. A pustular eruption.

empyocele (em′-pī-ō-sēl): A hydrocele in the scrotum; characterized by suppuration.

EMS: Emergency Medical Service; a federally funded program that provides funds for organizing and operating emergency medical services, and for training medical personnel in handling emergencies.

EMT: Abbreviation for Emergency Medical Technician (*q.v.*).

emulsify (ē-mul′-si-fī): To convert a substance into an emulsion by combining two solutions that do not normally mix, so that the result is a liquid containing particles in suspension.

emulsion (ē-mul′-shun): A fluid containing fat or oil particles in the state of subdivision and suspension, so that a smooth, milky white fluid results.

enamel (en-am′-el): The hard external covering of the crown of a tooth.

enanthem (en-an′-them), **enanthema** (en-an-thē′-ma]: An eruption on a mucous surface, *e.g.*, strawberry tongue in scarlet fever or Koplik's spots in measles.—enanthematous, adj.

enanthesis (en-an-thē′-sis): The skin eruption that is characteristic of certain general diseases, *e.g.*, scarlet fever.

enanthrope (en-an′-thrōp): A source of disease within the body; an autoinfection.

enantiopathy (en-an-ti-ōp′-a-thi): 1. A disease or pathological process that acts as a curative agent to another disease. 2. The curing of one disease by introducing another disease of an opposite nature.

enarthrosis (en-ar-thrō′-sis): A ball and socket joint such as the hip joint.

encanthis (en-can′-this): A small neoplasm or excrescence at the inner canthus of the eye.

encapsulation (en-kap-sū-lā′-shun): Enclosure within a capsule.

enceinte (on′-sant): Pregnant.

encelialgia (en-sē-li-al′-ji-a): Pain in any of the abdominal organs.

encelitis (en-se-li′-tis): Inflammation in any of the abdominal organs.

encephal-, encephala-, encephalo-: Combining forms denoting the brain.

encephalalgia (en-sef-a-lal′-ji-a): Pain in the head. Headache.

encephalasthenia (en-sef′-el-as-thē′-ni-a): Mental fatigue, particularly when of emotional origin.

encephalatrophy (en-sef-e-lat′-rō-fi): Atrophy of the brain.

encephalauxe (en-sef-a-lawk′-sē): Hypertrophy of the brain.

encephalemia (en-sef-a-lē′-mi-a): Congestion of the brain.

encephalic (en-se-fal′-ik): Relating to the structures within the cranium or to the brain alone.

encephalitis (en-sef-a-lī′-tis): Inflammation of the brain; may be a specific disease entity or occur as a sequel to another disease. Characterized by headache, malaise, fever, slowed mental and motor responses, and stuporous sleep. **ACUTE DISSEMINATED E.**, postinfection **E.** **ARBOVIRUS E.**, caused by an arborvirus such as Eastern equine or St. Louis equine. **EASTERN EQUINE E.**, see under **encephalomyelitis**. **E. AXIALIS DIFFUSA**, a form of **E.** occurring in children and adults, and characterized by destruction of the white matter of the brain; symptoms include progressive mental deterioration, bilateral spasticity, deafness, and blindness; also called Schilder's disease. **HERPES E., E.** caused by the herpes simplex virus; usually fatal. **E. LETHARGICA**, a sporadic and occasionally epidemic form of virus infection. Profound cerebral damage with cranial nerve palsies; stupor and delirium can occur. May be followed by alteration of personality or Parkinson's disease. **POSTINFECTION E.**, an acute infection of the central nervous system in persons recovering from an infectious disease, usually one caused by a virus. **POST-RUBEOLA E., E.** that usually develops within four to six days following the skin eruption; marked by sudden rise in temperature and drowsiness, stupor, neurological signs; often fatal. **POST-VACCINIAL E.**, acute **E.**, sometimes follows vaccination. **ST. LOUIS E.**, a viral infection of the central nervous system with symptoms resembling those of western equine **E.**, caused by a mosquito-borne arbovirus; occurs mostly in the late summer or early fall, chiefly in central and western U.S. **WESTERN EQUINE E.**, see under encephalomyelitis.—encephalitides, pl.; encephalitic, adj.

encephalocele (en-sef′-a-lō-sēl): Hernia of the brain with protrusion of the brain substance through an opening in the skull. Often associated with hydrocephalus when the protrusion occurs at a suture line.

encephalodialysis (en-sef′-a-lō-dī-al′-i-sis): Softening of the brain substance.

encephalodynia (en-sef′-a-lō-dī′-ni-a): Headache.

encephalogram (en-sef′-a-lō-gram): An x-ray picture of the contents of the skull. See pneumoencephalogram.

encephalography (en-sef-a-log′-ra-fi): Roentgenology of the skull contents, particularly of the brain. see pheumoencephalography.

encephaloid (en-sef′-a-loyd): Resembling the substance of the cerebrum. **E. CANCER**, encephaloma, a malignant tumor of the brain.

encephalolith (en-sef′-a-lō-lith): A concretion in the brain tissue or in one of the ventricles.

encephalology (en-sef-a-lol′-ō-ji): The scientific study of the brain.

encephaloma (en-sef-a-lō′-ma): A tumor within the brain.—encephalomata, pl.

encephalomalacia (en-sef′-a-lō-ma-lā′-shi-a): Softening of the brain.

encephalomeningitis (en-sef′-a-lō-men-in-jī′-tis): Inflammation of the brain and its meninges.

encephalomeningocele (en-sef′-a-lō-me-ning′-gō-sēl): Protrusion of the cerebral membranes and brain substance through a defect in the bones of the skull.

encephalomeningopathy (en-sef′-a-lō-men-in-gop′-a-thi): Pathology involving the brain and the meninges.

encephalomyelitis (en-sef′-a-lō-mī-e-lī′-tis): Inflammation of the brain and spinal cord. **EQUINE E.**, a viral disease transmitted by ticks and mosquitoes to horses and man; two forms occur in the U.S.; 1) **EASTERN EQUINE E.**, which occurs in eastern states, Canada, Mexico, and South America; characterized by stiff neck, fever, headache, vomiting; severe nervous system disorders may be a sequela; and 2) **WESTERN EQUINE E.**, which is less severe than the eastern variety; seen mostly in children and, in summer, in infants; occurs principally in the western states but also seen along the Atlantic coast and Gulf of Mexico. See also encephalitis.

encephalomyeloneuropathy (en-sef′-a-lō-mī′-e-lō-nū-rop′-a-thi): Pathology of the brain, spinal cord, and peripheral nerves.

encephalomyelopathy (en-sef′-a-lo-mī-e-lop′-a-thi): Disease affecting both the brain and spinal cord. **POSTINFECTION E., E.** that occurs secondarily to such common diseases as mumps, measles, chickenpox, influenza. **POSTVACCINIAL E., E.** arising as a complication in the reaction to vaccination for smallpox.

encephalomyocarditis (en-sef′-a-lō-mī-ō-kar-dī′-tis): Encephalitis associated with myocarditis; an acute febrile disease, usually affecting infants and children; caused by a variety of viruses.

encephalon (en-sef′-a-lon): The brain.

encephalonarcosis (en-sef′-a-lō-nar-kō′-sis): Stupor or coma caused by brain disease or lesion.

encephalopathy (en-sef′-a-lop′-a-thi): Any disease or dysfunction of the brain. **ALCOHOLIC E.**, see Wernicke's **E. HEPATIC E., E.** that occurs in patients with advanced liver disease; marked by nervous system disturbances, changes in behavior and consciousness which may proceed to confusion, lethargy, tremor, disorientation, stupor, coma; may also occur in patients having a portacaval shunt. **HYPERTENSIVE E., E.** marked by convulsions, coma; associated with malignant hypertension. **HYPOGLYCEMIC E., E.** induced by severe hypoglycemia as in overstorage of glycogen or disturbances in insulin secretion. **TRAUMATIC E., E.** that occurs in boxers and others subject to persistent trauma to the head; marked by headache, confusion, slowing of mental activity, and memory loss. **WERNICKE'S E.**, a condition caused by deficiency of vitamin B_1 (thiamine); commonly seen in chronic alcoholics, and characterized by delirium, various eye signs, paralysis of some of the eye muscles causing a squint or rhythmic jerking of the head when the patient tries to look to one side.

encephalopyosis (en-sef′-a-lō-pī-ō′-sis): A purulent inflammation or abscess of the brain.

encephalorrhagia (en-sef′-a-lō-rā′-ji-a): Hemorrhage from the brain or within it.

encephalosclerosis (en-sef′-a-lō-sklē-rō′-sis): Hardening of the brain.

encephalosepsis (en-sef′-a-lō-sep′-sis): Septic inflammation of the brain.

encephalosis (en-sef-a-lō′-sis): Any organic disease of the brain.

enchondroma (en-kon-drō′-ma): A benign cartilaginous tumor occurring in a part where cartilage is not normally found or within a bone near the epiphyseal line.—enchondromata, pl.; enchondromatous, adj.

enchondrosarcoma (en-kon′-drō-sar-kō′-ma): Chondrosarcoma (*q.v.*).

encopresis (en-kō-prē′-sis): Involuntary passage of feces not due to disease or organic defect. In children, often due to emotional problems.—encopretic, adj.

encounter group therapy: A type of therapy whereby patients meet in groups, designed to improve their orientation to reality and their relations with others. See also **sensitivity training.**

encyesis (en-sī-ē′-sis): Normal pregnancy.

encysted (en-sis′-ted): Enclosed in a cyst or sac or surrounded by a membrane.

end bulb: A term used to describe certain sensory nerve endings in some areas of the skin or mucous membrane.

end organ: An encapsulated structure containing the terminal part of a sensory nerve fibril in muscle tissue, skin, mucous membrane or a gland.

end plate: The ending of a motor nerve fiber in relation to skeletal muscle fibers. **MOTOR END PLATE,** a complex myoneural junction where the axon of a motor nerve fiber makes contact with striated muscle fibers by way of a synapse.

Endamoeba: See **Entamoeba.**

endaortitis (end-ā-ōr-ti′-tis): Inflammation of the membrane lining the aorta.

endareterectomy (end-ar-ter-ek′-tō-mi): Surgical removal of the innermost lining of an artery when it has become thickened by atheromatous plaque. **CAROTID E.**, surgical removal of atheromatous plaque from the intima of a carotid artery; may be done when transient ischemic attacks are thought to be due to such plaque; may involve both internal and external carotids. **CORONARY E.**, surgical removal of occluding material from the coronary artery.

endarterial (end-ar-tē′-ri-al): 1. Within an artery. 2. Pertinent to the intima of an artery.

endarteritis (end-ar-ter-ī′-tis): Inflammation of the tunica intima or lining coat of an artery. **E. OBLITERANS**, a form of **E**. in which the lumina of smaller vessels become obliterated.

endaural (end-awr′-al): Pertaining to the inner portion of the external auditory canal.

end-diastolic (dī-as-tol′-ik): Refers to the time period following diastole (end-diastole) just before the systolic contraction begins. **E. PRESSURE**, the pressure of the blood in the ventricles at end-diastole. **E. VOLUME**, the volume of blood in the ventricles just before the beginning of systole.

endemic (en-dem′-ik): Peculiar to a certain area; said of diseases that are habitually present within a given locality.—endemically, adv.; endemicity, n.

endemiology (en-dē-mi-ol′-ō-ji): The special study of endemic diseases.

endermic (en-der′-mik): Acting by absorption through the skin; an agent that acts by absorption through the skin.

endermosis (en-der-mō′-sis): Any eruptive disease of mucous membrane.

endo-: Combining form denoting within; inner.

endoaneurysmorrhaphy (en′-dō-an-ū-riz-mor′-a-fi): A surgical procedure for repairing an aneurysm; involves opening the aneurysmal sac and suturing together the internal openings of the vessel.

endoangiitis (en-dō-an-ji-ī′-tis): Inflammation of the intimal lining of a blood vessel; endophlebitis; endoarteritis.

endobiotic (en-dō-bī-ot′-ik): Pertaining to a parasite living in a host.

endobronchial (en-dō-brong′-ki-al): Within a bronchus. **E. TUBE,** a double lumen tube that can be inserted into the bronchus of one lung to permit deflation of the other lung for thoracic surgery; also may be used in administration of inhalation anesthetic.

endobronchitis (en-dō-brong-kī′-tis): Inflammation of the lining of the bronchi.

endocardial (en-dō-kar′-di-al): Pertaining to the endocardium. **E. FIBROELASTOSIS,** a heart disease of unknown cause; occurs mostly in infants; the lining of the heart chambers becomes thickened with elastic tissue, especially in the left ventricle, which impairs cardiac function.

endocarditis (en′-dō-kar-dī′-tis): Inflammation of the inner lining of the heart and/or the covering of the valves of the heart; most commonly due to rheumatic fever. **ABACTERIAL E., E.** that is not due to an invading organism; sometimes associated with lupus erythematosus. **ACUTE E.,** the nonbacterial **E.** that is often due to rheumatic fever. **ACUTE BACTERIAL E., E.** caused by pyogenic organisms, usually streptococcus, gonococcus, pneumococcus, or meningococcus; rapidly progressive; often fatal. **INFECTIVE E.,** infection of the endocardium; usually caused by a streptococcic, staphylococcic, or enterococcic organism; may occur in patients with congenital heart malformations or, more often, following valvular heart surgery. Also frequently occurs in patients having dental surgery and in those with infection of the periodontal membranes. Prophylaxis consists chiefly of preoperative administration of antibiotics. **MALIGNANT E.,** acute fulminating **E.;** usually associated with suppuration elsewhere in the body. **MARANTIC E.,** nonbacterial **E.,** usually associated with a neoplasm or other debilitating condition. **RHEUMATIC E.,** the **E.** of rheumatic fever, often involving the heart valves. **SUBACUTE BACTERIAL E.,** usually due to *Streptococcus viridans;* usually confined to the valves; of gradual onset; seen most often in young adults. **VALVULAR E., E.** that affects one or more of the heart valves. **VERRUCOUS E.,** vegetative **E.;** associated with formation of fibrinous clots on the endocardium and forming ulceration on the valves; often associated with lupus erythematosus.

endocardium (en-dō-kar′-di-um): The thin serous membrane lining the chambers of the heart and covering the surfaces of the heart valves. It is continuous with the lining of the vessels entering and leaving the heart.

endocervicitis (en′-dō-ser-vi-sī′-tis): Inflammation of the mucous membrane lining the cervix of the uterus; usually chronic. Also endotrachelitis.

endocervix (en-dō-ser′-vix): The mucous membrane lining of the cervix of the uterus.—endocervical, adj.

endochondral (en-dō-kon′-dral): Situated or occurring within cartilage; usually refers to the formation of bone within cartilage by the process of replacement.

endocolitis (en′-dō-kō-lī′-tis): Catarrhal inflammation of the mucous lining of the colon.

endocolpitis (en′-dō-kol-pī′-tis): Inflammation of the mucous membrane of the vagina.

endocranial (en-dō-kra′-ni-al): Within the cranium.

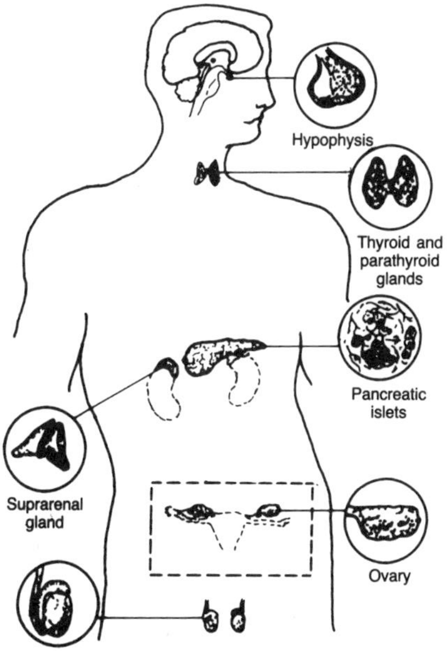

Endocrine glands

endocrine (en′-dō-krin): Secreting within; term applied to the ductless glands of the body whose secretions pass directly from the gland into the interstitial tissues, from which they are diffused into the blood or lymph to be carried to other parts of the body where they affect the functioning of other organs or parts. The opposite of exocrine (*q.v.*). **E. GLANDS** include the pineal, pituitary, thyroid, parathyroid, thymus, adrenals, ovaries, testes, and islands of Langerhans in the pancreas. **E. THERAPY,** treatment with **E.** preparations. **E. SECRETIONS,** those produced by the **E.** glands; they have important influences on the metabolic processes. **E. SYSTEM,** consists of all glands that deliver their secretions directly into the bloodstream.

endocrinology (en′-dō-kri-nol′-o-ji): The study of the ductless glands and their internal secretions.

endocrinoma (en′-dō-kri-nō′-ma): A tumor containing endocrine tissue that continues to function as the parent tissue but to an excessive degree.

endocrinopathy (en′-dō-kri-nop′-a-thi): Abnormality or disease of one or more of the endocrine glands, or abnormality of their secretions.

endocrinotherapy (en′-dō-krin-ō-ther′-a-pi): Treatment of disease by administration of endocrine substances.

endocytosis (en′-dō-sī-tō′-sis): The engulfing by a cell of particles that are too large to diffuse through the cell membrane, as occurs in phagocytosis.

endoderm (en′-dō-derm): The innermost of three layers of cells that form during the early development of the embryo; it gives rise to the epithelium of the digestive tract, liver, pancreas, urinary bladder and urethra, pharynx, auditory tube, larynx, trachea, bronchi, lungs, and the thyroid, parathyroid, and thymus glands, and the adenohypophysis.

Endodermophyton (en′-dō-der-mof′-i-ton): A genus of fungi, several species of which cause tinea in man; now usually called Trichophyton.

endodontics (en-dō-don′-tiks): The branch of dentistry that deals with diseases of the dental pulp and their treatment.

endodontium (en-dō-don′-shi-um): The pulp of a tooth.

endodontology (en′-dō-don-tol′-o-ji): The science of disorders of the dental pulp. Syn., endontia.

endoenteritis (en′-dō-en-ter-ī′-tis): Inflammation of the intestinal mucosa.

endoesophagitis (en′-dō-ē-sof-a-jī′-tis): Inflammation of the mucosal lining of the esophagus.

endogamy (en-dog′-a-mi): 1. In biology, sexual reproduction by conjugation of two gametes descended from the same ancestor cell. 2. In anthropology, the restriction of marriage to members of the same tribe, social group, or community.

endogastritis (en′-dō-gas-trī′-tis): Inflammation of the mucous lining of the stomach.

endogenic (en-dō-jen′-ic): Of inside origin; endogenous.

endogenous (en-doj′-e-nus): Originating within a structure, organ, or organism, as contrasted with exogenous.

endointoxication (en′-dō-in-tok-si-ka′-shun): Poisoning caused by an endogenous toxin.

endolymph (en′-dō-limf): The fluid contained in the membranous labyrinth of the internal ear.

endolysin (en-dol′-i-sin): An intracellular, leukocytic substance that destroys engulfed bacteria.

endometrial (en-dō-mē′-tri-al): Pertaining to or affecting the endometrium. **E. ASPIRATION,** use of a low-pressure suction apparatus to remove the endometrium and the products of conception. **E. CANCER,** a fairly common type of uterine cancer; usually an adenocarcinoma. **E. LAVAGE,** a procedure for obtaining endometrial cells for examination by injecting a solution of normal saline into the uterus as a lavage.

endometrioma (en′-dō-mē-tri-ō′-ma): A tumor containing shreds of misplaced endometrium; found most frequently in the ovary. Adenomyoma (*q.v.*). See **cyst** (chocolate).—endometriomata, pl.

endometriosis (en′-dō-mē-tri-ō′-sis): The presence of functioning endometrium in abnormal places both within and without the uterus; often the cause of abdominal and/or pelvic pain which becomes more severe at menstruation, and of an unusually heavy menstrual flow. Adhesions may form around these deposits and cause distortion of the pelvic organs and their functions. See **cyst, chocolate.**

endometritis (en-dō-mē-trī′-tis): Inflammation of the endometrium.

endometrium (en-dō-mē′-tri-um): The lining mucosa of the uterus.—endometrial, adj.

endomorph (en′-dō-morf): An individual whose body build differs from the normal in that the digestive viscera are large, there are accumulations of fat about the abdomen, the trunk and thighs are large and the extremities are tapering.—endomorphic, adj.

endomyocarditis (en′-dō-mī-ō-kar-dī′-tis): Inflammation of both the inner lining and muscular portions of the heart.

endomysium (en-dō-mis ′-i-um): The delicate connective tissue sheath that surrounds individual muscle fibers within a fasciculus and serves to support blood vessels and nerves that branch between the fibers.

endoneurim (en-dō-nū′-ri-um): The delicate, inner connective tissue surrounding the nerve fibers.

endoneuritis (en-dō-nū-rī′-tis): Inflammation of the endoneurium.

endoparasite (en-dō-par′-a-sīt): Any parasite living within its host.—endoparasitic, adj.

endoperiarteritis (en′-dō-per-i-ar-ter-ī′-tis): Inflammation of both the inner and outer coats of an artery.

endopericarditis (en′-dō-per-i-kar-dī′-tis): Inflammation of both the endocardium and the pericardium.

endoperimyocarditis (en′-dō-per-i-mī′-o-kar-dī′-tis): Inflammation of the endocardium, myocardium, and pericardium.

endophlebitis (en-dō-flē-bi′-tis): Inflammation of the intima of a vein.

endophthalmitis (en′-dof-thal-mī′-tis): Inflammation of any or all of the internal structures of the eye or of the ocular cavity and surrounding structures. May occur as a result of bacterial infection, perforating injury, or vascular disease, or as a complication of such infections as pneumonia or measles. **E. PHACOANAPHYLACTIA,** a form of uveitis caused by a hypersensitive reaction to lens protein that has escaped through the lens capsule or following cataract surgery; a chronic granulatomatous infection.

endophytic (en-dō-fit′-ik): Having a tendency to grow inward and proliferate within an organ or structure; often refers to tumors of the skin.

endoplasm (en′-dō-plazm): The central, more fluid portion of a unicellular organism, as distinguished from the ectoplasm (*q.v.*).

endoprosthesis (en′-dō-pros-thē′-sis): An artificial internal body part.

endorphin (en-dor′-fin): Any of several neuropeptides produced by the pituitary gland and widely distributed in the central nervous system; alpha, beta, and gamma **ENDORPHINS** have been isolated. **ENDORPHINS** have a molecular structure similar to that of morphine; they act as neruotransmitters and neuromodulators and have the effect of reducing pain. See also **enkephalin.**

endorrhachis (en-dō-rā′-kis): The spinal cord dura mater.

endosalpingitis (en′-dō-sal-pin-jī′-tis): Inflammation of the lining of either 1) a fallopian tube or 2) the eustachian tube.

endosalpinx (en-dō-sal′-pinks): The mucous membrane lining of the fallopian tubes; it is continuous with the lining of the uterus.

endoscope (en′-dō-skōp): A tubular, lighted instrument for visualization of the interior of body cavities or organs.—endoscopic, adj.; endoscopy, n.

endosepsis (en-dō-sep′-sis): Sepsis arising from some condition within the body.

endospore (en′-dō-spōr): A bacterial spore that has a purely vegetative function. It is formed by the loss of water and probable rearrangement of the protein of the cell, so that metabolism is minimal and resistance to environmental conditions, especially high temperature, desiccation and antibacterial drugs, is high; two genera that include pathogenic species that form spores are *Bacillus* and *Clostridium*.

endosteal (en-dos′-tē-al): 1. Pertaining to the

endosteum. 2. Located or occurring within a bone.

endosteitis (en′-dos-tē-ī′-tis): Inflammation of the endosteum (*q.v.*).

endosteoma (en-dos′-tē-ō′-ma): A benign tumor in the medullary canal of a bone.

endosteum (en-dos′-tē-um): The thin vascular connective tissue lining the medullary canal of a long bone.—endosteal, adj.

endothelial (en-dō-thē′-li-al): Pertaining to or resembling epithelium.

endothelioangiitis (en-dō-thē′-lē-ō-an-ji-ī′-tis): An inflammatory condition involving the endothelium of blood vessels in many organs; with fever, pericarditis, angiitis, and other symptoms resembling those of lupus erythematosus.

endotheliocyte (en-dō-thē′-li-ō-sīt): A macrophage (*q.v.*).

endotheliocytosis (en-dō-thē′-li-ō-sī-tō′-sis): An abnormal increase in the production of endotheliocytes.

endothelioid (en-do-thē′-li-oid): Resembling endothelium.

endothelioma (en′-dō-thē-li-ō′-ma): A tumor derived from the epithelial cells that make up the lining of blood or lymph vessels or serous cavities; may be benign or malignant.

endotheliosis (en′-dō-thē-li-ō′-sis): Overgrowth of endothelium (*q.v.*).

endothelium (en-dō-thē′-li-um): The very thin smooth vascular membrane lining of serous cavities, heart, blood and lymph vessels.—endothelial, adj.

endothrix (en′-dō-thriks): A fungal parasite that forms spores within the hair shaft.

endotoxemia (en-dō-tok-sē′-mi-a): A condition in which endotoxins are present in the bloodstream; may be a sign of impending shock.

endotoxicosis (en′-dō-tok-si-kō′-sis): Poisoning by an endotoxin.

endotoxin (en-do-tok′-sin): A toxin present in the cell wall of certain bacteria, caused chiefly by gram-negative organisms, which is freed only when the microorganism is broken down in the body; has a pyrogenic action and increases capillary permeability; associated with shock, thrombopenia, leukopenia. Opp. to exotoxin.—endotoxic, adj.

endotracheal (en-dō-trā′-kē-al): Within the trachea. **E. TUBE,** an airway catheter inserted through the nose or mouth into the trachea in tracheal intubation. See **intubation.**

endotracheitis (en′-dō-trā-kē-ī′-tis): Inflammation of the mucosa of the trachea.

endotrachelitis (en′-dō-trā-kel-ī′-tis): Inflammation of the membrane lining the uterine cervix; endocervicitis.

endovasculitis (en-dō-vas′-kū-lī′-tis): Inflammation of the intimal lining of a blood vessel.

enema (en′-e-ma): The injection of a liquid into the rectum, to be returned or retained. It can be further designated according to the function of the fluid: to promote evacuation of feces; to provide nutrients or medicinal substances; to introduce opaque material in x-ray examination of the lower intestinal tract.—enemata, pl.

energy (en′-er-ji): The capacity to do work; manifested in various forms such as motion, light, heat.

enervation (en-er-vā′-shun): 1. General weakness; loss of strength; lack of vigor or nervous energy. 2. Removal of a nerve or part of one.

engagement (en-gāj′-ment): In obstetrics, the entrance of the presenting part of the fetus into the superior pelvic strait. The beginning of the descent through the pelvic canal. Usually occurs about the fourth week before delivery and often accompanied by a sensation called lightening.

engorged (en-gorjd′): Distended or swollen with blood or other fluid; term is applied to a tissue, an organ, or a vessel.—engorgement, n.

engorgement (en-gorj′-ment): Congestion and distension of a tissue, organ, or vessel with fluid or other material.

engram (en′-gram): An enduring mark or trace. In psychology, a lasting impression made by an experience.

enhematospore (en-hem′-a-tō-spor): A spore of the malarial parasite that forms within the bloodstream. Also hematophore.

enkephalin (en-kef′-a-lin): Either of two pentapeptides normally found in the body, the brain in particular but also in the gastrointestinal tract and the pituitary gland; composed of five amino acids. The effect of enkephalins of the central nervous system derives from their combining with certain receptors to reduce the individual's perception of pain. See also **endorphin.**

enomania (ē-nō-mā′-ni-a): A mental disorder characterized by an uncontrollable desire for alcoholic drink; delirium tremens. Also oinomania.

enophthalmos (en-of-thal′-mus): Retraction of the eyeball within its orbit. Opp. to exophthalmos.

enostosis (en-os-tō′-sis): A bony growth within the medullary canal of a bone. See **exostosis.**

ensiform (en′-si-form): Sword-shaped. Term applied to the process at the lower end of the breast bone. Syn., xiphoid.

ENT: Abbreviation for ear, nose, and throat.

entad (en′-tad): Toward the center or interior; inwardly.

ental (en′-tal): Internal; inner; central.

entamebiasis (ent-a-me-bī′-a-sis): Infestation with a species of the Entamoeba; amebic dysentery.

Entamoeba (ent-a-mē′ba): A genus of protozoon parasites, some species of which affect man. **E. COLI,** nonpathogenic, infests the human intestinal tract. **E. GINGIVALIS,** infests the mouth about the gums and found in tartar on teeth; nonpathogenic. **E. HYSTOLYTICA,** pathogenic; causes amebic dysentery (*q.v.*).

enter-, entero-: Combining forms denoting intestine.

enteral (en′-ter-al): 1. Within the gastrointestinal tract. 2. Pertaining to the small intestine. **E. NUTRITION,** provides nutrition for those who are not able to ingest adequate nutrients orally but who are able to utilize them in the body; feedings are given through nasoduodenal, gastric, jejunostomy, or pharyngotomy tubes.

enteralgia (en-ter-al′-ji-a): Abdominal pain; cramps; colic.

enterectasis (en-ter-ek′-ta-sis): Distention or dilatation of the bowel.

enterectomy (en-ter-ek′-to-mi): Surgical removal of part of the small intestine.

enteric (en-ter′-ik): Pertaining to the intestine. **E. BACTERIA,** bacteria living in or isolated from the intestine. **E.-COATED,** refers to a pill or other medication that is coated with a substance that will not dissolve until it reaches the intestine. **E. FEVER,** includes typhoid and paratyphoid fever (*q.v.*).

enteritis (en-ter-ī′-tis): Inflammation of the intestine, the small intestine in particular.

enteroanastomosis (en′-ter-ō-a-nas-tō-mō′-sis): The surgical union of two parts of the intestine; term usually refers to the small intestine.

Enterobacter (en′-ter-ō-bak′-ter): A genus of the family *Enterobacteriaceae;* widely distributed in nature; **E. AEROGENES,** a species found in soil, sewage, water, dairy products, and intestinal canal of both humans and animals; often acts as an opportunistic pathogen.

Enterobacteriaceae (en′-ter-ō-bak-tēr-i-ā′-sē-ē): A large family of motile and nonmotile gram-negative bacteria which act on glucose to produce acid and gas; includes the *Escherichia coli, Salmonella, Shigella, Proteus,* and *Klebsiella* organisms.

enterobiasis (en-ter-ō-bī′-a-sis): Infestation with worms of the genus *Enterobius vermicularis* (*q.v.*), the human pinworm.

Enterobius vermicularis (en-ter-ō′bi-us ver-mik-ū-lar′is): A nematode which infests the small and large intestine. Threadworm; pinworm; seatworm. Found more often in children than adults. Presence in the rectum causes intense itching. Transmitted in the ova of the worm which is found in feces of infected persons. Prevalent among those whose environmental and personal hygiene are poor. Distribution is worldwide.

enterocele (en′-ter-ō-sēl): 1. Hernia of the intestine. 2. Prolapse of the intestine, sometimes into the upper posterior part of the vagina.

enterocentesis (en′-ter-ō-sen-tē′-sis): Surgical puncture of the intestine to withdraw gas or fluid.

enterocholecystostomy (en′-ter-ō-kō-le-sis-tos′-to-mi): Surgical creation of an opening from the gallbladder into the small intestine.

enteroclysis (en-ter-ok′-li-sis): The introduction of nutrient or medicinal fluid into the bowel; a high enema. Syn., proctoclysis.

enterococcus (en-ter-ō-kok′-us): A gram-positive encapsulated streptococcus that occurs in short chains and is relatively resistant to heat. It is found in the human intestine; sometimes is the causative organism in infections of the urinary tract, ear, and wounds and, more rarely, in endocarditis.

enterocolectomy (en′-ter-ō-kō-lek′-tō-mi): Surgical excision of parts of both the small intestine and the colon.

enterocolitis (en′-ter-ō-kō-lī′-tis): Inflammation of the mucous membrane lining of the intestines and the colon. **HEMORRHAGIC E., E.** characterized by hemorrhagic breakdown of the mucous lining of the intestinal mucosa. **NECROTIZING E.,** severe inflammation of the gastrointestinal tract; when it occurs in high risk neonates it is often fatal. **REGIONAL E.,** see Chron's disease. **PSEUDOMEMBRANOUS E.,** see colitis, pseudomembranous.

enterocolostomy (en′-ter-ō-kō-los′-to-mi): The surgical creation of an artificial opening between the small intestine and colon.

enterocutaneous (en′-ter-ō-kū-tā′-ne-us): Pertaining to the intestine and the cutaneous surface of the body, or to a communication between the two, as an **E.** fistula.

enterocyst (en′-ter-ō-sist): A cyst in the intestinal wall. Also enterocystoma.

enterocystocele (en-ter-ō-sis′-tō-sēl): A hernia involving both the urinary bladder and the intestine.

enterocystoma (en-ter-ō-sis-tō′-ma): A cystic tumor of the intestinal wall; enterocyst.

enterodynia (en-ter-ō-din′-i-a): Pain in the intestine.

enteroenterostomy (en′-ter-ō-en-ter-os′-to-mi): The surgical anastomosis of two parts of the intestine that do not normally adjoin each other.

enterogastritis (en′-ter-ō-gas-trī′-tis): Inflammation of the small intestine and the stomach.

enterogenous (en-ter-oj′-i-nus): Arising in the intestine.

enterohepatitis (en′-ter-ō-hep-a-tī′-tis): Inflammation of the intestine and the liver.

enterokinase (en-ter-ō-kī′-nās): An enzyme in intestinal juice. It converts inactive trypsinogen into active trypsin.

enterolith (en′-ter-ō-lith): An intestinal concretion.

enterolithiasis (en′-ter-ō-lith-ī′-a-sis): The presence of calculi or concretions in the intestine.

enterolysis (en-ter-ol′-i-sis): The surgical freeing of the intestine from adhesions.

enteromegaly (en-ter-ō-meg′-a-li): Enlargement of the intestine. See megacolon.

enteromycosis (en′-ter-ō-mī-kō′-sis): Any fungal disease of the intestine.

enteron (en′-te-ron): The gut, the small intestine in particular.

enteropathogenic (en′-ter-ō-path-ō-jen′-ik): Pertaining to or capable of producing disease in the intestine.

enteropathy (en-ter-op′-a-thi): Any pathology of the intestine. PROTEIN-LOSING E., excessive loss of serum protein through feces, particularly albumin, resulting in hypoproteinemia.

enteropexy (en′-ter-ō-pek-si): The surgical fixation of a part of the intestine to the abdominal wall.

enteroplasty (en′-ter-ō-plas-ti): Any plastic surgery on the bowel, but particularly that employed for enlarging the caliber of the bowel.

enteroplegia (en-ter-ō-plē′-ji-a): Paralysis of the intestine; see ileus.

enteroptosis (en-ter-op-tō′-sis): Descent or downward displacement of the intestines, usually associated with the downward displacement of other abdominal organs. Also called enteropsia, abdominal ptosis, visceroptosis.—enteroptotic, adj.

enterorrhagia (en-ter-ō-rā′-ji-a): Hemorrhage in or from the intestine.

enterorrhaphy (en-ter-or′-a-fi): Suture or repair of the intestine.

enterorrhexis (en-ter-ō-rek′-sis): Rupture of the intestine.

enterosepsis (en-ter-ō-sep′-sis): Intestinal toxemia, usually caused by putrefaction of intestinal content.

enterospasm (en′-ter-ō-spazm): Excessive contraction of the intestinal muscle.

enterostasis (en-ter-os′-ta-sis): Intestinal stasis; cessation or delay of the passage of intestinal contents.

enterostenosis (en′-ter-ō-ste-nō′-sis): A stricture or narrowing of a portion of the intestine.

enterostomy (en-ter-os′-to-mi): The surgical establishment of an artificial anus or opening into the intestine through the abdominal wall.

enterotomy (en-ter-ot′-o-mi): An incision into the intestine, the small intestine in particular.

enterotoxin (en-ter-ō-tok′-sin): A toxin produced in the intestine by certain species of bacteria and which produce symptoms associated with food poisoning.—enterotoxigenic, adj.

enterotropic (en-ter-ō-trop′-ik): Pertaining to or affecting the intestines.

enterovesical (en-ter-ō-ves′i-kal): Pertaining to the intestine and the urinary bladder.

enterovirus (en-ter-ō-vī′-rus): One of a group of more than 70 related viruses that were formerly classified as echovirus, coxsackievirus, and poliovirus, which enter the body through the alimentary tract and tend to invade the central nervous system. Recently, investigators have classified enteroviruses as a genus of picornoviruses (*q.v.*).

enterozoon (en-ter-ō-zō′-on): Any animal parasite that infects or inhabits the intestine.—enterozoa, pl.

enthesis (en′-the-sis): The use of metal or other inorganic material to replace lost or absent tissue.—enthetic, adj.

enthesitis (en-the-sī′-tis): Inflammation or disorder of the muscular or tendinous attachment to bone; caused by recurring muscle stress.

entity (en′-ti-tē): The existence of a thing or condition separate from its attributes and in contrast to them. In medicine, a distinct and separate disorder or disease.

entochondrostosis (en′-tō-kon-dros-tō′-sis): The development of bone within cartilage.

entoderm (en′-tō-derm): The innermost of the three primary layers of the embryo from which is derived the epithelial lining of the whole of the digestive tube except part of the mouth, pharynx, and rectum; the lining cells of the glands that empty into the digestive tube; the epithelium lining the respiratory tract and the auditory canal and part of the genitourinary tract; and part of the thyroid, thymus and parathyroid glands.—entodermal, adj.

entomology (en-tō-mol′-o-ji): The branch of biology that deals with the study of insects. MEDICAL E., the branch of medicine that deals with the study of insects that cause disease in man or serve as vectors of disease.

entomophobia (en-tō-mō-fō′-bi-a): A morbid dread of insects, mites, ticks, and other arthropoda.

entopic (en-top′-ik): Occurring in the correct place; opp. of ectopic (*q.v.*).

entoptic (ent-op′-tik): Pertaining to or occurring within the eyeball.

entoptoscopy (en-top-tos′-kō-pi): Examination of the interior of the eyeball.

entotic (ent-ō′-tik): Pertaining to or occurring within the inner ear.

entrails (en′-trāls): Intestines, or viscera; most often referring to those of animals.

entrapment syndrome: A condition caused by entrapment of a nerve in soft or hard tissue, characterized by pain in the part served by the involved nerve; also called compression neuritis.

entropion (en-trō′-pē-on): The turning inward of a margin or edge, particularly the inversion of an eyelid so that the lashes are in contact with the globe of the eye, occurring as a result of laxity of the structures supporting the eyelid.

entropy (en′-trō-pi): **1.** In physiology, a diminished capacity for adjusting to change, as occurs in the aging. **2.** The concept that all organized matter must degrade. **3.** The portion of energy in a system that cannot be converted to work.

enucleation (ē-nū-klē-ā′-shun): The removal of an organ or tumor in its entirety, as of an eyeball from its socket.—enucleate, v.

enuresis (en-ū-rē′-sis): Involuntary urination, especially bedwetting, when it is not due to any organic disease of the urinary organs. Habitually wetting oneself.

envenomation (en-ven-ō-mā′-shun): The injection of venom into the body through the puncture wounds of a snake or insect bite or sting.

environment (en-vī′-ron-ment): External surroundings. The total of all the conditions and forces that surround and act upon an organism or any of its parts.

environmental (en-vī-ron-men′-tal): Pertaining to the environment. **E. MANIPULATION,** in psychiatry, an attempt to help an individual by changing his environment so as to make it less stressful.

Environmental Protection Agency (EPA): An independent governmental agency that has responsibility for air and water quality, control of solid waste disposal, use of pesticides, radiation hazards, noise, and toxic substances. Conducts research on air pollution, promulgates standards, and enforces compliance with standards.

enzygotic (en-zī-got′-ik): Development from one zygote. **E. TWINS,** identical twins.

enzyme (en′-zīm): A complex organic compound, often a protein, produced by living cells, that acts specifically to accelerate or produce some chemical change without itself being changed. Each **E.** is specific for one particular chemical transformation only.—enzymic, enzymatic, adj.

enzymology (en-zī-mol′-ō-ji): The branch of chemistry dealing with the structure and function of enzymes.—enzymological, adj.; enzymologically, adv.

enzymolysis (en-zī-mol′-i-sis): Lysis that is activated by or caused by the action of an enzyme.

enzymopathy (en-zī-mop′-a-thi): Disturbance in the secretion or functional activity of an enzyme.

enzymuria (en-zī-mū′-ri-a): The presence of more than the normal amount of enzymes in the urine; seen in patients with renal damage including that which occurs in ischemia, neoplasms, transplant reactions, and following ingestion of nephrotoxic drugs.

eosin (ē′-ō-sin): A group of red-staining dyes used in histology and laboratory diagnostic procedures.

eosinopenia (ē-ō-sin-ō-pē′-ni-a): An abnormally small number of eosinophils per unit volume in the peripheral bloodstream.

eosinophil (e) (ē-ō-sin′-ō-fil): A cell having an affinity for eosin (*q.v.*). A type of white blood cell that constitutes about 1 to 4 percent of the total leukocytes in the blood and increases in number during allergic states and infestation with worms.

eosinophilia (ē-ō-sin-ō-fil′-i-a): An increase above normal in the number of eosinophils per unit volume in peripheral blood. **PULMONARY E.,** a transient condition usually due to worm infestation, but may also be produced by certain drugs. **SPUTUM E.,** the presence of an abnormal number of eosinophils in the sputum, a characteristic of asthma. **TROPICAL E.,** pulmonary **E.,** a type of **E.** occurring mainly in the tropics; may be associated with polyarteritis or asthma.

ep-, epi: Prefix denoting upon, above, over; beside; anterior; on the outside.

EPA: Abbreviation for Environmental Protection Agency.

ependyma (ep-en′-di-ma): The membrane lining the ventricles of the brain and the central canal of the spinal cord.—ependymal, adj.

ependymitis (ep-en-di-mī′-tis): Inflammation of the ependyma.

ependymoma (ep-en-di-mō′-ma): Neoplasm arising in the lining of the cerebral ventricles or central canal of the spinal cord. Occurs in all age groups. Clinically, it resembles astrocytoma (*q.v.*).

ephebiatrics (e-fē-bi-at′-riks): That branch of medicine that deals with the diseases of adolescents as compared with pediatrics and geriatrics.

ephebiatrist (e-fē-bī′-a-trist): A physician who specializes in the diseases of adolescents.

ephebic (e-fē′-bik): Pertaining to puberty or adolescence.

ephebology (ef-ē-bol′o-ji): The study of puberty, particularly the changes that occur during this period.

ephelis (ef-ē′-lis): A freckle.—ephelides, pl.

ephemeral (e-fem′-er-al): Fleeting; transient.

epiblepharon (ep-i-blef′-a-ron): A congenital anomaly in which an excess fold of skin on the lower eyelid causes the lashes to turn inward; seen in Down's syndrome and certain other abnormalities; to be differentiated from the epicanthal folds normal to Asiatics.

epicanthic fold: See epicanthus.

epicanthus (ep-i-kan′-thus): The congenital occurrence of a fold of skin that reaches from the root of the nose to the medial end of the eyebrow; may obscure the inner canthus and caruncle; a racial characteristic of certain ethnic groups.—epicanthal, epicanthic, adj.

epicardia (ep-i-kar′-di-a): The lower end of the esophagus between the diaphragm and the opening into the stomach.—epicardial, adj.

epicardial (ep-i-kar′-di-al): Pertaining to either 1) the epicardia, or 2) the epicardium.

epicardium (ep-i-kar′-di-um): The thin visceral or inner layer of the pericardium that immediately invests the heart.—epicardial, adj.

epicondyle (ep-i-kon′-dīl): A bony projection situated above a condyle on a bone.—epicondylar, adj.

epicondylitis (ep-i-kon-di-lī′-tis): Pain and tenderness at the outer side of the elbow due to injury of the lateral condyle of the humerus, resulting from violent twisting of the wrist, as often occurs in playing tennis. Also called tennis elbow; olecranon bursitis; lateral epicondylitis.

epicranium (ep-i-krān′-i-um): The scalp; that is, the muscle, skin, etc., that form the covering of the cranium.—epicranial, adj.

epicritic (ep-i-krit′-ik): Term applied to a set of nerve fibers in the skin and oral mucosa that enable one to discriminate fine variations in the sensations of touch, temperature, or pain, and to localize these sensations. The opposite of protopathic (*q.v.*).

epicureanism (ep-i-kūr-ē′-an-izm): A philosophy of life that emphasizes pleasure, the happiness of the moment, and instant gratification.

epicystitis (ep-i-sis-tī′-tis): Inflammation of the tissues surrounding the urinary bladder, including the peritoneum.

epicystotomy (ep-i-sis-tot′-o-mi): A suprapubic incision into the urinary bladder.

epidemic (ep-i-dem′-ik): 1. Simultaneously affecting many people in an area. Cf. endemic. 2. The occurrence in a community or region of a group of illnesses of a similar nature, in excess of normal expectancy, and derived from a common source. 3. Of, or pertaining to epidemics.

epidemic pleurodynia (ep-i-dem′-ik plū-rō-din′-i-a): An acute epidemic disease of viral origin, usually the Coxsackie B virus; characterized by acute paroxysmal pain in the lower chest and upper abdomen that increases on respiration, and headache, malaise, fever, aching limbs, sore throat.

epidemicity (ep-i-de-mis′-i-ti): The characteristic of being a community-wide and rapidly proliferating occurrence of disease.

epidemiologist (ep-i-dē-mi-ol′-o-jist): A person who specializes in epidemiology.

epidemiology (ep-i-dē-mi-ol′-o-ji): The scientific study of the factors that determine the causes, incidence, distribution and control of diseases and injuries in human populations, especially epidemic and endemic diseases.—epidemiological, adj., epidemiologically, adv.

epidermal (ep-i-der′-mal): Pertaining to or involving the epidermis.

epidermis (ep-i-der′-mis): The external, nonvascular layer of the skin; composed of several individual layers; the cuticle. Also known as the scarf skin.—epidermal, adj.

epidermitis (ep-i-der-mī′-tis): Inflammation of the epidermis or outer layer of the skin.

epidermodysplasia (ep-i-der′-mō-dis-plā′-zi-a): Faulty or incomplete development of the epidermis. **E. VERRUCIFORMIS**, a congenital defect characterized by verrucous lesions on the hands, feet, neck, or face; caused by a virus.

epidermoid (ep-i-der′-moyd): Resembling epidermis or epidermal cells. **E. CARCINOMA**, malignant epithelioma occurring in the skin. **E. CYST**, a cyst arising from aberrant epithelial cells, commonly occurring in subcutaneous areas as a steatoma or wen, but may also be seen in the skull, meninges, or brain.

epidermoidoma (ep′-i-der-moy-dō′-ma): A tumor involving the scalp, extradural space, and the upper part of the skull; usually benign.

epidermoma (ep-i-der-mō′-ma): Any growth or mass in the skin.

epidermomycosis (ep-i-der′-mō-mī-kō′-sis): Dermatitis caused by a fungus.

Epidermophyton (ep-i-der-mof′-i-ton): A genus of fungi that affects the skin and nails. **E. FLOCCOSUM**, the causative agent of several types of ringworm including ringworm of the scalp and athlete's foot.

epidermophytosis (ep-i-der′-mō-fī-tō′-sis): Infection with fungi of the genus Epidermophyton.

epidermosis (e-pi-der-mō′-sis): A skin disease which affects only the epidermis; characterized by decreased glandular secretion, water loss, degeneration of the cells of the dermis, thinning and wrinkling.

epidiascope (ep-i-dī′-a-skōp): An instrument used for projecting translucent or opaque pictures onto a screen.

epididymectomy (ep-i-did-i-mek′-to-mi): Surgical removal of the epididymis.

epididymis (ep-i-did′-i-mis): A small oblong

body attached to the posterior surface of the testis. Consists of the first, convoluted portion of the excretory duct of the testis; conveys the spermatozoa from the testis to the vas deferens.

epididymitis (ep-i-did-i-mī'tis): Inflammation of the epididymis (*q.v*); may occur following prolonged use of an indwelling catheter or occur as a complication of mumps, prostatitis, urethritis, syphilis, gonorrhea; symptoms include fever, pain in the inguinal area, local edema.

epididymo-orchidectomy (ep-i-did-i'-mō-or-kid-ek'-tō-mi): The surgical removal of a testis and epididymis.

epididymo-orchitis (ep-i-did'-i-mō-or-kī'-tis): Inflammation of the epididymis and the testis.

epidural (ep-i-dū'-ral): Upon or external to the dura mater. **E. BLOCK**, injection of the local anesthetic, usually in the lumbar or caudal region prior to rectal examination and surgery, a forceps delivery, or cesarean section. Currently used for crush injuries to the chest; the analgesia can be maintained for a week or more. **E. SPACE**, the space outside the dura mater of the brain and spinal cord.

epifolliculitis (ep'-i-fō-lik-u-lī'-tis): Inflammation of the hair follicles of the scalp.

epigastric (ep-i-gas'-trik): Pertaining to the epigastrium. **E. ANGLE**, the angle made by the xiphoid process and the body of the sternum.

epigastrium (ep-i-gas'-tri-um): The abdominal region lying directly over the stomach; the "pit" of the stomach.—epigastric, adj.

epiglottis (ep-i-glot'-is): The thin leaf-shaped flap of cartilage behind the tongue which, during the act of swallowing, covers the opening leading into the larynx.—epiglottic, adj.

epiglottitis (ep-i-glot-tī'-tis): Inflammation of the epiglottis. The acute form, which occurs mainly in children, may cause respiratory difficulty due to swelling of the epiglottis; other symptoms include croupy cough, stridulous breathing, cyanosis, and prostration.

epilation (ep-il-ā'-shun): Extraction or destruction of hair roots, *e.g.*, by coagulation necrosis, electrolysis, or forceps.—epilate, v.

epilatory (ē-pil'-a-tor-i): An agent that produces epilation.

epilemma (ep-i-lem'-ma): The outer sheath of very small nerves.

epilepsia (ep-i-lep'-si-a): Epilepsy.

epilepsy (ep'-i-lep-si): A recurrent paroxysmal disorder of cerebral function characterized always by variable clouding of consciousness, often associated with generalized convulsions, and due to an abnormal discharge of nerve impulses in the brain. **E.** can be classified on causation: 1) **SYMPTOMATIC E., E.** due to a recognized cause or agent, *e.g.*, cerebral tumor, trauma, or vascular abnormality; or 2) **IDIOPATHIC E., E.** of unknown cause; or on clinical features: 1) **GRAND MAL**—loss of consciousness with generalized convulsions; 2) **PETIT MAL**—clouding of consciousness with no generalized convulsions; or 3) **JACKSONIAN E.**, convulsions beginning in one muscle group and either remaining localized or else spreading in an orderly march to involve wider muscle groups, and which may then involve loss of consciousness; or according to age at onset: 1) **PRIMARY E., E.** with onset of seizures usually occuring in the first two years of life or later in adolescence; heredity is a factor in the etiology; 2) **SECONDARY E.**, which begins in childhood or after age 30; with many causative factors including brain tumor, trauma, infection, meningitis, encephalitis, exposure to toxic substances. **ABDOMINAL E.**, a rare form characterized by recurrent episodes of abdominal pain without the usual convulsions of epilepsy. **AKINETIC E.**, epileptic manifestations without movement and usually no loss of consciousness. **FOCAL E.**, minor recurrent seizures limited to one side of the body. **MYOCLONIC E.**, a hereditary **E.** which begins in childhood; characterized by sudden attacks of muscle clonus and shock-like jerks of a limb or the body; often occurs in the morning. **PSYCHOMOTOR E.**, convulsions follow soon after a head injury and may not recur, or convulsive attacks start a month or more after injury and are then likely to recur. **REFLEX E.**, a form of **E.** characterized by attacks that are brought on by an external stimulus. **SENILE E.**, includes several disorders that occur in the elderly; the person may not have seizures but usually has drop attacks. **TEMPORAL LOBE E.**, psychomotor **E.**, characterized by impaired consciousness, semi-purposeful movements of arms or legs, hallucinations. See status epilepticus under status.

epileptic (ep-i-lep'-tik): 1. A person affected with epilepsy. 2. Pertaining to epilepsy. **E. AURA**, premonitory subjective phenomena (tingling in the hand or visual or auditory sensations) that precede an attack of grand mal. **E. CRY**, the croak or shout heard from the epileptic person as he falls unconscious.

epileptiform (ep-i-lep'-ti-form): 1. Resembling epilepsy. 2. Descriptive of a convulsion that resembles the convulsions of epilepsy; accompanied by loss of consciousness.

epileptogenic (ep-i-lep-tō-jen'-ik): Causing epilepsy or an epileptic seizure.

epiloia (ep-i-loy'-a): A congenital familial abnormality of brain tissue resulting in a syndrome consisting of progressive mental deficiency, hypertrophic sclerosis of the brain, nodules on the floor of the lateral ventricles, seizures, congential tumors of the eye, sometimes growths in kidney or spleen. Also known as tuberous sclerosis. May be associated with epilepsy.

epimenorrhagia (ep-i-men-ō-rā′-ji- a): Too frequent and too excessive menstruation.

epimenorrhea (ep-i-men-ō-rē′-a): Reduction in the length of the menstrual cycle resulting in too frequent menstruation.

epimysium (ep-i-miz′-i-um): The external fibrous sheath of a skeletal muscle.

epinephrine (ep-i-nef′-rin): The chief hormone of the normal adrenal medulla; is also produced synthetically. A powerful vasopressor substance. Contracts arterioles of skin, mucuous membrane and viscera; dilates arterioles of skeletal muscles and brain; increases strength and rate of heart beat; increases heart output, blood pressure, blood sugar and metabolism; speeds blood clotting; relaxes bronchial muscles. Used therapeutically to control local bleeding as in epistaxis, and to relieve anaphylaxis, allergic conditions, asthmatic attacks, heart and circulatory failure, also in treatment of open-angle glaucoma. Also called adrenaline (in Great Britain).

epineurium (ep-i-nū′-ri-um): The connective tissue covering of a nerve trunk.

epiotic (ep-i-ot′-ik, ep-i-ō′-tik): Situated on or above the cartilage of the ear.

epipharynx (ep-i-far′-inks): Nasopharynx (*q.v.*).

epiphenomenon (ep-i-fe-nom′-e-non): An unexpected, or accidental event or condition occurring during the course of a disease; may or may not be related to the disease itself.

epiphora (ē-pif′-o-ra): Pathological overflow of tears onto the cheek. May be due to excessive secretion, obstruction, or narrowing of the lacrimal passages.

epiphysial, epiphyseal (ep-i-fiz′-i-al): Referring to or related to an epiphysis (*q.v.*). **E. FRACTURE,** the separation of the epiphysis from a long bone; results from injury. **E. PLATE,** the thin plate of cartilage between the shaft of a long bone and its epiphysis in children and young adults; it is the site of growth in bone length and when growth is completed it is replaced by bone, the resulting area being called the **EPIPHYSIAL LINE.**

epiphysiodesis (ep′-i-fiz-i-od′-e-sis): Premature ossification of an epiphysis resulting in cessation of bone growth. In surgery, the procedure of fixing a separated epiphysis to the diaphysis of the bone; done usually on children when the bones are of uneven length.

epiphysiolysis (ep′-i-fiz-i-ol′-i- sis): Abnormal separation of an epiphysis from the shaft of a bone.

epiphysis (ē-pif′-i-sis): The growing part of a bone, especially a long bone, that is separated from the end of the main shaft by a plate of cartilage; the latter disappears and becomes part of the bone when growth ceases. **SLIPPED E.,** displacement of an **E.,** especially the upper femoral; epiphysiolisthesis.—epiphyses, pl.; epiphysial, epiphyseal, adj.

epiphysitis (ē-pif-i-sī′-tis): Inflammation of an epiphysis.

epiphyte (ep′-i-fīt): A plant organism growing as a parasite on the body.

epiplocele (ē-pip′-lō-sēl): A hernia that contains omentum.

epiploenterocele (e-pip′-lō-en′-ter- ō-sēl): A hernia that contains both intestine and omentum.

epiploic (ep-i-plō′-ik): Related to or referring to the epiploon (*q.v.*).

epiplomphalocele (ep-i-plom-fal′-o-sēl): An umbilical hernia containing omentum.

epiploon (ē-pip′-lō-on): The greater omentum (*q.v.*).—epiploic, adj.

episacroiliac (ep′-i-sā-krō-il′- i-ak): Situated above the sacroiliac joint. **E. LIPOMA,** soft fleshy nodules occurring over the sacroiliac joint at the insertion of the erector muscles; a fairly common condition.

episclera (ep-i-sklē′-ra): Loose connective tissue between the sclera and conjunctiva.—episcleral, adj.

episcleral (ep-i-sklē′-ral): Situated on the outside of the sclera.

episcleritis (ep-i-sklē-rī′-tis): Inflammation of the tissues covering the sclera or of the outermost layers of scleral tissue.

episioperineoplasty (ē-piz′-i-ō-per-i-nē′-ō-plas-ti): Repair of a lacerated vulva and perineum by plastic surgery.

episiorrhagia (ē-piz-i-ō-rā′-ji-a): Hemorrhage from the vulva.

episiorrhaphy (ē-piz-i-or′-ra-fi): The surgical repair of a lacerated vulva or of an episiotomy after childbirth.

episiotomy (ē-piz-i-ot′-o-mi): Incision of the vulva made during the birth of a child when the vaginal orifice does not stretch enough and laceration of the perineum seems imminent.

epispadias (ep-i-spā′-di-as): A congenital anomaly in the male in which the urethral opening in the penis is on the dorsal side; occurs rarely in the female, when the opening is above the clitoris.

epispastic (ep-i-spas′-tik): 1. Causing blistering. 2. A blistering agent or vesicant.

episplenitis (ep-i-sple-nī′-tis): Inflammation of the capsule of the spleen.

epistasis (ē-pis′-ta-sis): 1. In genetics the supressive effect of one gene on another as occurs, *e.g.,* in albinism, in which the determining gene for pigmentation patterns is suppressed. 2. The control or stoppage of hemorrhage.

epistaxis (ep-i-stak′-sis): Bleeding from the nose.—epistaxes, pl.

episternum (ep-i-ster′-num): The manubrium or upper part of the sternum.

epistropheus (ep-i-strō′-fe-us): The axis; the second cervical vertebra.

epitendineum (ep′-i-ten-din′-ē-um): The fibrous sheath that covers tendons.

epithelial (ep-i-thē′-li-al): Pertaining to the epithelium. **E. PEARLS,** or **NESTS,** multiple rounded or oval, variously sized, aggregates of neoplastic epidermal material, frequently found in squamous cell carcinomata.

epithelialization (ep-i-thē′-li-al-ī-za′-shun): The growth of epithelium over a raw area; the final stage of healing. Also epithelization.

epithelioid (ep-i-thē′-li-oyd): Resembling epithelium.

epitheliolysin (ep′-i-thē-li-ol′-i-sin): A specific lysin in the blood serum that causes dissolution of epithelial cells.—epitheliolytic, adj.

epithelioma (ep-i-thē-li-ō′-ma): A malignant growth arising in epithelial tissue, usually the skin; a squamous cell carcinoma. **BASAL CELL E.,** skin cancer which often follows exposure to radium, radiation, or sunlight; starts as slow-growing nodules, sometimes pigmented with later ulceration that penetrates into the deep tissues; may be fatal. **SCROTAL E.,** chimney-sweep's cancer; caused by irritation due to coal soot.

epithelium (ep-i-thē′-li-um): The surface layer of cells covering cutaneous, mucous, and serous surfaces. It is classified according to the arrangement of the cells it contains as 1) simple squamous; 2) simple cuboidal; 3) simple columnar; and 4) pseudo-stratified columnar. **E.** protects underlying tissues from wear and tear and must be continually renewed; some epithelial cells are able to absorb certain substances; others have secretory or excretory functions.

epitrochlea (ep-i-trok′-lē-a): The medial epicondyle (*q.v.*) of the humerus.—epitrochlear, adj.

epityphlitis (ep-i-tif-lī′-tis): Appendicitis.

epizoon (ep-i-zō′-on): An animal parasite living on the outside of the host's body.—epizoa, pl. epizoic, adj.

eponychia (ep-ō-nik′-i-a): An infection of the fold of skin around the nail.

eponychium (ep-ō-nik′-i-um): The horny layer of skin attached to the margin of the nails.

eponym (ep′-o-nim): 1. One for whom something is named. 2. The name of something formed from or including a person's name, such as Cushing's syndrome.

epoophoron (ep-ō-of′-e-ron): A blind longitudinal duct appearing between the ovary and the fallopian tube; an embryonic remnant that corresponds to the epididymus in the male.

EPSDT: Early Periodic Screening, Diagnosis, and Treatment program, enacted into legislation in 1967; purpose is to provide health care for children who are on public assistance.

Epsom salt: Magnesium sulfate; formerly in wide use as a cathartic.

Epstein-Barr virus: Virus particles that resemble herpesvirus; associated with infectious mononucleosis; also thought to be a possible cause of Burkitt's lymphoma and nasopharyngeal carcinoma.

Epstein's pearls: Small yellowish white, slightly elevated cysts or masses seen on each side of the hard palate and sometimes on the gums in many newborns. [A. Epstein, Prague pediatrician. 1880-1965.]

epulis (ep-ū′-lis): A benign tumor growing on or from the gums.

epulosis (ep-ū-lo′-sis): A scarring over; cicatrization.

equation (ē-kwā′-zhun): An expression of equality of two things, or quantities; often involves the use of mathematical and/or chemical symbols.

equilibrium (ē′-kwi-lib′-ri- um): 1. A state of balance between forces or processes. 2. The normal, oriented state of the body in respect to its position in space, maintained through the labyrinthine sense. **ACID-BASE E.,** the state of the body when the acids and bases in body fluids are present in their normal ratio. **NITROGENOUS E.,** the condition of the body when the amount of nitrogen excreted is in the normal ratio to that taken in.

equinia (ē-kwīn′-i-a): A mild form of glanders (*q.v.*) in man; contracted from horses with glanders.

equinovalgus (ē-kwī′-nō-val′- gus): Talipes equinovalgus; elevation and outward rotation of the heel.

equinovarus (ē-kwī′-nō-var′- us): Talipes equinovarus; elevation and inward rotation of the heel; the most common form of clubfoot.

equinus (ē-kwī′-nus): Talipes equinus. See under talipes.

ER: Abbreviation for emergency room.

erasion (ē-rā′-zhun): Surgical removal of tissue by scraping. **E. OF A JOINT,** arthrectomy (*q.v.*).

Erb [William H. Erb, German neurologist. 1840-1921.]: **ERB'S PARALYSIS, ERB'S PALSY, ERB-DUCHENNE PALSY,** see under palsy. **ERB'S POINT:** a point 2 or 3 cm above the clavicle at the side of the neck where pressure on the brachial plexus gives rise to Erb's paralysis. **ERB'S SIGN,** 1) loss of the patellar reflex, an early sign of tabes dorsalis; or 2) increased excitablility to faradic or galvanic current; seen in tetany.

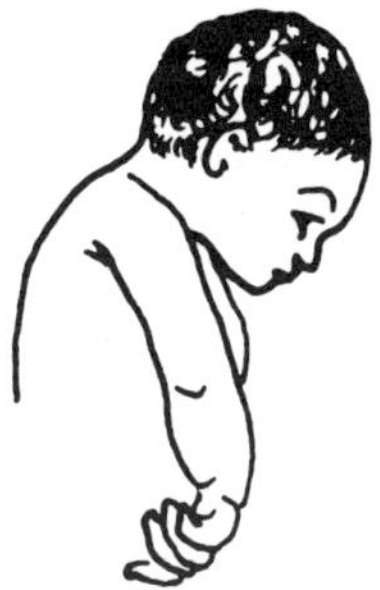

Erb's palsy

erectile (ē-rek′-tīl): Upright; capable of being elevated. **E. TISSUE,** highly vascular tissue, which, under stimulus, becomes rigid and erect from hyperemia.

erection (ē-rek′-shun): The condition achieved when erectile tissue is made rigid or elevated due to hyperemia. The enlarged, rigid penis of the male (or clitoris of the female) under stimulus of sexual excitement is said to be in a state of erection.

erector (ē-rek′-tor): A muscle that achieves erection of, or raises, a part.

erepsin (ē-rep′-sin): Old term for a proteolytic enzyme in succus entericus (*q.v.*).

erethism (er′-e-thizm): Heightened responsiveness of the nervous system.

erethisophrenia (er′-e-thiz-ō- frē′-ni-a): Abnormally heightened mental activity.

ERG: Abbreviation for electroretinogram.

erg: A unit of energy or of work.

ergasiomania (er-gas-i-ō-mā′-ni-a): 1. An abnormal desire to keep oneself continually working. 2. An unnatural eagerness to perform surgical operations. Also ergomania.

ergasiophobia (er-gas-i-ō-fō′-bi-a): 1. A morbid aversion to work. 2. Intense fear of performing surgical operations.

ergogram (er′-gō-gram): The graphic recording made by an ergograph.

ergograph (er′-gō-graf): An instrument that measures the amount of movement a muscle is capable of performing or the amount of work it is able to do; utilizes a weight or spring against which the muscle contracts.

ergography (er-gog′-ra-fi): The measurement of the output of effort in response to an electric stimulus as recorded in the tracing made by an ergograph.

ergometer (er-gom′-e-ter): An intrument for measuring the work done by muscular activity. **BICYCLE E.**, one used for measuring the energy expended while using a stationary bicycle.

ergometry (er-gom′-et-ri): Measurement of work done by muscles.—ergometric, adj.

ergonomics (er-gō-nom′-iks): The application of various biological disciplines in relation to man and his working environment.

ergosterol (er-gos′-ter-ol): A provitamin present in the subcutaneous fat of man; also found in plants and foodstuffs. On irradiation with sunlight or ultrviolet light it is converted into vitamin D_2 which has antirachitic properties.

ergot (er′-got): A fungus that is parasitic on rye. It is the source of several valuable alkaloids used in medicine; causes contraction of muscular coat of the arteries, raises blood pressure and contracts uterine muscle; widely used in control of postpartum hemorrhage. Also useful in treatment of certain vascular disorders including migraine headache.

ergotherapy (er-gō-ther′-a-pi): The treatment of disorders by muscular exercise.

ergotism (er′-got-izm): Chronic poisoning due to excessive or wrong use of ergot as a medicine or from eating food made from rye or wheat that was infected with the fungus; marked by muscle spasms, cerebrospinal symptoms and dry gangrene. Has been called St. Anthony's fire (*q.v.*).

Erlenmeyer flask: A flask with a cone-shaped body, a broad base, and a narrow neck; especially suitable for certain chemical procedures. [Emil Erlenmeyer, German chemist. 1825-1909.]

erode (ē-rōd′): To diminish or destroy gradually; to wear away.

erogenous (ē-roj′-e-nus) Descriptive of body areas or skin that are capable of arousing sexual excitement when stimulated, *e.g.*, the oral, anal, and genital areas. Also erotogenic.

eros (ē′-ros): 1. Physical love; sexual desire. 2. The Greek god of love. 3. In psychiatry, the life instinct, *i.e.*, the instinctive tendency toward self-preservation.

erosion (ē-rō′-zhun): 1. The superficial wearing away of tissue or a surface. 2. Loss of superficial epidermis. **CERVICAL E.**, ulceration of the superficial tissues at the squamocolumnar junction in the vaginal portion of the cervix.

erotic (ē-rot′-ik): Pertaining to sexual passion or interest; lustful.

erotica (ē-rot′-i-ka): Artistic or literary work that has an erotic theme or quality.

eroticism (ē-rot′-i-sizm): Sexual desire. In psychoanalysis any manifestation of the sexual instinct, specifically the heightened sexual response derived from stimulation of mucous membranes or special sense organs.

erotomania (ē-rot-ō-mā′-ni- a): Morbid preoccupation with erotic activites or imaginings.

erotophobia (ē-rot-ō-fō′-bi- a): Morbid fear of sexual love or aversion to its physical expression.

erratic (e-rat′-ik): 1. Wandering, said of pain or other symptoms. 2. Queer, eccentric.

erubescence (er-ū-bes′-ens): A reddening of the skin; a blush.—erubescent, adj.

eructation (e-ruk-tā′-shun): Noisy, oral expulsion of gas from the stomach. The act of belching.

eruption (ē-rup′-shun): 1. The act of becoming visible or breaking out. 2. The appearance of a rash or visible lesion on the skin due to disease; characterized by redness, prominence, or both.—erupt, v.

eruptive (ē-rup′-tiv): Pertaining to or characterized by eruption; appearing suddenly.

ERV: Abbreviation for expiratory reserve volume; see under respiratory.

erysipelas (er-i-sip′-e-las): An acute, contagious inflammatory cellulitis involving the skin and subcutaneous tissues; caused by a hemolytic streptococcus. The inflammation begins around a wound often too small to be noticed. The characteristic eruption is painful, red with small blebs, and has a raised edge. The disease is accompanied by fever and other severe constitutional symptoms. Sometimes called Saint Anthony's fire (*q.v.*).

erysipeloid (er-i-sip′-e-loid): A specific infective dermatitis resembling erysipelas, occurring primarily in persons who handle fish or meat. Usually confined to the hands but may become generalized and septicemic.

erythema (er-i-thē′-ma): Inflammatory redness of the skin. **E. AB IGNE,** a reddish mottling and macular eruption of the skin over the shins, as occurs in stokers, bakers, and others whose work exposes them to radiant heat, or those who sit too close to a fire or electric heater. **E. INFECTIOSUM,** a mild, non-febrile infection, probably viral, characterized by macropapular erythematous eruption; also called fifth disease and Sticker's disease. **E. MULTIFORME,** successive painless, toxic or allergic skin eruptions of short duration, appearing chiefly on the extremities; the lesions are violet-pink or dark red papules; see Stevens-Johnson syndrome. **E. NODOSUM,** an eruption of painful red nodules on the front of the legs; occurs in young women and is often accompanied by rheumatic pains; may be a symptom of many diseases including tuberculosis, acute rheumatism, gonococcal septicemia; also caused by certain drugs or food poisoning. **E. PERNIO,** chilblain (*q.v.*). **E. TOXICUM, E.** caused by allergic reaction to some substance, *e.g.*, a drug or a bacterial toxin; characterized by a generalized macular erythematous eruption. **E. TOXICUM NEONATORUM,** a self-limited condition occurring during the first few days of life; characterized by a temporary blotchy erythematous rash, sometimes papules or pustules; due to some allergy, often to mother's or cow's milk.—erythematous, adj.

erythr-, erythro-: Combining forms denoting: 1. Erythrocyte. 2. Red or redness.

erythrasma (er-i-thraz′-ma): A chronic skin infection, now thought to be caused by a bacterium; characterized by a reddish-brown eruption that occurs in the axilla, groin, inner surface of the thigh, and the pubic area; the patches desquamate but cause little or no discomfort.

erythredema (er-ith-rē-dē′- ma): A disease of infancy characterized by bluish-red swollen extremities, tachycardia, photophobia; cause unknown. Nervous irritability is extreme, leading to anorexia and disordered digestion, followed by multiple arthritis and muscular weakness. Syn., pink disease, Swift's disease, infantile acrodynia.

erythremia (er-i-thrē′-mi-a): A chronic form of polycythemia, characterized by an increase in the blood cells, especially the erythrocytes, and in blood volume; cause unknown. Also called erythrocythemia, polycythemia vera or rubra, and Osler's disease.

erythroblast (ē-rith′-rō- blast): An immature, nucleated red blood cell found in the red bone marrow and from which the erythrocytes are derived.—erythroblastic, adj.

erythroblastemia (ē-rith′-rō-blas-tē′-mi-a): The presence of abnormally large numbers of erythroblasts (*q.v.*) in the peripheral blood.

erythroblastosis (ē-rith′-rō-blas-tō′-sis): The presence of erythroblasts in the circulating blood. **E. FETALIS** or **NEONATORUM** is a hemolytic disease of the fetus or the newborn; occurs when the mother's blood is Rh negative, causing the development of antibodies against the fetus whose blood is Rh positive. Red blood cell destruction occurs with anemia, jaundice, hepatomegaly, splenomegaly, an excess of erythrocytes in the blood, and often generalized edema.

erythrochloropia (ē-rith′-rō-klō- rō′-pi-a): A form of color blindness in which only the colors red and green can be distinguished correctly.

erythroclasis (er-e-throk′-la-sis): The fragmentation of red blood cells.

erythrocyanosis (ē-rith′-rō-sī-a- nō′-sis): A condition characterized by swollen, bluish-red areas of discoloration on the skin that burn and itch. **E. FRIGIDA,** a vasoplastic disease in which there is hypertrophy of the arteriolar muscular coat; marked by bluish-red discoloration of the legs, especially of young women when exposed to cold.

erythrocyte (ē-rith′-rō-sīt): A non-nucleated, biconcave, disk-shaped blood cell containing an oxygen-carrying pigment, hemoglobin, which gives blood its red color. Produced in the marrow of spongy bone, at the ends of long bones, and in flat, irregular bones. Chief function is to carry oxygen to the cells of all the tissues of the body. Adult blood contains about five million erythrocytes per cubic millimeter; the average life of erythrocytes is about 120 days.

erythrocyte sedimentation rate: The rate at which red blood cells settle to the bottom of a glass tube within a given amount of time. The rate is increased in infections and conditions in which cell destruction occurs and decreased in abnormal morphology of red blood cells, as occurs in certain anemias, especially sickle-cell anemia, and in bleeding, congestive heart failure, and diseases of the bone marrow. Useful in diagnosing and following up on such illnesses as rheumatic fever, arthritis, and myocardial infarction. Abbreviated ESR.

erythrocythemia (ē-rith′-rō-sî- thē′-mi-a): Overproduction of red blood cells. This may be 1) a physiological response to the need for greater oxygenation of the tissues (congenital heart disease), and is referred to as erythrocytosis or secondary polycythemia; or 2) idiopathic, when the condition is called polycythemia vera; see polycythemia.—erythrocythemic, adj.

erythrocytolysis (ē-rith′-rō-sî- tol′-i-sis): Destruction or dissolution of red blood cells with escape of hemoglobin into the plasma.

erythrocytometer (ē-rith′-rō-sî- tom′-e-ter): An instrument for measuring or counting red blood cells.

erythrocytopenia (ē-rith′-rō-sî- tō-pē′-ni-a): Deficiency in the number of red blood cells.—erythrocytopenic, adj.

erythrocytosis (ē-rith′-rō-sî-tō′-sis): An increase in the red blood cells in the circulating blood resulting from a known cause; see erythrocythemia. STRESS E., a condition occurring in tense, anxiety-prone individuals; there is no increase in the red blood cell mass but a diminished plasma volume leads to an increase in peripheral hematocrit.

erythrocyturia (e-rith′-rō-sî-tū′-ri-a): The presence of red blood cells in the urine.

erythroderma (ē-rith′-rō-der′- ma): Excessive redness of the skin. Also erythrodermia.

erythrodermatitis (ē-rith′-rō-der-ma- tī′-tis): Reddening and inflammation of the skin.

erythrodontia (e-rith′-rō-don′-shi- a): A reddish discoloration of the teeth; seen in porphyria (*q.v.*).

erythrogenic (ē-rith-rō-jen′- ik): 1. Producing or causing a rash. 2. Producing red blood cells, or pertaining to their formation.

erythroid (er′-i-throyd): Of a red color.

erythroleukemia (e-rith′-rō-lū-kē′-mi-a): A malignant blood disorder characterized by the proliferation of erythroblasts and leukoblasts.

erythrolysis (er-i-throl′-i-sis): The dissolution or destruction of erythrocytes.

erythromelalgia (ē-rith′-rō-mel-al′-ji-a): A rare skin condition affecting chiefly both legs and feet and sometimes one or both hands; characterized by vasodilatation and a dusky red mottling discoloration of the affected parts which are very painful; cause unknown, but the condition is aggravated by exposure to heat and by exercise. Associated with polycythemia vera, nervous system disorder, gout. See also acrodynia.

erythromelia (ē-rith-rō-mē′- li-a): A painless condition in which the lower legs become erythematous accompanied by atrophy of the skin.

erythropenia (ē-rith-rō-pē′- ni-a): Deficiency in the number of red cells in the blood.

erythrophage (ē-rith′-rō-fāj): A phagocyte that engulfs and destroys red blood cells.

erythrophobia (ē-rith-rō-fō′-bi-a): 1. Abnormal fear of red colors. 2. Fear of blushing in public. 3. Morbid fear of the color red.

erythroplasia (ē-rith-rō-plā′-zi-a): A condition characterized by the formation of erythematous papules with ill-defined borders, at the junctions of mucous membrane with epithelium, chiefly at the anus, vulva, and mouth; when it occurs on oral mucous membrane it may be a sign of early cancer.

erythropoiesis (ē-rith′-rō-poi-ē′-sis): The production of red blood cells. Sec hemopoiesis.

erythropoietin (ē-rith′-rō-poy-ē′-tin): A substance found in many animals and man; secreted by the kidney, it circulates in the blood and is concerned with the stimulation and regulation of the production of erythrocytes.

erythropsia (er-i-throp′-si-a): An abnormality in vision in which the individual perceives all objects as red.

erythrorrhexis (ē-rith-rō-rex′- is): Fragmentation of red blood cells.

erythrosis (er-i-thrō′-sis): A condition marked by redness of the hair and beard along with ruddiness of the complexion.

erythrostasis (ē-rith-rō-stā′-sis): A condition due to stasis of the blood in the capillaries and hence stasis of the erythrocytes, which are then denied access to fresh plasma from which they would normally receive oxygen.

erythruria (er-i-thrū′-ri-a): Red discoloration of the urine.

eschar (es′-kar): A dry slough, as results from application of caustics, or from burns, especially second or third degree burns. See slough.—escharotic, adj.

escharectomy (es-ka-rek′-to-mi): The surgical removal of thick, tenancious slough or scar from a burned area; usually repeated every two to three days until the entire burned area has been cleared.

escharotic (es-ka-rot′-ik): 1. Any agent capable of producing an eschar. 2. Corrosive; caustic.

escharotomy (es-ka-rot′-o-mi): A surgical procedure for removing part of the eschar (*q.v.*) from a burned area; done to improve blood supply to areas distal to the burn by lessening the constriction caused by the eschar.

Escherichia (esh-e-rik′-i-a-): A genus of bacteria of the tribe Eschericheae; short gram-negative rods, nonmotile, widely distributed in nature. **E. COLI,** a natural inhabitant of the intestinal tract in man; usually nonpathogenic, but pathogenic strains frequently cause urinary tract infections, enteritis, peritonitis, cystitis, wound infections; also called colon bacillus.

eschrolalia (es-krō-lā′-li-a): Coprolalia (*q.v.*).

-esis: Suffix denoting action, condition, or process.

Esmarch's bandage: A rubberized roller bandage used to temporarily arrest the flow of blood in an extremity to create a bloodless field for surgery. [Johann Friedrich August von Esmarch, German military surgeon. 1823-1908.]

eso-: A combining form denoting within.

esocataphoria (es′-ō-kat-a-fō′-ri-a): A convergent squint with the eye turning downward and inward.

esoethmoiditis (es′-ō-eth-moy-dī′-tis): Inflammation of the mucous membrane lining of the ethmoid sinuses.

esogastritis (es-ō-gas-trī′-tis): Inflammation of the mucous membrane lining of the stomach.

esophagalgia (ē-sof-a-gal′-ji-a): Pain in the esophagus.

esophageal (ē-sof-a-jē′-al): Belonging or pertaining to the esophagus. **E. ATRESIA,** congenital failure of the lumen of the esophagus to develop fully. **E. DIVERTICULUM,** a circumscribed pouch-like protrusion from the wall of the esophagus. **E. HIATUS,** the opening in the diaphragm through which the esophagus passes before joining the stomach. **E. REFLUX,** see gastroesophageal r. under reflux. **E. PLEXUS,** a plexus surrounding the esophagus; made up of branches of the right and left vagus nerves and visceral fibers from the esophagus. **E. SPASM,** strong contractions of the muscles of the esophagus occurring after the individual swallows food; the contractions are not coordinated and do not propel the food toward the stomach; seen chiefly in the elderly. **E. SPEECH,** produced by the vibration of the column of air in the esophagus; used after removal of the larynx. **E. TEAR,** see Mallory Weiss syndrome. **E. TUBE,** a soft, flexible tube used for stomach lavage or forced feeding. **E. VARICES,** varices in the esophageal wall; see varix.

esophagectasia (ē-sof-a-jek-tā′-si-a): Dilatation of the esophagus.

esophagectomy (ē-sof′-a-jek′-to-mi): Excision of a portion of the esophagus.

esophagism (ē-sof′-a-jizm): Spasmodic stricture of the esophagus, due to contraction of the circular muscle fibers, causing dysphagia.

esophagitis (ē-sof-a-jī′-tis): Inflammation of the esophageal mucosa; may progress to ulceration, hemorrhage, and secondary infection. **PEPTIC E.,** caused by reflux of acid and peptin from the stomach; may be associated with hiatal hernia or duodenal ulcer; often occurs in the elderly; also called esophageal reflux.

esophagocardioplasty (ē-sof′-a-gō- kar′-di-ō-plas-ti): A plastic operation on the esophagus and the cardiac end of the stomach.

esophagocele (ē-sof′-a-gō-sēl): Hernia, diverticulum, or distention of the esophagus.

esophagoduodenostomy (ē-sof′-a-gō-dū-ō-dē-nos′-to-mi): The creation of a surgical anastomosis between the esophagus and the duodenum.

esophagodynia (ē-sof′-a-gō-din′-i-a): Pain in the esophagus.

esophagoenterostomy (ē-sof′-a-gō-en-ter-os′-to-mi): The surgical formation of an anastomosis between the esophagus and the intestine.

esophagogastrectomy (ē-sof′-a-gō-gas-trek′-to-mi): Removal of the distal end of the esophagus and the proximal part of the stomach.

esophagogastric (ē-sof′-a-gō-gas′-trik): Pertaining to the esophagus and the stomach.

esophagogastroduodenoscope (ē-sof′-a-gō-gas′-trō-dū-ō-dē′-nō-skōp): An instrument for examining the interior of the esophagus, stomach, and duodenum.

esophagogastroduodenoscopy (ē-sof′-a-gō-gas′-trō-dū-ō-dē-nos′-ko-pi): Examination of the esophagus, stomach, and duodenum with a long fiberoptic flexible scope.

esophagogastroscopy (ē-sof′-gō-gas-tros′-kō-pi): Examination of the esophagus and stomach with an endoscope.

esophagogastrostomy (ē-sof′-a-gō-gas-tros′-to-mi): The creation of an artificial communication between the esophagus and stomach. Also esophagogastroanastomosis.

esophagogram (ē-sof′-a-gō-gram): An x-ray view of the esophagus after the administration of a radiopaque substance.

esophagojejunostomy (ē-sof′-a-gō-jē-jū-nos′-to-mi): The surgical creation of an anastomosis between the esophagus and the jejunum.

esophagomalacia (ē-sof′-a-gō-ma-lā′-shi-a): Softening of the walls of the esophagus.

esophagomyotomy (e-sof′-a-gō-mî-ot′-o-mi): An incision through the muscular wall of the esophagus.

esophagoplasty (e-sof′-a-gō-plas-ti): Plastic

surgery for the repair of damage to the esophagus.

esophagoptosis (e-sof′-a-gop-tō′- sis): Relaxation of the esophageal walls and downward displacement of the esophagus.

esophagoscope (e-sof′-a-gō-skōp): An endoscope (*q.v.*) fitted with a light and lenses; used for examining the esophagus.

esophagoscopy (e-sof-a-gos′-kō-pi): The examination of the internal surface of the esophagus with an endoscopic type of instrument.

esophagospasm (e-sof′-a-gō-spazm): Spasm of the muscles of the esophagus.

esophagostenosis (e-sof′-a-gō-stē-nō′-sis): Constriction or stricture of the lumen of the esophagus.

esophagostomy (e-sof-a-gos′-to-mi): A surgically created fistula between the esophagus and the exterior; used temporarily for feeding after excision of some part of the throat, usually for cancer.

esophagotomy (e-sof-a-got′-o-mi): An incision into the esophagus.

esophagus (ē-sof′-a-gus): A musculomembranous canal or tube, about 9 or 10 inches long, that extends from the pharynx through the diaphragm to join the cardiac end of the stomach. Serves as a passage way for food.

esotropia (es-ō-trō′-pi-a): Convergent strabismus (*q.v.*); occurs when one eye fixes on an object and the other eye deviates inward. Opp. of exotropia—Syn., esophoria.

ESP: Abbreviation for extrasensory perception.

espundia (es-pun′-di-a): South American mucocutaneous leishmaniasis (*q.v.*). Causes ulceration of the legs with later involvement of the nose and throat. See leishmaniasis.

ESR: Abbreviation for erythrocyte sedimentation rate.

essence (es′-sens): 1. That which is the real nature of a thing and so the source of its particular qualities. 2. A solution of a volatile oil in alcohol.

essential (ē-sen′-shal): Of prime importance; indispensable. In medicine the term is often used to describe conditions of unknown origin, *e.g.*, essential hypertension.

EST: Abbreviation for electroshock therapy.

ester (es′-ter): Any organic compound formed by the combination of an acid and an alcohol with the elimination of water.

esterase (es′-ter-ās): An enzyme that acts as a catalyst in the hydrolysis of an ester (*q.v.*).

esterification (es′-ter-i-fi-kā′-shun): The reaction between an alcohol and an acid in which the removal of water results in the formation of an ester.

esthematology (es-them-a-tol′-o-ji): The study of the special senses and of the sense organs.

esthesia (es-thē′-zi-a): The capacity for feeling, sensation, or perception, as opposed to anesthesia.

esthesio-: A combining form denoting 1) sensation, feeling; 2) perception.

esthesiology (es-thē-zi-ol′-o-ji): The science of sensory phenomena.

esthesiometer (es-thēz-i-om′-e-ter): An instrument for measuring the sense of touch.

esthesioneurosis (es-thē′-zi-ō-nū- rō′-sis): Any neurosis with sensory manifestations such as anesthesia or hyperesthesia.

esthetic (es-thet′-ik): 1. Pertaining to sensation or feeling. 2. Pertaining to beauty.

estival (es′-ti-val): Pertaining to summer or occurring during the summer months.

estradiol (es-tra-dī′-ol): A steroid hormone, produced by the ovarian follicles and placenta; stimulates follicle growth, proliferation of the endometrium, and uterine contractions. Also influences the pituitary gland, stimulating production of gonadotropic hormones. Also prepared synthetically. Administered subcutaneously or intramuscularly.

estrin (es′-trin): Estrogen.

estrinization (es-trin-ī-zā′-shun): 1. Descriptive of the alterations that take place in the vaginal and uterine mucosa during estrus. 2. Treatment with estrogenic substances.

estriol (es′-trē-ōl): A naturally occurring estrogenic hormone secreted by the ovaries and found chiefly in the urine; makes up about 90 percent of the estrogen eliminated during pregnancy; it is synthesized by enzymes of the placenta and the adrenal gland of the fetus, hence measurement of the amount eliminated indicates the status of the placenta, the fetus, and the mother.

estrogen (es′-trō-jen): The collective name for the female sex hormones, whether natural or synthetic; in humans they are formed in the ovary, fetoplacental uterus, adrenal cortex, and testes. Estrogens are responsible for the development of secondary sex characteristics in the female and for the changes that occur in the genitalia during menstruation. They are used therapeutically in treating hormonal deficiencies, to suppress ovulation, to prevent lactation, and to ameliorate the symptoms of breast cancer. See also estrogenic.

estrogenic (est-rō-jen′-ik): Having the action of the female sex hormones. See estrogen. **E. HORMONES**, any of the substances secreted within the ovary that stimulate activity of the female sex organs; those produced in animals (mare) may be used in medicine when the normal supply is lacking or deficient. The active ingredient of the contraceptive pill.

estrus (es′-trus): The sexually receptive state in females. In humans, it occurs during that phase of the menstrual cycle when changes in the lining of the uterus prepare it for receiving the fertilized ovum, should conception occur.

ethacrynic acid (eth-a-krin′-ik): A diuretic drug.

ethanol (eth′-a-nōl): Ethyl alcohol (*q.v.*).

ether (ē′-ther): Thin, colorless, volatile, inflammable liquid; one of the oldest volatile general anesthetics.—Syn., diethyl ether, diethyl oxide, sulfuric ether.

ethical drugs: Drugs sold only by prescription.

ethics (eth′-iks): A code of moral principles that govern conduct. **NURSING E.**, the code governing the nurse's behavior, especially to her patients, visitors, and colleagues. It implies loyalty to the employing authority and to the profession.—ethical, adj.

ethisterone (ē-this′-ter-ōn): A steroid that resembles both progesterone and testosterone; used as a progestational agent. See progestational.

ethmoid (eth′-moid): 1. Sievelike; cribriform. 2. The sievelike bone that separates the nasal cavity from the brain; the olfactory nerves pass through perforations in it; contains small cavities called ethmoid sinuses.

ethmoidectomy (eth-moy-dek′-to-mi): Surgical removal of a part of the ethmoid bone, usually that forming the lateral nasal walls.

ethmoiditis (eth-moi-dī′tis): Inflammation of the ethmoid bone or sinuses.

ethnic (eth′-nik): Pertaining to a social group whose members share certain common qualities, especially cultural or physical characteristics, have common national origin, and speak a common language.—ethnicity, adj.

ethnocentrism (eth-nō-sen′-trizm): The attitude or belief that one's way of life is superior to all others.

ethnology (eth-nol′-o-ji): The science that deals with the races of mankind, their origins, distribution, relationships and characteristics.

ethology (eth-ol′-o-ji): The scientific study of 1) animal behavior; 2) the evolution of human behavior and character.—ethological, adj.

ethyl (eth′il): The univalent alcohol radical, present in many compounds, *e.g.*, ethyl alcohol and ethyl ether.

ethyl chloride (eth′-il klō′-rīd): A volatile general anesthetic for short operations, and a local anesthetic by reason of the intense cold produced when applied to the skin.

ethylene (eth′-i-lēn): A colorless, highly flammable, explosive gas used as an inhalation anesthetic, less frequently than formerly.

etiology (ē-ti-ol′-o-ji): The science that deals with causation of diseases and their modes of introduction into the host.—etiologic, etiological, adj.; etiologically, adv.

eu-: Combining form denoting 1) well, good; 2) well-being.

eubiotics (ū-bī-ot′iks): The science of hygienic living.

eucapnia (ū-kap′-ni-a): The condition in which the arterial carbon dioxide tension of the blood is optimal.

euchlorhydria (ū-klor-hī′- dri-a): The condition in which the amount of free hydrochloric acid in the gastric juice is normal.

eucholia (ū-kō′-li-a): The normal state of the bile in reference to quantity and quality.

eucrasia (ū-krā′-zi-a): The simultaneous existence of the normal qualities, functions, and chemical states of the body.

eudipsia (ū-dip′-si-a): Normal, ordinary thirst.

eugenics (ū-jen′-iks): The science dealing with those factors that tend to improve successive generations of the human race.—eugenic, adj.

euglycemia (ū-glī-sē′-mi-a): The normal amount of glucose in the circulating blood.

eunoia (ū-noy′-a): A normal mental state.

eunuch (ū′-nuk): A human male from whom the testes have been removed; a castrated male.

eunuchoidism (ū′-nuk-oyd-izm): Lack of masculine sex characteristics and sexual desire; due to a deficiency of androgen secretion which may, in turn, be due to lack of development or inadequate functioning of the testes.

euosmia (ū-oz′-mi-a): The condition of having a normal sense of smell.

eupepsia (ū-pep′-si-a): Normal digestion.

euphoria (ū-fō′-ri-a): A state of bodily comfort; well-being. In psychology, an exaggerated feeling of well-being, usually not justified by the circumstances.—euphoric, euphoretic, euphoriant, adj.

euphorigenic (ū-for-i-jen′-ik): Tending to produce a state of euphoria.

euplastic (ū-plas′-tik): Having the ability to heal readily.

euploid (ū′-ployd): Having the normal number of chromosomes.

eupnea (ūp-nē′-a): Normal easy respiration.

eupraxia (ū-prak′-si-a): The ability to perform perfectly movements involving coordination of muscles.

eurhythmic (ū-rith′-mik): 1. Harmonious development and relationship of the body parts. 2. Descriptive of a pulse beat that is regular.

eurhythmics (ū-rith′-miks): Harmonious body movements performed to music.

eurycephalic (ū′-ri-se-fal′-ik): Having a wide head.

eurygnathic (ū-rig-nath′-ik): Having a wide jaw.—eurygnathism, n.

eurysomatic (ū′-ri-sō-mat′-ik): Having a thick-set body.

eustachian (ū-stā′-ki-an): A canal, partly bony, partly cartilaginous, measuring 1 to 2 in.

in length, connecting the pharynx with the tympanic cavity. It allows air to pass into the middle ear, so that the air pressure is kept even on both sides of the eardrum. **E. CATHETER,** an instrument used for dilating the eustachian tube when it becomes blocked. **E. TUBE,** auditory tube; see under **auditory. E. VALVE,** the valve guarding the entrance of the inferior vena cava into the right atrium of the heart. [Bartolommeo Eustachius, Italian anatomist. 1520-1574.]

eustachitis (ū-sta-kī'tis): Inflammation of the mucous membrane lining of the eustachian tube.

eustress (ū'-stres): The body's response to a pleasant event or experience; the opposite of distress.

euthanasia (ū'-tha-nā'-zi-a): 1. An easy painless death. 2. The act of killing, or helping to kill, painlessly, a hopelessly ill or injured individual, as an act of mercy. **ACTIVE E.,** involves doing something that results in a person's death. **DIRECT E.,** involves an act intended to result in the death of an individual. **INDIRECT E.,** involves an act in which death is not the main intention. **INVOLUNTARY E.,** refers to **E.** carried out for patients who are comatose or otherwise unable to make decisions. **PASSIVE E.,** involves not doing something that might prevent death. **VOLUNTARY E.,** refers to **E.** produced with the person's knowledge and consent.

euthyroid (ū-thī'-royd): Pertaining to or characterized by normal thyroid function.—euthyroidism, n.

eutocia (ū-tō'-si-a): A natural and normal labor without any complications.

eutrophia (ū-trō'-fi-a): A normal state of nutrition.

evacuant (ē-vak'-ū-ant): An agent that promotes an evacuation, particularly of the bowel. **E. ENEMA,** fluid injected into the rectum that is intended to be returned, as distinct from retained.

evacuation (ē-vak'ū-ā'shun): 1. The act of emptying a cavity; generally refers to the discharge of fecal matter. 2. The material discharged from the rectum. 3. **SUCTION E.,** a procedure used to produce abortion of a fetus of less than 14 weeks gestation. 4. The production of a vacuum by removing the air from a closed container.

evagination (ē-vaj-i-nā'shun): An outpouching or protrusion of a layer or a part of an organ or of a tissue.

evanescent (ev-a-nes'-ent): Fleeting, unstable, unfixed, vanishing.

Evans formula: A solution consisting of 50 percent colloids and 50 percent lactated Ringer's solution.

evaporate (ē-vap'-o-rāt): To convert from the liquid or solid state to the gaseous state by conversion to vapor.—evaporation, n.

evaporating lotion: One which, applied as a compress, absorbs heat in order to evaporate, and so cools the skin.

eventration (ē-ven-trā'shun): 1. Protrusion of some of the contents of the abdomen through the abdominal wall. 2. Surgical removal of the contents of the abdominal cavity. **E. OF THE DIAPHRAGM,** a condition in which the muscular action of the diaphragm is defective, the left part being abnormally high and not moving during normal excursion. **UMBILICAL E.,** omphalocele, (*q.v.*).

eversion (ē-ver'-zhun): 1. A turning inside out or back upon itself, as the eversion of an eyelid to expose the conjunctival sac. 2. Turning inward of the ankle. 3. The position of a part when it is turned away from the midline of the body.—evert, v.

evisceration (ē-vis-e-rā'-shun): 1. Removal of the thoracic or abdominal organs. 2. Postoperative protrusion of viscera through a ruptured abdominal incision.

evolution (ev-ō-lū'-shun): 1. The process of continual, gradual and orderly growth and development or advance. 2. The theory that living things have developed to their present state by a series of changes that raised them from lower to higher orders of biological species.

evulsion (ē-vul'-shun): Forcible tearing away of a structure or a pulling out.

Ewing's tumor: Sarcoma involving the shaft of long bone before the twentieth year; arises in the medullary tissue; characterized by pain, fever, leukocytosis. Also called Ewing's sarcoma and endothelial myeloma. [James Ewing, New York pathologist. 1866-1943.]

ex-: Prefix denoting out, outside, outside of, outward, away from, lacking. Opp. to end-, endo-. Variants are e-, ef-.

exacerbation (eks-as-er-bā'-shun): Increased severity as of symptoms, or a flareup of symptoms that have subsided.

examination (eks-am-i-nā'-shun): The procedure of inspecting a patient to determine his physical condition and to aid in diagnosing his ailment. **PELVIC E.,** usually refers to examination of the female internal genitalia; see 2. under **bimanual. PHYSICAL E.,** examining the physical state of a person by inspection, palpation, percussion, and auscultation.

exania (ek-sā'-ni-a): Prolapse of the rectum.

exanthem (ek-san'-them): Exanthema (*q.v.*). **E. SUBITUM,** an acute, benign, febrile, probably viral noninfectious disease of infants and young children; characterized by three or four days of intermittent high fever followed by a maculopapular rash, mostly on the trunk and neck.

exanthema (eks-an-thē'-ma): 1. Any eruptive

disease such as measles. 2. A skin eruption.—examthematous, adj.

exanthesis (eks-an-thē′-sis): The coming out of a rash or eruption.

exanthrope (ek′-san-thrōp): A cause of disease that originates outside of the body.

exarteritis (eks-ar-ter-ī′tis): Inflammation of the external coat of an artery.

exarticulation (eks-ar-tik-ū-lā′-shun): 1. The amputation of a limb at a joint. 2. The removal of part of a joint.

excentric (eks-sen′-trik): Away from the center.

excernent (ek-ser′-nent): 1. Causing or promoting an evacuation or excretion. 2. An agent that causes or promotes an evacuation or excretion.

exchange list: See food exchange list.

exchange transfusion: See transfusion.

excipient (ek-sip′-i-ent): Any inert substance used to confer a desired consistency or to serve as a vehicle for a drug.

excise (ek′-sīz): To remove by cutting out or off.

excision (ek-sizh′-un): The act of removing a part by cutting out or off.

excitability (ek-sīt-a-bil′-i-ti): 1. The state of readiness of cells or an organism to respond to stimuli. 2. A state of being easily irritated.

excitation (ek-sī-tā′-shun): The act of stimulating an organ or tissue.

excitatory (ek-sīt′-a-tor-i): Tending to or able to excite or stimulate.

excitoglandular (ek-sī′tō-glan′dū-lar): Stimulating the increased secretion of a gland.

excitomotor (ek-sī-tō-mo′-tor): Stimulating or increasing muscular activity.

excoriation (eks-kō-ri-ā′-shun): Loss or removal of skin such as that produced by heat, moisture, scratching, scraping, burns, chemicals, or similar means. See abrasion.—excoriate, v.

excrement (eks′-kre-ment): Waste matter cast off by the body; usually refers to feces.

excrescence (eks-kres′-ens): Any abnormal protuberance or growth of the tissues; usually refers to surface outgrowths.

excreta (eks-krē′-ta): The waste matter which is normally discharged from the body, particularly urine and feces.

excrete (eks-krēt′): To separate and throw off from the body as waste matter.

excretion (eks-krē′-shun): The elimination of waste material from the body, and also the matter so discharged.—excretory, adj.; excrete, n; v.

excretory (eks′-kre-tō-ri): Pertaining to excretion. **E. SYSTEM,** term used to describe groups of organs that eliminate waste products from the body: urinary, digestive, and respiratory systems, and the skin.

excruciating (eks-krū′shi-āt-ing): 1. Agonizing or torturing, as pain. 2. Causing severe suffering.

excursion (eks-kur′-zhun): Any movement of a part of the body with the expectation that it will return to the original position, as the movement of the mandible from side to side or the movement of the diaphragm during respiration.

excurvation (eks-kur-va′-shun): An outward curving.

exdwelling drainage system: A system for collecting drainage material or a bodily excretion, such as urine, without inserting a tube into the organ or cavity; involves the use of a specially constructed apparatus that is attached to the skin and provides for collection in an appropriate container.

exencephaly (eks-en-sef′-a-li): A congenital anomaly marked by deficient formation of the cranium; the brain is exposed or extrudes through the skull.

exenteration (eks-en-te-rā′-shun): Evisceration. Removal of the viscera. **PELVIC E.,** the removal of pelvic organs, a radical operation for removal of malignant growths.

exenteritis (eks-en-ter-i′-tis): Inflammation of the serous covering of the intestine.

exercise (ek′-ser-sīz): Physical exertion engaged in for the purpose of improving one's health, correcting a deformity, or developing a particular skill. **ACTIVE E.,** voluntary muscular activity performed by one's own efforts. **ACTIVE ASSISTED E.,** exercise performed partly by a mechanical device or by a therapist, to increase range of motion or strength. **AEROBIC E., E.** performed while breathing continuously, as in dancing, walking, jogging, bicycling, swimming, playing tennis; advocated to promote cardiac fitness. **ANAEROBIC E.,** exercise or sport that requires short bursts of energy during which the person may "hold" his breath until the exercise is completed, the needed oxygen being released from various oxygen compounds in the body; such **E.** is limited to short periods of vigorous activity. **E. ELECTROCARDIOGRAM,** see Bruce treadmill test. **E. TOLERANCE TEST,** a test to determine the oxygen requirement of the mycoardium during exercise; helps in estimating the extent of coronary disease that may be present and to measure the person's capacity for exercise; may utilize the treadmill or the Master's two-step test. **ISOMETRIC E.,** exercises involving contraction of a muscle that has both ends fixed so that the muscle is tensed without its length being changed. **ISOTONIC E.,** exercise in which one end of the muscle is attached to a light weight which is lifted when the muscle shortens; the tone of the muscle does not change; opp. to isometric. **PASSIVE E.**, massage, manipulation, or movement of the body or parts of it, performed by another person, a machine, or other outside force without any effort on the part of the patient. **RANGE OF MOTION E.**, see range of motion. **RESISTIVE E.**, exercises against resistance of the therapist or a fixed object. **TCDB E.**, turning, coughing, deep breathing exercises. **UNDERWATER E.**, **E.** carried out under water where the movements of weakened muscles are facilitated by buoyancy. See also Buerger; Buerger-Allen; Kregel; yoga.

exfoliation (eks-fō-li-ā′-shun): The scaling off of tissue in layers, particularly of dead cells from the epidermis.—exfoliative.

exhalation (eks-ha-lā′-shun): The giving forth of a gas or vapor. In physiology, the breathing out of air from the lungs.

exhale (eks-hāl′): To breathe out; to force or let air out of the lungs.

exhaustion (eg-zaws′-chun): 1. Extreme weariness or fatigue. 2. Inability to respond to stimuli. 3. The using up of a supply of anything. **HEAT E.**, a condition caused by excessive heat, either from exposure to the sun or from working in hot places; characterized by prostration, subnormal temperatures, weakness, dehydration, and collapse.

exhibitionism (ek′-si-bish′-un-izm): Any kind of "showing off" or extravagant behavior to attract attention, including such perverted behavior as exposure of their genitalia, by males, for the purpose of obtaining sexual excitement and the desire to shock the victim who is usually female.—exhibitionist, n.

exhibitionist (ek′-si-bish′-un-ist): One who derives sexual stimulation or gratification from exposing parts of the body that are coventionally covered, the genitalia in particular, to someone of the opposite sex.

exitus (ek′-si-tus): Fatal termination of a disease; death.

exo-: Prefix denoting external, exterior, outside, outer, outer part.

exobiology (ek′-sō-bi-ol′-o-ji): The study of living organisms on planets other than the earth.

exocardia (ek-sō-kar′-di-a): Ectocardia (*q.v.*).

exocolitis (ek′-sō-kō-lī′-tis): Inflammation of the serous outer covering of the colon.

exocrine (ek′-sō-krēn): Term applied to glands that deliver their secretions to an epithelial surface either directly or through a duct, or to the secretions such glands produce. Opp. to endocrine (*q.v.*).—exocrinal, adj.

exodontics (ek-sō-don′-tiks): That branch of dentistry that deals with the extraction of teeth.

exoenzyme (ek-sō-en′-zīm): An enzyme that acts outside of the cell where it originated.

exogenous (eks-oj′-en-us): Of external origin.

exogomy (ek-sog′-a-mi): 1. Reproduction by union of two gametes of different ancestry. 2. Marriage outside of one's ethnic group.

exometritis (ek′-sō-mē-trī′-tis): Inflammation of the outer covering of the uterus.

exomphalos (eks-om′-fa-los): A congenital condition due to failure of the abdominal wall to develop properly; the abdominal viscera herniate through a gap in the umbilical region. Umbilical hernia.

exopathy (eks-op′-a-thi): A disease caused by something outside of the body.—exopathic, adj.

exophoria: See esophoria.

exophthalmic goiter (eks-of-thal′-mik goy′-ter): See exophthalmos and goiter.

exophthalmometer (ek-sof-thal-mom′-e-ter): An instrument for measuring the degree of exophthalmos (*q.v.*).

exophthalmos (ek-sof-thal′-mos): Abnormal protrusion of the eyeballs; most frequently occurs in hyperthyroidism. See goiter.—exophthalmic, adj.

exophylaxis (ek-sō-fī-lak′-sis): Protection of the body against entrance of disease or disease-causing organisms from without.

exophytic (ek-sō-fit′-ik): Growing outwardly. In oncology, refers to growth of a tumor on the exterior surface of the organ or structure where it originated.

exoserosis (ek-sō-ser-ō′-sis): The exudation or oozing of serum from the skin surface.

exoskeleton (ek-sō-skel′-e-ton): In vertebrates, applies to hard structures that develop on the exterior of the body. *e.g.*, hooves, nails, teeth, hair, etc.

exosmosis (eks-os-mo′-sis): Osmosis. The outward diffusion of a liquid through a membrane.

exostosectomy (eks-os-tō-sek′-to-mi): The surgical removal of an exostosis (*q.v.*). Also exostectomy.

exostosis (eks-os-tō′-sis): A benign bony outgrowth from the surface of a bone or tooth, forming a tumor. **SUBLINGUAL E.**, a bony outgrowth from under a nail, usually that of the great toe.

exotoxin (ek-sō-tok′-sin): A toxic product of living bacteria that is passed into the environment of the cell, becomes diffused and attacks specific tissues. The organisms causing diphtheria and typhoid fever produce exotoxins. Opp. to endotoxin.—exotoxic, adj.

exotropia (ek-sō-trō′-pi-a): Outward deviation of the visual axis of one eye. Also divergent strabismus, divergent squint, "walleye."

expanded role: In nursing, refers to a trend that began in the mid-1960's to utilize nurses in expanded roles, which resulted in the development of many (at least 24) specialty nursing roles all of which require education and knowledgeability beyond that required for basic nursing practice. Courses for such preparation are offered in many educational institutions; they lead to certification or to the Masters or higher degree in a particular nursing specialty. Many specialty groups have their own national organization that meets regularly, sponsors and conducts research, and sponsors an official publication. Professional nurses functioning in expanded roles include the primary care nurse, the clinical nurse specialist, and the nurse practitioner. The term may also refer to expansion in the degree of responsibility and accountability of the professional nurse for developing and carrying out care plans for clients in the health care system.

expansiveness (ek-span′-siv-nes): In psychiatry, behavior marked by euphoria, talkativeness, and an exaggerated sense of one's own importance.

expectorant (eks-pek′-to-rant): An agent that promotes or increases the expectoration of mucus or other exudate from the lungs, bronchi and trachea.

expectoration (ek-spek-tō-rā′- shun): 1. The elimination of secretion from the respiratory tract by coughing and spitting. 2. Sputum (*q.v.*).—expectorate, v.

expel (eks-pel′): To force out.

experiment (ek-sper′-i-ment): A procedure undertaken to 1) discover a fact, principle, or effect; 2) test a hypothesis; 3) illustrate a principle or point. A test or trial.

expiration (eks-pi-rā′-shun): 1. The act of breathing out air from the lungs. 2. Death.—expire, v.; expiratory, adj.

expiratory (eks-pī′-ra-tō-ri): Pertaining to expiration. **E. GRUNT**, grunting sound heard on expiration in comatose adults; may be a neurological reflex or caused by partial obstruction of the airway. In infants it is a sign of impending respiratory distress. **E. RESERVE VOLUME** (ESR), the amount of air that remains in the lungs after a maximum exhalation; for the normal adult, about 1200 cc. **E. RETARD,** a device that provides expiratory resistance sufficient to slow expiration.

expire (eks-pir′): 1. To exhale or breathe out. 2. To die.

explant (eks-plant′): To transfer tissue from the body to an artificial medium for growth, or the material so transferred.

exploration (eks-plō-rā′-shun): The act of exploring for diagnostic purposes, usually involving surgery or endoscopy.

expression (eks-presh′-un): 1. Expulsion by force, squeezing, or pressing out, as the placenta from the uterus, milk from the breasts, etc. 2. Facial reflection of feeling, mood, etc.

expulsion (eks-pul′-shun): The act of forcing out, as feces from the rectum or urine from the bladder.—expel, v.; expulsive, adj.

exsanguinate (ek-sang′-win-āt): To drain off blood.—exsanguination, n.; exsanguine, adj.

exsanguine (ek-sang′-win): Bloodless; anemic.

exsiccation (ek-si-kā′-shun): Dehydration; the process of drying.

exstrophy (ek′-strō-fi): The congenital turning inside out or eversion of a hollow organ such as the bladder.

ext.: Abbreviation for extract.

extended: E. CARE FACILITIES, refers to long-term care facilities that are equipped to provide skilled nursing care 24 hours a day for patients who need such care, particularly after being discharged from a hospital. **E. FAMILY,** one that includes aunts, uncles, grandparents, and other relatives in addition to the nuclear family.

extension (ek-sten′-shun): 1. Traction upon a fractured or dislocated limb. 2. The act of straightening a flexed limb or part.

extensor (ek-sten′-sor): A muscle which on contraction extends or straightens a part. Opp. to flexor.

exterior (eks-tēr′-i-or): The outside or outer part, or situated on or near the outside.

extern(e) (eks′-tern): A medical school graduate who is on the staff of a health care facility, usually a hospital, who assists with the medical and surgical care of patients in preparation for independent practice. In nursing, a graduate of a nursing education program who is in the transition period between school and employment as a professional nurse, and during which she receives clinical tutoring and guidance from a person with wide experience in nursing practice.—externship, n.

external: Of two parts, the one farther from the center of the body; on the outside or surface of the body. **E. CARDIAC MASSAGE,** see under cardiac. **E. HEMORRHAGE,** that in which blood escapes to the outside of the body; opposite to internal hemorrhage. **E. MALLEOLUS,** the prominence on the lateral side of the ankle formed by the rounded eminence on the lateral side of the fibula. **E. RESPIRATION,** the transport of oxygen from the atmosphere through the lungs to the alveoli, and of carbon dioxide from the lungs to the atmosphere. **E. ROTATION,** turning of the anterior surface of a limb outward or laterally.

external acoustic meatus: The tubular structure leading from the pinna of the external ear to the tympanic membrane. Also called external auditory canal.

external degree program: In nursing, refers to a program conducted by a college or university wherein a professional nurse can earn a baccalaureate degree, and sometimes a master's degree in nursing, through correspondence and study at home and spending a short time on the college campus before graduation. Some programs allow some college credit for graduates of diploma and associate degree programs and other educational experiences.

externship (ek′-stern-ship): In nursing, refers to a program which includes experience in a variety of settings; the objective is to help the advanced student nurse or recent graduate to adjust to the nursing practice setting.

exteroceptive (eks′-ter-ō-sep′-tiv): Pertaining to or activated by a stimulus to a sense receptor located at the surface of the body.

exteroceptor (eks′-ter-ō-sep′-tor): A sensory nerve terminal located in the skin or mucous membrane and that receives such external stimuli as heat, cold, pain, touch, taste, and smell.

extinction (ek-sting′-shun): In psychiatry, the weakening or cessation of a behavior pattern as a result of negative reinforcement. In neurophysiology, the loss of excitability by a nerve or by nervous tissue.

extirpation (ek-stir-pā′-shun): Complete removal or destruction of a part.

extortion (eks-tor′-shun): 1. Rotation of the eye away from the midline of the face. 2. Outward rotation of a limb or organ.

extra-: Prefix denoting outside of, beyond, without, or in addition to.

extra-articular (eks-tra-ar-tik′-ū-lar): Outside a joint.

extracapsular (eks′-tra-kap′-sū-lar): Outside a capsule, usually referring to the capsule of a joint.

extracardial (eks-tra-kar′-di-al): Outside the heart.

extracellular (eks-tra-sel′-ū-lar): Occurring outside a cell or cells. **E. FLUID,** found outside of cells; includes interstitial fluid, cerebrospinal fluid, and plasma; also called **E.** compartment.

extracorporeal (eks′-tra-kor-po-rē′-al): Pertains to something existing or taking place outside the body or unrelated to it. **E. CIRCULATION,** circulation of the blood outside the body as by a mechanical pump or pump-oxygenator, often done while surgery is being performed on the heart.

extract (eks′-trakt): A preparation obtained by evaporating a solution of a drug until it contains a predetermined proportion of the drug; the resulting preparation is several times stronger than the crude drug.

extraction (eks-trak′-shun): 1. The preparation of an extract. 2. The act or process of drawing or pulling out. **E. OF LENS,** surgical removal of the lens of the eye, **EXTRACAPSULAR E.,** being removal of the lens after rupturing its capsule, and **INTRACAPSULAR E.,** being removal of the lens within its capsule. **VACUUM E.,** the delivery of a fetus or extraction of uterine contents by application of a vacuum.

extractor (eks-trak′-tor): A surgical instrument used for removing a tooth, foreign object, or stone from the body.

extradural (eks-tra-dū′-ral): External to the dura mater (*q.v.*), or on the outer side of it.

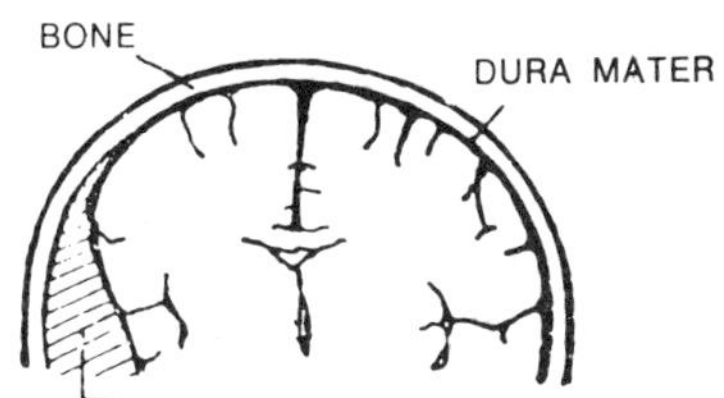

Extradural hematoma

extragenital (eks′-tra-jen′-i-tal): Not related to, originating in, or occurring on the genital organs. Occurring in areas apart from the genital organs. **E. CHANCRE,** the primary lesion of syphilis, occurring on the lip, breast, finger, etc.

extrahepatic (eks′-tra-hē-pat′-ik): Outside the liver, usually referring to disease affecting the liver but ocurring outside of it.

extramural (eks-tra-mū′-ral): Refers to something situated or occurring outside the walls of an organ.—extramurally, adj.

extraneous (eks-trā′-nē-us): 1. Originating, existing, or coming from outside of the organism. 2. Unessential; not vital.

extraocular (eks-tra-ok′-ū-lar) Adjacent to the eyeball but not within it.

extraperitoneal (eks′-tra-per-i-tō-nē′-al): Outside of the peritoneal cavity.—extraperitoneally, adv.

extrapleural (eks-tra-ploo′-ral): Outside the pleura, *i.e.*, between the parietal pleura and the chest wall. See plombage.

extrapulmonary (eks-tra-pul′-mo-na-ri): Outside of the lungs.

extrapyramidal (eks-tra-pi-ram′-i-dal): Outside of or independent of the pyramidal tracts; refers to other descending motor pathways. See pyramidal, motor fibers. **E. DISEASE,** characterized by disorders of movement such as tremor, rigidity, contractures, slowness, gait changes, flailing movements as seen in Parkinson's disease and Huntington's chorea.

extrasensory perception (eks-tra-sen′-so-ri per-sep′-shun): Thought transference. Term pertains to capacities or forms of perception of the thoughts or actions of others that are not dependent upon the five senses or explainable in relation to the senses. Abbreviated ESP.

extrasystole (eks′-tra-sis′-to-li): A premature beat that is independent of the regular pulse rhythm; the beat follows closely the preceding beat and is followed by a long pause before the next beat.

extrathoracic (eks'-tra-thō-ras'-ik): Outside the thoracic cavity.

extrauterine (eks-tra-ū'-ter-in): Outside the uterus. See ectopic pregnancy.

extravasation (eks-trav'-a-sā'-shun): An inadvertent escape of blood, lymph, intravenous infusions or medications from a vessel, or other natural enclosure, into the surrounding subcutaneous tissues.—extravasate, v.

extravascular (eks-tra-vas'kū-lar): Outside of a vessel or vessels.

extravenous (eks-tra-vē'-nus): Outside a vein.

extraventricular (eks-tra-ven-trik'ū-lar): Outside a ventricle; term usually refers to ventricles of the heart.

extraversion (eks'-tra-ver'-zhun): Extroversion (*q.v.*).

extravert (eks'-tra-vert): Extrovert (*q.v.*).

extremitas (eks-trem'-i-tas): In anatomy, a term used to designate a distal or terminal part of an organ or structure.

extremity (eks-trem'-i-ti): The terminal end of an elongated structure or thing. In anatomy, term refers to a distal or terminal position and is used to designate such parts as arm, leg, hand, foot.

extrinsic (eks-trin'-sik): Developing or having its origin at a site outside of the location where it is found or upon which it acts; often referring to muscle. E. FACTOR, Vitamin B_{12} (cyanocobalamin), which is normally present in the diet and absorbed from the gut; it is essential for normal hemopoiesis.

extro-; Prefix denoting outward, outside. Opp. to intro-.

extrophia (eks-trō'-fi-a): Exstrophy (*q.v.*).

extroversion (eks-trō-ver'-zhun): Turning outward; turning inside out; exstrophy. In psychology, the turning of one's thoughts to the external world and the focusing of one's interest on things outside oneself. Opp. of introversion.

extrovert (eks'-trō-vert): Used by Jung (*q.v.*) to describe one extreme of personality dimension. The person described as E. regulates his behavior in response to other people's attitude to him. He is sociable, a good mixer and interested chiefly in external things and the actions of others. Opp. of introvert.

extrude (eks-trood'): To force or push out of the position normally occupied, or to occupy such a position.—extrusion, n.

extubation (eks'tū-bā'shun): The removal of a tube that has been inserted into an organ or orifice, *e.g.*, a tracheostomy tube.

exudate (eks'-ū-dat): The matter that has passed through a vessel wall or membrane into surrounding space or tissue, or is deposited in the tissues; occurs in inflammation.

exudation (eks-ū-dā'-shun): The oozing out of serum and cells, mostly leukocytes, through unruptured walls of capillaries or venules.—exudate, n.; exude, v.

exumbilication (eks'um-bil-i-kā'shun): Abnormal protrusion of the navel.

exuviae (eks-ū'-vi-a): Something cast off from the body, as desquamated skin or slough.

eye: The organ of vision, located in the eye socket of the skull.

eye bank: An agency that collects and stores the corneas of human eyes for use in transplantation.

eye tooth: A canine tooth on either side of the upper jaw.

eyeball: The globe of the eye without any appendages such as the extrinsic muscles.

eyebrow: The area at the upper edge of the bony orbit that contains the eye, particularly the hairs covering it.

eyeground: The fundus of the eye as it is visible through the opthalmoscope (*q.v.*).

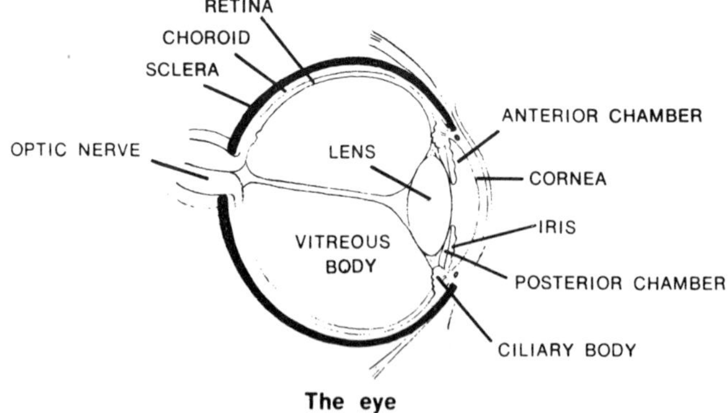

The eye

eyelash: One of the hairs that project from the edge of the eyelid.

eyelid: One of two movable folds of skin (upper and lower) that is continuous with the skin of the face, lined with conjunctiva (*q.v.*), and has a row of stiff hairs at the edge. See **meibomian gland, canthus.**

eye-minded (ī-mīnd′- ed): Descriptive of a person who remembers chiefly the impressions made on the eye.

eyepiece: Usually refers to the part of a microscope that the viewer looks into.

eyestrain: Fatigue of the eye from overuse, poor lighting, or an uncorrected defect in focusing.

F

F: Abbreviation for: 1. Fahrenheit. 2. Farad.

FA: Abbreviation for fatty acid.

FAAN: Fellow, American Academy of Nursing (*q.v.*).

fabella (fa-bel′-a): In anatomy, a small sesamoid bone that sometimes forms in the tendon at the head of the gastrocnemius muscle.

Faber's anemia: Iron deficiency anemia, often seen in association with achlorhydria; seen most often in women 30 to 50 years of age. Also called achlorhydric anemia.

Fabry's disease or syndrome: A rare condition seen mostly in men; characterized by small angiokeratomata over the entire body; other symptoms include vasomotor disturbances, enlarged heart, increased blood pressure, blood dyscrasias, edema. Angiokeratoma corporis diffusum. See angiokeratoma.

face: The anterior aspect of the human head, including the chin, mouth, cheeks, nose, and forehead. **F. LIFTING,** plastic surgery to restore youthful contours. **F. MASK,** 1) a mask made of several layers of folded gauze, worn over the nose and mouth by operating room and certain other health care personnel; 2) a device that fits over the nose and mouth, used in oxygen therapy to allow for variations in the concentration of oxygen in the inspired air. **PARKINSON'S F.,** the characteristic facies seen in persons with Parkinson's disease; see under facies. **F. PRESENTATION,** the position of the fetus when the face presents first in labor and delivery.

facet (fas′et): A small, smooth, flat surface on a bone. **ARTICULAR F.,** a small plane surface on a bone at a place where it articulates with another bone.

facet syndrome: Traumatic arthritis involving the facets of the vertebrae, marked by sudden onset; affects the lumbar spine particularly.

facetectomy (fas-e-tek′-to-mi): Excision of a facet of a bone, particularly of a vertebra.

facial (fā′-shul): Pertaining to the face. **F. NERVE,** one of the seventh pair of cranial nerves; supplies motor fibers to muscles used in facial expression, and to the salivary and lacrimal glands; supplies sensory fibers to the front two-thirds of the tongue. **F. NEURALGIA,** neuralgia (*q.v.*) in that part of the face supplied by the trigeminal (fifth cranial) nerve. **FACIAL PALSY,** Bell's palsy (*q.v.*). **F. PARALYSIS,** paralysis of the muscles supplied by the facial nerve. **F. SPASM,** muscular spasm on one side of the face or around the eye, irregular and not under conscious control.

-facient: Suffix denoting: 1. A person or agent that brings something about or initiates an action. 2. Making; causing.

facies (fā′-shi-ēz): An anatomical term used to designate a surface of a body structure or part, the expression on the face, or the face itself. **ABDOMINAL F.,** the expression seen in peritonitis; the skin is livid, the eyes sunken, and the lips dry. **ADENOID F.,** open-mouthed, vacant expression seen in children with enlarged adenoids. **F. HIPPOCRATICA,** the drawn, pale, pinched expression indicative of extreme prostration and approaching death. **MOON F.,** the round, full face seen in persons with Cushing's syndrome (*q.v.*); may also occur in those receiving corticosteroid therapy. **PARKINSON'S F.,** the masklike appearance seen in persons with Parkinson's disease; saliva may trickle from the corner of the mouth.

facilitation (fa-sil′-i-tā′-shun): The act of increasing the ease with which an action or function is carried out, *e.g.*, the reinforcement of a reflex action by impulses from some source other than a reflex center.

facio-: Combining form denoting face or relationship to the face.

faciocephalalgia (fa′-shi-ō-sef-a-lal′-ji-a): Neuralgic pain in the face and head.

faciolingual (fā′-shi-ō-ling′-gwal): Pertaining to the face and the tongue.

facioplasty (fā′-shi-ō-plas′-ti): Plastic surgery of the face.

facioplegia (fā′-shi-ō-plē′-ji-a): Facial paralysis.—facioplegic, adj.

factitious (fak-tish′-us): Artificial. **F. DISORDERS,** see Münchhausen's syndrome.

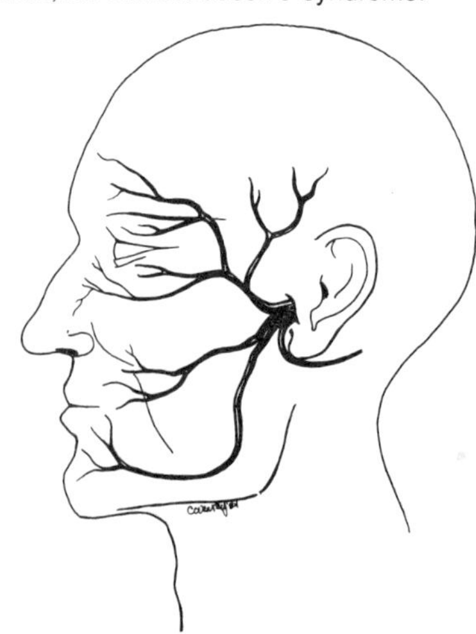

facial nerve distribution

factor (fak'tor): Something that contributes to the production of a result. *e.g.*, an agent, constituent, ingredient. In heredity, a gene; in nutrition a desirable ingredient or essential element, *e.g.*, a vitamin. **ANTIANEMIC F.**, vitamin B_{12} (cyanocobalamin). **ANTIHEMOPHILIC F.**, factor VIII. **ANTIHEMORRHAGIC F.**, vitamin K (*q.v.*). **ANTIRACHITIC F.**, ascorbic acid (*q.v.*). **ANTISTERILITY F.**, vitamin E (*q.v.*). **CLOTTING FACTORS**, 13 are identified and numbered I through XIII; essential for clotting or coagulation of blood. **EXTRINSIC F.**, vitamin B_{12} (cyanocobalamin). **FACTOR I**, fibrinogen (*q.v.*). **FACTOR II**, prothrombin (*q.v.*). **FACTOR III**, tissue thromboplastin; important in relation to activity of thromboplastin in clotting. **FACTOR IV.**, calcium; required in many phases of coagulation. **FACTOR V**, proaccelerin, the clotting factor essential for converting prothrombin to thrombin; found in plasma but not serum; heat and storage-labile; also called **LABILE F. FACTOR VI**, function indefinite. **FACTOR VII**, preconvertin, is concerned with a coagulation deficiency which results in a tendency to hemorrhage due to prolonged prothrombin time. **FACTOR VIII**, present in plasma, but not serum; participates in formation of thromboplastin; a deficiency is associated with hemophilia A, a hereditary hemorrhagic tendency; see Von Willebrand's disease. **FACTOR IX**, a precoagulant found in normal plasma; deficiency is associated with classic hemophilia B, a hereditary hemorrhagic tendency. **FACTOR X**, present in plasma and serum; deficiency may be inherited or be the result of anticoagulant therapy with certain drugs; also called **STUART-PROWER F. FACTOR XI**, an antecedent to plasma prothrombin and important in the functioning of the intrinsic factor. **FACTOR XII**, found in normal serum but deficient in individuals with hereditary bleeding disorders; necessary for rapid coagulation. **FACTOR XIII**, a fibrin stabilizing factor; necessary to fibrin in the formation of a firm clot. **HAGEMAN FACTOR**, factor XII. **INTRINSIC F.**, a mucoprotein secreted by the gastric glands; essential for the absorption of vitamin B_{12}; absent in pernicious anemia. **RH FACTOR**, see rhesus. **RHEUMATIC F.**, an immunoglobulin found in the blood serum of many individuals with rheumatic arthritis. **TRANSFER F.**, a **F.** occurring in some leukocytes that have been sensitized in one individual and that can apparently transfer the hypersensitivity to another individual in whom the leukocytes have not been sensitized.

Facts About Nursing: A publication of the American Nurses' Association, issued at intervals. Contains statistics about nurses, nursing service, nursing education and other topics of interest to nurses.

facultative (fak'-ul-tā-tiv): The ability to adjust and live under more than one set of environmental circumstances; said of bacteria.

faculty (fak'-ul-ti): 1. An inherent normal power, capability, function, or attitude; pertains chiefly to the human body or its parts, particularly in reference to mental endowments. 2. The teaching staff of an educational institution.

fae-: For words beginning thus see words beginning fe-.

Fahrenheit (far'-en-hīt): A thermometric scale; the freezing point of water is 32° and its boiling point 212°; the normal body temperature is 98.4°-98.6°. [Gabriel Fahrenheit, German physicist. 1686-1736.]

failure: Inability to perform a normal duty or expected action. **HEART F.**, sudden cessation of the heart's action.

failure-to-thrive syndrome: A condition of infants and young children characterized by malnutrition, faulty physical and emotional development, apathy, irritability, anorexia, sometimes vomiting and diarrhea; may be the result of underfeeding, congenital anomalies, infection, or disturbed mother-child relationship.

faint: 1. Weak; lacking in strength or in courage. 2. A swoon; a state of temporary unconsciousness. Syn., syncope.

fainting: Loss of consciousness due to lack of adequate blood to the brain.

Fairbank's splint: Used for treatment of Erb's palsy in infants. Baby's arm is immobilized in abduction and external rotation of the shoulder, flexion of the elbow to 90°, supination of the forearm, and extension of the wrist.

falciform (fal'-si-form): Sickle-shaped. **F. LIGAMENT**, a fold of peritoneum that separates the two main lobes of the liver.

fallectomy (fa-lek'-tō-mi): Salpingectomy (*q.v.*).

fallopian (fal-lō'-pi-an): **F. LIGAMENT**, the round ligament of the uterus. **F. TUBE**, one of two ducts that open out of the upper part of the uterus. Each measures about four inches. The distal ends lie near the ovary, are funnel-shaped and fimbriated, with one of the fimbriae reaching the ovary. The function is to carry the ova from the ovary to the uterus. [Gabriele Fallopius, 16th C. Italian anatomist.]

fallostomy (fal-os'-tō-mi): Salpingostomy (*q.v.*).

Fallot's tetralogy (fa-lōz'): Tetralogy of Fallot (*q.v.*).

fallout: Radioactive particles that result from a nuclear explosion and descend through the atmosphere.

false: Not true; not genuine. **F. LABOR**, painful contractions of the uterus that resemble those of true labor but without dilatation of the cervix. **F. NEGATIVE**, an incorrect result of a diagnostic or other test that indicates the absence of a finding or of a pathologic condition. **F. PAINS**, abdominal pains during pregnancy that are not true labor pains. **F. PELVIS,** that part of the pelvis above the pelvic brim. **F. POSITIVE,** an incorrect result of a diagnostic or other test that indicates the presence of a pathological condition that does not exist. **F. PREGNANCY,** unfounded preoccupation with thoughts of pregnancy and motherhood, intense desire to have a baby, sometimes accompanied by morning sickness, amenorrhea, and even enlarged breasts. **F. RIBS,** the lower five pairs of ribs, so called because they attach to the sternum by means of a cartilage rather than directly. **F. VOCAL CORDS,** see under vocal.

falx (falks): A sickle-shaped structure. **F. CEREBELLI,** the short process of the dura mater that extends from the occipital bone into the posterior notch between the two hemispheres of the cerebellum. **F. CEREBRI,** the fold of dura mater that separates the two cerebral hemispheres.

familial (fa-mil′ -i-al): Pertaining to the family, as of a disease affecting several members of the same family, or one that occurs in members of the same family in successive generations.

family: Any group of persons closely related by blood and certain other ties; may or may not be living under the same roof. **EXTENDED F.,** a nuclear **F.** plus blood-related others, *e.g.*, aunts, uncles, cousins, grandparents. **MATRIARCHAL F.,** one headed and dominated by a woman. **NUCLEAR F.,** consisting of only parents and their children living together. **ONE-PARENT F.,** one in which only one parent remains with the children. **PATRIARCHAL F.,** one headed by a man. **F. PLANNING,** is concerned with the avoidance of or spacing of pregnancies, with infertility, and with methods of effecting conception. **F. THERAPY,** see under therapy.

family health care unit: A care facility where primary health care is provided for families with the objective of identifying and treating unhealthful or pathologic conditions in individual family members, and in implementing preventive and other measures to improve and maintain the health of all members.

Family Nurse Practitioner: A primary care nurse who is prepared to give comprehensive, continuous, personalized care to patients at the point of entry into the health care system; to do patient assessments; to make nursing diagnoses, to carry out therapeutic measures in collaboration with a physician; and to give preventive, curative, and restorative care to patients from infancy to old age. Abbreviated FNP.

Fanconi's syndrome: A rare hereditary condition of two types: 1) characterized by various anomalies of the musculoskeletal and genitourinary systems, hypoplasia of the bone marrow and pancytopenia, and uneven brown skin discoloration; also called Fanconi's anemia and 2) characterized by short stature, osteomalacia and rickets, glycosuria, aminoaciduria, and the deposit of cystine in various parts of the body, including the liver, spleen, cornea, and bone marrow. Both types are known by several other names that are descriptive of the anomalies involved. [Guido Fanconi, Swiss pediatrician. 1882-.]

fang: In humans, the root of a tooth. In snakes, the hollow tooth through which venom is ejected.

fango (fang′ -gō): Volcanic mud, sometimes used as an external application in the treatment of rheumatism and other diseases of the joints and muscles.

fangotherapy (fang-gō-ther′ -a-pi): The therapeutic application of fango in the form of packs or baths.

fantasy (fan′ -ta-si): Imagination in which images or chains of images are directed by the desire or pleasure of the thinker, normally accompanied by a feeling of unreality; a normal process in childhood when learning to distinguish between wish and reality. Occurs pathologically in schizophrenia. Also spelled phantasy.—fantasize, v.

farad (far′ -ad): A unit of electrical capacity.—faradic, adj.

faradic (fa-rad′ -ik): Pertaining to rapidly alternating currents of induced electricity. **F. CURRENT,** an alternating current that is interrupted 80-100 times a second; has a tetanizing effect on muscle; used to stimulate paralyzed muscles.

faradotherapy (far′ -ad-ō-ther′ -a-pi): The use of faradic or induced electric current in treatment of diseased or paralyzed muscles.

Farber's disease: Disseminated lipogranulomatosis See lipogranulomatosis. [S. Farber, American pathologist. 1903–1973.]

farinaceous (far′ -i-nā′ - shus): Pertaining to cereal substances, *i.e.*, made of flour or grain. Starchy.

farmer's lung: A form of pneumoconiosis caused by sensitivity to the dust of moldy hay or grain, or moldy vegetable matter; characterized by fever, chills, cough, dyspnea, cyanosis, tachycardia. Recognized as an occupational disease. Also called farmer's asthma.

farmer's skin: See sailor's skin.

farsightedness: Hyperopia (*q.v.*).

fascia (fash′ -i-a): A connective sheath consisting of fibrous tissue and fat, which unites the skin to the underlying tissues. **DEEP F.,** forms a sheath for muscles, either separating them or holding them together; also invests such other deep structures as nerves and blood vessels. **SUPERFICIAL F.,** formed by the subcutaneous tissue; contains fat, small arteries and branches of nerves; is loosely attached to the deep **F. F. LATA,** the strong, tough **F.** that envelops the muscles of the thigh.—fasciae, pl.; fascial, adj.

fascial (fash′-i-al): Pertaining to a fascia.

fascicle (fas′i-k′l): Fasciculus (*q.v.*)

fascicular (fa-sik′-ū-lar): 1. Pertaining to a fasciculus. 2. Arranged in a bundle.

fasciculation (fa-sik-ū-lā′-shun): 1. The formation of fasciculi; see fasciculus. 2. The uncoordinated contraction or twitching of several groups of muscle fibers that are all supplied by the same motor neuron; may be indicative of any one of several nutritional or neurologic disorders; also occurs as a side effect of certain drugs. When it occurs in heart muscle it is called fibrillation.

fasciculus (fa-sik′-ū-lus): A small bundle, as of nerve or muscle fibers. Also called fascicle.—fasciculi, pl.; fascicular, adj.

fasciectomy (fash-i-ek′-tō-mi): Excision of a fascia or of strips of fascia.

fasciitis (fash-i-ī′-tis): Inflammation of fascia.

Fasciola (fa-sī′-o-la): A genus of flukes of the *Trematoda* class that infest the liver of certain animals and occasionally are transmitted to man through certain snails that feed on infected water plants.

fasciolopsiasis (fas′-i-ō-lōp-sī′-a-sis): The condition of being infested with the flukes of the genus of nematodes called *Fasciolopsis*. **F. BUSKI**, a large intestinal fluke, found in eastern and southern Asia; transmitted to man by infected water plants and other vegetation.

fasciorrhaphy (fash-i-or′-a-fi): Suturing of a torn or cut fascia.

fascioscapulohumeral (fas′-i-ō-scap′- ū-lō-hūm′-er-al): Pertinent to the face, scapula, and upper arm. **F. MUSCULAR DYSTROPHY**, Landouzy-Dejerine dystrophy; see under dystrophy.

fasciotomy (fash-i-ot′-o-mi): Incision of a fascia.

fast: 1. To abstain from eating. 2. To be resistant to destruction or to staining, said of bacteria.

fastidious (fas-tid′-i-us): In microbiology, pertains to an organism that is difficult to grow under ordinary laboratory conditions.

fastidium (fas-tid′-i-um): Repugnance or aversion to food or to eating. Squeamishness.

fastigium (fas-tij′-i-um): 1. The highest point of a fever; the period of full development of a disease. 2. The highest point in the roof of the fourth ventricle of the brain.

fasting blood sugar test: A test for diagnosis of a glucose metabolism disorder; requires the patient to fast for 12 hours before the test.

fat: 1. Plump, stout, obese. 2. The oily substance that makes up most of the cell content of adipose tissue. 3. An oil of animal or vegetable origin, either solid or liquid. **POLYUNSATURATED F.**, refers to fats that have many unsaturated chemical bonds and which tend to be liquid at room temperature; these fats are found in corn, cottonseed, soybean, and safflower oils, and in fish and poultry. **SATURATED FATS**, tend to be solid at room temperature; they are found in meats, chocolate, butter, cheese, cream, whole milk.—fatty, adj.

fat embolism syndrome: A condition caused by the lodgement of a fat embolus in the pulmonary circulation; symptoms resemble those of adult respiratory distress syndrome; an emergency situation requiring immediate correction.

fat soluble: Usually refers to the vitamins A, D, E, and K, which are soluble in fat but not in water.

fatal (fā′-tal): Causing death; deadly.

fatigue (fa-tēg′): The feeling of weariness and of reduced capacity for mental or physical work, usually resulting from prolonged or excessive labor or exertion. In physiological experiments on muscle the term is used to denote diminishing reaction to stimuli.—fatigability, n.; fatigable, adj.

fatty acid: Any organic acid that will combine with glycerine to form fat, especially oleic, palmitic, and stearic acids. Obtainable from most plants and animals. Used by the tissues as a major source of energy. **ESSENTIAL F.A.**, an unsaturated **F.A.** that cannot be formed in the body; must be supplied by the diet. **SATURATED F.A.**, not capable of absorbing any more hydrogen; palmitic and stearic are the most common of this group; found in products of both animal and vegetable origin including dairy products; beef, lamb, veal, and pork; coconut and palm oils, and chocolate. Diets heavy in these products have been found to be associated with high serum cholesterol levels. **UNSATURATED F.A.** (essential **F.A.**), capable of absorbing more hydrogen; linoleic and arachidonic are the most common of this group; found in fowl and fish; olive and safflower oils; sunflower seeds and cottonseeds; soybeans; walnuts, peanuts, cashew nuts, almonds, and pecans. Diets high in unsaturated **F.A.** have been found to be associated with low serum cholestrol levels.

fatty degeneration: Degeneration (*q.v.*) of tissues which results in appearance of fatty droplets in the cytoplasm: found especially in diseases of liver, kidney and heart.

fauces (faw′-sēz): The space between the mouth and the pharynx, bounded above by the soft palate, below by the tongue. **PILLARS OF THE F.**, anterior and posterior, lie laterally and enclose the tonsil.—faucial, adj.

faucitis (faw-sī′-tis): Inflammation of the fauces.

faveolate (fā-vē′-ō-lāt): Pitted; honeycombed in appearance.

faveolus (fā-vē′-ō-lus): A depression or small pit.

favism (fā′-vizm): Hemolytic anemia; thought to be a sensitivity reaction to certain groups of drugs as well as to fava beans (broad beans) or the pollen from the fava bean plant. Characterized by headache, abdominal pain, vomiting, diarrhea, fever, prostration.

favus (fā′-vus): A type of ringworm in which suppurating yellow, cup-shaped crusts form around the hair follicles on the scalp; collectively, they resemble a honeycomb in appearance, have a characteristic odor, leave permanent scars and result in alopecia.

FBS: Abbreviation for fasting blood sugar (test) (*q.v.*).

FCCU: Abbreviation for family-centered care unit.

FDA: Abbreviation for Food and Drug Administration, an administration within the U.S. Department of Health and Human Services.

Fe: Chemical symbol for iron.

fear: An unpleasant, strong emotion occurring in response to recognition of danger or a threat; apprehension, dread, alarm. When carried to morbid excess it is called a phobia (*q.v.*). Fear was accepted as a nursing diagnosis by the Fourth National Conference on the Classification of Nursing Diagnoses.

febri-: Combining form denoting fever.

febricant (feb′-ri-kant): Causing or producing fever. Also febrifacient, febrific.

febricide (feb′-ri-sīd): An agent that reduces or destroys fever.

febricula (fe-brik′-ū-la): A slight temporary elevation of body temperature, of indefinite origin.

febrifacient (feb′-ri-fā′-shent): Producing fever.

febrific (feb-rif′-ik): Producing fever.

febrifuge (feb′-ri-fūj): An agent that reduces fever.

febrile (feb′-ril): Feverish; accompanied by fever, or having a fever. **F. ALBUMINURIA,** albuminuria that is due to fever. **F. SEIZURE,** a generalized convulsive seizure induced by sudden elevation in temperature; usually occurring in children between six months and five years of age; thought to be due to underdevelopment of the body's capacity to adjust to sudden changes in the body temperature.

fecal (fē′-kal): Relating to feces. **F. IMPACTION,** an accumulation of hardened feces in the rectum or sigmoid colon, resulting from prolonged constipation and which is immovable by normal intestinal activity. **F. VOMITING,** the vomiting of fecal matter; often a sign of intestinal obstruction.

fecalith (fē′-ka-lith): A concretion formed in the bowel from fecal matter.

fecaloid (fē′-ka-loyd): Resembling feces.

fecaloma (fē′-ka-lō′-ma): A tumor-like mass of feces accumulated in the rectum.

fecaluria (fē′-ka-lū′-ri-a): The presence or evidence of fecal matter in the urine.

feces (fē′-sēz): The waste matter excreted from the bowel, consisting of indigestible cellulose, unabsorbed food, mucus, intestinal secretions, water, and bacteria. Also called stool or defecation.—fecal, adj.

feculent (fek′-ū-lent): 1. Foul. 2. Having sediment. 3. Pertaining to, containing, or of the nature of feces.

fecundate (fē′kun-dāt): 1. To fertilize; to impregnate. 2. To render fertile.

fecundation (fē′-kun-dā′-shun): Impregnation. Fertilization.

fecundity (fē-kun′-di-ti): 1. Pronounced fertility; the power to reproduce offspring in large numbers. 2. The innate physiological ability of an individual to produce offspring, as opposed to fertility.

Federal Register: Daily official governmental publication. Publishes proposed regulations for administration of legislation passed by Congress and invites comments from interested parties. Later, the final regulations which have the force of law are published.

feeblemindedness (fē-b'l-mīnd′-ed-nes): Obsolete term for mental retardation.

feedback: In general, all information resulting from a process. In nursing, the results of planned nursing interventions in the form of information that can be applied to the control and improvement of patient care. See also biofeedback.

feeding: The giving or taking of food. **DEMAND F.,** feeding an infant when he indicates he is hungry rather than on a set schedule. **F. TUBE,** a tube for introducing food into the stomach. **FORCED F.,** giving food by force when the patient refuses to eat. **INTRAVENOUS F.,** feeding by introducing liquid food into a vein. **NASOGASTRIC F.,** gavage; introducing feedings into the stomach via the nose, pharynx, and esophagus. **TRANSPYLORIC F.,** feeding of a special formula through a tube positioned through the nares into the stomach, then into the duodenum or jejunum; used for feeding neonates or small infants when necessary, or sometimes adults after surgery. **TUBE F.,** introducing food via tube into the stomach, duodenum or rectum. See hyperalimentation.

fee-for-service: A system of payment for health care services wherein the charge is based on the particular service rendered.

feeling: 1. The sense of touch. 2. The awareness of the sensations produced by the special sense organs. 3. An emotion or mental state that is recognized as pleasurable or unpleasurable.

Fehling's solution (fā′-lings): An alkaline, copper solution used chiefly to detect presence and amount of sugar in a specimen. [Hermann von Fehling, German chemist. 1812-1885.]

Feingold diet: Consists of a high protein, low carbohydrate allowance and eliminates all artificial colorings and flavorings and certain other food additives; useful in treatment of hyperkinetic children.

Feldenkrais exercises: A system of exercises aimed at improving posture and movement. The person doing them concentrates on breathing and the relationship of the body to the environment. Usually taught in groups; sometimes called "awareness through movement."

feldscher (feld'sher): An old term now used mainly in Russia and other European countries to describe medical workers who are trained at several different levels, from village medical helper to medical assistant, and who provide primary care. Several U.S. medical schools have programs for training such persons who are called "physician's assistants."

fellatio (fe-lā'-shi-ō): Insertion of the penis into the mouth of another person, male or female. Oral coitus.

Fellow of the American Academy of Nursing (FAAN): See American Academy of Nursing.

felon (fel'-un): A purulent infection involving the end of a finger, usually near the nail, usually follows a minor penetrating wound. Whitlow.

Felty's syndrome: A combination of adult rheumatoid arthritis and hypersplenism, often accompanied by pigmented spots on the skin of the legs, by anemia, thrombocytopenia, and granulocytopenia, leukopenia, splenomegaly.

female (fē'-māl): 1. Pertinent to the sex that produces the ovum and becomes pregnant. 2. A person of the female sex. **F. PSEUDOHERMAPHRODITISM**, a condition in which the external genitalia are male but the internal genitalia are entirely female.

femaleness (fē'-māl-nes): The anatomic and physiologic features of a female that are concerned with procreation and nurturance of offspring.

feminine (fem'-i-nin): Pertaining to the qualities and role behavior of a female apart from her procreative and nurturant capacities.

feminism (fem'-i-nizm): 1. Femaleness. 2. The possession of feminine traits and characteristics by the male. 3. The social movement for equality of women.

feminization (fem'-i-nī-zā'-shun): 1. The normal development of female traits and characteristics. 2. The development of female characteristics in a male, *e.g.*, high-pitched voice, female type of breast.

femoral (fem'-or-al): Pertaining to the femur or to the thigh as a whole. **F. ARTERY**, the main blood vessel supplying blood to the leg. **F. CANAL**, a conical canal, about 1.25 cm in length, situated in the region between the anterior superior spine of the ilium and the symphysis pubis; a frequent site of hernia. **F. HERNIA**, see under hernia. **F. NERVE**, originates in the lumbar plexus; enervates the muscles of the front of the thigh, and the leg, hip, and knee joints. **F. PULSE**, the pulse of the femoral artery which may be felt in the groin. **F. VEIN**, the large vein in the upper two-thirds of the thigh.

femorocele (fem'-o-rō-sēl): Femoral hernia. See hernia.

femoropopliteal (fem'-or-ō-pop-li-tē'-al): Pertaining to the femur and the popliteal space, or to the femoral and popliteal arteries. **F. BYPASS**, the insertion of a vascular prosthesis between the femoral and popliteal arteries to bypass an obstructed segment.

femorotibial (fem'-o-rō-tib'-i-al): Pertaining to the femur and the tibia.

femur (fē'-mur): The thigh bone; the longest and strongest bone in the body extending from the hip to the thigh. Also called the thigh bone.—femora, pl.; femoral, adj.

fenestra (fe-nes'-tra): 1. A window-like opening. 2. An aperture or opening cut into a plaster of Paris bandage or cast to give access for inspection, relieve pressure, or give skin care. **F. OVALIS**, the oval window, an oval opening between the middle and inner ear. Below it lies the **F. ROTUNDA**, round window, a round opening in the wall between the middle and inner ear.

fenestrated (fen'-es-trāt-ed): Pierced by one or more openings, *e.g.*, the cribriform plate of the ethmoid bone.

fenestration (fen-es-trā'-shun): 1. Perforation. 2. The surgical procedure of creating a new opening in the labyrinth of the inner ear to restore hearing in persons with otosclerosis.

ferment (fer-ment', fer'-ment): 1. To undergo fermentation (*q.v.*). 2. Any substance that causes other substances to undergo fermentation.

fermentation (fer-men-tā'-shun): The chemical changes brought about by the action of enzymes or ferments on complex carbohydrates, usually accompanied by the liberation of heat and gas. Excellent examples are the making of cheese and wine.

fern test: A test for ovulation. Mucus from the cervix during the preovulatory phase will show a fern-like pattern when dried and examined under a microscope. After ovulation this pattern disappears.

ferning: The presence of a fern pattern in a dried specimen of mucus from the uterine cervix before ovulation. In pregnancy, ferning is an indication of the presence of amniotic fluid in the vagina following premature rupture of the membranes.

ferr-, ferri-, ferro-: Combining forms denoting or pertaining to iron.

ferretin (fer′-i-tin): An iron protein complex formed in the intestinal mucosa and stored in the liver, spleen, and bone marrow; essential for hematopoiesis.

ferric (fer′-ik): Pertaining to iron. **F. AMMONIUM** citrate, an iron preparation sometimes used in treatment of anemia. **F. CHLORIDE,** a water or tincture preparation of iron that is sometimes used as a styptic or as an astringent in treatment of skin disorders.

ferrotherapy (fer′-ō-ther′-a-pi): The therapeutic use of iron and its compounds.

ferrous (fer′-rus): Pertaining to divalent iron, as of its salts and compounds.

ferruginous (fe-roo′-ji-nus): 1. Containing iron. 2. Of the color of iron rust.

fertile (fer′-til): Fruitful; not sterile or barren; capable of conceiving and bearing young.—fertility, n.

fertility (fer-til′-i-ti): The ability of a man to impregnate a woman or of a woman to conceive and give birth to a live infant. **F. PLANNING,** see family planning. **F. RATE,** the number of live births per 1000 women of child-bearing age (15-44) in a specific population.

fertilization (fer′ti-lī-zā′shun): The impregnation of an ovum by a spermatozoon. Conception.

fervescence (fer-ves′-ens): An increase in a fever or in body temperature.

fester (fes′-ter): To ulcerate, generate pus, or suppurate superficially.

festinating (fes′-tin-ā-ting): Accelerating; hastening. **F. GAIT,** see under gait.

festination (fes-ti-nā′-shun): An involuntary hastening in gait as seen in paralysis agitans and some other nervous system disorders.

fetal (fē′-tal): Pertaining to a fetus (*q.v.*). **F. ALCOHOL SYNDROME,** a group of features seen in newborns whose mothers are alcoholics; consists of low birth weight, poor growth pattern, failure to thrive, and mental retardation. **F. CIRCULATION,** see under circulation.

fetation (fe-tā′-shun): 1. Pregnancy. 2. The formation and development of a fetus.

feticide (fē′-ti-sīd): The intentional killing or destruction of an embryo or fetus in utero.

fetid (fet′-id): Having an offensive odor; stinking.

fetish (fet′-ish): An inanimate object that is believed to have magical or supernatural power, or that is worshipped or regarded with unreasonable devotion.

fetishism (fet′-ish-izm): 1. The worship of an inanimate object as a substitute for, or symbol of, a loved person. 2. The displacement of the natural erotic interest from a human to an inanimate object. In psychiatry, a form of sexual deviation in which the person feels a strong attachment for an inanimate object usually associated with the other sex, or uses a nonhuman object for sexual arousal.

fetishist (fet′-ish-ist): A person who derives sexual pleasure from an inanimate object.

fetography (fē-tog′-ra-fi): X ray of the fetus in utero.

fetology (fē-tol′-o-ji): A branch of medicine that deals with the diagnosis of abnormalities in the fetus and the treatment of certain pathological conditions in the unborn child. Embryatrics.

fetometry (fē-tom′-e-tri): Estimation of the size of the fetus in utero, particularly of the size of the head.

fetoplacental (fē′-tō-pla-sen′-tal): Pertaining to the fetus and the placenta.

fetoprotein (fē-tō-prō′-tē-in): A fetal antigen that may also be found in adults. **ALPHA-FETOPROTEIN,** when increased in the fetus as shown by amniocentesis, may be diagnostic of neural tube defects; may also appear in the serum of persons with certain liver diseases, inculding malignancies. **BETA-FETOPROTEIN,** a protein found in fetal liver; may also be found in the liver of adults with some liver diseases; is identical with ferritin (*q.v.*).

fetor (fē′-tor): Offensive odor; stench. **F. EX ORE,** bad breath; halitosis. **F. HEPATICUS,** the peculiar breath odor noticed in patients with terminal liver disease; due to exhalation of sulfur containing substances formed in the intestine by bacterial action on sulfur-containing amino acids.

fetoscope (fē′-tō-skōp): A stethoscope for auscultating the fetal heartbeat.

fetoscopy (fē-tos′-ko-pi): A technique for examining the external surface of the fetus, whereby a cannula is inserted through the abdominal and uterine walls and a fine needlescope with a fiberoptic light is introduced into the amniotic sac; photographs can be taken and such abnormalities as spina bifida and anencephaly can be detected; blood samples and biopsies can be taken; done between the 14th and 16th weeks of pregnancy.

fetus (fē′-tus): An unborn child. In the human, the term usually refers to the unborn child from the end of the seventh week after gestation when all of the internal and external organs are present and are undergoing further development, until birth. **CALCIFIED F.,** a **F.** that has died but remained in the uterus and become calcified. **MUMMIFIED F.,** a dead fetus that has taken on the characteristics of a mummy. **F. PAPYRACEUS,** a mummified dead **F.** pressed flat by the presence of a growing twin.

FEV: Abbreviation for forced expiratory volume.

fever (fē′-ver): 1. An elevation of body temperature above normal (37°C; 98.6°F). Syn.—pyrexia. 2. Designates some infectious condition, *e.g.*, paratyphoid fever, scarlet fever, etc. **FEVER BLISTER**; herpes simplex of the lip. **F. OF UNDETERMINED ORIGIN, F.** that persists for weeks or months, often exceeding 101°F.; of obscure origin; abbreviated FUO; also referred to as pyrexia of undetermined origin. **HECTIC F., F.** that occurs daily and tends to rise in the afternoon; seen in tuberculosis and septicemia. **F. THERAPY**, see under therapy. (For special fevers see the nouns.)

fiat (fī′-at): Literally, let there be made. A term used in prescription writing.

fiber (fī′-ber): A slender, elongated, threadlike structure.—fibrous, adj. **NERVE F.**, a slender process of a neuron, particularly from an axon; may vary in length up to several feet; see ganglion, neuron, plexus.

fiberoptic (fī-ber-op′-tik): Refers to the fine, flexible, coated glass or plastic tubes of the fiberscope that have special refractive properties, making it possible to visualize body parts not previously visible, such as the esophagus, stomach, bronchus, bladder and rectum. Combined with the laser beam, the **F.** endoscope is useful in controlling gastrointestinal bleeding.

fiberoptics (fī-ber-op′-tiks): The technique and procedure for observing the interior of a cavity or organ by using a fiberscope, which has glass or plastic fibers with special optical properties.

fiberscope (fī′-ber-skōp): An instrument made of flexible glass, embodying light, an eyepiece and a photographic device; it provides a valuable diagnostic tool, as it permits close examination of the bronchial tree, stomach, esophagus, duodenum, and part of the jejunum as well as parts of the large bowel. Also used for doing biopsies.—fiberoscopy, adj.

fibr-, fibro-: Combining forms denoting 1) fiber; 2) fibrous tissue; 3) fibrin.

fibremia (fī-brē′-mi-a): The presence of fibrin in the blood.

fibril (fī′-bril): A component filament of a fiber, as of a muscle or nerve. A small fiber.—fibrillar, fibrillary, adj.

fibrillation (fi-bri-lā′-shun): Uncoordinated, rapid, quivering contraction of muscle, referring usually to **ATRIAL F.** in the myocardium wherein the atria beat very rapidly and not in synchronization with the ventricular beat. The result is a total irregularity in the pulse rhythm. **VENTRICULAR F.**, similar to atrial **F.** and resulting in rapid, wavering, and ineffectual contraction of the ventricle, seen most often in association with organic heart disease, such as hypertension, thyrotoxicosis, mitral valve disorder, rheumatic heart disease.

fibrillolysis (fī-bril-ol′-i-sis): The dissolution of fibrils.

fibrin (fī′-brin): An elastic, threadlike, insoluble protein that forms the matrix on which a blood clot is formed. Derived from soluble fibrinogen of the blood by the catalytic (enzymatic) action of thrombin.—fibrinous, adj.

fibrin foam: An absorbable spongy material made of human fibrin and used to arrest hemorrhage in neurosurgery particularly, and in hemophilic patients.

fibrinase (fi′-brin-ās): Factor XIII; see under factor.

fibrinogen (fī-brin′-ō-jen): A soluble protein of the blood from which is produced the insoluble protein called fibrin (*q.v.*) essential to blood coagulation. Also called plasminogen. See Factor I under Factor.

fibrinogenopenia (fī-brin′-ō-jen- ō-pē′-ni-a): Lack of blood plasma fibrinogen. May be congenital or due to liver disease. Fibrinopenia. Hypofibrinogenemia.

fibrinolysin (fī′-bri-nol′-i-sin): An enzyme produced by certain bacteria and which causes the destruction of fibrin, thereby aiding in the dissolution of blood clots. Thought to dissolve the fibrin that occurs in tissues after minor injuries. Also called plasmin.

fibrinolysis (fī′-bri-nol′-i-sis): The digestion or dissolution of fibrin by various enzymes and mechanisms.—fibrinolytic, adj.

fibrinolytic (fī′-bri-nō-lit′-ik): 1. Pertaining to fibrinolysis. 2. A drug that dissolves blood clots.

fibrinopurulent (fī′-bri-nō-pū′-rū-lent): Characterized by the presence of both fibrin and pus.

fibrinosis (fī′-bri-nō′-sis): An excess of fibrin in the blood.

fibrinuria (fī-brin-ū′-ri-a): The presence of fibrin in the urine.

fibroadenoma (fī′-brō-ad-e-nō′-ma): A benign tumor containing fibrous and glandular tissue. Often occurs as a breast tumor in women under 30; the mass is firm, movable, well defined; appears suddenly and may become very large; biopsy confirms the diagnosis.

fibroadenosis (fī′-brō-ad-e-nō′-sis): A condition characterized by the development of nodular non-neoplastic tissue in the breast.

fibroblast (fī′-brō-blast): A large stellate cell from which connective tissue arises, including fibrous tissues, tendons, aponeuroses, and other supporting connective tissues; also commonly seen in developing tissues and tissue that is undergoing repair. Syn., fibrocyte.—fibroblastic, adj.

fibroblastoma (fī′-brō-blas-tō′-ma): A tumor arising from the ordinary connective tissue cells or from fibroblasts.

fibrocarcinoma (fī′-brō-kar-si- nō′-ma): A carcinoma that contains fibrous elements.

fibrocartilage (fī′-brō-kar′-ti-lij): Cartilage containing fibrous tissue, found especially in the intervertebral disks.

fibrochondritis (fī′-brō-kon-drī′-tis): Inflammation of fibrocartilage.

fibrochondroma (fī′-brō-kon-drō′-ma): A benign tumor of cartilaginous tissue which contains a considerable amount of fibrous tissue.

fibrocyst (fī′-brō-sist): A fibroma that has undergone cystic degeneration with the cyst becoming the predominant component of the lesion.

fibrocystic (fī-brō-sis′-tik): Pertaining to a fibrocyst. **F. DISEASE OF BONE,** cysts may be solitary or generalized. The latter condition, when accompanied by decalcification of bone, is due to hyperparathyroidism. **F. DISEASE OF THE BREAST,** mastitis characterized by the formation in the female breast of cysts that contain straw-colored fluid; usually occurs at or near menopause. **F. DISEASE OF THE PANCREAS,** see mucoviscidosis; iontophoretic sweat test.

fibrocystoma (fī-brō-sis-tō′-ma): A benign neoplasm characterized by cysts within a fibrous stroma; develops from glandular epithelium.

fibrocyte (fī′-brō-sīt): See fibroblast.—fibrocytic, adj.

fibroelastic (fī-brō-ē-las′-tik): Containing both fibrous and elastic elements.

fibroelastosis (fī′-brō-ē-las-tō′-sis): An overgrowth of fibroelastic tissue. **ENDOCARDIAL F.,** hypertrophy of the left ventricle wall and thickening of the fibroelastic coat of the endocardium; the capacity of the left ventricle may be reduced or increased; symptoms include dyspnea, cyanosis, anorexia.

fibroepithelioma (fī′-brō-ep-i- thē-li-ō′-ma): A skin tumor consiting of fibrous tissue and basal cells of the epidermis; may develop into basal cell carcinoma.

fibroid (fī′-broyd): 1. Being fibrous in nature. 2. A benign tumor originating in smooth muscle tissue often found in the endometrium in multiparous women between 30 and 50 years of age, and which tends to regress at menopause; may occur singly or as multiple firm, round, encapsulated tumors. Most common symptoms are a feeling of dragging in the pelvis; pain and irregular spotting and/or excessive bleeding may occur. Also called fibroma uteri and leiomyoma uteri.

fibroidectomy (fī′-broid-ek′- tō-mi): Surgical removal of a uterine fibroid.

fibrolymphoangioblastoma (fī′-brō- lim′-fō-an′-ji-ō-blas-tō′- ma): A fibrous tumor of the breast; it is hard and freely movable although somewhat adherent to the skin.

fibroma (fī-brō′-ma): An irregularly shaped, firm, slow growing, benign tumor composed chiefly of fibrous or fully developed connective tissue; usually painless; a fibroid. **JUVENILE NASOPHARYNGEAL F.,** a benign neoplasm of the nasopharynx; most often seen in young males.

fibromasarcoma (fī-brō′-ma-sar- kō′-ma): A rare malignant tumor derived from fibroelastic (fibrocystic) cells. **F. OF THE BONE,** occurs in long bones of young adults; prognosis usually poor.—fibromasarcomata, pl.; fibrosarcomatous, adj.

fibromatosis (fī-brō-ma-tō′- sis): A condition in which several fibromata develop at the same time; they may be quite widely distributed throughout the body.

fibromuscular (fī′brō-mus′kū-lar): Pertaining to or consisting of fibrous and muscle tissue.

fibromyitis (fī′-brō-mī-ī′-tis): Inflammation of the muscles, followed by degeneration of the muscular fibers.

fibromyoma (fī′-brō-mī-ō′-ma): A benign tumor consisting of fibrous and muscle tissue.—fibromyomata, pl; fibromyomatous, adj.

fibromyositis (fī′-brō-mī-ō-sī′-tis): Any of a large group of acute or chronic disorders characterized by inflammation of muscles, overgrowth of connective tissues, and stiffness of the joints.

fibroneuroma (fiī′-brō-nū-rō′-ma): A tumor that has the elements of both a fibroma and a neuroma.

fibro-osteoma (fī′-brō-os-tē-ō′-ma): A tumor that has the characteristics of both a fibroma and an osteoma.

fibroplasia (fī-brō-plā′-zi-a): The formation of fibrous tissue; occurs in the healing of wounds; usually implies an abnormal increase of fibrous tissue. **RETROLENTAL F.,** the presence of fibrous tissue in the vitreous, from the retina to the lens, causing blindness. Noticed shortly after birth, more commonly in premature babies who have had continuous oxygen therapy.—fibroplastic, adj.

fibroplastic (fī-brō-plas′- tik): Giving origin to or producing fibrous tissue.

fibrosarcoma (fī′-brō-sar-kō′-ma): A sarcoma that develops from fibroblasts; begins with small skin nodules and metastasizes early.

fibrose (fī′-brōs): 1. The forming of fibrous tissue. 2. Fibrous.

fibrosis (fī-brō′-sis): The formation of fibrous tissue in an organ or part; usually refers to excessive formation as part of a reparative process. It is the cause of adhesions of the peritoneum and other serous tissues. **CYSTIC F. OF THE PANCREAS,** see cystic. **F. OF THE LUNGS,** the formation of scar tissue in the stroma of the lungs following an infection or inflammation. **PERIGLOMULAR F.,** the deposition of collagen in Bowman's capsule, *q.v.* under nephron. **PUL-**

MONARY F., progressive **F.** of the walls of the alveoli resulting in severe dyspnea; the acute form may be rapidly fatal.

fibrositis (fī′-brō-sī′-tis): Inflammation of the white fibrous tissue, especially that of some of the muscles. Syn., muscular rheumatism. See Bornholm disease, lumbago, pleurodynia.

fibrositis syndrome: A painful condition that may occur at certain points of fascial and tendinous attachment of muscles to bones or may be widespread in areas of tissue supplied by cervical and lumbar segments of the spinal nerves; in addition to pain, there may be diffuse stiffness, paresthesia, muscle contraction, headache, restless sleep.

fibrothorax (fī′ brō-thō′- raks): A condition in which the two layers of the pleura adhere to each other. It may result from fibrosis of the pleural space associated with trauma, tuberculous effusion, or emphysema.

fibrotic (fī-brot′-ik): Characterized by or pertinent to fibrosis.

fibrous (fī′-brus): Consisting of, containing, or like fibers. **F. TISSUE,** a type of connective tissue that is made up of strong, tough, white fibers; forms tendons, ligaments and fascia.

fibula (fib′-ū-la): One of the longest and thinnest bones of the body; situated on the outer side of the leg and articulating at the upper end with the lateral condyle of the tibia and at the lower end with the lateral surface of the talus (astragalus) and tibia.—fibular, adj.

Fick principle: States that an indirect measure of cardiac output per minute can be obtained by comparing the amount of oxygen consumed per minute to the amount of oxygen absorbed by each mililiter of blood as it passes through the capillaries of the lungs. See also cardiac output under cardiac.

field (fēld): A limited area; an open space. **F. OF HEARING,** the space within which sounds are audible. Also called auditory field. **F. OF VISION,** the entire area in which objects can be seen by the fixed eye.

fifth disease: Erythema infectiosum; see under erythema.

fight or flight reaction: 1. In physiology, the response of the sympathetic nervous system and the adrenal medulla to stress, which results in alterations in metabolism and blood flow that, in turn, promote preservation of the individual in emergency situations. 2. In psychiatry, the response of the individual to stress; he may fight by striving to adjust, or flee by taking refuge in a psychosis, which allows him to ignore the stressful circumstance.

filaceous (fi-lā′-shus): Made up of small fibers or filaments.

filament (fil′-a-ment): A delicate fiber or threadlike structure.—filamenta, pl.; filar, filamentous, adj.

Filaria (fi-lā′-ri-a): A generic term formerly loosely applied to members of the superfamily Filarioidea; includes several types of nematode worms that may infest man and invade the circulatory and lymphatic systems, serous cavities, or connective tissue.

filariasis (fil-a-rī′-a-sis): Infestation with a nematode parasite of the superfamily Filarioidea which enters the body through the bite of a mosquito or other insect and infests the lymphatic system causing blocking of the lymph vessels resulting in swelling and pain in the limbs. See elephantiasis.

filaricide (fi-lar′-i-sīd): An agent that destroys filaria.—filaricidal, adj.

Filarioidea (fī-lar-i-oy′-dē-a): A superfamily of parasitic threadlike nematode worms found mainly in the tropics and sub-tropics and in the Orient, several varieties of which may infest humans.

filial (fil′-i-al): Pertaining to or relating to a son or daughter.

filiform (fil′-i-form): Thread-like. **F. PAPILLAE,** small projections ending in several minute processes; found on the tongue.

filipuncture (fil′-i-pung′- chur): Insertion of a coil of wire thread, etc., into an aneurysm to produce coagulation of contained blood.

film badge: A small packet device containing x-ray sensitive film, worn by individuals exposed to ionizing radiation in their work, for estimating the amount of radiation to which they have been exposed.

filter (fil′-ter): 1. To screen out or strain the solids from a substance by passing it through a device that will hold back the solids larger than a certain size while letting the liquid pass. 2. Any substance or device that screens or strains out certain suspended particles. In radiotherapy the term applies to a sheet of metal that lets certain rays pass through while holding others back. **F. PAPER,** a coarse-grained paper used for filtering solutions. **F. PASSING VIRUS,** see virus.

filterable (fil′-ter-a-b′l): Capable of passing through a filter. **F. VIRUS,** a pathogenic agent that is so small it passes through the pores of the finest filter available.

filtrate (fil′-trāt): That part of a solution that has passed through a filter.

filtration (fil-trā′-shun): The process of straining through a filter. The act of passing fluid through a porous medium. **F. UNDER PRESSURE,** occurs in the kidneys, due to pressure of the blood in the glomeruli.

filum (fī′-lum): Any filamentous or threadlike structure. **F. TERMINALE,** a strong, fine cord blending with the spinal cord above, and the periosteum of the sacral canal below; the terminal end of the spinal cord.

fimbria (fim′-bri-a): A fringe or frond resembling a frond of a fern, especially one of the fondlike processes at the end of a fallopian tube.—fimbriae, pl.; fimbrial, fimbriate, fimbriated. adj.

fimbriectomy (fim′-bri-ek′-to-mi): The surgical excision of the fimbriated portion of a fallopian tube.

finger: A digit of the hand. **CLUBBED F.**, swelling of the terminal phalanx of digits that occurs in many persons with heart or lung disease. **F. COT**, see under cot. **INDEX F.**, that nearest the thumb. **F. READING**, Braille reading; see Braille. **F. SPELLING**, a method of communication between deaf people; the letters of the alphabet are formed by various positions of the hands and fingers. **F. STALL**, **F.** cot. **TRIGGER F.**, one that locks when flexed so it can be opened only with difficulty, making a snapping noise; due to chronic tenosynovitis. **WEBBED F.**, one that is joined to another by a fold of skin.

fingeragnosia (fing′-ger-ag-nō′-si- a): Loss of ability to recognize or identify the fingers on one's hands.

finger-finger test: A test for cerebellar function; the patient is asked to stretch his arms out to the sides and then bring the tips of the index fingers together; normally the motion is carried out smoothly and accurately.

finger-nose test; A test for cerebellar function. The patient extends his arm to one side and then slowly tries to touch the end of his nose. Test is conducted in several ways, all involving touching the end of the nose.

fingerprint: The impression made when the ends of the fingers are inked and then pressed on a piece of paper. Used for identification purposes as no two persons have the same pattern of ridges in the skin at the ends of the fingers.

fingersweep: A technique utilized before administering the abdominal thrust maneuver to a choking or unconscious patient; the curved index finger of one hand is inserted at the side of the cheek and quickly passed over the back of the throat and sides of the cheek to remove any food or other object that may be obstructing the airway.

FiO_2: Fractional inspired oxygen; the percentage of oxygen inspired and delivered to the respiratory tract.

fire damp: A gas, largely methane, that forms in mines; explosive when mixed with air; potentially lethal.

first aid: The immediate treatment given to a person who is injured or who becomes suddenly ill, before the doctor arrives or medical treatment can be obtained.

first intention healing: See under healing.

first pass effect: In pharmacokinetics, refers to the rate of inactivation of orally given drugs that is brought about by the action of enzymes in the intestine and in the liver, making it necessary sometimes to give a higher dose initially than would be required if the drug were given parenterally.

Fishberg concentration test: A kidney function test in which the specific gravity of urine is determined after the patient has abstained from liquids for 12 hours.

fish-skin disease: Ichthyosis (*q.v.*).

fission (fish′-un): The action of splitting. In biology, the reproduction of a cell by simple division into two approximately equal parts. In nuclear physics, the splitting of the nucleus of the atom, causing the release of great quantities of energy.

fissiparous (fi-sip′-a-rus): Reproducing by fission.

fissure (fish′-ur): A split, crack, or groove in tissue; may be structural and normal or abnormal. **ANAL F.**, or **FISSURE IN ANO**, a crack or linear ulcer on the margin of the anus; causes severe pain on defecation; usually treated surgically. **LONGITUDINAL F.**, separates the right and left hemispheres of the cerebrum. **PALPEBRAL F.**, the opening between the eyelids. **F. OF ROLANDO**, see rolandic. **F. OF SYLVIUS**, see Sylvius.

fissured tongue: A tongue in which there are deep furrows in the mucous membrane. Also called scrotal tongue.

fistula (fis′-tū-la): An abnormal tube-like communication between two body surfaces or cavities, or between an internal organ and the surface of the body, *e.g.*, a gastrocolic **F.** between the stomach and the colon, or a colostomy between the colon and the abdominal surface. **ABDOMINAL F.**, one leading from an abdominal viscus to the exterior. **ANAL F.**, fistulo in ano. **ARTERIOVENOUS F.**, an abnormal communication between an artery and a vein. **CIMINO-BRESCIA F.**, a **F.** created between a cephalic vein and the radial artery; made to provide a mode of entry to the circulation for dialysis. **COLONIC F.**, a **F.** between the intestine and the skin of the abdomen or between the colon and another hollow organ. **FECAL F.**, a **F.** that opens onto the surface of the body; it discharges feces. **F. IN ANO**, a deep slit in the skin around the anus; often a sequela to perineal abscess. **INTESTINAL F.**, an abnormal passage into the intestine; may refer to one surgically created. **PANCREATIC F.**, 1) an opening from the pancreas to the surface of the body; may be created in certain gastric or duodenal operations; or 2) a surgically created internal passage from the pancreas to the small intestine or gallbladder. **RECTOVAGINAL F.**, a fistulous opening between the rectum and vagina. **TRACHEAL F.**, an abnormal passage opening into the trachea. **TRACHEOESOPHAGEAL F.**, a communication channel between the trachea and the esophagus; a serious congenital anomaly requiring immediate surgery. **VESICOINTESTINAL F.**, a fistulous communication between the urinary bladder and the intestine. **VESICOVAGINAL F.**, a fistulous opening between the urinary bladder and the vagina.—fistular, fistulous, adj.; fistulae, pl.

fistulectomy (fis-tū-lek′-tō-mi): Excision of a fistula.

fistulization (fis-tū-lī-zā′- shun): 1. The surgical creation of a fistula (*q.v.*) 2. The process of becoming a fistula. Also fistulation.

fistulous (fis′-tū-lus): Resembling a fistula.

fit: Convulsion (*q.v.*). Inappropriate, sudden attack of motor or psychic activity, or both. Typical episode involves patient in involuntary and paroxysmal muscular movements (writhing), associated with loss of consciousness. See epilepsy.

Fitz-Hugh-Curtis syndrome: A condition in which gonococcal salpingitis is associated with upper quadrant pain and inflammation of the liver; to be distinguished from hepatitis.

fix: To fasten firmly. See fixation.

fixation (fik-sā′-shun): 1. The act of fastening something into a fixed position, often by suturing. 2. The condition or state of being fixed in a certain position. 3. In microscopy, a method of treating material to be examined so as to preserve it or to make possible a more thorough examination. 4. In personality development, the arrest of development at a level short of maturity; may result in unnatural behavior, *e.g.*, excessive emotional attachment for a parent. 5. In optics, the direct focusing of one or both eyes so that the image falls on the fovea centralis. **COMPLEMENT F.**, when antigen and homologous antibody unite to form a complex, complement may unite with such a complex, and this is referred to as **F. SKELETAL F.**, a method of treating fractures that are difficult to treat by traditional means; utilizes a rigid metal plate or apparatus that holds the bones in alignment; when applied to the surface of the body it is called **EXTERNAL F.**, when surgically applied directly to the bone it is called **INTERNAL F.**

fixative (fik′-sa-tiv): An agent that hardens and preserves specimens for laboratory study.

fixator (fiks-ā′-ter): Name given to the apparatus used to immobilize fractures without casting when there is skin loss or injury, or in compound fractures.

fl dr: Abbreviation for fluidram.

fl oz: Abbreviation for fluid ounce.

flaccid (flak′-sid, flas′-id): Soft, flabby, not firm; term is often used to describe muscles that have lost all or part of their tone. Also sometimes used to describe a certain type of personality. See paralysis.—flaccidity, n.

flagella (fla-jel′-a): Plural of flagellum (*q.v.*).

flagellant (flaj′-e-lent): 1. Pertaining to flagella. 2. One who practices flagellation. 3. Pertaining to a stroking maneuver in massage.

flagellate (flaj′-e-lāt): Having flagella. See flagellum.

flagellation (flaj-e-lā′-shun): 1. A massage manuever consisting of whipping the skin with the fingers. 2. A sadistic or masochistic act in which one or both partners derive pleasure from whipping.

flagellum (fla-jel′-um): A fine hair-like appendage capable of lashing movement. Characteristic of spermatozoa, certain bacteria and protozoa; used for locomotion.—flagella, pl.

flail (flāl): Refers to flaccidity or lack of normal control over a part. **FLAIL CHEST**, see under chest. **FLAIL JOINT**, one that is excessively mobile and cannot be controlled due to paralysis of the muscles that control its movements.

flank: That part of the trunk of the body that lies between the lowest ribs and the ilia.

flap: A piece of skin or soft tissue of varying size, shape, and thickness that has been detached from the underlying tissue but left attached at some point to retain its own circulation; used in various plastic operations and to cover the end of bone after amputation of a part. **SKIN F.**, refers to a true flap of skin created by a curved incision, leaving a portion attached.

flare (flār): Diffuse reddening of an area around an injury or an infected area.

flask: A bottle with a narrow neck; has many laboratory uses.

flatfoot: A congenital or acquired condition in which the arch of the instep is depressed so that the entire sole of the foot touches the ground when one is standing or walking. See talipes.

flatulence (flat′-ū-lens): Gastric and intestinal distension with air or gas.—flatulent, adj.

flatus (flā′-tus): Gas or air in the stomach or intestines. **F. BAG**, a bag attached to a rectal tube which may drain into a vented container that may or may not contain water. **F. TUBE**, a rectal tube; see under rectal.

flatworm: Any worm belonging to the phylum *Platyhelminthes,* including tapeworms and flukes.

flaxseed (flaks′-sēd): The seed of flax; used medicinally as an emollient and cathartic.

fld: Abbreviation for fluid.

flea (flē): A blood-sucking wingless parasitic insect of the order Siphonaptera; it may act as host and transmit such diseases as typhus and plague. Its bite leaves a portal of entry for infection. **HUMAN F.**, Pulex irritans. **RAT F.**, Xenopsylla cheopis, transmitter of plague (*q.v.*).

flesh: The soft tissues of an animal or human body, especially the muscle tissue. **GOOSE F.**, cutis anserina (*q.v.*). **PROUD F.**, the excessive growth of granular tissue in a wound.

fletcherism (fletch′-er-izm): A way of eating that includes taking small bites or amounts of food at a time and chewing excessively; a certain number of "chews" is assigned to each type of food, the theory being that the completely broken down food substances are more readily digested and absorbed.

flex: 1. Bend. 2. To move a joint so that the two parts it connects are brought closer together.

flexibilitas cerea (flek-si-bil′-i-tas-sē′-rē-a): Literally, waxy flexibility. A condition of generalized hypertonia of muscles found in catatonic schizophrenia. When fully developed, the patient's limbs retain positions in which they are placed, remaining immobile for hours at a time. Occasionally occurs in hysteria, as hysterical rigidity.

flexibility (flek-si-bil′-i-ti): The ability to change, bend, or conform. **WAXY F.**, see cerea flexibilitas.

flexion (flek′-shun): 1. The act of bending. 2. The condition of being bent. 3. The movement of certain joints so as to decrease the angle between the two parts it connects, as in bending the elbow. Opp. of extension.

Flexner Report: A study by Abraham Flexner [U.S. educator, 1860-1959] of 155 medical schools in the U.S. and Canada. Published in 1910. Initiated reforms in medical education and in laws concerning the practice of medicine in U.S. and Canada.

Flexner's bacillus (*Shigella flexneri*): A pathogenic gram-negative rod bacterium, which is the most common cause of bacillary dysentery epidemics, and sometimes infantile gastroenteritis. It is found in the feces of cases of dysentery and carriers, from whence it may pollute food and water supplies, or be transferred by contact.[Simon Flexner, American pathologist. 1863-1946.]

flexor (flek′-sor): A muscle which on contraction flexes or bends a part. Opp. to extensor.

flexure (flek′-sher): A bend. **HEPATIC F.**, the bend between the ascending and transverse colon on the right side near the liver. **SIGMOID F.**, the S-shaped bend at the lower end of the descending colon, at its juncture with the rectum below. **SPLENIC F.**, the bend at the junction of the transverse and descending parts of the colon on the left side near the spleen.—flexural, adj.

flight of ideas: Sometimes seen in acute mania when a patient talks continually and repeatedly changes his line of thought.

floaters (flō′-ters): Opaque specks in the vitreous space that float across the visual field and cast moving shadows on the retina; may be congenital or due to degenerative changes in the vitreous or retina.

floating: In anatomy, an organ that is out of, or has become detached from, its normal position in the body. **FLOATING KIDNEY**, see nephroptosis. **FLOATING RIBS**, a name sometimes given to the 11th and 12th pairs of ribs because they are not attached to the sternum.

floccillation (flok-si-lā′-shun): Carphology (*q.v.*).

flocculation (flok-ū-lā′- shun): The coalescence of colloidal particles in suspension resulting in their aggregation into larger discrete masses, which are often visible to the naked eye.

flocculent (flok′-ū-lent): Containing flaky or downy shreds of material.

flocculus (flok′-ū-lus): A small tuft; may apply to a structure in the body or to a material such as wool or cotton.

flooding: 1. In psychiatry, behavior therapy in which treatment of phobias consists of repeated exposure to the worst possible phobic situations, progressing from fantastic to real life situations. Also called implosion. 2. Bleeding profusely as from the uterus following childbirth.

"floppy" baby: Descriptive of an infant with respiratory distress syndrome (*q.v.*); rapid respirations, grunting expirations, retraction of the sternum and ribs are prominent signs.

floppy mitral valve syndrome: A structural alteration of the mitral valve leading to stretching and weakness of the cusps of the valve which allows some of the blood to leak back into the left atrium when the heart pumps instead of being pushed through the aorta. Also called Barlow's syndrome.

flora (flō′-ra): The collective plant life of a certain area. In human physiology, the bacterial and fungal life that normally inhabits an area. **INTESTINAL F.**, the bacteria normally found in the intestinal canal. **NORMAL F.**, refers to flora that normally inhabit certain areas of the body without causing infection.

florid (flor′-id): 1. Having a bright red color. 2. A flushed appearance of the skin, especially of the face.

flotation pad: A device consisting of a rubber bag filled with water that fits over the entire mattress; used in prevention of decubitus ulcers by relieving pressure on susceptible areas.

flow chart: A chronological record in graph or tabular form that reflects ongoing observations; used to follow a patient's progress when rapid changes in condition are occurring. Observations usually recorded are temperature, pulse rate, blood pressure, respirations, reflexes. May also be used in clinics and physician's offices to follow changes in a patient's weight, blood pressure, etc. Also called flow sheet.

flowmeter (flō′-mē-ter): A device that monitors the flow of oxygen and other gases and liquids.

flu: Abbreviation for influenza (*q.v.*).

fluctuate (fluk′-tū-āt): 1. To change from time

to time or to vary irregularly. 2. To move with wave-like motion or to undulate.

fluctuation (fluk-tū-ā′-shun): A wave-like motion felt on digital examination of an organ or structure containing fluid.—fluctuant, adj.

fluid (floo′-id): A substance composed of particles that may change their relative positions but do not separate from the mass, and which is capable of flowing. **AMNIOTIC F.**, see under amniotic. **EXTRACELLULAR F.**, the interstitial **F.** plus the blood plasma; constitutes about 20 percent of body weight. **EXTRAVASCULAR F.**, all body fluid that is outside the blood vessels; constitutes about 50 percent of body weight. **F. BALANCE**, see under balance. **INTERSTITIAL F.**, that which is in the spaces between the cells; constitutes about 16 percent of body weight. **INTRACELLULAR F.**, that which is inside the cells. **PLEURAL F.**, the minute amount of **F.** between the visceral and parietal pleura. **PROSTATIC F.**, the whitish **F.** secreted by the prostate gland; a constituent of semen. **SEMINAL F.**, semen. **SYNOVIAL F.**, the clear fluid that serves as a lubricant for joints and bursae.

fluid dram: A unit of liquid measure (apothecaries' system) equal to 60 minims, ⅛ fluid ounce, or approximately 1 teaspoonful. In the metric system it equals 3.7 cc. Also fluidram.

fluid ounce: In liquid measure 8 fluidrams (apothecaries' system); 29.57 cc (metric system).

fluidextract (floo-id-eks′- trakt): A liquid preparation of a plant drug in which 1 cc contains the equivalent of 1 gram of the crude drug. The solvent is usually alcohol.

fluke (flook): A small, flat, unsegmented trematode worm that may be parasitic to animals and to man, particularly in tropical countries.

fluor albus (floo-or al′-bus): Leukorrhea (*q.v.*).

fluorescein (floo-ō-res′-ē-in): The red crystalline powder that is used in eye drops to detect foreign bodies in the eye and lesions of the cornea. **F. ANGIOGRAPHY**, multiple photographs of the retina taken at definite intervals after sodium **F.** has been injected into the antecubital vein; the flow of the dye is traced through the retina and the choroid.

fluorescence (floo-ō-res′-ens): The property of emitting radiation, usually visible light, as a result of having absorbed the radiation from another source.

fluorescent (floo-ō-res′-ent): Having the property of emitting electromagnetic radiation following absorption of radiation from some other source. **F. ANTIBODY TEST**, a rapid sensitive laboratory test which, among other uses, can be used to detect the presence of streptococci that cause rheumatic fever. **F. SCREEN**, one that gives temporary visualization of a structure when it is interposed between the subject and a source of x rays. **FLUORESCENT TREPONEMAL ANTIBODY ABSORPTION TEST**, a test performed on cerebrospinal fluid to confirm the diagnosis of neurosyphilis; abbreviated FTA-ABS.

fluoridate (floo-or′-i-dāt): To add fluorine salts to a community water supply to aid in control of dental caries.

fluoridation (floo-or-i-dā′-shun): The addition of fluorine salts to water; term usually refers to treatment of the water supply of a community as a public health measure to reduce the incidence of dental caries; the dilution is usually 1:1,000,000. See fluorine.

fluoride (floo′ or-īd): A compound of fluorine and another element; the form of fluorine used as an additive to drinking water to prevent caries. Also applied directly to the teeth.

fluoridize (floo-or′-i-diz): 1. To add fluoride to the drinking water. 2. To apply a fluoride to the teeth as a preventive measure against the formation of caries.

fluorine (floo′-or-rēn): A non-metallic gaseous element; in the human body it is found chiefly in bones and teeth. When present in natural water supply, it tends to reduce dental decay; in excess it gives a mottled appearance to the teeth. See fluoridation.

fluoroentgenography (floo′-ō-rent-gen-og′-ra-fi): The photography of images on a fluorescent screen. Also called fluorography, photofluorography.

fluorometer (floo-or-om′-e-ter): A device for detecting and measuring fluorescence.

fluoroscope (floo-or′ ō-skōp): A device for immediate projection of an x-ray image on a fluorescent screen for visual examination of the deeper structures of the body.

fluoroscopy (floo-ō-ros′-ko-pi): X-ray examination by means of a fluorescent screen; commonly called screening.—fluoroscopic, adj.

fluorosis (floo-or-ō′-sis): A condition caused by excessive intake of a fluoride substance; characterized by brittleneess of bones, discoloration and mottling of the teeth; may occur when the water supply of a community contains an excessive amount of natural fluoride.

flush: A sudden reddening of the skin, especially of the face and neck. **HECTIC F.**, redness of the cheeks seen as a characteristic of certain chronic infections, *e.g.*, pulmonary tuberculosis. **HOT FLUSH**, lay term for sudden reddening of the face and a subjective feeling of heat experienced by women during menopause.

flutter: A rapid pulsation or vibration; tremulousness; said especially of the heart. **ATRIAL F.**, a type of cardiac arrhythmia in which the atrial contractions may reach 250-400 per minute, but remain rhythmic and of uniform strength; the ventricular rate is usually about 150; this pattern produces saw-tooth waves in the ECG; it is a manifestation of underlying heart disease involving particularly the coronary arteries. **OCULAR F.**, spontaneous horizontal oscillations of the eye during fixation; often associated with cerebellar pathology. **VENTRICULAR F.**, rapid ventricular tachycardia with the ECG showing no distinct QRS or T waves.

flux: 1. An excessive flow of any of the body secretions. 2. Diarrhea. **BLOODY F.**, dysentery.

FNP: Abbreviation for Family Nurse Practitioner (*q.v.*).

focal (fō′-kal): Limited to one area; localized. **F. INFECTION**, one localized more or less in one site, from which it spreads to other parts of the body. **F. SEIZURE**, an epileptic seizure due to irritation of a localized area of the brain; usually there is no loss of consciousness.

focus (fō′-kus): 1. A point at which rays converge; said of light and sound waves. 2. The area of the body where disease or a morbid process is localized.—foci, pl.; focal, adj.

foe-: For words beginning thus see words beginning fe-, e.g., fetus.

folacin (fō′-la-sin): Folic acid (*q.v.*).

folate (fō′-lāt): A salt of folic acid. Folates are present in natural foods; they act as coenzymes.

fold: A thin margin or doubling of tissue, or a plica. See plica.

Foley catheter: See under catheter.

foliate (fō′-li-āt): Shaped like a leaf.

folic acid (fō′-lik): A water-soluble constituent of the vitamin B complex; found in certain nuts, leafy plants, yeast, liver, kidney. Has antianemic properties, and in conjunction with vitamin B_{12} is important in formation of red blood cells in the bone marrow. Effective in preventing sprue, and pernicious and megaloblastic anemia; is commonly deficient in the average diet.

folie (fō-lē′): Old term for psychosis or insanity. **FOLIE A DEUX**, a situation in which two closely related persons have the same thoughts, ideas, and delusions. **FOLIE DU DOUTE**, term referring to an individual who has spells of doubting, brooding, and of constantly changing his or her mind, making it impossible to arrive at decisions.

folk medicine: The nonprofessional practice of medicine by individuals not trained in medical science and who use procedures and remedies that are based on tradition and, often, on superstition; many of the remedies they use are of plant origin and the recipes for preparation of the medications are kept secret by the "medicine men or women."

follicle (fol′-ik'l): 1. A small secreting sac. 2. A simple tubular gland. **GRAAFIAN F.**, a minute vesicle in the stroma of the ovary containing a single ovum. **HAIR F.**, the tubular oil-secreting invagination of epithlium in which the hair grows. **OVARIAN F.**, graafian **F. PILOSEBACEOUS F.**, the hair follicle with its attached oil gland.

follicle-stimulating hormone: A hormone of the anterior pituitary lobe which stimulates the graafian follicles of the ovary, promotes maturation of the follicle and liberation of estrin (*q.v.*). In the male it stimulates the production of spermotozoa through stimulation of the epithelium of the seminiferous tubules. Abbreviated FSH.

follicular (fō-lik′-ū-lar): Pertaining to a follicle, or follicles. **F. CYST**, a cyst developing in a follicular space, as in the ovary. **F. HORMONE**, estrogen produced in the ovarian follicle. **F. TONSILLITIS**, see under tonsillitis.

folliculitis (fō-lik-ū-lī′tis): Inflammation of a follicle; usually refers to infection around the hair follicles. **F. BARBAE**, infection of the hair follicles of the beard with formation of papules and pustules; also called ringworm of the beard and barber's itch. **F. DECALVANS**, an alopecia (*q.v.*) of the scalp characterized by pustulation and scars.

folliculoma (fō-lik-ū-lō′-ma): An ovarian tumor that arises in the epithelium of the Graafian follicle.

folliculosis (fō-lik-ū-lō′-sis): A chronic disorder characterized by an abnormally increased number of lymph follicles.

fomentation (fō′-men-tā′- shun): A hot, wet application used to reduce pain or inflammation. When the skin is intact, strict cleanliness is observed (medical **F.**); when the skin is broken, asceptic technic is observed (surgical **F.**). See stupe.

fomite (fō′-mit): Any article that has been in contact with infection and is capable of transmitting same.—formites, pl.; also fomes.

fontanel, fontanelle (fon′-ta-nel′): Any one of the six spaces ("soft spots") between the converging cranial bones in which ossification is not complete at birth. The diamond-shaped **ANTERIOR F.** lies at the junction of the frontal and parietal bones; it usually closes at about the eighteenth month of life. The triangular-shaped **POSTERIOR F.** lies at the junction of the occipital and parietal bones; it usually closes at about the second month of life. The two **ANTEROLATERAL**

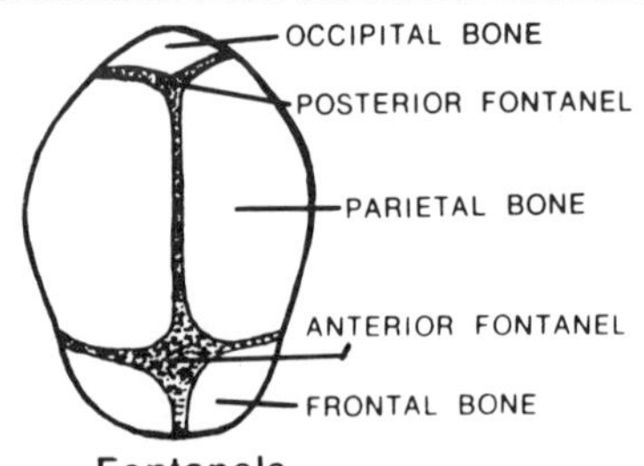

Fontanels

F.S lie at the junction of the frontal, parietal, temporal, and sphenoid bones; they usually close at about the third month of life. The two POSTEROLATERAL F.S. lie at the junction of the parietal, occipital, and temporal bones; they do not usually close until the second year of life.

Food and Drug Administration (FDA): A federal agency (now in the Department of Health and Human Services) established in 1938; is charged with the duty of inspecting and passing on the purity and potency of foods and drugs offered for sale in the U.S; regulates research in drugs and pharmaceuticals; conducts research on biological sera and vaccines. A "watchdog" agency responsible for ensuring that foods, drugs, and cosmetics sold in the U.S. are safe, fulfill their stated functions, and are correctly labeled and packaged and are in accordance with the body of law that has developed from the Pure Food and Drug Act of 1906 and the Federal Food, Drug, and Cosmetic Act of 1938, as well as the Controlled Substances Act of 1965.

food exchange list: Any of several lists of foods and the quantities of each that will provide the same number of calories and the same amount of nutritive value. Useful in planning regular diets as well as diets for persons requiring special diets. The main groups on the list are milk, vegetables, bread, meat and fats.

Food For Freedom Program: A federal agency concerned with nutrition; provides food for the world's needy from U.S. agricultural surpluses.

food groups: A reference to food lists that have been called The Basic Four, *i.e.*, meats, milk, fuits and vegetables, breads and cereals; well-planned meals will contain foods from each classification.

food intolerance: Inability of the body to digest certain foods due to lack of an enzyme necessary to their digestion and metabolism; to be differentiated from food allergy. See also celiac disease.

food poisoning: Characterized by vomiting, with or without diarrhea, resulting from eating food contaminated with chemical poison, preformed bacterial toxin, or live bacteria.

Food Stamp Program: A federal program designed to assist individuals and families with low incomes to increase their food-purchasing power by providing stamps that can be exchanged for food at certain stores; persons over age 60 can use the stamps to pay for home-delivered meals.

foot: That portion of the lower leg that is below the ankle. The sole or bottom is called the plantar surface; the top side is called the dorsal surface. ATHLETE'S F., tinea pedis (*q.v.*). DROP F., or FOOTDROP, inability to dorsiflex the foot, as in severe sciatica and nervous conditions affecting lower lumbar regions of the cord; sometimes results from failure to protect feet from pressure of bedclothing. MADURA F., see mycetoma. TRENCH F., immersion F., so called because it occurs among soldiers in trenches; also occurs in frostbite and other conditions of exposure when there is local deprivation of blood supply.

foot candle: A unit of illumination on a surface that is one foot from a light source of one candle and equal to one lumen per square foot.

foot-and-mouth disease: An acute, highly infectious viral disease of cattle, transmissible to man, causing a vesicular eruption of the mucous membranes of the mouth and nose and of the skin of the interdigital spaces; other symptoms include headache, fever, malaise.—Syn., aphthous fever.

footboard: A device made of wood or other firm material to be placed at the foot of the bed to prevent the patient from slipping down in bed, to keep the weight of bedclothes off the feet, and to keep the feet at right angles to the leg in order to maintain good posture and prevent foot drop.

footdrop: See drop foot under foot.

footling: In obstetrics, refers to a presentation of the feet foremost.

footprint: An ink impression of the sole of the foot. Used in maternity hospitals or wards as a means of identification of newborn infants.

foramen (fō-rā′ men): A natural hole or opening. Generally used with reference to a bone or a membranous structure. F. OF MAGENDIE, an opening in the roof of the fourth ventricle of the brain for the passage of cerebrospinal fluid into the subarachnoid space. F. MAGNUM, the opening in the occipital bone through which the spinal cord passes and becomes continuous with the medulla oblongata. F. OF MUNRO, a communication between the lateral and third ventricles of the brain; also called intraventricular F. F. OF MORGAGNI, a small gap on either side of the diaphragm between the sternal and costal portions through which the superior epigastric blood vessels and some lympatics pass. NUTRIENT F., any of the channels through which nutrient-carrying vessels enter the medullary cavity of long bones. OBTURATOR F., an aperture situated in the anterior portion of the innominate bone. F. OVALE, the fetal communication between the left and right atria; closes at birth. VERTEBRAL F., the space in the vertebrae through which the spinal cord passes. F. SPINOSUM, an opening in the great wing of the sphenoid to accomodate the middle meningeal artery.—foramina, pl.

forced expiratory volume: The volume of gas exhaled over a given time period while performing forced vital capacity determination. Abbreviated FEV.

forced vital capacity: The maximal amount of gas that can be expelled from the lungs following a maximal inspiration with an expiration as forceful and rapid as possible. Abbreviated FVC.

forceps (for′-seps): Surgical instruments with two opposing blades which are used to grasp or compress tissues, swabs, needles, and many other surgical appliances. The two blades are controlled by direct pressure (tong-like), or by handles (scissor-like). **KELLY F.**, a surgical instrument used to clamp large blood vessels. **OBSTETRIC F.**, used to help extract the infant's head from the birth canal.

forearm (for′-arm): That part of the arm that is between the elbow and the wrist. Antebrachium.

forebrain (for′-brān): The part of the embryonic brain that develops into the telencephalon and diencephalon.

foreconscious (for-kōn′-shus): Information not usually within consciousness but which can be recalled voluntarily; preconscious.

forefinger: The index finger, *i.e.*, the one next to the thumb.

forefoot (for′-foot): The front or fore part of the foot.

foregut (for′-gut): The embryonic structure from which most of the small intestine, stomach, liver, esophagus, lung, and pharynx develop.

forehead (for′-hed): The anterior part of the cranium that is above the eyes; the brow.

foreign body: Any substance or object lodged in a place in the body where it does not belong.

foremilk (for′milk): Colostrum (*q.v.*).

forensic medicine (for-en′-sik): 1. The relationship and influence of law on the practice of medicine. 2. The use of autopsy findings and medical facts in trials for murder or deaths from suspicious causes. See medical jurisprudence.

foreplay (for′-plā): Sexual stimulation preceding and leading to sexual intercourse.

foreskin (for′-skin): The prepuce or skin covering the glans penis.

forewaters (for′-wat-erz): In pregnancy the chronic discharge of a watery fluid resembling amniotic fluid from the vagina, with no indication of rupture of the membranes. Hydrorrhea gravidarum.

formaldehyde (fó-mal′-de-hīd): A colorless, pungent, irritating gas that has disinfectant and germicidal properties. Used in the gas form and also in solution. See formalin.

formalin (for′-ma-lin): Approximately a 40 percent solution of formaldehyde. Used mainly for room disinfection and for fixing and preserving pathological specimens.

formic acid (for′-mik as′-id): An organic acid found naturally in ants and other insects as well as in some plants, *e.g.*, nettles.

formicant (for′-mi-kant): Producing a sensation resembling that of ants crawling on the skin. **F. PULSE**, a feeble small pulse resembling the movements of ants.

formication (for-mi-kā′-shun): The hallucination or illusion that insects, particularly ants, are running over the body or under the skin. Occurs in persons with nerve lesions, particularly in the regenerative phase.

formiciasis (for-mis-ī′-a-sis): The condition of having been bitten by ants.

formula (for′-mū-la): 1. A prescription. 2. Recipe for an infant's artificial feeding, or the feeding itself. 3. A simplified statement of a general fact or rule expressed in figures, symbols, or simple language. 4. A rule or method of doing something, especially something done regularly and automatically. 5. An expression of the composition of a compound by symbols and figures that show the proportions of the various constituents.

formulary (for′-mū-lar-i): A collection of formulas, recipes, prescriptions. **NATIONAL F.**, a book issued periodically by the American Pharmaceutical Association, containing standards for pharmaceuticals that are not included in the U.S. Pharmacopeia.

fornicate (for′-ni-kāt): To have sexual intercourse with a person to whom one is not married.—fornication, n.

fornix (for′-niks): An arch-shaped structure or space, often referring to the space between the vaginal wall and the cervix of the uterus. **CONJUNCTIVAL F.**, the line of reflection of the conjunctiva from the eyelids into the eyeball.—fornices, pl.

fortified (for′-ti-fīd): In nutrition, refers to the addition of substances intended to make food more nutritious.

fossa (fos′a): In anatomy, a depression, hollow, pit, or furrow. **ANTECUBITAL F.**, the hollow at the front of the elbow; also called cubital **F. CORONOID F.**, the hollow at the distal end of the humerus; it accommodates the coronoid process of the ulna in flexion. **HYPOPHYSEAL F.**, a deep depression in the middle of the sella turcica; it contains the pituitary gland. **ILIAC F.**, the large smooth concave area occupying most of the inner surface of the wing of the ilium. **INTERCONDYLAR F.**, lies between the medial and lateral condyles of the lower end of the femur. **OLECRANON F.**, a depression on the posterior surface of the humerus into which the olecranon of the ulna fits when the arm is extended. **F. OVALIS CORDIS**, a depression on the right side of the interatrial septum of the heart; it represents the remains of the fetal foramen ovale. **POPLITEAL F.**, the space at the back of the knee; contains blood vessels and nerves. **SUPRACLAVICULAR F.**, a depression on the surface of the body just above and behind the clavicle and lateral to the tendon of the sternocleidomastoid muscle.—fossae, pl.

fossette (fos-set′): 1. A small deep ulcer of the cornea. 2. A small depression.

"fossy" jaw: See phosphonecrosis.

Foster frame: A turning frame similar to the Stryker frame (*q.v.*); used particularly in the care of patients with spine or spinal cord injury and those who have had Harrington rod instrumentation; consists of two stretcher-like parts that hold the patient horizontally between them and allow for turning without injury to the spine.

Foster Grandparents Program: A program sponsored by the federal Administration on Aging; recruits and trains older people to care for needy institutionalized children. Workers are reimbursed for out-of-pocket expenses, are paid a minimum wage, and usually work 4 hours 5 days a week.

Fothergill's operation: An operation to correct prolapse of the uterus by fixation of the uterine ligaments. [William Fothergill, English gynecologist. 1865-1926.]

foulage (foo-lazh′): A movement in massage consisting of kneading and pressing the muscles; also called petrissage.

fourchette (foor-shet′): A membranous fold connecting the posterior ends of the labia minora.

Fournier's disease: Gangrene of the genitalia, the scrotum in particular.

four-point gait: See under crutchwalking.

fovea (fō′-vē-a): A small depression or fossa, particularly the fovea centralis retinae in the macula lutea of the retina, the site of most distinct vision.

foveate (fō′-vē-āt): Pitted; having depressions on the surface.

foveation (fō-vē-ā′shun): The formation of pitted scars, as may occur in smallpox or chickenpox.

foveola (fō-vē′ō-la): A very small depression or pit.

Fowler's position: The position in which the patient's head or the head of the bed is raised 18-20 inches above the level. The knees are flexed and supported by a pillow. Aids abdominal and pelvic drainage and useful in aiding breathing in respiratory disorders. Also called semisitting position.

foxglove (foks′-glov): See digitalis.

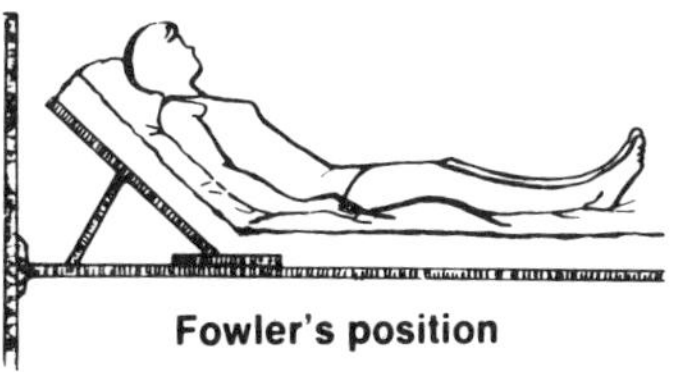

Fowler's position

Fr: 1. Abbreviation for French scale. 2. Chemical symbol for francium.

frac dos: Fractional or divided doses. Also fract. dos.

fractional sterilization: Sterilizing material by submitting it to temperatures of 100°C on three or four successive days to kill the spores that may develop in the periods between heatings. Also called intermittent sterilization.

fractional test meal: A method of examining the gastric contents by withdrawing samples at intervals after a standard meal, and subsequently submitting them to chemical analysis.

fractionation (frak-shun-ā′shun): 1. In chemistry, the separation of a substance into its component parts. 2. In radiation, the division of a total dosage of radiation into smaller doses given at preset intervals.

fracture (frak′cher): A break in the continuity of a bone, epiphyseal plate, or joint surface. AVULSION F., results from forceful contraction of a muscle, which causes a fragment of bone to be torn loose at the tendinous insertion of the muscle. BARTON'S F., dorsal dislocation of the carpus on the radium, with fracture of the dorsal articular surface of the radius. BASOCERVICAL F., F. at the base of the femoral neck. BENNETT'S F., F. of the first metacarpal, often the result of a fall or a fight. BLOWOUT F., F. of the floor of the bony orbit of the eye, caused by direct blunt trauma to the eyeball, which causes increase in intraorbital pressure. BOXER'S F., impacted F. of the necks of the fourth and fifth metacarpals, caused by striking the knuckles on a hard object. BURSTING F., a F. with many fragments occuring most often in the first cervical vertebra. BUTTERFLY F., a F. in which wedge-shaped segments split off laterally so that the fracture looks like a butterfly with outspread wings. CHAUFFEUR'S F., F. of the distal radial styloid, caused by twisting or snapping type of injury; these were formerly caused by cranking a car. CHIP F., a F. in which a chip of bone is separated from a bony process. CLOSED F., a F. with no break in the skin. COLLES F., F. of the lower end of the radius giving a typical dinner-fork deformity. COMMINUTED. F., one which has multiple fracture lines. COMPLETE F., the bone is broken completely. COMPLICATED F., in addition to the F. there is injury to the surrounding organs and/or structures. COMPRESSION F., usually occurs in the lumbar region, due to hyperflexion of the spine; the anterior vertebral bodies are crushed together. COMPOUND F., the skin is broken, allowing communication of the broken ends of bone with the atmosphere; also called OPEN F. COTTON'S F., F. of the ankle involving the medial, lateral, and posterior malleoli. DEPRESSED F., the fragmented bone presses on and may penetrate an underlying structure, as the lung; usually refers to skull or rib F.

DISPLACED F., the bone fragments are no longer in anatomical alignment. **DOUBLE F.**, segmented **F.** of a bone in two places. **EPIPHYSEAL F.**, a **F.** that involves the cartilaginous growth plate of a bone. **FATIGUE F.**, a stress **F.** resulting from strenuous physical activity over a short period of time. **FISSURE F.**, a crack in the surface of a long bone. **GALLEAZZI'S F.**, **F.** in the lower part of the shaft of the radius, with dislocation of the distal end of the ulna. **GOSSELIN'S F.**, a V-shaped **F.** of the distal end of the tibia. **GREENSTICK F.**, an incomplete **F.**, occurring in children; also called hickory-stick or willow-stick **F.**; the periosteum on one side of the bone remains intact. **IMPACTED F.**, one end of the bone is driven into the other. **INCOMPLETE F.**, the bone is only cracked and fissured. **INTERTROCHANTERIC F.**, a **F.** between the greater and lesser trochanters of the femur. **LEFORT'S F.**, bilateral horizontal **F.** of the maxilla; classified as Type I, II, or III according to the location and extent of the **F.** and what other facial bones are involved. **LINEAR F.**, a lengthwise **F.**, usually of a long bone; it implies no displacement. **MARCH F.**, **F.** in the shaft of the second or third metatarsal; caused by excessive marching. **MULTIPLE F.**, two or more lines of fracture in the same bone. **MONTEGGIA F.**, **F.** in the upper shaft of the ulna with dislocation of the head of the radius. **NIGHT-STICK F.**, an undisplaced **F.** of the shaft of the ulna caused by a direct blow. **OBLIQUE F.**, a **SLANTED F.**, of the shaft of a long bone. **OCCULT F.**, one that is not detected by x ray; hidden. **PARATROOPER'S F.**, **F.** of the malleolus and/or the margin of the posterior tibia. **PATHOLOGIC F.**, one caused by osteoporosis or other local disease of the bone. **POTT'S F.**, **F.** of the distal end of the fibula and the tibial malleolus, often accompanied by dislocation of the tarsal bones and injury to ligaments with lateral displacement of the foot. **SECONDARY F.**, occurs in a bone weakened by disease. **SIMPLE F.**, closed **F.**, not compound, with the ends of the bone in proper alignment. **SMITH'S F.**, **F.** of the lower end of the radius near the joint, with displacement of the lower fragment. **SPIRAL F.**, one in which the fracture line is spiral in shape; also called **TORTION F.** when it is caused by a twisting force. **SPONTANEOUS F.**, one occurring without force. **SPRINTER'S. F.**, **F.** of the antero-inferior spine of the ilium, with a fragment of the bone being pulled by muscular violence as at the start of a sprint. **STABLE F.**, one that can be reduced and can be maintained with a cast or splint. **STELLATE F.**, a **F.** with a central point of injury from which several fracture lines radiate. **STIEDA'S F.**, **F.** of the internal condyle of the femur. **STRESS F.**, caused by repeated or prolonged stress on a bone. **T-F.**, intercondylar **F.**, shaped like a T. **TEARDROP F.**, a **F.** of the anterior lip of the body of a cervical vertebra; shaped like a teardrop. **TRANSVERSE F.**, the line of fracture goes across a long bone at right angles to

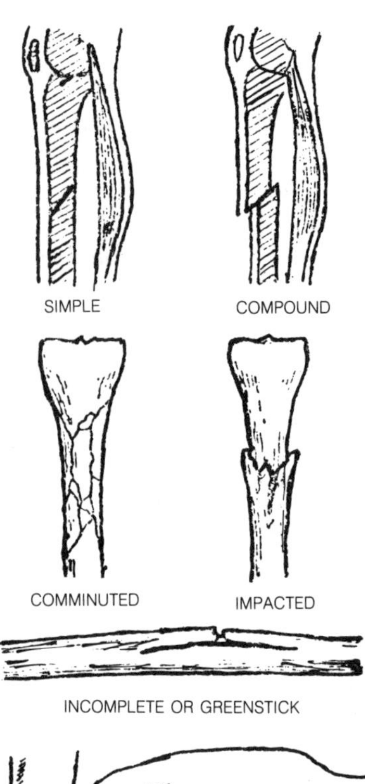

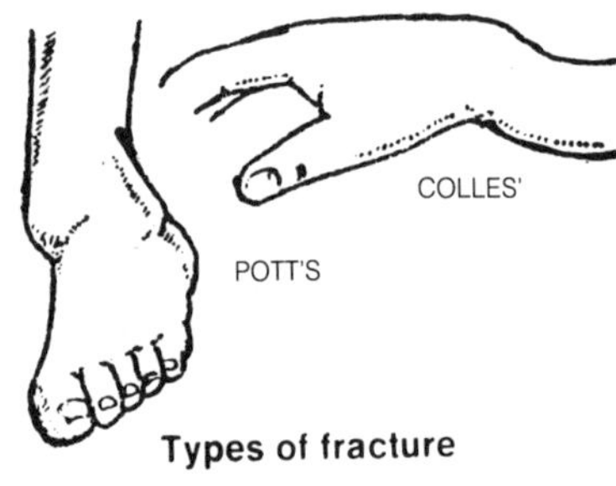

Types of fracture

its length. **UNSTABLE F.**, a **F.** that cannot be held in reduction by splinting or traction without internal fixation. **UNUNITED F.**, failure to form a bridge of callus at the ends of a fractured bone; the ends become fragmented and a false joint results. **Y-F.**, an intercondylar **F.** shaped like a Y. **WEDGE F.**, a compression **F.** of a vertebra. **WILLOW F.**, **GREENSTICK F. WILSON'S F.**, an interarticular **F.** on the palmer side of an interphalangeal joint.

fracture-dislocation: Fracture of a bone accompanied by dislocation of the bone from its normal position in a joint.

fragilitas (fra-jil′-i-tas): Brittleness. **F. CRINIUM,**

brittleness of the hair. **F. OSSIUM,** congenital disease characterized by abnormal fragility of bone, multiple fractures and a china-blue discoloration of the sclera. **F. SANGUINIS,** fragility of the red blood cells. **F. UNGUIUM,** abnormal brittleness of the nails.

fragility (fra-jil′-i-ti): Brittleness; the tendency to break down or disintegrate. **F. OF THE BLOOD** refers to the increased tendency of the red blood cells to break down under certain conditions.

fragmentation (frag-men-tā′shun): The division or breaking into small pieces or parts.

frambesia (fram-bē′zi-a): Yaws (*q.v.*)

frambesioma (fram-bē-zē-ō′-ma): The large protruding nodule that is the primary lesion in yaws; called the mother yaw.

frame: See Balkan, Bradford, Foster, Stryker.

Framingham Study: A long-term project, begun in the 1950s, which initially included half of the middle-aged people in Framingham, Massachusetts, to examine the epidemiology of cardiovascular disease. It is the longest-running and most comprehensive project of its kind in medical history and was the first American study to demonstrate that antihypertensive drug therapy could reduce high blood pressure. It has revealed the roles that cholesterol, high blood pressure, cigarette smoking, obesity, lack of exercise, stress, EKG abnormalities, and other factors play in cardiovascular disease and has shown that heart disease is not an inevitable consequence of age but rather is largely the result of how people live.

Franceschetti syndrome: Mandibulofacial dystosis (*q.v.*).

Francisella: A genus of nutritionally fastidious gram-negative rods; belongs to the family *Brucellacaea*. *F. tularensis*, the causative organism of tularemia in wild animals; may be transmitted to man by contaminated water, by blood-sucking insects, or through handling infected animals; also called *Pasteurella tularensis*. See tularemia.

francium (fran′-si-um): A radioactive element. Formerly called virginium.

frank: Obvious; unmistakable; evident.

Frank-Starling principle: Based on the observation that muscle tension is increased when its resting length is increased, and that, in the heart, the tension created by contraction of the cardiac muscle in systole is reflected in the end-diastolic volume by increased stroke output or work.

fraternal twins: Twins that have developed from the fertilization of two ova; may or may not be of the same sex or identical in appearance. Dizygotic twins.

FRC: Abbreviation for functional residual capacity; the sum of the reserve volume and the expiratory reserve volume.

freakout (frēk′-owt): Term used by drug abusers to describe loss of mental control leading to panic following the use of certain drugs.

freckle (frek′l): A small brownish spot on the skin, often due to exposure to sunlight. **MELANOTIC F.,** a macule that develops on the skin of older people; of uneven brownish pigmentation. In some cases the focus of malignant melanoma. Also called Hutchinson's freckle.

Fredet-Ramstedt operation: Surgical correction of congenital stenosis of the pylorus. Pyloromyotomy. Also called Ramstedt's operation.

free association: In psychoanalysis, the verbalization of any thoughts or feelings that come to mind without selection or repression of any kind.

Free-standing ambulatory surgical center: A health care facility existing independently of a hospital, where surgical services are provided for ambulatory patients.

freezing: 1. Frostbite. 2. The use of freezing temperatures to produce temporary anesthesia, *e.g.*, spraying the skin with liquid carbon dioxide snow or the use of ice bags. When used for therapeutic purposes, it is called cryotherapy.

Freiberg's disease: Osteochondritis of the second metatarsal head. [Albert Henry Freiberg, American orthopedic surgeon. 1868–1940.]

Frei's disease: Lymphogranuloma venereum; see under lymphogranuloma.

Frejka splint (frā′-ka): Used to correct congenitally dislocated hips. Consists of a pillow stuffed with kapok and held in position between the baby's legs by a special garment, with straps that are placed over the baby's shoulders and pinned securely; It is applied over the regular diaper. The baby's legs are maintained in a position of abduction and flexion, and with the head of the femur articulating with the acetabulum. Also called Frejka's pillow splint.

fremitus (frem′-i-tus): A vibration that can be felt by resting the fingers on the chest or certain other parts of the body. It is diminished in some respiratory diseases and increased in certain other pathological conditions such as tumor or consolidation. **TACTILE F.,** vibration that can be felt by palpation on the chest wall over the trachea and bronchi; produced by the spoken voice. **VOCAL F.,** vibration of vocal sounds heard on auscultation of the chest; is decreased in emphysema, pulmonary edema and other pathologic conditions marked by pleural effusion.

frenal (frē′-nal): Pertaining to any frenum.

French chalk: Talc (*q.v.*).

French scale: Scale used in sizing catheters

and certain other tubular instruments. It is a measure of the outside diameter, each unit being roughly equivalent to 0.33 millimeters; can be converted by dividing by 3. French sized catheters 16 to 18 are commonly used for adults.

frenectomy (fre-nek′-to-mi): The excision of a frenum.

frenetic (fre-net′-ik): Wild. excited, frantic, frenzied.—frenetically, adv.

Frenkel's exercises: Exercises for persons with tabes dorsalis, to teach muscle and joint sense in order to restore lost coordination. [Heinrich Frenkel, Swiss neurologist. 1860-1931.]

frenotomy (fre-not′-o-mi): Surgical severance of a frenum, particularly for tongue-tie.

frenulum (fren′-ū-lum): A small frenum (*q.v.*). F. CLITORIDIS, a F. formed by the union of the folds of the labia minora on the under surface of the glans clitoris. F. LINGUAE, the vertical fold of mucous membrane under the tongue. F. PREPUTII PENIS, the fold of tissue on the under side of the penis that connects with the prepuce.

frenum (frē′-num): A small fold of mucous membrane from a more or less fixed part extending to two movable parts which checks or limits their movement. See frenulum.

frenzy (fren′-zē): Violent, abnormal, compulsive excitement or agitation.

frequency: 1. The rate of regular recurrences in a given time, *e.g.*, the heartbeat. 2. In electricity, the number of alternations per second in an alternating current. 3. In vital statistics, the number of occurrences of a recognized disease entity per unit of time in a specific population. 4. The number of vibrations per minute made by a sound wave; expressed in cycles per second (cps) or Herz. 5. The felt need to urinate more often than normally.

Freud (froyd): The originator of psychoanalysis and the psychoanalytical theory of the causation of neuroses. He first described the existence of the unconscious mind, censor, repression, and the theory of infantile sexuality, and worked out in detail many mental mechanisms of the unconscious which modify normal and account for abnormal human behavior. [Sigmund Freud, Austrian psychiatrist. 1856–1939.]

freudian (froyd′-ē-an): Pertaining to Freud (*q.v.*) or his doctrines.

friable (frī′-a-b'l): Easily crumbled; readily pulverized.—friability, n.

fricatives (frik′-a-tivs): Sounds produced when breath is forced through a constricted passageway, as are the sounds of *f, v, z, ch, t*.

friction (frik′-shun): Rubbing. F. MURMUR, heard through the stethoscope when two rough or dry surfaces rub together, as occurs in pleurisy and percarditis. F. BURN, a wound caused by strenuous rubbing or friction; also called brush burn. PERICARDIAL F. RUB, see under rub. PLEURAL F. RUB, see under rub.

Friedländer's bacillus: *Klebsiella pneumoniae;* see under Klebsiella.

Friedreich's ataxia: A rare progressive familial disease with symptoms beginning in childhood, in which there develops a sclerosis of the sensory and motor columns in the spinal cord, with consequent muscular weakness and staggering (ataxia), impairment of speech and lateral curvature of the spine. Also called hereditary cerebellar ataxia. [Nikolas Friedreich, German neurologist. 1825–1882.]

Friedreich's disease: Myoclonus multiplex; see under myoclonus.

Fried's rule: A rule for calculating dosages of drugs for infants; age of the infant in months multiplied by the average dose, divided by 150.

$$\frac{\text{age in months} \times \text{adult dose}}{150} = \text{infant dose}$$

frigid (frij′-id): 1. Lacking desire for sexual intercourse. 2. Unable to achieve orgasm during sexual intercourse. 3. Temperamentally unresponsive.

frigidity (fri-jid′-i-ti): Lack of normal sexual desire or response; usually refers to the female; often a symptom of psychoneurotic disorder.

frigolabile (frig′-ō-lā′-bīl): Having the tendency to be destroyed by low temperatures; said of microorganisms.

frigostable (frig′-ō-stā′-b'l): Resistant to destruction by low temperatures.

frigotherapy (frig′-ō-ther′-a- pi): The use of low temperatures or of cold in the treatment of disease; cryotherapy.

frog: F. BREATHING, a type of breathing taught to patients with respiratory difficulty to help free them from dependence on mechanical breathing aids such as the respirator. Air is forced down the throat by the tongue. F. PLASTER, conservative treatment of a congenital dislocation of the hip, whereby the dislocation is reduced by gentle manipulation and both hips are immobilized in plaster of Paris, both limbs abducted to 80 degrees. F. POSITION, see under position.

Fröhlich's syndrome: A group of symptoms caused by damage to the pituitary gland and hypothalamus, including adiposity, sexual infantilism, excessive somnolence and, occasionally, diabetes insipidus. Also called dystrophia adiposogenitalis. [Alfred Fröhlich, Viennese neurologist. 1871-1953.]

Froin's syndrome: A condition in which the cerebrospinal fluid below a lesion shows xanthochromia, hyperglobulinemia, and spontaneous clotting, and very few, if any, cells.

frolement (frōl-mon'): 1. A rustling sound heard on auscultation in pericardial disease. 2. A massage maneuver consisting of very light friction with the hands.

frontad (fron'-tad): Toward the front.

frontal (fron'-tal) 1. Pertaining to the front or anterior part of an organ or of the body. 2. The bone of the forehead. **F.SINUS,** a cavity at the inner aspect of each orbital ridge on the **F.** bone. **F. SUTURE,** the line of union between the two halves of the frontal bone.

frontal lobe syndrome: A syndrome occurring after lobotomy or injury to the frontal area of the brain; symptoms include behavioral changes, lessened self-control, emotional dullness, lack of energy, mental deterioration with loss of ability to concentrate, impulsiveness, and aggression.

Frontier Nursing Service: Founded in 1923. Purpose: to provide health care to people in approximately 1000 square miles of eastern Kentucky through a home health agency, rural clinics, a 40-bed hospital, a primary care center, and the Frontier School of Mid-wifery and Family Services. Address, Hyden, KY 41749.

frontoparietal (fron'-tō-pa-rī'-e-tal): Pertaining to the frontal and parietal bones.

frontotemporal (fron'-tō-tem'-pō- ral): Pertaining to the frontal and temporal bones.

frost: A deposit resembling frozen vapor. **UREA F.**, the deposit of salt crystals on the skin following the evaporation of sweat in urhydrosis (*q.v.*). Also called uremic frost.

frostbite (frost'-bīt): Freezing of the skin and superficial tissues resulting from exposure to extreme cold. The fingers, toe, nose and ears are most frequently affected. The lesion is similar to a burn and may become blistered, with deep-seated destruction of tissue and possible development of gangrene.

frottage (frō-tahzh'): 1. A rubbing movement in massage. 2. Obtaining sexual satisfaction by rubbing or pressing against another person; may occur in crowded situations.

frotteur (frō-tūr'): One who obtains sexual pleasure from frottage (*q.v.*).

frozen: **F. SECTION,** section cut from frozen tissue for histologic examination, *e.g.*, that removed from the body during surgery and examined immediately for possible malignancy. **F. SHOULDER,** disability of the shoulder joint in which there is limited abduction and rotation of the arm; results from a fibrositis (*q.v.*) of unknown origin; initial pain is followed by stiffness which lasts several months; as the pain subsides exercises are intensified until full recovery is gained.

fructose (fruk'-tōs): A monosaccharide found with glucose in plants. It is the sugar in honey and is a constituent of cane sugar. Syn., levulose.

fructose-6-phosphate: An intermediate product in the metabolism of fructose.

fructosuria (fruk'-tō-sū'-ri-a): The presence of frucrose in the urine; due to a metabolic disorder.

frustration (frus-trā'- shun): The condition of emotional tension resulting when forces outside oneself block or thwart the performance of acts which, if carried out, would result in satisfaction or gratification of specific needs or desires.

FSH: Abbreviation for follicle-stimulating hormone.

FTA-ABS test: Abbreviation for fluorescent treponemal antibody absorbtion test. See under fluorescent.

FTT: Abbreviation for failure to thrive.

fuchsin (fook'-sin): A dark red dye which has antifungal properties; also used as a component of a staining fluid.

Fuch's dystrophy: See under dystrophy.

-fugal: Combining form denoting 1) passing from, driving away; 2) relieving or dispelling.

fugitive (fū'-ji-tiv): Wandering; transient. Descriptive of certain inconstant symptoms.

fugue (fūg): An attempt to escape from reality. A period of loss of memory as to identity but with retention of habits, skills, and mental faculties; sometimes involving flight from familiar surroundings. During the fugue, the patient may appear to act in a purposeful manner, but after recovery he has no memory of what occurred during the state although earlier events are remembered. Occurs in schizophrenia, hysteria; sometimes after an epileptic seizure.

fulgurant (ful'-gū-rant): Suddenly severe and agonizing. A darting, momentary pain.

fulgurate (ful'-gū-rāt): 1. To come and go quickly, like a flash of lightning. 2. To destroy tissue by electricity.—fulguration, n, fulgurize, v.

fulguration (ful-gū-rā'shun): The destruction of tissue by means of a high-frequency electric current applied with a metal point. See electrodessication.—fulgurate, fulgurize, v.

full term: Mature—when pregnancy has lasted 40 weeks.

fulminating (ful'-mi-nā-ting): Developing quickly with great severity, characterized by a severe course and an abrupt termination. Also called fulminant.—fulminate, v.

fumes: Vapors, particularly those that are irritating.

fumigant (fū'-mi-gant): A substance which emits fumes for fumigation (*q.v.*).

fumigation (fū-mi-gā'-shun): Disinfection by exposure to the fumes of a vaporized disinfectant. Now used primarily for destroying insects and rodents.

fuming (fū′-ming): Smoking; emitting a visible vapor, usually unpleasant.

function: 1. The special work performed by an organ or structure in its normal state. 2. To perform a special work or action.

functional: 1. Pertaining to function. 2. Describing a disorder of the function but not the structure of an organ or system. 3. In psychiatry, a disorder of neurotic origin, *i.e.*, psychogenic, without primary organic disease. **F. ASSESSMENT,** an assessment of a person's ability to function physically, mentally, emotionally, and socially, within his or her environment, and to carry out the activities of self-maintenance. **F. DISEASE,** a disorder in which the function of an organ or part is disturbed but there is no evidence of structural disease. **F. RESIDUAL CAPACITY,** the volume of air in the lungs at rest, that is, the amount remaining in the lungs at the end of a normal quiet respiration; it equals the sum of respiratory reserve volume and residual volume. Abbreviated FRC.

functionalism (funk′-shun-a-lizm): The branch of psychology that deals with the function of mental processes, particularly the role played by the intellect, emotions, and behavior of a person in his adaptation to his environment.

fundal (fun′dal): Pertaining to a fundus.

Fundamentals of Nursing: Refers to a course of instruction given early in the nursing course. It provides an introduction to the principles and practice of nursing through an understanding of the basic needs of patients and of nurses' responses to these needs, as well as practice in developing the skills required for carrying out the various nursing procedures and activities.

fundectomy (fun-dek′-tō-mi): The surgical removal of the fundus of an organ, *e.g.*, the fundus of the stomach or the uterus. Also fundusectomy.

fundoplication (fun′dō-pli-kā′shun): Plication (folding) of the fundus of the stomach around the esophagus; usually done to relieve gastrointestinal reflux.

fundus (fun′-dus): The basal portion of a hollow structure; the part that is farthest from the opening. **F. OF THE EYE,** the inside of the back part of the eye seen by looking through the pupil. **F. OF THE UTERUS,** that part which is above the points of insertion of the fallopian tubes.—fundal, adj.; fundi, pl.

funduscope (fun′-dus-scōp): An instrument for examining the fundus of the eye; an ophthalmoscope.

funduscopy (fun-dus′-kō-pi): The examination of the interior of the eyeball with an ophthalmoscope.

fundusectomy (fun-dū-sek′-to-mi): Excision of the fundus of an organ, most often that of the stomach.

fungal (fung′-gal): Relating to or caused by a fungus; fungous.

fungate (fung′-gāt): 1. To grow rapidly or to granulate rapidly. 2. To assume a fungus-like form. 3. To produce fungus-like growths.

fungemia (fun-jē′-mi-a): 1. The presence of fungi in the circulating blood. 2. A fungal infection that is carried by the bloodstream.

fungicide (fun′-ji-sīd): An agent that is lethal to fungi.—fungicidal, adj.

fungiform (fun′-ji-form): Resembling a mushroom in shape.

fungistasis (fun-ji-stā′-sis): The inhibition or prevention of the growth of fungi.

fungistat (fun′ji-stat): An agent that inhibits the growth of fungi. Also fungistatic.

fungoid (fung′-goid): Resembling a fungus; usually referring to a heavy growth on the surface of the body.

fungous (fung′-gus): Having the characteristics of a fungus.

fungus (fung′-gus): A low form of vegetable life including mushrooms, toadstools, molds, and many microscopic organisms that live on organic matter; a few are capable of producing disease in man.—fungi, pl.; fungoid, fungous, adj. See also actinomycosis, ringworm, tinea pedis.

funic (fū′-nic): Pertaining to the umbilical cord. **F. SOUFFLE,** the purring sound heard over the pregnant uterus; it has the same frequency as the fetal heart beat.

funicle (fū′-ni-k'l): Funiculus (*q.v.*).

funicular (fū-nik′-ū-lar): Pertaining to the spermatic or to the umbilical cord. **F. PROCESS,** the part of the tunica vaginalis that covers the spermatic cord.

funiculitis (fū-nik′-ū-lī′tis): Inflammation of a funiculus, the spermatic cord in particular.

funiculus (fū-nik′ū-lus): A cord-like structure. **F. UMBILICALIS,** the umbilical cord.

funiform (fū′-ni-form): Resembling a cord or rope; rope-like.

funis (fū′-nis): A cord; the umbilical cord in particular.

funnel breast: A congenital deformity in which the breastbone is depressed toward the spine (pectus excavatum). May also be seen in patients with rickets. Also called funnel chest.

funny bone: Lay term for a place at the back of the elbow that responds with a tingling sensation when struck; it is the place where the ulnar nerve passes over the medial condyle of the humerus.

FUO: Abbreviation for fever of unknown or undetermined origin.

furcal (fur′-kal): Forked.

furfur (fūr′-fur): 1. A scaly desquamation. 2. Dandruff.

furfuraceous (fūr-fū-rā′-shus): 1. Resembling dandruff. 2. Composed of small desquamated scales.

furor (fū′-ror): Fury; madness; rage. Violent angry outbursts.

furrow: In anatomy, a groove or crease.

furuncle (fū′-rung-k'l): An acute, painful, circumscribed inflammatory lesion of the skin and subcutaneous tissue, usually caused by infection of a hair follicle with the *Staphylococcus aureus;* suppuration occurs with the formation of a central core that is eventually discharged. It has but one opening for drainage in contrast to a carbuncle (*q.v.*). A boil.

furunculosis (fū-rung′-kū-lō′-sis): The condition of being afflicted with furuncles.

furunculous (fū-rung′-kū-lus): Resembling a furuncle, or boil.

furunculus orientalis (fū-rung′-kū-lus- o-ri-en-tā′-lis): Oriental sore (*q.v.*).

fusiform (fū′-zi-form): Resembling a spindle; round in the middle and tapering at both ends. **F. BACILLI**, found in the mouth, gums, and fauces in cases of Vincent's angina (*q.v.*).

fusion (fū′-zhun): In surgery, the introduction of bony ankylosis in joints when it is desirable to immobilize them. **BINOCULAR F.**, the fusion of two separate images of an object into one clear image, as occurs in binocular vision. **SPINAL F.**, the surgical procedure of joining two or more of the vertebrae by bone grafts to immobilize part of the spinal column; used in cases of arthritis, severe trauma, herniated disk, or tuberculosis of the spine.

Fusobacterium fusiforme (fū-zō-bak-tēr′-i-um fū-zi-fōr′-mē): A genus of anaerobic gram-negative bacteria found in the normal mouth, intestine, and genitalia, and in necrotic lesions. Also the causative organism in Vincent's angina.

fusospirillosis (fū′-zō-spī′-ri- lō′-sis): Vincent's angina (*q.v.*).

fusospirochetosis (fū-zō-spī′-rō-kē-tō′-sis): Infection with both fusiform and spirochetal organisms, which occurs in Vincent's angina, lung abscesses, vulvovaginitis (*q.v.*), and balanitis (*q.v.*).—fusospirochetal, adj.

fusostreptococcicosis (fū-zō-strep′- tō-kok-si-kō′-sis): An infection caused by fusiform bacteria and streptococci.

FVC: Forced vital capacity; the maximum amount of air that can be expelled during a specific time after a deep inspiration.

Fx: Abbreviation for fracture.

G

G or g: Abbreviation for gram(s).

γ: Symbol for the Greek letter gamma (*q.v.*).

G suit: A pressure suit used by test pilots to prevent blacking out at high speeds of travel in aircraft. Has been used experimentally to control intra-abdominal bleeding in patients with aortic aneurysm or other types of abdominal trauma; it is applied below the diaphragm where it causes compression of the vascular beds, shunts blood to the structures above, and tends to squeeze shut a wound in the aorta or elsewhere in the large vessels. Also sometimes used in treatment of hypotension.

GA: Abbreviation for: 1. Gastric analysis. 2. General anesthesia.

Ga: Chemical symbol for gallium (*q.v.*).

GABA: Abbreviation for gamma aminobutyric acid (*q.v.*).

gadfly (gad′-flī): Any of the several bloodsucking flies of the genus *Tabanus,* including horseflies and deerflies; they deposit their eggs under the skin, causing swelling and the development of lesions resembling boils; they may also transmit certain diseases including anthrax.

Gaffkya (gaf′-ki-a): A genus of *Micrococcaceae.* **G. TETRAGENA,** a micrococcus found in mucous membranes of the respiratory tract in man, occasionally pathogenic. [Georg Gaffky, German bacteriologist. 1850–1918.]

gag: 1. A device that is placed between the teeth to keep the mouth open. 2. To prevent one from speaking. 3. To retch or attempt to vomit. **GAG REFLEX,** the contraction of the constrictor muscle of the pharynx when the back of the pharynx or the soft palate is touched; also called pharyngeal reflex.

gait: A manner of walking. **ATAXIC G., G.** in which the foot is raised high, then brought down suddenly. **CEREBELLAR G.,** reeling, staggering, lurching **G. CRUTCHWALKING G.,** see under crutchwalking. **FESTINATING G.,** seen in patients with paralysis agitans and other nervous disorders; the person takes short, increasingly rapid steps, often on tiptoe. **PARKINSONIAN G.,** seen in parkinsonian patients; the body is held rigid with the head bent forward while the person takes short, mincing steps interrupted by sudden uncontrolled propulsive movements. **SCISSOR G., G.** in which the legs cross each other in progression. **SLAPPING G.,** a **G.** in which the feet are wide apart, raised high and slapped down while the person's gaze is fixed on the floor to guide placement of the feet. **SPASTIC G.,** a stiff, shuffling **G.** with the legs held closely together. **STAGGERING G.,** a reeling, uncertain **G.** resembling that of an intoxicated person. **SWING-THROUGH G.,** a crutch-walking **G.**; the person advances his crutches and then swings the legs through to the same point. **TABETIC G.,** ataxic **G.** Tandem **G., G.** with one heel placed directly in front of the toes of the other foot in walking; used as a test of the person's ability to control motor activity. **TRENDELENBURG G.,** see under Trendelenburg.

galact-, galacto-: Combining forms denoting: 1. Milk. 2. Galactose.

galactacrasia (gal-ak′-ta-krā′-zi-a): An abnormality in the constituents of breast milk.

galactagogue (ga-lak′-ta-gog): 1. An agent that induces or increases the flow of milk. 2. Increasing the flow of milk. Also galactogogue.

galactic (ga-lak′-tik): 1. Pertaining to or resembling milk. 2. An agent that increases the flow of milk.

galactidrosis (ga-lak′-ti-drō′-sis): The excretion of sweat resembling milk.

galactin (ga-lak′-tin): An old term for prolactin (*q.v.*).

galactocele (ga-lak′-tō-sēl): 1. A cyst in the mammary gland containing milk; due to occlusion of a milk duct. 2. A hydrocele that contains a milky fluid.

galactography (gal-ak-tog′-ra-fi): Mammography depicting the ductal system of the breast.

galactoid (ga-lak′-toyd): Resembling milk.

galactokinase (ga-lak′-tō-kī′-nās): An enzyme that is involved in the metabolism of galactose.

galactophagous (gal′-ak-tof′-a-gus): Subsisting on a diet of milk.

galactophlebitis (ga-lak′-tō-flē-bī′-tis): Phlegmasia alba dolens ("milk leg"); see under phlegmasia.

galactophore (ga-lak′-tō-fōr): A milk duct.

galactophoritis (ga-lak′-tō-fō-rī′-tis): Inflammation of a milk duct.

galactophthisis (ga-lak-tof′ thi-sis): Old term for a condition of emaciation and general weakness thought to be caused by excessive flow of milk or prolonged nursing.

galactophygous (gal-ak-tof′-i-gus): Arresting or diminishing the flow of milk.

galactopoieses (ga-lak′-tō-poy-ē′-sis): The production and secretion of milk.—galactopoietic, adj.

galactopyra (ga-lak′-tō-pī′-ra): Milk fever.

galactorrhea (ga-lak-tō-rē′-a): 1. Excessive flow of milk. 2. Continued flow of milk after a child has been weaned. 3. Spontaneous, excessive flow of milk in the absence of a recent pregnancy.

galactoschesis (ga-lak-tos′-ke-sis): Suppression of the secretion of milk.

galactose (ga-lak′-tōs): A monosaccharide found with glucose in lactose or milk sugar; it is converted into glycogen in the liver.

galactose tolerance test: A test of the carbohydrate tolerance of the liver to determine whether the liver is functioning normally.

galactosemia (ga-lak′-tō-sē′-mi-a): 1. A congenital metabolic disorder, beginning in infancy, in which galactose is present in the blood causing a toxic effect that is particularly damaging to the liver and brain. Symptoms include vomiting, malnutrition, jaundice, poor weight gain. 2. The presence of galactose in the circulating blood.

galactosis (ga-lak-tō′-sis): The secretion of milk.

galactostasis (ga-lak-tos′-ta-sis): Lessening or cessation of milk secretion.

galactosuria (ga-lak′-tō-sū′-ri-a): The presence of galactose in the urine.

galactotherapy (ga-lak′-tō-ther′-a-pi): 1. Treatment by milk diet; refers particularly to breast feeding of the newborn. 2. Giving medicinal treatment to a nursing infant by giving the drug to the mother; part of the drug is excreted in the milk.

galacturia (ga-lak-tū′-ri-a): Passing of urine that has a milky appearance.

galea aponeurotica (gal′-ē-a a-pon-ū-rot′-i-ka): An aponeurosis of the scalp; connects the frontal and occipital parts of the occipitofrontalis muscle. Also called aponeurosis epicranialis.

galeanthropy (gal-ē-an′-thrō-pi): The mental delusion that one has become a cat.

galeophobia (gal-ē-ō-fō′-bi-a): Abnormal dislike or fear of cats.

galeropia (gal-er-ō′-pi-a): A visual condition characterized by unusual clearness of vision.

gall: Bile.

gallbladder (gawl′-blad-der): A pear-shaped bag on the right underside of the liver. Between meals it concentrates and stores bile; during digestion it releases the bile into the duodenum where it acts on fats. **G. SERIES,** x-ray examination of the gallbladder for diagnostic purposes.

gallipot (gal′-i-pot): A small pot for storing ointments or lotions.

gallium (gal′-i-um): A rare metallic chemical element; has been used in scanning to evaluate presence of active infection in the kidney, in localizing neoplasms, and in detecting perinephritic and psoas abscesses. **RADIOACTIVE G.,** an isotope of **G.,** used in treatment of neoplasms of bone.

gallon (gal′-un): Four quarts, liquid measure; in the metric system; 3.785 liters.

gallop: See under rhythm.

galloping consumption: An old colloquial term for rapidly fatal tuberculosis.

gallstone (gawl′-stōn): A stone or concretion consisting of crystalline cholesterol that forms within the gallbladder or bile ducts, often multiple and faceted. Cholelith.

Galton system: An identification system based on fingerprints; the imprints of the ten fingers are made in a definite order on a card.

galvanic (gal-van′-ik): Pertaining to a direct current of electricity, particularly that produced by a battery. **G. SKIN RESPONSE,** easily measured skin changes in response to various stimuli; used in many experimental studies.

galvanism (gal′-van-izm): Treatment by galvanic electric current. **DENTAL G.,** a phenomenon experienced when dissimilar metals have been used in dental fillings or to replace missing teeth; an electric current is created, causing sharp painful shocks to the involved teeth; may cause inflammation of the tooth pulp.

galvanocauterization (gal′-va-nō-kaw′-ter-ī-zā′-shun): The use of a wire heated by galvanic current to destroy tissue.

galvanocontractility (gal′-va-nō-kon-trak-til′-i-ti): The ability of a muscle to contract when stimulated by a direct current of electricity.

galvanogustometer (gal′-va-nō-gus-tom′-e-ter): A galvanic apparatus used in tests to determine the taste threshold for various substances.

galvanometer (gal-va-nom′-e-ter): An instrument for measuring the strength of an electric current.

galvanotherapy (gal′-va-nō-ther′-a-pi): Treatment by means of direct or galvanic current.

galvanotonus (gal′-va-not′-ō-nus): Tonic muscle contraction occurring in response to galvanic stimulation.

gam-, gamo-: Combining forms denoting relationship to marriage or sexual contact.

gamasoidosis (gam-a-soy-dō′-sis): Infestation with mites of the order *Acarina* (formerly called *Gamasidae*); also called Gambian sleeping sickness or Gambian trypanosomiasis. See trypanosomiasis.

gamete (gam′-ēt): 1. A mature male or female reproductive cell; see ovum, spermatozoon. 2. The sexual form of the malarial parasite during its existence in the stomach of the mosquito.

gametocide (ga-mē′-tō-sīd): An agent that destroys gametes, particularly those of malarial organisms.—gametocidal, adj.

gametocyte (ga-mē′-tō-sīt): An undifferentiated cell from which gametes are produced. Often refers to the sexual stage of the malarial parasite in blood, which may produce gametes after being taken in by the mosquito host.

gametogenesis (gam′-e-tō-jen′-e-sis): The formation and development of gametes.

Gamgee (gam′-jē): A surgical dressing of absorbent cotton enclosed in a fine gauze mesh.

gamma: The third letter in the Greek alphabet; sometimes used in scientific nomenclature to designate the third in a series. **G. RADIATION,** radiation from radioactive cobalt; has been used to replace x ray in treatment of malignancies; large doses are used to sterilize instruments and dressings. **G. RAYS,** electromagnetic radiation similar to x rays but with greater penetrating power.

gamma globulin (gam′-ma glob′-ū-lin): A broad general term for the chemically extracted fraction of human plasma, made up of proteins, that contains immunoglobulins having specific antibody activity against a variety of viruses, specifically the immunoglobulins A, D, E, G, and M. May be used in temporary protection against various infections including measles and hepatitis. **GAMMA-A GLOBULIN,** an immunoglobulin that comprises about 10 percent of the antibodies in human plasma; the chief immunoglobulin in tears, saliva, colostrum, and intestinal fluid.

gamma-aminobutyric acid (GABA) (gam′-ma-am′-i-nō-bū-tir′-ik): An amino acid found in brain tissue; found also in yeast, green plants, and certain bacteria. Considered a neurotransmitter and thought to be implicated in several psychiatric and neurologic conditions, chiefly Huntington's chorea.

gammacism (gam′-a-sizm): Inability to pronounce consonants correctly, *g* and *k* in particular.

gammaglobulinopathy (gam′-a-glob′-ū-lin-op′-a-thi): Any abnormality of the gamma globulins in the blood.

gamma-glutamyl transpeptidase (gam′-ma-glū-tam′-il trans-pep′-ti-dās): An enzyme found chiefly in the kidney, liver, and pancreas, but also in lesser amounts in the prostate, salivary glands, brain, and heart. Elevated levels are seen in liver damage; laboratory determinations are useful in diagnosis. Also of medicolegal significance in investigations of rape, because seminal fluid contains high concentrations of it. Abbreviated GGTP.

gammopathy (gam-mop′-a-thi): A disorder characterized by abnormally increased levels of gamma globulins in the blood; may be seen in myeloma, macroglobulinemia, Hodgkin's disease, and lymphatic leukemia. Also called gammaglobulinopathy and immunoglobulinopathy.

Gamna's disease: Slow progressive enlargement of the spleen; splenomegaly.

gamogenesis (gam-ō-jen′-e-sis): Sexual reproduction.

gampsodactyly (gamp-sō-dak′-til-i): Claw-foot; a claw-like deformity of the toes.

gangli-, ganglio-: Combining forms denoting ganglion.

ganglial (gang′-gli-al): Pertaining to a ganglion.

gangliectomy (gang-gli-ek′-to-mi): The excision of a ganglion. Also ganglionectomy.

ganglioblast (gang′-gli-ō-blast): An embryonic cell from which the cerebrospinal ganglia develop.

gangliocyte (gang′-gli-ō-sīt): A ganglion cell; a neuron in which the body of the cell lies outside of the brain and spinal cord.

gangliocytoma (gang′-gli-ō-sī-tō′-ma): A tumor made up of ganglion cells.

ganglioglioma (gang′-gli-ō-glī-ō′-ma): A central nervous system tumor containing nerve cells and many ganglion cells.

ganglioma (gang-li-ō′-ma): See ganglioneuroma.

ganglion (gang′-gli-on): 1. A semi-independent, organized mass of nerve cell bodies outside the brain and spinal cord, forming a subsidiary nerve center that receives and sends out nerve fibers, *e.g.*, the ganglionic masses forming the sympathetic nervous system. 2. A cystic tumor on a tendon or aponeurosis; sometimes on the back of the wrist due to strain, such as excessive piano practice. 3. An enlargement on the course of a nerve such as is found on the receptor nerves before they enter the spinal cord. 4. An enlarged lymphatic gland. **GASSERIAN G.,** is deeply situated within the skull, on the sensory root of the fifth cranial nerve. It is involved in trigeminal neuralgia.—ganglia, pl.; ganglionic, adj.

ganglionectomy (gang′-gli-ō-nek′-to-mi): Surgical excision of a ganglion; usually of a dorsal root ganglion, to control intractable pain; also called gangliectomy.

ganglioneuroblastoma (gang′-gli-ō-nū′-rō-blas-tō′-ma): A tumor composed of ganglioneuromatous and neuroblastomatous material; see neuroblastoma, ganglioneuroma.

ganglioneuroma (gang′-gli-ō-nū-rō′-ma): A firm encapsulated benign neoplasm made up of nerve fibers and ganglionic cells, often with foci of calcification.

ganglionic (gang-gli-on′-ik): Pertaining to a ganglion or of the nature of ganglia.

ganglionitis (gang′-gli-ō-nī′-tis): Inflammation of a ganglion.

ganglioside (gang′-glē-ō-sīd): General term for a number of galactose-containing cerebrosides (*q.v.*) found in the tissues of the central nervous system.

gangliosidosis (gang′-gli-ō-sī-dō′-sis): An inborn error of metabolism affecting lipid storage in the body, with the result that glycosides accumulate in the tissues of the nervous system. Characterized by poor physical development, skeletal deformities, enlargement of the liver, anorexia, progressive mental deterioration.

gangrene (gang′-grēn): Death of part of the tissues of the body. Usually the result of inadequate blood supply, but occasionally due to direct injury (traumatic **G.**) or infection (gas **G.**, for example). Deficient blood supply may result from pressure on blood vessels (*e.g.*, tourniquets, thigh bandages, or swelling of a limb); from obstruction within healthy vessels; from frostbite when the capillaries become blocked; from spasm of a vessel wall; or from thrombosis due to disease of the vessel. **ARTERIOSCLEROTIC G.**, dry **G.** of the extremities due to failure of the terminal circulation in patients with arteriosclerosis. **DIABETIC G.**, **G.** that occurs in the course of diabetes mellitus, usually as a result of a slight injury; may be of the dry or moist variety. **DRY G.**, occurs when circulation of the blood through the affected part is inadequate; usually starts in the toes; tissues become shrunken and black. **EMBOLIC G.**, follows the cutting off of blood supply by an embolism. **GAS G.**, results from the infection of a dirty lacerated wound by anaerobic organisms, usually *Clostridium welchii;* the gas that forms spreads through the muscles, so they give a crackling sound when touched; formerly a serious problem in wartime wounds. **MOIST G.**, a form of **G.** in which the necrosed tissue is soft and moist due to decomposition caused by putrefactive bacteria. **SENILE G.**, arteriosclerotic **G.**

gangrenous (gang′-gre-nus): Pertaining to or of the nature of gangrene.

Ganser's syndrome: A syndrome complex, usually of hysteric origin; characterized by inappropriate actions, hallucinations, absurd answers to questions, and disturbances of consciousness. Term often used to describe behaviors of prisoners who wish to mislead others in regard to their mental state. Also called fake insanity, hallucinatory mania, prison psychosis, depressive pseudodementia.

Gardnerella vaginitis: A vaginal infection, often caused by the *Gardnerella vaginale*; characterized by a thin, frothy, grayish discharge with a foul odor; usual treatment includes use of antibiotics and treatment of the sexual partner. Formerly called *Haemophilus* vaginitis.

Gardner's syndrome: Familial polyposus (*q.v.*) of the colon, which may become malignant, with the presence of supernumerary teeth, tumor formations in bone, sebaceous cysts, and deformities of the skull.

gargle: 1. The act of washing the throat by tipping back the head and holding liquid at the back of the throat while forcing expired air through it. 2. The liquid material used to gargle, usually medicated.

gargoylism (gar′-goyl-izm): Rare congenital mucopolysaccharide disorder of metabolism with recessive or sex-linked inheritance. Characterized by skeletal abnormalities, dwarfism, coarse features, heavy ugly facies, enlarged liver and spleen, mental subnormality. Also called lipochondrodystrophy, Hunter syndrome, Hurler syndrome, and Hunter-Hurler syndrome.

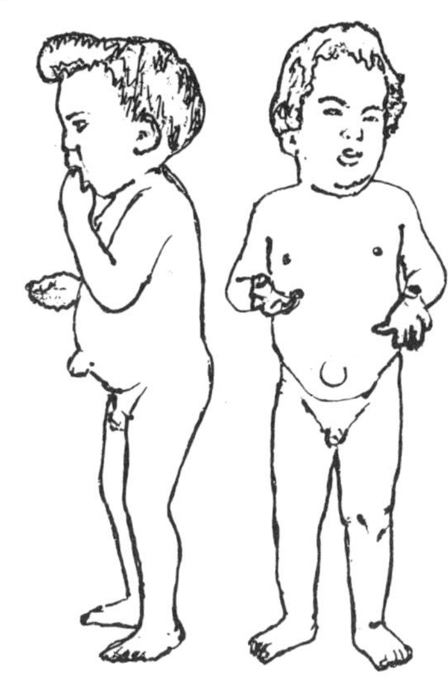

Gargoylism

Gärtner's bacillus: *Salmonella enteritidis*. A motile gram-negative rod bacterium, widely distributed in domestic and wild animals, particularly rodents, and sporadic in man as a cause of food poisoning. [August Gärtner, German bacteriologist. 1848–1934.]

gas: 1. One of the three states of matter. It retains neither shape nor volume when released but expands so that it is evenly distributed in whatever container or area it is released into. 2. Any gas that is utilized for lighting or heating an area. 3. In wartime, to release a poisonous gas into a specific area. 4. In criminology, to execute a person by administering a poisonous gas. **BLOOD GASES**, a term used to express the clinical determination of the partial pressures of oxygen and carbon dioxide exchange in the circulating blood. **G. EMBOLUS**, the presence of small bubbles of gas in the blood which occlude the smaller vessels; a disorder frequently affecting deep sea divers; aeroembolism. **G. GANGRENE**, see under **gangrene**. **LAUGHING G.**, nitrous oxide, a gas anesthetic which sometimes causes a patient to experience an amusing delirium before the anesthetic has become fully effective. **MARSH G.**, methane (*q.v.*). **METHANE G.**, a gas that develops in marshy places and mines; it results from the decay of organic matter; it is colorless, odorless and inflammable. **MUSTARD G.**, a poisonous gas developed for use in warfare. **G. POISONING**, see asphyxia and carbon monoxide. **TEAR G.**, a gas that irritates the mucous membranes, particularly the conjunctiva, causing a heavy flow of tears.

gas exchange impaired: Accepted as a nursing diagnosis by the Fourth National Conference on the Classification of Nursing Diagnoses.

gasp: 1. To catch one's breath audibly in response to shock or emotion. 2. To breathe with difficulty through the open mouth.

gasserectomy (gas-er-ek′-to-mi): Surgical excision of the gasserian ganglion (*q.v.*).

gasserian ganglion (gas-sē′-ri-an): A large flattened ganglion of the sensory root of the 5th cranial nerve (trigeminal); located in a cleft in the dura mater over the anterior part of the temporal bone; gives off the ophthalmic and maxillary nerves and part of the mandibular nerve.

gaster (gas′-ter): The stomach.

gastr-, gastri-, gastro-: Combining forms denoting: 1. The stomach. 2. The ventral area.

gastralgia (gas-tral′-ji-a): Pain in the stomach. Also gasteralgia.

gastrectasia (gas-trek-tā′-zi-a): Dilatation of the stomach.

gastrectomy (gas-trek′-to-mi): Removal of a part or the whole of the stomach. **PARTIAL G.**, the commonest operation carried out for peptic ulcer; also referred to as **SUBTOTAL G. TOTAL G.**, carried out only for cancer of the stomach.

gastric (gas′-tric): Pertaining to the stomach. **G. ANALYSIS**, analysis of gastric contents for diagnostic purposes; patient is given a meal and specimens are withdrawn at intervals during digestion in the stomach. **G. GAVAGE**, introduction of a feeding through a tube that is passed from the mouth into the stomach. **G. HORMONE**, see gastrin. **G. INFLUENZA**, a term used when gastrointestinal symptoms predominate. **G. JUICE**, juice secreted by the glands in the mucous lining of the stomach; the two main ingredients are pepsin and hydrochloric acid. **G. LAVAGE**, a washing out of the stomach. **G. SUCTION**, intermittent or continuous suction to keep the stomach empty after abdominal operations. **G. PARTITIONING**, the surgical creation of a smaller pouch and a smaller stoma; sometimes done in treatment of morbid obesity. **G. TUBE**, a rubber tube for introducing food into the stomach or for washing out the stomach. **G. ULCER**, see under ulcer.

gastricism (gas′-tri-sizm): Any gastric disorder.

gastrin (gas′-trin): A hormone secreted by the gastric mucosa on entry of food, which causes a further flow of gastric juice, and helps to stimulate the secretion of bile and pancreatic enzymes.

gastritis (gas-tri′-tis): Inflammation of the mucous membrane lining the stomach; may be acute or chronic. The acute form is usually due to viral or bacterial infection, ingestion of alcohol or certain drugs including aspirin; symptoms include nausea, vomiting, and gastric pain. The chronic form usually indicates the presence of some pathological condition, *e.g.*, peptic ulcer or cancer. **ATROPHIC G., G.** that is characterized by atrophy of parts of the gastric mucosa; likely to be associated with gastric achlorhydria.

gastroanastomosis (gas′-trō-a-nas-tō-mō′-sis): The surgical creation of a passageway between two pouches of stomach for the relief of a condition described as hourglass stomach.

gastroblennorrhea (gas′-trō-blen-ō-rē′-a): Excessive secretion of gastric mucus.

gastrocele (gas′-trō-sēl): Hernia of part of the stomach.

gastrocnemius (gas-trok-nē′-mi-us): The large two-headed muscle of the calf of the leg.

gastrocolic (gas-trō-kol′-ik): Pertaining to the stomach and the colon. **G. REFLEX**, sensory stimulus arising on entry of food into the stomach, resulting in strong peristaltic waves in the colon.

gastrocolitis (gas′-trō-kō-lī′-tis): Inflammation of the stomach and colon.

gastrocoloptosis (gas′-trō-kō-lop-tō′-sis): Downward displacement of the stomach and colon.

gastrocolostomy (gas′-trō-kō-los′-to-mi): The surgical creation of an anastomosis between the stomach and the colon.

gastrocolotomy (gas′-trō-kō-lot′-o-mi): An incision into the stomach and colon.

gastrocutaneous (gas′-trō-cū-tā′-nē-us): Pertaining to both the stomach and the skin, or pertaining to a communication between the stomach and the skin, as a fistula.

gastroduodenal (gas′-trō-dū′-ō-dē′-nal): Pertaining to the stomach and duodenum.

gastroduodenitis (gas′-trō-dū′-ō-de-nī′-tis): Inflammation of the stomach and the duodenum.

gastroduodenoscopy (gas′-trō-dū′-ō-dē-nos′-ko-pi): Examination of the stomach and duodenum, usually by means of a gastroscope passed through the esophagus.

gastroduodenostomy (gas′-trō-dū′ ō-de-nos′-to-mi): A surgical anastomosis between the stomach and the duodenum.

gastrodynia (gas-trō-din′-i-a): Pain in the stomach.

gastroenteralgia (gas′-trō-en-ter-al′-ji-a): Pain in the stomach and intestine.

gastroenteric (gas′-trō-en-ter′-ik): Pertaining to the stomach and intestines; gastrointestinal.

gastroenteritis (gas′-trō-en-ter-ī′-tis): Inflammation of mucous membranes of stomach and small intestine; although sometimes the result of dietetic error, the cause is usually a bacterial or viral infection, or food poisoning. **EPIDEMIC NEONATAL G.**, of insidious onset; usually caused by various strains of Escherichia coli, and usually develops after first week of life; symptoms include listlessness, pallor, watery yellow stools, and dehydration.

gastroenteroanastomosis (gas′-trō-en′-ter-ō-a-nas-to-mō′-sis): The surgical creation of an anastomosis between the stomach and intestine.

gastroenterocolitis (gas′-trō-en′-ter-ō-kō-lī′-tis): Inflammation of the stomach, small intestine, and colon.

gastroenterologist (gas′-trō-en-ter-ol′-ō-jist): A physician who specializes in diseases of the digestive tract.

gastroenterology (gas′-trō-en-ter-ol′-o-ji): The branch of medicine concerned with the physiology and pathologic conditions of the stomach, intestines, and accessory organs of digestion.—gastroenterological, adj.

gastroenteropathy (gas′-trō-en-ter-op′-a-thi): Any disease of the stomach and intestine.—gastroenteropathic, adj.

gastroenteroptosis (gas′-trō-en-ter-op-tō′-sis): Prolapse or downward displacement of the stomach and part of the intestine.

gastroenterostomy (gas′-trō-en-ter-os′-to-mi): The surgical creation of an anastomosis between the stomach and the small intestine, most often the jejunum.

gastroenterotomy (gas′-trō-en-ter-ot′-o-mi): An incision into both the stomach and intestine.

gastroesophageal (gas′-trō-ē-sof′-a-jē′-al): Pertaining to the stomach and esophagus. **G. REFLUX**, see under reflux. **G. VARICES**, enlarged and tortuous blood vessels of the stomach and esophagus.

gastroesophagitis (gas′-trō-ē-sof-a-jī′-tis): Inflammation of the stomach and the esophagus.

gastroesophagostomy (gas′-trō-ē-sof-a-gos′-to-mi): The surgical formation of an artificial passageway from the esophagus into the stomach.

gastrogastrostomy (gas′-trō-gas-tros′-to-mi): The surgical removal of part of the stomach and anastomosis of the two remaining parts. May be done to relieve a condition known as hourglass stomach.

gastrogavage (gas-trō-ga-vazh′): The introduction of food directly into the stomach via a tube through an opening in the wall of the stomach.

gastrogenic (gas-trō-jen′-ik): Originating in the stomach.

gastrograph (gas′-trō-graf): An instrument that records the peristaltic movements of the stomach.

gastrohelcosis (gas′-trō-hel-kō′-sis): Ulcer of the stomach.

gastrohepatic (gas′-trō-hē-pat′-ik): Pertaining to the stomach and the liver.

gastrohepatitis (gas′-trō-hep-a-tī′-tis): Inflammation of the stomach and the liver.

gastrohydrorrhea (gas′-trō-hī′-drō-rē′-a): The secretion by the stomach of a large quantity of watery fluid containing little hydrochloric acid or gastric enzymes.

gastrohysterectomy (gas′-trō-his-ter-ek′-to-mi): See abdominohysterectomy.

gastrohysterotomy (gas′-trō-his-ter-ot′-o-mi): An incision through the abdominal wall into the uterus, as in a cesarean section.

gastroileac (gas-trō-il′-e-ak): Pertaining to the stomach and the ileum. **G. REFLEX**, change in the motility of the ileum that results from the entrance of food into the stomach, causing the ileocecal valve to open.

gastroileitis (gas′-trō-il-ē-ī′-tis): Inflammation of the stomach and the ileum.

gastroileostomy (gas′-trō-il-ē-os′-to-mi): The surgical creation of an anastomosis between the stomach and the ileum.

gastrointestinal (gas′-trō-in-tes′-ti-nal): Pertaining to the stomach and intestine. **G. TRACT**, the stomach and intestine considered as a continuous structure.

gastrojejunostomy (gas′-trō-je-joo-nos′-to-mi): A surgical anastomosis between the stomach and the jejunum.

gastrolavage (gas-trō-la-vazh′): Washing out of the stomach.

gastrolith (gas′-trō-lith): A calculus or stone formed in the stomach.

gastrology (gas-trol′-ō-ji): The scientific study of the stomach and its diseases.

gastrolysis (gas-trol′-i-sis): The operation of freeing the stomach of adhesions.

gastromalacia (gas′-trō-ma-lā′-shi-a): Abnormal softening of the stomach walls.

gastromegaly (gas′-trō-meg′-a-li): Abnormal enlargement of the stomach or of the abdomen.

gastropancreatic (gas′-trō-pan-krē-at′-ik): Pertaining to the stomach and pancreas.

gastropancreatitis (gas′-trō-pan-krē-a-tī′-tis): Inflammation of the stomach and the pancreas.

gastroparesis (gas′-trō-pa-rē′-sis): Paralysis of the stomach. **G. DIABETICUM**, a condition occurring in patients with diabetes; there is delay in emptying the stomach contents, resulting in a feeling of fullness after eating only a small amount of food; nausea; and vomiting.

gastropathy (gas-trop′-a-thi): Any disease of the stomach.—gastropathic, adj.

gastroperitonitis (gas′-trō-per-i-tō-nī′-tis): Inflammation of the stomach and the peritoneum.

gastropexy (gas′-trō-peks-si): Surgical fixation of a displaced stomach to the wall of the abdomen or some other structure.

gastrophrenic (gas-trō-fren′-ik): Pertaining to the stomach and diaphragm.

gastroplasty (gas′-trō-plas-ti): Any plastic operation on the stomach; may refer to surgery to reduce the size of the gastric pouch.

gastroplication (gas′-trō-pli-kā′-shun): An operation for the treatment of dilated stomach by pleating the wall.

gastroptosis (gas-trō-tō′-sis): Downward displacement of the stomach.

gastropylorectomy (gas′-trō-pī′-lō-rek′-tō-mi): Excision of the pyloric end of the stomach. Pylorectomy.

gastrorrhagia (gas-trō-rā′-ji-a): Hemorrhage from the stomach.

gastrorrhea (gas-trō-rē′-a): Excessive secretion of mucus or gastric juice by the stomach.

gastrorrhexis (gas-trō-rek′-sis): Rupture of the stomach.

gastroschisis (gas-tros′-ki-sis): A congenital fissure in the abdominal wall, which remains open; the defect usually occurs laterally to the umbilicus on the right side, usually with protrusion of the viscera.

gastroscope (gas′-trō-skōp): An endoscope for viewing the interior of the stomach. See endoscope.—gastroscopic, adj.

gastroscopy (gas-tros′-kō-pi): Examination of the interior surface of the stomach with a fiberoptic endoscope.

gastrospasm (gas′-trō-spazm): Spasmodic contraction of the walls of the stomach.

gastrosplenic (gas-trō-splen′-ik): Pertaining to the stomach and the spleen.

gastrostenosis (gas-trō-sten-ō′-sis): A reduction in the size of the stomach.

gastrostomy (gas-tros′-tō-mi): A surgically established fistula between the stomach and the exterior abdominal wall; usually for artificial feeding.

gastrotomy (gas-trot′-ō-mi): Incision into the stomach.

gastrotropic (gas′-trō-trōp′-ik): Having an effect upon the stomach.

gastrotympanites (gas′-trō-tim-pa-nī′-tēz): Distention of the stomach with gas.

gastroxynsis (gas-trok-sin′-sis): Excessive secretion of hydrochloric acid by the stomach; hyperchlorhydria. Also gastroxia.

gastrula (gas′-troo-la): An embryo in an early stage of development when it consists of two cellular layers, which are the primary ectoderm and entoderm.

Gatch bed: See under bed.

gate control theory: The theory that impulses going over afferent nerve fibers in the spinothalamic tract to the brain can be interrupted or altered as they pass by special cells (T cells) along the tract, thus preventing the person from experiencing the sensations produced in response to touch, temperature, and such noxious stimuli as pain.

Gaucher's disease (gō′-shāz): A rare familial disorder of fat metabolism; due to an enzyme deficiency, occurring chiefly in Jewish children of Ashkenazi descent. It is characterized by pain in the back or limbs, anemia, bone destruction, marked enlargement of the lymph nodes, spleen, and liver, and internal bleeding or white cell deficiency that may result in a fatal infection. Almost always fatal in children. Diagnosis follows sternal puncture and the finding of Gaucher cells (distended with lipoid). [Phillippe Charles Ernest Gaucher, French physician. 1854–1918.]

gauge (gāj): An instrument with a graduated scale for measuring a dimension of a structure or substance.

gauze (gawz): A thin open-mesh material used in all surgical procedures and for making surgical and other dressings. **TUBULAR G., G.** prepared in tubular form and applied with a special applicator; particularly useful for finger dressings.

gavage (ga-vazh′): Forced feeding through a tube that is passed into the stomach through the nose, pharynx, and esophagus.

gay: Popular term for a person who is a homosexual.

Gay Lussac's law: Charles' law (*q.v.*).

GB series: Abbreviation for gallbladder series, an x-ray procedure to determine whether the gallbladder can fill and empty properly.

GC: Abbreviation for gonococcus; gonorrhea; gonorrheal. Also written Gc.

gegenhalten (gā′-gen-hal-ten): Paratonic rigidity, see paratonia. A form of passive involuntary resistance to movement; the patient is unable to relax his muscles evenly when the arms or legs are being held by another person, and his walking may be characterized by going and stopping; occurs in persons with certain cerebral cortical disorders.

Gehrig's disease: A popular name for amyotrophic lateral sclerosis (see sclerosis); so called because it was fatal to an American baseball hero, Lou Gehrig.

Geiger counter: A device for detecting and

registering radioactivity. Also Geiger-Müller counter.

geisoma (gī-sō′-ma): The eyebrows, or the supraorbital ridges (*q.v.*).

gel (jel): A substance consisting of a liquid and a colloid, the mixture being more solid than liquid in form. See colloid.

gelasmus (je-laz′-mus): Hysterical or maniacal laughter.—gelasmic, adj.

gelate (jel′-āt): To convert into a gel.

gelatin (jel′-a-tin): The protein-containing, glue-like substance obtained by boiling bones, skin and other animal tissues. Used in various ways in pharmaceutical preparations, as a bacteriological culture medium, and as a food.—gelatinoid, gelatinous, adj.

gelatinase (je-lat′-i-nās): An enzyme found in bacteria, molds, yeasts; acts to liquefy gelatin.

Geller-Gesner tables: A set of tables published periodically showing the leading causes of death.

Gelle's test: A hearing test to determine whether a person has a conductive hearing loss. It tests the mobility of the stapes.

gelose (jel′-ōs): Agar (*q.v.*).

gelosis (jel-ō′-sis): A hard mass in tissues, especially in a muscle.

gemellipara (jem-el-lip′-a-ra): A woman who has given birth to twins.

gemellology (jem-el-ol′-o-ji): The scientific study of twins and twinning.

geminate (jem′ i-nāt): Occurring in pairs.

geminus (jem′-i-nus): A twin.

-gen: Combining form denoting an agent that produces or generates.

gen-; geno-: Combining forms denoting production.

gena (jē′-na): The side of the face; the cheek.—genal, adj.

gender (jen′-der): Sex. The category to which a person is assigned in terms of male or female.

gene (jēn): The factor in the chromosome that is responsible for the determination and transmission of hereditary characteristics. Genes are capable of self-reproduction and occur typically in pairs, occupying definite places on the chromosomes, one being found on the chromosome received from the father and one on that received from the mother. Genes are composed, in general, of deoxyribonucleic acid (DNA) and protein, and are the smallest unit of heredity, there being one for each physical or biochemical characteristic. **DOMINANT G.**, one that is capable of transmitting its characteristics regardless of whether it is present in the chromosomes of the other parent. **RECESSIVE G.**, one that will transmit its characteristics only if it is present in the chromosomes of both parents.—genetic, genic, adj.

genera (jen′-e-ra): Plural of genus (*q.v.*).

general: Said of a disease that affects all or many parts of the body. **G. ANESTHETIC**, see anesthetic. **G. PARESIS**, see paresis. **G. PRACTITIONER**, a physician who engages in the general practice of medicine, as opposed to being a specialist.

generation (jen-er-ā′-shun): 1. A group of individuals who came into being at approximately the same time and who have some experience, attitude, or belief in common. 2. The time period, usually about 30 years, between the genesis of one generation and the next. 3. The process of producing offspring; procreation.

generative (jen′-er-at-iv): Pertaining to generation or reproduction.

generic (je-ner′-ik): 1. Pertaining to a genus (*q.v.*). 2. Distinctive. 3. Not protected by patent or trademark; said of drugs.

generic nursing program: An education program that prepares students for professional nursing; often used to distinguish baccalaureate degree programs from masters or practitioner programs.

genesiology (jen-ē-si-ol′-ō-ji): 1. Genetics (*q.v.*). 2. The study of reproduction.

genesis (jen′-e-sis): The production, generation, or origin of a substance, organism, or other entity.

genetic (je-net′-ik): 1. Relating to origin or reproduction. 2. Inherited or produced by a gene. 3. Relating to the science of genetics. **G. CODE**, the form in which genetic information is transmitted; the characteristics in genes that are passed from one generation to the next. **G. COUNSELING**, counseling of prospective parents in regard to risks, diagnostic procedures available, and possible occurrence of congenital or inherited disorders in a family; involves chromosomal studies of both prospective parents.

geneticist (je-net′-i-sist): A scientist who specializes in genetics.

genetics (je-net′-iks): The study of heredity. **BEHAVIOR G.**, the branch of psychology that deals with the influence of heredity on behavior.

genetotrophic (je-net-ō-trōf′-ik): Pertaining to nutritional problems that are hereditary in nature.

Geneva Convention: An agreement between European nations signed in Geneva, Switzerland in 1864, and later adopted by other nations, specifying that prisoners of war, the sick, wounded and dead, as well as those caring for them, would be humanely treated. The founding of the International Red Cross Society was a direct outcome of this meeting.

genial (jē′ni-al): In anatomy, pertaining to the chin.

-genic: Combining form denoting: 1. Forming, producing, produced by, formed from. 2. Of or relating to a gene. 3. Suitable for production or reproduction.

genicular (je-nik′-ū-lar): Pertaining to the knee.

geniculate (je-nik′-ū-lāt): Bent, in the way the knee is bent. **LATERAL G. BODY,** a nuclear mass in the posterior thalamic zone that receives auditory impulses and relays them to the appropriate area in the cortex. **MEDIAL G. BODY,** a flattened area in the posterior of the thalamus that receives impulses from the retina and relays them to the appropriate area in the cortex. See geniculum.

geniculum (je-nik′-ū-lum): A knee-like bend in a small structure.

genioplasty (jē′-ni-ō-plas-ti): Plastic surgery on the chin.

genital (jen′-it-al): Pertaining to the organs of generation. **G. HERPES,** see herpesgenitalis under herpes. **G. STAGE,** according to Freud, the stage in human psychosexual development, from about the second to the sixth year, when the child is interested in his genitals and when infantile masturbation is common.

genitalia (jen-i-tā′-li-a): The organs of generation. **EXTERNAL G.,** the reproductive organs that are not located within the pelvic cavity. **INTERNAL G.,** the reproductive organs that are contained within the pelvic cavity. See penis, vagina.

genito-: Combining form denoting the genital organs.

genitocrural (jen′-it-ō-kroo′-ral): Pertaining to the genital area and the leg.

genitoplasty (jen′-i-tō-plas-ti): Plastic surgery on the genital organs.

genitourinary (jen-it-ō-ū′-rin-a-ri): Pertaining to the reproductive and urinary systems or to the organs of those systems.

genoblast (jē′-nō-blast): The nucleus of a fertilized ovum.

genocide (jen′-ō-sīd): The systematic killing or destruction of an entire population, ethnic group, or tribe.

genodermatosis (jen′-ō-der-ma-tō′-sis): Any congenital skin disorder or malformation involving the skin.

genogram (jen′-ō-gram): An outline of family history in which each member of a group gives his own family history; helps both the individual and the social investigator to visualize the family structure and to gain perspective on an individual in light of successive events in his background.

genome (jē′-nōm): 1. The genetic makeup of a species. 2. The human genetic complement of 23 pairs of chromosomes, 22 of which appear in both sexes; the 23rd is the sex chromosome, which is identified as XX in the female and XY in the male.

genotype (jen′-ō-tīp): 1. The entire inherent genetic endowment of an individual. 2. A group of organisms in which all members have the same genetic constitution.—genotypically, adj.

-genous: A suffix denoting produced by, resulting from, or arising in.

gentian violet: A dye derived from coal tar; widely used as a stain in biological and histological laboratories and as a topical anti-infective, antifungal, and anthelmintic agent.

genu (jē′-nū): 1. The knee. 2. Any knee-like structure. **G. VALGUM,** knock knee. **G. VARUM,** bowleg. **G. RECURVATUM,** backward curvature of the knee joint.—genua, pl.; genicular, adj.

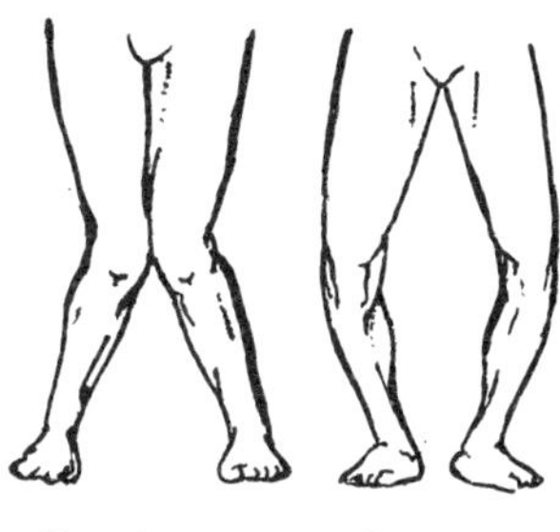

G. valgum G. varum

genucubital (jen-ū-kū′-bit-al): Pertaining to the knees and the elbows.

genupectoral position (jen-ū-pek′-tor-al): Pertaining to the knees and the chest. **G. POSITION,** the knee-chest position; see under position.

genus (jē′-nus): A classification ranking between family (higher) and species (lower).

geomedicine (jē′-ō-med′-i-sin): The branch of medicine that deals with the influence of environment and climate on health and disease.

geophagia (jē-ō-fā′-ji-a): The habit of eating earth, clay, or similar unsuitable substance. Also called geophagism and geophagy.

geotrichosis (jē′-ō-tri-kō′-sis): Infection by a fungus; sites most frequently affected are the lungs, mouth, and intestine.

geotropism (jē-ot′-rō-pizm): The influence of gravity on growth. Also called geotaxis.

ger-; gerat-; Combining forms denoting old age.

geratic (je-rat′-ik): Pertaining to old age.

geratology (jer-a-tol′-ō-ji): Gerontology (*q.v.*).

geriactivist (jer-i-ak′-tiv-ist): A recently coined term used to describe an older person who is himself active in the causes of the elderly.

geriatric (jer-ē-at′-rik): Pertaining to advanced age or to the elderly.

Geriatric Nursing: A journal published by the American Journal of Nursing Company since

1980. The articles deal with the common diseases, disabilities, and living problems of the elderly and ways of meeting their special needs. The magazine also carries news items, book reviews, and drug information.

geriatrician (jer-i-a-trish′-an): A physician who specializes in the care of the elderly.

geriatrics (jer-i-at′-riks): The branch of medical science that deals with the application of the knowledge of aging in providing care for the elderly with all kinds of physical and mental illnesses.

germ (jurm): 1. A small bit of living substance capable of developing into a new individual. 2. Any microorganism, particularly a pathogenic bacterium. 3. The part of a cereal grain that is separated from the starchy part in the milling process, *e.g.*, wheat germ. 4. A beginning. 5. One of three layers of cells in the embryo from which the organs and structures of the body develop (ectoderm, mesoderm, entoderm).

germ cell: A sexual reproductive cell; an ovum or spermatazoon in any stage of its development.

germ plasm: The protoplasm of the germ cell (*q.v.*); it contains the hereditary material of the cell.

German measles: See rubella.

germicide (jer′-mi-sid): An agent that kills germs (pathogenic bacteria).—germicidal, adj.

germinal (jer′min-al): 1. Pertaining to a germ. 2. Pertaining to a reproductive cell.

germination (jer-min-ā′-shun): In physiology, the development of a fertilized ovum into an embryo.

gero-, geronto-: Combining forms denoting old age or aging.

gerocomia (jer-ō-kō′-mi-a): 1. The medical care and hygiene of the old. 2. The care of old men.

geroderma (jer-ō-der′-ma): Thickening and wrinkling of the skin when associated with old age.

gerodontics (jer-ō-don′-tiks): The dental problems of the elderly.

gerogenesis (jer-ō-jen′-e-sis): Pertains to the conditions, both normal and pathological, that occur as the body ages, or to the various theories of aging.

geromarasmus (jer′-ō-ma-raz′-mus): Atrophy and wasting of the body in the elderly.

geromorphism (jer-ō-morf′-izm): Premature aging or senility.

geront-; geronto-: Combining forms denoting old age.

gerontal (jer-on′-tal): 1. Pertaining to the aged. 2. Pertaining to old men.

gerontic (jer-on′-tik): Pertaining to both geriatrics and gerontology.

geronting (jer-on′-ting): The psychological process of aging as expressed by the individual's ability to influence and manipulate his or her environment so as to achieve the highest possible quality of life.

gerontologic (jer′-on-tō-loj′-ik): Of or pertaining to the study of gerontology. **G. MEDICINE,** the branch of medicine dealing with the medical treatment of age-related diseases and disorders occurring in the elderly. **G. NURSING,** nursing practice that is concerned with the study of the aging process, geriatric nursing, and nursing research in health care of the elderly. Education for practice as a gerontologic nurse practitioner is offered in several American gerontology centers located in university settings.

gerontology (jer-on-tol′-ō-ji): The scientific study of the aging processes and the problems of the aging; a multidisciplinary field that draws its content and methods from biology, medical science, psychology, sociology, philosophy, political science, economics, education, and social services. **BIOLOGICAL G.,** the biology of longevity, aging, and death.

gerontophilia (jer-on-tō-fil′-i-a): Excessive love of older people.

gerontophobia (jer-on-tō-fō′-bi-a): 1. Dislike or fear of old age. 2. Pathologic fear of old people.

gerontopia (jer-on-tō′-pi-a): Improvement of near vision in older persons, often a sign of incipient cataract; often called "second sight."

gerontotherapeutics (jer-on′-tō-ther-a-pū′-tiks): The branch of medical science that deals with treatment of the aged.

gerontotherapy (jer-on′-tō-ther′-a-pi): Management of the disorders of the elderly.

gerontoxon (jer-on-tok′-son): An area of degeneration around the outer circumference of the cornea creating a grayish or white ring. Also called arcus senilis and arcus cornealis.

gerophysiatric (jer′-ō-fiz-i-at′-rik): Pertaining to the use of physical agents in the treatment of geriatric patients. See physiatrics.

gerophysiatrist (jer′-ō-fiz-i-at′-rist): A physician who utilizes physical agents in the treatment of disorders and diseases of the elderly. See physiatrics.

geropsychiatrist (jer′-ō-si-kī′-a-trist): A geriatrician who cares for elderly persons with mental illnesses. Also called psychogeriatrician.

geropsychiatry (jer′-ō-si-kī′-a-tri): The branch of psychiatry that deals with presenile or senile mental diseases or disturbances.—geropsychiatric, adj.

Gerstmann's syndrome: A condition characterized by right-left disorientation, finger agnosia, agraphia; due to a lesion in the dominant cerebral hemisphere.

gestalt (ge-stalt): A school of psychology founded in Germany by Dr. Frederick Perls; holds that objects that come to mind are perceived as total configurations arising from the interrelations of their component parts and cannot be split into separate parts; and that the word gestalt means "integrated unit," hence individuals are treated as complete functional units in their particular setting and condition.

gestation (jes-tā′-shun): 1. Pregnancy. 2. The development of an individual from conception to birth.

gestational age (jes-tā′-shun-al): The age of a conceptus, computed from the first day of the mother's last menstrual period, expressed in weeks.

gestosis (jes-tō′-sis): Any toxic disorder of pregnancy.

-geusia: Combining form denoting taste, or the sense of taste.

GFR: Abbreviation for glomerular filtration rate. See glomerular filtrate under glomerular.

GH: Abbreviation for growth hormone.

Ghon's focus: The initial lesion in tuberculosis of the lung in children, occurring as a small focus of infection in lung tissue and associated with enlargement of lymph nodes in the hilum and mediastinum; usually heals spontaneously. Also called Ghon tubercle. [Anton Ghon, Czechoslovakian pathologist. 1866–1936.]

ghost surgery: A term given to a former practice in which surgery was performed by someone other than the one the patient thought had done it.

GI: Abbreviation for gastrointestinal.

giant cell tumor: See osteoclastoma.

Giardia lamblia (ji-ar′-di-a): A flagellated beet-shaped organism that attaches itself to the intestinal wall; usually does not cause pathology but may cause giardiasis (*q.v.*). *Lamblia intestinalis.*

giardiasis (ji-ar-dī′-a-sis): Infection with the protozoan *Giardia* lamblia; usually there are no definite symptoms, but occasionally the organism gives rise to diarrhea and dysentery. Transmitted by foods, water, and lack of handwashing among caregivers and others. Incubation period may be as short as 5 days or as long as 25 days. Symptoms include sudden onset of violent diarrhea, abdominal cramps; nausea and vomiting, low grade fever, chills. Attacks may be of short duration or may last as long as several weeks.

gibberish (jib′-er-ish): Incoherent, unintelligible language.

gibbosity (gib-bos′-i-ti): A humped back, or the condition of being humpbacked.—gibbus, n.; gibbous, adj.

giddiness (gid′-i-nes): An unpleasant sensation resembling dizziness.

Giemsa's stain: An azure dye commonly used for staining blood smears for examination for the presence of Negri bodies, malarial organisms, protozoa, spirochetes, and various other parasitic microorganisms; also useful for doing differential leukocyte counts.

Gierke's disease: Glycogenosis (*q.v.*).

gigantism (gī′-gan-tizm): An abnormal overgrowth, especially in height. May be associated with anterior pituitary tumor if the tumor develops before fusion of the epiphyses. ACROMEGALIC G., pituitary G. FETAL G., excessive size of the fetus or newborn; may be seen in offspring of diabetic mothers, when it is called *fetoprotein diabetica;* see Beckwith-Wiedemann syndrome. PITUITARY G., that due to excessive pituitary secretion; occurs before puberty.

gigantoblast (jī-gan′-tō-blast): An unusually large red blood cell.

gigantomastia (jī-gan′-tō-ō-mas′-ti-a): The condition of having unusually large breasts.

gigantosoma (jī-gan-tō-sō′-ma): Abnormally large size of the body; gigantism.

Gigli's saw: A flexible wire saw used in cranial and other bone operations.

Gilbert's disease: An inborn error of bile metabolism; associated with mild jaundice, malaise, abdominal pain. Also referred to as Gilbert's syndrome.

Gilles de la Tourette syndrome (zhēl′ de la too-ret′): A relatively rare condition characterized by progressively violent tics or jerks of muscles of the face, shoulder, and extremities; by compulsive acts, echolalia, explosive obscene utterances, grunting, barking, or hissing. Usually begins between the ages of 2 and 14 years. [Gilles de la Tourette, French neurologist, 1857–1904.]

Gilliam's operation: A method of correcting retroversion of the uterus by shortening the round ligaments. [David Tod Gilliam, American gynecologist. 1844–1923.]

ginger (jin′-jer): The dried rhizome of a tropical plant; sometimes used in medicine in treatment of colic and flatulence. POWDERED G. ROOT, prepared in capsules for use by travelers to avoid air, car, or other motion sickness.

gingiva (jin′-ji-va): The gum; the dense fibrous tissue covered with mucous membrane into which the teeth are set.—gingivae, pl.; gingival, adj.

gingivalgia (jin-ji-val′-ji-a): Diffuse pain in the gingivae.

gingivectomy (jin-ji-vek′-to-mi): Excision of a portion of the gum, usually for pyorrhea.

gingivitis (jin-ji-vī′-tis): Inflammation of the gingivae; often the result of poor oral hygiene with the formation of bacterial plaque. DESQUAMATIVE G., a condition sometimes seen in menopausal women and older people; a gray necrotic membrane forms on the gingivae and eventually sloughs off; usually chronic.

gingivoglossitis (jin′-ji-vō-glos-sī′-tis): Inflammation of the gingivae and of the tongue. See also stomatitis.

gingivolabial (jin′-ji-vō-lā′-bi-al): Pertaining to the gingivae and the lips; or the angle formed at the line of their junction.

gingivoplasty (jin′-ji-vō-plas′-ti): Plastic surgery on the gingivae.

gingivostomatitis (jin′-ji-vō-stō-ma-tī′-tis): Inflammation of both the gingivae and the oral mucosa usually seen in young children; often due to a herpesvirus infection.

ginglymus (jin′-gli-mus): A hinge joint (*q.v.*).—ginglimoid, adj.

girdle (ger′-dl): 1. A belt. 2. An encircling structure or part. **G. PAIN,** a constricting pain around the waist region, occurring in tabetic persons. **PELVIC G.,** comprises the two innominate bones, sacrum, and coccyx. **SHOULDER G.,** comprises the two clavicles and scapulae.

Girdlestone: [G. R. Girdlestone, English surgeon. 1881–1950.] **G'S. ARTHROPATHY,** the insertion of a partial or total artificial hip joint. **G'S. OPERATION,** a surgical procedure for draining a seriously infected hip joint.

girth (gerth): Circumference, particularly of the abdomen.

glabella (gla-bel′-la): A smooth prominence on the frontal bone at about the level of the upper margin of the orbit of the eye; the bridge of the nose.—glabellar, adj.

glabellar tap sign (gla-bel′-ar): Elicited by rhythmic tapping on the glabella with the finger; normally the person responds by blinking, which stops when the tapping stops; the parkinsonian patient continues to blink or the eyelids begin to contract spasmodically.

glabrous (glā′-brus): Smooth; hairless.

gladiate (glā′-di-āt): Sword-shaped.

gladiolus (gla-dī′-ō-lus): The blade-like middle portion of the sternum.

glairy (glā′-ri): Slimy, albuminous; like the white of egg.

gland: An organ, structure or group of cells capable of manufacturing a fluid substance 1) to be eliminated from the body, or 2) to be used in some part of the body other than the place it is made. **LYMPHATIC G.,** (node) does not secrete but is concerned with filtration of the lymph. See endocrine, exocrine.—glandular, adj.

glanders (glan′-derz): A contagious, febrile, ulcerative disease communicable from horses, mules, and asses to man through ingestion, inhalation, skin abrasions, or via the conjunctiva; symptoms include headache, backache, vomiting, prostration, myalgia, purulent inflammation of mucous membranes, and the development of ulcerative skin nodules. The causative organism is *Pseudomonas mallei*.

glandula (glan′-dū-la): A small gland.

glandular (glan′-dū-lar): 1. Pertaining to or resembling a gland. 2. Pertaining to the glans penis. **G. FEVER,** see infectious mononucleosis.

glans (glanz): The bulbous termination of the clitoris and penis.

Glasgow Coma Scale: A neurological evaluation tool based on eye, motor, and verbal responses; the various responses are given a number value on the scale, and the patient's state of responsiveness is expressed in the total of the number values; the lowest possible score is 3 and the highest is 15.

Glasgow's sign: A systolic murmur that is heard over the brachial artery in patients with an aneurysm of the aorta.

glass arm: Lay term for irritation of the long head of the biceps brachii muscle.

glaucoma (glaw-kō′-ma): A condition of the eye in which vision is lost due to increased intraocular pressure when the rate of absorption of the fluid within the eye is slower than the rate of production; may be acute or chronic, causing damage to the retina and optic nerve, hardening of the globe of the eye, and blindness if undetected or untreated; the classic symptom is seeing halos around lights. The cause may not be known, but the disorder may follow a blow on the head, emotional stress, diabetes, sudden dilatation of the pupil; heredity may also be involved. **G.** occurs most often in people over 40 years of age, but is also seen in young children. Not considered curable but can be kept from progressing through treatment. **HEMORRHAGIC G.,** caused by retinal hemorrhage. **NARROW-ANGLE** or **CLOSED-ANGLE G.,** increased intraocular pressure due to blocking of the angle of the anterior chamber by fibrous bands; of sudden onset; characterized by intense pain, blurring or loss of vision, redness of the conjunctiva; may become chronic with permanent closure of the angle; surgical treatment is necessary to drain off the rapidly building pressure and prevent damage to the optic nerve. **WIDE-ANGLE** or **OPEN-ANGLE G.,** increased intraocular pressure of insidious onset; the angle remains open but the filtration of intraocular fluid is diminished, leading to increased pressure, often with eventual loss of vision; treated with eye drops and oral medication.

glaucomatous (glaw-kō′-ma-tus): Pertaining to glaucoma. **G. CUP,** a depression in the optic disk occurring in glaucoma.

gleet: A chronic urethral discharge in the male; usually mucoid in character; may occur as a sequela of gonorrheal infection.

glenohumeral (glē-nō-hū′-mer-al, glen-ō-): Pertaining to the glenoid cavity of the scapula and the humerus.

glenoid (glē'noyd, glen'oyd): Resembling a pit or socket, particularly the cavity on the scapula into which the head of the humerus fits to form the shoulder joint. **G. FOSSA,** the depression in the temporal bone in which the condyle of the lower jaw rests.

glia (glī' -a): The non-nervous supporting tissue of the brain and spinal cord; the neuroglia.

-glia: Combining form denoting neuroglia in which the elements are of a particular kind or size, *e.g.*, microglia.

gliadin (glī' -a-din): A protein derived from the gluten of grains, such as wheat, rye, and oats.

glial (glī' -al): Pertaining to glia or neuroglia.

gliding: A smooth, continuous movement. **G. JOINT,** a synovial joint in which the movement is limited as to plane, as occurs in the wrist or ankle joints.

glioblastoma (glī-ō-blas-tō' -ma): A general term for malignant forms of astrocytoma. **G. MULTIFORME,** a rapidly growing, highly malignant tumor, occurring chiefly in the cerebral hemispheres.

gliocyte (glī' -ō-sīt): A neuroglial cell.

gliocytoma (glī-ō-sī-tō' -ma): Glioma (*q.v.*).

gliogenous (glī-oj' -e-nus): Formed by or produced by glial cells.

glioma (glī-ō' -ma): An infiltrative neoplasm, usually malignant, that arises in the neuroglia, often in the cerebral hemispheres or spinal cord of adults. The tumor has no well defined border; it blends into the surrounding tissues, making complete excision almost impossible. One form occurring in the retina is hereditary. **ASTROCYTIC G.,** see astrocytoma. **EPENDYMAL G.,** see ependymoma. **GANGLIONIC G.,** see neuroblastoma. **OPTIC NERVE G.,** a slow-growing neoplasm of the optic nerve or chiasm, beginning with visual loss; later symptoms include bulging of the eyeball, strabismus, and loss of eye movement.—gliomatous, adj.

gliomatosis (glī-ō-ma-tō' -sis): Overdevelopment of the neuroglia, particularly in the spinal cord; may refer to a sizeable neoplasm.

gliomyoma (glī-ō-mī-ō' -ma): A tumor of nerve and muscle tissue.—gliomyomata, pl.

gliosis (glī-ō' -sis): A condition marked by the presence of tumors or overgrowth in the neuroglia.

glissonitis (glis-sō-nī' -tis): Inflammation of Glisson's capsule. (*q.v.*):

Glisson's capsule: The connective tissue sheath that surrounds the liver, covers it and the blood vessels that enter it, and follows the blood vessels into the liver, dividing it into lobes and lobules. [Francis Glisson, English physician and anatomist. 1579–1677.]

glitter cells: Leucocytes that, when viewed under the microscope, appear to have granules that move about and have a sparkling appearance.

globin (glō' -bin): A protein that combines with hematin to form hemoglobin.

globule (glob' -ūl): A small spherical mass.—globoid, globular, adj.

globulin (glob' -ū-lin): A fraction of serum or plasma protein. **ANTIHEMOPHILIC G.,** factor VIII; see under factor. **ANTILYMPHOCYTIC G.,** a purified serum produced in animals; used in combatting rejection reaction in organ transplantation. **GAMMA G.,** human **G.** prepared from convalescent serum; contains antibodies against certain bacterial and viral infections; used in prevention and treatment of measles, poliomyelitis, and several other infections. **HYPERIMMUNE G., G.** prepared from serum of patients recently recovered from certain viral diseases including those caused by herpesviruses and hepatitis B, and by certain encephalitides and zoonoses.

globulinuria (glob' -ū-lin-ū' -ri-a): The presence of globulin in the urine.

globulolysis (glob-ū-lol' -i-sis): Destruction of red blood cells.—globulolytic, adj.

globus hystericus (glō' -bus his-ter' -ik-us): Subjective feeling of a lump in the throat; of neurotic origin. Can also include difficulty in swallowing and is due to tension of muscles of deglutition. Occurs in hysteria, anxiety states and depression. Sometimes follows slight trauma to throat, *e.g.*, scratch by foreign body.

globus pallidus (glō' -bus pal' -li-dus): The pale smaller and more medial part of the lentiform nucleus of the corpus striatum of the brain.

glomangioma (glō-man-ji-ō' -ma): A benign vascular tumor, singular or multiple, arising from a conglomeration of small blood vessels of the skin, occurring chiefly on the digits; usually small, bluish in color, and either painless or extremely painful.

glomectomy (glō-mek' -to-mi): The excision of a glomus (*q.v.*).

glomerular (glō-mer' -ū-lar): Pertaining to a glomerulus (*q.v.*). **G. FILTRATE,** the non-protein filtrate of plasma produced by the malpighian corpuscles of the kidney and that passes into the lumen of Bowman's capsule (*q.v.*). **G. FILTRATION RATE,** the rate at which the kidney filters fluid from the circulating blood; measured in volume per unit of time, either minutes or hours.

glomerulitis (glō-mer-ū-lī' -tis): Inflammation of the glomeruli of the kidney.

glomerulonephritis (glō-mer' -ū-lō-nē-frī' -tis): A term used in nonsuppurative acute or chronic disease of the kidney, primarily of the glomeruli. In children and young persons **ACUTE G.** often follows streptococcal infections, marked by hematuria, hypertension, edema, and proteinuria; the prognosis is good. In older persons, the disease is marked by malaise, nausea, joint pain, proteinuria, hypertension, and pulmonary complications; all symptoms are more severe than in children and the prognosis is somewhat less favorable. **POSTINFECTIOUS G.**, acute **G.**, often follows streptococcal infections but may also follow infections caused by staphylococcal and pneumococcal organisms.

glomerulopathy (glō-mer-ū-lop′-a-thi): Any disease condition of the glomeruli of the kidney.

glomerulosclerosis (glō-mer′-ū-lō-sklē-rō′-sis): Fibrosis of the glomeruli of the kidney, the result of inflammation. **INTERCAPILLARY G.**, is a common pathological finding in persons with diabetes mellitus.—glomerulosclerotic, adj.

glomerulus (glō-mer′-ū-lus): A coil of minute arterial capillaries held together by scanty connective tissue. It invaginates the entrance of a uriniferous tubule in the kidney cortex.—glomerular, adj; glomeruli, pl.

glomus (glō′-mus): In anatomy, a small encapsulated globular body containing many arterioles that are connected to veins, and having a rich nerve supply, especially sensory receptors, *e.g.*, the **G. CAROTICUM**, situated behind the carotid artery at its bifurcation. **G. TUMOR**, a neoplasm of unknown cause; consists of a slightly elevated, rounded, firm, nodular mass, occurring chiefly in the skin; generally seen on distal ends of fingers and toes and in the nailbed; treatment is surgical removal.

glos-, glosso-: Combining forms denoting: 1. The tongue. 2. Language.

glossa (glos′-a): The tongue.—glossal, adj.

glossalgia (glos-al′-ji-a): Pain in the tongue.

glossectomee (glos-ek′-tō-mē): A person who has undergone a glossectomy.

glossectomy (glos-ek′-tō-mi): Amputation of all or part of the tongue.

glossitis (glos-ī′-tis): 1. Inflammation of the tongue. 2. Cellulitis of the tongue. **MOELLER'S G.**, see papillitis.

glossocele (glos′-ō-sēl): Edema and swelling of the tongue, resulting in its protrusion from the mouth.

glossocoma (glō-sok′-ō-ma): Retraction of the tongue.

glossodynia (glos-ō-din′-i-a): Pain in the tongue; may be acute or chronic and due to inflammation or the presence of an ulcer.

glossohyal (glos-ō-hī′-al): Pertaining to the tongue and the hyoid bone.

glossolabial (glos-ō-lā′-bi-al): Relating to the tongue and the lips.

glossolalia (glos-ō-lā′-li-a): Unintelligible talk; gibberish.

glossoncus (glo-sonk′-us): Any swelling of the tongue, including the presence of a neoplasm.

glossopathy (glos-op′-a-thi): Any disease of the tongue.

glossopharyngeal (glos′-ō-fa-rin′-jē-al): Pertaining to the tongue and pharynx. **G. BREATHING**, frog breathing (*q.v.*). **G. NERVE**, one of the 9th pair of cranial nerves; has motor fibers that go to the parotid gland and sensory fibers for the sensations of touch, temperature, and pain from the back of the tongue, tonsils, and pharynx; and taste from the back one-third of the tongue. **G. NEURALGIA**, a condition marked by pain in the tongue and throat; seen most often in the elderly.

glossopharyngeolabial (glos′-ō-fa-rin′-jē-ō-lā′-bi-al): Pertaining to the tongue, pharynx, and lips.

glossopharyngeum (glos′-ō-fa-rin′-jē-um): The tongue and pharynx considered together.

glossophytia (glos-ō-fit′-i-a): Black tongue. Blackish to yellow, furlike painless patches at the back of the tongue; often due to a fungal infection.

glossoplasty (glos′-ō-plas-ti): Plastic surgery on the tongue.

glossoplegia (glos-ō-plē′-ji-a): Paralysis of the tongue.

glossoptosis (glos-op-tō′-sis): Retraction or downward displacement of the tongue.

glossopyrosis (glos-ō-pī-rō′-sis): A burning sensation in the tongue, from whatever cause.

glossotrichia (glos-ō-trik′-i-a): Hairy tongue; the papillae become greatly elongated; sometimes occurs after sucking antibiotic lozenges.

glottal (glot′-al): Pertaining to the glottis.

glottic (glot′-ik): Pertaining to 1) the glottis; 2) the tongue.

glottis (glot′-is): The part of the larynx that is concerned with voice production. See vocal cords and rima glottidis.—glottides, pl.; glottic, adj.

glottitis (glot-ī′-tis): Inflammation of the glottic part of the larynx.

glove and stocking disease: See glove and stocking anesthesia under anesthesia.

gluc-, gluco: Combining forms denoting glucose.

glucagon (gloo′-ka-gon): Hormone produced in alpha cells of pancreatic islets of Langerhans. Causes breakdown of glycogen into glucose, thus preventing blood sugar from falling too low during fasting.

glucagonoma (gloo′-ka-gon-ō′-ma): A tumor of the glucagon-secreting cells of the pancreas; symptoms include excessive production of glucagon, stomatitis, redness and blistering of the skin, anemia, weight loss, and the tendency to metastasize.

glucocorticoid (gloo′-kō-kor′-ti-koyd): Any steroid hormone that promotes gluconeogenesis (*i.e.*, the formation of glucose and glycogen from protein) and antagonizes the action of insulin. Occurs naturally in the adrenal cortex as cortisone and hydrocortisone; also produced synthetically. **G. INSUFFICIENCY,** see Addison's disease.

glucogenesis (gloo-kō-jen′-e-sis): The formation in the body of glycogen from the breakdown of glucose.—glucogenic, adj.

gluconeogenesis (gloo′-kō-nē′-ō-jen′-e-sis): Glyconeogenesis (*q.v.*).

glucose (gloo′kōs): Dextrose or grape sugar. A common and important monosaccharide, present in most fruits. The chief end product of the digestion of carbohydrates and the form in which they are absorbed from the gastrointestinal tract. A normal constituent of blood and other fluids of the body. The chief source of energy in the body. Excess over what is needed or utilized by the body is stored in the form of glycogen or in body tissues as fat.

glucose tolerance test: Useful in the diagnosis of diabetes mellitus and other causes of glycosuria. Serial collections of blood are estimated for blood glucose following the oral or intravenous administration of glucose, and urine samples are simultaneously tested for glucose.

glucoside (gloo′-kō-sīd): Any of a group of natural vegetable substances that decomposes into glucose and another substance; many have medicinal properties with specific uses in medicine.

glucosuria (gloo-kō-sū′-ri-a): The presence of an abnormal amount of glucose in the urine.

glucuronic acid (gloo-kū-ron′-ik): A product formed in the oxidation of glucose.

glucuronidase (gloo-kū-ron′-i-dās): An enzyme that acts as a catalyst in the hydrolysis of glucuronides; occurs in the liver, spleen, and endocrine glands.

glucuronide (gloo-kū′-ron-īd): A compound resulting from the interaction of glucuronic acid with a phenol, an alcohol, or an acid containing the carboxyl group (COOH).

glue-sniffing: The inhalation of fumes from epoxy glue; initial stimulation of the central nervous system is followed by depression. The effect of the inhalation is enhanced when the glue is poured into a plastic bag that is placed over the nose and mouth.

glutamic acid decarboxylase (gloo-tam′-ik as′-id dē-kar-boks′-i-lās): An enzyme affecting regulation of the neurotransmitter, gamma-aminobutyric acid, which is markedly reduced in Huntington's chorea.

glutamic oxaloacetic transaminase (gloo-tam′-ik oks′-a-lō-a-se′-tik trans-am′-i-nās): An enzyme that catalyzes the transfer of the amino group of glutamic acid to oxaloacetic acid; tests for measuring the levels of this enzyme in the blood serum give useful information in diagnosing myocardial infarction and certain liver diseases. Found in varying concentrations in heart and skeletal muscle, liver, pancreas, and kidney tissue. Abbreviated GOT.

glutamic-pyruvic transaminase (gloo-tam′-ik pī-roo′-vik trans-am′-i-nās): An enzyme found in high concentrations in the liver, and in lesser amounts in the kidney, heart, and muscle tissue; used in laboratory tests for diagnosis of liver disease. Essential in the hydrolysis of protein. Abbreviated GPT.

glutamine (gloo′-ta-mēn): An amino acid found in certain proteins, blood, and other tissues; on hydrolysis it yields glutamic acid and ammonia.

glutaraldehyde (gloo-ta-ral′-de-hīd): A compound used for fixing a tissue specimen for examination by electronmicroscopy; it preserves very fine details.

glutathione (gloo-ta-thī′-ōn): A tripeptide that has been isolated from yeast, liver, and muscle; thought to be important in cellular respiration.

gluteal (gloo′-tē-al): Pertaining to the buttocks. **G. FOLD,** the crease between the posterior thigh and the buttock. **G. REFLEX,** contraction of the gluteal muscles from stimulation of the skin over them.

gluten (gloo′-ten): A protein constituent of wheat and several other grains; used commercially for making adhesives. **G. ENTEROPATHY,** adult celiac disease; see under celiac.

gluteofemoral (gloo′-tē-ō-fem′-o-ral): Pertaining to the gluteal muscles and the femur.

gluteus (gloo′-tē-us): **G. MAXIMUS,** the largest and most superficial of the three large muscles that form the buttock. **G. MEDIUS,** the middle of the muscles that form the buttock. **G. MINIMUS,** the innermost of the muscles that form the buttock.

glutinous (gloo′-ti-nus): Viscid; adhesive; sticky.

glutitis (gloo-tī′-tis): Inflammation of the gluteal muscles.

glyc-, glyco-, gluco-: Combining forms denoting glycogen.

glycase (glī′-kās): An enzyme that converts maltose to maltodextrin and dextrose.

glycemia (glī-sē′-mi-a): The presence of glucose in the blood.

glycerin (e) (glis′-er-in): A clear, syrupy liquid prepared synthetically or obtained as a by-product in soap manufacture. It has a hygroscopic action. Widely used in pharmaceutical preparations as a solvent or vehicle for drugs in syrups, lozenges, suppositories. Useful as an emollient (*q.v.*).

glycerol (glis′-er-ol): Glycerin (*q.v.*).

glycerophosphate (glis′-er-ō-fos′-fāt): Any salt of glycerophosphoric acid; several of them are used in compounding so-called "nerve tonics."

glycine (glī′-sēn): A nonessential amino acid; the simplest of the amino acids; found widely distributed in animal and plant proteins; also prepared synthetically; has some uses in medicine.

glycinemia (glī-si-nē′-mi-a): The presence of glycine in the blood.

glycinuria (glī′-sin-ū′-ri-a): Excretion of glycine in the urine. Associated with mental subnormality.

glycocalyx (glī′-kō-kā′-lix): The glycoprotein and polysaccharide covering surrounding many of the body cells.

glycocholic acid (glī′-kō′-kol-ik): An acid found in bile.

glycogen (gli′-kō-jen): The form into which glucose is converted by insulin for storage in the body; when it is needed it is converted to monosaccharides, providing an immediate source of energy. See **glycogen storage disease.**

glycogen storage disease: Any of a group of disorders caused by an inborn error of metabolism and occurring chiefly in childhood. Types I through VI have been recognized, each caused by a different metabolic defect and having different characteristics: Type I, von Gierke's disease; Type II, Pompe's disease; Type III, Cori's disease; Type IV, Andersen's disease, Type V, McArdle's disease; Type VI, Hers' disease.

glycogenase (glī′-kō-jen-ās): An enzyme necessary for the conversion of glycogen into glucose.

glycogenesis (glī-kō-jen′-e-sis): The synthesis or formation of glycogen from glucose or other monosaccharides.—glycogenetic, adj.

glycogenolysis (glī-kō-je-nol′-i-sis): The conversion of glycogen into glucose.

glycogenosis (glī′-kō-je-nō′-sis): A chronic metabolic disorder of childhood leading to increased storage of glycogen, particularly in the kidney and liver. Leads to enlargement of liver, glycogen myopathy, hypoglycemia.

glycogeusia (glī-kō-gū′-si-a): A sweet taste in the mouth.

glycokinase (glī-kō-kī′-nās): An enzyme that, in the presence of ATP (*q.v.*), catalyzes the conversion of glucose to glucose-6-phosphatate.

glycolysis (glī-kol′-i-sis): The enzymatic, anaerobic breakdown of glucose or other carbohydrate in the body, with the formation of lactic acid or pyruvic acid and the release of energy. **AEROBIC G.**, a kind of fermentation in which the potential energy in polysaccharides is activated during such functions as muscle contraction.

glycometabolism (glī′-kō-me-tab′-ō-lizm): The utilization of sugar in the body.—glycometabolic, adj.

glyconeogenesis (glī′-kō-nē-ō-jen′-e-sis): The formation of sugar from protein or fat when there is lack of available carbohydrate.

glycopenia (glī-kō-pē′-ni-a): A deficiency of sugar in the body tissues.

glycopexis (glī-kō-pek′-sis): The fixation and storage of glycogen in the liver.—glycopexic, adj.

glycophilia (glī-kō-fil′-i-a): A condition characterized by the production of hyperglycemia following the ingestion of a small amount of sugar.

glycoprotein (glī-kō-prō′-tē-in): Refers to a class of proteins that contain a carbohydrate group (conjugated proteins); they include the mucins, the mucoids, and chondroproteins.

glycoptyalism (glī-kō-tī′-al-izm): Glycosialia (*q.v.*).

glycorrhachia (glī-kō-rā′-ki-a): The presence of glucose in the cerebrospinal fluid.

glycosemia (glī-kō-sē′-mi-a): Glycemia (*q.v.*).

glycosialia (glī′-kō-sī-ā′-li-a): The presence of sugar in the saliva.

glycosialorrhea (glī′-kō-sī′-a-lō-rē′-a): The secretion of an excessive amount of saliva that contains sugar.

glycoside (gli′-kō-sīd): A complex natural substance composed of a sugar with another compound, particularly as found in some plants, *e.g.*, digitalis, strophanthus, and others. The non-sugar fragment is sometimes of therapeutic value.

glycosometer (glī-kō-som′-e-ter): An instrument for measuring the proportion of sugar in the urine.

glycostatic (glī′-kō-stat′-ik): Tending to maintain a constant level of glycogen in the body tissues.

glycosuria (glī-kō-sū′-ri-a): The presence of an abnormal amount of sugar in the urine.

glycuresis (glī-kū-rē′-sis): The normal appearance of glucose in the urine following a carbohydrate meal.

glycuronic acid (glī-kū-ron′-ik): An acid formed by oxidation during animal metabolism; found in urine in combination with several other substances.

glycyrrhiza (glis-i-rī′-za): Licorice or licorice root; the dried roots of *Glycyrrhiza glabra;* used in several pharmaceutical preparations.

Gm; gm: Gram. G. and g. are also used.

gnath-, gnatho: Combining forms denoting jaw.

gnathalgia (nath-al′-ji-a): Pain in the jaw.

gnathic (nath′-ik): Pertaining to 1) the jaw, or 2) the alveolar processes.

gnathitis (nath-ī′-tis): Inflammation of the jaw.

gnathodynamometer (nath′-ō-dī-na-mom′-e-ter): An instrument used to determine the biting force of the jaws.

gnathodynia (nath-ō-din′-i-a): Pain in the jaw.

gnathology (na-thol′-ō-ji): The study of the mastication process.

gnathoplasty (nath′-ō-plas-ti): Plastic surgery of the jaw.

gnathoschisis (nath-os′-ki-sis): Congenital cleft in the upper jaw, as occurs in cleft palate.

gnosia (nō′-si-a): The faculty of being able to perceive and recognize objects and persons.

-gnosis: Combining form denoting recognition; knowledge.

gnotobiotics (nō′-tō-bī-ot′-iks): The science of producing and raising germ-free animals such as chickens, guinea pigs, rabbits, monkeys, and swine, which are useful in research studies of disease production, immunity, antibody formation, etc., or studies that utilize such animals.—gnotobiotic, adj.

GNP: Abbreviation for Geriatric Nurse Practitioner.

goblet cells: Special secreting cells, shaped like a goblet, found in the mucous membranes, particularly in the stomach, intestines, and respiratory tract; they secrete mucus.

Goeckerman method: A method of treating psoriasis whereby tar is applied to the entire body, which is then irradiated with ultraviolet light and later bathed to remove scales; takes 21 days to complete.

goiter (goy′-ter): A chronic enlargement of the thyroid gland, causing a swelling in front of the neck; may be due to iodine deficiency in the diet, tumor, inflammation, or hyper- or hypofunction of the thyroid gland. **ADENOMATOUS G.**, one in which the gland becomes firm and enlarges more on one side than the other; it may grow slowly and then enlarge greatly during middle age; may become toxic or not. **COLLOID G.**, the gland enlarges and becomes soft due to collection of gelatinous matter in the follicles. **ENDEMIC G.**, occurs in certain areas of the world where the food and water do not contain the normal amount of iodine, but the goiters are usually of the simple type. **EXOPHTHALMIC G.**, gland may or may not enlarge; excess of thyroid hormone is secreted, leading to physical symptoms such as nervousness, loss of weight, profuse sweats, accelerated pulse, psychic disturbances, increased basal metabolism, fine muscle tremor, and exophthalmos (*q.v.*). Also called Graves' disease. **LYMPHADENOID G.**, diffuse enlargement of the thyroid; of unknown cause; marked by epithelial changes and lymphoid hyperplasia. Also called struma lymphomatosa. **MULTINODAL G., G.** in which there are several enlarged colloid lobules; occurs most often in women. **NONTOXIC G.**, simple **G.**, not accompanied by any of the symptoms seen in exophthalmic goiter; due to an enlargement of the gland in response to iodine insufficiency in the diet; may disappear spontaneously. **SUBSTERNAL G.**, enlargement chiefly of the lower part of the isthmus of the thyroid, only slightly palpable or not at all. **TOXIC G.**, exophthalmic **G.**

goitrogen (goy′-trō-jen): Any agent causing goiter.

goitrogenic (goy-trō-jen′-ik): Pertaining to or producing goiter.

gold: A solid yellow metallic element; its salts are used therapeutically in treatment of rheumatoid arthritis. **RADIOACTIVE G.**, used in treatment of certain types of cancer and as a diagnostic scintiscanning agent.

Golden Olympics: An annual sports contest for persons 55 years of age or older.

Goldmark Report: See Nursing and Nursing Education in the United States.

Goldthwaite: GOLDTHWAITE'S BELT, a wide belt with a metal support; for treating back injuries. **G'S. SIGN**, pain occurring in the sacroiliac region when the leg is held straight and flexed at the hip; a sign of sprain of the sacroiliac ligaments. **G'S. STRAP**, a support strap used in treating an injured foot. [Joel Goldthwaite, American orthopedic surgeon. 1866–1961.]

golfers' elbow: A condition comparable to tennis elbow (*q.v.*), with the affected area being the medial condylar region of the humerus; treatment is as for tennis elbow.

Golgi bodies (gol′-jē): Also Golgi apparatus. An anastomosing network of delicate fibrils found near the nucleus in the cytoplasm of nearly all cells. [Camillo Golgi, Italian histologist. 1843–1926.]

gomphiasis (gom-fī′-a-sis): The abnormal loosening of the teeth.

gomphosis (gom-fō′-sis): An immovable joint, where a conical eminence fits into a socket, *e.g.*, a tooth, or the styloid process of the temporal bone.

gon-: Combining form denoting: 1. Semen or seed. 2. Relationship to the knee.

gonad (gō′-nad): One of the essential sex glands of the male or female. See ovary, testis.—gonadal, adj.

gonad-, gonado-: Combining forms denoting a gonad (*q.v.*).

gonadectomy (gōn-a-dek′-tō-mi): Excision of a testis or ovary.

gonadogenesis (gon′-a-dō-jen′-e-sis): The development of the gonads in the embryo.

gonadopathy (gon-a-dop′-a-thi): Any disease of the gonads.

gonadotherapy (gon′-ad-ō-ther′-a-pi): Treatment by the use of gonadal hormones or extracts.

gonadotrophic (gon′-ad-ō-trō′-fik): Gonadotropic (*q.v.*).

gonadotropic (gon′-ad-ō-trō′-pik): Having an affinity for influencing or stimulating the gonads; often refers to the two secretions of the anterior pituitary, *i.e.*, the follicle stimulating hormone and the luteinizing hormone.

gonadotropin (gon′-ad-ō-trō′-pin): Any gonad-stimulating hormone. **HUMAN CHORIONIC G.**, produced in the placenta during the first trimester of pregnancy, reaching a peak in 15 to 18 days following the first missed menses, then declining; its function is to stimulate growth and secretion of the corpus luteum and thus help to maintain the pregnancy; may be demonstrated in the urine and blood; tests for its presence are reliable tests for pregnancy. Also may be used in treatment for underdevelopment of the sex glands.

gonagra (gon-ag′-ra): Gout in the knee. Formerly called gonatagra.

gonalgia (gō-nal′-ji-a): Pain in the knee.

gonangiectomy (gon′-an-ji-ek′-to-mi): Excision of the vas deferens or part of it. Syn., vasectomy.

gonarthritis (gon-ar-thrī′-tis): Inflammation of the knee or knee joint.

gonarthromeningitis (gon-ar′-thrō-men-in-jī′-tis): Inflammation of the synovial membrane of the knee joint.

gonarthrotomy (gon′-ar-throt′-o-mi): Incision into the knee joint.

gonatocele (gō-nat′-ō-sēl): A swelling or tumor of the knee.

gonecystis (gon-e-sis′-tis): A seminal vesicle (*q.v.*).

gonecystitis (gon′-e-sis-tī′-tis): Inflammation of a seminal vesicle.

gonecystolith (gon-e-sis′-tō-lith): A concretion in a seminal vesicle.

goneitis (gon-ē-ī′-tis): Inflammation of the knee.

gonepoiesis (gon-e-poy-ē′-sis): The formation of semen.

goniometer (gō-ni-om′-e-ter): An instrument for measuring angles, *e.g.*, the angle of the mandible. Also used for measuring range of motion in degrees and to test for labyrinthine disease by determining the patient's sense of balance.

gonioplasty (go-ni-ō-plas′-ti): A surgical technique for widening a narrow angle in narrow angle glaucoma; may utilize the laser beam.

goniopuncture (gō′-ni-ō-punk′-tur): An operation for glaucoma in which a knife is inserted through the cornea, across the anterior chamber, and through the opposite corneoscleral wall.

gonioscope (gō′-ni-ō-skōp): An instrument for examining the angle of the anterior chamber of the eye.—gonioscopic, adj.

gonioscopy (gō-ni-os′-kop-i): Measuring or examining the angle of the anterior chamber of the eye with a gonioscope.

goniotomy (gō-ni-ot′-o-mi): Operation for glaucoma. Incision is through the anterior chamber angle to the canal of Schlemm.

gonitis (gō-nī′-tis): Inflammation of the knee.

gonoblennorrhea (gon′-ō-blen-ō-rē′a): Gonorrheal conjunctivitis.

gonococcal complement fixation test: A specific serological test for the diagnosis of gonorrhea.

gonococcemia (gon-ō-kok-sē′-mi-a): The presence of gonococci in the bloodstream.

gonococcicide (gon-ō-kok′-si-sīd): An agent that kills gonococcic organisms.

gonococcus (gon-ō-kok′-us): *Neisseria gonorrhoeae;* a gram-negative, encapsulated diplococcus, usually occurring in pairs; the causative organism of gonorrhea.—gonococci, pl.; gonococcal, adj.

gonorrhea (gon-ō-rē′-ah): An infectious disease of venereal origin caused by the *Neisseria* gonorrhoeae organism; the incubation period is two to five days. Chief manifestations in the adult male are purulent urethritis and dysuria; in the adult female urethritis and endocervicitis; often spreads to the fallopian tubes and the periotoneum. In rare cases the infection is carried by the bloodstream to the heart, joints, or other structures. In children the infection is usually accidental and may occur as 1) ophthalmia neonatorium, acquired during passage through the birth canal, or 2) gonococcal valvovaginitis in girls before puberty and acquired through nonsexual contact with an infected adult.

gonorrheal (gon-ō-rē′-al): Resulting from or caused by gonorrhea. **G. ARTHRITIS**, a manifestation of gonorrheal infection. **G. CONJUNCTIVITIS**, severe purulent conjunctivitis that causes scarring of the cornea and possible blindness. **G. OPHTHALMIA**, one form of ophthalmia neonatorum. **G. SALPINGITIS**, see pelvic inflammatory disease under pelvic.

gony-: Combining form denoting relationship to the knee.

gonycampsis (gon′-i-kamp′-sis): An abnormal bend or curvature of the knee.

gonycrotesis (gon-i-krō-tē′-sis): Knock-knee. Genu valgum.

gonyectyposis (gon′-i-ek-ti-pō′-sis): Bowlegs. Genu varum.

gonyocele (gon′-i-ō-sēl): Synovitis of the knee joint.

gonyoncus (gon-ē-ong′-kus): Tumor of the knee.

Good Samaritan laws: Laws that protect health professionals from civil or criminal liability when they give emergency care to accident or disaster victims. Many states have enacted such laws.

Goodell's sign: Softening of the cervix of the uterus; considered evidence of pregnancy. [W. Goodell, American gynecologist. 1829–1894.]

Goodenough's Draw-a-Person Test: A test for assessing the intelligence of children 3 to 10 years of age.

Goodpasture's syndrome: A serious glomerulonephritis affecting mostly young men; associated with or preceded by pulmonary problems, hemoptysis, anemia, hematuria, proteinuria, and hypertension; rapidly progressive and often fatal. Hemodialysis is used in treatment and, sometimes, kidney transplant.

gooseflesh: Cutis anserina. Roughness of the skin produced by the erection of papillae when the arrectores pilorum muscles attached to the sides of the hair follicles contract under stimulation, usually cold or fear. Also called goose bumps, goose pimples

GOT: Abbreviation for glutamic oxaloacetic transaminase.

gouge (gowj): A chisel with a grooved blade for removing bone.

gout (gowt): A metabolic disorder stemming from biochemical defects in purine metabolism; uric acid is overproduced and retained in the body, and sodium urate crystals are deposited around the joints and other places in the body. Characterized by redness, swelling, pain, and inflammation of the joints, particularly in the great toe; and by hyperuricemia and the formation of stones in the urinary collecting system and tract. Frequently said to be due to heavy eating of rich foods and consumption of alcohol, but may also be familial in origin. TOPHACEOUS G., G. involving an increasing number of joints, including the ankle, knee, and elbow; tophaceous deposits of sodium urate form in subacutaneous and periarticular tissues, the pinna of the ear, along the tendons of fingers and toes, and in bursae.—gouty, adj.

Gower's sign: Unequal contraction of the pupils in reaction to light; an early sign of tabes dorsalis.

GP: Abbreviation for a general practitioner; usually refers to a physician.

GPT: Abbreviation for glutamic pyruvic transaminase.

gr: Abbreviation for grain.

graafian follicle: See under follicle.

gracile (gras′-il): Slender or delicate.

gracilis (gras′-il-is): G. MUSCLE, the long slender muscle at the inner side of the thigh.

graduate (grad′-ū-āt): A pitcher-shaped vessel marked with lines at different levels; used for measuring liquids.

Graefe's knife (grā′-fes): Finely pointed knife with narrow blade, used for making incision across anterior chamber of the eye prior to removal of a cataract. [Albrecht von Graefe, German ophthalmologist. 1828–1870.]

graft: A tissue or organ that is transplanted to another part of the body of the same animal (autograft), or to another animal of the same species (homograft), or to another animal of a different species (heterograft). AUTOGENOUS G., an autograft. BONE G., a piece of bone, usually taken from the tibia (or supplied by a bone bank), and used elsewhere in the body of the individual or a donee. BYPASS G., a G. utilizing a synthetic tube to create a diversion in the bloodstream to bypass an obstructed or weakened blood vessel. CORNEAL G., the transplantation of healthy corneal tissue to a defective cornea. FULL-THICKNESS G., a G. utilizing a full thickness of skin and the subcutaneous tissue. ISOGRAFT, tissue or an organ transplanted from one identical twin to the other. NERVE G., replacement of a segment of a defective nerve with a section from a sound one. PATCH G., a G. of living tissue used to close an incision made in a vein to enlarge its lumen. PEDICLE G., a flap of skin and subcutaneous tissue attached to a pedicle. PINCH G., a small thin piece of skin obtained by lifting it with a needle and slicing it off. SPLIT-THICKNESS G., a skin G. utilizing only part of the skin thickness. THIERSCH G., utilizes small thin split strips of epidermis with part of the dermis; also called Ollier-Thiersch G. and Ollier G.

Graham's law: States that the relative rate of diffusion of any two gases is inversely proportional to the square roots of their densities.

grain: The unit of weight in the apothecaries' system; equivalent to about 1/15 of a gram in the metric system. (Sometimes abbreviated gr, but it is advisable to spell it out.)

-gram: Combining form denoting 1) something written down, 2) something drawn, 3) a recording.

gram, gramme: The unit of weight in the metric system; equivalent to 15.432 grains in the apothecaries' system. Equal to one thousandth of a kilogram.

gram molecular weight: The molecular weight of a compound expressed in grams.

gram molecule: The weight of a substance expressed in grams, the number of grams being equivalent to the molecular weight of the substance; *e.g.*, the molecular weight of hydrogen is 2, therefore a gram molecule of hydrogen weighs 2 grams. Also called gram mole.

gram-negative: See under Gram's stain.

gram-positive: See under Gram's stain.

Gram's stain: A bacteriological stain for differentiation of microorganisms. First, a violet stain is applied, followed by an application of iodine solution; then the material is decolorized by alcohol or an acetone solution, and a counter-stain, safranin, is applied. Organisms that retain the violet color are called gram-positive and those that appear as rose-pink due to discoloration of the first stain are called gram-negative. Also called Gram's method. [Hans Christian Gram, Danish physician. 1853–1938.]

gran mal (grahn mal): Major epilepsy; see epilepsy. **GRAND MAL SEIZURE,** characterized by loss of consciousness, generalized convulsions, frothing at the mouth, cyanosis of the face; usually preceded by an aura.

grandiosity (gran-di-os′-i-ti): In psychiatry, a condition characterized by delusions of grandeur, wealth, importance, or influence.—grandiose, adj.

Grandparents for Tots program: A voluntary organization in which elderly people spend time with children in orphanages or day care centers.

Grantly Dick-Read method: See Read method.

granular (gran′-ū-lar): Made up of, marked by the presence of, or resembling granules.

granulase (gran′-ū-lās): An enzyme that splits starch into dextrin and maltose.

granulation (gran-ū-lā′shun): The outgrowth of new capillaries and connective tissue cells from the surface of an open wound that is not healing by first intention (*q.v.*). **G. TISSUE,** the young, soft tissue formed by granulation.

granule (gran′-ūl): A grain, or a very small distinct mass.

granuloblast (gran′-ū-lō-blast): An immature granulocyte.

granulocyte (gran′-ū-lō-sīt): Any cell containing granules; refers particularly to neutrophils, eosinophils, or basophils that contain granules in their protoplasm; constitute 60 percent of all leukocytes; their function is to engulf and kill invading bacteria by means of a chemical substance formed in the granules.

granulocytopenia (gran′-ū-lō-sī-tō-pē′-ni-a): Decrease of granulocytes in the blood but not to a degree sufficient to warrant the term agranulocytosis (*q.v.*).

granulocytopoiesis (gran′-ū-lō-sī-tō-poy-ē′-sis): The formation or production of granulocytes.

granulocytosis (gran′-ū-lō-sī-tō′-sis): The presence of an abnormally large number of granulocytes in the circulating blood.

granuloma (gran-ū-lō′-ma): A tumor formed of granulation tissue. **G. ANNULARE,** a **G.** characterized by hard reddish nodules that enlarge progressively until a ring is formed; chronic and self-limited; usually seen on the extremities. **EOSINOPHILIC G.,** a benign chronic proliferative process in bone with many eosinophilic cells present, producing one or more bone lesions. **G. INGUINALE,** one of the venereal diseases in which lesions form on the genitals and in the inguinal regions. **PYOGENIC G., G.** characterized by a fungating growth with the granulations consisting of masses of pyogenic organisms; also called **SEPTIC G. SWIMMING POOL G.,** a granulomatous lesion that may develop in abrasions sustained in swimming pools; usually heals spontaneously but slowly; thought to be caused by *Mycobacterium balnei*. **WEGENER'S G.,** a rare serious variant of polyarteritis nodosa, marked by the formation of granulomata in the nose and mouth, which ulcerate causing pain, erosion of bone, renal problems, and development of pulmonary nodules.

granulomatosis (gran′-ū-lō-ma-tō′-sis): A condition characterized by the formation of multiple granulomas in bones and elsewhere. **LYMPHOMATOID G.,** a type of **G.** that resembles leprosy; the lesions have the features of both lymphoma and granuloma. **WEGENER'S G.,** a form of **G.** marked by progression and lesions in the respiratory tract, arteriolitis, and inflammation of most of the body organs.

granulomatous (gran-ū-lom′-a-tus): Resembling a granuloma.

granulopenia (gran′-ū-lō-pē′-ni-a): A decreased number of granulocytes in the circulating blood.

granulosa cells (gran-ū-lō′-sa): Modified epithelial cells that surround the ovum in a follicle; after ovulation they are transformed into granular cells of the corpus luteum.

grape sugar: Dextrose or glucose.

graph (graf): A diagram or curve presenting clinical or experimental data in pictorial form that shows relationships between sets of data.

-graph: Combining form denoting 1) something written; 2) an instrument for writing, recording, or transmitting.

graphanesthesia (graf′-an-es-thē′-zi-a): The inability of one whose eyes are closed to identify words, letters, or numbers traced on the skin; may be indicative of a cortical lesion.

graphesthesia (graf′-es-thē′-zi-a): The ability of one whose eyes are closed to identify words, numbers, or figures traced on the skin.

graphology (graf-ol′-o-ji): The scientific study of handwriting for clues as to an individual's character, aptitudes, and temperament.

graphomotor (graf-ō-mō′-tor): Pertaining to the movements required in writing.

graphorrhea (graf-ō-rē'-a): The writing of a stream of meaningless words or phrases.

graphospasm (graf'-ō-spazm): Writer's cramp; cramping and pain in the muscles of the hand and forearm caused by writing for long periods of time.

-graphy: Combining form denoting 1) writing; 2) a writing on a particular subject.

grasp reflex: The grasping motion exhibited by the fingers or toes in response to stimulation by stroking the palm or sole.

grass: Street term for cannabis or marijuana.

grattage (gra-tazh'): The scraping or brushing of a surface to stimulate healing, or to remove granulations as in treatment of glaucoma.

grave (grāv): Severe; serious; life-threatening.

gravel: Minute stones or sandy deposit occurring in the gallbladder or urinary bladder.

Graves' disease: Hyperthyroidism; see thyrotoxicosis. [Robert James Graves, Irish physician. 1797–1853.]

gravid (grav'-id): Pregnant.

gravida (grav'-i-da): A pregnant woman. Gravida I designates the first pregnancy, gravida II the second, and so on.

gravidarum (grav-id-ar'-um): Literal translation is "of the pregnant." **G. STRIAE,** the purplish longitudinal marks that occur on the skin of the lower abdomen during the later weeks or months of pregnancy.

gravidism (grav'-i-dizm): The state of being pregnant.

gravitational (grav-i-tā'-shun-al): Subject to the force of gravity. **G. ULCER,** varicose ulcer (*q.v.*).

gravity (grav'-i-ti): Weight. **SPECIFIC G.,** the weight of a substance compared with that of an equal volume of water.

Grawitz's tumor: Renal cell carcinoma; hypernephroma. [Paul Albert Grawits, German pathologist. 1850–1932.]

gray matter: Nervous system tissue consisting mostly of cell bodies of neurons and unmyelinated nerve fibers; of grayish color. Occurs in the cortex of the brain, the basal ganglia, and the central H-shaped portion of the spinal cord.

Gray Panthers: Organized in the mid-70s; composed of both older and younger people working together for social change, particularly with respect to some of the problems of the elderly, *e.g.*, housing, health care, financial status.

greater: 1. **GREATER MULTANGULAR,** synonym for the trapezium, one of the bones of the wrist. 2. **GREATER OMENTUM,** see under omentum. 3. **GREATER TROCHANTER,** the larger of the two processes of the femur at the point where the neck joins the shaft; it projects medially and laterally and serves as a site for the attachment of muscles including the gluteal muscles. 4. **GREATER VESTIBULAR GLANDS,** see Bartholin's glands.

green sickness: Chlorosis (*q.v.*).

green soap: A soft gelatinous soap; prepared as a tincture in a two to one solution with alcohol, used for cleansing skin before surgery.

greenstick fracture: See fracture.

grenz rays (grentz): Roentgen rays with wavelengths of from one to 10 Ångstroms; often used in x-ray therapy for skin conditions, because of their light penetration.

Grey Turner's sign: Discoloration of the skin in the area of the loin, which occurs in hemorragic pancreatitis.

grid: A chart with horizontal and perpendicular lines on which curves may be plotted. **WETZEL G.,** a chart on which weight, height, and other factors of growth and development are plotted; used for evaluating physical fitness of young and adolescent children.

grief (grēf): The normal emotional reaction of deep distress, caused by the loss of a loved one or of a treasured object, usually self-limited. Phases of the grief process have been described as 1) numbness or shock, accompanied by disbelief in the grievous event; 2) protest and yearning, accompanied by anger and longing; 3) disorganization, accompanied by chaos, despair, and depression; and 4) reorganization, characterized by acceptance of the event and making plans to resolve the crisis it created. **ANTICIPATORY G.,** grieving that occurs prior to an actual loss either by death or separation from a loved person or object.

Griess's test: A test for detecting the presence of nitrites in the urine as a method of identifying gram-negative enteric bacteria in it.

grieving, dysfunctional: Accepted as a nursing diagnosis by the Fourth National Conference on the Classification of Nursing Diagnoses.

grinders (grīn'-derz): The molars or "double" teeth.

grinders' asthma: See under asthma.

grip: Influenza. Also grippe, la grippe.

gripe (grīp): 1. Colic. 2. A sharp, spasmodic intestinal pain.

gristle: Cartilage (*q.v.*).

grocer's itch: An eczema due to sensitivity to flour, sugar, chocolate, cinnamon, etc.

groin: The junction, or the area of the junction, of the thigh with the abdomen.

groove: In anatomy, a long narrow depression, especially one in a bone or tooth substance.

gross: 1. Large or coarse. 2. Seen as a whole, without fine details. 3. Visible without the use of a microscope.

group: A number of persons or things gathered closely together and forming a recognizable unit. **GROUP PRACTICE,** an arrangement whereby two or three physicians practice together, sharing office space and often secretarial help; the advantages include ease of consultation and the convenience of covering for each other. **GROUP PSYCHOTHERAPY,** see group therapy under therapy .

grouping: Blood grouping. See blood groups.

growing pains: Pains in the musculoskeletal system, the limbs particularly, during youth; thought by some to be rheumatic in origin; other causes that have been suggested are postural defects, emotional problems, muscle fatigue.

growth: 1. Normal progressive development or normal increase in size of any organism. 2. An abnormal increase in size of cells or of tissue, as in a tumor. **G. FACTOR,** any substance such as hormones that promote growth. **G. HORMONE,** a secretion of the anterior part of the pituitary gland that promotes growth and helps to regulate the metabolism of proteins, fats, and carbohydrates.

gruel (groo′-el): A cereal that is cooked or diluted with water, milk, or broth; may be used in liquid diets or for tube feedings.

grunt: A deep gutteral sound in the chest; usually signifies chest pain, as in pneumonic conditions, rib fracture, and neonatal respiratory distress syndrome.

gryposis (grī-pō′-sis): An abnormal curvature. **G. PENIS,** chordee (*q.v.*). **G. UNGUIUM,** abnormal curvature of the nails.

GSW: Abbreviation for gunshot wound.

gt: Abbreviation for *gutta* [L.], meaning drop. Plural, gtt for *guttae*.

GTT: Abbreviation for glucose tolerance test.

GU: Abbreviation for genitourinary.

guaiac test (gwī′-ak): A test for the presence of occult blood in the feces.

guarana (gwa-ra′-na): An astringent prepared from the seeds of a Brazilian tree (*Paullinia cupana*); used as treatment for diarrhea.

gubernaculum (goo-ber-nak′-ū-lum): A fibrous connecting cord between two structures.

Guillain-Barre syndrome (gē-yan′-bar-rā′): A neurologic syndrome; cause unknown but thought to be due to a virus; symptoms include pain, tenderness, and progressive weakness and flaccidity of muscles, ascending paralysis; chief laboratory finding is an increase in protein in the cerebrospinal fluid without accompanying increase in the cell count. Also called idiopathic polyneuritis, acute febrile polyneuritis, infectious polyneuritis.

guillotine (gil′-o-tēn): A surgical instrument for excision of the tonsils.

guilt (gilt): In psychiatry, unconscious **G.** consists of mental reactions that are initiated by unconscious punishment fantasies; suffering that results from gratification of, or drive toward, gratification of a repressed wish.

Guinea worm: A genus of nematodes parasitic to man, found especially in Africa and India; transmitted to humans through infected water; the long thread-like worm burrows through the skin and into the subcutaneous and muscular tissues. *Dracunculus medinensis.*

gullet (gul′-let): The tube by which food passes from the mouth to the stomach; includes the pharynx and esophagus.

gum: 1. The dried sap from certain trees and shrubs, insoluble in ether or alcohol, but mixes with water to form a viscid mass. 2. The gingiva, the fleshy tissue that covers the alveolar processes of the jaw.

gumboil: An abscess on a gum (gingiva); may be due to infection of a tooth, injury, or tooth decay; may rupture spontaneously or require incision.

gumma (gum′-a): A localized area of soft, gummy, vascular, granulation tissue, such as is seen in the later stages (tertiary) of syphilis; may occur in almost any tissue. Obstruction to the blood supply results in necrosis, and gummata near the surface of the body tend to break down, forming chronic ulcers in such places as the nose, lower leg, and palate which heal slowly and probably are not infectious.—gummata, gummas, pl.; gummatous, adj.

gurgling (gur′-gling): A coarse sound heard when auscultating over a large cavity or when there is a large amount of secretion in the trachea.

gurney (ger′-nē): A wheeled stretcher or cart.

gustation (gus-tā′-shun): 1. The act of tasting. 2. The sense of taste.

gustatory (gus′-ta-tor-i): Pertaining to the sense of taste.

gut: 1. The intestines, (informal). 2. Suture material made from the intestine of sheep.

Guthrie test: A legally accepted test for the presence of phenylketonuria in newborns in those states that require testing for the disease; a drop of blood is obtained by heel prick and examined for the presence of phenylalanine; should be done before the eighth day postnatal. Some states require two tests, one before the infant leaves the hospital and another at two weeks of age. [S. Guthrie, American pediatrician. 1916–.]

gutta (gut′-a): A drop. **G. PERCHA,** a waterproof material, formerly much used for surgical drains, among other purposes; now largely replaced by synthetics.

guttate (gut′-āt): 1. Having small, usually colored, spots or drops. 2. Drop-shaped.

guttatim (gut-tā′-tim): Drop by drop.

guttur (gut′-ter): The throat.—guttural, adj.

gymnastics (jim-nas′-tiks): Physical exercises that may be simple or complicated, ranging from calisthenics to acrobatics and performed with or without special equipment; may be done for prophylactic, curative, or corrective purposes.

gymnophobia (jim-nō-fō′-bi-a): Morbid dread of viewing a naked body.

gyn-, gyne-, gynec-, gyneco-, gyno: Combining forms denoting 1) woman; 2) female reproductive organs.

gynae-: For words beginning thus see words beginning gyn-.

gynandrism (gī-nan′-drizm, ji-nan): Female pseudohermaphroditism. See **pseudohermaphroditism.**

gynandromorphism (gī-nan-drō-mor′-fizm, ji-nan): An abnormality in which certain parts of an individual have both female and male characteristics.—gynandromorphous, adj.

gynatresia (gī-na-trē′-zi-a, ji-nan): The occlusion of part of the female genital tract, particularly the vagina.

gynecic (gī-nē′-sik, ji-nan): Pertaining to women.

gynecogen (gin′-e-kō-jen, ji′-ne): Any substance such as a hormone that stimulates the development of female characteristics.

gynecography (gin-e-kog′-ra-fi): Roentgenography of the female reproductive organs after the introduction of air into the peritoneal cavity and with the patient in the knee-chest position; the film shows the shape and size of the ovaries.

gynecoid (gin′-e-koyd, jī′-ne): Resembling a woman, or having female characteristics; refers especially to a pelvis that is shaped like a female pelvis.

gynecologic (gin-e-kō-loj′-ik, jī′-ne): 1. Affecting or relating to the female reproductive tract. 2. Related to gynecology.

gynecologist (gin-e-kol′-ō-jist, jī-ne): A physician who specializes in gynecology.

gynecology (gin-e-kol′-ō-ji,jī-ne): The branch of medicine that deals with disorders of the female genital tract.

gynecomania (gin-e-kō-ma′-ni-a, jī′-ne): Satyriasis (*q.v.*); excessive sexual desire in a male; may be of psychologic origin. Also called satyromania.

gynecomastia (gin-e-kō-mas′-ti-a, jī-ne): Excessive enlargement of the male mammary glands.

gynecopathy (gin-e-kop′-a-thi, jī-ne): Any disease peculiar to women.

gynephobia (gin-e-fo′-bia, jī-ne): Morbid dread of, or aversion of, women.

gyniatrics (gin-i-at′-riks, jī-ni): Treatment of the diseases of women.

gynoplasty (gin′-ō-plas-ti, jī′-no): Plastic or reconstructive surgery of female reproductive organs.

gypsum (jip′-sum): Plaster of Paris (calcium sulphate).

gyrate (jī′-rāt): 1. To revolve. 2. Twisted into a spiral or ring shape.

gyrectomy (jī-rek′-to-mi): Surgical removal of a gyrus (*q.v.*) from the surface of the cortex of the brain.

gyrus (jī′-rus): Convolution. Term is used specifically to describe the tortuous elevations on the surface of the cortex of the brain; these elevations are separated from each other by shallow grooves called sulci and deep grooves called fissures.—gyri, pl.

H

H: Symbol for hydrogen.

h: Abbreviation for hour(s).

habilitate (ha-bil′-i-tāt): To clothe, equip, educate or train the handicapped or the physically or mentally disabled to function better in their environment.—habilitation, n.

habit: 1. A constant automatic response to a given situation, acquired by frequent repetition; when applied to thoughts, thinking habits become attitudes that influence behavior patterns. 2. The repeated, steady use of addictive drugs or narcotics. **H. SPASM,** sudden, rapid, twitching, coordinated movement of muscles of a certain area, habitually repeated, voluntary at first, becoming involuntary. **H. TRAINING,** teaching a child to acquire certain habits that will enable him to adjust to his environment as he grows, primarily habits related to eating, dressing, sleeping, and elimination.

habitual (ha-bit′-ū-al): 1. Formed or established, by frequent repitition. 2. Usual, frequent, steady, much seen or done, or used. **H. ABORTION,** abortion occuring spontaneously three or more times, always before the 20th week of a pregnancy.

habituation (ha-bit-ū-ā′-shun): The act or process of becoming accustomed to a stimulus or environment. **DRUG H.,** psychological dependence on a drug when there is no physical need for it; the craving for the pleasurable or desirable effects of a drug is usually followed by its compulsive use. Usually there is no tendency to increase the dose and, on this basis, **H.** is often differentiated from drug addiction.

habitus (hab′-i-tus): The physical characteristics of a person, particularly the tendency to develop some disease or such fault as an inborn error of metabolism.

hacking (hak′-ing): 1. Short, chopping blows; a maneuver used in massage. 2. Short, dry, interrupted coughing.

haem (hēm): Heme (*q.v.*).

haem-: For words beginning thus see words beginning hem-.

Haemophilus (hē-mof′-i-lus): See Hemophilus.

Hageman factor: Factor XII. See under factor.

Hagie pin: A pin used in surgical treatment of fracture of the hip.

Haglund's disease: Achilles' bursitis; see under bursitis.

hahnemannian (hah-ne-man′-i-an): Relating to Hahnemann or to the doctrine of homeopathy which he taught. See homeopathy.—hahnemannism, n.

hair: Thread-like filament present on all parts of human skin except the palms, soles, lips, glans penis and that surrounding the terminal phalanges. Also the aggregation of such filaments, especially on the scalp. Consists of a shaft and a bulb-like root. **EXCLAMATION-MARK H.,** the broken off stump found at the periphery of spreading bald patches in alopecia areata; atrophic thinning of the hair shaft gives this characteristic shape—hence its name. **H. CELLS,** usually pertains to the hairs in the organ of Corti in the inner ear; they function as receptors for the sensation of sound. **H. FOLLICLE,** see under follicle. **H. PULLING,** trichotillomania. **H. TRANSPLANTATION,** the surgical process of transplanting hair follicles from one part of the scalp to another, a time-consuming technique that is sometimes used to correct baldness.

hairball: Trichobezoar (*q.v.*).

hairy tongue: A condition in which the filiform papillae of the tongue become enlarged and discolored, due to the presence of bacteria and food pigments. May also occur as a side effect of certain antibiotics.

halation (ha-lā′-shun): Blurring of vision caused by strong light or illumination coming from the direction in which one is looking.

halazone (hal′-a-zōn): A white powder containing chlorine, useful in disinfecting drinking water.

Haldane effect: The amount of carbon dioxide that can be carried by the blood as carbinohemoglobin decreases when the PO_2 of the blood increases. [John S. Haldane, British physiologist. 1860–1936.]

half life: 1. The time it takes the radioactivity of a substance to decay to one-half its original value. 2. In pharmacology, the time it takes for the concentration of a drug to decrease by one-half in the blood serum; used to determine the optimum dosing interval to provide the person with therapeutic but nontoxic dosage.

halfway house: A special residence for individuals who do not need full-time hospital care but are not yet ready to return to independent community living, or who are not able to behave in a manner acceptable to the community at large.

halibut liver oil: A very rich source of vitamins A and D. The smaller dose required makes it more acceptable than cod liver oil.

halitosis (hal-i-tō′-sis): Bad breath. Often due to poor oral hygiene, but may also be caused by oral infections, dental problems, certain foods, alcohol, smoking, systemic disease.

Hall-Stone ring: An intrauterine contraceptive device.

hallucination (ha-lū′-si-nā′-shun): A sensory experience of something that does not exist; unique to the individual; occurs without any true sensory stimulus but regarded by the person as real. May be auditory, gustatory, olfactory, kinetic, tactile, or visual. A common symptom in severe schizophrenia and confusional states; may be induced by drugs, alcohol, or stress. **COMMAND H.,** H. in which the person is "commanded" by imaginary voices to perform certain acts. **HYPNAGOGIC H.,** occurs at a time between sleep and wakefulness. **KINESTHETIC H.,** involves a false perception of the sensation of movement. **LILLIPUTIAN H.,** H. of small objects or animals, often rapidly moving. **SENSORY H.,** involves a mental impression of sensory vividness without any external stimulation; includes H.'s of taste, smell, hearing, vision. **VISCERAL H.,** involves visceral sensations,—hallucinatory, adj.

hallucinogen (ha-lū′-si-nō-jen): An agent, drug, or specifically, a chemical such as mescaline or LSD, that is capable of altering the perception of sensations such as sight, sound, and touch, and of producing hallucinations.

hallucinogenic (ha-lū′-si-nō-jen′-ik): 1. Pertaining to a stimulus that creates the impression that one is having a hallucination. 2. Pertaining to hallucinogens.

hallucinosis (ha-lū′-si-nō′-sis): A psychosis in which the patient is grossly hallucinated, although in a state of clear consciousness. Usually a subacute state of delirium; the predominant symptoms are auditory, gustatory, or visual illusions and hallucinations. **ALCOHOLIC H.,** that occurring in chronic alcoholism.

hallus (hal′-us): Hallux (*q.v.*).

hallux (hal′-uks): The great toe. **H. DOLOROSUS,** pain in the great toe, especially when walking, often associated with flatfoot. **H. FLEXUS,** hammertoe involving the great toe. **H. RIGIDUS,** ankylosis and progressive loss of motion in the great toe joint, may be due to arthritis, trauma, or deformity. **H. VALGUS,** lateral deviation of the great toe, as in a bunion. **H. VARUS,** inward deviation of the great toe.

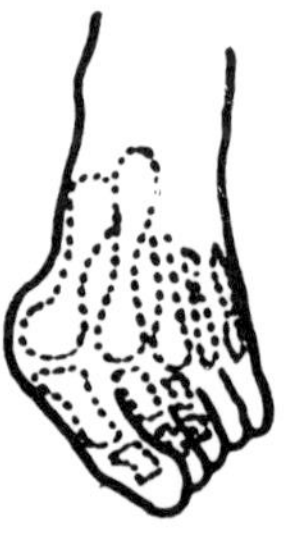

Hallux valgus

halo (hā′-lō): A circle of light, particularly the flashing colored circles seen around lights by patients with glaucoma. **H. TRACTION,** see under traction.

halogen (hal′-ō-jen): Any one of a family of elements that includes bromine, chlorine, fluorine, and iodine.

halothane (hal′-ō-thān): A clear, colorless, non-explosive liquid used as an inhalation anesthetic.

Halsted's operation: 1. Radical mastectomy including removal of the supraclavicular lymph nodes; done for cancer of the breast, see also mastectomy. 2. Radical surgery for correction of inguinal hernia.

hamartome (ham-ar-tō′-ma): A malformation that resembles a neoplasm but is caused by faulty development of an organ. There is an abnormal arrangement or proportion of the elements normally found in the particular location; the malformation grows at the same rate as normal tissues grow.—hamartomatous, adj.

hamate (ham′-āt): The medial bone in the second row of wrist bones. Also hamatum.

hammer: The hammer-shaped bone of the middle ear; the malleus. **PERCUSSION H.,** a rubber-headed hammer used to tap various parts of the body to produce sounds for diagnostic purposes. **REFLEX H.,** a rubber-headed hammer for tapping tendons, muscles or nerves to elicit reflexes during physical examination.

hammertoe: A claw-like deformity of the foot in which there is permanent hyperextension of the first phalanx and plantar flexion of the second and third phalanges. May be congenital or the result of hallux valgus (*q.v.*) or too tight shoes.

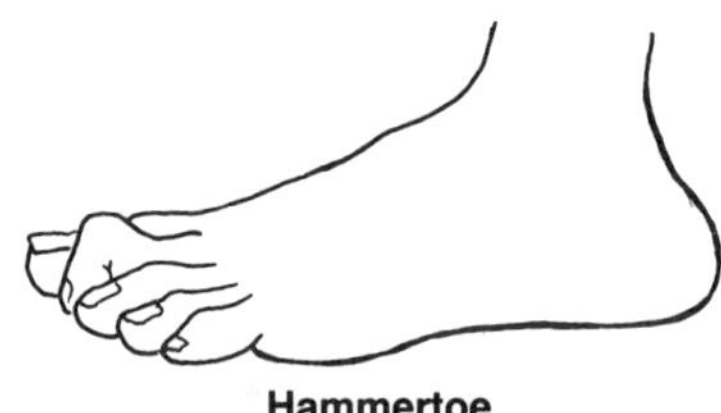

Hammertoe

hamstring: Name given to 1) the tendons on either side of the popliteal space; 2) the three muscles on the posterior aspect of the thigh; their function is to flex the leg at the knee and to adduct and extend the thigh; they are the semimembranous, senitendinous, and biceps femoris muscles.

hamulus (ham′-ū-lus): In anatomy, a hook-shaped process, usually of bone.

hand roll: A roll of cloth or cylinder-shape object held in the hand to counteract the tendency to remain contracted and closed or loosely open and flaccid. The objective is to prevent contractures by keeping the hand in a functional position.

handedness: A tendency to prefer to use one or the other hand in all voluntary motor acts, depending on cerebral dominance, *i.e.*, in a right-handed person the left side of the cerebrum is dominant, and vice versa.

hand-foot syndrome: A condition seen in patients with sickle cell hemoglobinopathy. There is painful swelling of the hands and feet, occuring at about two years of age; in older persons other joints are affected; caused by an impairment in circulation to the metacarpal and metatarsal bones.

handicap: 1. Pertains to the interference a particular disability creates in a person's efforts to perform the activities inherent in a given life area. 2. A physical or mental disability or impairment; may be congenital due to impairment of normal function, or to a static condition of a disease or disorder.

Hand-Schüller-Christian disease or **syndrome:** Generalized lipid histiocytosis of bones; an inborn error of fat metabolism. Occurs chiefly in children and young adults; marked by exophthalmos, bone defects, growth retardation, otitis media, yellowish skin, loss of teeth; development of diabetes insipidus. Associated with mental retardation.—Syn., histiocytosis. Also called Schüller-Christian disease, Schüller's disease, Christian disease, and Letterer-Siwe disease.

hanging drop: A method of preparing microorganisms for microscopic study. A drop of liquid containing the microorganisms is suspended from a cover glass over a depression in a glass slide.

hangnail (hang′-nāl): A narrow strip of skin, partly detached from the nail fold.

hangover: Popular term for the headache, nausea, thirst, fatigue, irritability, and other unpleasant after-effects, usually occurring in the morning, after overindulgence of alcoholic beverages or other central nervous system depressants.

Hanot's disease (an′-ōz): Hypertrophic cirrhosis of the liver with jaundice, splenomegaly, and fever. [Victor Charles Hanot, French physician. 1844–1896.]

Hansen's disease: Leprosy (*q.v.*). [Gerhard H. A. Hansen, Norwegian physician. 1841–1912.]

haploid (hap′-loid): Having half the number of chromsomes normally carried by the particular cell or cells.

hapten (hap′-ten): The part of an antigenic molecule that determines its specific immunologic character and potential.

haptoglobins (hap-tō-glō′-binz): Globulins that bind any free hemoglobin in the blood plasma and then allow it to be excreted in the urine; increased in any inflammatory disease and in patients on steroid therapy; decreased in hemolysis, severe liver disease, and infectious mononucleosis.

hard palate: the "roof" of the mouth.

hardening: HARDENING OF THE ARTERIES, arteriosclerosis (*q.v.*).

harelip: A congenital defect in the lip; a fissure extending from the margin of the lip to the nostril; may be single or double, and is often associated with cleft palate.

harlequin color change: A condition sometimes seen in normal newborns, especially the immature. A transient redness of the skin that develops on the side on which the baby is lying; the coloration stops abruptly at the midline.

Harrington rod: Part of the Harrington distraction system for correcting scoliosis; consists of a rigid rod that is wedged beneath the lamina of the vertebrae at either end of the curve on the concave side and then forcibly opened to the degree possible during a fusion operation; the rod remains in situ.

Harrison: [Edward Harrison, London physician. 1766–1838.] HARRISON'S GROOVE, a groove that extends laterally from the xiphoid process of the sternum and corresponding to the line of attachment of the diaphragm; seen in rickets. HARRISON'S SULCUS, pigeon-breast deformity seen in asthma when the sternum is pushed forward and a groove forms along the line of the 6th rib; may be reversible.

Harrison Narcotics Licensing Act: Usually referred to as the Harrison Narcotics Act, a federal law enacted in 1915, which imposes strict regulations on the purchase, possession, sale, or prescription of narcotics such as cocaine, morphine, opium; requires that physicians and hospitals keep accurate records of all narcotics purchased and dispensed. Violations are punishable by heavy fines, imprisonment, or both.

Hartmann's solution: A saline solution containing sodium lactate; used in treating acidosis. Lactated Ringer's solution.

Hartnup disease: A disease believed to be due to an inborn error of protein metabolism. Associated with mental subnormality. Characterized by red scaly rash following exposure to sunlight, cerebellar ataxia, emotional instability, excessive excretion of indican.

Harvard Criteria for Death: See under death.

Harvard Medical School Project Omega: An institute for the study of death and dying.

Harvey, William: Noted English physician; discovered how the blood circulates in the body; expounded his theory of circulation in 1628. [1578–1657.]

Harvey-Rand-Rittler plates: Any one of several polychromatic plates used in assessing color vision.

hasheesh: Hashish (*q.v.*).

Hashimoto's disease: A condition in which the thyroid gland is infiltrated with lymphocytes, resulting in destruction of the parenchyma and mild hypothyroidism. Occurs in middle-aged females mostly, and is a result of being sensitized to one's own thyroid protein, thyroglobulin. Also called Hashimoto's thyroiditis, struma lymphomatosa, and lymphadenoid goiter. See autoimmunization. [H. Hashimoto, Japanese surgeon. 1881–1934.]

hashish (hash′-ēsh): Cannabis indica (*q.v.*).

Hassall's corpuscle: A characteristic, rounded body in the medulla of the thymus gland; it is considered to be the source of thymosin, which has some of the properties of a hormone. Also called Hassall's body.

haunch: The hip and buttock.

haustration (haws-trā′-shun): 1. Haustrum (*q.v.*). 2. The formation of a haustrum.

haustrum (haw′-strum): One of the sacculations in the colon; these sacculations or pouches are caused by the longitudinal bands along the colon that are slightly shorter than the gut itself,—haustra, pl.; haustral, adj.

haversian (ha-ver′-shan): H. SYSTEM, the makeup of compact bone. Consists of a central canal that contains blood vessels, lymphatics, nerves; lamellae (*q.v.*) arranged around the canal; spaces between the lamellae are called lacunae; and the fine channels are called canaliculi, which bring nutrients and oxygen to the osteocytes. H. CANALS, see above. [Clopton Havers, English physician. 1650–1702.]

hay fever: A seasonal form of allergic rhinitis in which the release of histamine in response to exposure to a pollen, or other antigen to which the individual is sensitive, results in irritation of the conjunctiva and the mucous membranes of the upper respiratory tract.

Haygarth's nodes: Swelling of joints (exostoses) sometimes seen in the fingers of patients suffering from arthritis. [John Haygarth, English physician. 1740–1827.]

Hb, hb: Abbreviations for hemoglobin.

HB_sAg: Abbreviation for hepatitis-B surface antigen. See Australia antigen.

HBIG: Abbreviation for hepatitis-B immune globulin.

HbO_2: Chemical formula for oxyhemoglobin.

HBV: Abbreviation for hepatitis-B virus.

HCFA: Abbreviation for Health Care Financing Administration.

HCG: Abbreviation for Human chorionic gonadotropin, obtained from the placenta. HCG TEST, a serology test using anti-HCG, which will show the presence or absence of HCG in the serum; a positive test result is a reliable indicator of pregnancy.

hct: Abbreviation for hematocrit. Also written HCT.

head: 1. The uppermost structure of the body, containing the brain and organs of hearing, speech, smell, and taste. 2. The superior or uppermost part of an organ or structure. 3. A rounded eminence on a bone that articulates with another bone at a joint. H. NOISES, see tinnitus.

head box: A device that fits loosely around the head; used in oxygen therapy for babies and small children to confine oxygen-rich atmosphere.

head halter: See halter traction, under traction.

headache: Pain in the head. Often accompained by nausea, as in migraine H. Of many types; described both as to location and quality of the pain: frontal, one-sided, top-of-the-head, sharp, dull, pulsating or throbbing, steady, intermittent, depressing. May be hereditary or familial, and of sudden or gradual onset. Causes include worry, lack of sleep, fatigue, hunger, tension, anxiety, high blood pressure, epilepsy, indigestion, constipation, liver and kidney disorders, allergy, eye disorders, sinusitis, fever, onset of a communicable disease, intake of certain foods, *e.g.*, chocolate, or premenstrual tension. CLUSTER H., migrainous neuralgia; occurs in clusters, with attacks several times a day for days or weeks, followed by long headache-free periods; the intense pain is unilateral, located in the eye region, and accompanied by coryza, tearing, flush, and constricted pupil. OCULAR H., results from a pathological or functional disorder of one or more ocular structures. MIGRAINE H., see migraine. SICK H., migraine H. SINUS H., caused by congestion and edema of the nasal and paranasal mucous membranes; may be related to allergens, infection, or some anatomical anomaly. TENSION H., due to habitual overwork or emotional strain. TRACTION H., caused by stretching of intracranial structures by a space-occupying lesion. VASCULAR H., migraine H.

headward acceleration: In aerospace travel, the acceleration of the body forward following the direction of the head; this causes the blood to rush from the head downward in the body.

Heaf multiple puncture test: A test for tuberculosis that utilizes a stainless steel disk with four prongs or tines, precoated with tuberculin, a purified protein derivative of tubercle bacilli; when the tines are pressed against the volar surface of the forearm; they penetrate the outer layer of skin. The test is said to be positive if a hard raised red spot develops around the puncture area. Also called tine test.

healing (hē′-ling): Curing. The natural process of getting well or of repair of disordered body parts or tissues. **H. BY FIRST INTENTION,** occurs when the edges of a clean wound are accurately held together and heal with the minimum of scarring and deformity. **H. BY SECOND INTENTION,** occurs when the edges of a wound unite after the formation of granular tissue. **H. BY THIRD INTENTION,** occurs when granular tissue fills the wound cavity, followed by the formation of scar tissue.

health: The state of an individual who enjoys physical, mental, and social well-being, in the absence of disease or other abnormal condition.

health assessment: An evaluation of a person's state of health based on data obtained from the health history and the physical examination.

health behavior: Any health maintenance activity that is undertaken by an individual who believes himself to be healthy, as opposed to illness behavior, which refers to activities undertaken by one who has symptoms of illness.

health care: A service sought by people who need help for physical or emotional problems. **H.C. INSTITUTIONS,** institutions devoted to the care of the sick, aged, or infirm; includes hospitals, convalescent homes and hospitals, health clinics, nursing homes, extended care facilities, home health agencies, health maintenance organizations. **PRIMARY H.C.,** includes ambulatory care, treatment of acute illnesses and disabilities, management of common chronic disorders, guidance and counseling to individuals and families, preventive measures.

health care delivery system: A complex group of agencies and services the purpose of which may be to prevent illness by focusing on wellness and health; to provide treatment for health problems; or to provide supportive or rehabilitative care. The patient may utilize services from one or more agencies at different times or at the same time.

Health Care Financing Administration (HCFA): Established in 1981 as an Administration within the Department of Health and Human Services. Provides funds for nursing home care and assistance to nursing home facilities; administers the Medicare and Medicaid programs.

health care team: A group of health care professionals working both independently and collaboratively in providing health care to patients; may include physicians, nurses, social workers, various therapists.

health history: Data obtained from the patient, his family, and other sources regarding his present and past physical and psychological health; used in diagnosing his present illness and in planning his care and followup.

Health Maintenance Organization (HMO): A form of group practice by physicians and allied personnel. The HMO Act of 1973 (Title XIII of the U.S. Public Health Service) provided for funding and outlined services to be provided including physician care and diagnostic and treatment services, often also including services in such specialty areas as dentistry, ophthmalology, audiology, and psychiatry. Subscribers pay a premium set in advance of services and a small fee when services are required. The emphasis throughout is on the maintenence of health and continuity of care.

hearing: 1. The special sense that enables one to perceive sound. 2. The ability to perceive the sensation of sound. **H. LOSS,** inpairment in ability to hear, sometimes within only certain frequencies. May be 1) **CONDUCTIVE LOSS,** due to damage to the conducting mechanism of the ear, usually by a congenital malformation or an obstruction, or may be the result of infection; 2) **MIXED LOSS,** consisting of both conductive and sensorineural loss; or 3) **SENSORINEURAL LOSS,** due to damage to the organ of Corti (*q.v.*), the cochlear nerve, or the auditory branch of the acoustic nerve. **H. TEST,** any test of one's ability to hear, usually by means of an audiometer or tuning fork. **RESIDUAL H.,** the amount of hearing that a hard-of-hearing person has retained.

hearing aid: Any of several types of devices worn in or near the external auditory canal to improve hearing. The type which is worn on the body has a receiver that is worn in the external auditory canal and is connected by an electric cord to a case containing a microphone, amplifier, transmitter, and battery. Many all-in-the-ear types are available.

heart: The hollow muscular organ that pumps blood through the body; situated behind the sternum, lying obliquely between the two lungs. It weighs 8 to 12 ounces in the female and 10 to 12 ounces in the male. The heart is made up of four chambers, the right and left atria and the right and left ventricles. The muscular heart wall has three layers: the outer serous layer, the epicardium; the middle muscular layer, the myocardium; and the inner membranous layer, the endocardium. The flow of blood into, out of, and through the heart is controlled by valves. The heart is enclosed in a fibroserous sac, the epidardium, and the space between it and the pericardium is called the pericardial cavity. **H. ARREST,** cardiac arrest, see under cardiac. **HEART ATTACK,** see myocardial infarct, under infarct. **H. CATHETERIZATION,** see under catheterization. **H. FAILURE,** sudden fatal stoppage of the heartbeat as may occur in coronary thrombosis; when it is the result of failure to maintain adequate circulation in all parts of the body there is congestion of blood in the portal and pulmonary circulations, and then it is called congestive heart failure. **H. MASSAGE,** cardiac massage; see under cardiac. **H. MURMUR**, see murmur. **H. RATE**, the number of times the heart beats per minute. **H. SOUNDS**, four sounds heard over the heart area are recognized; the first sound (lub), S_1, is dull and prolonged; it coincides with the closing of the mitral and tricuspid valves and the beginning of ventricular systole. The second sound (dup), S_2, coincides with the closing of the aortic and pulmonary valves and the beginning of the filling of the atria. The third sound is dull, weak, and low-pitched; may be heard most clearly over the apex; is often compared to the sound of Ken-tuk′-kē; is caused by the rapid filling of the ventricles and may be normal in children and adults; may also indicate some cardiac pathology, hypertension or congestive heart failure. The fourth sound is heard best at the apex during atrial contraction and may or may not be considered pathological. When the third and fourth sounds are considered pathological, they are referred to as gallop. See also gallop, click, murmur, thrill. **HEART STROKE VOLUME**, see under volume. **H. VALVES**, the valves that control and regulate the flow of blood through and from the heart; they are the atrioventricular (mitral and tricuspid), aortic, and pulmonary valves.

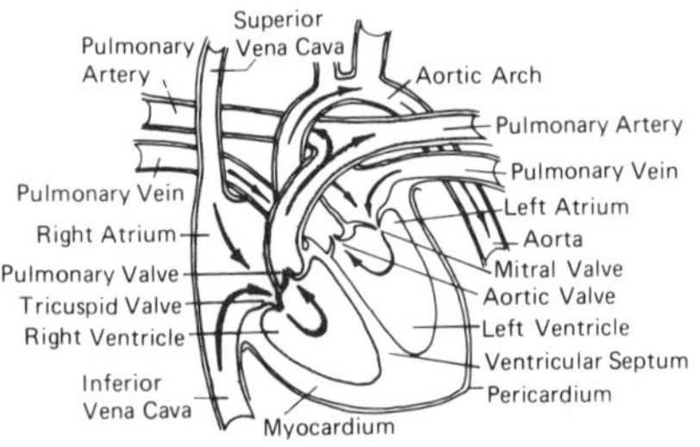

Cross section of heart

heart block: Partial or complete inhibition of the conduction of the electrical impulse from the atrium to the ventricle of the heart. The cause may be an organic lesion or a functional disturbance. In its mildest form it can only be detected electrocardiographically, while in its complete form the ventricles beat at their own intrinsic rate uninfluenced by the atria. Usually described according to degree; first degree block, **B.**, all impulses from the atria reach the ventricles but only after lengthy delay at the A-V node; second degree block, some but not all of the impulses from the atria reach the ventricles; third degree block, all conditions for A-V conduction are present but conduction does not take place. **ATRIOVENTRICULAR B.**, delay or interruption in conduction of impulses through the A-V node and bundle of His; heart block. **BUNDLE BRANCH B.**, complete or incomplete blockage of conduction in either right or left branch of the bundle of His (*q.v.*), or of both branches. **COMPLETE HEART B.**, a blockage of conduction of all atrial impulses in the heart, often refers specifically to atrioventricular block. **CONGENITAL HEART B.**, present at birth; due to defective development of the conduction tissues of the heart. **HEMIBLOCK**, of either the anterior or posterior branch of one of the fascicles of the left branch of the bundle of His. **INTRA-ATRIAL B.**, interference with conduction through the atria. **INTRAVENTRICULAR B.**, delayed conduction through the ventricles or the myocardium. **MOBITZ TYPE I BLOCK**, impulses from the atria to the ventricles are delayed for increasingly longer periods of time until finally one impulse is not conducted at all and then the cycle starts over again. May be caused by certain drugs or be associated with myocardial infarction; sometimes hereditary. Usually transient and may not require treatment. **MOBITZ TYPE II BLOCK**, the block between the atria and ventricles is in one of the bundle branches; may be congenital but usually associated with the use of certain drugs or due to the effects of myocardial infarction, or of sclerosing, on the conduction system. **MONOFASCICULAR B.**, a slowing of conduction velocity or a block in a fascicle of the right or left bundle branch. **SINUS B.**, a block in the conduction system between the sinoatrial node and the atria; results in a complete cardiac cycle being stopped. See also Wenckebach phenomenon.

heartburn: A vague scalding or burning sensation felt behind the sternum, usually associated with acid regurgitation after eating; caused by incompetence of the sphincter muscle at the lower end of the esophagus; usually follows ingestion of fatty foods, caffeine, or nicotine; may be relieved by ingestion of certain medicinal substances, antacids in particular. Also called pyrosis and waterbrash.

heart-lung machine: A mechanical pump used in heart surgery; it shunts the blood from the venous circulation through the machine where it is oxygenated, and returns it to the arterial circulation.

heat: 1. The form of energy that produces a sensation of warmth opposed to cold. 2. To expose a substance, or the body, to a source of heat that characteristically causes an increase in the temperature of the substance or the body. 3. The sensation of an increase in temperature. **H. CRAMPS**, spasms of voluntary muscles; usually occur in otherwise healthy persons following exercise during hot weather; due to loss of sodium chloride and water through excessive sweating. **H. EXHAUSTION**, collapse, with or without loss of consciousness, suffered in conditions of heat and high humidity, resulting largely from loss of fluid and salt by sweating; if the surrounding air becomes saturated, heat stroke will ensue, characterized by pallor, cold clammy skin, rapid pulse, normal or subnormal temperature. **H. FLASH,** a sudden transitory sensation of warmth; may involve the entire body; occurs as a symptom during menopause. **LATENT H.,** excess body heat that is used up in the evaporation of sweat. **H. PRODUCTION,** in the body, is accomplished chiefly by metabolism. **RADIANT H., H.** applied to the surface of the body from a source of infrared radiation. **SENSIBLE H.,** heat that results in a rise in temperature of a body when absorbed. **SPECIFIC H.,** the heat required to raise the temperature of 1 gram of a substance 1 degree as compared to that required to raise the temperature of water through 1 degree. **PRICKLY H., H. RASH,** see miliaria. **H. STROKE,** a serious condition produced by prolonged exposure to excessive temperatures; symptoms include hot, dry skin, headache, dizziness, rapid pulse, high fever; in severe cases coma and death may ensue; see h. exhaustion. **H. SYNCOPE,** dizziness, fatigue and sudden faintness after exercising in the heat; accompanied by weak pulse, sweaty pale skin, decrease in blood pressure; recovery follows removal from direct heat. **H. OF VAPORIZATION,** the amount of heat needed to convert water into steam over and above that needed to bring it to the boiling point; this amount is released when steam is reconverted into water.

heat labile: Thermolabile (*q.v.*).

hebephrenia (hē-be-frē′-ni-a): A type of schizophrenia (*q.v.*) most often seen in adolescents; characterized by silly, uncoordinated, meaningless behavior; giggling; superficial mannerisms; incoherent talk; delusions.

Heberden: 1. **H'S.** disease; angina pectoris. 2. **H'S. NODES,** small osseous swellings at terminal phalangeal joints occurring in many types of arthritis. [William Heberden, English physician. 1710–1801.]

hedonism (hē′-don-izm): Excessive devotion to pleasure, so that a person's conduct is determined by an unconscious drive to seek pleasure and avoid unpleasant things.

heel spur: A bony projection on the heel, caused by deposit of calcium during healing of chronic injury to the plantar fascia of the calcaneus (*q.v.*).

heelcord: Achilles tendon, see under Achilles.

Hegar's sign: Marked softening of the cervix in early pregnancy. [Alfred Hegar, German gynecologist. 1830–1914.]

Heidelberg arm: An artificial arm that is activated by means of carbon dioxide released from a cylinder.

Heimlich maneuver: An emergency procedure for dislodging an object in the trachea that is choking a person. The rescuer stands behind the person who may be standing or sitting, wraps his arms about the victim, makes a fist with one hand, places it on the person's abdomen above the navel and below the rib cage, grasps the fist with the other hand and makes a quick upward thrust against the victim's abdomen causing the diaphragm to contract and force a column of air up against the obstruction. The maneuver may have to be repeated several times. If the person is lying down, the rescuer kneels beside the person and executes the same maneuver except that the heel of the hand is used instead of the fist. Also called abdominal thrust maneuver and the hug of life. [Henry J. Heimlich, American thoracic surgeon. 1920–.]

Heinz bodies: Small, round, oval, or irregularly shaped particles of denatured hemoglobin sometimes found in red blood cells; they indicate potential instability of the cells.

helcoplasty (hel′-kō-plas-ti): Plastic surgery or repair of tissues damaged by ulcers, utilizing healthy skin grafts.

helcosis (hel-kō′-sis): Ulceration; ulcer formation.

heli-, helio-: Combining forms denoting 1) sun, sunlight; 2) solar energy.

helicotrema (hel′-i-kō-trē′-ma): The passage that connects the scala tympani and the scala vestibuli at the apex of the cochlea.

heliosensitivity (hē′-li-ō-sen-si-tiv′-i-ti): Sensitivity to the sun's rays.

heliosis (hē-li-ō′-sis): Sunstroke.

heliotherapy (hē′-li-ō-ther′-a-pi): Treatment by exposure of the body to the sun's rays.

helium (hē′-li-um): A colorless, odorless, tasteless, inert gas. Sometimes used in medicine as a diluent for other gases.

helix (hē′-liks): 1. The curved fold forming most of the rim of the external ear. 2. A coiled structure. **WATSON-CRICK H.,** a double **H.** in which each chain contains information specifying the other chain; it represents the manner in which the genetic factors in DNA (deoxyribonucleic acid) reproduce themselves.

Heller's operation: Cardiomyotomy, a surgical procedure for relieving stenosis of the cardiac sphincter.

Heller's test, Heller's ring test: A test for albumin in the urine. Urine is dropped gently down the side of a test tube containing nitric acid; if an opaque white layer forms at the point of junction of the two liquids, the urine contains albumin.

helminth (hel′-minth): A general term for a worm or wormlike parasite, particularly one found in the intestine.—helminthoid, adj.

helminth-, helmintho-: Combining forms denoting worms.

helminthagogue (hel-min′-tha-gog): See anthelmintic.

helminthiasis (hel-min-thī′-a-sis): Infestation with parasitic intestinal worms.

helminthology (hel-min-thol′-o-ji): The study of parasitic intestinal worms.

heloma (hē-lō′-ma): A corn or callosity on the hand or foot.

hem-, hema-, hemat-, hemo-: Combining forms denoting blood.

hemachromatosis: Hemochromatosis (*q.v.*).

hemacyte: Hemocyte (*q.v.*).

hemacytometer (hē′-ma-sī-tom′-e-ter): Hemocytometer.

hemadynamometer: Hemodynamometer (*q.v.*).

hemafecia (hem-a-fē′-si-a, hē-ma-): Blood in the feces.

hemagglutination (hē′-ma-gloo′-ti-nā′-shun, hem′-a-): Clumping of red blood cells; may be caused by antibodies or viruses.

hemagglutinin (hē′-ma-gloo′-ti-nin, hem′-a): A substance that agglutinates (clumps) red blood cells.

hemagogue (hem′-a-gog, hē′-ma-): An agent that promotes the flow of blood, especially the menstrual flow.

hemangiectasis (hē-man-ji-ek′-ta-sis, hem-an-): Dilatation of the blood vessels.

hemangioblastoma (hē-man′-ji-ō-blas-tō′-ma, hem-an-): A tumor of immature blood vessels, especially of the capillaries of the cerebellum; may be associated with polycythemia.

hemangioma (hē-man′-ji-ō′-ma): A benign lesion of blood vessels that may occur in any part of the body. When it occurs in the skin it may be called a birthmark, port wine stain, or strawberry mark. **CAVERNOUS H.**, a benign tumor made up of large thin-walled blood vessels.—hemangiomatoma, pl.; hemangiomatous, adj.

hemangiosarcoma (hē-man′-ji-ō-sar-kō′-ma): A malignant neoplasm composed of anaplastic cells derived from the blood vessels; highly progressive and infiltrative.

hemarthrosis (hēm-ar-thrō′-sis, hē′-mar): The extravasation of blood into a joint or the synovial cavity of a joint.

hematemesis (hē′-ma-tem′-e-sis, hem′-a-): Vomiting of blood; vomitus has bright red color when the hemorrhage is recent; "coffee-ground" color indicates blood has been in the stomach long enough to be acted on by the gastric juice.

hematin (hem′-a-tin, hē′-ma-): An iron-containing constituent of hemoglobin. Heme (*q.v.*).

hematinic (hēm-a-tin′-ik, hē′-ma-): 1. Pertaining to hematin. 2. Any substance required for the production of red blood cells and their constituents. 3. An agent that improves the quality of red blood cells and hemoglobin.

hematobilia (hē′-ma-tō-bil′-i-a, hem′-a-): A pathological condition in which there is blood in the bile ducts. Often the result of trauma to the liver.

hematoblast (hē′-ma-tō-blast, hem′-a-): 1. A primitive cell from which a blood cell develops. 2. An immature erythrocyte.

hematocele (hē′ma-tō-sēl, hem′a): 1. A swelling filled with blood. 2. An effusion of blood into a body cavity or a sac, particularly into the sac that covers the testes.

hematochezia (hē′-ma-tō-kē′-zi-a, hem′-a-): The presence of blood in the stools.

hematochromatosis (hē′-ma-tō-krō-ma-tō′-sis, hem′-a-): Staining of tissues with blood pigment. See hemochromatosis.

hematochyluria (hē′-ma-tō-kī-lū′-ri-a, hem′-a-): The presence of both blood and chyle in the urine.

hematocolpos (hē′-ma-tō-kōl′-pōs, hem′-a): Accumulation of menstrual blood in the vagina; sometimes due to imperforate hymen. See cryptomenorrhea.

hematocrit (hē-mat′-ō-krit): 1. The term commonly used to express the percentage of the volume of red blood cells in the blood; abbreviated hct. 2. The calibrated tube, the centrifuge, or the procedure used to determine the percentage volume of red cells in the blood.

hematocyst (hē-mat′-ō-sist, hem′a-tō): 1. A cyst containing blood. 2. Effusion of blood into the urinary bladder.

hematocyte (hē-mat′-ō-sīt, hem′-a-tō): A blood corpuscle; hemocyte.

hematocytometer: Hemacytometer (*q.v.*).

hematocytopenia (hē′-ma-tō-sī-tō-pē′-ni-a): A deficiency or decrease in the cellular content of the blood.

hematocytosis (hē′-ma-tō-sī-tō′-sis, hem′-a-): An increase on the cellular content of the blood.

hematocyturia (hē′-ma-tō-sī-tū′-ri-a, hem′-a-): The presence of red blood cells in the urine.

hematogenesis (hē′-ma-tō-jen′-e-sis, hem′-a-): The formation of blood or blood cells.

hematogenous (hē-ma-toj′-e-nus, hem′-a-): 1. Concerned with the formation of blood. 2. Carried by the bloodstream. 3. Derived from or produced by blood.

hematoid (hē′-ma-toyd, hem′-a): Resembling blood.

hematologist (hē-ma-tol′-ō-jist, hem′-a): A physician who specializes in the study of blood and blood dyscrasias.

hematology (hē-ma-tol′-o-ji, hem′-a-): The science dealing with the formation, composition, functions, and diseases of the blood and the morphology of the blood-forming organs.—hematological, adj.; hematologically, adv.

hematolysis (hē-ma-tol′-i-sis): Hemolysis (*q.v.*).

hematoma (hē-ma-tō′-ma, hem′-a-): A localized mass of blood, usually clotted, within a tissue or body part; caused by a break in a blood vessel. EPIDURAL H., a collection of blood between the dura mater and the skull; may also be referred to as EXTRADURAL H., INTRACRANIAL H., one within the cranium; usually due to loss of venous integrity. H. OF THE BREAST, occurs as a result of trauma; may be mistaken for malignant tumor. SUBDURAL H., occurs between the dura mater and the arachnoid; may involve one or both hemispheres of the brain; usually due to trauma but may also be seen in certain blood dyscrasias; signs and symptoms may vary with the patient's age, but usually include depressed consciousness; severe headache, possibly hempilegia.

hematometra (hē′-ma-tō-mē′-tra, hem′-a): An accumulation of blood (or menstrual fluid) in the uterus.

hematomphalocele (hē′-ma-tom-fal′-ō-sēl, hem′-a-): An umbilical hernia that contains blood.

hematomyelia (hē′-ma-tō-mī-ē′-li-a, hem′-a-): Hemorrhage into the substance of the spinal cord.

hematomyelitis (hē′-ma-tō-mī-e-lī′-tis, hem′-a-): Acute inflammation of the spinal cord with bloody effusion.

hematopenia (hē′-ma-tō-pē′-ni-a): Deficiency of blood.

hematophilia: Hemophilia (*q.v.*).

hematopoiesis (hē′-ma-tō-poy-ē′-sis, hem′-a-): Hemopoiesis (*q.v.*).

hematorrhachis (hē-ma-tor′-a-kis, hem′-a-): Hemorrhage into the spinal canal.

hematosalpinx (hē′-ma-tō-sal′-pinks, hem′-a-): An accumulation of blood in the fallopian tube: most often occurs in association with ectopic pregnancy.

hematosepsis (hē′-ma-tō-sep′-sis, hem′-a-): Septicemia (*q.v.*).

hematotoxin (hē′-ma-tō-toks′-in, hem′-a-): Any substance that causes the destruction of red blood cells. Also called hemotoxin.

hematozoa (hē′-ma-tō-zō′-a, hem′-a-): Animal parasites living in the blood stream.—hematozoon, sing.

hematuria (hē-ma-tū′-ri-a, hem′-a-): The presence of red blood cells in the urine; caused by bleeding in any part of the urinary tract. GROSS H., that which can be observed without the use of microscopy. MICROSCOPIC H., that which can be demonstrated only by the use of the microscope.

heme (hēm): The pigment-carrying nonprotein portion of hemoglobin. Formerly called hematin.

hemeralopia (hem′-er-a-lō′-pi-a): Defective vision in a bright light with ability to see more distinctly in a dim light; day blindness.

hemi-: Prefix denoting 1) half of, or one-half; 2) affecting half of an organ or part.

hemiachromatopsia (hem′-i-a-krō-ma-top′-si-a): Color blindness in one half the visual field of each eye.

hemialgia (hem-i-al′-ji-a): Pain affecting only one side of the body.

hemianalgesia (hem′-i-an-al-jē′-zi-a): Loss of sensitivity to pain in one side of the body.

hemianesthesia (hem′-i-an-es-thē′-zi-a): Loss of sensation on one side of the body; unilateral anesthesia.

hemianopia (hem-i-a-nō′-pi-a): Blindness or defective vision in one half of the field of vision, occurring in persons suffering from hemiparesis. BITEMPORAL H., blindness on the temporal side of the field of vision in one or both eyes. HOMONYMOUS H., H. that affects half of the visual fields of both eyes. Also called heminopsia, hemianopia.

hemiatrophy (hem-i-at′-ro-fi): Atrophy of one half or one side of the body or of an organ or part. H. FACIALIS, a congenital condition, or a manifestation of scleroderma (*q.v.*), in which the structures on one side of the face are shrunken.

hemiballismus (hem-i-bal-iz′-mus): Sudden, violent jerking movements on one side of the body, resulting from a brain lesion and occurring on the side of the body opposite to the lesion. Also hemiballism.

hemiblock (hem′-i-block): A block in either the anterior or posterior division of the left branch of the bundle of His.

hemibrachia (hem-i-brā′-ki-a): The congenital absence of one arm.

hemicardia (hem-i-kar′-di-a): A congenital anomaly in which 1) one lateral half of the heart is lacking, or 2) two of the four normal chambers of the heart are lacking.

hemicellulose (hem-i-sel′-ū-lōs): A general name for a group of indigestible polysaccharides which resemble cellulose but are more soluble; may be used to increase bulk in the diet.

hemichorea (hem′-i-kō-rē′-a): Choreiform movements limited to one side of the body. See chorea.

hemicolectomy (hem′-i-kō-lek′-to-mi): Removal of approximately half the colon.

hemicorporectomy (hem′-i-kor-po-rek′-to-mi): Amputation above the brim of the pelvis, including the lower extremities and all of the tissues and organs of the pelvic area. A radical operation that has been performed in a few cases of inoperable cancer and war injuries in which there is extensive destruction of tissue of and below the pelvis.

hemicrania (hem-i-krā′-ni-a): 1. Unilateral headache, as in migraine 2. Congenital anomaly in which the cerebrum has not developed properly.

hemidiaphoreses (hem′i-dī-a-fō-rē′sis): Profuse sweating on only one side of the body.

hemidiaphragm (hem-i-dī′-a-fram): 1. One lateral half of the diaphragm. 2. Deficient muscular development of one lateral half of the diaphragm. 3. Paralysis of only half of the diaphragm.

hemidysesthesia (hem′-i-dis-es-thē′-zi-a): A disorder of sensation affecting only one side of the body.

hemidystrophy (hem-i-dis′-trō-fi): A condition of underdevelopment of one side of the body.

hemigastrectomy (hem′-i-gas-trek′-to-mi): Removal of half or part of the stomach.

hemiglossectomy (hem′-i-glos-sek′-to-mi): Surgical removal of one side or part of the tongue.

hemihypesthesia (hem′-i-hī-pes-thē′-zi-a): Lowered sensitivity in one lateral half of the body.

hemilaryngectomy (hem′-i-lar-in-jek′-to-mi): Surgical removal of one half of the larynx.

hemilateral (hem-i-lat′-er-al): Pertaining to or affecting one lateral half of the body or of an organ.

hemimandibulectomy (hem′-i-man-dib-ū-lek′-to-mi): Resection of one half of the mandible.

heminephrectomy (hem′-i-nef-rek′-to-mi): Surgical excision of part of a kidney.

hemiparaplegia (hem′-i-par-a-plē′-ji-a): Paralysis of one side of the lower half of the body, or of one lower extremity.

hemiparesis (hem-i-pa-rē′-sis): A slight paralysis or muscular weakness of one half of the body or face.—hemiparetic, adj.

hemipelvectomy (hem′-i-pel-vek′-to-mi): Surgical removal of an entire leg and the hip bone on that side.

hemiplegia (hem-i-plē′-ji-a): Paralysis of one side of the body, usually resulting from a cerebrovascular accident on the opposite side. **FACIAL H., H.** affecting one side of the face but not the rest of the body. **FLACCID H., H.** in which the muscles of the affected side lose their tone and tendon reflexes are lost. **SPASTIC H., H.** in which the muscles of the affected side are spastic and the tendon reflexes are increased.

hemisacralization (hem′-i-sā-kral-ī-zā′-shun): The fusion of the fifth lumbar vertebra to the uppermost segment of the sacrum on one side only.

hemisphere (hem′-i-sfēr): Half of a sphere or half of any spherical structure or organ; term commonly applied to either half of the cerebrum or the cerebellum.

hemihypertrophy (hem′-i-hī-per′-trō-fi): A congenital anomaly in which one half of the body is overdeveloped.

hemivertebra (hem-i-ver′-te-bra): A congenital anomaly in which one lateral half of a vertebra fails to develop completely.—hemivertebrae, pl.

hemoagglutination: Hemagglutination (*q.v.*).

hemoagglutinin: Hemagglutinin (*q.v.*).

hemoblast (hē′-mō-blast): An immature blood cell; a blood platelet.

hemochezia (hē-mō-kē′-zi-a): The discharge of blood from the rectum, especially bright red blood.

hemochromatosis (hē′-mō-krōm-a-tō′-sis): A congenital error in iron metabolism; excessive deposits of iron in the pancreas and liver resulting in bronze discoloration of the skin; may occur in patients with diabetes mellitus or cirrhosis of the liver, and in patients who have received iron compounds over a period of time. See hemosiderosis. Syn., bronze diabetes.—hemochromatic, adj.

hemochromometer (hē′-mō-krō-mom′-e-ter): An apparatus for estimating the percentage of hemoglobin in the blood; a colorimeter.

hemocidal (hē-mō-sī′-dal): 1. Destructive to red blood cells. 2. An agent that destroys red blood cells.

hemoclastic (hē-mō-klas′-tik): Pertaining to or causing destruction of red blood cells.

hemoconcentration (hē′-mō-kon-sen-trā′-shun): Relative increase of volume of red blood cells to volume of plasma, usually due to loss of the latter. May occur in such conditions as shock, burns, diabetes mellitus. The degree of concentration is determined by a hematocrit (*q.v.*).

hemocyte (hē′mō-sīt): 1. A blood corpuscle. 2. Any blood cell.

hemocytolysis (hē′-mō-sī-tol′-i-sis): Destruction of blood cells.

hemocytometer (hē′-mo-sī-tom′-e-ter): An apparatus for determining the number of blood corpuscles in a measured amount of blood.

hemodialysis (hē′-mō-dī-al′-i-sis): A process of removing metabolic waste products, other poisons, and excess fluids from the blood and replacing essential blood constituents by a process of diffusion through a semi-permeable membrane. Such a technique is used in the artificial kidney. The patient's blood is diverted from a blood vessel by cannula and tubing into a dialysis machine where it is treated and then returned to the patient's circulation by another cannula inserted into a different vessel. May be used in treatment of acute or chronic renal failure, drug overdosage, hepatic coma, or other situation in which the natural kidney function is inadequate.

hemodialyzer (hē-mō-dī'a-lī-zer): A machine for hemodialysis (*q.v.*). Artificial kidney.

hemodilution (hē'-mō-dī-lū'-shun): A condition in the blood in which the ratio of blood cells to plasma is reduced. It is the first step in the reconstitution of the blood after severe blood loss. Also a natural occurrence during pregnancy.

hemodynamics (hē'-mō-dī-nam'-iks): Study of the movement of blood in the body and of the forces and mechanisms involved.

hemodynamometer (hē'-mō-dī-na-mom'-e-ter): An apparatus for measuring blood pressure.

hemoglobin (hē-mō-glō'-bin): The oxygen-carrying coloring matter in the red blood cells. It is composed of an iron-containing substance called heme (*q.v.*) combined with globin. Has the reversible function of combining with and releasing oxygen. See oxyhemoglobin. **SICKLE CELL H.**, the hemoglobin found in sickle cell anemia; see under anemia.

hemoglobinemia (hē'-mō-glō-bi-nē'-mi-a): Free hemoglobin in the blood plasma. **PAROXYSMAL H.**, hemolysis occurring during sleep; usually associated with intramuscular thrombosis, a rare condition.

hemoglobinometer (hē'-mō-glō-bi-nom'-e-ter): An instrument for estimating the percentage of hemoglobin in the red blood cells.

hemoglobinopathy (hē'-mō-glō-bi-nop'-a-thi): Any disease caused by an abnormality of the hemoglobin; many are caused by inherited erythrocytic deficits, e.g., sickle cell anemia.

hemoglobinuria (hē'-mo-glō-bin-ū'-ri-a): The presence of free hemoglobin in the urine. **MALARIAL H.**, blackwater fever (*q.v.*). **PAROXYSMAL NOCTURNAL H.**, see Machiafavi-Micheli syndrome.

hemoid (hē'-moyd): Resembling blood.

hemolith (hēm'-o-lith): A concretion or stone in the wall of a blood vessel.

hemolymphangioma (hē'-mō-lim-fan-ji-ō'-ma): A tumor that is composed of blood vessels and lymph vessels.

hemolysin (hē-mol'-i-sin): Any agent or condition that causes disintegration of red blood cells by liberating their hemoglobin.

hemolysis (hē-mol'-i-sis): Laking; disintegration of red blood cells with liberation of contained hemoglobin. May be caused by bacterial toxins, antibodies, immune bodies, various chemical agents, freezing or heating, venom of various snakes, hypotonic salt solution. Causes reddish discoloration of urine. See anemia, hemoglobinemia.—hemolytic, adj.; hemolyze, v.

hemolytic (hē-mō-lit'-ik): 1. Pertaining to hemolysis. 2. Being able to cause hemolysis. **H. ANEMIA**, see under anemia. **H. DISEASE OF THE NEWBORN**, see erythroblastosis fetalis. **H. STREPTOCOCCI**, see under streptococcus.

hemolytic-uremic syndrome: An acute condition occurring chiefly in infants, characterized by bloody diarrhea, hemolytic anemia, thrombocytopenia, and azotemia; cause unknown; sometimes follows respiratory infection. Most frequent cause of renal failure in children.

hemometra (hē-mō-mē'-tra): See hematometra.

hemopathy (hē-mop'-a-thi): Any disease or disorder of the blood, or of blood formation.

hemoperfusion (hē'-mō-per-fū'-zhun): The passing of blood over a sorbent material to remove a toxic substance; activated charcoal is often used.

hemopericardium (hē'-mō-per-i-kar'-di-um): The presence of blood in the pericardial sac.

hemoperitoneum (hē'-mō-per-i-tō-nē'-um): The presence of blood in the peritoneal cavity.

hemophagia (hē-mō-fā'-ji-a): Phagocytosis (*q.v.*) of red blood cells.

hemophilia (hē-mō-fil'-i-a): An inherited bleeding disease found only in males and transmitted through carrier females, who are daughters of affected males. Under special genetic circumstances, females with **H.** may be produced. Patient is subject to prolonged bleeding following even minor injuries. **CLASSIC H., HEMOPHILIA A.**, due to deficiency in activity of Factor VIII. **HEMOPHILIA B**, Christmas disease, is due to deficiency of activity of Factor IX. See also Von Willebrand's disease.

hemophiliac (hē-mō-fil'-i-ak): 1. Pertaining to hemophilia. 2. A person afflicted with hemophilia.

hemophilic (hē-mō-fil'-ik): 1. Pertaining to hemophilia. 2. Blood-loving; said of microorganisms.

Hemophilus (hē-mof'-i-lus): A genus of bacteria; small gram-negative rods that vary greatly in shape; strict parasites that require the presence of certain accessory substances in the blood for their growth; found in the respiratory tracts of vertebrates and often associated with acute and chronic diseases such as influenza, whooping cough, pinkeye. See Ducrey's bacillus. **H. AEGYPTIUS**, the causative agent of catarrhal conjunctivitis (pinkeye). **H. INFLUENZAE TYPE B**, the causative agent of such serious pyogenic infections as meningitis, pneumonia, otitis media, croup, and bacteremia, particularly in children; early symptoms may be mistaken for those of a common cold; sequelae may include deafness, partial paralysis, and mental retardation. **H. VAGINALIS,** see under Gardnerella vaginale. Also spelled Haemophilus (British).

hemophobia (hē-mō-fō′-bi-a): Morbid dread of blood.

hemophthalmia (hē-mof-thal′-mi-a): Bleeding into the eyeball. Also hemophthalmus.

hemopneumothorax (hē′-mō-nū-mō-thor′-aks): The presence of blood and air in the pleural cavity causing compression of lung tissue.

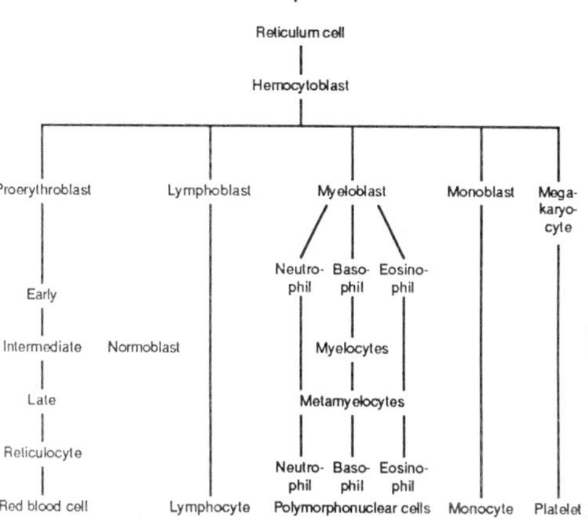

hemopoiesis (hē′-mō-poy-ē′-sis): The formation and development of the various types of blood cells.

hemopoietic (hē′-mō-poy-et′-ik): 1. Pertaining to the formation of blood cells. 2. An agent that affects the production of blood cells. **H. SYSTEM,** the tissues concerned with the production of blood, including the lymphatic tissues and bone marrow.

hemoproctia (hē-mō-prok′-shi-a): Hemorrhage from the rectum.

hemoptysis (hē-mop′-tis-is): The coughing up of blood or blood-stained sputum.—hemoptyses, pl.

hemorrhage (hem′-or-rij): The escape of copious amounts of blood from a vessel by diapedesis through a vessel wall or by direct outflow through a break in vessel walls. The terms **ARTERIAL H., VENOUS H.,** and **CAPILLARY H.** designate the type of vessel from which it escapes. **PRIMARY H.** occurs at the time of surgery or injury. **SECONDARY H.** may also occur after surgery or injury but after a considerable time has elapsed. **ACCIDENTAL ANTEPARTUM H.,** bleeding from separation of a normally situated placenta after the 28th week of pregnancy. The term placental abruption is now preferred. **ANTEPARTAL H.,** vaginal bleeding before the onset of labor. **BRONCHIAL H.,** hemoptysis. **CEREBRAL H., H.** into the substance of the cerebrum. **CONCEALED H.,** internal **H. EXTRADURAL H.,** extravasation of blood into the space between the skull and the dura mater. **GASTRIC H., H.** into the stomach. **INTERNAL H., H.** with the extravasated blood remaining in one of the organs or cavities of the body. **INTRACEREBRAL H. H.** within the substance of the brain. **INTRAPARTAL H.,** occurs during labor. **MASSIVE H.,** loss of a large amount of blood in a short time. **NASAL H.,** epistaxis. **PETECHIAL H.,** bleeding from small capillaries into the skin, forming petechiae. **POSTMENOPAUSAL H.,** vaginal blood loss after menopause; requires immediate attention; may indicate presence of a malignancy. **POSTPARTAL H.,** excessive bleeding within 24 hours after giving birth. **PULMONARY H.,** hemoptysis. **REACTIONARY H.,** a surgical complication that may occur in the first 12 to 24 hours after surgery; caused by dislodgement of an insecure or loose suture. **SUBARACHNOID H.,** bleeding into the space between the arachnoid and the pia mater. **SUBDURAL H.,** bleeding into the space between the dura mater and the arachnoid.—hemorrhage, v.; hemorrhagic, adj.

hemorrhagic (hem-ō-raj′-ik): Pertaining to or marked by hemorrhage. **H. DISEASE OF THE NEWBORN,** a tendency to bleeding in the neonatal period; results from deficiency of vitamin K and prolonged prothrombin time; erythroblastosis fetalis (*q.v.*). **H. PURPURA,** purpura hemorrhagica (*q.v.*).

hemorrheology (hem′-ō-rē-ol′-ō-jē): The study of blood flow and of the properties of the vessels through which it flows.

hemorrhoid (hem′-o-royd): Varicosity of a vein in the rectal area. **EXTERNAL H.,** one outside of the anal sphincter covered with skin. **INTERNAL H.,** one inside the anal sphincter covered with mucous membrane.

hemorrhoidal (hem-o-royd′-al): 1. Pertaining to hemorrhoids. 2. Applied to nerves and blood vessels in the anal region.

hemorrhoidectomy (hem′-o-royd-ek′-to-mi): Surgical removal of hemorrhoids.

hemosalpinx (hē-mō-sal′-pinks): Hematosalpinx (*q.v.*).

hemosiderin (hē-mō-sid′-er-in): A glycoprotein containing iron; found in the liver and most other tissues; excess amounts sometimes occur in pathological conditions.

hemosiderosis (hē′-mō-sid-er-ō′-sis): A condition in which hemosiderin accumulates in the tissues; occurs in diseases in which there is marked destruction of red blood cells; may be associated with several types of anemia, chronic infection, malnutrition; often affects the kidney and lung.

hemospermia (hē-mō-sper′-mi-a): The discharge of blood-stained semen.

hemostasis (hē-mō-stā′sis, hē-mos′ta-sis): 1.

Arrest of bleeding. 2. Stagnation of blood within its vessel, due to interruption of its flow.

hemostat (hē′-mō-stat): 1. An agent that arrests bleeding. 2. An instrument for constricting a blood vessel to stop or control the flow of blood.

hemostatic (hē-mō-stat′-ik): 1. An agent that arrests bleeding. 2. Having the effect of arresting bleeding.

hemothorax (hē-mō-thō′-raks): The presence of bloody fluid in the pleural cavity.

hemotympanum (hē′-mō-tim′-pa-num): The presence of blood in the middle ear.

Hemovac drainage system: A closed drainage system involving the use of a suction apparatus attached to a drainage tube; used to evacuate fluid that may accumulate in an operative site following surgery, *e.g.*, a mastectomy.

Hendon arm: A prosthesis for children; powered by carbon dioxide.

Henle: LOOP OF H., see under nephron.

Henoch-Schönlein syndrome: Henoch-Schönlein purpura; see under purpura.

Henry's law: States that when the temperature is constant, the solubility of any gas in a liquid is almost directly proportional to the pressure of the liquid; is applied in cases of nitrogen narcosis in deep sea divers.

hepar (hē′-par): The liver.—hepatic, adj.

heparin (hep′-a-rin): A naturally occurring acid substance in several body tissues, especially the liver; it tends to prevent blood from clotting. In pharmacy, a preparation made from the livers or lungs of cattle, usually given by intravenous injection to inhibit coagulation of the blood; widely used in prevention and treatment of thrombosis.

heparin lock: A device used for the intermittent administration of medications that are to be given intravenously; it consists of a scalp vein needle attached to a length of tubing that has a self-sealing diaphragm at the end; after the venipuncture, the needle is secured to the skin by its skin flaps; following an administration of medication a weak heparin solution is put into the needle and tubing to keep the line open.

heparinize (hep′-ar-i-nīz): To treat with administration of heparin for the purpose of increasing the clotting time of the blood.—heparinization, n.

hepat-, hepatico-, hepato-: Combining forms denoting liver.

hepatectomy (hep-a-tek′-to-mi): Excision of part of the liver.

hepatic (hē-pat′-ik): Pertaining to the liver. H. COMA, see under coma. H. DUCTS, right and left, unite to form the common hepatic duct which joins the cystic duct from the gallbladder to form the common bile duct. H. ENCEPHALOPATHY, see under encephalopathy. H. FAILURE occurs when the liver is unable to carry out its normal functions due to damage from acute viral hepatitis, poisonings, or states of low cardiac output; clinical signs include jaundice; ascites; edema; abnormal blood chemistry; tendency to spontaneous hemorrhage, often into the gastrointestinal tract and skin; and coma. H. FLEXURE, see flexure. H. VIRUS, type A causes infectious hepatitis which affects mostly the young, drug addicts, and those in low socioeconomic groups; and type B which causes serum hepatitis and is usually transmitted by blood transfusion.

hepaticocholedochostomy (hē-pat′-i-kō′-kō-lē-dō-kos′-to-mi): End-to-end union of the severed hepatic and common bile ducts.

hepaticoduodenostomy (hē-pat′-i-kō-dū′-ō-de-nos′-to-mi): The surgical creation of a new opening between the bile duct and the duodenum.

hepaticoenteric (hē-pat′-i-kō-en-ter′-ik): Pertaining to the liver and the intestine.

hepaticoenterostomy (hē-pat′-i-kō-en-ter-os′-to-mi): The surgical establishment of an artificial communication between the hepatic duct and the intestine.

hepaticojejunostomy (hē-pat′-i-kō-jē-ju-nos′-to-mi): Anastomosis of the hepatic duct to a loop of proximal intestine.

hepaticolithotripsy (he-pat′-i-kō-lith′-o-trip′sē): The crushing of a calculus in the hepatic duct.

hepaticostomy (hē-pat-i-kos′-to-mi): The establishment of a permanent fistula into the hepatic duct for the purpose of drainage.

hepatitis (hep-a-tī′-tis): Inflammation of the liver. Two main types are described: hepatitis A and hepatitis B. HEPATITIS A (infectious H.), caused by the hepatitis type A virus; is spread by the oral-fecal route; gives rise to epidemics in schools and among the armed forces, and is of worldwide distribution; is marked by jaundice occurring after an influenza-like illness, malaise, nausea, vomiting, clay-colored stools, and the presence of bilirubin in the urine; confers indefinite immunity. HEPATITIS B (serum H.), caused by hepatitis B virus; may be transmitted by contaminated needles, blood, mucous membranes (sexual intercourse), or ingestion of contaminated food; has long incubation period and long duration; characterized by increase in SGOT and SGPT levels and increased bilirubin in the blood; may be acute, chronic, or recurrent; produces carriers in 10 percent of patients. ALCOHOLIC H., occurs as a sequela of alcoholism. CHOLANGIOLITIC H., inflammation of the bile ducts and obstructive jaundice. CHRONIC H., persistent H., H. involving inflammation of the liver, sometimes cirrhosis, and may follow viral H. ENZOIC H., Rift Valley fever (*q.v.*). EPIDEMIC H., infectious H. FULMINANT H., acute H., may cause death from acute yellow atrophy of the liver. HOMOLYGOUS H., symptoms as for infectious **H.** but is caused by a B or SH virus and spread by contact, blood transfusion, or serum therapy, or by improperly sterilized needles or instruments; incubation period is 6 weeks to 6 months; can be severe, even fatal; an estimated 2 to 3 percent of the adult world population are carriers. **INFECTIOUS H.,** hepatitis A. **NEONATAL H.,** occurs soon after birth; cause often unknown; tends to be chronic and fatal. **TRANSFUSION H.,** usually caused by viral **H.**, type B. **SERUM H.,** hepatitis B. **VIRAL H.,** may be caused by **H.**A, or **H.**B virus, or **NON**-A or **NON**-B virus.

hepatitis B surface antigen: Formerly called Australian antigen because originally found in the serum of Australian aborigines. Carried in patients with liver disease, including those who develop hepatitis after many blood transfusions; also carried in dirty syringes. Has been found in city areas frequented by alcoholics and drug addicts. Blood banks now screen for this antigen.

hepatization (hep'a-tī-zā'shun): Pathological changes in the tissues, which cause them to resemble liver. Occurs in the lungs in the exudative stages of lobar pneumonia.

hepatobiliary (hep'-a-tō-bil'-i-ar-i): Pertaining to the liver and the bile or bile ducts. **H. SYSTEM,** composed of the liver, the hepatic duct system, the gallbladder, cystic duct, and common bile duct.

hepatocele (hep'-a-tō-sēl): A hernia or protrusion of a part of the liver through the diaphragm or the abdominal wall.

hepatocellular (hep'-a-tō-sel'-ū-lar): Pertaining to, or affecting liver cells.

hepatocholangeitis (hep'-a-tō-kō-lan-jē-ī'-tis): Inflammation of the liver and the biliary ducts.

hepatocirrhosis (hep'-a-tō-si-rō'-sis): Cirrhosis of the liver.

hepatocystic (hep'-a-tō-sis'-tik): Pertinent to the liver and gallbladder.

hepatocyte (hep'-a-tō-sīt): One of the cells of the epithelial type that make up most of the liver substance.

hepatoduodenal (hep'-a-tō-dū-ō-dē'-nal): Pertaining to the liver and the duodenum.

hepatogenous (hep-a-toj'-e-nus): Originating in the liver.

hepatolenticular (hep'-a-tō-len-tik'-ū-lar): Pertaining to the liver and the lenticular nucleus; see under nucleus. **H. DEGENERATION,** a rare inherited disorder due to a defect in metabolism of copper; characterized by a pigmented ring (Kayser-Fleischer ring) at the outer border of the cornea, cirrhosis of the liver, enlarged spleen, rigidity and contractures of muscles, dysphagia, progressive weakness, degeneration of the lenticular nucleus, and psychic disturbances; also called Wilson's disease.

hepatolith (hep'-a-tō-lith): A concretion within the liver.

hepatologist (hep-a-tol'-ō-jist): A physician who specializes in hepatology.

hepatology (hep-a-tol'-ō-ji): The study of the liver.

hepatoma (hep-a-tō'-ma): Primary carcinoma of the liver.

hepatomegaly (hep'a-tō-meg'a-li): Enlargement of the liver.

hepatopancreatic (hep'-a-tō-pan-krē-at'-ik): Pertaining to the liver and the pancreas. **H. AMPULLA,** see ampulla of Vater, under ampulla.

hepatorenal syndrome: Term originally used to describe death from hepatic and renal failure after cholecystectomy for prolonged obstructive jaundice. Now used to describe liver and kidney failure from any cause occurring simultaneously, and resulting from infection, dehydration, hemorrhage, or shock.

hepatorrhea (hep'-a-tō-rē'-a): Excessive formation or flow of bile from the liver.

hepatorrhexis (hep'-a-tō-rek'-sis): Rupture of the liver.

hepatosplenomegaly (hep'-a-tō-splē-nō-meg'-al-i): Enlargement of the liver and the spleen.

hepatotherapy (hep'-a-tō-ther'-a-pi): The treatment of disease by the administration of animal liver or liver extract.

hepatotomy (hep-a-tot'-ō-mi): An incision into the liver.

hepatotoxic (hep-a-tō-tok'-sik): Having an injurious effect on liver cells.

hepatotoxicity (hep'-a-tō-tok-sis'-i-ti): The quality of being toxic to the cells of the liver.

hepatotoxin (hep'-a-tō-tok'-sin): 1. Any substance that is destructive of or injurious to the liver cells. 2. A toxic substance elaborated in the liver.

hept-, hepta-: Combining forms denoting 1) seven; 2) division into seven units.

heptadactylia (hep'-ta-dak-til'-i-a): The condition of having seven toes or fingers on one hand or foot.

herbicide (erb'-i-sīd): Any substance used to inhibit the growth of undesirable plants or weeds.

hereditary (he-red'-i-ter-i): Inherited; capable of being inherited. **H. DISEASE,** a disorder passed from parent to child through genes; may be recessive or dominant; may not be observable at birth. Predisposition to certain diseases is also a hereditary trait; may or may not be detectable at birth.

heredity (hē-red'-i-ti): 1. The genetic factor responsible for the persistence of particular characteristics in successive generations. 2. The physical and mental components that are transmitted from parent to offspring at conception. 3. The transmission of particular traits and characters from parents to offspring.

heredofamilial (her′-e-dō-fa-mil′-i-al): Refers to a disease that occurs in more than one member of a family and is probably inherited.

Hering-Breuer reflex: See under **reflex**.

heritability (her′-it-a-bil′-i-ti): The quality of being inheritable.

heritable (her′-it-a-b'l): Capable of being inherited.

hermaphrodite (her-maf′-rō-dīt): An individual possessing both ovarian and testicular tissue. Such a person may approximate either the male or female type, but is usually sterile from imperfect development of the gonads.

hermaphroditism (her-maf′-rō-dit-izm): The condition in which both ovarian and testicular tissue exist in the same individual. Also hermaphrodism.

hermetic (her-met′-ik): Airtight.—hermetically, adv.

hernia (her′-ni-a): Rupture. The protrusion of an organ or part of an organ, through an abnormal aperture in the structure containing it; commonly the protrusion of an abdominal organ through a gap in the abdominal wall. Weakness of the wall may be caused by injury, general debilitation, old age, lifting, tumor, increased pressure from coughing. **CEREBRAL H.** protrusion of brain substance through the skull, usually occurs after surgery for brain tumor. **DIAPHRAGMATIC H.**, protrusion through the diaphragm, most commonly involving the stomach at the esophageal opening. **FEMORAL H.**, protrusion of intestine through the femoral canal, alongside the femoral vessels as they pass into the thigh. **HIATAL H.**, diaphragmatic **H. INCISIONAL H.**, may occur after abdominal surgery when there is a breakdown of sutures in the deep layers of tissue; may be caused by wound infection. **INGUINAL H.**, protrusion of a sac of peritoneum through the inguinal canal, alongside the spermatic cord in the male. **IRREDUCIBLE H.**, one that cannot be reduced by manual manipulation. **OBTURATOR H.**, one through the obturator foramen; occurs rarely, usually in women. **POPLITEAL H., H.** of the synovial membrane at the back of the knee; occurs when the capsule is weakened by arthritis or infection; baker's cyst. **REDUCIBLE H.**, one that can be corrected by manual manipulation. **RICHTER'S H.**, one in which only a part of the intestinal wall is within the hernial sac. **STRANGULATED H.**, one in which the blood supply to the herniated part is impaired; usually due to constriction by surrounding tissues or structures. **UMBILICAL H.**, protrusion of part of the intestine through the umbilical scar area. **VAGINAL H.**, a hernia into the vagina. **VENTRAL H.**, a hernia through the abdominal wall.

herniated (her′-ni-ā-ted): 1. Having a hernia. 2. Descriptive of a structure that protrudes like a hernia. **H. DISK**, an intervertebral disk in which the nucleus pulposus has ruptured through the surrounding fibrocartilage; most often occurs in the lumbar area; may cause pressure on spinal nerves, causing severe pain; also called slipped disk and ruptured intervertebral disk.

herniation (her-ni-ā′-shun): 1. Formation of a hernia. 2. A hernia.

hernioplasty (her′-ni-ō-plas-ti): An operation for hernia, in which an attempt is made to prevent recurrence, by refashioning the structures to give greater strength.—hernioplastic, adj.

herniorrhaphy (her-ni-or′a-fi): An operation for hernia, in which the weak area is reinforced by some of the patient's own tissues, or by some other material.

herniotomy (her-ni-ot′-o-mi): An operation to cure hernia by the return of its contents to their normal position, and the removal of the hernial sac.

heroic (he-rō′-ik): Severe or extreme; said of extraordinary medical or surgical measures taken to save life.

heroin (her′-ō-in): A highly addictive white crystalline powder derived from opium; favored by drug addicts. Formerly used as a narcotic, analgesic, and cough remedy; cannot be legally manufactured or sold in the U.S.

herpangina (herp-an-jī′-na): A brief febrile illness in children, characterized by the formation of minute vesicles and ulcers at the back of the mouth around the fauces; caused by a coxsackivirus.

herpes (her′-pez): Name given to conditions that are caused by any one of five closely related herpesviruses and that are characterized by vesicular eruptions on the skin and mucous membranes of the facial and genital areas and by the ability to remain quiescent in the body until triggered by some event such as exposure to sunlight (herpes simplex, HSV-1) or a stressful event (genital herpes, HSV-2). **H. GENITALIS** (HSV-2), infectious recurring herpes of the genitalia; very contagious; transmitted by sex-

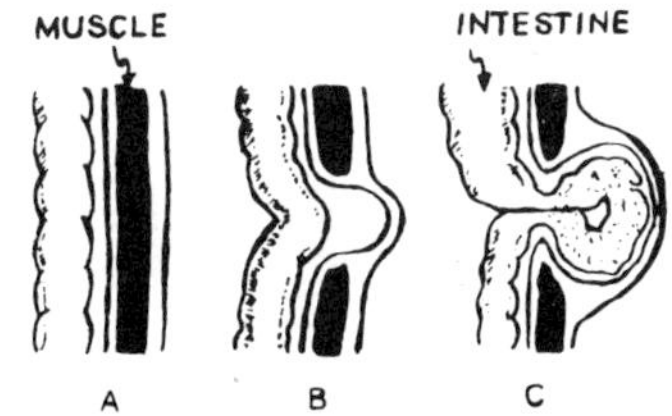

Formation of hernia. A, normal. B, simple hernia. C, strangulation of loop of intestine.

ual intercourse; occurs in epidemics. Accompanied by fever, regional adenopathy, dysuria, possibly inflammation of the meninges of the brain and spinal cord. In women, the vesicles may develop into painful ulcers on the vulva, vaginal mucosa, perianal skin, and groin; other symptoms include vaginal discharge and sometimes neurological symptoms. In men, the lesions usually occur on the glans penis and scrotum. No known cure; treatment is symptomatic. Also called **H.** progenitalis. **H. SIMPLEX (HSV-1),** is characterized by the formation of blisters chiefly along the borders of the lips and external nares. Also called "fever blister." **VARICELLA-ZOSTER, VIRUS** appears as 1) chickenpox (*q.v.*), or 2) herpes zoster. **H. ZOSTER,** is characterized by the eruption of vesicles that follow the course of a nerve, and severe pain; usually unilateral; also called shingles; fairly common in the elderly. **H. ZOSTER OPHTHALMICUS,** a herpetic virus infection of the ophthalmic division of the trigeminal nerve ganglion; often accompanied by vesicular eruption along the ophthalmic branch of the nerve; may result in uveitis, glaucoma, keratitis. **ZONA FACILIS,** herpes of the face. See also Epstein-Barr virus; cytomegalovirus; hepatic keratitis under keratitis.

herpesvirus (her′-pez-vī′-rus): See herpetoviridae.

herpetic (her-pet′-ik): Pertaining to herpes. **H. NEURALGIA,** severe pain sometimes associated with herpes zoster; it follows the course of the affected nerve.

herpetiform (her-pet′-i-form): Resembling herpes.

Herpetoviridae (her′-pe-tō-vir′-i-de): A group of similar viruses formerly referred to as herpesvirus; includes herpes simplex virus, varicella-zoster virus, cytomegalovirus, and Epstein-Barr virus.

Hers disease: Glycogen storage disease, Type VI. A rare hereditary condition characterized by the storage of large amounts of glycogen in the liver and hepatomegaly.

hertz (herts): In physics, a unit of frequency in a periodic process, equal to one cycle per second. Used in audiometry. Also known as cycle per second.

Herxheimer's reaction: A reaction that sometimes takes place when penicillin treatment for syphilis is begun: characterized by fever and irritating skin lesions.

hesperidin (hes-per′-i-din): Functions as vitamin P (*q.v.*). See citrin.

heter-,hetero-: Combining forms denoting 1) different; 2) other then usual; 3) containing several kinds.

heterecious (het-er-ē′-shus): Pertaining to an organism that lives upon one host in one stage of its development and upon another in the next stage.

heterocellular (het′-er-ō-sel′-ū-lar): Made up of different kinds of cells.

heterochromia (het′-er-ō-krō′-mi-a): A difference in the color of two anatomical parts that are normally of the same color, *e.g.*, the iris of the eye.

heterogeneous (het′-er-ō-jē′-nē-us): Made up of ingredients or constituents that are dissimilar.

heterogenesis (het′-e-rō-jen′-e-sis): Reproduction in which successive generations differ in character from the preceding generation.

heterogenous (het-er-oj′-e-nus): 1. Of unlike origin. 2. Not originating within the body. Opp. to autogenous (*q.v.*).

heterograft (het′-er-ō-graft): A graft of tissue from an individual of a species other than that of the recipient.

heterohypnosis (het′-er-ō-hip-nō′-sis): Hypnosis that is induced by the hypnotist as opposed to self-hypnosis.

heterokaryon (het′-er-ō-kar′-ē-on): A cell with two or more nuclei, each with a different genetic makeup.

heterokaryosis (het′-er-ō-kar-ī-ō′-sis): The formation of or the state of containing heterokaryons.

heterokinesia (het′-er-ō-kī-nē′-si-a): Movements that are the opposite of what the patient is told to make.

heterolateral (het-er-ō-lat′-er-al): Pertaining to or situated or occurring on the opposite side.

heterologous (het-er-ol′-o-gus): 1. Of different origin; from a different species. 2. Pertaining to or consisting of tissue that is not normal to that part of the body.

heterometropia (het′-er-ō-me-trō′-pi-a): A condition in which the degree of refraction is not the same in the two eyes.

heteromorphosis (het′-er-ō-mor-fo′-sis): The development of tissue or an organ that is different from the normal type, especially that which occurs in regeneration of tissue or of a structure that was destroyed or removed.

heteromorphous (het′-er-ō-mor′-fus): Differing in shape or structure from the normal type.

heteronymous (het-er-on′-i-mus): Having different names that are indicative of correlation, *e.g.*, male, female. **H. HEMANIOPIA,** loss of vision in the inner or outer halves of the field of vision.

heterophasia (het-er-ō-fā′-zi-a): A speech disorder in which the person says one thing but means another.

heterophil (het′-er-ō-fil): A granular leukocyte of varying sizes and staining characteristics.

heterophilic (het′-er-ō-fil′-ik): Refers to a microorganism, cell, or tissue that stains with a stain other than the one usually used.

heterophoria (het′-er-ō-fō′-ri-a): Failure of the visial axes of the two eyes to remain in parallel position after the removal of a functional stimulus; one eye may deviate toward the other or away from the other.

heterophthalmia (het′-er-of-thal′-mi-a): A difference in the color of the two eyes.

heteroplasia (het′-er-ō-plā′-zi-a): The development of tissue in a place where it is not normally found or in a place where another type of tissue is normally found.

heteroplasty (het′-er-ō-plas-ti): Plastic surgery using a graft from an individual of another species, or a synthetic material that is not organic.—heteroplastic, adj.

heteropsia (het-er-op′-si-a): Unequal vision in the two eyes.

heterosexual (het′-er-ō-seks′-ū-al): Relating to or characterized by heterosexuality (*q.v.*).

heterosexuality (het′-er-ō-seks-ū-al′-i-ti): Sexual attraction toward those of the opposite sex.

heterosome (het′-er-ō-sōm): A sex chromosome.

heterotopia (het′-er-ō-tō′-pi-a): The presence of tissue or an organ in a place where it is not normally located.

heterotransplant (het′-e-rō-trans′-plant): Xenograft (*q.v.*).

heterotrichosis (het′-er-ō-trī-kō′-sis): Growth of hair of different colors on the body. **H. SUPERCILIORUM,** difference of color in the two eyebrows.

heterotrichous (het-er-ot′-ri-kus): Having cilia that are irregular in size, shape, and distribution. See cilia.

heterotropia (het′-er-ō-trō′-pi-a): Strabismus (*q.v.*).

heterozygote (het-e-rō-zī′-gōt): In biology, refers to an organism or an individual in which one or more pairs of genes are unlike in regard to a given characteristic; the gene that produces its effect in the presence of the other is called dominant and the other is called recessive. See gene; allelomorph.—heterozygous, adj.

hexachlorophene (heks-a-klō′-rō-fēn): An antiseptic used on the skin, as a bacteriostatic; and in some bactericidal soaps.

hexadactylism (hek′-sa-dak′-til-izm): The presence of six fingers on one hand or six toes on one foot.

hexosamine (hek-sos′-am-in): A nitrogenous sugar in which a hydroxyl group has replaced an amine group; glucosamine is an important hexosamine.

hexose (hek′-sōs): A class of monosaccharides ($C_6H_{12}O_6$). The two chief hexoses are glucose and fructose; others are mannose and galactose.

Hg: Symbol for mercury; also sometimes for hemoglobin.

Hgb, hgb: Abbreviations for hemoglobin.

hiatus (hī-ā′-tus): A space or opening. See hernia.—hiatal, adj.

hibernation (hī′-ber-nā′-shun): The winter sleep of some animals. **ARTIFICIAL H.,** lowering of the body temperature of human beings by the external application of cold packs (ice, etc.) in combination with drugs to control shivering. It reduces the oxygen requirements of vital tissues, and is used mainly in the treatment of head injuries and in cardiac surgery. Syn., hypothermia (*q.v.*). See refrigeration.

hibernoma (hī′-ber-nō′-ma): A benign tumor of adipose tissue. So called because its color is like that of the brown fat organs of hibernating animals.

hibokusha (hi-bō-kū′-sha): Describes survivors who are keenly aware of harboring a condition that will cause their death; refers particularly to Hiroshima survivors.

hiccough, hiccup (hik′-up): An involuntary inspiratory spasm with sudden closure of the glottis and contraction of the diaphragm resulting in a short inspiratory cough.

hidradenitis (hī-drad-e-nī′-tis): Inflammation of a sweat gland. **H. AXILLARIS, H.** suppurativa of the axilla. **H. SUPPURATIVA,** chronic **H.** with malodorous pus formation, affecting chiefly the apocrine glands.

hidradenoma (hī-drad-e-nō′-ma): A benign sweat-gland tumor.

hidrorrhea (hī-drō-rē′-a): Profuse sweating.

hidroschesis (hī-dros′-ke-sis): The suppression of sweat.

hidrosis (hī-drō′-sis): 1. Sweat secretion. 2. Excessive sweating.

hidrotic (hī-drot′-ik): 1. Having the ability to cause sweating. 2. Any agent that causes sweating; diaphoretic (*q.v.*).

H_2O: Chemical formula for water.

H_2O_2: Chemical formula for hydrogen peroxide.

high blood pressure: Blood pressure that is above the normal range. See blood pressure, hypertension.

Highmore: **ANTRUM OF HIGHMORE;** the maxillary sinus; see under antrum.

Hill-Burton Act: Name commonly used for the Hospital Survey and Construction Act of 1946. Provided for improvement in the ratio of hospital beds to population and for upgrading all hospital facilities and standards. Amendments provided for funds to improve existing facilities in all areas. Schools of nursing benefited as well as hospitals.

hilum (hī′-lum): Hilus (*q.v.*).

hilus (hī′-lus): A depression on the surface of an organ where vessels, ducts, etc., enter and leave.—hilar, adj.; hili, pl.

hindbrain (hīnd′-brain). See rhomboencephalon.

hindgut (hīnd′-gut): The embryonic structure from which the colon is formed.

hinge joint: A synovial articulation that allows for movement in only one plane. Syn., ginglymus.

Hinton test: A widely used macroscopic flocculation test for syphilis. [W.A. Hinton, American bacteriologist. 1883–1959.]

hip: The lateral part of the body on either side between the waist and the thigh. **H. BONE,** the os coxae, a large, stable, irregular bone, one on either side of the body, which together form the pelvic girdle and to which the lower extremities are attached; consists of three parts, the ilium, ischium, and pubis; also called the innominate bone. **TOTAL HIP REPLACEMENT,** a surgical procedure in which the natural hip socket (the acetabulum) is replaced with a polyethylene cup and the head of the femur with a stainless steel ball-and-socket appliance; also called a hip implant.

hippocampus (hip-pō-kam′-pus): One of two curved bands, about 5 cm in length, consisting of a special type of cortex, on the floor of the inferior horn of the lateral ventricle on each side of the brain. It is an important functional part of the limbic system (*q.v.*). Also called Ammon's horn.

Hippocrates (hi-pok′-ra-tēz): Famous Greek physician and philosopher (460 to 370 B.C.) who established a school of medicine at Cos, his birthplace. He is often termed the Father of Medicine.

Hippocratic oath: An oath based on one attributed to Hippocrates and required of his students, which has been the ethical guide of the medical profession ever since. It has been adapted for nurses and is often repeated by nursing students at their graduation exercises.

hippuria (hip-pū′-ri-a): An excess of hippuric acid in the urine.

hippuric acid (hip-ū′rik as′id): An acid formed in the body by synthesis in the liver, and in the kidney; is excreted in the urine; its salts have some therapeutic uses.

hippus (hip′-us): Abnormal spasmodic rhythmic contraction and dilation of the pupil independently of illumination or any other external stimulus.

hircus (hur′-kus): 1. A hair of the axilla. 2. The odor of the axilla.

Hirschprung's disease: Megacolon. Congenital hypertrophy and massive enlargement of the colon. The affected part is sometimes removed surgically. [Harold Hirschprung, Danish physician. 1830–1916.]

hirsute (hur′-sūt): Being hairy or shaggy.

hirsutism (hur′-sū-tizm): Excessive hairiness, especially in women, or the growth of hair in unusual places.

Hirudo (hi-roo′-dō): A genus of leeches, including the species sometimes formerly used in medicine.

His (hiss): See bundle of His.

hist-, hista-, histio-, histo-: Combining forms denoting relationship to tissue.

histaminase (his-tam′-i-nās): An enzyme that is widely distributed in body tissues and that inactivates histamine (*q.v.*).

histamine (his′-ta-mēn): A naturally occurring chemical substance in body tissues which, in small doses, has profound and diverse actions on muscle, blood capillaries, and gastric secretion. Its sudden excessive release from the tissues, into the blood is believed to be the cause of the main symptoms and signs in anaphylaxis (*q.v.*).—histaminic adj.

histidase (his′-ti-dās): An enzyme found in the liver.

histidine (his′-ti-dēn): An essential amino acid which is widely distributed and is present in hemoglobin. It is a precursor of histamine.

histidinemia (his′-ti-di-nē′-mi-a): A rare hereditary disorder of metabolism in which there is an increase in the amount of histidine in the blood; often accompanied by speech disorders, slow growth, mild mental retardation.

histiocyte (his′-tē-ō-sīt): A tissue cell; a macrophage found in connective tissue.

histiocytoma (his′-tē-ō-si-tō′-ma): A tumor that contains histiocytes.

histiocytosis (his′-tē-ō-sī-tō′-sis): A condition marked by an excessive number of histiocytes in the blood. **HISTIOCYTOSIS X,** a group of diseases characterized by proliferation of histiocytes; includes Letterer-Siwe disease and eosinophilic granuloma of bone.

histioma (his-ti-ō′-ma): Histoma (*q.v.*).

histochemistry (his-tō-kem′-is-tri): The study of the chemical components of cells and/or tissues; involves use of specific staining techniques, reagents, and tests, and microscopy.

histocompatibility (his′-tō-kom-pat-a-bil′-i-ti): 1. The ability of the cells or tissue of a graft that enables the graft to be accepted and become functional following transplantation to another organism. 2. The quality of transfused blood cells to survive and remain functional in the donee without immunological interference.

histodiagnosis (his′-tō-dī-ag-nō′-sis): Diagnosis that is based on microscopic findings in tissue or cells.

histodialysis (his′-tō-dī-al′-sis): Disintegration of tissue.

histology (his-tol′-o-ji): Microscopic study of the structure of cells and tissues.—histological, adj.; histologically, adv.

histolysis (his-tol′-i-sis): Disintegration of organic tissue.—histolytic, adj.

histoma (his-tō′ma): A benign tumor composed of cells and tissue that are very similar to those of the area where it arises, *e.g.*, a fibroma.

histopathology (his′-tō-pa-thol′-o-ji): The study of microscopically visible changes in diseased cells or tissue.

histoplasmin (hist-ō-plaz′-min): A preparation made from a culture of *Histoplasma capsulatum* for injection subcutaneously in a test for the presence of histoplasmosis. Also used in studies to determine the geographical distribution of the fungus *Histoplasma capsulatum*.

histoplasmosis (his′-tō-plaz-mō′-sis): A widespread infectious systemic disease caused by infection with the fungus *Histoplasma capsulatum* and involving the reticulo-endothelial system; may produce varying clinical pictures but usually produces fever, emaciation, splenomegaly, anemia, leukopenia and pulmonary symptoms; transmitted by spores of the organism in soil dust; often occurs in epidemics.

histrionic (his-tri-on′-ik): Refers to theatrical or hysterical behavior such as uncontrolled weeping or laughing and other kinds of attention-getting actions.

HIV: Abbreviation for Human Immunodeficiency Virus (*q.v.*).

hives (hīvs): Nettle-rash; urticaria (*q.v.*).

HMO: Abbreviation for Health Maintenance Organization (*q.v.*).

H_2O: Chemical formula for water.

H_2O_2: Chemical formula for hydrogen peroxide.

hoarse (hors): Harsh or grating; said of the voice; hoarseness, n.

hobnail liver: Descripting the appearance of the liver in one form of cirrhosis; the surface of the liver is covered with small nodules while the body of the organ is shrunken and hard.

Hodgkin's disease: Lymphadenoma. Progressive, painless, virtually fatal disease in the reticulo-endothelial system, shown in generalized enlargement of the lymphatic glands and splenomegaly; of unknown cause. Other features are recurring fever, anemia, and occasionally cutaneous manifestations. Also called lymphosarcoma, lymphadenoma, anemia lymphatica, malignant lymphoma, [Thomas Hodgkin, English physician. 1798–1866.]

Hoffa's disease: Hypertrophy of the infrapatellar pad of fat, due to trauma; causes localized pain, especially in weight-bearing or walking.

Hoffman's sign: May be elicited in patients with upper motor neuron lesions. The patient's hand is held with fingers extended and pressure is applied to the nail of the middle finger; the thumb adducts and the other fingers flex.

hol-, holo-: Combining forms meaning 1) all or entire; or 2) denoting relationship to the whole.

holandric (hōl-an′-drik): Pertaining to characteristics that are transmitted only through the male of the species.

holarthritis (hol-ar-thrī′-tis): Arthritis in all or many of the joints; polyarthritis.

holism, wholism (hō′-lizm): The philosophical concept that an entity in nature consists of a unified whole that is separate from and more than the sum of its separate parts. In health care, refers to the approach that incorporates the concept that the individual is a unified entity that is independent of and more than the sum of all the factors in his or her environment.

holistic, wholistic (hō-lis′-tik): Of or pertaining to the theory of holism. **H. HEALTH CARE,** the utilization of health care plans that incorporate the body-mind-spirit approach by taking into consideration the effects of the social, economic, physical, psychological, and spiritual aspects of the individual's life on his or her present illness. **H. NURSING,** nursing in which care plans, actions, and interventions are planned on an understanding of the uniqueness of the individual and which consider the influence of the external and internal environmental factors on the individual's illness.

Hollenhorst bodies or plaques: Small pieces of atheromatous plaques that have broken off and become lodged as emboli in retinal vessels; an indication of a serious cardiovascular problem.

hollow-back: See under back.

Holmgren's test: A test for color perception; the patient is given a skein of wool and asked to match it with one from a group of skeins of several colors.

holoendemic (hōl′-ō-en-dem′-ik): Refers to a disease that affects practically all of the inhabitants of a particular area.

hologram (hōl′-ō-gram): The negative produced on a photographic plate in a type of lensless photography that utilizes the laser beam; a three-dimensional image.

hologynic (hōl′-ō-jin′-ik): Pertaining to characteristics that are transmitted only through the female.

holosystolic (hōl′-ō-sis-tol′-ik): Lasting throughout the systolic phase of the heartbeat; said of murmurs caused by valvular insufficiency or ventricular septal defect.

Holter monitor: A cardiac monitor worn around the waist or on the shoulder of patients undergoing cardiac rehabilitation; usually worn for 24 hours only to identify any arrhythmias or to assess the effectiveness of antiarrhythmic drugs.

Holter pump: A motor-driven device designed to deliver an accurate volume of parenteral fluid or medication.

Holtzman inkblot technique: A technique similar to the Rorschach technique utilizing inkblots to test for disorders of thought and emotion.

hom-, homo-: Combining forms denoting 1) alike, similar. one and the same, corresponding in structure or type; 2) from or of the same species.

Homans' sign: Pain in the calf muscles when the foot is passively dorsiflexed, with the patient lying flat on the bed; indicative of incipient or established venous thrombosis of the leg. [John Homans, American surgeon. 1877–1954.]

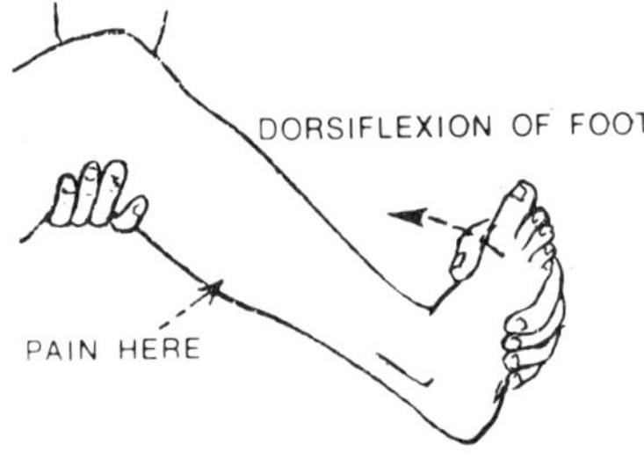

Homans' sign

home care coordinator: Usually a nurse from a community agency, who is responsible for the planning and administration of home nursing care services.

home health aide: A nonprofessional health care giver who assists the patient at home with his personal care, prepares nutritious meals and special diets, helps the patient to use a wheel chair or walker; accompanies patient to the doctor, or in outdoor exercise and walking.

home health care: Skilled nursing and rehabilitation services, including assistance with the activities of daily living; provided primarily by nonprofit agencies, *e.g.*, Visiting Nurse Associations.

homemaker services: General housekeeping services needed to maintain a person at home; provided by community or private agencies; the purpose is to reduce the use of nursing homes. Duties include giving simple health care, doing housekeeping chores, laundry, and errands; and preparing meals.

homeo-: Combining form denoting the same, alike, similar, unchanging.

homeodynamics (hō′-mē-ō-dī-nam′-iks): The process by which an individual maintains emotional balance in the presence of stressors that have the potential for disturbing one's emotional and/or physical stability.

homeomorphus (hō′-mē-ō-mor′-fus): Of similar shape and structure but not of the same composition.

homeopathy (hōm-ē-op′-a-thi): A method of treating disease by prescribing minute doses of drugs which, in maximum dose, would produce symptoms of the disease. First adopted by Hahnemann.—homeopathic, adj. [Christian Friedrich Samuel Hahnemann, German physician. 1775–1843.]

homeoplasia (hō-mē-ō-plā′-zi-a): The growth of new tissue that is similar to the adjacent tissue.

homeostasis (hō′-mē-ō-stā′-sis, -os′-ta-sis): The state of relative stability or equilibrium of the internal environment of the body, including the various functions, such measurable conditions as blood pressure, temperature, heart rate, etc., and the chemical composition and reactions of tissues and fluids; or the physiological process by which this stasis is maintained.

homeotherapy (hō-mē-ō-ther′-a-pi): Prevention or treatment of a pathological condition by use of a substance or product that is similar to, or identical with the agent that caused the condition.

homicide (hom′-i-sīd): Killing of a human being; manslaughter; murder. A murder.

homocystine (hō-mō-sis′-tin): An amino acid containing sulfur; produced synthetically.

homocystinuria (hō′-mō-sis-tin-ū′-ri-a): Excretion of homocystine (a sulfur-containing amino acid, homologue of cystine) in the urine.

homoeroticism (hō′-mō-ē-rot′-i-sizm): Homosexuality. Eroticism directed toward another of the same sex.

homogenate (hō-moj′-e-nāt): A substance produced by homogenization (*q.v.*).

homogeneous (hom-ō-jē′-nē-us): Of the same kind; of the same quality or consistency throughout.

homogenization (hō-moj′-en-ī-zā′-shun): The process of breaking down and blending the particles of a substance with those of another substance with which it is not normally miscible to form a uniform suspension or emulsion.—homogenize, v.

homogenize (hō-moj′-e-nīz): To reduce the particles of a substance so that they are uniformly small and evenly distributed throughout the substance.

homogenous (hō-moj′-e-nus): 1. Having a structural resemblance because of having a common progenitor. 2. Having a like nature, *e.g.*, a bone graft from another human being.

homogentisic acid (hō′-mō-jen-tis′-ik as′-id): Found in urine of persons with alkaptonuria (*q.v.*), an intermediate product in the oxidation of tryosine and phenylalanine. Formerly called glycosuric acid.

homograft (hō′-mō-graft): A tissue or organ that is transplanted from one individual to another of the same species.

homolateral (hō-mō-lat′-er-al): On the same side.—homolaterally. adv.

homologous (hō-mol′-ō-gus): Corresponding in origin and structure, but not necessarily in function.

homologue (hom′-ō-log): 1. A part or organ of the body that is similar in structure to another part or organ. 2. Any part of an organ or structure of an animal that is similar in structure to that of another animal but which may differ in function.

homonymous (hō-mon′-im-us): In anatomy, being in the same relation or having corresponding halves. See hemianopia. In language, having two names or meanings.

homophilic (hō-mō-fil′-ik): Descriptive of an antibody that reacts with, or has affinity for, a specific antigen.

homophobia (hōm-ō-fō′-bi-a): Fear of homosexuals, of one's own homosexual tendencies, or of being considered a homosexual.

homophonia (hō-mō-fō′-ni-a): A speech defect characterized by lack of ability to produce vocal sounds, resulting in whispering speech.

homoplasty (hō′-mō-plas-ti): Surgical replacement of lost parts or tissue by similar parts or tissue from another of the same species.

homosexual (hō-mō-seks′-u-al): 1. Relating to the same sex. 2. An individual who exhibits homosexuality (*q.v.*). 3. A person who has an erotic inclination toward those of the person's own gender.

homosexual panic: An extreme anxiety reaction experienced by heterosexual or homosexuals due to conflicts involving gender identity, fear of being identified as homosexual, or fear of sexual attack by a person of the same sex.

homosexuality (hō′-mō-seks-ū-al′-i-ti): 1. Sexual attraction for or erotic relationship with persons of one's own sex. In psychiatry, the term may be used in relation to the period of development when attraction to the same sex is a normal manifestation. FEMALE H., lesbianism (*q.v.*).

homothermal (hō-mō-ther′-mal): Descriptive of organisms that maintain a constant temperature in spite of changes in the temperature of the environment. Denoting warm-blooded animals.

homotransplantation. (hō′-mō-trans-plan-tā′-shun): Transfer of tissue or organ to a member of the same species. Syn., homograft.

homozygosis (hō-mō-zī-gō′-sis): The formation of a zygote by the union of like gametes.

homozygote (hō-mō-zī′-gōt): An individual produced by the union of two gametes of identical genetic composition.—homozygous, adj.

homunculus (hō-mung′-kū-lus): 1. A midget. 2. A small scale model of the human body or a part of it. 3. A miniature human body, once thought to preexist as such in the sperm or ovum.

honeycomb lung: Descriptive of the change that occurs in fibrosing alveolitis when the advancement of the disease causes solidification of the alveoli and the air spaces consist mainly of dilated bronchioles.

hookworm: Any one of a number of parasitic nematode worms (including Ancylostoma and Uncinaria) that infest the intestinal tract of man; transmitted by feces. H. DISEASE, a chronic debilitating disease, characterized by severe anemia; caused by the blood-sucking hookworm, which enters the body through the skin, usually that of the feet. The disease is found mostly in warm areas where disposal of feces is inadequate and people do not wear shoes.

hordeolum (hor-dē′-ō-lum): A stye. A purulent inflammation of one or more of the sebaceous glands of the eyelid; may be external, occurring on the skin at the edge of the lid; or internal, occurring on the conjunctival surface of the lid.

hormone (hor′-mōn): A specific chemical substance manufactured in a gland or organ in the body and carried by the blood or lymph to another organ or tissue, where it acts as a stimulant or accelerator of an involuntary and self-regulating process. Many hormones are secreted by ductless glands. See also endocrine.—hormonic, hormonal, adj.

hormone replacement therapy: The administration of hormones prepared in drug form as a substitute for those hormones that the body no longer produces or which have been lost through surgery; replacement must be continued throughout life.

hormonopoiesis (hor′-mō-nō-poy-ē′-sis): The production of hormones.—hormonopoietic, adj. Also hormopoiesis.

hormonoprivia (hor′-mōn-ō-priv′-i-a): Old term for a pathological condition caused by lack of one or more hormones.

hormonotherapy (hor′-mō-nō-ther′-a-pi): Treatment with hormones.

Horner's syndrome: A condition caused by unilateral paralysis of cervical sympathetic nerves; characterized by constriction of the pupil, slight ptosis of the upper eyelid, sinking in of the eyeball, anhidrosis, and vasodilatation over the affected side of the face. [Johann Friedrich Horner, Swiss ophthalmologist. 1831–1886.]

horse serum: Serum obtained from a horse immunized against a specific organism or its toxins.

Horton's syndrome: Severe headache with pain in the eye, temple, neck, and face; nasal discharge; tearing. Due to release of histamine in the body. To be differentiated from migraine. [Bayard Taylor Horton, American physician. 1895–.]

hospice (hos′-pis): 1. Any shelter for the poor, the sick, orphan children, or travelers. 2. Today, the term usually refers to an institution or a set of services designed to improve the quality of life for the terminally ill and their families. The focus is on symptomatic relief and psychosocial support for the patient and his family. May be free standing, associated with a hospital, or based in the patient's home.

hospital: An institution that is devoted to the diagnosis, treatment, and rehabilitation of persons who are mentally or physically ill or injured. **BASE H.**, a military hospital at a large military base that receives the wounded from smaller hospital units nearer the fighting front. **COMMUNITY H.**, any nongovernmental short-term general or special **H. DAY H.**, one that patients attend daily, returning to their homes at night; recreational and occupational therapy are often provided; used mostly for psychiatric and geriatric patients. **FIELD H.**, a first aid station near the fighting front. **GENERAL H.**, 1) a large civilian hospital that cares for medical/surgical, obstetrical, and emergency patients and has a resident staff of physicians; or 2) a military hospital of 1000 or more beds. **GOVERNMENTAL H.**, a public hospital under the control of local, state or federal government. **ISOLATION H.**, a **H.** for care of patients with contagious disease. **LONG-TERM H.**, a **H.** in which the average length of stay is 30 or more days. **MATERNITY H.**, a **H.** for women in childbirth. **NIGHT H.**, one for patients who are able to go to work during the day but return to the **H.** at night because they require treatment or some other service that cannot be provided elsewhere; used mostly by psychiatric patients. **OPEN H.**, may be either 1) a mental **H.** with unlocked windows and doors; or 2) any **H.** to which physicians who are not on the **H.** staff may send their patients and direct their care and treatment. **PRIVATE** or **PROPRIETARY H.**, a **H.** owned and operated by an individual or corporation for profit. **SHORT-TERM H.**, a **H.** in which the average length of stay is less than 30 days. **SMALL H.**, a **H.** with less than 100 beds or less than 4000 admissions a year. **VETERANS ADMINISTRATION H.**, a **H.** built at government expense and controlled and managed by the Veterans Administration; cares for veterans of U.S. wars and retired service men and women. **VOLUNTARY H.**, a **H.** supported by voluntary contributions and managed by a board of managers, often voluntary and non-salaried.

hospital-caused infection: See nosocomial.

hospitalization (hos′-pi-tal-ī-zā′-shun): Placement of an individual in a hosptial for observation, diagnostic tests, or treatment for some disease or disorder.

host: 1. An organism that receives a transplant of tissue from another organism. 2. In biology, the organic structure upon which a parasite lives or grows. **INTERMEDIATE** or **INTERMEDIARY H.**, one in which a parasite passes its larval or cystic stage.

hot: 1. Having a relatively high temperature. 2. Term is used colloquially to describe something that is charged with electricity or that contains dangerous radioactive material. **H. FLASH**, a phenomenon usually associated with the menopause, and due to vasodilation of the vessels of the head and neck particularly; accompanied by a visible flush and sweating, and sometimes, a feeling of suffocation.

hourglass contraction: A circular constriction in the middle of a hollow organ (usually the stomach or uterus), dividing it into two portions.

house: 1. **H. PHYSICIAN:** a physician who cares for hospital patients under the supervision of the medical and surgical staffs; usually a resident or an intern. 2. **H. STAFF:** the interns, externs, and residents of a hospital who care for patients under the direction of the general staff. 3. **H. SURGEON**, the senior member of the surgical staff who cares for patients of an attending surgeon when the latter is not available.

housemaid's knee: Prepatellar bursitis. A traumatic condition in which there is marked swelling of the bursa in front of the patella, the result of kneeling.

Houston's folds or **valves:** The crescent-shaped transverse folds of mucous membrane found in the rectum.

Howell-Jolly bodies: Small round basophilic particles that may be seen in the red blood cells of patients with anemia or leukemia, or following splenectomy.

Hoyer patient lifter: A hydraulic apparatus with a sling; used for lifting heavy patients, or those in casts, in and out of bed. See mechanical lift.

H & P: Abbreviation for history and physical examination.

HPFSH: Abbreviation for human pituitary follicle stimulating hormone.

hr: Abbreviation for hour.

HRA: Health Resources Administration. A federal agency responsible for health planning, research, evaluation, and development of health resources and needs, including manpower and facilities as well as the collection and dissemination of health data.

HRIG: Abbreviation for human rabies immunoglobulin; preferred to ARS (*q.v.*), which is estimated to cause serum sickness in 15% of children and 40% of adults.

h.s.: Abbreviation for *hora somni* [L.], meaning hour of slumber; sleep; bedtime.

HSA: Health Services Administration: A federal agency responsible for improvement in the delivery of health care services to the American people.

HSV-2: Herpes simplex virus, type 2. See under herpes.

HTLV-I: Human T-cell leukemia-lymphoma virus: A virus that has been implicated in the occurrence of some cancers of white blood cells; rare in the U.S.; quite common in Japan, Africa, South America and the Caribbean. May be transmitted through sexual contact, transfusion, and by pregnant women to fetuses.

Hubbard tank: A large tank used in physical therapy, especially for underwater exercises. Also used for underwater treatment of patients with extensive burns.

huffing: Forced expiration; a technique used in chest physical therapy.

hug of life: The Heimlich maneuver (*q.v.*).

Huhner's test: A test involving post-coital examination of mucus from the cervical canal to determine the number and motility of the sperm.

human chorionic gonadotropin: See gonadotropin, chorionic. Abbreviated HCG.

human growth hormone: A secretion of the anterior part of the hypophysis; promotes growth and directly influences the metabolism of fats, proteins, and carbohydrates in the body. Can be produced artificially for treatment in disorders that interfere with normal growth.

human immunodeficiency virus: Virus thought to cause AIDS.

human placental lactogen: A protein hormone elaborated by the placenta; its actions resemble somewhat those of the pituitary growth hormone and prolactin.

humectant (hū-mek′-tant): 1. A substance that promotes the retention of moisture. 2. Moist.

humerus (hū′-mer-us): The bone of the upper arm, between the elbow and shoulder joint; it articulates with the glenoid cavity of the scapula at the proximal end and with the radius and ulna at the distal end.—humeral, adj.; humeri, pl.

humidification (hū-mid′-i-fi-kā′-shun): The process of moistening air; in respiration, by moisture from the mucous membrane lining the respiratory tract.

humidifier (hū-mid′i-fi-er): An apparatus for adding humidity to the air in a specific area.

humidity (hū-mid′-it-i): The amount of moisture in the atmosphere as measured by a hygrometer. **POSITIVE H.**, the actual amount of vapor present in the air; expressed in grains per cubic foot. **RELATIVE H.**, the ratio of the amount of moisture present in the air to the amount which would saturate it (at the same temperature). **H. TENT**, an enclosure placed over the patient, or just over the head, when administering humidity in the form of a mist.—humidification, n.

humor, humour (hū′-mor): Any normal fluid or semi-fluid of the body. **AQUEOUS H.**, the fluid filling the anterior and posterior chambers in front of the optical lens. **VITREOUS H.**, the gelatinous mass filling the interior of the eyeball from the lens to the retina.

humoralism (hū′-mor-al-ism): An ancient doctrine, now obsolete, that the human body is made up of four humors, and that health and temperament are determined by changes in these humors which were identified as blood, phlegm, choler (yellow bile) and melancholy (black bile).

humpback, hunchback: Kyphosis (*q.v.*).

hunger (hun′-ger): A longing, desire, or urgent need, especially for food. **AIR H.**, see air. **H. PAIN**, epigastric pain, which is relieved by taking food; associated with duodenal ulcer.

Hunner's ulcer: A lesion in the bladder wall characterized by dysuria that is relieved by voiding; occurs in chronic interstitial nephritis; is difficult to detect.

Hunter-Hurler syndrome: An inherited form of mucopolysaccharidosis, but the symptoms are less severe; closely resembles Hurler's syndrome (*q.v.*).

hunterian chancre: The hard sore of primary syphilis. [John Hunter, Scottish anatomist. 1728–1793.]

Huntington's chorea or disease: See under chorea.

Hunt's syndrome: 1. A condition characterized by intention tremor, which begins in an extremity and gradually increases in intensity as more parts of the body become involved. 2. A condition resulting from a viral infection of the seventh cranial nerve; signs and symptoms include herpes zoster, facial paralysis, otalgia. Also called Ramsay-Hunt syndrome.

HUP: Abbreviation for Hospital Utilization Program.

Hurler's syndrome: An inherited disorder of metabolism marked by skeletal deformities, causing a grotesque appearance, gargoylism, mental retardation, enlarged liver and spleen. Mucopolysaccharidosis (*q.v.*).

Hutchinson-Gilford syndrome: Premature aging in juveniles; marked by accelerated growth, severe atherosclerosis, hyperlipidemia, collagen disorders.

Hutchinson's teeth: Defect of the upper central incisors which is regarded as part of the facies of the congenital syphilitic person. The central incisors (second dentition) are broader at the gum than at the cutting edge and each shows an elliptical notch in the lower edge; the lateral incisors are pegged. [Jonathan Hutchinson, English surgeon. 1828–1913.]

HVP-77: An attenuated vaccine based on a rubella virus strain called HVP-77 (high virus passage of the 77th level); first developed in 1965 and licensed for production in the U.S. in 1969; used to produce active immunity against rubella (German measles).

Hx: Abbreviation for history.

hyaline (hī'a-līn -lēn): Like glass; transparent. **H. MEMBRANE,** see under membrane. **H. MEMBRANE DISEASE** or **H. MEMBRANE SYNDROME,** see respiratory distress syndrome under respiratory.

hyalitis (hī-al-ī'-tis): Inflammation of the optical vitreous humor or its enclosing membrane.

hyaloid (hī'-a-loyd): Resembling hyaline; glassy. **H. MEMBRANE,** the transparent capsule enclosing the optical vitreous humor.

hyaluronic acid (hī'-al-ū-ron'-ik): A polysaccharide that occurs as a gelatinous substance in the intercellular spaces, especially of the skin; it holds the cells together.

hyaluronidase (hī'-al-ū-ron'-i-dās): An enzyme found in some pathogenic bacteria, sperm and some venoms; it breaks down hyaluronic acid (*q.v.*) and thus increases the permeability of tissues. When injected subcutaneously, it promotes the absorption of fluid; given with or immediately before a subcutaneous infusion. See hyaluronic acid.

hybrid (hī'-brid): The offspring of parents belonging to different but closely allied races, cultures, species, or genotypes.

hydatid (hī'-da-tid): 1. Any cyst-like structure. 2. The cyst formed by a tapeworm and found in various parts of the body, especially the liver. It may rupture and give rise to daughter cysts. See Echinococcus.

hydatid disease (hī'-da-tid): An infection caused by the larval forms of tapeworms of the genus Echinococcus, characterized by the formation of multiple expanding cysts.

hydatidiform (hī-da-tid'-i-form): Resembling a hydatid cyst. **H. MOLE,** see mole.

hydr-, hydra-, hydro-: Combining forms denoting: 1. Water, or water-loving organism. 2. Hydrogen.

hydragogue (hī'-dra-gog): 1. A purgative which produces a watery evacuation of the bowel. 2. Producing a watery discharge, particularly from the intestines.

hydramnios (hī-dram'-ni-os): An excess of amniotic fluid.

hydranencephaly (hī'-dran-en-sef'-a-li): Congenital absence, or partial absence, of some or all of the cerebral hemispheres, with the space they would normally occupy being filled with cerebrospinal fluid.

hydrargyrum (hī-drar'-ji-rum): Mercury or quicksilver.

hydrarthrosis (hī-drar-thrō'-sis): A collection of watery fluid in a joint cavity. **INTERMITTENT H.,** appears periodically, develops spontaneously, lasts a few days, and disappears. The joint may be normal between attacks, Affects young women mostly; may be due to an allergy.

hydrate (hī'-drāt): 1. A compound made up of water in chemical union with another substance. 2. To combine with or take up water.—hydration, n.

hydration (hī-drā'-shun): The union or combining of water with another substance.

hydraulic lift: A mechanical device for lifting a completely helpless person from the bed to a stretcher, wheel chair, toilet, etc.

hydremia (hī-drē'-mi-a): A relative excess of plasma volume compared with the red cell volume of the blood; it is normally present in late pregnancy.—hydremic, adj.

hydriatic (hī-dri-at'-ik): Pertaining to hydrotherapy.

hydrion (hī'-drī-on): Hydrogen in the ionized form.

hydroa (hī-drō'-a): A skin condition marked by the eruption of vesicles or bullae; dermatitis herpetiformis (*q.v.*). **H. AESTIVALE,** a vesicular or bullous skin disease of children; the vesicles appear upon reddened patches of the skin. It may recur every summer; affects exposed parts and probably results from photosensitivity; often associated with porphyrinuria (*q.v.*). **H. VACCINIFORME** is a more severe form of **H. ESTIVALE** in which scarring occurs.

hydrocarbon (hī'-drō-kar'-bon): Any compound that contains only hydrogen and carbon.

hydrocele (hī'-drō-sēl): A swelling due to accumulation of serous fluid, especially in the tunica vaginalis of the testis, or along the spermatic cord. **COMMUNICATING H.** a **H.** in which the tunica vaginalis testis is filled with fluid and connects directly with the peritoneal cavity.

hydrocelectomy (hī'-drō-sē-lek'-to-mi): The incision of a hydrocele and drainage of fluid from within the scrotal sac.

hydrocephalus (hī'-drō-sef'-a-lus): Literally, water on the brain. An excess of cerebrospinal fluid within the ventricles of the brain or within the subdural spaces; usually a congenital condition but may also result from injury, infection, tumor, or developmental anomalies. The head enlarges, the brain atrophies, and mental weakness follows. **COMMUNICATING H.,** a **H.** in which there is no obstruction in the ventricles and the cerebrospinal fluid passes into the spinal canal but is not absorbed. **EXTERNAL H., H.** in which the fluid is mainly in the subarachnoid space. **INTERNAL H., H.** in which the fluid excess is mainly in the ventricles of the brain. **NONCOMMUNICATING H., H.** in which there is a block in the passage from the ventricles of the brain where the cerebrospinal fluid is produced and the subarachnoid space from which it is absorbed.—hydrocephalic, adj.

hydrochloric acid (hī-drō-klor′-ik): A colorless compound of hydrogen and chlorine; it is caustic and has an escharotic effect when undiluted. Also secreted by the stomach lining and normally present in gastric juice in 0.2 percent solution.

17 hydrocortiocosteroids (hi′-drō-kor′-ti-kō-stē′-royds): The metabolites or breakdown products of hydrocortisone, cortisone, and small amounts of aldosterone; their presence is increased in the urine of patients with Cushing's syndrome, adrenal cancer, polycystic ovaries, some adrenal tumors, and in late pregnancy; and decreased in Addison's disease and hypopituitarism.

hydrocortisone (hī′-drō-kor′-ti-sōn): The pharmaceutical name for the adrenocortical steroid commonly called cortisol; used for its anti-inflammatory action.

hydrocyanic acid (hī′-drō-sī-an′-ik): An extremely dangerous acid, obtained from the stones of peaches and other fruits, used as an exterminant for rodents and other insects. Inhalation of very small amounts will cause death. Also called prussic acid.

hydrogel (hī′-drō-jel): A gel in which water is the dispersion medium. See **gel**.

hydrogen (hī′-drō-jen): A colorless, odorless, flammable gas, explosive when mixed with air; found in all organic compounds and water. The lightest element known. **H. ION CONCENTRATION,** a measure of the acidity or alkalinity of a solution, expressed as *p*H and ranging from *p*H 1 to 14, 7 being approximately neutral; the lower numbers denote acidity, the higher ones alkalinity. **H. PEROXIDE** (H_2O_2), an oxidizing agent used for cleansing wounds.

hydrogen peroxide test: A test for the presence of blood in a fluid; is positive if bubbles arise when a 20 percent solution of hydrogen peroxide is added.

hydrogenation (hī′-drō-jen-ā′-shun): The addition of hydrogen to a compound, especially to an unsaturated fat or fatty acid, causing soft fats and oils to be solidified.

hydrogymnastics (hī′-drō-jim-nas′-tiks): Active therapeutic exercises done in or under water. Also called hydrokinesitherapy.

hydrolabyrinth (hī′drō-lab′i-rinth): An excess of fluid (endolymph) in the inner ear.

hydrology (hī-drol′-o-ji): The study of water and its uses.

hydrolysate (hī-drol′-i-sāt): The product of hydrolysis. **PROTEIN H.,** the amino acids resulting from splitting the protein molecule by an acid, alkali, or enzyme.

hydrolysis (hī-drol′-is-is): The splitting of a substance into more simple substances by the addition of water.—hydrolytic, adj.; hydrolyze, v.

hydroma (hī-drō′-ma): Hygroma (*q.v.*).

hydromassage (hī′-drō-ma-sazh′): Massage by a whirlpool device or some other form of moving water.

hydrometer (hī-drom′-et-er): An instrument for determining the specific gravity of a liquid as compared to that of an equal volume of water.

hydrometra (hī-drō-mē′-tra): A collection of watery fluid or mucus within the uterus.

hydrometrocolpos (hī′-drō-mē′-trō-kōl′-pos): A condition marked by the collection of watery fluid in the uterus and vagina.

hydromyelia (hī′-drō-mī-ē′-li-a): An increased amount of fluid in the expanded central part of the spinal cord.

hydronephrosis (hī′-drō-nē-frō′-sis): Distension of the kidney pelvis with urine, from obstructed outflow. If unrelieved, pressure eventually causes atrophy of kidney tissue and impaired renal function.—hydronephrotic, adj.

hydropathy (hī-drop′-a-thi): The use of water both internally and externally in treatment of disease, particularly the unscientific use of water as compared with hydrotherapy.

hydropericarditis (hī′-drō-pe-ri-kar-dī′-tis): Pericarditis with serous effusion.

hydropericardium (hī′-drō-pe-ri-kar′-di-um): Fluid in the pericardial sac in the absence of inflammation. Can occur in heart and kidney failure.

hydroperitoneum (hī′-drō-pe-ri-tō-nē′-um): Ascites (*q.v.*).

hydrophilia (hī-drō-fil′-i-a): The property of readily absorbing and holding water.—hydrophilic, adj.

hydrophilic (hī-drō-fil′-ik): 1. Having the property of readily absorbing water; water soluble. 2. A substance that is attracted to water and readily absorbs it.

hydrophobia (hī-drō-fō′-bi-a): 1. Morbid fear of water. 2. Spasm of the muscles of swallowing, particularly liquids, as occurs in patients with rabies; results in aversion to water. 3. Rabies (*q.v.*).

hydropneumothorax (hī′-drō-nū-mō-thō′-raks): Pneumothorax further complicated by effusion of fluid in the pleural cavity. Often tubercular.

hydrops (hī′-drops): Dropsy; an abnormal accumulation of serous fluid in the body tissues or a body cavity. **ENDOLYMPHATIC H.,** Meniére's syndrome. **H. FETALIS,** severe form of erythroblastosis fetalis; infants are often dead at delivery.—hydropic, adj.

hydrorrachis (hī-dror′-a-kis): More than the normal amount of cerebrospinal fluid between the spinal cord and its membranes.

hydrorrhea (hī-drō-rē′-a): Copious watery discharge from any organ or part. **H. GRAVIDARUM,** the intermittent discharge of a clear fluid from the uterus during the last months of pregnancy.

hydrosalpinx (hī-drō-sal′-pinks): Distension of the fallopian tube with watery fluid, often the end result of an infection.

hydrosis (hī-drō′-sis): Hidrosis (*q.v.*).

hydrostatic (hī-drō-stat′-ik): Pertaining to the study of hydrostatics. **H. PRESSURE,** in physiology, the pressure exerted by blood and other body fluids. **H. TEST,** one that indicates a live birth if, in post mortem, the infant's lungs float in water; obsolete.

hydrostatics (hī-drō-stat′-iks): The branch of physics that deals with the study of liquids at rest and of the forces exerted by and on them.

hydrotherapist (hī′-drō-ther′-a-pist): One trained in the use of hydrotherapy (*q.v.*).

hydrotherapy (hī′-drō-ther′-a-pi): Treatment of disease by the scientific application of water externally; hydrotherapeutics.—hydrotherapeutic, adj.

hydrothorax (hī′-drō-thō′-raks) The presence of serous fluid in the pleural cavity. May be caused by famine, edema, heart failure, renal disorders.

hydroureter (hī′-drō-ū-rē′-ter): Abnormal distension of a ureter with urine; may be caused by stricture, the presence of a stone, or a new growth.

hydroureteronephrosis (hī′-drō-ū-rē′-ter-ō-nef-rō′-sis): Distention and dilatation of one or both kidneys and ureters with urine or other watery fluid; due to an obstruction in outflow.

hydrouria (hī-drō-ū′-ri-a): An increase in the water content of urine while the amount of solids remains normal or is reduced.

hydrous (hī′-drus): Describes a substance containing chemically-bound water.

hydroxybutyric acid (hī-drok′si-bū-tir′ik): An intermediate product formed during fat metabolism; one of a group of compounds called collectively ketone or acetone bodies, which are found in the urine of patients with ketosis.

hydroxyl (hī-drok′-sil): The univalent group OH, consisting of a hydrogen atom linked with an oxygen atom; when combined with certain other radicals, hydroxides are formed.

hydroxyl group (hī-drok′-sil): The OH group in an organic compound.

hydroxyproline (hī-drok′-si-prō′-lin): An amino acid produced in the digestion of certain proteins, including collagens.

hydruria (hī-drū′-ri-a): Polyuria (*q.v.*). See diabetes insipidus.

Hygeia (hī′-jē-a): In Greek mythology, the daughter of Aesculapius (*q.v.*), and the goddess of health.

hygiene (hī′-jēn): The science dealing with health and its maintenance. **COMMUNITY H.,** embraces all measures taken to supply the community with pure food and water, good sanitation, housing, etc. **INDUSTRIAL H.** (occupational **H.**), includes all measures taken to preserve the individual's health while at work. **MENTAL H.,** deals with the establishment of healthy mental attitudes and emotional reactions. **OCCUPATIONAL H.,** industrial **H. ORAL H.,** deals with the proper care of the mouth and teeth for the maintenance of health. **PERSONAL H.,** deals with those measures taken by the individual to preserve his own health. **PUBLIC H.,** community **H. SOCIAL H.,** deals with sex education, marriage, family relations, and the promotion of sexual health.—hygienic, adj.

hygienist (hī′-ji-en-ist): One who specializes in the science of health. **DENTAL H.,** one trained to give dental prophylactic treatment.

hygr-, hygro-: Combining forms denoting moisture, humidity, or relationship to water.

hygroma (hī-grō′-ma): A cyst, bursa or sac filled with watery fluid. **CYSTIC H.,** a cystic swelling containing watery fluid, usually situated in the neck, and present at birth.—hygromata, pl.; hygromatous, adj.

hygrometer (hī-grom′-et-er): An instrument for measuring the amount of moisture in the air. See humidity.

hygrophobia (hī′-grō-fō′-bi-a): Abnormal fear of water or liquids.

hygroscopic (hī′-grō-skop′-ik): Readily absorbing water, *e.g.*, glycerin.

hymen (hī′-men): A membranous, perforated structure partially covering the vaginal entrance. **IMPERFORATE H.,** a congenital condition leading to hematocolpos. See cryptomenorrhea.—hymenal, adj.

hymenectomy (hī-me-nek′-to-mi): Surgical excision of the hymen.

hymenotomy (hī-me-not′-o-mi): Surgical incision of the hymen.

hyoid (hī′-oyd): A U-shaped bone at the root of and supporting the tongue.

hypacusis (hī-pa-kū′-sis): Slightly impaired hearing. Also hypacusia.

hypalgesia (hī-pal-jē′-zi-a): Decreased sensitiveness to pain. Also hypalgia; hypoalgesia.—hypalgesic, adj.

hypamnion (hī-pam′-ni-on): A deficiency of amniotic fluid.

hypemia (hī-pēm′-i-a): Lack of blood supply to a part.

hyper: Prefix denoting: 1. Excessive; above normal. 2. Located above.

hyperabduction syndrome: Erythema, numbness, and paresthesia accompanied by pain coursing down the arm and weakness of the hand; due to abduction of the arm for long periods of time, as occurs during sleep or in some occupations that cause a stretching of the nerves and vessels of the brachial plexus.

hyperacidaminuria (hī′-per-as′-id-am-i-nū′-ri-a): An excess of amino acids in the urine.

hyperacidity (hī′-per-a-sid′-i-ti): Excessive acidity. See **hyperchlorhydria.**

hyperactivity (hī′-per-ak-tiv′-i-ti): Excessive activity or restlessness as may sometimes be seen in children with minimal brain dysfunction.

hyperacusis (hī′-per-a-kū′-sis): 1. Abnormal acuteness of hearing. 2. Painful sensitivity to sounds. Also hyperacusia.

hyperadiposis (hī′-per-ad-i-pō′-sis): Excessive fatness.

hyperadrenalism (hī′-per-a-drē′-nal-izm): A condition in which the adrenal cortex secretes abnormally large amounts of glucocorticoid, mineralocorticoid, estrogen, or androgen; may occur without apparent cause or may be due to excessive administration of the adrenal cortical hormones. See **Cushing's disease.**

hyperadrenocorticism (hī′-per-a-drē′-nō-kor′-ti-sizm): Cushing's syndrome (*q.v.*).

hyperalbuminemia (hī′-per-al-bū-mi-nē′-mi-a): Abnormally high percentage of albumin in the blood.

hyperaldosteronism (hī′-per-al-dos′-ter-o-nizm): Excessive secretion of aldosterone, causing disturbance of electrolyte metabolism; may be primary as in Conn's syndrome or secondary to another disease condition such as hypertension, heart failure, cirrhosis, low serum potassium levels, hypoproteinemia, muscular weakness.

hyperalgesia (hī′-per-al-jē′-zi-a): Excessive sensitivity to pain. Also hyperalgia.—hyperalgesic, adj.

hyperalimentation (hī′-per-al-i-men-tā′-shun): Administration or ingestion of more than the optimal amount of nutrients; may be a temporary therapy or permanent for patients whose absorptive capabilities are inadequate. Usually refers to administration through an indwelling catheter in the subclavian vein; the solution given contains the substances for complete nutrition when the patient cannot take these via the usual route; has been used for patients with such conditions as esophageal obstruction, ulcerous conditions, cancer of different parts of the digestive tract and accessory organs, enteritis, ulcerative colitis, burns, pancreatitis, and acute renal, hepatic, or respiratory failure. **ENTERAL H.,** the special nutrient formula is introduced into the intestine through a tube that is inserted through the nose and passed to the small intestine.

hyperammonemia (hī′-per-am-mō-nē′-mi-a): 1. An increase in the level of ammonia in the blood. 2. An inborn error of metabolism in which there are high levels of ammonia in the blood and cerebrospinal fluid; manifested by lethargy, slurred speech, weak pulse, ataxia, gastrointestinal symptoms, and coma; if untreated, death may ensue.

hyperammonuria (hī′per-am-mō-nū′ri-a): Increased excretion of ammonia in the urine.

hyperamylasemia (hī′-per-am′-i-lā-sē′-mi-a): The presence of an abnormally large amount of amylase in the blood serum; occurs in acute pancreatitis.

hyperandrogenism (hī′-per-an-droj′-en-izm): The state characterized by or resulting from oversecretion of androgens.

hyperaphia (hī-per-ā′-fi-a): Abnormal acuteness of the sense of touch.

hyperasthenia (hī′-per-as-thē′-ni-a): Extreme weakness.—hyperasthenic, adj.

hyperbaric (hī-per-bar′-ik): At greater pressure, specific gravity, or weight than normal. **H. OXYGEN CHAMBER,** sealed cylinder containing oxygen under pressure. Accommodates patient, attendant, and equipment. In some units surgery can be performed, as anaerobic organisms and their ability to produce toxins are adversely affected by oxygen, so oxygen saturated tissues respond better to radiotherapy. **H. OXYGEN TREATMENT** has been suggested for treatment of burns, refractory osteomyelitis, cerebral edema, soft tissue infections, peripheral vascular disease, gas gangrene, carbon monoxide poisoning, and any other condition in which the oxygen content of the blood is deficient.

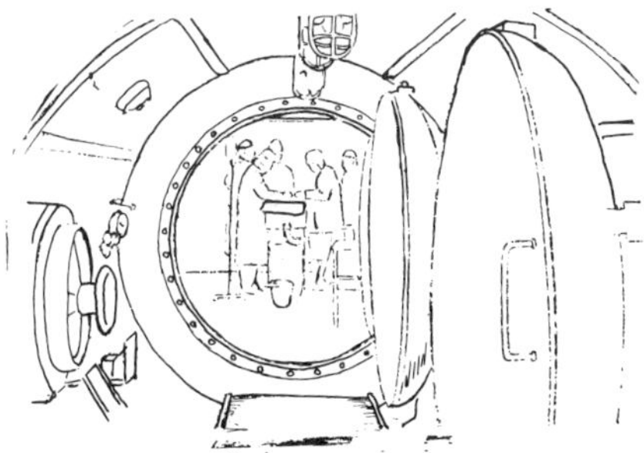

Hyperbaric oxygen chamber

hyperbicarbonatemia (hī′per-bī-kar′bō-na-tē′mi-a): The presence of an excessive amount of bicarbonate in the circulating blood.

hyperbilirubinemia (hī′-per-bi-li-roo-bi-nē′-mi-a): Excessive bilirubin in the blood, resulting in jaundice.—hyperbilirubinemic, adj.

hypercalcemia (hī′-per-kal-sē′-mi-a): An excessive amount of calcium in the circulating blood; occurs in osteoporosis, hyperparathyroidism, and other conditions marked by resorption of bone.

hypercalciuria (hī′-per-kal-si-ū′-ri-a): Greatly increased calcium excretion in urine, as seen in hyperparathyroidism. Of importance in pathogenesis of nephrolithiasis. **IDIOPATHIC H.**, H. for which there is no known metabolic cause.

hypercapnia (hī-per-kap′-ni-a): Excessive amounts of carbon dioxide in the circulating blood.—hypercapnic, adj.

hypercarbia (hī-per-kar′-bi-a): Hypercapnia (*q.v.*).

hypercatabolism (hī′per-ka-tab′ō-lizm): An abnormally increased rate of catabolism.—hypercatabolic, adj.

hypercellular (hī-per-sel′-ū-lar): Characterized by an abnormally large number of cells or an increase in the number of cells present.—hypercellularity, n.

hyperchloremia (hī′-per-klō-rē′-mi-a): Excessive amounts of chloride in the circulating blood.—hyperchloremic, adj.

hyperchlorhydria (hī′-per-klor-hid′-ri-a): Excessive hydrochloric acid in the gastric juice.—hyperchlorhydric, adj.

hypercholesterolemia (hī′-per-ko-les′-ter-ōl-ē′-mi-a): Excessive cholesterol in the blood. Predisposes to atheroma and gallstones. Also found in myxedema.—hypercholesterolemic, adj.

hyperchromatism (hī′-per-krō′-ma-tizm): 1. Excessive pigmentation of the skin. 2. A condition in which certain parts of a cell accept more than a normal amount of stain. 3. An increased amount of chromatin in the nuclei of cells.

hyperchromia (hī′-per-krō′-mi-a): 1. Hyperchromatism (*q.v.*). 2. An increase in the normal amount of hemoglobin in the red blood cells.

hyperchylia (hī′-per-kī′-li-a): Excessive secretion of gastric juice.

hypercoagulability (hī′-per-kō-ag′-ū-la-bil′-i-ti): The state of being more than normally coagulable; usually refers to the blood.

hypercorticism (hī′-per-kor′-ti-sizm): Hyperadrenocorticism (*q.v.*).

hypercortisolism (hī′-per-kor′-ti-sol-izm): A condition characterized by excessive secretion of hydrocortisone (cortisol) by the adrenal cortex, as occurs in Cushing's syndrome.

hypercryalgesia (hī′-per-krī-al-jē′-zi-a): Abnormal sensitiveness to cold. Also hyperesthesia.

hypercythemia (hī′-per-sī-thē′-mi-a): An abnormal number of red blood cells in the circulating blood.

hypercytosis (hī′-per-sī-tō′-sis): An abnormal increase in the number of cells in the circulating blood; term is sometimes used synonymously with leukocytosis (*q.v.*).

hyperdactylia (hī′-per-dak-til′-i-a): The presence of more than the usual number of fingers or toes. Also hyperdactyly and hyperdactylism.

hyperdipsia (hī′-per-dip′-si-a): Intense, relatively temporary thirst.

hyperdynamia (hī′-per-dī-nā′-mi-a): Excessive strength or activity of muscles.

hyperemesis (hī′-per-em′-e-sis): Excessive vomiting. **H. GRAVIDARUM**, the pernicious vomiting of pregnancy.

hyperemia (hī-per-ē′-mi-a): Excess of blood in an area. **ACTIVE H.**, caused by an increased flow of blood to a part. **PASSIVE H.** occurs when there is restricted flow of blood from a part.—hyperemic, adj.

hyperendemic (hī′-per-en-dem′-ik): Refers to a disease that is present in a community at all times and with a high incidence rate.

hyperesthesia (hī′-per-es-thē′-zi-a): Excessive sensitiveness of the skin or another special sense organ.—hyperesthetic, adj. Cf. anesthesia.

hyperextension (hī′-per-ek-sten′-shun): Over-extension of a limb or part, *i.e.*, extreme or excessive straightening of a limb beyond its normal limit.

hyperfibrinogenemia (hī′-per-fī′-brin-ō-je-nē′-mi-a): An excess of fibrinogen in the circulating blood.

hyperflexion (hī′-per-flek′-shun): Excessive flexion of a limb or part beyond its normal limit.

hypergalactia (hī′-per-ga-lak′-shi-a): Excessive secretion of milk.

hypergammaglobulinemia (hī′-per-gam-ma-glob′-ū-lin-ē′-mi-a): An excess of gammaglobulin in the blood plasma.

hypergeusia (hī-per-gū′-si-a): Abnormal acuteness of the sense of taste.

hyperglobulinemia (hī′-per-glob′-ū-lin-ē′-mi-a): An increase in the concentration of globulin in the blood serum or plasma.

hyperglycemia (hī′-per-glī-sē′-mi-a): An excessive amount of glucose in the circulating blood; hyperglycosemia.—hyperglycemic, adj.

hyperglyceridemia (hī′-per-glis′-er-i-dē′-mi-a): An excessive amount of glycerides in the circulating blood, a normal condition following a meal high in lipids but becomes abnormal if it persists.

hyperglycosuria (hī′-per-glī-cō-sū′-ri-a): The persistent excretion of glucose in the urine in much greater amounts than is usually observed in glycosuria.

hypergonadism (hī′-per-gon′-a-dizm): A condition characterized by overgrowth and precocious sexual development due to increased secretion of gonadal hormones.

hyperhemolytic (hī′-per-hē-mō-lit′-ik): Pertaining to or the cause of excessive hemolysis.

hyperhidrosis (hī′-per-hī-drō′-sis): Excessive sweating.—hyperhidrotic, adj.

hyperimmune (hī′-per-im-mūn′): The condition of having large quantities of antibody in the serum.

hyperinflation (hī′-per-in-flā′-shun): Overdistention of an inflatable structure such as the lung.

hyperinsulinemia (hī′-per-in′-sū-li-nē′-mi-a): A condition of the blood wherein there is an excessive amount of insulin present.

hyperinsulinism (hī′-per-in′-sū-lin-izm): A condition caused by excessive secretion of insulin, which causes an abnormally low blood sugar concentration; may be due to pathology of the pancreas, overdosage of insulin, or obesity; may also occur in infants of diabetic mothers. Characterized by intermittent or continuous loss of consciousness, with or without convulsions. Sometimes called insulin shock.

hyperinvolution (hī′-per-in-vo-lū′-shun): Reduction to below normal size, as of the uterus after parturition.

hyperirritability (hī′-per-ir-i-ta-bil′-i-ti): Pathologically extreme response to a slight stimulus.

hyperkalemia (hī′-per-ka-lē′-mi-a): Excessive potassium in the circulating blood; may be caused by renal pathology, adrenal insufficiency, oral or intravenous intake in excessive amounts; symptoms include flaccidity of muscles, shallow respirations, depression of myocardium, arrhythmias.

hyperkeratosis (hī′-per-ker-a-tō′-sis): 1. Overgrowth of the horny layer of the skin. 2. Overgrowth of the cornea. **EPIDERMOLYTIC H.**, a hereditary disease characterized by formation of blisters and erythema; at birth the skin is covered with thick hard scales that are shed and then reform. **H. SUBLINGUALIS, H.** occurring in the nail bed.—hyperkeratotic, adj.

hyperketonuria (hī′-per-kē′-tō-nū′-ri-a): Excessive secretion of ketone bodies in the urine.

hyperkinesia (hī′-per-kī-nē′-si-a): Excessive movement; abnormal restlessness, or excessive muscular activity. Also hyperkinesis.—hyperkinetic, adj.

hyperkinetic (hī′-per-kī-net′-ik): Characterized by or pertaining to hyperkinesia (*q.v.*). **H. SYNDROME**, a form of minimal brain dysfunction (*q.v.*) characterized by excessive energy and motor activity, emotional instability, distractibility, lack of fear; seen mostly in children with brain injuries or mental defect.

hyperleukocytosis (hī′-per-lū′-kō-sī-tō′-sis): An increase in the number of leukocytes in the blood greater than that usually seen in leukocytosis.

hyperlipemia (hī′per-līp-ē′mi-a): An excess of one or more of the lipemic substances in the blood, particularly cholesterol and triglycerides; may be a primary condition in disorders of metabolism or secondary as occurs in diabetes mellitus.

hyperlipidemia (hī′-per-lip-i-dē′-mi-a): Hyperlipemia.

hyperlipoproteinemia (hī′-per-lip-o-prō′-tē-in-ē′-mi-a): A disorder of fat metabolism characterized by the presence of more than the normal amount of lipoproteins in the circulating blood; associated with a large group of inherited and acquired disorders in which large amounts of lipoproteins and cholesterol appear in the blood.

hypermagnesemia (hī′-per-mag-ne-sē′-mi-a): An abnormally high level of magnesium in the blood serum, occurs most often in people who habitually take large amounts of antacid drugs containing magnesium.

hypermastia (hī′-per-mas′-ti-a): 1. Abnormal increase in the size of the mammary gland. 2. The presence of supernumerary mammary glands.

hypermelanosis (hī′-per-mel-a-nō′-sis): Excessive melanin pigmentation.

hypermenorrhea (hī′-per-men-ō-rē′-a): Prolonged or abnormally profuse menses recurring at regular intervals.

hypermetabolism (hī′-per-me-tab′-ō-lizm): An abnormal increase in the utilization of food materials by the body, resulting in the production of excessive heat. Characteristic of thyrotoxicosis.—hypermetabolic, adj.

hypermetropia (hī′-per-mē-trō′-pi-a): Hyperopia (*q.v.*). Syn., far-sightedness; long-sightedness.

hypermnesia (hī-perm-nē′-zi-a): Unusual power of memory with extraordinary ability to remember names, dates, and specific details of experiences.

hypermobility (hī′-per-mō-bil′-i-ti): Excessive mobility, referring particularly to increased range of motion of joints.

hypermotility (hī′-per-mō-til′-i-ti): Increased motility or movement, as peristalsis.

hypermyotonia (hī′-per-mī-ō-tō′-ni-a): Excessive muscle tone.

hypermyotrophy (hī′-per-mī-ot′-rō-fi): Unusual development of muscle tissue.

hypernatremia (hī′-per-nā-trē′-mi-a): An unusually high level of sodium in the blood. May occur either when an excessive water loss follows an excessive water intake, or in diabetes insipidus.—hypernatremic, adj.

hypernephroma (hī′-per-ne-frō′-ma): Grawitz tumor. A malignant neoplasm of the kidney.—hypernephromata, pl.; hypernephromatous, adj.

hypernoia (hī-per-noy′-a): Excessive mental activity.

hypernutrition (hī′-per-nū-trish′-un): Overfeeding, or the effects of it.

hyperonychia (hī′-per-ō-nik′-i-a): Excessive growth of the nails.

hyperopia (hī′-per-ō′-pi-a): A condition in which the rays of light entering the eye are focused behind the retina; usually due to a flattening of the eyeball from front to back. Farsightedness.—hyperopic, adj. Syn., hypermetropia.

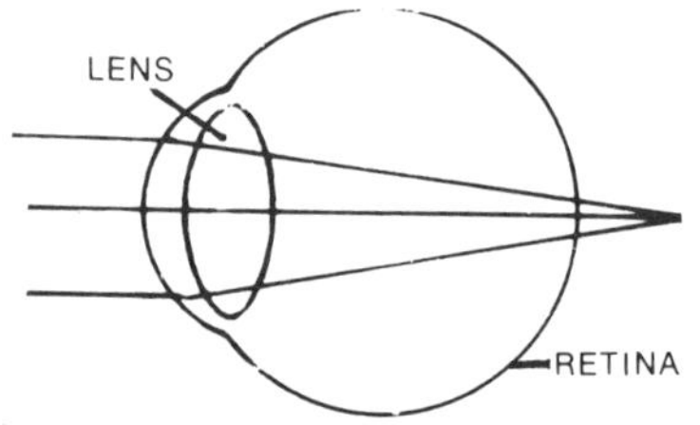

Hyperopia

hyperorality (hī′-per-ō-ral′-i-ti): An extremely strong tendency to touch everything with the mouth.

hyperorexia (hī′-per-ō-rek′-si-a): Excessive appetite. Bulimia.

hyperosmia (hī-per-oz′-mi-a): An abnormally high sensitiveness to odors.—hyperosmic, adj.

hyperosmolar (hī′-per-oz-mō′-lar): Pertaining to a solution with osmotic pressure greater than that of normal blood plasma.—hyperosmolarity, adj.

hyperostosis (hī′-per-os-tō′-sis): Thickening or overgrowth of bone. Exostosis.

hyperoxaluria (hī′-per-ok-sa-lū′-ri-a): A genetic disorder of metabolism marked by the appearance of excess amounts of oxalic acid in the urine; a common cause of nephrolithiasis and nephrocalcinosis in children.

hyperoxemia (hī′-per-ok-sē′-mi-a): A condition in which the blood is excessively acid.

hyperoxia (hī-per-ok′-si-a): An excess of oxygen in the tissues or the system.—hyperoxic, adj.

hyperparathyroidism (hī′-per-par-a-thī′-royd-izm): A condition due to overaction of the parathyroid glands resulting in loss of calcium from the bones and an increase in serum calcium levels; may result in osteitis fibrosa cystica with decalcification and spontaneous fracture of bones.

hyperperistalsis (hī′-per-pe-ri-stal′-sis): Excessive peristalsis, with very rapid passage of food through the gastrointestinal tract; most often due to diffuse infection of the peritoneum.

hyperphagia (hī′-per-fā′-ji-a): Overeating.

hyperphasia (hī′-per-fā′-zi-a): Excessive talkativeness.

hyperphenylalaninemia (hī′-per-fen′-il-al-a-ni-nē′-mi-a): A condition in which the blood levels of phenylalanine are abnormally high; seen in premature and full-term infants; may be associated with phenylketonuria (*q.v.*); symptoms may include aminoaciduria, jaundice, splenomegaly, cataracts, cerebral and liver damage.

hyperphoria (hī′-per-fō′-ri-a): The tendency for one eye to turn upward.

hyperphosphatemia (hī′per-fos-fa-tē′mi-a): Excess of phosphates in the blood.

hyperphosphaturia (hī′-per-fos-fa-tū′-ri-a): An increased amount of phosphates in the urine.

hyperphrenia (hī-per-frē′-ni-a): 1. Excessive mental activity. 2. An unusually high intellect.

hyperpiesis (hī-per-pī-ē′-sis): High blood pressure of unknown origin, especially essential hypertension (*q.v.*).

hyperpigmentation (hī′-per-pig-men-tā′-shun): Increased or excessive pigmentation of a tissue or part. **H.** of the skin, may be due to exposure to sunlight, use of certain drugs, or adrenal insufficiency.

hyperpituitarism (hī′-per-pi-tū′-i-ta-rizm): Overactivity of the anterior lobe of the pituitary, producing gigantism or acromegaly.

hyperplasia (hī′-per-plā′-zi-a): Excessive formation of cells resulting in overgrowth of tissue. **CONGENITAL ADRENAL H.**, a group of disorders caused by enzymatic defects that result in excessive secretion of the adrenal androgens; the congenital form of adrenogenital syndrome (*q.v.*). **GINGIVAL H.**, enlargement of the gums until they cover portions of the teeth.—hyperplastic, adj.

hyperplastic (hī′-per-plas′-tik): 1. Pertaining to hyperplasia. 2. Overgrown.

hyperpnea (hī′-perp-nē′-a): Rapid, deep, labored breathing; panting; gasping.—hyperpneic, adj.

hyperpotassemia (hī′-per-pot-a-sē′-mi-a): Increased potassium in the blood, a condition that, theoretically, can cause heart block, cardiac arrest, and muscle paralysis. Syn., hyperkalemia.—hyperpotassemic, adj.

hyperprolactinemia (hī′-per-prō-lak′-tin-ē′-mi-a): An excess of prolactin in the blood, a normal condition in lactating women, but otherwise abnormal; may be associated with pituitary tumors; often accompanies amenorrhea.

hyperproteinemia (hī'-per-prō'-tē-in-ē'-mi-a): More than the normal amount of protein in the circulating blood.

hyperpsychosis (hī'-per-sī-kō'-sis): Excessive mental activity.

hyperpyrexia (hī'-per-pī-rek'-si-a): Extremely high fever. **MALIGNANT H.**, a rare, often fatal, possibly hereditary condition usually affecting young people; marked by high fever and muscular rigidity; most often seen in postoperative patients who have been given certain drugs.

hyperreflexia (hī'-per-rē-flek'-si-a): Exaggeration of the deep tendon reflexes. **AUTONOMIC H.**, exaggerated sympathetic response to noxious stimuli applied below the level of a spinal cord lesion.

hyperreflexic (hī'-per-rē-flek'-sik): Spastic or hypertonic, or pertaining to hyperreflexia. **H. BLADDER**, see neurogenic bladder under neurogenic.

hyperresonance (hī'-per-rez'-o-nans): Greater than normal resonance heard on percussion of the chest, particularly in patients with emphysema and pneumothorax (*q.v.*).—hyperresonant, adj.

hypersalivation (hī'-per-sal-i-vā'-shun): Increased secretion of saliva.

hypersensitivity (hī'-per-sen-si-tiv'-i-ti): A state of being unduly sensitive to a stimulus or an allergen (*q.v.*).—hypersensitive, adj.

hypersexuality (hī'-per-seks-ū-al'-i-ti): Abnormal increase in sexual drive.

hypersomnia (hī'-per-som'-ni-a): A condition in which one sleeps for long periods of time but is normal in the intervals between sleeping.—hypersomniac, n.; adj.

hypersplenism (hī'-per-splen'-izm): A condition in which there is increased hemolytic activity of an enlarged spleen; there may be refractory anemia, leukopenia, or thrombocytopenia, in spite of active bone marrow.

hypersteatosis (hī'-per-stē-a-tō'-sis): Excessive secretion by sebaceous glands.

hypersthenia (hī-per-sthē'-ni-a): Excessive or abnormal strength or tonicity of muscles.

hypertelorism (hī'-per-tel'-or-izm): 1. Greater than normal width between two paired parts or organs. 2. Genetically determined cranial anomaly (low forehead and pronounced vertex) associated with mental subnormality. **OCULAR H.**, greater than normal space between the eyes.

hypertension (hī'-per-ten'-shun): 1. Transient or persistently high blood pressure, by custom referring to blood pressure readings in which either or both systolic and diastolic pressure readings are significantly higher than the mean for the population. 2. Persistent elevation of blood pressure that is over 140 systolic and 90 diastolic. (WHO definition.) **H.** is a symptom rather than a disease and the cause is often unknown, but it may indicate change in the condition of the blood vessels or the heart muscle, or a kidney disorder; it is likely to increase during periods of emotional stress and decrease during periods of rest and sleep. **H.** is not usually considered curable, but can be controlled by appropriate medication. **ESSENTIAL H.**, that which occurs without preexisting disease or demonstrable change in kidneys, heart, or blood vessels; also sometimes called primary or benign **H.**; symptoms include headache, dizziness, tinnitus, nosebleed, fainting **MALIGNANT H.**, usually develops at a comparatively early age, runs a rapid course, and has a poor prognosis. **PORTAL H.**, abnormally high blood pressure in the portal venous system; often seen in cirrhosis of the liver. **PULMONARY H.**, increased blood pressure within the pulmonary circulation. **RENAL H.**, that due to damaged or defective kidney function. **RENOPARENCHYMAL H.**, that due to disease of the renal parenchyma; cause obscure; usually chronic and bilateral. **RENOVASCULAR H.**, that resulting from interference with blood supply to the kidney.

hypertensive (hī'-per-ten'-siv): 1. Pertaining to, affected with, or characterized by hypertension. 2. A person affected with hypertension. **H. CRISIS**, a sudden rise in blood pressure to measurements over 200/120 mmHg; occurs most often in patients who have not been treated or who have stopped taking prescribed medications. **H. ENCEPHALOPATHY**, a condition occurring in persons with advanced arterial hypertension; symptoms include headache, vomiting, somnolence, and sometimes convulsions. **H. HEART DISEASE**, a condition characterized by enlarged ventricles, altered pulse rate, nocturnal dyspnea. **H. RETINOPATHY**, see under retinopathy.

hyperthecosis (hī'-per-thē-kō'-sis): Hyperplasia of the graafian follicles of the ovaries.

hyperthelia (hī'-per-thē'-li-a): The presence of one or more supernumerary nipples.

hyperthermalgesia (hī'-per-ther-mal-jē'-si-a): Abnormal sensitiveness to heat.

hyperthermia (hī'-per-ther'-mi-a): 1. Extremely high temperature; hyperpyrexia. 2. A method of treating disease by raising the temperature of the body, either by external applications, the introduction of disease organisms into the body, or the injection of foreign proteins. See thermodialysis. **MALIGNANT H.**, a rare complication of anesthesia; the temperature rises very rapidly, with muscular rigidity, cardiac arrhythmia, circulatory collapse, and often coma and death.

hyperthrombinemia (hī'-per-throm-bin-ē'-mi-a): A condition characterized by an abnormally high level of thrombin in the circulating blood.

hyperthymia (hī'-per-thī'-mi-a): 1. An overactive mental state with a tendency to perform impulsive acts. 2. Oversensitiveness. 3. Cruel or foolhardy behavior as sometimes seen in patients with mental disorders.

hyperthyroidism (hī'-per-thī'-roy-dizm): Thyrotoxicosis (*q.v.*).

hypertonia (hī'-per-tō'-ni-a): Abnormally increased tone in a muscular structure.—hypertonic, adj.; hypertonicity, n.

hypertonic (hī'-per-ton'-ik): 1. Having hypertonia (*q.v.*). 2. Having an osmotic pressure greater than a solution used for comparison, *e.g.*, normal saline has a greater osmotic pressure than normal physiological (body) fluids.—hypertonicity, n.

hypertonus (hī'-per-tō'-nus): Hypertonia.

hypertoxic (hī'-per-tok'-sik): Very poisonous.

hypertrichiasis (hī'-per-tri-kī'-a-sis): Excessive hairiness. May be congenital or acquired; may occur in women at menopause, and in patients with Cushing's disease, acromegaly, or thyrotoxicosis.

hypertrichosis (hī'-per-tri-kō'-sis): Hypertrichiasis (*q.v.*).

hypertriglyceridemia (hī'-per-trī-glis'-er-i-dē'-mi-a): An excessively high level of triglycerides in the blood.

hypertrophy (hī-per'-trō-fi): Increase in the bulk of a tissue or structure; due to increase in size of the cells, not to tumor formation; usually the result of functional activity, *e.g.*, the **H.** of a muscle. Hypertrophia.—hypertrophic, adj.

hyperuresis (hī'-per-ū-rē'-sis): Old term for polyuria (*q.v.*).

hyperuricemia (hī'-per-ū-ri-sē'-mi-a): Excessive uric acid in the blood. Characteristic of gout.—hyperuricemic, adj.

hyperuricuria (hī'-per-ū-ri-kū'-ri-a): Excess of uric acid in the blood.

hypervascular (hī-per-vas'-kū-lar): Containing an abnormally large number of blood vessels.—hypervascularity, n.

hyperventilation (hī'-per-ven-ti-lā'-shun): 1. Over-breathing; more than 20 inspirations per minute. 2. A state in which there is a decrease of carbon dioxide in the blood as a result of rapid and deep breathing; symptoms may include dizziness, confusion, and muscle cramps. **H. SYNDROME**, rapid and labored breathing, as occurs in persons affected with depression or anxiety, leading to alkalosis.

hyperviscosity (hī'-per-vis-kos'-i-ti): The state of being excessively glutinous, sticky, or viscous.

hyperviscous (hī'per-vis'kus): The condition of being abnormally viscous. See **VISCOUS**.

hypervitaminosis (hī'per-vī'ta-min-ō'sis): Any condition arising from an excess ingestion of vitamins; large overdoses of vitamin A and D may cause pathological conditions. Water-soluble vitamins apparently do not accumulate in the body in sufficient quantities to cause pathological conditions.

hypervolemia (hī'-per-vō-lē'-mi-a): An abnormal increase in the volume of blood circulating in the body. Plethora (*q.v.*).—hypervolemic, adj.

hypesthesia (hī'pes-thē'-zi-a): Hypoesthesia (*q.v.*).

hypha (hī'-fa): One of the filaments that make up the mycelium (*q.v.*) of a fungus.—hyphae, pl.

hyphema (hī-fē'-ma): The presence of blood in the anterior chamber of the eye, usually due to an injury.

hyphemia (hī-fē'-mi-a): A deficiency of blood; oligemia.

hyphidrosis (hip-hid-rō'-sis): A decrease in the secretion of sweat.

hypn-, hypno-: Combining forms denoting: 1. Sleep. 2. Hypnosis or hypnotism.

hypnagogic (hip-na-goj'-ik): Producing sleep or induced by sleep. In psychiatry, refers to hallucinations that occur during the period just before falling asleep.

hypnagogue (hip'-na-gog): An agent that induces sleep. A hypnotic.

hypnoanalysis (hip'-nō-a-nal'-a-sis): Psychoanalysis with the patient under hypnosis (*q.v.*).

hypnolepsy (hip'-nō-lep-si): Uncontrollable, abnormal drowsiness.

hypnosis (hip-nō'-sis): A state resembling sleep, brought about by the hypnotist utilizing the mental mechanism of suggestion. **H.** can be used to produce painless labor and dental extractions; is occasionally utilized in minor surgery and in psychiatric practice.—hypnotic, adj.; hypnotize, v.t.

hypnotherapy (hip'-nō-ther'-a-pi): Treatment by prolonged sleep or hypnosis.

hypnotic (hip-not'-ik): 1. Pertaining to hypnotism. 2. A drug that produces sleep.

hypnotism (hip'-nō-tizm): 1. The process of inducing a condition in which a person appears to be asleep but is susceptible to suggestion and carries out commands. 2. The study or practice of hypnosis.

hypo: Hypodermic (colloq.).

hypo-: Prefix denoting: 1. Deficient; less than normal. 2. Located beneath or below.

hypoacidity (hī'-pō-a-sid'-i-ti): Less than normal acidity; usually refers to acidity of the gastric juice.

hypoactivity (hī'-pō-ak-tiv'-i-ti): Abnormally diminished activity; said of glands, nerves, muscles, or of the entire organism.

hypoacusis (hī′-pō-a-kū′-sis): Hearing impairment.

hypoadrenalism (hī′-pō-a-drē′-na-lizm): The condition of reduced adrenocortical function; adrenal insufficiency.

hypoadrenocorticism (hī′-pō-a-drē′-nō-kor′-ti-cizm): A condition characterized by a decrease in the activity of the adrenal gland; Addison's disease.

hypoalbuminemia (hī′-pō-al-bu-min-ē′-mi-a): An abnormally low amount of albumin in the circulating blood.—hypoalbuminemic, adj.

hypoaldosteronism (hī′-pō-al-dos′-ter-ō-nizm): Deficient production of aldosterone; characterized by hypotension and excess secretion of salt; often associated with hypoadrenalism.

hypobaric (hī′pō-bar′ik): 1. Referring to atmospheric pressure that is significantly lower than usual. 2. Referring to an anesthetic in solution that has a lower specific gravity than that of cerebrospinal fluid.

hypobaropothy (hī′pō-bar-op′a-thi): A condition caused by diminished air pressure or decrease in oxygen in the air. Examples are altitude sickness, mountain sickness, aviator's sickness, caisson disease (*q.v.*).

hypobulia (hī′-pō-bū′-li-a): Abnormal weakness of the will.—hypobulic, adj.

hypocalcemia (hī′-pō-kal-sē′-mi-a): Abnormally low levels of calcium in the circulating drug; occurs in such conditions as hypoparathyroidism, inadequate intake of calcium, vitamin D deficiency, kidney and pancreatic pathology; chief symptoms are tetany of the hands, feet, tongue and lips, and cardiac arrhythmias. See **tetany**.

hypocalciuria (hī′-pō-kal-si-ū′-ri-a): An abnormal diminution in the amount of calcium excreted in the urine.

hypocapnia (hī-pō-kap′-ni-a): Less than the normal amount of carbon dioxide in the circulating blood.—hypocapnic, adj.

hypocarbia (hī-pō-kar′-bi-a): Hypocapnia (*q.v.*).

hypocellular (hī-pō-sel′-ū-lar): Characterized by an abnormally low number of cells or a decrease in the number of cells present.—hypocellularity, n.

hypochloremia (hī′-pō-klō-rē′-mi-a): Less than the normal amount of chlorides in the circulating blood. A form of alkalosis.—hypochloremic, adj.

hypochlorhydria (hī′-pō-klor-hid′-ri-a): Less than the normal amount of hydrochloric acid in the gastric juice.—hypochlorhydric, adj.

hypochlorite (hī-pō-klō′-rīt): Any salt of hypochlorous acid. Such salts are easily decomposed to yield active chlorine, and have been widely used on that account in treating wounds, *e.g.*, Dakin's solution.

hypochloruria (hī′-pō-klōr-ū′-ri-a): The excretion of abnormally small amounts of chlorides in the urine.

hypocholesteremia (hī′-pō-kō-les′-ter-ē′-mi-a): Less than the normal amount of cholesterol in the blood.

hypochondria (hī-pō-kon′-dri-a): A fixed mental attitude involving the erroneous conviction that the body or an organ is diseased. Excessive anxiety about one's health; common in depressive and anxiety states.—hypochondriac, adj.

hypochondriac (hī-pō-kon′-dri-ak): 1. One suffering from hypochondria (*q.v.*). 2. Pertaining to the hypochondrium (*q.v.*). 3. Pertaining to hypochondriasis (*q.v.*).

hypochondriasis (hī-pō-kon-drī′-a-sis): Constant conscious or unconscious preoccupation with the state of one's health, a role often adopted to get attention and to manipulate friends and relatives; in some cases there are actual physical illnesses, but the majority of illnesses reported have no pathological basis. Also called hypochondria.

hypochondrium (hī-pō-kon′-dri-um): The upper lateral regions (right and left) of the abdomen, just below the lower ribs.—hypochondria, pl.; hypochondriac, adj.

hypochromia (hī-pō-krō′-mi-a): 1. Deficiency in coloring or pigmentation. 2. Less than the normal percentage of hemoglobin in the red blood cells.—hypochromic, adj.

hypochylia (hī-pō-kī′-li-a): Deficiency in the amount of gastric juice secreted.

hypodactyly (hī-pō-dak′-til-i): Less than the normal number of fingers or toes. Also called hypodactylia and hypodactylism.

hypodermic (hī-pō-der′-mik): 1. Below the skin; subcutaneous. 2. An injection into or under the skin. 3. A small syringe with a hollow needle used for injecting drugs or other agents into or under the skin.—hypodermically, adv.

hypodermis (hī-pō-der′-mis): The layer of tissue lying immediately beneath the corium of the skin (*q.v.*).

hypodermoclysis (hī-pō-der-mok′-li-sis): The injection of a large amount of fluid, usually saline solution, into the subcutaneous tissues; a procedure formerly much used following hemorrhage or surgical shock when the patient could not be given fluids by mouth, intravenously, or by rectum.

hypodipsia (hī-pō-dip′-si-a): Abnormally diminished sensation of thirst.

hypoesthesia (hī′-pō-es-thē′-zi-a): Abnormally diminished sensitiveness of a part.

hypofibrinogenemia (hī′-pō-fī′-brin-ō-je-nē′-mi-a): Abnormally low levels of fibrinogen in the circulating blood.

hypofunction (hī′-pō-funk′-shun): Diminished or inadequate function.

hypogalactia (hī-pō-ga-lak′-shi-a): Less than normal secretion of milk.

hypogammaglobulinemia (hī′-pō-gam-ma-glob′-ū-li-nē′-mi-a): Decreased gamma globulin in the blood; may be acquired or congenital; several types are identified, all of which are characterized by immunoficiency (*q.v.*). See **immune response** under **immune**.

hypogastric (hī-pō-gas′-trik): Refers to the area immediately below the stomach. See **region, abdominal**.

hypogastrium (hī′-pō-gas′-tri-um): That area of the anterior abdomen which lies immediately below the umbilical region. It is flanked on either side by the iliac regions.- hypogastric, adj.

hypogenitalism (hī-pō-jen′-i-tal-izm): Underdevelopment of the genitalia.

hypogeusia (hī-pō-gū′-zi-a): Abnormally diminished sense of taste. Also hypogeusesthesia.

hypoglossal (hī-pō-glos′-al): Situated under the tongue. **H. NERVE,** one of the twelfth pair of cranial nerves; the fibers arise in the medulla and go to the muscles of the tongue.

hypoglycemia (hī′-pō-glī-sē′-mi-a): Abnormally low blood glucose levels; usually due to insulin overdose, dietary mismanagement, or an abnormal secretion of insulin, but may also result from anxiety, excitement, overactivity; symptoms include excessive perspiration, delirum, possibly coma. **H.** is sometimes produced intentionally in treatment of schizophrenia. **POSTPRANDIAL H.,** occurs in normal persons following the ingestion of a meal high in carbohydrates; a sharp insulin release is followed by a fall in the blood glucose level; called also reactive glycemia.

hypoglycemic (hī′-pō-glī-sē′-mik): Pertaining to hypoglycemia. **H. AGENT,** a drug or substance that lowers the glucose content of the blood; of two main types: 1) a drug that lowers the blood glucose and controls the various metabolic effects of the diabetes, *e.g.*, the sulfonylureas; and 2) a drug that assists patients who have some capacity to produce their own insulin to control their blood glucose *e.g.*, the biguanides. **H. CRISIS** or **SHOCK,** see **insulin shock**.

hypoglycorrhachia (hī′-pō-glī-kō-rāk′-i-a): A condition in which the glucose level in the cerebrospinal fluid is below normal; may be indicative of meningeal infection.

hypogonadism (hī-pō-gō′ na-dizm): Diminished internal secretion by the testes or ovaries; may be due to organic defect or to lack of adequate stimulation by the anterior lobe of the hypophysis.

hypohidrosis (hī′-pō-hī-drō′-sis): Abnormally decreased secretion of sweat.

hypoinsulinism (hī′-pō-in′-sū-lin-izm): Deficient secretion of insulin by the pancreas; results in hyperglycemia.

hypokalemia (hī′-pō-ka-lē′-mi-a): Abnormally low level of potassium in the blood. Symptoms are variable but may include muscle weakness and fatigue, nausea and/or vomiting, paralytic ileus, constipation or diarrhea, apnea, shallow breathing, respiratory arrest, arrhythmias. May be due to administration of potent diuretics or steroids, loss of body fluids by vomiting or diarrhea, or decreased intake of dietary potassium.

hypokinesia (hī′-pō-kī-nē′-si-a): Abnormally decreased motor activity or function.

hypokinetic (hī′-pō-kī-net′-ik): Characterized by or pertaining to hypokinesia (*q.v.*). **H. SYNDROME,** a form of minimal brain dysfunction (*q.v.*) in which motor activity is decreased.

hypoleukocytosis (hī′-pō-lū′-kō-sī-tō′-sis): Less than the normal number of leukocytes in the circulating blood. Syn., leukocytopenia.

hypomagnesemia (hī′-pō-mag-ne-sē′-mi-a): Decreased magnesium content in the blood; may occur concurrently with hypercalcemia.

hypomandibulosis (hī′-pō-man-dib-ū-lō′-sis): Underdevelopment of the mandible.

hypomania (hī-pō-mā′-ni-a): A mild form of manic depressive illness; the patient's moods fluctuate between elation and irritation, euphoria and depression. **ACUTE H.,** may be accompanied by the delusions or hallucinations that are characteristic of certain types of schizophrenia.

hypomanic disorder (hī-pō-man′-ik): An atypical bipolar disorder in which a patient who previously had a depressive epidode has a minor manic epidode that is not serious enough to be classed as bipolar II.

hypomastia (hī-pō-mas′-ti-a): Abnormal smallness of the breasts.

hypomenorrhea (hī′-pō-men-ō-rē′-a): Less than the normal amount of uterine bleeding at regular intervals; the period of flow may be the same or less than normal time.

hypometabolism (hī′-pō-me-tab′-ō-lizm): An abnormal decrease in the body's utilization of food materials with resulting diminution in the production of heat; low metabolic rate. Characteristic of myxedema.—hypometabolic, adj.

hypomnesis (hī-pom-nē′-sis): Impaired memory.

hypomotility (hī′-pō-mō-til′-i-ti): Decreased or insufficient movement of any part, *e.g.*, the stomach or intestines. Hypokinesis.

hypomyotonia (hī′pō-mī-o-tō′ni-a): Abnormally low muscular tonicity.

hyponatremia (hī′-pō-na-trē′-mi-a): Abnormally low concentration of sodium in the blood plasma; symptoms include muscle weakness, fatigue, possibly convulsions. May be 1) **DILUTIONAL**, when it results from the intake of large amounts of water as is sometimes seen in schizophrenic and alcoholic patients or in those receiving excessive water enemas or electrolyte-free intravenous solutions, or 2) **DEPLETIONAL**, when it is due to inappropriate use of diuretics, loss of body fluids, adrenal insufficiency, or renal disease.—hyponatremic.

hyponatruria (hī'-pō-na-trū'-ri-a): Abnormally low level of sodium in the urine.

hyponychium (hīpō-nik'i-um): The thickened epidermis that lies at the free end of a nail.—hyponychial, adj.

hypo-osmolarity (hī'-pō-oz-mō-lar'-i-ti): Syn., hypotonicity. A solution exerting a lower osmotic pressure than another is said to have hypo-osmolarity with reference to it. In medicine the comparison is usually made with normal plasma.

hypoparathyroidism (hī'-pō-par-a-thī'-royd-izm): The condition produced by undersecretion or removal of the parathyroid glands; the serum calcium level is decreased, resulting in tetany (*q.v.*).

hypopepsia (hī-pō-pep'-si-a): Impaired digestion, particularly when it is due to deficient secretion of pepsin.

hypoperfusion (hī'-pō-per-fūzh'-un): Lack of adequate perfusion of the tissues with blood, due to decreased blood volume or inability of the heart to pump effectively.

hypopharynx (hī'-pō-far'-inks): The part of the pharynx below and behind the aperture into the larynx and extending to the esophagus. Correctly called the laryngopharynx.

hypophoria (hī-pō-fō'-ri-a): A state in which the visual axis of one eye is lower than that of the other.

hypophosphatasia (hī'-pō-fos-fa-tā'-zi-a): A deficiency of alkaline phosphatase in the blood, as occurs in rickets. Sometimes occurs as an inborn error of metabolism and results in skeletal deformities, defective tooth development, and osteomalacia.

hypophosphatemia (hī'-pō-fos-fa-tē'-mi-a): Decreased phosphates in the blood.—hypophosphatemic, adj.

hypophosphaturia (hī'-pō-fos-fa-tū'-ri-a): Reduced excretion of phosphates in the urine.

hypophrenia (hī-pō-frē'-ni-a): Feeblemindedness.—hypophrenic, adj.

hypophyseal (hī-pō-fiz'-ē-al): Pertaining to a hypophysis, particularly the pituitary gland.

hypophysectomy (hī'-pof-i-sek'-to-mi): Surgical removal of the pituitary gland. **TRANSSPHENOID H.**, a **H.** performed through the sphenoid bone, a procedure that makes it possible for the posterior lobe of the pituitary gland to retain its function.

hypophysis (hī-pof'-i-sis): Any outgrowth or process. **H. CEREBRI**, the small oval-shaped gland lying in the pituitary fossa of the sphenoid bone and connected to the under surface of the brain by a stalk; the pituitary gland.—hypophyseal, adj.

hypopiesis (hī'-pō-pī-ē'-sis): Abnormally low pressure.

hypopigmentation (hī'-pō-pig-men-tā'-shun): Decreased or poor pigmentation.

hypopituitarism (hī'-pō-pi-tū'-i-tar-izm): Pituitary gland insufficiency, especially of the anterior lobe. Absence of gonadotrophins leads to failure of ovulation, uterine atrophy, amenorrhea. Loss of trophic hormones to other endocrines produces mental inertia, laziness, weakness, lack of sweating, sensitivity to cold, oliguria, loss of pubic and axillary hair, hypoglycemia, pale skin, depigmentation of mammary areolae and perineum. Can result from postpartum infarction of the pituitary gland.

hypoplasia (hī-pō-plā'-zi-a): Defective or incomplete development of any tissue or organ due to a decrease in cell formation. **CONGENITAL ADRENOCORTICOID H.**, caused by a defect in adrenal function, with absence or decrease in secretion of hydrocortisone; results in anomalies and abnormal development of reproductive organs, abnormal growth patterns, excessive hairiness, and skin pigmentation.

hypopnea (hī-pop'-nē-a): An abnormal decrease in the rate and depth of respirations. Opp. to hyperpnea.

hypopotassemia (hī'pō-pō-ta-sē'mi-a): Hypokalemia (*q.v.*).

hypoproteinemia (hī-pō-prō'-tē-in-ē'-mi-a): A deficiency of protein in the blood plasma, often the result of dietary deficiency or excessive excretion (albuminuria).—hypoproteinemic, adj.

hypoprothrombinemia (hī'-pō-prō-throm'-bin-ē'-mi-a): Deficiency of prothrombin in the blood, which retards its clotting ability. See vitamin K and jaundice.—hypoprothrombinemic, adj.

hypoptyalism (hī'-pō-tī'-al-izm): Deficient secretion of saliva. Also hyposalivation.

hypopyon (hī-pō'pi-on): A collection of pus in the anterior chamber of the eye.

hyporeactive (hī'-pō-rē-ak'-tiv): Having less than normal response to stimuli.

hyporeflexia (hī'-pō-rē-flek'-si-a): A condition of weakened reflexes.

hyposalivation (hī'-pō-sal-i-vā'-shun): An abnormal decrease in the secretion of saliva; hypoptyalism.

hyposecretion (hī-pō-sē-krē'-shun): Deficient rate or amount of secretion.

hyposensitive (hī-pō-sen'-si-tiv): Having a deficient response to stimuli.

hyposensitiveness (hī-pō-sen′-si-tiv-nes): Subnormal sensitiveness in which 1) responses to stimuli are lessened or delayed; or 2) there is greater than normal power of resistance to a pathogenic agent.

hyposensitization (hī′-pō-sen-si-tī-zā′-shun): Reduction of the sensitiveness of an individual, especially to allergens; usually achieved by repeated injections of small amounts of the particular allergen.

hyposexuality (hī′-pō-seks-ū-al′-i-ti): Deficient in sexuality.

hyposmia (hī-poz′-mi-a): Abnormally decreased sensitiveness to odors.

hyposomnia (hī-pō-som′-ni-a): Insomnia (*q.v.*).

hypospadias (hī-pō-spā′-di-as): A congenital malformation in which the male urethra opens on the under surface of the penis, that of the female opens into the vagina instead of externally from the bladder. Also hypospadia.—hypospadiac, adj.

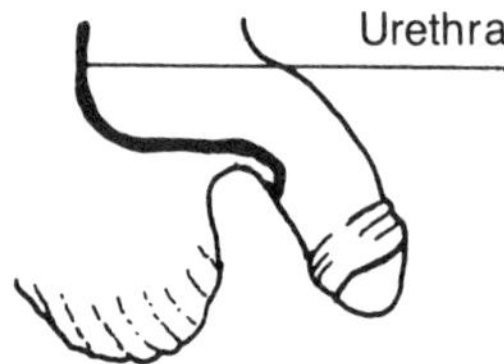

Hypospadias

hypostasis (hi-pos′-ta-sis): 1. Congestion of blood in a part; due to impaired circulation. 2. The formation or deposit of a sediment resulting from impairment of flow of blood or other body fluid.

hypostatic (hī-pō-stat′-ik): 1. Caused by or pertinent to hypostasis (*q.v.*). 2. Abnormally static; said of certain inherited characteristics that are hidden or suppressed by other characteristics. H. CONGESTION, see congestion. H. PNEUMONIA, see pneumonia.

hyposthenia (hī′-pos-thē′-ni-a): Bodily weakness.—hyposthenic, adj.

hyposthenuria (hī-pos-the-nū′-ri-a): The secretion of urine that is of lower than normal specific gravity; often associated with chronic nephritis.

hypostosis (hip-os-tō′-sis): Deficient development of bone.

hypotension (hī-pō-ten′-shun): Lowered blood pressure, primary or secondary. May result from a decrease in cardiac output, total blood volume, or peripheral resistance, or from an endocrine disturbance, hemorrhage, fever, shock, Addison's disease, or drug toxicity. A person is said to be hypotensive when the systolic pressure is below 110 mmHg and the diastolic pressure is below 70 mmHg. ESSENTIAL H., may exist without apparent cause; seen most often in women and the undernourished. ORTHOSTATIC H., a fall in blood pressure that occurs when a person stands up after being in a supine position, or stands erect for a long time; also called postural hypotension.

hypotensive (hī-pō-ten′-siv): 1. A drug or agent that lowers blood pressure. 2. A person suffering from hypotension. 3. Characterized by low blood pressure.

hypothalamus (hī′-pō-thal′-a-mus): Below the thalamus. The part of the midbrain nearest to the pituitary gland; important because the nuclei of this region control the body temperature, visceral activities, sleep, water balance, and the metabolism of fats and carbohydrates; also important in emotional and motivational behavior.—hypothalamic, adj.

hypothenar eminence (hī′-pō-thē′-nar): The eminence on the ulnar side of the palm below the little finger.

hypothermia (hī-pō-ther′-mi-a): 1. A temperature below normal body temperature (below 98.6° F, or 37° C). 2. Artificially induced H. (86° F or 30° C) can be used in the treatment of head injuries and in cardiac surgery. It reduces the oxygen consumption of the tissues and thereby allows greater and more prolonged interference of normal blood circulation. H. OF THE NEWBORN, failure of the newborn child to adjust to external cold; may be associated with infection. ACCIDENTAL H., unexpected drop in body temperature; develops over a period of time, usually in old people in a cool but not cold environment; the temperature will continue to fall and death will result unless there is a change in the environment. H. BLANKET, 1) a covering used to conserve the body heat of a person suffering from hypothermia, or 2) a blanket that has built-in hollow coils carrying cold water and alcohol or other cooling solution kept in circulation by a pump; used to reduce prolonged high fever or for its anesthetic action on patients undergoing brain or heart surgery. NEONATAL H., precipitous fall in body temperature within an hour of birth; the common causes are prematurity and hypoxic brain damage.

hypothesis (hī-poth′-e-sis): A theory or an assumption made for the sake of argument, or as a basis for action to be taken.

hypothrepsia (hī-pō-threp′-si-a): Malnutrition. See athrepsia.

hypothrombinemia (hī′-pō-throm-bin-ē′-mi-a): A deficiency of thrombin in the blood; resulting in a tendency toward bleeding.

hypothyroidism (hī′-pō-thī′-royd-izm): A group of symptoms caused by deficiency of thyroid secretion; characterized by low metabolic rate, slowing of all bodily functions, fatigue, lethargy, hoarseness, intolerance of cold, constipation, weight gain, rough skin; occurs most often in women. **INFANTILE H.**, may result from agenesis of the thyroid gland or inadequate intake of iodine by the mother during pregnancy. See cretinism; myxedema.

hypotonia (hī-pō-tō′-ni-a): 1. Flaccid muscle tone or muscle weakness. When present at birth the infant is referred to as "floppy." 2. Lack of tone in the muscle walls of arteries. 3. Reduced tension, as in the eyeball.

hypotonic (hī-pō-ton′-ik): 1. Having a low osmotic pressure; less than isotonic. 2. Lacking in tone, tension, strength. **H. SOLUTION**, a solution having an osmotic pressure lower than that of physiologic saline.

hypotrichosis (hī-pō-tri-kō′-sis): Presence of less than the usual amount of hair.

hypotrophy (hī-pot′-ro-fi): Progressive degeneration of cells and tissues with loss of function.

hypotropia (hī-pō-trō′-pi-a): Strabismus characterized by permanent downward deviation of the axis of one eye.

hypouresis (hī′-pō-ū-rē′-sis): Reduced output of urine.

hypouricuria (hī′pō-ū-ri-kū′ri-a): Less than the normal amount of uric acid in the urine.

hypoventilation (hī′-pō-ven-ti-lā′-shun): 1. Diminished breathing or underventilation. 2. Less than the normal amount of air entering the lungs; results in less oxygen reaching the alveoli than the body needs for normal metabolism, and an elevation of the carbon dioxide content of the blood, thus causing hypoxemia and hypercapnia.

hypovitaminosis (hī′-pō-vī-ta-min-ō′-sis): A deficiency of one or more of the essential vitamins. Less severe than avitaminosis (*q.v.*).

hypovolemia (hī′-pō-vō-lē′-mi-a): An abnormal decrease in the amount of blood circulating in the body. Opp. to hypervolemia.—hypovolemic, adj.

hypovolemic (hī′-pō-vō-lē′-mik): Pertaining to or characterized by hypovolemia. **H. SHOCK**, shock caused by a reduced amount of blood in circulation, as may occur in perforating wounds, burns, or other types of trauma.

hypoxemia (hī-pok-sē′-mi-a): Less than the normal amount of oxygen in the arterial blood.—hypoxemic, adj.

hypoxia (hī-pok′-si-a): Diminished amount of oxygen in the tissues. **ANEMIC H.**, due to a decrease or alteration in the hemoglobin content of the blood. **HISTOLYTIC H.**, the condition existing when the cells' ability to utilize required amounts of oxygen is impaired. **HYPOXIC H.**, due to a reduced amount of arterial oxygen, caused by interference with the passage of oxygen over the alveolar membrane. **ISCHEMIC H.**, is due to inadequate perfusion of the tissues with blood. **STAGNANT H.**, a condition in which the oxygen tension in peripheral vessels is less than normal while that in the arterial blood is normal; occurs in congestive heart failure, shock, and when venous return is interfered with.

hypoxin (hī-poks′-in): A deficiency of oxygen at the cellular or tissue level.

hypsarrhythmia (hip′-sa-rith′-mi-a): Term applied to a condition in infants that is characterized by a distinct abnormality in the electrogram and usually associated with metal retardation; often accompanied by spasms or quivering.

hyster-, hyster-: Combining forms denoting: 1. Hysteria. 2. Uterus.

hysteralgia (his′-ter-al′-ji-a): Pain in the uterus.

hysterectomy (his-te-rek′-to-mi): Surgical removal of the uterus. **ABDOMINAL H.**, effected via a lower abdominal incision. **RADICAL H.**, Wertheim's **H.** (*q.v.*). **SUBTOTAL H.**, removal of the uterine body, leaving the cervix in the vaginal vault. **TOTAL H.**, complete removal of the uterine body and the cervix. **VAGINAL H.**, effected through the vagina. **WERTHEIM'S H.**, total removal of the uterus, the adjacent lymphatic vessels and glands, and a cuff of the vagina. See also panhysterectomy.

hysteria (his-tēr′-i-a): A psychoneurosis or neurosis characterized by a physical disorder such as blindness or paralysis, brought on by psycholgical rather than organic disorder. Marked by conversion of anxiety into such symptoms as nervousness, uncontrollable laughing, crying, convulsions, intense muscular activity, psychic disorders. **CONVERSION H.**, a condition in which hysteria is used to symbolize intrapsychic conflict.

hysterical (his-ter′-i-kal): Related to or affected with hysteria (*q.v.*). **H. CONVULSIONS**, see hysteroepilepsy. **H. NEUROSIS**, see hysteria. **H. PSYCHOSIS**, in psychiatry, refers to acute episodes marked by sudden violent behavior or reaction in a person of hysterical personality; see personality.

hysterics (his-ter′-iks): An uncontrollable fit of laughing or crying, or both. See hysteria.

hysterocele (his′-ter-ō-sēl): A hernia of the uterus.

hysteroepilepsy (his′-ter-ō-ep′-i-lep-si): A form of hysteria characterized by seizures that occur only in the presence of other persons, imitate true epilepsy in nature, and terminate abruptly; usually associated with an emotional situation. Also called pseudoepilepsy.

hysterography (his′-te-rog′-ra-fi): 1. X-ray examination of the uterus. 2. The procedure of making a graphic record that shows the strength of uterine contractions during labor.—hysterograph, hysterogram, n.; hysterographical, adj.; hysterographically, adv.

hysterolaparotomy (his′-ter-ō-lap-a-rot′-o-mi): A hysterectomy done through the abdominal wall.

hysteromyoma (his′-ter-ō-mī-ō′-ma): A myoma (*q.v.*) of the uterus.

hysteromyomectomy (his′-ter-ō-mī-ō-mek′-tō-mē): Surgical removal of a myoma (*q.v.*) from the uterus.

hysteropathy (his-ter-op′-a-thi): Any disease or disorder of the uterus.

hysteropexy (his′-ter-ō-pek-si): Fixation of a displaced or abnormally placed uterus; may be fastened to the vaginal or abdominal wall.

hysteroptosis (his′-ter-op-tō′-sis): Prolapse of the uterus.

hysterorrhaphy (his-ter-or′-ra-fi): Surgical repair of a lacerated uterus.

hysterosalpingectomy (his′-ter-ō-sal-pin-jek′-to-mi): Excision of the uterus and usually both uterine tubes (oviducts).

hysterosalpingography (his′-ter-ō-sal-ping-gog′-ra-fi): X-ray examination of the uterus and tubes after injection of a contrast medium utilizing a tight fitting cervical cannula; the x rays taken during the procedure will show the size and site of any blockage in a tube as well as the size and shape of the uterine cavity.—hysterosalpingogram, n.

hysterosalpingo-oophorectomy (his′-ter-ō-sal′-ping-gō-ō′-of-o-rek′-to-mi): Removal of the uterus, fallopian tubes, and ovaries.

hysterosalpingostomy (his′-te-rō-sal-ping-gos′-to-mi): Anastomosis between an oviduct and the uterus.

hysteroscope (his′-ter-ō-skōp): An instrument used in visual examination of the uterine cervix and cavity.

hysteroscopy (his-ter-os′-kō-pi): Examination of the uterus by means of a hysteroscope (*q.v.*).

hysterotomy (his-ter-ot′-o-mi): Incision into the uterus. **ABDOMINAL H.**, a surgical procedure in which the contents of the uterus are evacuated; most often done during the second trimester when the patient is to be sterilized as well.

hysterotrachelorrhaphy (his′-ter-ō-trak-el-or′-a-fi): Repair of a lacerated cervix.

hysterotraumatism (his′-ter-ō-traw′-ma-tizm): Traumatic hysteria that may follow severe injury.

Hz: Herz (*q.v.*).

I

I: The chemical symbol for iodine.

I^{131}, I^{132}: Radioactive isotopes of iodine.

-ia: Suffix often used in naming diseases or pathological conditions.

ianthinopsia (ī—an-thi-nop′-si-a): A defect in vision in which the individual sees all objects as violet.

-iasis: A combining form denoting: 1. Morbid condition; disease produced by something specific, *e.g.* amebiasis. 2. Disease having the characteristics of a specific thing, *e.g.*, elephantiasis.

iatric (ī-at′-rik): Denoting or referring to medicine or a physician.

-iatrics: Combining form denoting a special field of medical practice.

-iatrist: A combining form denoting a physician, *e.g.*, psychiatrist.

iatro-: Combining form denoting relationship to a physician or to medicine, *e.g.*, iatrogenic.

iatrochemistry (ī-at-rō-kem′-is-tri): The treatment of disease by chemical agents.

iatrogenesis (ī-at-rō-jen′-e-sis): The inadvertent development of a secondary illness or condition through medical or surgical treatment for a primary disorder.—iatrogenic, adj.

-iatry: Combining form denoting medical treatment, healing.

IC: Abbreviation for inspiration capacity.

ICD: Abbreviation for: International Classification of Diseases of the World Health Organization.

ICDA: International Classification of Diseases. Adapted for Use in the United States; widely used in hospital record departments.

ICEA: Abbreviation for International Childbirth Education Association.

ice-water test: A test for reflex activity of the bladder following spinal cord injury; ice cold sterile saline is introduced into the bladder with a straight catheter; if the catheter is expelled the test is considered positive.

ICF: Abbreviation for intermediate care facility.

ichnogram (ik′-nō-gram): An imprint of the soles of the feet: a footprint.

ichor (ī′-kor): A thin, watery discharge, as from a raw wound or ulcer.—ichorous, adj.

ichthio-: Combining form denoting fish, fishy, or fish-like.

ichthyoid (ik′-thi-oyd): Fish-shaped; fish-like.

ichthyosis (ik-thi-ō′-sis): A congenital chronic condition of keratin formation in which the skin becomes rough, dry, and scaly over the entire body, the hair is lusterless, and cold weather causes intense itching; also called fish skin or alligator skin. **I. CONGENITA NEONATORUM,** a severe form of **I.** in the newborn; the skin and mucuous membranes of the body are thickened, dry, and cracked; the skin may peel off; the eyelids may be everted; the fetus may be stillborn or die soon after birth; also called harlequin fetus because of the bizare effect produced by the cracking of the skin. **I. VULGARIS,** a form of **I.** that is inherited as an autosomal dominant trait; onset is in childhood; characterized by fine scales on most of the body; tends to improve with age. **SEX-LINKED I., I.** that appears at birth or soon thereafter; seen only in males; marked by the presence of large brown scales on most of the body except the face, palms, and soles; does not improve much with age.

ichthyotoxin (ik-thi-ō-tok′-sin): A poisonous substance found in the blood serum of the eel. The term is often applied to any toxic substance derived from fish.

ichythyotoxism (ik-thi-ō-toks′-izm): Any toxic condition derived from eating contaminated fish.

ICN: Abbreviation for International Council of Nurses (*q.v.*).

ICP: Abbreviation for: 1. Infection control practitioner. 2. Intracranial pressure.

ictal (ik′-tal): Pertaining to a stroke or seizure, *e.g.*, an acute epileptical seizure.

icteric (ik-ter′-ik): Pertaining to or affected with jaundice.

icterus (ik′ter-us): Jaundice. **I. GRAVIS,** acute yellow atrophy (see **acute**). **I. GRAVIS NEONATORUM,** one of the clinical forms of hemolytic disease of the newborn (erythroblastosis fetalis, *q.v.*). **I. NEONATORUM,** the normal, or physiological jaundice occurring in the first week of life as a result of destruction of hemoglobin in excess of the infant's needs.

icterus index (ik′-ter-us in′-deks): An index, expressed in units, representing the bilirubin concentration in the blood plasma; used in diagnosis of jaundice. The normal range is 4-6 units.

ictus (ik′-tus): A stroke or blow; a sudden attack or fit; an epileptic seizure.

ICU: Abbreviation for intensive care unit (*q.v.*). **ICU PSYCHOSIS,** see under **psychosis**.

I & D: Abbreviation for incision and drainage.

ID: Abbreviation for: 1. Identification. 2. Intradermal.

id: In psychoanalysis, that part of the unconscious mind that consists of a system of primitive urges (instinctual drives), including sexuality and aggression, and that persists unrecognized into adult life as the source of basic desires operating for self-gratification; man's inner drives.

ID disk: An identification system whereby a microdisk carrying the individual's Social Security number is bonded to a rear molar; the S.S. number is filed in a central computer registry which also has on file identifying information and the person's medical history. Useful in locating lost or kidnapped children, retarded individuals, the disoriented or aphasic elderly, and disaster victims.

ideation (ī-dē-ā'shun): The process concerned with the highest function of awareness, the formation of ideas. It includes thought, intellect, and memory.

idée fixe (ē-dā-fēks'): A fixed idea, an obsession; a delusion.

identical twins: Monozygotic twins; two offspring developed from a single fertilized egg. They are always of the same sex and commonly much alike in appearance. See binovular, uniovular.

identification (i-den'ti-fi-kā'shun): In psychology, the way in which personality is formed by modeling it on a chosen person, *e.g.*, identification with the parent of the same sex in helping to form one's sex role, or identification with a person of one's own sex, as in the hero worship of adolescence.

identification band or **bracelet:** A band that is placed on the wrist or ankle when a patient enters a hospital and worn throughout the hospital stay; the patient's name and other identification information is on it.

identity (ī-den'-ti-ti): The group of characteristics that distinguish an individual from others. **I. CRISIS,** loss of the sense of one's self and inability to adopt the role one perceives as being expected; is most likely to occur when one moves from one age group to another, as during adolescence or as one grows older and one's status in the community changes.

ideology (ī'dē-ol'o-ji): 1. The science that deals with the development of ideas. 2. The ideas or manner of thinking that characterize a group or an individual.

ideomotor (ī'dē-o-mō'tor): Descriptive of automative muscular activity that is aroused by thoughts or ideas such as moving the lips while reading silently. Agitated movements of parts of the body resulting from mental agitation.

idio-: Combining form denoting: 1. Self-produced, self-producing, arising within the self 2. Separate, distinct, peculiar.

idiocy (id'i-ō-si): Extreme mental deficiency, usually congenital but may follow disease or injury during childhood; due to incomplete or abnormal development of the brain. See amaurotic familial idiocy, mongolian, and Down's syndrome.

idioglossia (id'-ē-ō-glos'-si-a): Any form of invented speech that is unique to the individual but is incomprehensible to others except in close siblings or twins in whom it often develops.

idiographic (id'-i-ō-graf'-ik): In research, refers to a study of events or subjects in which a great deal of data is acquired from a few people, perhaps only one. Opp. of nomothetic (*q.v.*).

idiopathic (id'i-ō-path'ik): 1. Self-originated; of unknown cause. 2. Relating to a peculiar individual characteristic.

idiopathy (id-i-op'-a-thi): A pathologic state of unknown or spontaneous origin.—idiopathic, adj.

idiophrenic (id'-i-ō-fren'-ik): Related to or originating solely in the mind.

idiosyncrasy (id'i-ō-sin'kra-si): A peculiar variation of constitution or temperament. Unusual individual response to certain drugs, proteins, etc., whether administered by injection, ingestion, inhalation, or contact.

idiosyncratic reaction (id-i-ō-sin-krat'-ik): A reaction that is completely different from the one expected: usually refers to drugs which may produce a reaction that is completely opposite to the one which the drug was expected to produce.

idiot: A severely mentally deficienct person who ranks lowest in the grades of mental deficiency, has an IQ of below 25, is unable to use language meaningfully, avoid ordinary dangers, or be a productive member of society. **MONGOLIAN I.,** one who exhibits monogolism (*q.v.*).

idiot savant (id'-i-ot-sa-vant'): A person who is in general mentally retarded and cannot perform the simplest tasks, but who displays unusual brilliance or aptitude in some special area, *e.g.*, music or mathematics.

idioventricular (id'-i-ō-ven-trik'ū-lar): Pertaining to the cardiac ventricles and not affecting the atria.

IgG: The symbol for immunoglobulin G, which comprises about 80 percent of the serum antibodies in the adult.

IH: Abbreviation for infectious hepatitis; see under hepatitis.

ILCD: Abbreviation for International List of Causes of Death.

ileal (il'-ē-al): Pertaining to or involving the ileum. **I. BYPASS,** the formation of an anastomosis between a part of the ileum and a part farther on; decreases the area for absorption; sometimes done in treatment of obesity. **I. CONDUIT,** a surgically constructed passageway for urine in which a section of the ileum is separated from the rest of the bowel and one end is closed; the two ureters are attached to this segment which serves as a bladder; the unclosed end is brought to the surface of the abdominal wall in a stoma where the urine is collected in a special bag. Also called ileal bladder, ileal loop, and ileal loop diversion.

ileectomy (il-ē-ek′-to-mi): Surgical excision of the ileum.

ileitis (il-ē-ī′-tis): Inflammation of the ileus, characterized by ulceration, possible formation of adhesions, pain in the umbilical area and right lower quadrant, vomiting, alternating constipation and diarrhea. **REGIONAL I.**, acute or chronic **I.**, marked by diarrhea, anemia, abdominal pain, grayish or brownish colored stools; may give rise to intestinal obstruction. Also called Chron's disease.

ileo-: A combining form denoting the ileum.

ileocecal (il′ē-ō-sē′kal): Pertaining to the ileum and the cecum. **I. VALVE**, the sphincter muscle that guards the opening between the ileum and the large intestine, allowing material to pass from small to large intestine, but not in the reverse direction.

ileocecostomy (il′-ē-ō-sē-kos′-to-mi): The creation of an anastomosis between the ileum and the cecum. Also called cecoileostomy.

ileocolic (il′-ē-kol′-ik): Pertaining to the ileum and the colon.

ileocolitis (il′-ē-ō-kō-lī′-tis): Inflammation of the mucous membrane of the ileum and the colon.

ileocolostomy (il′-ē-ō-kō-los′to-mi): The creation of an anastomosis between the ileum and the colon; usually the transverse colon. Most often done to bypass an obstruction or inflammation of the cecum or ascending colon.

ileocystoplasty (il′ē-ō-sis′tō-plas-ti): Operation to increase the capacity of the urinary bladder. See colocystoplasty.—ileocystoplastic, adj.

ileoileostomy (il′-ē-ō-il-ē-os′to-mi): The surgical creation of an anastomosis between two parts of the ileum.

ileojejunitis (il′-i-ō-jē-jun-ī′-tis): Inflammation of the jejunum and part or all of the ileum; usually chronic; may lead to stenosis of the bowel.

ileoproctostomy (il′-ē-ō-prok-tos′-to-mi): An anastomosis between the ileum and the rectum; used when disease extends to the sigmoid colon. Also called ileorectostomy.

ileorectal (il-ē-ō-rek′-tal): Pertaining to the ileum and the rectum.

ileosigmoidostomy (il′ē-ō-sig-moy-dos′to-mi): An anastomosis between the ilium and the sigmoid colon; used when most of the colon has to be removed.

ileostomate (il-ē-os′-tō-māt): A person who has undergone surgery for the creation of an ileostomy.

ileostomy (il-ē-os′-to-mi): A surgically made fistula between the ileum and the surface of the anterior abdominal wall; usually a permanent form of artificial anus when the whole of the large bowel has to be removed, *e.g.*, in severe ulcerative colitis. **I. BAGS**, rubber or plastic bags worn on the body to collect the liquid discharge from the ileum.

ileoureterostomy (il′-ē-o-ū-rēt-er- os′to-mi): Transplantation of the lower ends of the ureters from the bladder to an isolated loop of small bowel which, in turn, is made to open on the abdominal wall. See bladder.

ileum (il′-ē-um): The lower three-fifths of the small intestine, lying between the jejunum and the cecum; about 12 feet long.—ileal, adj.

ileus (il′-ē-us): Intestinal obstruction. Usually restricted to paralytic as opposed to mechanical obstruction and characterized by abdominal distention, vomiting, fever, and dehydration. **MECONIUM I.**, occurs in the newborn; due to blockage of the bowel by thick meconium; usually an indication of fibrocystic disease (*q.v.*). **PARALYTIC I.**, an intestinal obstruction that may result from hypokalemia, toxemia, or trauma, especially that caused by handling during abdominal surgery; characterized by intense pain and abdominal distention. **SPASTIC I.**, obstruction resulting from persistent contraction of the intestinal muscles.

ili-, ilio-: Combining forms denoting relationship to the ilium or flank.

iliac (il′-i-ak): Pertaining to the ilium. **I. ARTERY**, the large artery that transports blood to the pelvis and the legs.

iliococcygeal (il′i-ō-kok-sij′i-al): Pertaining to the ilium and the coccyx.

iliofemoral (il′-i-ō-fem′-or-al): Pertaining to the ilium and the femur.

iliopectineal (il′-i-ō-pek-tin′-ē-al): Pertaining to the ilium and the pubis. **I. LINE**, an anatomical landmark consisting of a bony ridge that begins on the inner surface of the pubis and continues across the ilium to the sacrum; it separates the lesser pelvis below from the greater pelvis above.

iliopubic (il′-i-ō-pū′-bik): Pertaining to the ilium and the pubis. **I. EMINENCE**, a ridge on the hipbone where the ilium and the pubis unite; also called iliopectineal eminence.

iliosacral (il′-i-ō-sā′-kral): Pertaining to the ilium and the sacrum.

iliosciatic (il′i-ō-sī-at′ik): Pertaining to the ilium and the ischium.

iliotibial (il′-i-ō-tib′-i-al): Pertaining to the ilium and the tibia or extending between them.

iliotrochanteric (il′i-ō-trō-kan-ter′ik): Pertaining to the ilium and the greater trochanter of the femur.

ilium (il′-i-um): The large, flaring, lateral, and uppermost of the three bones that compose the innominate (hip) bone; it is a separate bone in fetal life. The flank.—iliac, adj.

illegitimate (il-lē-jit′-i-mat): Born out of wedlock.

illiopsoas (il′-i-ō-sō′-as): Pertaining to the iliacus and psoas muscles.

illness: Disease, sickness, or the condition of being in poor health, either physicially or mentally.

illuminism (i-lū′-mi-nizm): A state occurring in certain psychoses in which the person has delusions of communicating with supernatural beings.

illusion (i-lū′-zhun): 1. A sensory experience that is different from reality, causing the individual to misidentify a sensation, *e.g.*, of sight, whereby a white sheet is mistaken for a ghost; an apparition. 2. The state of being deceived. 3. A false impression, or misconception of a sensory stimulus, often with difficulty in focusing and with increased color vision and hearing acuity, and disturbance of depth perception. 4. A perception that does not give the true character of an object; may be normal as in certain optical illusions, or abnormal as occurs in insanity.

illusionogenic (i-lū′-zhun-ō-jen′-ik): Usually pertains to illusion-producing drugs.

IM: Abbreviation for intramuscular; intramuscularly.

image (im′-ij): 1. A reasonably accurate representation or imitation of a person or thing, *e.g.*, a statue. 2. An optical picture transferred to the brain by the optic nerve. 3. A mental representation of a precept, or a thing, not actually present but that is recalled by memory or created by imagination, as a taste or smell. See also **afterimage**.

imagery (im′-ij-ri): Imagination. The recall of mental images of various types depending on the special sense organs involved when the images were formed. In behavior therapy, imagery is used as a technique by which the person is conditioned to recall or imagine pleasant situations or experiences that counter feelings or memories that are unpleasant or painful.

imago (i-mā′-gō): 1. The sexually mature adult form of an insect. 2. A memory, usually of someone loved during childhood, which has become altered over time, and may not be correct. 3. An image or shadow.

imagocide (i-mā′-gō-sīd): An agent that kills adult insects, especially mosquitoes.

imbalance (im-bal′-ans): Want of balance. Lack of equality of power between opposing forces, especially between muscles and particularly the ocular muscles. Term is also used in reference to lack of balance between the endocrine secretions, as well as to describe an abnormal balance of fluids and electrolytes in the body.

imbecile (im′-be-sil): An old term for one afflicted with mental deficiency of intermediate grade, *i.e.*, between the grades of idiot and moron; the IQ is between 25-30, and the mental age between 3 and 7. Such an individual is mentally retarded, yet capable of some education and training.—imbecility, n.

imbibition (im-bi-bish′-un): The absorption of a liquid by a solid without causing any chemical change.

imbrication (im-bri-kā′shun): Overlapping. The closing of a wound with layers of overlapping tissue.

immature (im-a-tūr′): Not fully developed or grown. **I. INFANT,** one of less than 37 weeks gestation.—immaturity, n.

immedicable (im-med′-i-ka-bl): Not curable.

immersion (i-mer′-zhun): The plunging of a body or part into a fluid. **I. FOOT,** a condition resulting from long exposure to cold and dampness, or of actual immersion of the feet in water causing damage to the skin, blood vessels, and nerves; also called trench foot.

immiscible (i-mis′i-b'l): Not capable of being mixed with something else.

immobility (im-mō-bil′-i-ti): Inability to move separate parts of the body (especially the limbs or the whole body) easily and without pain.

immobilization (im-mō′-bi-lī-zā′shun): The act of making immovable. In medicine or surgery, the act of making a normally movable limb or part immovable by splints, bandages, surgical procedures, etc.—immobilize, v.t.

immune (im-ūn′): 1. Not susceptible to a particular infection. 2. A sensitivity reaction that indicates immunity following exposure to an antigen. **I. BODY,** antibody (*q.v.*). **I. REACTION,** that which causes a body to reject a transplanted organ. **I. RESPONSE,** specifically altered reactivity of the body following exposure to an antigen, and which is manifested as antibody production, cell-mediated immunity, or immunological tolerance; term is often used synonymously with **I.** reaction. **I. SYSTEM,** a complex system that is involved with maintaining homeostasis in which potentially harmful invading organisms are inactivated or eliminated, mutated cells that may become malignant are destroyed, and toxins are neutralized; also called immune defense system.

immunity (im-ū′-ni-ti): A state of relative resistance to a disease. Immunity can be **NATURAL** (acquired from inherited qualities) or it can be **ACQUIRED,** actively or passively, naturally or artificially. **ACTIVE IMMUNITY** is acquired naturally during a disease (infectious), or artificially by vaccination with dead or living organisms of the disease. Such immunity is long lasting. **PASSIVE I.** is acquired naturally when maternal antibodies pass to the child via the placenta or the milk, or artificially by administering immune sera containing antibodies obtained from animals or human beings. **ARTIFICIAL PASSIVE I.** is more temporary than active **I.** A simple classification based on the way immunity is produced, lists four types: 1. Artificial active **I.**, produced by the introduction of *antigens* into the body. 2. Artificial passive **I.**, produced by the introduction into the body of *antibodies*. 3. Natural active **I**, produced by having the disease. 4. Natural passive **I**, acquired by heredity.

immunization (im'ū-nī-za'shun): The process of making an individual immune, or of becoming immune. **TRIPLE ANTIGEN I.**, immunization with a mixed vaccine containing diphtheria toxoid, tetanus toxoid, and pertussis vaccine; usually one dose is given at age 4 weeks and repeated at age 10 weeks; produces active immunity against diphtheria, tetanus, and pertussis. See also **vaccination**.

immunochemistry (im'ū-nō-kem'is-tri): The special branch of chemistry that deals with immunologic phenomena, antigens, and antibodies.—immunochemical, adj.

immunocompetence (im'ū-nō-kom'pe-tens): The competence or ability to develop an immune reaction or response, *e.g.*, the production of antibodies.

immunocyte (im'ū-nō-sīt): A lymphoid cell that can react with an antigen to produce antibody.

immunodeficiency (im'-ū-nō-dē- fish'-ensi): A deficiency in the immune response of the body.

immunodepression: See **immunosuppression.**

immunodiagnosis (im'ū-nō-dī-ag-nō'sis): Diagnosis based on the reactions of blood serum to antigens.

immunoelectrophoresis (im'-ū-nō-ē- lek'-trō-fō-rē'-sis): A technique for distinguishing proteins from one another on the basis of their electrophoretic mobility and their specific immune reactions. See **electrophoresis.**

immunofluorescence (im'ū-nō-floo-ō-res'ens): A method of detecting the location of an antigen or an antibody in tissue by exposing it to the particular antigen or antibody that has been labeled with a fluorescent compound.

immunogenesis (im'ū-nō-jen'e-sis): The process of producing immunity.—immunogenetic, adj.

immunogenetics (im'ū-nō-jen-et'iks): A branch of genetics that is concerned with the study of immunology, including the inheritance of genetic factors that control an individual's immune response and the transmission of these factors to offspring.

immunogenicity (im'ū-nō-jen-is'i-ti): The ability to produce immunity. Antigenicity.

immunoglobulins (im'ū-nō-glob'ū-lins): Syn., gamma globulins (*q.v.*).

immunohematology (im'-ū-nō-hē-ma-tol'-o-ji): A branch of the science of hematology that deals with antigen-antibody reactions and other phenomena related to the pathogenesis of blood dyscrasias.

immunology (im-ū-nol'-o-ji): The special branch of medicine that deals with the body's natural defense systems and of immunity to disease.

immunopathology (im'-ū-nō-path-ol'-o-ji): 1. The study of the phenomena associated with immunity. 2. Abnormal immune reaction, as when a person becomes sensitized.

immunoprophylaxis (im'-ū-nō-prō-fi- lak'-sis): The prevention of disease by the use of vaccine to produce immunity.

immunosensitivity (im'ū-nō-sen-si-tiv'i-ti): The state produced by immunopathology (*q.v.*).

immunosuppression (im'-ū-nō-sū-presh'un): Modification of the body's immune response so that its reaction to a foreign substance is diminished; may be produced by any one of several immunosuppressive agents; including drugs, radiation, and antilymphocytic serum. Used to enhance the survival of allografts.

immunosuppressive (im'-ū-nō-sū-pres'-iv): 1. Pertaining to immunosuppression. 2. An agent that prevents the occurrence of an immune reaction; used therapeutically following organ transplant and in treatment of autoimmune disease.

immunotherapy (im'ū-nō-ther'a-pi): 1. Passive immunity conferred on one individual by administration of serum containing antibodies formed by another individual. 2. Therapy utilizing chemicals, drugs, or x rays for suppressing immunological reactions in the body.

immunotransfusion (im'-ū-nō-trans-fū'-zhun): Transfusion of blood from a donor previously rendered immune by repeated inoculations with a given agent from the recipient.

impacted (im-pak'-ted): Firmly wedged or pressed together so as to be immovable; said of a fracture when the jagged ends of bone are wedged together; of feces in the rectum; of a fetus in the uterus; of a tooth in its socket; or of a calculus in a duct.—impaction, n.

impaction (im-pak'-shun): Compressed material in a confined space, as hardened feces in the colon.

impairment (im-par'-ment): A physical or anatomical loss, deterioration, or weakening; due to disease or trauma.

impalpable (im-pal'-pa-b'l): Not palpable. Incapable of being felt by touch (palpation).

impatent (im-pā′-tent): Closed or obstructed; not patent.

impedance (im-pēd′-ans): Opposition to the flow of an alternating current. **ACOUSTIC I.**, interference with the passage of sound waves.

imperforate (im-per′-fō-rāt): Lacking a normal opening. **I. ANUS**, absence of an opening from the rectum. **I. HYMEN**, a fold of mucous membrane at the vaginal entrance, which has no natural outlet for the menstrual fluid.

impermeable (im-per′-mē-a-b'l): Penetrable; not permitting passage, as of a fluid through a membrane.

impetigo (im-pe-tī′-gō): A common, acute, imflammatory skin disease, highly contagious, characterized by pustules that rupture and become crusted, usually appearing around the mouth and nostrils; most often caused by staphylococci or streptococci, or a combination of both. **I. CONTAGIOSA**, a highly contagious form of **I.**, commonest on the face and scalp; starts with a small red spot, quickly develops into rapidly spreading, superficial vesicles that rupture; the escaped serum dries into honey-colored gummy crusts. **I. HERPETIFORMIS**, a rare form of **I.** occurring in pregnant women; characterized by pustules on the trunk and thighs, vomiting, fever, delirium, prostration; potentially fatal.

impinge (im-pinj′): To encroach or press upon.

implant (im′-plant) 1. To insert or to graft. 2. Any material that is implanted into a host's intact tissues; for example, a metal pin, electronic device, mucous or bony tissue, or certain drugs. Drugs administered in this way provide for slow, steady release over a definite period of time; examples include 1) the use of testosterone in treatment of carcinoma of the breast; 2) deoxycortone acetate (DOCA) in Addison's disease; 3) insulin in diabetes; 4) certain drugs for treatment of bronchial asthma; 5) certain contraceptives. **INTRAOCULAR I.**, a plastic lens placed in the anterior and posterior chamber of the eye as a substitute for a lens extraction for cataract. **PENILE I.**, a relatively new procedure to counteract impotence; several devices are available, including a sponge-filled silicone rod, and inflatable prostheses.

implantation (im-plan-tā′-shun): 1. The insertion of living cells or solid materials into the tissues, as in a) surgical implantation of radium, solid drugs, or a pacemaker; or b) accidental implantation of tumor cells in a wound. 2. The attachment of the fertilized ovum to the epithelial lining of the uterus.

implosion (im-plō′-zhun): In psychiatry, treatment by exposing the patient to his severest phobias, first in imagination, then in actual life situations. Also called imaginative flooding. See **flooding**.

impotence (im′-pō-tens): Lack of sexual power, by custom referring to the inability of the male to have an erection or to ejaculate following an erection; may be due to a physiological or psychological condition.

impotent (im′-pō-tent): 1. Barren or sterile. 2. Unable to copulate.—impotence, n.

impregnate (im-preg′-nāt): Fill. Saturate. Render pregnant.

impulse (im′-puls): 1. A sudden uncontrollable urge to act without deliberation. 2. A sudden push or communicated force.—impulsive, adj.

IMV: Abbreviation for intermittent mandatory ventilation.

in-: A prefix denoting: 1. Into, in, inside, on, toward. 2. Non-; not. Appears as il before l; ir before r; and im- before m, p, and b.

in articulo mortis (in ar-tik′ū-lō mor′tis): At the moment of death.

in extremis (in-eks-trē′-mis): At the point of death.

in loco parentis (in lō′-ko pa-ren′-tis): A Latin term meaning "in absence of the parents" which is invoked by school authorities and other responsible persons when a person who is under legal age requires medical care or surgery and the parents are not available to sign permissions or make decisions about treatment.

in situ (in sī′-tū): In the normal or natural place; in the correct position; undisturbed by neighboring tissues.

in utero: Within the uterus; unborn.

in vitro (vē′-trō): In glass, as in a test tube. Outside of the living body.

in vivo (vē′-vō): In living tissue or in a living body.

inaccessibility (in′-ak-ses-i-bil′-i- ti): In psychiatry, denotes absence of patient response.

inactivate (in-ak′-ti-vāt): To destroy the active principle or the biological activity of an agent or a substance.—inactivation, n.

inanimate (in-an′-i-māt): 1. Not alive. 2. Bereft of life or consciousness. 3. Dull, inert, stolid.

inanition (in-a-nish′-un): Exhaustion and wasting from lack of food or from lack of proper assimilation of food. **I. FEVER**, occurs during the first few days of life; high fever with rapid weight loss and restlessness; also called dehydration fever.

inappropriate antidiuretic hormone syndrome: A syndrome characterized by hyponatremia and water intoxication, caused by elevated blood levels of antidiuretic hormone; may be associated with hypoalbuminemia, major trauma, the use of certain drugs, or decreased blood volume which may result from hemorrhage, decreased cardiac output, or dehydration; treated by administration of sodium chloride, diuretics, and fluid restriction.

inarticulate (in-ar-tik'ū-lāt): 1. Not jointed. 2. Said of speech that is not intelligible. 3. Not able to speak distinctly or clearly. 4. Inability to express oneself in speech.

inassimilable (in-a-sim'-i-la-b'l): Not capable of absorption and appropriation by the body for nourishment.

inborn (in'-born): Descriptive of physical and mental characteristics that are present at birth and that have developed or been implanted while the fetus was in utero. Innate.

inborn error of metabolism: A disorder resulting from a defect in the genetic material; most commonly involves the chemical processes involved in metabolism as occurs in phenylketonuria in infants, and in diabetes mellitus, cystic fibrosis, sickle cell anemia, Down's syndrome, goiter. Also called genetotrophic disease and enzymopathy.

incarcerated (in-kar'-ser-āt-ed): In medicine, the abnormal imprisonment of a part, as in a hernia that is irreducible, or a pregnant uterus that is held beneath the sacral promontory.

incendiarism (in-sen'-di-ar-izm): An obsession for setting fires. Pyromania.

incest (in'-sest): Sexual intercourse between near kin, whose marriage is prohibited by law.

incidence (in'-si-dens): The rate of occurrence of an event or of a condition, *e.g.*, the number of new cases of a specific disease occurring in a population over specified time, usually one year.

incident report: A required report to the administrative staff of a health care unit regarding the occurrence of any injury to a patient or visitor; cardiac arrest; error of omission or commission of meals, medications, or treatments; theft or loss of a patient's belongings; or any other untoward event involving a patient.

incipient (in-sip'-i-ent): Initial, beginning, or in early stages; often said of symptoms.

incise (in-sīz'): To cut or cut into.

incision (in-sizh'-un): A cut or wound produced by cutting into body tissue, using a sharp instrument.—incise, v.; incisional, adj.

incisors (in-sī'-zers): The eight front cutting teeth, four in each jaw.

incisure (in-sī'-zhur): In anatomy, a notch, groove, or fissure.

inclusion bodies: Minute particles found in the cells of tissues that are affected by a virus, *e.g.*, the virus of smallpox or measles. They are stainable and vary (in size, appearance, and quantity) with different diseases.

incoherent (in-kō-hēr'-ent): 1. The state or fact of being confused, disjointed, inconsistent, rambling, incongruous, or without proper sequence. 2. Being unable to express oneself in an intelligible and understandable manner.—incoherence, n.; incoherently, adj.

incompatibility (in'-kom-pat-i-bil'-i-ti): In medicine and pharmacology, a situation in which two substances cannot be used together without producing undesirable reaction. Usually refers to the bloods of donor and recipient in transfusion, when antigenic differences in the red cells result in reactions such as hemolysis and agglutination. See **blood groups.** May also refer to tissue transplants that are rejected by the recipient because certain antibody factors involved are not compatible.

incompetence (in-kom'-pe-tens): 1. Inadequacy to perform a natural or required function, often said of cardiac valves. 2. Inability to manage one's own affairs properly and, often, the inability to tell right from wrong.—incompetency, n.; incompetent, adj.

incontinence (in-kon'-ti-nens): Inability to control the evacuation of any excretory product, particularly urine and feces; may be due to loss of sphincter control or to a cerebral or spinal lesion. **DRIBBLING I.**, continuous outflow of urine; may be associated with neurologic pathology. **FECAL I.**, inability to postpone defecation; due to loss of control of the anal sphincter; may be caused by ulcerative colitis, disorders of the central nervous system, impaction, cancer, muscular deficiency. **NOCTURNAL I.**, enuresis (*q.v.*). **OVERFLOW I.**, dribbling of urine from a fully distended bladder; due to an obstruction or to damage to pelvic nerves. **PARADOXICAL I.**, dribbling of urine due to chronic retention or a flaccid bladder. **STRESS I.**, of urine, occurs when intra-abdominal pressure is raised, as in coughing or sneezing; due to relaxation or incompetence of the sphincter muscle of the urethra, or injury to the pelvic floor. **TRUE I.**, of urine, occurs when there is a fistulous connection between the urinary and genital tracts, usually between the bladder and the vagina. **URGE I.**, of urine, occurs when a hypertonic bladder contracts strongly even when there is only a small amount of urine in it; the urge to void is followed immediately by voiding.

incontinent (in-kon'-ti-nent): Inability to resist yielding to normal impulses, such as the sexual impulse, or normal urges such as the urge to defecate or urinate.

incoordination (in'-kō-or-di-nā'-shun): 1. Inability to produce smooth, harmonious muscular movements. 2. Failure of organs to work together harmoniously.

incrustation (in'-krus-tā'-shun): The formation of a scab on a wound.

incubate (in'-kū-bāt): To promote the growth of microorganisms by placing them in an incubator (*q.v.*).

incubation (in'kū-bā'shun): In medicine, the maintenance of organisms in conditions that are optimal for their growth and reproduction. **I. PERIOD,** the time that elapses between entry of infection and the appearance of the first symptom of disease.

incubator (in′-kū-bā-ter): A temperature-regulated apparatus in which: 1) premature or delicate babies may be placed; 2) microorganisms can be cultivated.

incubus (ing′-kū-bus): A suffocating or stifling dream; nightmare.

incudectomy (ing-kū-dek′-to-mi): Surgical removal of the incus.

incus (ing′-kus): The central one of the chain of three small bones of the middle ear, taking its name from the Latin for anvil, which it resembles in shape.

Independent Nurse Practitioner: See nurse practitioner.

independent variable: In research, a variable that can be controlled by the investigator and measured as to its effect on the condition or topic under investigation.

index: 1. The second finger; the pointer. 2. The ratio of measurement (size, capacity, or function) of one substance, thing, or part of a thing compared with a standard that is fixed after a series of observations and usually represented as 1 or 100.

Index Medicus: A compilation of medical journal articles published throughout the world, listed by author and subject; published monthly by the U.S. National Library of Medicine, and as a cumulative index at the end of each year.

Indian Health Service: A federally sponsored service of the Health Services Administration, consisting of hospitals, health centers, and field clinics and their personnel, which serve half a million American Indians and Alaskan natives.

Indian hemp: Cannabis indica (*q.v.*). Hashish.

indican (in′-di-kan): A potassium salt formed from the decomposition of tryptophan in the intestinal tract and found in the urine and sweat.

indicanuria (in′di-kan-ū′ri-a): The presence of more than the normal amount of indican in the urine. See indole.

indicator (in′-di-kā-ter): In chemistry, a substance used to make visible the completion of a chemical reaction.

indigenous (in-dij′-e-nus): Native to a certain locality or country.

indigestion (in-di-jes′-chun): Dyspepsia. Lack or failure of digestion (*q.v.*).

indirect contact: Refers to the transfer of infection by such conveyers as milk, water, air, contaminated hands, and inanimate objects.

indisposition (in-dis-pō-zi′shun): In medicine, a slight or temporary illness, malaise.

individuation (in′di-vid-ū-ā′shun): The process of developing individual parts or characteristics of a whole that become increasingly distinct and independent.

indole (in′-dōl): A product of intestinal putrefaction: it is oxidized to indoxyl in the liver and excreted in urine as indican. See indicanuria.

indolent (in′-dō-lent): Lazy, sluggish, inert. In medicine, a sluggish ulcer that is generally painless and slow to heal.

induction (in-duk′-shun): The act of bringing on or causing to occur, as applied to anesthesia and labor. **I. PERIOD,** the period between the starting of anesthesia and the time the state necessary for performing surgery is achieved.

inductive reasoning: The process of reasoning from a part to a whole, or from particular to general. Opp. of deductive reasoning (*q.v.*).

induration (in-dū-rā′-shun): 1. A hard swollen area beneath the surface of the skin. 2. The hardening of tissue as in hyperemia, infiltration by neoplasm, etc. **BRAWNY I.,** inflammatory thickening and hardening of tissue.—indurated, adj. **BROWN INDURATION OF THE LUNG,** a condition of firmness and brown color of the lung which is associated with hemosiderin-pigmented macrophages in the alveoli; due to long-standing congestion occurring with heart disease.

Industrial Hygienist: A health professional whose work involves being in charge of environmental control of toxic chemicals and physical agents that are associated with work operations, working with others on accident prevention programs, and conducting education programs for workers in regard to occupational safety and health; works closely with the occupational health nurse and other professionals on the occupational health team to see that the recommendations of the Occupational and Safety Health Act (OSHA) are carried out in industrial situations.

indwelling (in′-dwel-ling): Pertaining to a drainage or feeding tube, or a catheter, that is fastened in position and allowed to remain fixed for a period of time. See Foley catheter.

inebriation (in-ē′brē-ā′shun): Drunkenness.

inebriety (in-ē-brī′-e-ti): Habitual drunkenness.

ineffective individual coping: A nursing diagnosis accepted by the Fourth Conference on the Classification of Nursing Diagnoses.

inert (in-ert′): 1. Slow, sluggish, inactive; having no physical or mental activity. 2. Term used to denote drugs that have no pharmaceutical or therapeutic action.

inertia (in-er′-shi-a): Lack of activity or force, physical or mental. **I. UTERI,** sluggishness of uterine muscles during labor; may be primary due to constitutional weakness, or secondary due to exhaustion from frequent and forcible contractions.

infant (in′-fant): A child less than two years of age; in law, a person under the age of 21, but in criminal law, anyone under the age of 14. **PREMATURE I.**, one born before term but capable of life; one who weighs less than 5.5 pounds at birth and is born 29-36 weeks after conception. **I. RESPIRATORY DISTRESS SYNDROME**, acute difficulty in breathing; seen most often in premature infants, those delivered by cesarean section, or those born of diabetic mothers; see under respiratory distress syndrome.

infant Hercules syndrome: Adrenogenital syndrome. A condition in a male child in whom an excessive amount of androgens is produced, causing great acceleration of physical and sexual growth.

infant mortality rate: The number of children per 1000 live births in a specific area who die during the first year of life.

infanticide (in-fan′-ti-sīd): The killing of an infant.

infantile (in′-fan-tīl): Pertaining to an infant. Childish. **I. UTERUS**, term used to describe a uterus that is undeveloped or underdeveloped.

infantile amaurotic idiocy: A group of inherited disorders seen mostly in children of East European ancestry; age of onset and progression varies. Characterized by hypotonia, blindness, convulsions, intellectual deterioration, and the appearance of a cherry-red spot on the macula lutea. Syn., Tay-Sachs disease. See also idiocy.

infantile autism: A chronic disorder that develops before the age of 30 months; more common in boys; characterized by aversion to expressions of affection, signs of possible deafness, lack of language development, performance of ritualistic motor acts, lability of mood.

infantile paralysis: See poliomyelitis.

infantilism (in-fan′-ti-lizm): 1. A condition in which childish physical, intellectual, and emotional characteristics persist into adolescence and adult life; may be idiopathic or the result of underdevelopment of certain organs or systems of the body. 2. A condition of psychologic origin occurring in adults that is characterized by the use of childish patterns of speech and voice.

infarct (in′-farkt): The area of tissue, organ, or part that dies when the end artery supplying it, or the vein that carries blood from it, is occluded, *e.g.*, in the kidney or heart; a common complication of subacute endocarditis. **MYOCARDIAL I.**, see infarction, myocardial.

infarction (in-fark′-shun): 1. Formation of an infarct. 2. Death of a section of tissue because the blood supply has been shut off. **CEREBRAL I.**, ischemia of a part of the brain due to lack of blood supply in an area of distribution of one of the cerebral arteries. **MYOCARDIAL I.**, necrosis of part of the myocardium as a result of lack of blood supply to that part, as occurs in coronary thrombosis. **PULMONARY I.**, necrosis of a localized area of the lung due to obstruction of the blood supply, as occurs in pulmonary embolism.

infect (in-fekt′): To cause infection; to contaminate with disease-producing organisms.

infection (in-fek′-shun): 1. The successful invasion, establishment, and growth of microorganisms in a degree sufficient to cause symptoms of disease in the host. 2. The condition produced by the introduction and growth of microorganisms in the tissues of the body. **AIRBORNE I.**, one transmitted by the air, *e.g.*, organisms transmitted from one person to another by droplets discharged in coughing or sneezing. **COMMUNITY-ACQUIRED I.**, one due to a pathologic organism common in the community. **CONCURRENT I.**, one occurring at the same time as another. **CONTAGIOUS I.**, one that is communicable by contact with a person suffering from it, or with articles the ill person has handled. **CROSS I.S**, those transmitted to each other by persons with differing infections. **DIRECT CONTACT I.**, one caused by direct transmission from one person to another, as by kissing. **DROPLET I.**, airborne **I.** **ENDOGENOUS I.**, one transferred from a body site where the organism is commensal to another site where it acts as a pathogen. **EXOGENOUS I.**, one transmitted from sources outside the body, such as infected materials or people; enters by ingestion, inhalation, or inoculation. **FOCAL I.**, one confined to one part of the body. **INDIRECT CONTACT I.**, one transmitted by inanimate objects that have been contaminated by one suffering from it. **MASS I.**, one produced by invasion of a large number of a disease-producing organism. **MIXED I.**, one occurring concurrently with one or more others caused by different organisms; seen in abscesses. **NOSOCOMIAL I.**, one acquired by a person while a patient in a health-care institution. **PYOGENIC I.**, one due to a pus-producing organism. **SECONDARY I.**, one **I.** imposed upon another. **SLOW VIRUS I.**, an **I.** caused by any of several viruses that remain in the body for a long time before symptoms appear; now thought to be causative in certain rare degenerative diseases, Alzheimer's disease, subacute sclerosing panencephalitis, multiple sclerosis, and certain types of diabetes. **SUBCLINICAL I.**, one not severe enough to have clinical symptoms. **URINARY TRACT I.**, bacterial infection of the kidney, collecting system of the kidney, or the bladder, or of all of these; usually caused by *Escherichia coli*. **VIRAL I.**, may be caused by any one of a score of viruses that are pathogenic to humans and that may enter the body through the skin, respiratory or digestive tract, or by transfusion, and that may or may not confer immunity to the particular virus.

infection control committee: A multidisciplinary group in a health care facility organized for the purpose of developing, maintaining, and monitoring a program of infection control; members usually include representatives from the facility's administration, medical staff, housekeeping staff, dietary service, nursing service, medical laboratory, and operating room. It is responsible for setting policies, developing protocols, conducting surveillance programs, and educating personnel.

infection control practitioner: Usually a professional nurse with experience in nursing, a good understanding of microbiology, and knowledge of epidemiology; functions as an independent agent directly under the hospital administrator; is involved in investigating, implementing, and enforcing infection control measures in the facility.

infectious (in-fek'-shus): 1. Communicable; capable of being transmitted by direct or indirect contact. 2. Denoting a disease caused by a specific, pathogenic organism and capable of being transmitted to another individual. **I. HEPATITIS,** an endemic type of hepatitis caused by hepatitis A virus. **I. MONONUCLEOSIS,** see mononucleosis.

infective (in-fek'-tiv): 1. Relating to an infection. 2. Infectious.—infectivity, n.

inferior (in-fē'-ri-or): In anatomy, denotes lower, beneath, or below a point of reference. **I. VENA CAVA,** main vein returning blood to the right atrium of the heart from the trunk and lower extremities.

inferiority complex: See under complex.

infertile (in-fer'-til): Unable to conceive or to maintain a pregnancy; term is not usually applied until a person has engaged in sexual intercourse for a year or longer.

infertility (in'-fer-til'-i-ti): Lack of ability to reproduce; not necessarily irreversible.

infest (in-fest'): To occupy a site and dwell on the surface of the body, usually by macroscopic parasites, as opposed to dwelling within the body. *i.e.*, to infect.

infestation (in-fes-tā'-shun): The presence of such animal parasites as insects, ticks, fleas, mites, lice, or worms in or on the body.—infest, v.

infibulation (in-fib-ū-lā'-shun): The act of buckling or fastening; may refer to the procedure of fastening the edges of a wound together by a clasp. May also refer to the ancient practice of stitching or otherwise fastening the labia majora to prevent sexual intercourse.

infiltrate (in-fil'-trāt): 1. To permeate a substance by penetrating the spaces between the particles of a tissue or of a substance. 2. Cells or material that passes into body tissues by infiltration.

infiltration (in'fil-trā'shun): Penetration of the surrounding tissues by a fluid, as from an intravenous line, or by some other foreign substance; the leaking or oozing of a fluid into the tissues. **I. ANESTHESIA,** analgesia produced by infiltrating the tissues with a local anesthetic.

infirm (in-firm'): Weak or feeble, either physically or mentally, because of old age or illness.

infirmary (in-fir'-ma-ri): A hospital, usually small, especially one in a school or other institution.

infirmity (in-fir'-mi-ti): An unhealthy or debilitated condition of body or mind.

inflamed (in-flāmd'): Hot and swollen; affected with inflammation (*q.v.*).

inflammation (in-fla-mā'-shun): The protective, characteristic chemical or physical reaction of living tissues to injury, infection or irritation; characterized by pain, swelling, redness and heat.—inflammatory, adj.

inflation (in-flā'shun): In medicine, the distention of a part with liquid or gas.

influenza (in-floo-en'-za): An acute, highly contagious infection, marked by inflammation of the nasopharynx and respiratory tract, fever, prostration, muscular and neurologic pains, gastrointestinal disturbances, headache, and depression; primarily caused by a filterable virus and occurring in epidemic and pandemic form. Syn., la grippe, the grip, flu.—influenzal, adj.

informed consent: See under consent.

infra-: Prefix denoting a position or status under or below the part named in the word to which it is joined.

infraclavicular (in'fra-kla-vik'ū-lar): Below the clavicle.

infradiaphragmatic (in'fra-dī-a-frag-mat'ik): Below the diaphragm.

infraorbital (in'fra-or'bit-al): Below or on the floor of the orbital cavity.

infrared rays: Long, invisible rays beyond the red end of the visible spectrum. Used therapeutically for the production of heat in tissues.

infrasound (in'-fra-sownd): Vibration of the same nature as sound waves but below the frequency range that is audible to the human ear.

infraspinous (in-fra-spī'nus): Below a spine, *e.g.*, of the scapula.

infrasternal (in-fra-ster'-nal): Below the sternum. **I. NOTCH,** the slight depression in the anterior abdominal wall that overlies the xiphoid process of the sternum.

infraversion (in'-fra-ver'-zhun): The downward rotation of one or both eyes.

infriction (in-frik'-shun): The application of a medicated substance to the skin using friction.

infundibulum (in-fun-dib'-ū-lum): Any funnel-shaped passage or structure; often refers to the pituitary stalk, which connects the pituitary gland to the hypothalamus.—infundibula, pl.; infundibular, adj.

infusion (in-fū′-zhun): 1. An aqueous solution containing the active principle of a drug, made by steeping the crude drug in water. 2. Fluid other than blood, flowing by gravity into the body. **INTRAVENOUS I.,** usually refers to the intravenous administration of more than 100 ml of a fluid substance. **I. PUMP,** a device for injecting a specific amount of fluid within a specific time span. See amniotic fluid infusion under amniotic.

ingestant (in-jes′-tant): A substance that is taken into the body through the mouth or digestive system; usually refers to nutrients.—ingesta, pl.

ingrown toenail: A nail whose edges have grown into the tissue on either side of it, causing inflammation and pain.

inguinal (ing′-gwi-nal): Pertaining to the groin. **I. CANAL,** a tubular opening through the lower part of the anterior abdominal wall, parallel to and a little above the I. (Poupart's) ligament. It measures 1.5 in. In the male it contains the spermatic cord; in the female, the uterine round ligaments. **I. HERNIA,** one occurring through the internal abdominal ring of the I. canal. **I. LIGAMENT,** a strong cord of fibrous tissue that extends from the anterior superior iliac spine to the pubic spine; forms a firm edge of the abdominal wall across the groin; Poupart's ligament.

inhalant (in-hā′-lant): 1. That which is inhaled; may be something in the atmosphere or a medication. 2. A substance that occurs as an inhalant or one that is used medicinally as an inhalant.

inhalation (in-ha-lā′-shun): 1. The act of breathing in of air, or of a vapor. 2. A medicinal or treatment substance that is inhaled, such as a gas anesthetic, water vapor, etc.

inhalator (in′-hal-ā-tor): A device for assisting in the inhalation of a gas or spray, as for providing oxygen or mixture of oxygen and carbon dioxide for resuscitation.

inhale (in-hāl′): To draw in breath; to inspire.

inhaler (in-hā′-ler): 1. An apparatus that provides for the breathing in of medicinal substances. 2. An apparatus that can be worn to prevent breathing in dust, smoke, dirt, etc. 3. An atomizer. **METERED DOSE.,** a device used in administering medications to the bronchial tree that ensures the medication gets to the desired part of the airway.

inherent (in-hēr′-ent): Innate; inborn.

inheritance (in-her′-i-tans): The process of acquiring characters or qualities by transmission from parent to offspring, or the characters and qualities so acquired.

inherited (in-her′-i-ted): Descriptive of mental and physical characteristics that one has received from one's parents; inborn.

inhibition (in′-hi-bish′-un): Loss or partial loss of function or activity, due to restraint, arrest, or being held back. In psychiatry, the restraint of a function or activity as a result of mental (psychic) influences, *e.g.*, failing to "speak up" for fear of making unimportant or incorrect statements.

inhibitor (in-hib′-i-tor): A substance or agent that interferes with a physiological function or a chemical reaction.

inion (in′-i-on): The most prominent external protruberance of the occipital bone.

inject (in-jekt′): To force into. In medicine, to force fluid, gas, air, or other substance into tissue, a cavity, or an organ of the body.

injectable (in-jek′-ta-b'l): 1. Capable of being injected. 2. A substance that can be injected.

injected (in-jek′-ted): 1. Congested; with full vessels. 2. Forced in by injection (*q.v.*).

injection (in-jek′-shun): 1. The act of introducing a fluid (under pressure) into the tissues, a vessel, cavity or hollow organ. (Air can be injected into a cavity. See pneumothorax.) 2. The substance injected. See hypodermic, intra-arterial, intracutaneous, intradermal, intramuscular, intrathecal, intravascular, intravenous, subcutaneous. 3. Congestion; referring especially to dilatation of vessels in the vascular bed.

injury: A nursing diagnosis accepted by the Fourth National Conference on the Classification of Nursing Diagnoses.

injury, potential for: (in′-jer-i): A wound or damage to a person or thing, specifically any disruption to the continuity of body tissue that may or may not involve the skin. **BIRTH I.,** the impairment of a body function as a result of some damage to the child during the birth process.

inkblot test: See Rorschach test.

inlet (in′-let): A means of entrance, particularly to a body structure. **PELVIC I.,** the upper limit of the pelvic cavity.

innate (in-āt′): Inborn; dependent on genetic constitution; congenital; hereditary; inherent.

inner ear: See ear.

innervation (in′-er-vā′- shun): The nerve supply to or in a part.

innidiation (i-nid-i-ā′shun): The development of cells within a tissue to which they have been carried by lymph or the bloodstream.

innocent (in′-ō-sent): Benign; not malignant; apparently not harmful.

innocuous (i-nok′-ū-us): Harmless.

innominate (i-nom′-i-nāt): Unnamed. **I. ARTERY,** the largest branch of the aortic arch; it divides into the right common carotid and the right subclavian arteries. **I. BONE,** one of the bones forming the pelvis; it is composed of the ilium, ischium and pubis; the os innominatum.

I. VEINS, formed by the union of the subclavian and internal jugular veins on either side.

innoxious (i-nok′-shus): Not harmful.

inoculate (in-ok′-ū-lāt): To introduce a disease-producing agent or an antigenic material into the body for the purpose of creating immunity, treating a disease, or making a diagnosis.

inoculation (in-ok′-ū-lā′-shun): 1. Introduction of material (usually vaccine) into the tissues, often done to create immunity by giving the person a mild form of the disease. 2. Introduction of microorganisms into culture medium for propagation.

inoculum (in-ok′-ū-lum): The microorganism or other material used in an inoculation.—inocula, pl.

inoperable (in-op′-er-a-b'l): Describing a condition that under other circumstances could be relieved or cured by surgery, but that, because of the location or advanced stage of the pathology, surgery would be either ineffective or unsafe.

inorganic (in′-or-gan′-ik): Neither animal nor vegetable in origin. In chemistry, the term refers to compounds that do not contain carbon.

inositol (in-ō′-si-tol): A member of the vitamin B_2 complex.

inotropic (in-ō-trŏp′-ik): Having an effect on the contractility of muscle tissue, usually referring to drugs, some of which have a weakening negative effect while others have a positive strengthening effect.

inpatient: A person who receives food and lodging in a hospital or other institution while receiving treatment or undergoing tests.

inquest (in′-qwest): A legal inquiry, held by a coroner, into the cause of sudden or unexpected death.

insane (in-sān′): 1. Of unsound or deranged mind. Usually implies inability to manage one's own affairs or conduct oneself in a socially acceptable manner. 2. Relating to insanity.

insanitary (in-san′-i-ter-i): Unclean to such a degree as to be injurious to health.

insanity (in-san′-i-ti): Old term for severe mental illness. In law, the term is used to designate the degree of mental illness that renders a person incapable of conduct or judgment that is legally regarded as normal.

insecticide (in-sek′-ti-sīd): An agent that kills insects.—insecticidal, adj.

insemination (in-sem-in-ā′-shun): Introduction of semen into the vagina, normally by sexual intercourse. **ARTIFICIAL I.**, instrumental injection of semen into the female genital tract.

insensible (in-sen′-si-b'l): Without sensation or consciousness. Too small or gradual to be perceived, as **I.** perspiration (*q.v.*). **I. LOSS,** usually refers to loss of fluids from the body in ways that cannot be measured by ordinary means, *e.g.*, in sweat.

insertion (in-ser′-shun): 1. The act of setting or placing in. 2. The attachment of a muscle to the bone it moves.

inservice education: Planned continuing education for personnel already employed by an institution.

insidious (in-sid′-i-us): Having an imperceptible commencement, as of a disease with a late manifestation of definite symptoms.

insight (in′-sīt): Clear and immediate understanding; keen discernment. In psychiatry, means: 1) knowing that one is emotionally ill; 2) a developing knowledge of one's present attitudes and past experiences and the connection between them.

insolation (in-sō-lā′-shun): 1. Sunstroke. 2. Treatment of disease by exposure to the sun's rays.

insoluble (in-sol′-ū-b'l): Incapable of being dissolved.

insomnia (in-som′ni-a): Sleeplessness, especially when chronic, or difficulty in falling asleep or remaining asleep during the period when sleep occurs normally.

inspection (in-spek′-shun): Examination of persons or things by the eye.

inspersion (in-sper′-shun): The act of sprinkling, as with a powder or a fluid.

inspiration (in-spi-rā′shun): The drawing of air into the lungs; inhalation.—inspire, v.; inspiratory, adj.

inspiratory (in-spī′-ra-to-ri): Pertaining to inspiration, or breathing in. **I. CAPACITY,** the sum of respiratory reserve volume and tidal volume. **I. RESERVE VOLUME,** the maximum amount of air that can be exhaled after exhalation of the tidal volume.

inspire (in-spīr′): To breathe in; inhale.

inspirometer (in′-spī-rom′-e-ter): An instrument for measuring the amount of air inspired.

inspissated (in-spis′āt-ed): Thickened by evaporation, absorption, or dehydration.

inspissation (in′-spis-sā′-shun): The process of drying or thickening a substance by evaporating its vaporizable constituents.

instability: 1. Lack of stability or support; insecure support. 2. Lack of purpose; changeableness in beliefs or opinions.

instep (in′-step): The arch of the foot on the dorsal surface.

instillation (in′-sti-lā′-shun): The pouring, drop by drop, of a fluid into a body cavity or opening, *e.g.*, the conjunctival sac or external auditory meatus.—instill, v.

instinct (in′stinkt): An inborn tendency, present in all normal members of a species, to act in a certain way that is usually helpful and beneficial, *e.g.*, **PATERNAL I.**, the **I.** to protect children. **HERD I.**, the urge to copy standards of thinking and behavior of a group.—instinctive, adj.; instinctively, adv.

insufficiency (in-su-fish′-en-sē): The condition of being unable to perform an allotted duty or function. Term is used to describe failure to function properly of such organs and parts as the heart, cardiac valves, liver, stomach, kidney, adrenal or thyroid glands, muscles.

insufflation (in′-sū-flā′-shun): The act of blowing into; often refers to blowing air into the lungs of the newborn; blowing a powder, gas, or vapor into a body cavity; or blowing air along a tube (eustachian or fallopian) to establish patency.—insufflate, v.

insula (in′sū-la): An island, particularly the islands of Langerhans in the pancreas or the island of Reil, a triangular area of the cerebral cortex. See island.

insulation (in-sū-lā′-shun): The surrounding of a body or a space with non-conducting material to prevent the escape or entrance of radiant energy, electricity, sound or heat; also, the material so used.

insulin (in′sū-lin): A pancreatic hormone produced in the islet (beta) cells of the islands of Langerhans, secreted into the bloodstream in response to glucose in the blood; promotes utilization of glucose, synthesis of protein, and the formation and storage of neutral lipids. The hormone is obtained from animals and prepared commercially in several forms and strengths which vary in their speed, length, and potency of action, and which are used in treatment of diabetes mellitus; most forms are given subcutaneously. Insulin is now also produced by bacteria via genetic engineering. Excess dosage results in hypoglycemia and insulin shock; inadequate dosage results in hyperglycemia and diabetic ketoacidosis

insulin pump: A device that is powered by batteries and worn by patients with diabetes; it is programmed to deliver a set amount of insulin at regular intervals; is connected to the infusion site, which is usually on the abdomen. The patient can control the amount of insulin delivered when blood sugar tests indicate the need for change in dosage.

insulin shock: A condition resulting from severe hypoglycemia caused by overdose of insulin, insufficient intake of food, or excessive physical exertion; symptoms include sweating, chills, pallor, hunger, thirst, extreme nervousness and fear, fainting, possibly convulsions; treatment consists of immediate intake of sugar or intravenous injection of glucose. Also called hypoglycemic crisis or shock.

insulinase (in′-sū-lin-ās): An enzyme in the liver that is capable of inactivating insulin.

insulinoma (in′-sū-lin-ō′-ma): Adenoma of the islands of Langerhans in the pancreas. Also insuloma.

insulitis (in′-sū-lī′-tis): Inflammation of the islands of Langerhans.

insult (in′-sult): 1. An injury or trauma. 2. To injure or traumatize.

insusceptibility (in′su-sep-ti-bil′i-ti): Immunity. The incapability of becoming infected with a specific pathogen.

intake (in′tāk): In medicine, usually refers to substances taken into the body, by mouth or otherwise, and expressed in amounts such as cc's of fluid intake, or caloric content of food intake. **I. WORKER**, one who takes initial information about an individual who is being admitted to a hospital or other health care facility.

integument (in-teg′-ū-ment): A covering, especially the skin.—integumentary, adj.

integumentary (in-teg-ū-men′-ta-ri): Relating to the integument of the body. **I. SYSTEM**, the skin and its appendages—the hair, nails, sweat glands, sebaceous glands, and mammary glands.

intellect (in′-te-lekt): The power or facility of reasoning, thinking, and understanding; intelligence.

intellectualize (in-tel-lek′-tū-a-līz): To examine or analyze rationally; to reason.

intelligence (in-tel′-i-jens): The ability to comprehend or understand relationships, to think, to solve problems, and to adjust to new situations. Inborn mental ability. **I. QUOTIENT**, or IQ, the ratio of mental age to chronological age; obtained by dividing the mental age by the chronological age and multiplying the result by 100. **I. TESTS**, Tests designed to determine one's level of intelligence or mental age.

intensive care syndrome: See ICU psychosis under ICU.

intensive care unit: A special area in a hospital, where critically ill patients who need close observation and frequent ministrations can be cared for by highly qualified, specially trained staff working under the best possible conditions. Some hospitals provide an intermediate intensive care unit for patients who do not require intensive care nursing but are not yet ready to return to a general care unit.

intention: A natural process of healing involving the union of the edges of a wound. **FIRST I.**, healing of a wound by immediate union and scar formation without granulation or suppuration. **SECOND I.**, healing of a wound after suppuration, by union of the two granulated surfaces and formation of a larger scar than forms in healing by first intention. **THIRD I.**, healing of a wound with extensive granulation and the formation of a still larger scar. **I. TREMOR**, see tremor.

inter-: Prefix denoting among, between, together, within, in the midst.

interaction (in-ter-ak′-shun): A mutual or reciprocal action or influence. In pharmacotherapeutics, the modification of the action of one drug by one or more other drugs; may be detrimental or beneficial to the patient. **I.** may also occur between a drug and certain foods.

Interagency Council on Library Resources for Nursing: An advisory council composed of representatives of agencies and organizations having an active interest in library resources for nurses. Founded in 1960, its objective is to promote development and use of better library sources for nurses and to provide broader library services for nurses. Address, Librarian, American Journal of Nursing Company, 555 W. 57th St., New York, N.Y. 10019.

interarticular (in-ter-ar-tik′ū-lar): 1. Between two articulating surfaces. 2. Between two joints.

interatrial (in-ter-ā′-tri-al): Between the two atria of the heart.

intercapillary (in-ter-kap′-i-lā-ri): Between or among capillaries.

intercellular (in-ter-sel′-ū-lar): Between the cells of a structure.

intercerebral (in′-ter-ser′-e-bral): Located between or connecting the two cerebral hemispheres.

interclavicular (in-ter-kla-vik′-ū- lar): Between the clavicles.

interconception period: The period between pregnancies.

intercondylar (in-ter-kon′-di-lar): Between condyles, *e.g.*, the intercondylar notch at the lower posterior end of the femur.

intercostal (in-ter-kos′-tal): Between the ribs. **I. MUSCLES,** those located between the ribs. **EXTERNAL I. MUSCLES,** those that act to increase the size of the thoracic cavity. **INTERNAL I. MUSCLES,** those that act to decrease the size of the thoracic cavity during breathing. **I. SPACE,** the space between two adjacent ribs.

intercourse (in′-ter-kōrs): Communication; interchange or exchange. **SEXUAL I.,** coitus.

intercurrent (in-ter-kur′-ent): Intervening, interrupting or occurring in the midst of a process. Said of a second disease arising in a person already suffering from one disease.

interferon (in-ter-fēr′on): A class of small soluble glycoproteins produced naturally in most body cells in response to viral infections; discovered in 1957 and still under investigation. Called the body's first line of defense against infections, especially viral infections. Interferon is not in itself antiviral but is thought to initiate RNA and protein synthesis, yielding a new protein that has an antiviral effect and prevents further spread of the infection; also appears to be effective against certain bacteria, protozoa, and rickettsias, and in certain types of cancer.

interictal (in′-ter-ik′-tal): Between attacks or paroxysms, *e.g.*, epileptic seizures.

interlobar (in-ter-lō′-bar): Between the lobes of an organ, *e.g.*, interlobar pleurisy.

interlobular (in-ter-lob′-ū-lar): Located or occurring between lobules of an organ.

intermediate care: Care of patients beyond the acute stage of their illness and prior to the phase of long-term care.

intermediate care facility: A nursing home or area of a hospital that provides care and observation between hospital and home for patients who no longer require care in a skilled nursing facility. Most of the intermediate facilities provide rehabilitation services and emphasize self-care.

intermenstrual (in-ter-men′-stroo-al): Between menstrual periods.

intermittent (in-ter-mit′ent): Occurring at intervals; characterized by periods of complete cessation of activity. **I. CLAUDICATION,** see claudication. **I. FEVER,** one in which the symptoms of the disease disappear between attacks of fever, as occurs in malaria and undulant fever. **I. INFUSION SET,** an apparatus that delivers intravenous solution into a vein at preset intervals; heparin lock. **I. POSITIVE PRESSURE BREATHING,** (IPPB), a useful technique when weaning a patient from a respirator; the patient breathes spontaneously while still on the respirator which delivers a breath of air or oxygen at set intervals which are gradually lengthened until the patient is breathing entirely on his own. **I. PULSE,** one in which there is an absence of beat at intervals. **I. VENTILATION,** may be 1) mandatory, whereby the patient breathes at his normal rate but is helped by a respirator that is set to deliver a certain volume of air at a preset rate, or 2) demand, the same as mandatory except that the ventilator is set to deliver a certain amount of air at the patient's respiratory rate.

intermuscular (in-ter-mus′-kū-lar): Situated between muscles.

internal (in-ter′-nal): Located or occurring on the inside. **I. EAR,** that part of the ear that comprises the vestibule, semicircular canals, and the ossicles. **I. ENVIRONMENT,** the extracellular fluid that immediately surrounds the cells of the body. **I. HEMORRHAGE,** bleeding into a cavity or organ of the body. **I. SECRETIONS,** those produced by the ductless (endocrine) glands and passed directly into the bloodstream; hormones.—internally, adj.; internality, n.

internalization (in-ter′-nal-ī-zā′-shun): The unconscious adoption, as one's own, of another's values, characteristics, and attitudes.

International Classification of Diseases (ICD): The official list of disease categories, issued by the World Health Organization. **ICDA** is the adaptation of this list for use in the U.S., prepared by the U.S. Public Health Service.

International Council of Nurses (ICN): A federation founded in 1899, the oldest health care association in the world. Ninety-four nations are now members; meets every four years. Purpose is to develop the highest level of health for all peoples of the world; to improve the status and competency of nurses; to improve the standards of nursing care; to promote the development of strong national nursing organizations; and to serve as the authoritative voice for nurses internationally. Publishes the International Nursing Review. Address, 37 rue de Vermont, 1202 Geneva, P.O. Box 42, 1211 Geneva, Switzerland

International Nursing Index: Published quarterly, with a cumulative annual volume, by the American Journal of Nursing Company in cooperation with the National Library of Medicine. Indexes over 260 nursing journals and organizations and agencies interested in nursing, arranged by country.

International Red Cross (IRC): A worldwide voluntary relief organization founded in Switzerland in 1864, largely through the efforts of Henri Dunant, who had visited the battlefields of the Crimean War and had seen the great need for care for wounded soldiers. The original purpose of the IRC was to aid the wounded and other victims of war but its activities now include disaster relief and the sponsorship of many health-related and social programs. The national Red Cross Societies and the Red Crescent Societies of Moslem countries make up the international organization. The American Red Cross was founded in 1882, largely through the efforts of Clara Barton, and was officially recognized by Congress in 1905. See also Red Cross.

International System of Units: A system consisting of a complete coherent list of physical units of measurement of activity or potency of certain substances, often a hormone, enzyme, vitamin, or antibiotic; used in scientific or technological work; based on the metric system plus units of time, electric current, temperature, and luminous quality; recommended for universal use by the General Conference on Weights and Measures.

International Unit: A unit of measurement in the International System of Units; the amount of a specified substance that produces a specific biological effect and which has been adopted for universal use by the International Conference for Unification of Formulae.

intern (e) (in'-tern): A medical school graduate who often lives within the hospital and who is receiving a year of postgraduate training in the care of medical and surgical patients preliminary to becoming licensed to practice. Cf. extern. In nursing, an advanced or recently graduated student who is getting practical clinical experience under the supervision of experienced workers in preparation for entering practice as a professional nurse.—internship, n.

interneuron (in'-ter-nū'-ron): An internuncial neuron. See internuncial.

internist (in-tern'-ist): A physician who is a specialist in internal medicine, as differentiated from surgery, obstetrics, etc.

internship (in'-tern-ship): In nursing, an education program for graduate nurses, and sometimes for senior student nurses, with the objective of improving the nurse's clinical performance and helping her to adjust to the role of staff nurse.

internuncial (in-ter-nun'-shi-al): Between neurons. Referring to a neuron that connects two other neurons in a neural pathway.

interoceptor (in'-ter-ō-sep'- tor): A sensory nerve terminal or end organ situated in the walls of organs or in viscera and which responds to stimuli that arise within the body.—interoceptive, adj.

interossei (in-ter-os'-sē-ī): Small muscles that insert on the phalanges of the hands and feet.

interosseous (in-ter-os'-ē- us): Lying between bones, as some muscles and ligaments.

interpersonal: Usually refers to forces or relationships between people.

interphalangeal (in'-ter-fa-lan'-jē- al): Between two phalanges.

interrupted: Lacking continuity; broken at intervals. **I. STERILIZATION,** that which is done at intervals in order to allow any spores to develop in the periods between applications of the procedure. **I. SUTURES,** a technique of closing a wound with stitches that are each made with a separate piece of suture material.

interscapular (in-ter-skap'-ū-lar): Situated between the scapulae.

interseptum (in-ter-sep'-tum): The diaphragm.

intersex (in'ter-seks): A congenital condition in which the sex of the individual is not clear. Two types are recognized: 1) true hermaphrodism, in which the individual possesses a mixture of both male and female gonads; and 2) pseudohermaphrodism, which occurs in individuals whose gonads are either basically male or female, but whose external genitalia did not develop accordingly in embryonic life. See hermaphrodite.

intersexuality (in'ter-seks-ū-al'i-ti): The possession of both male and female characteristics. See Turner's and Klinefelter's syndrome.

interspinous (in-ter-spī'-nus): Between spinous processes, especially those of the vertebrae.

interstice (in-ter′-stis): A small gap or space in a tissue or structure.

interstitial (in-ter-stish′-al): 1. Related to or situated in the interstices of a tissue or part. 2. Distributed throughout the connective tissue. **I. FLUID**, see under **fluid**.—Syn., intercellular.

interstitium (in-ter-stish′-i-um): The supporting framework between organs that binds them together; may consist of various kinds of intercellular connective tissue, fibers, and so on.

intertrigo (in-ter-trī′gō): A superficial irritating inflammation occurring where folds of skin overlap; lack of evaporation of sweat causes chafing, redness, itching, and sometimes maceration.—intertriginous, adj.

intertrochanteric (in′-ter-trō-kan-ter′-ik): Between trochanters, particularly the greater and lesser trochanters of the femur.

interval (in′-ter-val): The space between two objects or the time between two occurrences.

intervention: Planned action to alter or correct an undesirable condition or situation.

interventricular (in-ter-ven-trik′-ū- lar): Between ventricles, as those of the brain or heart.

intervertebral (in-ter-ver′te-bral): Between two adjacent vertebrae, as disks or foramina. **I. DISK**, a flattened cartilaginous disk lying between vertebrae, preventing friction and absorbing shock; it is spoken of as ruptured when accident or strain causes the soft central part of the disk to protrude through the surrounding ligament.—see **nucleus, prolapse.**

intestinal (in-tes′-tin-al): Of or pertaining to the intestine. **I. JUICE**, succus entericus, secreted by the intestine; its function is to complete the hydrolysis of carbohydrates and proteins; consists of water, salts, and the enzymes enterokinase, peptidase, maltase, sucrase, lactase, and lipase. **I. OBSTRUCTION**, stoppage of the passage of food or feces through the intestine; may be due to physical blockage, lack of peristalsis, adhesions, tumors, stricture, volvulus, strangulation; symptoms include intense localized pain, vomiting, constipation, abdominal distention.

intestine (in-tes′-tin): The bowel; that part of the alimentary canal that extends from the pyloric end of the stomach to the anus. The **SMALL I.**, is separated from the stomach by the pyloric valve, is about 20 ft. in length, and consists of the duodenum, jejunum, and ileum, in that order. Between the small **I.** and the large **I.** is the ileocecal valve. **LARGE I.**, about 6 ft. in length, is composed of the cecum, colon (ascending, transverse, and descending), and rectum, in that order. The function of the intestine is to complete digestion of foods, and to allow for absorption of digested food material, by blood and lymph vessels, through its walls, and to eliminate waste products of digestion.—intestinal, adj.

intima (in′-tim-a): The internal coat of a blood vessel.—intimal, adj.

intolerance (in-tol′-er-ans): 1. Inability to bear pain or discomfort. 2. In medicine, an idiosyncrasy (*q.v.*) to certain drugs, etc.

intortion (in-tor′-shun): 1. Inward rotation of the eye so that it moves toward the nose. 2. Inward rotation of a body part.

intoxicant (in-tok′-si-kant): An agent that decreases the individual's control over mental and physical functioning and causes intoxication.

intoxication (in-tok-si-kā′-shun): 1. The pathological state of being poisoned by alcohol, a drug, or any toxic substance that gains entrance to the body. 2. The state of being intoxicated, usually referring to the condition produced by overindulgence in alcohol; drunkenness. **WATER I.**, see under **water.**

intra-: Prefix denoting within, on the inside, internal, between the layers of.

intra vitam (vī′-tam): During life.

intra-abdominal (in′-tra-ab-dom′-i-nal): Inside the abdomen.

intra-amniotic (in′-tra-am-ni-ot′-ik): Within, or into, the amniotic fluid or amnion. **I. INJECTION**, the injection of hypertonic saline solution into the amniotic sac to produce abortion; usually done after the 14th week of gestation.

intra-aortic (in′-tra-ā-or′-tik): Within the aorta. **I. BALLOON PUMP**, a device consisting of a balloon attached to the end of a catheter that is inserted into the aorta via a skin incision, and connected to an external pump mechanism that alternately inflates the balloon during diastole and deflates it during systole. May be used to correct ventricular failure by increasing aortic blood pressure and the flow of blood through the coronary arteries.

intra-arterial (in′-tra-ar-tē′-ri-al): Within an artery.—intraarterially, adj.

intra-articular (in′-tra-ar-tik′-u-lar): Within a joint.

intra-atrial (in-tra-ā′-tri-al): Within either or both of the atria of the heart.

intrabronchial (in-tra-brong′ki-al): Within a bronchus.

intracanalicular (in′-tra-kan-a-lik′ū-lar): Within a canaliculus. **I. FIBROADENOMA**, a benign proliferative breast tumor often reaching a size that causes distortion of the glands and ducts within the tumor; also called **I.** myxoma. **I. SARCOMA**, a proliferative breast tumor in which there is great increase in size of the mammary gland due to modular proliferation of the connective tissue; also called cystosarcoma phyllodes.

intracapsular (in-tra-kap′sū-lar): Within a capsule, *e.g.*, that of the lens or of a joint. Opp. to extracapsular.

intracardiac (in-tra-kar′-di-ak): Within the heart.

intracartilaginous (in′tra-kar-ti-laj′i-nus): Within a cartilage.

intracatheter (in-tra-kath′-e-ter): Refers to a plastic tube inserted into or to be inserted into a vein; usually spoken of as **intracath.**

intracavitary (in-tra-kav′i-tā-ry): Within a cavity.

intracellular (in′-tra-sel′-ū-lar): Within a cell. Opp. to extracellular. **I. FLUID,** fluid within the cell walls.

intracerebral (in-tra-ser′e-bral): Within the cerebrum. **I. STEAL,** refers to a situation in which blood drains from one area of the cerebrum because of lowered cerebrovascular resistance in another area.

intracorpuscular (in′-tra-kor-pus′-kū-lar): Within a corpuscle.

intracostal (in-tra-kos′-tal): Refers to the inner surface of the ribs.

intracranial (in-tra-krā′-ni-al): Within the skull.

intractable (in-trak′-ta-b′l): Obstinate; refractory. Resistant to treatment; not easily cured.

intracutaneous (in′tra-kū-tā′nē-us): Within the skin tissues. **I. TEST,** involves introducing an antigen between the layers of the skin and evaluating the reaction this causes.

intracytoplasmic (in′tra-sī-tō-plaz′mik): Within the cytoplasm of a cell.

intradermal (in-tra-der′-mal): Within the skin. Often refers to an injection into or between the skin layers.—intradermally, adj.

intraductal (in-tra-duk′-tal): Within a duct.

intradural (in-tra-dū′-ral): Within the dura mater, *e.g.,* hemorrhage.

intragastric (in-tra-gas′-trik): Within the stomach. **I. TUBE FEEDING,** utilized when it is necessary to assure that the patient receives adequate fluids and foods, and to give extra proteins; introduced via a nasogastric tube inserted through the pharynx and esophagus into the stomach.

intrahepatic (in-tra-he-pat′ik): Within the liver.

intralobular (in-tra-lob′-ū-lar): Within a lobule, as the vein draining a hepatic lobule.

intraluminal (in-tra-lū′-min-al): Within the hollow of a tubelike structure.—intraluminally, adv.

intramedullary (in′tra-med′ū-lar-i): 1. Within the medulla oblongata or the spinal cord. 2. Within the marrow cavity of a bone or the bone marrow. **I. NAIL,** a nail or metal rod inserted into the intramedullary canal of a long bone to provide internal fixation. It extends on both sides of the fracture, thus holding the two parts of the fractured bone in proper position for healing.

intramembranous (in-tra-mem′bran-ous): Within a membrane or between membranes. Descriptive of a type of bone formation that differs from endochondral bone formation.

intramural (in-tra-mū′-ral): Within the layers of the wall of a hollow tube or organ.—intramurally, adv.

intramuscular (in-tra-mus′kū-lar): Within or into the substance of a muscle, as an intramuscular injection.—intramuscularly, adj.

intranasal (in-tra-nā′-zal): Within the nasal cavity.—intranasally, adv.

intranatal (in-tra-nā′-tal): At the time of birth. Syn., intrapartum (*q.v.*).—intranatally, adv.

intraocular (in′-tra-ok′-ū-lar): Within the globe of the eye. **I. PRESSURE,** the pressure of the fluid within the eye, as measured by a tonometer. **I. LENS TRANSPLANT,** the substitution of an artificial lens for one that has to be removed, usually for cataract.

intraoperative (in′-tra-op′-er-a-tiv): During the time of an operation.

intraoral (in′-tra-ō′-ral): Within the mouth, as an intraoral appliance.—intraorally, adv.

intraorbital (in-tra-or′-bi-tal): Within an orbit, as of the eye.

intraosseous (in-tra-os′-ē-us): Within or into the substance of a bone.

intrapartum (in-tra-par′-tum): During labor or delivery, as asphyxia, hemorrhage, or infection.—intrapartal, adj.

intraperitoneal (in′tra-per-i-tō-nē′al): Within the peritoneal cavity.

intraplacental apoplexy (in′-tra-pla-sen′-tal ap′-ō-plek-si): See **Couvelaire's uterus.**

intrapleural (in-tra-ploo′-ral): Within, or going into, the pleural cavity.—intrapleurally, adv.

intrapsychic (in′-tra-sī′-kik): Refers to that which takes place within the psyche or mind of the individual and which is not involved in one's exchanges with other persons.

intrapulmonary (in-tra-pul′-mo-nar-i): Within the lungs, as **I.** pressure.—intrapulmonic, adj.

intraretinal (in-tra-ret′-i-nal): Within the retina.

intraspinal (in-tra-spī′-nal): Within, or going into, the spinal canal, as **I.** anesthesia.—intraspinally, adv.

intrasplenic (in′tra-splen′ik): Within the spleen.

intrastitial (in-tra-stish′-al): Within the cells of a tissue.

intrasynovial (in-tra-si-nō′vi-al): Within a synovial membrane or sac.

intrathecal (in-tra-thē′-kal): Within a sheath. Within or going under or between the meninges of the brain or spinal cord, as an injection. **I. THERAPY,** the introduction of a therapeutic agent into the spinal subarachnoid space.—intrathecally, adj.

intrathoracic (in′-tra-thō-ras′-ik): Within, or occurring within, the cavity of the thorax.

intratracheal (in-tra-trā′kē-al): Within, or going into or through the trachea. **I. ANESTHESIA,**

the administration of an anesthetic through a special tube passed down the nose or mouth into the trachea.—intratracheally, adv.

intrauterine (in-tra-ū′-ter-in): Being or occurring within the uterus. **INTRAUTERINE CONTRACEPTIVE DEVICE (IUD),** a device placed within the uterus to prevent conception. The most commonly used IUD is the T 380A, marketed in the U.S. as ParaGard, a T-shaped plastic device with copper affixed to the horizontal arms and stem of the T, which is inserted high into the uterus and removed via a minor surgical procedure; it is effective for four years.

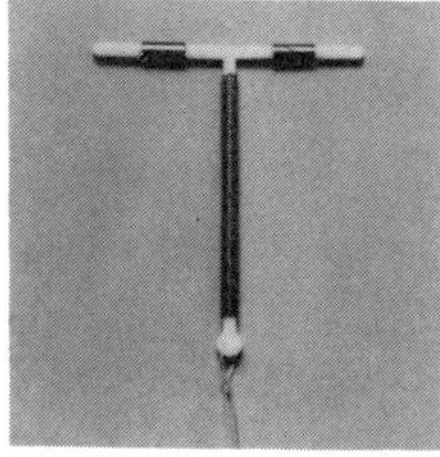

Model T 380A, ParaGard

intravaginal (in-tra-vaj′-i-nal): Within the vagina.—intravaginally, adv.

intravasation (in-trav-a-zā′-shun): The introduction of foreign or abnormal matter into a blood vessel.

intravascular (in-tra-vas′-kū-lar): Within a vessel, especially within a blood vessel or lymphatic.

intravenous (in-tra-vē′-nus): Within, or going directly into a vein or veins. **I. INFUSION,** see under infusion. **I. PYELOGRAM,** see under pyelogram.

intraventricular (in-tra-ven-trik′-ū-lar): Within, or going into a ventricle of the brain or heart.

intravitreous (in-tra-vit′-rē-us): Into or within the vitreous.

intrinsic (in-trin′-sik): Inherent or inside; from within; real; innate; natural. Often used in reference to certain muscles, *e.g.*, certain eye muscles **I. FACTOR,** a glycoprotein secreted by the gastric mucosa; essential for the satisfactory absorption of vitamin B_{12}.

intro-: Prefix denoting into, within, inward, inwardly, to or on the inside.

introitus (in-trō′-it-us): Any opening in the body; an entrance to a cavity, particularly the vagina.

introjection (in-trō-jek′-shun): In psychiatry, an unconscious defense mechanism whereby a person identifies with another loved or hated person or object.

intromission (in-trō-mish′-un): The act of putting one part of the body, or an instrument, into another; usually refers to the act of putting the penis into the vagina.

introspection (in-trō-spek′-shun): The act of looking inward to one's thoughts and feelings; self-examination.—introspective, adj.

introversion (in-trō-ver′-shun): 1. Reclusiveness. 2. The tendency to be overly concerned with one's thoughts, to be reflective rather than overtly expressive. 3. The turning "outside in" of a part, more or less completely, as invagination.—introvert, n., introverted, adj.

introvert (in′-trō-vert): 1. To turn one's thoughts inward toward one's own mental processes. 2. A person who is self-centered and introspective, and who tends to be thoughtful, self-sufficient, and interested more in his own thoughts and feelings than in those of others. Tends to withdraw in social situations and to be a poor mixer. Opp. to extrovert (*q.v.*).

intubation (in-tū-bā′-shun): The insertion of a tube into an organ or passage, usually through the nose or mouth, into a part of the body, especially a canal and particularly the trachea or intestine. **DUODENAL I.,** a procedure for instilling barium into the duodenum prior to fluoroscopy. **ENDOTRACHEAL I., I.** done to maintain an airway by keeping the trachea open to administer anesthesia, or to restore patency in cases of obstruction.

intuition (in-tū-ish′-un): The quality or state of having quick insight or immediate comprehension or of having untaught knowledge.

intumescence (in′-tū-mes′-ens): 1. A swelling or prominence on the body. 2. The enlarging or swelling of a part, particularly as a reaction to heat.—intumesce, v.i.; intumescent, adj.

intussusception (in′-tus-sus-sep′-shun): A condition in which one part of the bowel slips or telescopes into the part immediately adjacent (invaginates). It occurs most commonly in infants and most frequently at the junction of the ileum and the cecum; causes obstruction. Usual therapy is surgery. **ILEOCECAL I., I.** in which the ileocecal valve prolapses into the cecum. **ILEOCOLIC I., I.** in which the ileum prolapses into the colon.

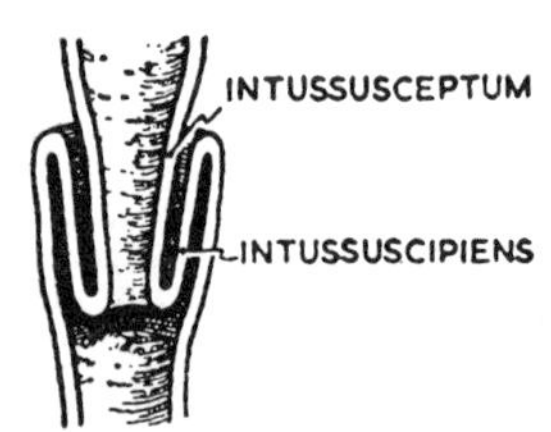

intussusceptum (in′-tus-sus-sep′-tum): The invaginated portion of an intussusception.

intussuscipiens (in′-tus-sus-sip′-i-ens): The receiving portion of an intussusception.

inulin (in′-ū-lin): A tasteless vegetable starch that occurs in some plants; yields levulose on hydrolysis; is used as a diagnostic agent in some kidney function tests.

inunction (in-ungk′-shun): Annointing. The act of rubbing an oily or fatty substance that contains a drug into the skin for therapeutic purposes, or a sustance so used.—inunct. v.t.

invagination (in-vaj′-i-nā′-shun): The act or condition of being ensheathed; a pushing inward; telescoping; forming a pouch.—invaginate, v.t.

invalid (in′-va-lid): Weak, sickly. A person who is chronically disabled by some infirmity or illness but not completely incapacitated.

invasion (in-vā′-zhun): 1. The entry of bacteria into the body. 2. The beginning or onset of a disease. 3. The spreading of a malignancy into surrounding tissue.

invasive (in-vā′-siv): 1. Tending to invade healthy surrounding tissues; said of neoplasms or microorganisms. 2. Referring to a procedure that involves penetration of an organ or deeper tissues of the body. **I. MONITORING,** monitoring of conditions existing within the body, utilizing devices that are placed within the body. **I. PRESSURE MONITORING,** direct measurement of blood pressure, pulmonary artery pressure, venous pressure, or intracranial pressure; a cannula is inserted into the pressure source and connected to a transducer, which converts the pressure into an electric signal that can be seen on a monitor. **I. PULMONARY DISORDERS,** caused by inflammation resulting from infection or tumor development; characterized by chest pain, dyspnea, cough, hemoptysis, anorexia, fatigue, debilitation.

inversion (in-ver′-zhun): 1. A turning inside out, upside down, outside in, or in any direction that is the reverse of normal. 2. Position in which a part is turned toward the midline of the body. 3. Outward turning of the ankle. 4. Supination. In obstetrics, **I.** of the uterus, an obstetric emergency that may follow delivery; may also be caused by the uterus attempting to expel a tumor. 5. A deviant or abnormal psychosocial preference leading to anti-social behavior, *e.g.*, pedophilia, bestiality.

invert (in′-vert): In psychiatry, a homosexual individual. **I. SUGAR,** the mixture of glucose and fructose obtained by hydrolyzing sucrose.

invertase (in′-ver-tās): A sugar-splitting enzyme in intestinal juice. Also called sucrase.

invertebrate (in-ver′-te-brāt): An animal without a backbone.

inverted (in-ver′-ted): Turned upside down, inward, or any direction contrary to normal.

invertin (in′-ver-tin): Invertase (*q.v.*).

invest (in-vest′): To surround or enclose in a membrane or sheath.

inveterate (in-vet′-er-at): Chronic; recurring; obstinate or resistant to therapy.

involucrum (in-vo-lū′-krum): 1. An enveloping membrane or sheath. 2. A sheath of new bone, which forms around necrosed bone, in such conditions as osteomyelitis.

involuntary (in-vol′-un-ta-ri): Independent of the will, as the smooth muscle of the abdominal organs. **I. SMOKING,** the inhalation of cigarette smoke by non-smokers; also called passive smoking.

involution (in-vō-lū′-shun): 1. The normal shrinkage of an organ after fulfilling its functional purpose, *e.g.*, the uterus after labor. 2. The period of progressive alteration in the body after middle age when glandular activity lessens and degenerative changes set in. 3. The menopause.

involutional (in-vō-lū′-shun-al): Pertaining to involution. **I. MELANCHOLIA,** a term descriptive of agitated depression occurring in women during the menopause; characterized by agitation, insomnia, irritability.

I & O: Abbreviation for intake and output.

iodide (ī′-ō-dīd): A compound of iodine with another element or radical, *e.g.*, potassium iodide.

iodine (ī′-ō-dēn): A nonmetallic element with several industrial and medicinal uses; obtained chiefly from seaweed. **I.** is also found in the body, chiefly in the form of thyroglobulin in the thyroid gland; protein-bound iodine (PBI) is estimated in thyroid investigations. **LUGOL's SOLUTION,** a 5 percent aqueus solution of iodine given orally in thyrotoxicosis, usually for preoperative stabilization. **RADIOACTIVE I.** (I^{131}), used in investigation and treatment of thyrotoxicosis. **I. TEST,** a test for starch; when **I.** is added to a compound containing starch a deep blue color is produced; the color disappears when the substance is heated and reappears when it is cooled. **TINCTURE OF I.,** a 2 to 5 percent solution of iodine in alcohol, used as an antiseptic and disinfectant for small wounds.

iodism (ī′-ō-dizm): Poisoning by prolonged or excessive use of iodine or iodides; symptoms are those of a common cold, with excessive secretion of saliva, sore gums, rash. Treated by withdrawing the medication.

iodize (ī′-ō-dīz): 1. To treat with iodine or an iodide. 2. To impregnate with iodine, as table salt.—iodized, adj.

iodoform (ī-ō′-dō-form): A lemon-yellow, volatile, crystalline, chemically produced substance containing iodine; used as a topical antiseptic for skin and mucous membrane, usually in the form of impregnated gauze.

iodophor (ī-ō′-dō-for): A disinfectant in which the active ingredient is iodine; used as a skin disinfectant in surgical scrubs, but its primary use is in veterinary medicine.

iodopsin (ī-ō-dop̄′-sin): A protein substance which, with vitamin A, is a constituent of visual purple present in the retinal cones and important in daylight vision.

ion (ī′-on): An atom, or group of atoms, that has either a positive or negative charge of electricity and which, in electrolysis, passes to one pole or the other.

ionization (ī-on-ī-zā′-shun): 1. The breaking up of a substance into its component ions when in solution. 2. Treatment whereby ions of various substances, *e.g.*, zinc, chlorine, iodine, histamine, are introduced into the skin by means of a constant electrical current.

iontophoresis (ī-on′-tō-fō-rē′-sis): The introduction,, through the skin,, of ions of various salts for therapeutic purposes; accomplished by electrical means.

iontophoretic sweat test (ī′-on-tō-fō-ret′-ik): A test for fibrocystic disease of the pancreas; pilocarpine is introduced into the skin, usually of the forearm or thigh by means of an electric current, to stimulate the sweat glands; measurement of the electrolyte concentration in the sweat is a diagnostic procedure.

iopanoic acid (ī-ō-pan-ō′-ik): A radiopaque medium used in radiography of the gallbladder.

IP: Abbreviation for intraperitoneal.

ipecac (ip′-e-kak): The dried roots and rhizome of a Central and South American tree; used in medicine as an emetic and in expectorants. Ipecacuanha.

IPPA: Abbreviation for inspection, palpation, percussion, and auscultation.

IPPB: Abbreviation for intermittent positive pressure breathing. See under **intermittent**.

IPPV: Abbreviation for intermittent positive pressure ventilation, a temporary measure to ensure adequate ventilation, *e.g.*, in treating patients with asthma, until other therapies can bring an acute attack under control; usually administered by endotracheal intubation along with sedatives and muscle relaxants.

ipsilateral (ip-si-lat′-er-al): Situated or appearing on the same side, or affecting the same side.—ipsilaterally, adv.

IQ: Abbreviation for intelligence quotient.

ir-: See **in-**.

IRCU: Abbreviation for intensive respiratory care unit.

IRDS: Abbreviation for infant respiratory distress syndrome, see under **respiratory distress syndrome**.

irid-, iridio-: Combining forms denoting the iris of the eye.

iridectomy (ir-i-dek′to-mi): Excision of part of the iris, thus enlarging the pupil or creating an artificial one.

iridencleisis (ir′-i-den-klī′-sis): An operation for decreasing the intraocular pressure in glaucoma.

iridium (i-rid′-i-um): A hard white metal used as an alloy to confer rigidity to platinum. **IRIDIUM-192,** a radioactive isotope of iridium, used in treatment of certain cancers.

iridocele (ir′i-dō-sēl): Protrusion of part of the iris through a defect or wound in the cornea.

iridocyclitis (ir′-i-dō-sī-klī′-tis): Inflammation of the iris and ciliary body.

iridodialysis (ir′-i-dō-dī-al′-i-sis): A separation of the iris from its ciliary attachment, often a result of trauma.

iridodonesis (ir′-i-dō-dō-nē′-sis): Quivering movements of the iris; seen in patients with aphakia (*q.v.*).

iridokinesis (ir′-i-dō-kī-nē′-sis): Contraction and expansion of the iris of the eye as it contracts and dilates the pupil.

iridology (ī-ri-dol′ō-ji): A study of the markings and changes in color that are said to occur in the iris in the course of systemic disease, the assumption being that every organ of the body has a representative area in the iris.

iridoplegia (ir′i-dō-plē′ji-a): Paralysis of the sphincter of the iris, with resulting inability of the pupil to contract or dilate.

iridoptosis (ir′-i-dop-tō′-sis): Prolapse of the iris.

iridotomy (ir′-i-dot′-om-i): A small incision into the iris, as in the operation to create an artificial pupil. **LASER I.,** utilized in treatment of glaucoma.

iris (ī′-ris): The colored circular membrane forming the anterior one-sixth of the middle coat of the eyeball. It consists of two layers of muscle and is perforated in the center by an opening called the pupil. Contraction of its muscle fibers regulates the amount of light entering the eye. **I. BOMBÉ,** bulging forward of the iris due to pressure of aqueous behind it when posterior adhesions are present.—irides, pl.; iridal, iridian, iridic, adj.

iritis (ī-rī′-tis): Inflammation of the iris, often with pain, tearing, photophobia, decreased vision, irregular pupils; due to local or systemic infection.

iron: A common metallic element found in some soils and waters and in certain minerals. Present in the body in small amounts, most of it in the red blood cells; important in the physiological process of transporting oxygen to the tissues. Some of it is stored in liver, spleen, or bone marrow, but since a certain amount is excreted in feces, it must be supplied daily in the diet. Some of its salts are used in treating various forms of anemia. **I. LUNG,** a device used to force air in and out of the lungs when the nerves controlling chest muscles fail to act, as occurs in poliomyelitis. See **respirator**.

iron deficiency anemia: See under **anemia**.

irradiation (ir-rā′dē-ā′shun): 1. Subjection of a patient to the action of such rays as those of heat, light, radium, etc. for diagnostic or therapeutic purposes. 2. Subjection of a substance, especially a food, to certain rays, *e.g.*, ultraviolet, to increase its vitamin potency. 3. A spreading out, as of nerve impulses.—irradiate, v.

irrational (ir-rash′un-al): Term refers to the lack of one's usual clarity of thought and speech, and control of voluntary actions. Unreasonable.

irreducible (irrē-dūs′i-b'l): 1. Term applied to a hernia, fracture, or dislocation that is not capable of being brought into the desired position; opp. of reduction (*q.v.*). 2. Incapable of being made smaller or less in amount. 3. In chemistry, incapable of being made simpler or reduced. **I. HERNIA,** one in which the contents of the sac cannot be returned to the appropriate cavity without surgical intervention.

irreversible (ir-rē-ver′si-b'l): Not capable of being reversed; said of a disease or process from which recovery is not possible.

irrigate (ir′-i-gāt): To cleanse a body area by flushing with a fluid.

irrigation (ir-i-gā′-shun): In medicine, the washing out of a body cavity or part with a continuous stream of water, or other fluid, for therapeutic purposes.—irrigate, v.

irritable (ir′i-ta-b'l): In medicine, capable of responding to stimuli; responding easily to stimuli.—irritability, n.

irritable bowel syndrome: A collection of symptoms, including tenderness over the small intestine and the ascending and transverse colon; also, alternating constipation, diarrhea, and normal bowel movements; anxiety; fatigue; dysuria; excessive secretion of mucus; bloating. Also called spastic colon and irritable colon syndrome.

irritant (ir′-i-tant): Any agent that causes irritation (*q.v.*).—irritative, adj.

irritation (ir-i-tā′-shun): 1. The normal response of a muscle or nerve to a stimulus. 2. An exaggerated response of a nerve or tissue to stimulus. 3. Greater than normal response of tissues to injury or trauma.

IRV: Abbreviation for inspiratory reserve volume; see under inspiratory.

ischemia (is-kē′mi-a): Local temporary reduction of blood supply of an area due to obstruction in the blood vessels supplying the area or to vasoconstriction. **MYOCARDIAL I.,** inadequate blood supply to the myocardium due to coronary artery disease.—ischemic, adj.

ischemic (is-kē′-mik): Pertaining to or affected by ischemia (*q.v.*). **I. CONTRACTURE,** see Volkmann's ischemia. **I. HEART DISEASE,** caused by reduced blood supply to the myocardium; usually due to obstruction of flow in the coronary arteries. **I. STROKE,** see transient ischemic attack.

ischi-, ischio-: Combining forms denoting the ischium.

ischial (is′ki-al): Pertaining to the ischium. **I. SPINE,** one that lies above the ischial tuberosity and divides the greater and lesser sciatic notches. **I. TUBEROSITY,** the body of the ischium; the part of the pelvis that the trunk rests on when one is sitting.

ischiocavernosus (is′-ki-ō-kav-er-nō′-sus): One of a pair of muscles of the female pelvic floor, extending from the ramus of the ischium on each side of the clitoris to the tuberosity of the ischium.

ischiofemoral (is-ki-ō-fem′-o-ral): Pertaining to the ischium and the femur. **I. LIGAMENT,** a wide, strong ligamentous band in the hip joint, extending from the ischium to the greater trochanter of the femur.

ischiorectal (is-ki-o′rek′tal): Pertaining to both the ischium and the rectum. **I. REGION,** the region at the posterior part of the pelvic outlet, between the ichshium and the rectum.

ischium (is′-ki-um): The lower, heavy, posterior part of the innominate bone of the pelvis; the bone on which the body rests when sitting.—ischia pl.; ischial, adj.

ischo-: Combining form denoting suppression or relationship to suppression.

ischocholia (is-kō-kō′-li-a): Suppression of bile formation or failure of the bile to reach the intestine. Also ischolia.

ischuria (is-kū′-ri-a): Retention or suppression of urine.

Ishihara's test: A test for color vision; consists of a series of plates with dots of differing sizes and colors.

island: In anatomy, a group of cells or a mass of tissue, separated in some way, or marked off, from surrounding tissue. **I.S OF LANGERHANS,** clusters of special cells scattered throughout the pancreas; they secrete insulin (*q.v.*), which pours directly into the bloodstream. **I. OF REIL,** see insula.

islet (ī′-let): An island, as one of the islands of Langerhans.

iso-: Prefix or combining form denoting equal, like, uniform, homogenous.

isochronous (ī-sok′-rō-nus): Occurring during the same time period or passing through the same phases at the same time.

isocoria (ī′-sō-kō′-ri-a): Equality in the size of the two pupils.

isocortex (ī′-sō-kor′teks): Neocortex (*q.v.*).

isodactylism (ī-sō-dak′til-izm): A condition in which all of the fingers are of approximately the same length.

isoenzyme (ī′sō-en′zīm): One of a group of enzymes occurring in a given species that have similar catalytic characteristics but differing other physical properties. Also isozyme.

isograft (ī′-sō-graft): A graft of tissue that has been obtained from another individual of the same species. Also called isotransplant.

isohemagglutinin (ī′-sō-hē-ma-gloo′-tin-in): A hemagglutinin in one person's blood serum that will agglutinate another person's red blood cells.

isoimmunization (ī′sō-im-ū-nī-zā′shun): The development in an individual of antibodies in response to antigens from another individual of the same species, *e.g.*, the development of anti-Rh agglutinins in the blood of an Rh-negative person who has been given an Rh-positive transfusion, or who is carrying an Rh-positive fetus.

isolate (ī′-sō-lāt): 1. To set oneself apart. 2. To place alone. 3. To quarantine.

isolation (ī-sō-lā′shun): The act of setting a person with an infectious disease apart from those who do not have the disease. **I. TECHNIQUE,** measures and precautions taken to prevent the spread of infection from a patient in isolation to others. **REVERSE I.,** the use of strict isolation technique to protect the patient from infection caused by organisms in the environment, or that may be carried into the unit by caretakers or through articles used in the patient's care; the precautions are taken when entering the unit instead of when leaving it after giving care. May involve the use of laminar air flow (*q.v.*). Also called protective isolation.

isolation amentia (ī-sō-lā′-shun a-men′-shi-a): Mental retardation due to isolation of an individual from normal contacts; in the elderly, often due to blindness or deafness.

Isolette (ī-sō-let′): An incubator for premature babies, providing accurate control of humidity, temperature, and oxygen supply, made so that the infant can be cared for without being taken out of it.

isologous (ī-sol′o-gus): 1. Pertaining to any one or both of two compounds that are similar in structure but have differing compositions. 2. Characterized by an identical genotype (see 2. under genotype). **I. TRANSPLANT,** a tissue transplant between identical twins.

isomers (ī′sō-merz): Compounds made up of the same elements but in different arrangements of their atoms, which gives them different physical or chemical properties, although the elements are present in the same proportions.

isometric (ī-sō-met′rik): Of equal length or dimensions. In physiology, a muscle contraction that occurs without shortening of the muscle, as it is fixed at both ends, but with increase in tone of the muscle fibers. **I. EXERCISE,** active muscular exercise in which the muscle contraction does not reduce its length, due to the force exerted by an opposing muscle at the same time.

isometropia (ī-sō-me-trō′-pi-a): The condition of having equal and like refraction in both eyes.

isomorphous (ī-sō-mor′-fus): Having the same form or shape.

isopropyl alcohol (ī′-sō-prō′-pil): An alcohol similar to, but more toxic than ethyl alcohol; used in manufacture of cosmetics and medicinal preparations for external use. Rubbing alcohol contains about 70 percent isopropyl alcohol in water.

isorrhea (ī-sō-rē′ah): Water equilibrium, *i.e.*, the amount of water output is equal to the amount of water intake.

isosensitization (ī′sō-sen-sit-ī-zā′shun): See autosensensitization.

isosexual (ī′sō-seks′ū-al): 1. Characteristic of or referring to the same sex. 2. Pertaining to the existence of the characteristics of both sexes in an individual.

isosthenuria (ī-sos′-the-nū′-ri-a): A state in chronic renal disease characterized by the maintenance of a constant osmolality of the urine, regardless of the osmotic pressure of the blood; the specific gravity remains fixed, usually around 1.010, regardless of fluid intake; seen in arteriosclerosis, hydronephrosis, and glomerulonephritic kidney disease.

isotherapy (ī′-sō-ther′-a-pi): Treatment of a disease by administering its active causal agent, as is done in the treatment for prevention of rabies. Term also used to describe treatment of a disease organ with that organ or extract of it, *e.g.*, liver disease treated with liver extract.

isotonic (ī′-sō-ton′-ik): 1. Having equal tension; applied to any solution that has the same osmotic pressure as blood. **I. SALINE,** (syn., normal saline), 0.9 percent solution of salt in water. 2. Descriptive of muscular contraction that takes place without significant increase in tone but with shortening of the fibers. Opp. of isometric.

isotope (ī′-sō-tōp): One of two or more forms of the same element that have identical chemical properties but differing physical properties. Isotopes with radioactive properties emit their excess energy in three forms—alpha rays, beta rays, and gamma rays; they are used in medicine for research, diagnosis, and treatment of disease. **I. SCAN,** see radioisotope scan under radioisotope.

isovaleric acid (ī′sō-val-er′ik): A colorless substance with a disagreeable odor and taste; found in tobacco and several other plants; used in the manufacture of certain pharmaceuticals.

isthmus (is′-mus): In anatomy, a connecting part between two larger parts. **I. UTERI,** the constricted part of the uterus where the cervix and body of the uterus join.

itch: A name given to a wide variety of skin conditions that arouse a sensation of pricking or stinging and an intense desire to scratch or rub the affected part. May be caused by the itch mite, by exposure to irritating plant oils, or by substances handled in certain occupations; allergic or neurogenic reactions are among many other causes.—itch, v.; itchiness, n.; itchy, itching, adj.

-ite: Suffix denoting: 1. "Of the nature of"; a native of. 2. Adherent, follower. 3. A salt or an ester of an acid with a name ending in -ous.

-itis: Suffix denoting disease, usually inflammatory.—itises, itides, pl.

IU: Abbreviation for International Unit.

IUCD: Abbreviation for intrauterine contraceptive device. See under **intrauterine.**

IUD: Abbreviation for intrauterine device.

IV: Abbreviation for intravenous, intravenously.

IV push: The injection of a medication directly into a vein; may be done with a hypodermic needle, via a heparin lock, or through intravenous tubing; the drug is absorbed instantly.

IVH: Abbreviation for intravenous hyperalimentation. See **hyperalimentation.**

IVP: Abbreviation for intravenous pyelogram.

ivy bleeding time: The time it takes for bleeding from a small puncture wound made in the forearm to stop.

ivy poisoning: Dermatitis caused by exposure to a toxic oil contained in the poison ivy plant. Also often used to describe dermatitis caused by exposure to such plant oils as those of poison oak and sumac.

J

J: Symbol for joule (*q.v.*).

J point: Refers to the point where the QRS complex of the electrocardiogram meets the T segment.

J receptors: Sympathetic vagal nerve endings located deep in the parenchyma of the lung; thought to respond to the presence of pulmonary embolism or pulmonary edema.

jacket: In medicine, a fixed bandage or covering for a part of the body, especially the thorax or trunk; sometimes made of plaster of Paris. STRAIT J., a shirt-like garment with long sleeves used to restrain an irrational or violently disturbed person.

jackknife rigidity: The clasp-knife phenomenon (*q.v.*).

jacksonian epilepsy: See epilepsy. [John Hughlings Jackson, English neurologist. 1835–1911.]

Jacquemier's sign (zhak'-mē-ās): Blueness of the vaginal muscosa seen in early pregnancy. [Jean Marie Jacquemier, French obstetrician. 1806–1879.]

jactitation (jak'-ti-tā'- shun): Excessive restlessness; constant turning or tossing about as seen in patients with high fever or serious illness.

Jaeger chart: A chart for testing near vision; uses a series of different sizes of printers' type. Also called Jaeger's test types. [Edward Jaeger von Jastthal, Austrian oculist. 1818–1911.]

Jakob-Creutzfeldt disease: A progressive, usually fatal nervous system disorder, of unknown cause but thought to be of metabolic origin; begins with neurasthenia followed by weakness and stiffness of the extremities, unsteady gait, choreoathetoid movements, apathy, confusion, and progressive dementia. The brain cells atrophy and the gray matter becomes spongy. A disease of middle and old age. Also Creutzfeldt-Jakob disease.

jalap (jal'-ap): The dried root of a Mexican plant; has purgative properties.

JAMA: Journal of the American Medical Association. See American Medical Association.

jamais vu (zha'-mā-voo): Literally, never having seen. A psychic phenomenon in which the patient feels an absolute stranger in surroundings with which he is normally familiar; usually due to a lesion in the temporal lobe or to epilepsy.

Janeway's lesions: Circumscribed, slightly raised, erythematous, hemorrhagic, nodular or macular lesions; usually painless and occurring on the palms and soles; may be symptomatic of subacute bacterial endocarditis or mycotic aneurysm.

jargon (jar'-gon): 1. Unintelligible or confused speech. 2. The technical terms used by specialists working in a particular field of knowledge.

jaundice (jawn'dis): A condition characterized by a raised level of bilirubin in the blood (hyperbilirubinemia); due to deposition of bile pigments resulting from obstruction in bile passageways, excess destruction of red blood cells, or disturbance in liver function. Minor degrees are detectable only chemically and are most often referred to as LATENT J. Major degrees are recognized by yellow skin, sclerae and mucosae and are referred to as OVERT or CLINICAL J. J. may be due to 1) obstruction anywhere in the biliary tract (obstructive J.) 2) excessive hemolysis of red blood cells (hemolytic J.); or 3) toxic or infective damage of liver cells (hepatocellular J.). ALCHOLURIC J., J. without bile in the urine; usually reserved for congenital hemolytic anemia, a familial disease characterized by abnormally fragile, small, spheroid cells that hemolyze readily. Congenital spherocytosis. HEMOLYTIC J., occurs in erythroblastosis fetalis or from excessive transfusion reactions. HEPATIC J., occurs in cirrhosis, and in infectious, viral, and toxic hepatitis. HEPATOCELLULAR J., J. due to impaired function or destruction of liver cells. INFECTIOUS OR INFECTIVE J., most commonly due to a virus. J. OF THE NEWBORN, icterus neonatorum (*q.v.*). MALIGNANT J., acute yellow atrophy of the liver; see under acute. OBSTRUCTIVE J., occurs when a gallstone becomes lodged in the bile duct leading from the gallbladder thus preventing the flow of bile into the duodenum. PHYSIOLOGIC J. OF THE NEWBORN, yellowness of the skin and sclera, and hyperbilirubinemia; seen in some neonates; usually mild and disappears in 7 to 14 days.

jaundiced (jawn'-disd): Of a yellowish color; marked by jaundice.

jaw: Either the maxillary or mandibular bone, which together form the bony framework of the mouth into which the teeth are set.

jawbone: Either the maxilla (upper jaw) or mandible (lower jaw).

jaw-winking syndrome: See Marcus Gunn syndrome.

JCAH: Abbreviation for Joint Commission on Accreditation of Hospitals (*q.v.*).

jejun-, jejuno-: Combining forms denoting jejunum.

jejunal (jē-joo'-nal): Of or pertaining to the jejunum. J. ULCER, an ulcer in the mucous membrane lining the jejunum.

jejunectomy (jē-joo-nek′ -to-mi): Surgical excision of the jejunum, or part of it.

jejunitis (jē-joo-nī′tis): Inflammation of the jejunum.

jejunocecostomy (jē-joo′ -nō-sē- kos′ -to-mi): The surgical creation of an anastomosis between the jejunum and the cecum.

jejunocolostomy (jē-joo′ -nō-kō-los′ -to-mi): The surgical creation of an anastomosis between the jejunum and the colon.

jejunogastric (jē-joo′ -nō-gas′ trik): Pertaining to the jejunum and the stomach.

jejunoileal shunt (jē-joo′ -nō-il′ -ē-al): A bypass procedure in which the upper jejunum is anastomosed to the terminal part of the ileum, and a blind loop is created; done for patients who are morbidly obese, to decrease the available area for absorption of food in the intestine.

jejunoileitis (jē-joo′ -nō-il-ē-ī′ -tis): Inflammation of the jejunum and the ileum.

jejunoileostomy (jē-joo′ -nō-il-ē- os′ -to-mi): The surgical creation of a passage between the jejunum and a noncontinuous part of the ileum.

jejunoileum (jē-joo′nō-il′ē-um): The part of the small intestine between the duodenum and the cecum.—jejunoileal, adj.

jejunojejunostomy (jē-joo′ -nō-jē- joo-nos′ -to-mi): The surgical creation of an anastomosis between two parts of the jejunum.

jejunostomy (jē-joo-nos′ -to-mi): A surgically made fistula between the jejunum and the anterior abdominal wall; used temporarily for feeding in cases where passage of food through the stomach is impossible or undesirable.

jejunotomy (jē-joo-not′o-mi): An incision into the jejunum.

jejunum (jē-joo′num): That part of the small intestine between the duodenum and the ileum. It is about 8 ft. in length.—jejunal, adj.

Jellineck's sign: The brownish pigmentation, particularly of the upper eyelids, seen in hypoparathyroidism.

jelly: A semi-solid gelatinous substance. **K. Y. JELLY,** trade name for a lubricating jelly. **WHARTON'S J.,** the gelatinous substance that makes up the basic substance of the umbilical cord.

Jenner, Edward: English physician; in 1796 developed the method of preventing smallpox by inoculation with cowpox vaccine. [1815–1898.]

jerk: A sudden involuntary muscular movement; a reflex. Describes certain reflex actions that follow tapping or striking a muscle or tendon, *e.g.*, knee jerk.

Jervell and Lange-Nielsen syndrome: A condition occurring in certain congenitally deaf children; characterized by sudden attacks of syncope, ventricular fibrillation, and electrocardiographic anomalies.

Jesuits' balsam: Compound tincture of benzoin. See benzoin.

Jesuits' powder or bark: See Peruvian bark.

jet injection: The administration of medication by injection, intrasubcutaneously or subcutaneously, using a device that injects the fluid with great velocity and penetrates the skin painlessly.

Jewett brace: A brace for providing extension of the spinal column; consists of a metal frame with vinyl padding that fits over the sternum, symphysis pubis, and small of the back.

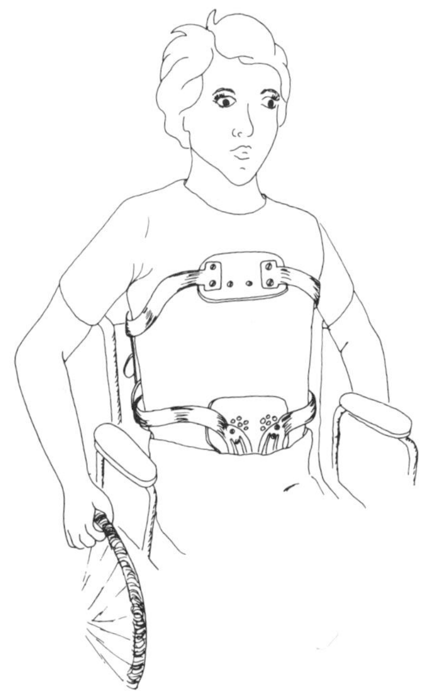

Jewett brace

jigger (jig′ -ger): (*Tunga penetrans*) A flea, prevalent in the tropics. It burrows under the skin to lay its eggs, causing intense irritation. Secondary infection is common.

Jimson weed: *Datura stramonium*. A poisonous herb, now naturalized, with rank-smelling foliage and large white trumpet-shaped flowers; the drug stramonium (used in treatment of asthma) is derived from the leaves, which are also burned, powdered, and smoked; intoxicating in large doses. Other constituents are scopolamine and hyocyamine.

JOD: Abbreviation for juvenile onset diabetes. See diabetes.

jogging: Running at a slow even pace.

jogger's heel: A painful traumatic condition of the heel, caused by repeatedly striking the heel forcefully on the ground or a hard surface when jogging.

joint: The articulation or connection of two or more bones for mobility and stability; consists of two cartilage-covered articular surfaces, a synovial membranous sac, and a capsule that thickens and becomes a ligament; provides for flexion, extension, abduction and adduction. Three main designated classes are: 1) SYNARTHROSES (fibrous), consisting usually of two bones bound together by fibrous material when little movement is desirable; further classified as a) SUTURA, *e.g.*, the sutures of the skull: b) SYNDESMOSES, *e.g.*, the union of the distal ends of the tibia and fibula; and c) GOMPHOSES, *e.g.*, the articulation of the teeth in the gums; and 2) CARTILAGINOUS, in which two bones connected by cartilage allow for limited motion, *e.g.*, the joints between the ribs and the sternum; further classified as a) SYNCHONDROSES (as between the epiphyses and diaphyses of the long bones, in which the opposing surfaces are eventually converted into bone); and b) SYMPHYSES, which are connected by a disk of fibrocartilage (as in the pubis, where the disk remains unossified throughout life); and 3) DIARTHROSES or SYNOVIAL, which are freely moveable joints, *e.g.*, the hip and elbow joints.

joint capsule: The fibrous sheath that encloses a synovial joint.

joint cavity: The closed space in a synovial joint formed by synovial membrane that contains synovial fluid.

Joint Commission on Accreditation of Hospitals (JCAH): Formed in 1951 by the American College of Surgeons, the American College of Physicians, the American Medical Association, the American Hospital Association, and the Canadian Medical Association (no longer a member). It sets standards, conducts examinations, and accredits hospitals that meet the standards. JCAH accreditation is required of hospitals for participation in Medicaid and Medicare programs. Standards include those for physical design, management, staff organization, and various hospital services, including those for nursing. It publishes an accreditation manual which is updated periodically, outlining the requirements for accreditation, and which is used by the assessment teams that inspect the hospitals applying for accreditation. See accreditation.

joint mouse: A small, loose, often calcified concretion in a synovial joint cavity.

joule (jool): Term used in nutritional science for calorie. It denotes the quantity of heat released when food is utilized in the body. One large scale calorie (kilocalorie) equals 4.184 kilojules. JOULE'S EQUIVALENT, the mechanical equivalent of the amount of heat or energy expended in raising one pound of water 1 degree Fahrenheit; 772 foot pounds. [J.P. Joule, English physicist. 1818–1889.]

jowl: The fleshy hanging part under the lower jaw.

jugal (jū′-gal): Relating to the cheek, the zygomatic bone in particular.

jugular (jug′-ū-lar): Pertaining to the throat. J. VEINS, two veins passing down either side of the neck.

jugulum (joo′-gū-lum): The neck or throat.

juice: Any fluid from a body tissue; succus. DIGESTIVE J., secreted by the glands in the walls of the small intestine; *succus entericus*. GASTRIC J., secreted by glands in the stomach walls; *succus gastricus*. PANCREATIC J., secreted by the pancreas; discharged into the duodenum; *succus pancreaticus*.

jumping Frenchmen of Maine: Refers to a rare, bizarre, familial disease affecting only males of French-Canadian ancestry; characterized by episodes in which the individual makes a single violent jump following certain stimuli—sounds, touch, or sudden movements; often accompanied by echolalia; cause unknown.

junction: The point or line where two parts meet.—junctional, adj.

junctional (junk′shun-al): Pertaining to a junction. J. RHYTHM, a cardiac rhythm for which the pacemaker is in the atrioventricular junctional tissues. J. TACHYCARDIA, an arrhythmia with a heartbeat of 140 to 220 per minute, for which the impulse arises in the atrioventricular node or in the atrioventricular tissues.

Jung: Carl Gustav Jung, Swiss psychiatrist. [1875–1961.] Founder of the school of analytic psychology. See jungian psychology under psychology.

jungian: Relating to or characteristic of C.G. Jung, his theories, methods, or doctrines. See under psychology.

jungle fever: 1. Malaria (*q.v.*). 2. Yellow fever (*q.v.*):

junket (jun′-ket): Milk predigested by the addition of rennet. Formerly, curds and cream.

jurisprudence (jur-is-prū′-dens): The science or philosophy of law. MEDICAL J., see under medical.

jury mast: An upright bar inserted into a plaster of Paris jacket to support the head in spinal fracture, or in spinal disease, as Pott's disease.

justo minor pelvis: A pelvis that is like the normal female pelvis in every way except that it is in miniature. All pelvic measurements are in the correct proportion but diminished.

juvenile (joo′-ve-nil): Pertains to childhood, immaturity, or youth. J. KYPHOSIS, Scheuerman's disease (*q.v.*). J. MUSCULAR DYSTROPHY, limb-girdle muscular dystrophy, see under dystrophy. J.-ONSET DIABETES, see under diabetes. J. OSTEOMALACIA, rickets. J. RHEUMATOID ARTHRITIS, see Still's disease.

juxta-: Combining form denoting situated near.

juxta-articular (juks′ta-ar-tik′ū-lar): Near a joint.

juxtaglomerular (juks′-ta-glō-mer′-ū-lar): Adjacent to or near the glomerulus. **J. APPARATUS**, a cuff of tissue surrounding the arteriole leading into the glomerulus. **J. CELLS**, cells found within the cuff of the apparatus surrounding the arteriole that supplies the glomerulus; their function is unknown.

juxtamedullary (juks′ta-med′ū-lar-i): Pertaining to the part of the kidney cortex that is adjacent to the medulla.

juxtapose (juks′-ta-pōz): To place side by side.

juxtaposition (juks′ta-pō-zish′un): Side by side; adjacent; apposition; close at hand.

K

K: Chemical symbol for potassium.

Kahler's disease: Multiple myeloma; see under **myeloma.**

kaif (kif): An Arabic term for a dreamy state of tranquility induced by certain drugs.

kakidrosis (kak-i-drō'-sis): Extremely unpleasant smelling sweat.

kakosmia (kak-oz'-mi-a): 1. An offensive odor. 2. Perception of an unpleasant odor that does not exist. Also spelled cacosmia.

kakotrophy (kak-ot'-rō-fi): Undernutrition. Also spelled cacotrophy.

kala-azar (ka'-la a-zar'): An often fatal generalized form of leishmaniasis occurring in the tropics; symptoms include anemia, fever, hepatomegaly, splenomegaly and wasting. It is caused by the parasite *Leishmania donovani* and is spread by the sand fly.

kalemia (ka-lē'mi-a): The presence of potassium in the blood. Also spelled kaliemia.

kalimeter (ka-lim'-i-ter): A device for measuring the alkalinity of a substance. Alkalimeter.

kaliopenia (kal-i-ō-pē'-ni-a): An insufficiency of potassium in the body.—kaliopenic, adj.

kaliuresis, kaluresis (kal-i-ū-rē'-sis, kal-ū-rē'-sis): The presence of potassium in the urine.

kaliuretic, kaluretic (kal-i-ū-ret'-ik, kal-ū-ret'-ik): 1. Pertaining to kaliuresis. 2. An agent that promotes kaliuresis.

kallidin (kal'-i-din): A kinin liberated by the action of kallikrein on a globulin in the blood plasma; of two varieties, K.-I and K.-II. They increase capillary permeability.

kallikrein (kal-li-krē'-in): One of several proteolytic enzymes present in blood plasma, salivary glands, lymph glands, pancreas, urine, and lymph. It acts on a globulin in blood plasma to release kinins, such as bradykinin, from kininogens.

kallikreinogen (kal-i-krī'-nō-jen): The precursor of kallikrein, normally present in the blood plasma.

Kandahar sore: Cutaneous leishmaniasis; see **leishmaniasis.**

Kanga pants: A garment made with a detachable absorption pad that can be removed when soiled without changing the entire garment; used by incontinent geriatric patients.

kangaroo ligature: Suture material made from the tendon from kangaroo tail.

kaolin (kā'-ō-lin): Powdered dehydrated aluminum silicate; used internally as an absorbent in the treatment of diarrhea and externally as a protective application that absorbs moisture.

kaolinosis (kā'ō-lin-ō'-sis): A form of pneumoconiosis caused by inhalation of particles of kaolin.

Kaposi: [Moritz K. Kaposi, Hungarian dermatologist. 1837–1902.] **KAPOSI'S DISEASE,** a rare condition marked by dermatosis, discoloration of the skin that may give rise to keratosis, ulcers, neoplastic growth, and a fatal termination; usually starts in childhood. **KAPOSI'S SARCOMA,** a malignant neoplasm of the skin marked by the development of purplish nodules or papules on the skin, lymphadenectomy, excessive weight loss, and immune deficiency; see **acquired immune deficiency syndrome. KAPOSI'S VARICELLIFORM ERUPTION,** a viral skin infection occurring in the presence of another skin disease such as eczema or herpes simplex.

karaya (ka-rā'-a): A vegetable gum with nonirritating and protective qualities; used especially for sealing ostomy appliances to the skin; also sometimes used as a laxative.

Kardex (kar'-deks): A card filing system of record keeping on which data regarding the patient, her condition, treatment, and so on, are recorded; it provides a temporary concise summary of pertinent information for quick reference.

Kartagener's syndrome: A hereditary condition in which dextrocardia is present along with bronchiectasis and sinusitis.

kary-, karyo-: Combining forms denoting the nucleus of a cell.

karyochrome (kar'-i-ō-krōm): A nerve cell with a nucleus that takes a stain easily but has few, if any, Nissl bodies.

karyoclasis (kar-i-ok'-la-sis): the breaking down of a cell nucleus, an early stage in necrosis.

karyocyte (kar'-i-ō-sīt): Any nucleated cell; usually refers to a young red blood cell.

karyogenesis (kar-i-ō-jen'-e-sis): The formation of a cell nucleus.

karyokinesis (kar'i-ō-kī-nē'sis): Equal division of nuclear material, as occurs in cell division.

karyolymph (kar'-i-ō-limf): The clear fluid part of a cell nucleus in which the other elements are dispersed.

karyolysis (kar-i-ol'-i-sis): The dissolution or destruction of a cell nucleus.—karyolytic, adj.

karyomegaly (kar-i-ō-meg'a-li): Abnormal enlargement of the nucleus of a cell.

karyon (kar'-i-on): Nucleus of a cell.

karyoplasm (kar'-i-ō-plazm): The protoplasm

of a cell that is contained within the nucleus, *i.e.*, the nucleoplasm.

karyopyknosis (kar'i-ō-pik-nō'sis): Shrinkage of a cell nucleus with condensation of the chromatin content.

karyorrhexis (kar-i-ō-rek'-sis): Fragmentation of the chromatin mass in the nucleus of a cell, a stage in necrosis that precedes karyolysis.

karyosome (kar'-i-ō-sōm): The spherical mass of chromatin in the cell nucleus.

karyotheca (kar-i-ō-thē'-ka): The membrane around the nucleus of a cell.

karyotype (kar'-i-ō-tīp): The total chromosomal makeup of the nucleus of a single cell as to number, size, shape, and location of the centromere, and which is characteristic of an individual, species, or other grouping.

Kashin-Beck disease: A slowly progressive form of osteoarthritis of the peripheral joints and spine, occurring chiefly in young children in Eastern Siberia and Northern China; caused by eating fungus-contaminated grain.

katabolism (ka-tab'ō-lizm): Catabolism (*q.v.*).

katathermometer (kat'a-ther-mom'e-ter): A pair of wet and dry alcoholic thermometers for measuring the cooling and drying powers of the atmosphere; can be used in estimating the amount of moisture that evaporates from the body and the subsequent decrease in body temperature.

Katz-Wechtel sign: A change in the QRX complexes as shown on the electrocardiogram; indicates a defect in the ventricular septum.

Kawasaki's disease: A rare, acute, arthritis-like disorder, first described in 1967; endemic in Japan; usually occurs in children under two years of age, more often in boys than girls. Cause and mode of transmission not known; may be a sequel to a viral infection. Symptoms include a rash of red flat spots followed by desquamation, especially of the fingertips; sore throat, conjunctivitis, cervical lymphadenopathy, and, in 30 percent of cases, cardiac complications. Also called mucocutaneous lymph node syndrome.

Kayser-Fleischer ring: A ring of gray-green to red-gold color at the outer margin of the cornea; seen in hepatolenticular degeneration (*q.v.*).

kcal: Kilocalorie. Also abbreviated kgcal and C. The quantity of energy required to raise the temperature of one kilogram of water 1°C. Has 1000 times the value of a small calorie. Also known as large caloric.

Keeley cure: A method of treatment for the alcohol or opium habit. [Leslie E. Keeley, American physician. 1834-1900.]

Kegel's exercise: An exercise regimen for tightening certain perineal muscles to improve the ability to retain urine; it utilizes the squeezing action of stop-and-go voiding of urine. Also called pubococcygeus exercise.

Kehr's sign: Radiating shoulder pain occurring when the diaphragm is irritated by blood in the peritoneal cavity; may be a sign of ruptured spleen.

Kell blood group system: First described in 1946. Red blood cells that are antibodies to the K antigen; have been observed in infants with hemolytic disease of the newborn and in association with hemolytic transfusion reactions. Also referred to as K or k blood group system. Thought by some to be next in importance to the ABO and Rh groups.

Keller's operation: Arthroplasty of the metatarsophalangeal joint of the great toe, for removal of the bursa and for treatment of exostosis; bunionectomy.

Kelly forceps: See under forceps.

Kelly or Kelly's pad: A special inflatable rubber and fabric pad that is placed under a patient to protect a chair, bed, or operating table.

keloid (kē'-loyd): An overgrowth of scar tissue, consisting of a shiny, firm, usually elevated, benign, thickened mass of fibrous tissue forming at the site of a burn, skin wound, or surgical incision; has a predilection for the face and trunk; may produce a constriction deformity. Most common in blacks.

keloidosis (kē'-loy-dō'-sis): A condition marked by the formation of keloids.

keloma (kē-lō'-ma): A keloid.

kelotomy (kē-lot'-o-mi): An operation for the relief of strangulated hernia.

kelp: Any of several varieties of marine algae widely used as food in the Orient; formerly the chief source of iodine and potassium salts.

Kempner rice diet: A special diet consisting mainly of rice plus fruits and sugar; has been used in treatment of hypertension and kidney disease.

Kennedy's syndrome: Retrobulbar optic neuritis, a condition usually seen in tumors of the frontal lobe or sphenoid crest; symptoms include optic nerve atrophy, unilateral blindness, sometimes anosmia. Also called Foster Kennedy syndrome. [Robert Foster Kennedy, American neurologist. 1884–1952.]

Kenny method, treatment: A method of treating patients with anterior poliomyelitis to prevent paralysis; involves the use of hot wet packs, positioning, and muscle reeducation. [Sister Elizabeth Kenny, Australian nurse. 1886–1952.]

Kent's bundle: A muscular bundle which, in some people, forms a direct connection between the atrial and ventricular walls.

kerat-, kerato-: Combining forms denoting: 1. The cornea. 2. Horny tissue.

keratalgia (ker-a-tal'-ji-a): Pain in the cornea.

keratectasia (ker-a-tek-tā′-zi-a): Protrusion of the cornea.

keratectomy (ker-a-tek′-to-mi): Removal of a portion of the cornea.

keratiasis (ker-a-tī′-a-sis): The presence of horny warts on the skin.

keratin (ker′-a-tin): A relatively insoluble protein found in all horny tissue; a principal constituent of the epidermis, where it serves to waterproof and toughen the skin. In pharmacology, used to coat pills given for their intestinal effect, since keratin can withstand the action of gastric juice.

keratinization (ker′a-tin-ī-zā′shun): 1. The formation of keratin in body tissues. 2. The development of a horny quality in tissues by the excess formation of keratin; occurs as a pathological process in vitamin A deficiency.

keratinize (ker′-a-tin-īz): To become horny.

keratinocyte (ke-rat′-in-ō-sīt): The epidermal cell which synthesizes keratin in the skin.

keratinous (ke-rat′-in-us): Horny.

keratitis (ker-a-tī′-tis): Inflammation of the cornea. **ACNE ROSEACEA K.**, severe **K.** associated with acne roseacea of the eyelids and cornea. **HERPETIC K.**, **K.** characterized by simultaneous appearance with herpes simplex; fairly common in the elderly. **INTERSTITIAL K.**, marked by deposits in the corneal substance giving it a hazy ground glass appearance; associated with congenital syphilis. **K. NUMMULARIS**, a benign, slowly developing type of **K.** in which deposits in the cornea form into circles with sharply defined areas, surrounded by less dense areas forming a halo.

keratoacanthoma (ker′a-tō-ak′an-thō′ma): A rapidly growing firm skin nodule, usually singular, appearing on hairy parts of the body, especially on exposed areas; has a dome-shaped center of keratotic material; resembles squamous cell carcinoma. Usually occurs in sun-damaged skin, but may also be due to exposure to tars and mineral oil products.

keratocele (ker′-a-tō-sēl): Hernial protrusion of Descemet's membrane, the innermost layer of the cornea.

keratocentesis (ker′-a-tō-sen-tē′-sis): Surgical puncture of the cornea.

keratochromatosis (ker′a-tō-krō-ma-tō′sis): Discoloration of the cornea.

keratoconjunctivitis (ker′a-tō-kon-junk′ti-vī′tis): Inflammation of the cornea and conjunctiva. **ACTINIC K.**, inflammation of the conjunctiva and the cornea; may be caused by exposure to ultraviolet radiation or to repeated flashes of light; symptoms include pain, tearing, and photophobia. **EPIDEMIC K.**, long lasting, highly contagious **K.**, presents as an acute follicular conjunctivitis with periauricular and submaxillary adenitis, irritation of the conjunctiva, and photophobia. **K. SICCA**, **K.** that is associated with lacrimal deficiency. See Sjögren's syndrome.

keratoconus (ker′-a-tō-kō′-nus): An inherited, degenerative, noninflammatory condition marked by conical protrusion of the central part of the cornea; usually bilateral; results in astigmatism. Seen more often in women. May be associated with Down's syndrome. In advanced cases the cornea becomes scarred and a corneal transplant is required.

keratocyte (ker′-a-tō-sīt): One of the flattened cells between the lamellae of the cornea, with branching processes that communicate with those of other cells.

keratoderma (ker′a-tō-der′ma): Hypertrophy of the horny layer of the skin (stratum corneum), marked by the appearance of cone-shaped horny lesions, affecting primarily the palms and soles. **K. BLENNORRHAGICUM**, characterized by pustular, crusted, cone-shaped lesions on the palms and soles; may be associated with gonorrheal arthritis. **K. CLIMACTERICUM**, occurs in menopausal women; marked by lesions on the hands and feet; may be associated with obesity.

keratogenesis (ker′-a-tō-jen′-e-sis): The formation of horny growths.

keratogenous (ker-a-toj′-e-nus): Causing formation of horny tissue.

keratoglobus (ker′a-tō-glō′bus): Prominent globular protrusion of the cornea; seen in congenital glaucoma.

keratohelcosis (ker′a-tō-hel-ko′sis): Ulceration of the cornea.

keratoid (ker′-a-toyd): 1. Hornlike. 2. Resembling corneal tissue.

keratoiritis (ker′-a-tō-ī-rī′-tis): Inflammation of the cornea and the iris.

keratoleukoma (ker′-a-tō-lū-kō′-ma): Areas of white opacity in the cornea.

keratolysis (ker-a-tol′-i-sis): 1. Shedding of the epidermis. 2. A congenital anomaly characterized by the periodic shedding of skin.—keratolytic, adj.

keratoma (ker-a-tō′-ma): An overgrowth of horny tissue. Callosity.—keratomata, pl.

keratomalacia (ker′a-tō-ma-lā′shi-a): Softening of the cornea with possible ulceration; frequently caused by lack of vitamin A.

keratome (ker′-a-tom): A knife used in surgery on the cornea. Keratotome.

keratometer (ker-a-tom′-e-ter): An instrument for measuring the curvature of the surface of the cornea; used in fitting contact lenses.

keratomycosis (ker′-a-tō-mī-kō′-sis): A fungal disease of the cornea.

keratonyxis (ker′-a-tō-nik′-sis): Surgical puncture of the cornea, as in the procedure of needling the lens in treatment of soft cataract.

keratopathy (ker-a-top′-a-thi): Any disease of the cornea.—keratopathic, adj.

keratoplasty (ker′-a-tō-plas-ti): Corneal grafting. Replacing of unhealthy corneal tissue with healthy tissue obtained from a donor.—keratoplastic, adj.

keratoprosthesis (ker′-a-tō-pros-thē′-sis): An acrylic plastic corneal implant that replaces an area of the cornea that has become opaque.

keratorrhexis (ker′-a-tō-reks′-is): Rupture of the cornea; may be caused by trauma or be due to ulceration.

keratoscleritis (ker′-tō-sklē-rī′-tis): Inflammation of the cornea and the sclera.

keratoscope (ker′-a-tō-skōp): An instrument for examining the cornea.

keratose (ker′-a-tōs): Horny.

keratosis (ker-a-tō′-sis): Thickening or overgrowth of the horny layer of the skin, such as a callosity or wart. **ACTINIC K.**, slowly developing wartly lesions in areas that are long exposed to sunlight; affects chiefly the middle-aged and elderly; potentially malignant; also called senile keratosis, solar keratosis, keratoderma. **ARSENICAL K.**, precancerous hard, wart-like lesions seen in persons who have received medications containing arsenic or been long exposed to pesticides, dyes, or other substances containing arsenic; may not appear until 10 years after exposure. **K. FOLLICULARIS,** a rare congenital condition marked by areas of symmetrical crusting and papular growths on the trunk, axillae, face, and scalp. **K. NIGRICANS,** acanthus nigricans; see under acanthus. **K. PALMARIS ET PLANTARIS,** (tylosis), a congential thickening of the horny layer of the palms and soles. **K. SENILIS,** dry, harsh condition of the skin seen in the aged; also descriptive of the pigmented elevated papules seen in the skin of patients long exposed to sunlight. **SEBORRHEIC K.**, a coarse waxy benign neoplasm of the skin characterized by the formation of multiple shiny tan to brown dome-shaped lesions of varying size; usually develops in middle life. **SPLAR K.**, chronic dermatitis on exposed areas; due to long exposure to sunlight; also called peasant's neck. **SOLAR K.**, actinic k.—keratoses, pl.; keratotic, adj.

keratotomy (ker-a-tot′-o-mi): A surgical incision into the cornea.

kerion (kē′-ri-on): A boggy suppurative swelling, often associated with ringworm of the scalp.

keritherapy (ker-i-ther′-a-pi): Treatment of burns and denuded skin surfaces by the external use of liquid paraffin.

Kerley lines: Horizontal step-ladder-like lines appearing on chest x-rays, indicating thickened interlobular septa due to edema or fibrosis.

kernicterus (ker-nik′-ter-us): A serious form of icterus neonatorum; caused by high levels of bilirubin in the blood, bile staining, and widespread destructive lesions in various parts of the brain; may result in severe neurological defects; often a sequel to erythroblastosis fetalis (*q.v.*).

Kernig's sign (ker′nigs): Inability to straighten the leg at the knee joint when the thigh is flexed at right angles to the trunk. Occurs in meningitis. [Vladimir Kernig, Russian physician. 1840–1917.]

Kerr-Mills bill: Passed in 1961; provided for federal matching funds to states that license nursing homes and carry out inspection of the facilities.

keto acid: A chemical compound that is both an acid and a ketone. See ketone.

ketoacidosis (kē′-tō-as-i-dō′-sis): Acidosis accompanied by an increase of acetone bodies in the blood; due to incomplete metabolism of fatty acids; commonly seen in diabetes mellitus, starvation, pregnancy, or after ether anesthesia. **DIABETIC K.**, due to insulin deficiency, characterized by dehydration, electrolyte depletion, hyperpnea, acetone odor to the breath, dry mouth and hyperglycemia, followed by glycosuria and polyuria and, possibly, death.

ketoaciduria (ke′-to-as-i-dū′-ri-a): The presence of excessive keto acids in the urine.

ketogenesis (kē-tō-jen′-i-sis): The production of ketone bodies. See acetone bodies.

ketogenic (kē-tō-jen′-ik): Producing or capable of producing ketone bodies. **K. DIET**, consists of foods that cause a ketogenic state as a result of changes in the acid-base balance, *i.e.*, large amounts of fats and minimal amounts of protein; used in treatment of epilepsy.

ketohexose (kē-tō-hek′-sos): A monosaccharide that contains a six-carbon chain and a ketone group.

ketolysis (kē-tol′-i-sis): The dissolution or splitting up of acetone or ketone bodies.—ketolytic, adj.

ketone (kē′-tōn): Any organic compound that contains the carbonyl group CO. The product of incomplete oxidation of fat in the body; when present in the bloodstream **K.**'s upset the acid-base balance of the body and produce ketosis. See acetone bodies.

ketone bodies: Acetone, acetoacetic acid, and b-hydroxybutyric acid; normal products of metabolism of lipids and pyruvate in the liver, occurring in increased amounts in the blood and urine of persons with certain conditions, *e.g.*, pregnancy, starvation, and diabetic acidosis.

ketonemia (kē-tō-nē′mi-a): An excess of ketone bodies in the blood as occurs in starvation or diabetes mellitus.

ketonuria (kē-tō-nū′-ri- a): Excessive ketone bodies in the urine.—ketonuric, adj.

ketosis (ke-tō′-sis): A condition that arises when incomplete oxidation of fatty acids results in an accumulation of ketone bodies in the blood; symptoms include drowsiness, headache, and deep respirations. A complication of diabetes mellitus and of starvation when it is the result of decreased carbohydrate intake.—ketotic, adj.

ketosteroids (kē-tō-stē′roidz): Steroid hormones that contain a keto group, formed by the addition of an oxygen molecule to the basic ring structure. The 17-**K.** (which have this oxygen at carbon 17) are produced by the adrenal cortex and excreted in normal urine; they are present in excess in overactivity of the adrenal glands and the gonads, and in renal and ovarian tumors; hyper- or hyposecretion is indicative of an endocrine disorder.

kg: Abbreviation for kilogram.

kibe (kib): 1. An ulcerated chilblain. 2. A crack in the skin due to exposure to cold.

Kidd blood group: Red blood cell antigens that react with antibodies designated anti-Jk[a], first found in the mother of an infant with erythroblastosis; occasionally cause transfusion reactions or erythroblastosis fetalis.

kidney (kid′-ni): One of two bean-shaped organs, situated on the posterior abdominal wall, behind the peritoneum in the lumbar region, one on either side of the vertebral column. Function is to secrete urine. **ARTIFICIAL K.**, a popular name for an apparatus that is used for removing from the blood, while it is circulating outside of the body, the same elements normally removed by the kidneys. **FLOATING K.**, one that is misplaced and more or less freely movable. **HORSESHOE K.**, a congenital malformation in which the **K.** has the shape of a horseshoe. **K. STONE**, a calculus (*q.v.*) that forms, usually in the pelvis of the kidney, composed mostly of calcium oxalate. When small, calculi may pass down through the ureters and bladder and cause agonizing pain as they pass through the urethra. **POLYCYSTIC K.**, a hereditary condition characterized by the formation of multiple cysts on both kidneys.

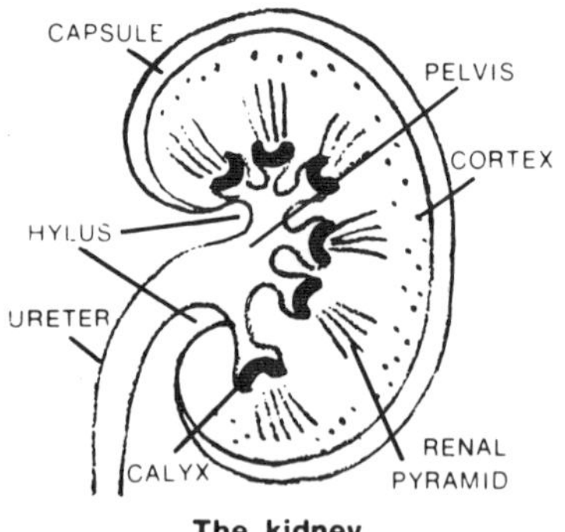

The kidney

kidney basin: An emesis basin that is kidney-shaped.

kidney function tests: Various tests for measuring renal function, all requiring careful collection of urine specimens. Some of those in common use are: paraaminohippuric acid clearance test for measuring renal blood flow; creatinine clearance test for measuring glomerular filtration rate; ammonium chloride test for measuring tubular ability to excrete hydrogen ions; urinary concentration and dilution tests for measuring tubular function.

Kienbach's disease or atrophy: Osteochondrosis (*q.v.*) of the lunate bone of the wrist; marked by pain, loss of grip, limitation of motion. [Robert Kienbach, Austrian roentgenologist. 1871–1953.]

Kiernan's spaces: Triangular spaces in the liver formed by the invagination of Glisson's capsule (*q.v.*); they contain the larger branches of the portal vein, hepatic artery, and the hepatic duct.

Kiesselbach's area: An area on the anterior inferior part of the nasal septum; often the site of epistaxis.

killer cells: Lymphocytes developed in the bone marrow that, in the presence of an antibody, attack certain cells directly.

Killian's operation: The removal of a part of the frontal bone to allow for drainage from a suppurating frontal sinus.

kilo-: Combining form denoting one thousand; used chiefly in names of units in the metric system.

kilocalorie (kil′-ō-kal-o-ri): Large calorie; see under calorie.

kilogram (kg) (kil′-ō-gram): One thousand grams; equivalent to 2.2 pounds avoirdupois.

kiloliter (kl) (kil′-ō-lē-ter): One thousand liters; equivalent to 264.18 gallons.

kilometer (km) (ki-lom′-e-ter): One thousand meters; five-eighths of a mile.

kilovolt (kv) (kil′-ō-vōlt): One thousand volts.

Kimmelstiel-Wilson syndrome: A condition that occurs in diabetics of long standing when glomerulosclerosis has occurred; characteristic signs are hypertension, edema, proteinuria, and renal failure.

kin-, kine-, kinesi-, kinesio-, kino-: Combining forms denoting motion, action.

kinanesthesia (kin-an-es-thē′zi-a): Loss of the sense of movement.

kinase (kī′nās): An enzyme activator. Syn., coenzyme. See enterokinase, thrombokinase.

kinekard (kin′-e-kard): A polypeptide substance in blood plasma; stimulates the muscles of the heart and blood vessels and inhibits activity of smooth muscles of the intestine.

kinematics (kin-e-mat′-iks): The science of motion of the body and of the body parts.

kinematograph (kin-e-mat′-ō-graf): A device for showing pictures of objects in motion; a moving picture camera.

kinemia (kī-nē′-mi-a): The cardiac output. See under **cardiac.**

kinemometer (kī-nē-mom′-e-ter): An electromagnetic device used to measure the reflex time of a tendon reflex.

kineplastic surgery: Operative measures utilized in amputations whereby certain muscle groups are isolated and utilized to work certain modified prostheses.

kinescope (kin′-e-skōp): An instrument used in testing ocular refraction.

kinesia (kī-nē′-si-a): Motion sickness.

kinesialgia (kī-nē′-si-al′-ji-a): Pain caused by muscular movements.

kinesiatrics (kī-nē′-si-at′-riks): The therapeutic use of active or passive movements; movement therapy. Kinesitherapy.

kinesics (kī-nē′-siks): The study of nonverbal bodily activity in communication, including posture, facial expression, and body movements.

kinesiology (kī-nē-si-ol′-o-ji): The science or study of human motion.

kinesis (kī-nē′-sis): Physical movement.

kinesitherapy (kī-nē′-si-ther′-a-pi): Treatment by massage and therapeutic exercises. Kinesiatrics.

kinesthesia (kin-es-thē′-zi-a): Muscle sense; perception of movement, weight, and position.—kinesthetic, adj. Also kinesthesis.

kinesthesiometer (kin′es-thē′zi-om′-e-ter): An instrument for measuring proprioception (*q.v.*).

kinetic (kī-net′-ik): Pertaining to, or producing, motion.

kinetism (kin′-e-tizm): The ability to consciously initiate and perform movement.

kinetocardiogram (ki-nē′-tō-kar′-di-ō-gram): A graphic representation of the chest wall vibrations and pulsations caused by the acitivity of the heart; a diagnostic tool.

kinetogenic (ki-nē-tō-jen′-ik): Causing or resulting in movement.

kinetoplasm (ki-nē′-tō-plazm): The chromophilic substance present in the nerve cells only at the time the cells begin to perform their specific functions.

kinetosis (ki-nē-tō′-sis): Any illness due to motion.

kinin (kī′-nin): Any of a group of several peptides that appear to have a direct action on the blood vessels, cause contraction of smooth muscle, act as hypotensives, increase capillary permeability, and have certain other properties in common. **VENOM K.,** found in the venom of snakes. **WASP K.,** found in the venom of wasps. See also **bradykinin.**

kink: Angulation. An unnatural bend, twist, or angle in a structure, particularly in a duct or tube.

kinked carotid syndrome: A strong arterial pulsation felt just above the right clavicle; occurs chiefly in older women with systolic hypertension; to be differentiated from carotid aneurysm.

kinky hair syndrome or **disease:** A sex-linked inherited disorder characterized by early onset, light kinky hair, developmental abnormalities, and early death; cause unknown. Also called Menkes' syndrome.

kinomometer (kin-ō-mom′-e-ter): An instrument for measuring the degree of motion in a joint.

kinotoxin (kin-ō-tok′-sin): Toxin produced by fatigue.

kinurenine (kin-ū-ren′-in): An intermediate product in the conversion of tryptophan to niacin (*q.v.*).

kiotomy (kī-ot′-o-mi): Excision of the uvula or part of it.

Kirschner's wire (kirsch′-ner): A wire drilled into a bone to apply skeletal traction. [Martin Kirschner, German surgeon. 1879-1942.]

kiss of life: A method of artificial respiration in which the exhaled breath of the operator inflates the patient's lungs. Mouth-to-mouth, mouth-to-nose, and mouth to nose and mouth are the methods used. Also called mouth-to-mouth resuscitation.

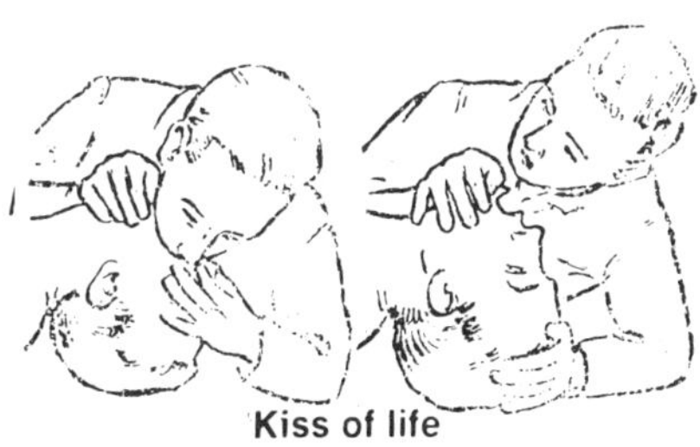
Kiss of life

kissing: **K. DISEASE,** infectious mononucleosis (*q.v.*). **K. ULCER,** an ulcer caused by pressure of apposing parts.

KJ, kj: Abbreviations for knee jerk.

Klebsiella (kleb-si-el′-ah): A genus of the family *Enterobacteriaceae;* anaerobic, nonsporeforming, gram-negative rods which may or may not be pathogenic; found in the respiratory, intestinal, and urogenital tracts; may be the causative agent in bronchitis, sinusitis, and certain pneumonias. **K. PNEUMONIAE,** Friedländer's bacillus; a large gram-negative rod bacterium occassionally found in the upper respiratory tract; may be the cause of lobar pneumonia and other inflammations of the respiratory tract.

Klebs-Loeffler bacillus: (*Corynebacterium diphtheriae*) A clinicolaboratory term for the diphtheria bacillus named after the discoverers of the organism. [Edwin Klebs, German bacteriologist. 1834–1913. Friederich A. J. Loeffler, German bacteriologist. 1852–1915.]

kleptolagnia (klep′-tō-lag′-ni-a): Sexual gratification derived from the act of stealing.

kleptomania (klep′-tō-mā′-ni-a): Compulsive stealing due to mental disturbance, usually of the obsessional neurosis type.

kleptomaniac (kelp′-tō-mā′-ni-ak): 1. Pertaining to kleptomania. 2. A person who is a compulsive thief.

Klinefelter's syndrome: A condition associated with abnormality of the sex chromosomes; in most instances the cells have an extra X chromosome. The individual appears to be male but has large breasts, small genitalia, atrophied testes, and is sterile; genetic female, pragmatic male. Frequently recognized in sterility clinics. [Harry F. Klinefelter, American physician. 1912–.]

Klippel-Feil syndrome: A condition occurring in infants with congenital hemivertebra (*q.v.*); the neck is short and its movement is limited due to either a reduction in the number of cervical vertebrae or to fusion.

Klumpke's paralysis: Atrophic paralysis affecting the forearm.

Klüver-Bucy syndrome: A rare syndrome that sometimes follows bilateral temporal lobectomy; characterized by psychic blindness or hyperactivity to visual stimuli, depressed emotional reactions, lack of sexual inhibitions.

kneading (nēd′-ing): A movement used in massage.

knee: The hinge-joint formed by the lower end of the femur and the head of the tibia. **K. JERK,** a reflex contraction of the relaxed quadriceps muscle elicited by a tap on the patellar tendon; usually performed with the lower femur supported from behind, the knee bent and the leg limp. Persistent variation from normal usually signifies organic nervous disorder. **HOUSEMAID'S K.,** inflammation of the prepatellar bursa. **KNOCK–K.,** abnormal closeness of the knees while the ankles are abnormally far apart; genu valgum. See valgus.

kneecap: The patella (*q.v.*).

knee-chest position: Genupectoral position; see under position.

knee replacement: A surgical procedure in which diseased surfaces within the knee joint are removed and replaced with a hinged prosthesis that is cemented to the femur and tibia; usually done to relieve pain and to restore loss of range of motion due to osteoarthritis or some other pathological condition.

knife: In surgery, any cutting instrument.

knismogenic (nis-mō-jen′-ik): Causing a tickling sensation.

knit (nit): Term used to describe the growing together of the ends of bones after a fracture.

knock-knee: A condition in which the legs curve inward at the knees and the ankles are far apart; often the result of rickets in childhood. See genu valgum.

knuckle (nuk′ l): The dorsal aspect of any of the joints between the phalanges and the metacarpal bones, or between the phalanges.

Koch, Robert. [German physician and bacteriologist. 1843–1910.] **KOCH'S BACILLUS,** *mycobacterium tuberculosis,* the causative organism of tuberculosis. **KOCH'S POSTULATES,** a list of requirements that an organism must meet before it can be considered the cause of a disease; also called Koch's law.

Koch-Weeks bacillus: A small, gram-negative rod; the cause of infective conjunctivitis (pinkeye).

Köhler's disease: 1. Osteochondritis of the navicular bone. 2. Osteochondritis of the second or third metatarsal head. [Alban Köhler, German physician, 1874–1947.]

Kohlrausch's folds: Horizontal folds of the rectal mucosa; rectal valve. Syn. Houston's valves.

koilo-: Combining form denoting hollowed, depressed, concave.

koilonychia (koy-lō-nik′-i-a): Spoon-shaped nails, characteristic of iron deficiency anemia.

koilorrhachic (koy-lō-rak′-ik): Having a spinal column in which the lumbar vertebrae curve anteriorally.

koilosternia (koy-lō-ster′-ni-a): Funnel breast (*q.v.*).

kola (kō′ la): The dried cotyledons of the *Cola* species of plants; contain caffeine, theobromine, and cotalin; used in medicine as a nerve and heart stimulant.

kolp-, kolpo-: See words beginning colp-.

konio-: See words beginning conio-.

Koplik's spots: Small, bluish-white spots, each surrounded by a bright red ring, that appear bilaterally on the mucous membrane inside the mouth, opposite the juncture of the molars, during the first 10 days of measles; they appear before the rash and are diagnostic. [Henry Koplik, American pediatrician. 1858–1927.]

Kopp's asthma (kops az′-ma): Spasm of the glottis in children under two; thought to be due to enlarged thymus gland.

kopr-, kopra-: See words beginning copr-, corpra-.

Korean hemorrhagic fever: Caused by a togovirus, endemic in Korea; spreads directly from animals to man. Symptoms include prostration, chills and fever, headache and backache, conjunctivitis, severe proteinuria, and, in severe cases, shock and renal failure.

Korotkoff's sounds: The sounds heard through a stethoscope placed over the brachial artery below the pressure cuff of the sphygmomanometer during the procedure for determining the blood pressure. [Nicolai Korotkoff (Korotkov), Russian physician. 1874–1920.]

Korsakoff's psychosis or syndrome: A chronic condition that follows delirium and toxic states. Often due to alcoholism or dietary deficiencies. The consciousness is clear and alert, but the patient is disoriented as to time and place, especially for recent events; hallucinates and often confabulates to fill in the gaps in memory. Afflicts more men than women in the 45–55 age group. Also called alcoholic dementia, cerebropathica psychica toxaemia, chronic alcoholic delirium, polyneuritic psychosis. [Sergei S. Korsakoff, Russian neurologist. 1853–1900.]

kosher (kō′ sher): Clean or fit to eat according to Judaic dietary laws. Term is used to describe food that is prepared according to Jewish law.

koumiss (koo′ -mis): Fermented milk. Also kumiss, kumyss.

Kr: Chemical symbol for krypton.

Krabbe's disease: Globoid cell leukodystrophy; a rapidly progressing hereditary disease with onset early in infancy; symptoms include stupor, apathy, vomiting, rigidity, fretfulness, blindness, dysphagia, and mental retardation; death usually occurs within a year of onset.

kraurosis (kraw-rō′ -sis): Progressive atrophy, shrinking, and sclerosing of the skin. **K. VULVAE,** a degenerative condition of dryness, itching, and atrophy of the vaginal introitus associated with postmenopausal lack of estrogen; may be precancerous; often occurs in conjunction with leukoplakia. **K. OF THE PENIS,** see balanitis xerotica obliterans under balanitis.

Krebs cycle: A cyclic series of reactions in the metabolism of fats, carbohydrates, and proteins in which enzymes act as catalysts in the formation of acetate, which in turn is oxidized into carbon dioxide and water with the release of energy.

Krönig's isthmus: A narrow area of resonance heard both anteriorally and posteriorally when percussing the apices of the lungs just above the clavicles; also called Krönig's fields, and Krönig's area.

Krukenberg's tumor: A secondary malignant tumor of the ovary, usually bilateral. The primary growth is usually in the stomach. [Friedrich Ernst Krukenberg, German pathologist. 1871–1946.]

kry-, kryo-: See cry-, cryo-.

krymotherapy (krī′mō-ther′a-pi): See crymotherapy.

krypton (krip′ -ton): A gaseous element occurring in small amounts in the atmosphere.

Kuf's disease: A hereditary disorder of lipid metabolism, with symptoms developing in adolescence or early life; marked by dementia, seizures, ataxia, and sometimes retinal pigmentation. Syn., late juvenile amaurotic familial idiocy. See sphingolipidosis.

Kugelberg-Welander disease: A hereditary disease marked by slowly progressive muscle weakness and wasting, beginning in the lower extremities and pelvic girdle, with onset usually between 2 and 17 years of age; evidence of lower motor neuron disease. Also called juvenile muscular atrophy.

Kupffer's cells: Large intensely phagocytic cells found in the lining of the sinusoids of the liver.

Küntscher nail: See under nail.

kuru (koo′ -roo): A chronic, progressive degenerative disorder of the central nervous system, of viral origin; found among natives of certain areas in New Guinea; most cases occur in women and children; characterized by tremor, ataxia, strabismus, dementia, and usually death within a year of onset.

Kussmaul: [Adolph Kussmaul, German physician, 1822–1902.] **K.'S APHASIA,** voluntarily refraining from speaking, as practiced by certain individuals suffering from a psychosis or insanity. **K. RESPIRATIONS,** paroxysms of deep inspirations with sighing expirations, often a forerunner of diabetic acidosis and coma; also called air hunger and Kussmaul-Kien respirations. **K.'S SIGN,** seen when the neck veins distend rather than collapse with inspiration; may occur in patients with cardiac tamponade and constrictive pericarditis.

kwashiorkor (kwa-shi-or′ -kor): A nutritional disorder of infants and young children when the diet is persistently deficient in essential protein. Most common in Africa. Characteristic features are anemia, wasting, dependent edema, fatty liver, changes in hair color, delayed wound healing; often accompanied by parasitic or viral infections. Untreated, it progresses to death.

K.Y. jelly: A sterile, lubricating jelly.

kymatism (kī′ -ma-tizm): Quivering of the muscles or a twitching of an isolated segment of a muscle.

kymograph (kī′ -mō-graf): An apparatus for recording movements, *e.g.,* of muscles, columns of blood. Used in physiological experiments.—kymographic, adj.; kymographically, adj.

kymoscope (kī′ -mō-skōp): An apparatus for measuring variations in pulse wave and in blood flow and pressure.

kyphorachitis (kî-fō-ra-kî-tis): A rachitic deformity involving both the thorax and the spine and marked by an anteroposterior hump.

kyphos (kī′-fos): The "hump" of an individual with kyphoscoliosis.

kyphoscoliosis (kī′-fō-skō-li-ō′-sis): A backward and lateral curvature of the spine; seen in Scheuermann's disease (*q.v.*), in which there is necrosis of the epiphyses of the vertebrae.

kyphosis (kī′-fō′-sis): An excessive backward convex curvature of the spine, usually in the thoracic region. Also called Pott's curvature, humpback, and hunchback. See also **Pott's disease.**

kyrtorrhachia (kir-tō-rak′-ik): Old term for a curved lumbar spine characterized by a backward concavity.

kysthoptosis (kis-thop-tō′-sis): Prolapse of the vagina; colpoptosis.

L

L: 1. Abbreviation for left. 2. Symbol for liter.

L & A: Light and accommodation; refers to reactions of pupils of the eyes.

la belle indifference: Lack of concern for the implications of one's disability; seen in patients with hysterical neuroses. See **hysteria**.

la grippe (la grip): Influenza (*q.v.*).

La Leche League International: Founded in 1956 by a group of women in Illinois; purpose is to provide women with knowledge of how to achieve satisfying and satisfactory breast feeding of their infants; stresses a primolactic style of lactation and a longer duration of nursing with gradual weaning.—See **lactation**.

labia (lā′-bi-a): Lips. **L. MAJORA,** two large liplike folds extending from the mons veneris to encircle the vaginal opening. **L. MINORA,** two smaller folds lying within the **L.** majora.—labium, sing; labial, adj.

labile (lā′-bīl): Unstable, readily changed, as happens to many drugs when in solution. In psychology, emotionally unstable.

lability (la-bil′-i-ti): Instability. **EMOTIONAL L.,** rapid change in mood; frequently occurs in the elderly with mental disorders or following stroke, when the patient's emotional reactions may include anxiety, anger, frustration, denial of illness, depression, disorientation, childishness.

labio-: Combining form denoting relationship to a lip or lips.

labioglossolaryngeal (lā′bi-ō-glos′ō-la-rin′jē-al): Relating to the lips, tongue, and larynx. **L. PARALYSIS,** a nervous system disease characterized by progressive paralysis of the lips, tongue, and larynx.

labioglossopharyngeal (lā′bi-ō-glos′ō-fa-rin′jē-al): Relating to the lips, tongue, and pharynx.

labiomancy (lā′-bi-ō-man-si): Lip reading.

labium (lā′-bi-um): Lip. In anatomy, a term descriptive of a fleshy structure that forms a border or edge of a part. Sing. of labia (*q.v.*).

labor: The act of giving birth to a child; parturition. The first stage lasts from onset until there is full dilatation of the cervical os; the second, until the baby is delivered; the third, until the placenta is expelled. **COMPLICATED L.,** that in which convulsions, hemorrhage or some other untoward event occurs. **DRY L.,** that which occurs after most of the amniotic fluid has been expelled. **INDUCED L.,** that which is brought on by mechanical or other extraneous means. **FALSE L.,** uterine contractions that occur before the onset of true **L. PREMATURE L.,** that which occurs after the fetus is viable but before the gestation period is complete, that is, between the 28th and 37th weeks of pregnancy.

labrum (lā′-brum): In anatomy, a lip, brim, or edge. **ACETABULAR L.,** the ring of fibrocartilage attached to the rim of the acetabulum, increasing its depth. **GLENOID L.,** The ring of fibrocartilage attached to the glenoid cavity of the scapula, increasing its depth.—labra, pl.

labyrinth (lab′i-rinth): An intricate communicating passageway, particularly the tortuous cavities of the internal ear. **BONY L.,** that part which is directly hollowed out of the temporal bone. **MEMBRANOUS L.,** the membrane which loosely lines the bony labyrinth.—labyrinthine, adj.

labyrinthectomy (lab-i-rin-thek′-to- mi): Surgical removal of part or the whole of the labyrinth of the internal ear.

labyrinthitis (lab-i-rin-thī′- tis): Inflammation of the labyrinth of the ear. Syn., otitis interna (*q.v.*).

labyrinthotomy (lab-i-rinth-ot′-o-mi): A surgical incision into the labyrinth of the ear.

lac (lak): Any liquid with a whitish, milky appearance.

lacerated (las′-er-āt-ed): Torn.—lacerate, v.

laceration (las-er-ā′-shun): A wound made by tearing, with a blunt object; the edges are torn and ragged.—lacerate, v.

lacrimal (lak′-ri-mal): Pertaining to tears. **L. APPARATUS,** consists of the structures that secrete tears and drain them from the surface of the eyeball: lacrimal glands, ducts, sac, and nasolacrimal ducts. **L. BONE,** a tiny bone at the inner side of the orbital cavity. **L. DUCT,** connects **L.** gland to upper conjunctival sac. **L. GLAND,** situated above the upper outer canthus of the eye; secretes tears. **L. SAC,** situated in a groove in the **L.** bone at the upper end of the

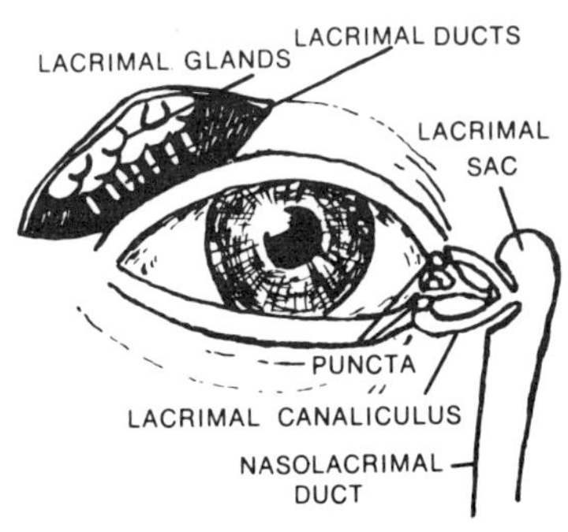

Lacrimal apparatus

nasolacrimal duct. **NASOLACRIMAL DUCT,** extends from the **L.** sac to the inferior meatus of the nose.

lacrimation (lak-ri-mā′-shun): An outflow of tears; weeping.

lacrimator (lak′-ri-mā-tor): A substance that increases the flow of tears.

lacrimonasal (lak-ri-mō-nā′- zal): Pertaining to the lacrimal and nasal bones and ducts.

lacrimotomy (lak-rim-ot′-o-mi): Incision of a lacrimal gland, duct, or sac.

lact-, lacti-, lacto-: Combining forms denoting relationship to 1) milk; 2) lactose.

lactacidemia (lak-tas-i-dē′-mi-a): The presence of lactic acid in the blood.

lactagogue (lak′-ta-gog): Galactagogue (*q.v.*).

lactalbumin (lac′-tal-bū′-min): An albumin found in milk; resembles serum albumin. It is the more easily digested of the two milk proteins. See caseinogen.

lactase (lak′-tās): A sugar-splitting enzyme of intestinal juice; it splits lactose into glucose (dextrose) and galactose.

lactated Ringer's solution: Ringer's solution to which sodium lactate has been added; it is administered intravenously to replentish fluids and electrolytes and to create a condition of alkalinity in the body. See Ringer's solution.

lactation (lak-tā′-shun): Secretion of milk. Suckling; the period during which the child is nourished from the breast. **PRIMOLACTIC L., L.** in which the infant is allowed frequent and unlimited opportunity to nurse; weaning is slow, beginning at about six months. **MIMELACTIC L., L.** in which the infant is allowed to be at breast only at specified times and for a limited time; weaning begins at about three months.

lacteal (lak′-tē-al): 1. Resembling or pertaining to milk. 2. Any one of the beginning lymphatic ducts in the intestinal villi that take up split fats and convey them to the cisterna chyli (*q.v.*).

lactescent (lak-tes′-ent): 1. Milky in appearance. 2. Secreting milk or a fluid resembling milk.

lactic (lak′-tik): Pertaining to milk. **L. ACID,** an acid formed by the action of certain bacteria on lactose and responsible for the souring of milk; in the body, this acid is found in muscles during exercise. **L. ACIDOSIS,** a condition in which lactic acid accumulates in the tissues; occurs in association with circulatory failure, hypotension, and hypoxia.

lactic acid dehydrogenase (lak′-tik as′- id dē-hī-droj′-e-nas): An enzyme widely distributed in the tissues of mammals; it catalyzes the dehydrogenation of lactic acid to pyruvic acid; measuring the level present in the blood is useful in diagnosing myocardial infarction. Abbreviated LHD. Also called lactate dehydrogenase.

lactiferous (lak-tif′-er-us): Conveying or secreting milk. **L. DUCTS,** ducts that carry the secretion of the mammary gland; they open on the nipple.

lactifuge (lak′-ti-fūj): Any agent that suppresses milk secretion.—lactifugal, adj.

Lactobacillus (lak-tō-ba-sil′-us): A genus of bacteria of the family *Lactobacillaceae,* occurring as gram-positive rods that are active in fermenting carbohydrates, with the production of acid; found in dairy products, beer, wine, sour dough, mash, grain and meat products, fruits and fruit juices; seldom pathogenic. **L. ACIDOPHILUS,** ferments the sugars in milk producing lactic acid; found in milk and in the feces of bottle-fed infants. **L. BULGARICUS,** the species that ferments milk to produce yoghurt.

lactocele (lak′-tō-sēl): Galactocele (*q.v.*).

lactoferrin (lak-to-fer′-in): An iron-binding protein found in human milk, tears, saliva, and the secretions of the respiratory and intestinal tracts; prevents bacteria from metabolizing iron and assists antibodies to resist certain infectious diseases.

lactoflavin (lak′-tō-flā-vin): Riboflavin (*q.v.*).

lactogen (lak′ tō-jen): Any substance that promotes lactation. **HUMAN PLACENTAL L.,** a hormone secreted by the placenta until delivery of the fetus; promotes lactation and growth; also called placental growth hormone.—lactogenic, adj.

lactogenesis (lak-tō-jen′-e-sis): The establishment of the secretory state in the mammary glands.

lactogenic (lak-tō-jen′-ik): Stimulating milk production; milk producing.

lactogenic hormone (lak-tō-jen′-ik hor′-mōn): Prolactin (*q.v.*).

lactose (lak′-tōs): Milk sugar; a disaccharide that is less soluble and less sweet than ordinary sugar. Used in infant feeding to increase the carbohydrate content of diluted cow's milk.

lactosuria (lak′-tō-sū′-ri- a): The presence of lactose in the urine.—lactosuric, adj.

lactotherapy (lak′-tō-ther′-a- pi): Treatment by milk diet. Galactotherapy. If the patient is a nursing infant, the drug is given to the mother and secreted in the milk.

lactotropin (lak-tō-trō′-pin): Prolactin (*q.v.*).

lactulose (lak′-tū-lōs): A white crystalline sugar ($C_{12}H_{22}O_{11}$), produced synthetically; used as a cathartic.

lacuna (la-kū′-na): A small depression or hollow, or a space between cells; sinus.—lacunae, pl.; lacunar, adj.

lacunar (la-kū′-nar): Pertaining to a lacuna. **L. STROKES,** small strokes resulting from damage to vessels scattered throughout the brain.

Ladin's sign: An area of elasticity that develops just above the cervix on the anterior wall of the uterus; can be felt on palpatation through the vagina as early as the fifth week of pregnancy; increases in size as the pregnancy progresses.

Laennec's cirrhosis: See under **cirrhosis.**

lag: 1. The time that elapses between the application of a stimulus and the response. 2. To move or progress unusually slowly, or to fall behind.

lagophthalmos (lag′-of-thal′-mos): A condition marked by inability to close the eye completely. Also lagophthalmia.

Laki-Lorland factor: Coagulation factor XIII. Fibrin stabilizing factor; its action is important in enabling fibrin to form a firm blood clot.

laking of blood (lā′-king): Hemolysis (*q.v.*).

lalling (lal′-ing): 1. A form of stammering in which babbling makes speech almost unintelligible; infantile speech. 2. Pronouncing *r* like *l*.

Lamaze method: A method of education for natural childbirth through a series of classes in which the pregnant woman and her partner are trained in controlled breathing and neuromuscular exercise; partner remains throughout labor.

lambda (lamb′-da): The point in the skull where the sagittal and lambdoidal sutures meet.

lambdoidal suture (lam-doyd′-al): The line of union between the occipital and parietal bones.

Lamblia intestinalis: *Giardia lamblia* (*q.v.*).

lambliasis (lam-blī′-a-sis): Infestation with the parasite *Giardia lamblia* (*q.v.*). Can be symptomless, or can produce persistent desentery and occasionally steatorrhea.

lamella (la-mel′-a): 1. A thin plate-like scale or partition. 2. A gelatin-coated disk containing a drug; it is inserted under the eyelid. 3. Any of the tiny circular plates of bone between the Haversian systems in compact bone.—lamellae, pl.; lamellar, adj.

lamina (lam′-in-a): A thin plate or layer, usually of bone.—laminae, pl.

lamina cribrosa sclerae: The perforated portion of the sclera through which the axons of the ganglion cells of the retina pass.

laminar air flow (lam′-i-nar): Air is introduced at high speed on one side of the patient's room and extracted at the opposite side, to remove organisms from the vicinity of the patient; used after organ transplant and in special care units, when it is necessary to protect the patient from exposure to infection.

Laminaria (lam-i-nā′-ri-a): A genus of kelp from which several varieties of alginates are derived; see **alginate.**

laminectomy (lam-i-nek′-to-mi): Removal of laminae of one or more vertebrae—to expose the spinal cord and meninges. Most often performed in lumbar region, for removal of degenerated intervertebral disk.

laminogram (lam′-i-nō-gram): An x-ray photograph of a selected layer of the body obtained by sectional radiography.

laminography (lam-i-nog′-ra-fi): Body section roentgenography. A special x-ray technique used to show in detail the structures at a certain plane of the body while dimming or obliterating the details of structures in other planes.

lance (lans): 1. A short, two-edged knife; also called lancet. 2. To incise with a knife, as a boil or abscess.

Lancefield's groups or classification: A serological classification of hemolytic streptococci into groups A to O, according to their antigenic actions. Most streptococci that are of major importance to human health are in Group A; strains from Group F and nonpathogenic strains from G and H may also be found in the human throat; those from the other groups are found in certain foods and lower animals or animal products. [Rebecca Craighill Lancefield, American bacteriologist. 1875–1981.]

lancet (lan′-set): A small, sharp two-edged surgical knife.

lancinating (lan′-si-nā′-ting): Sharp, cutting, tearing; term used to describe a certain type of pain.

Landau reaction or response: When a normal infant is held suspended in the air, with the examiner's hands supporting him around the chest, the infant raises his head and extends his legs; then, when the head is flexed, the leg muscles lose their tone; the "floppy" infant will not give this response while the hypertonic infant will give an exaggerated response.

Landry's disease: A form of paralysis that starts in the legs, ascends gradually to the arms, chest, and trunk, and then progresses to the circulatory and respiratory centers.

Landsteiner: [Karl Landsteiner, Austrian biologist in the U.S. 1868–1943.] Landsteiner's classification, see **blood groups.**

Langerhans' islands: See **island.** [Paul Langerhans, German pathologist. 1847–1888.]

languor (lan′-ger): Listlessness; lack of vigor.

lanolin (lan′-ō-lin): Wool fat containing 30 percent of water. **ANHYDROUS L.,** the fat obtained from sheep's wool. It is used in ointment bases, as such bases can form water-in-oil emulsions with aqueous constituents, and are readily absorbed by the skin.

lanugo (lan-ū′-gō): The fine down or hair on the fetus from about the fifth month until birth. Also sometimes used to describe fine, downy hair on a child or adult.

Lanz tube: A tracheostomy tube that has a semi-rigid cannula, a low-pressure cuff, an exterior pressure valve, and a control balloon.

laparo-: Combining form denoting relationship to the 1) loin or flank; 2) the abdominal wall, particularly an incision into it.

laparohysterectomy (lap′-a-rō-his-ter-ek′-to-mi): Removal of the uterus through an incision in the abdominal wall.

laparoscope (lap′a-rō-skōp): A lighted instrument used for viewing the interior of the abdomen and for performing certain surgical procedures.

laparoscopy (lap-a-ros′-ko-pi):The insertion of a laparoscope through a small abdominal incision for diagnostic purposes, lysis of adhesions, or tubal division. In tubal division, the laparoscope is inserted through a small incision near the navel, and the fallopian tubes are located, cauterized, and separated; the operation takes little time and the patient is not incapacitated for long.

laparotomy (lap-a-rot′-o-mi): Surgical opening into the flank; term commonly used to describe any opening into the abdominal wall.

LaPlace's law: States that the pressure produced in the ventricles of the heart depends on the size and shape of the heart as well as the tension produced by the ventricular myocardium when it contracts.

lardaceous (lar-dā′-shus): Waxy or fatty; resembling lard.

large-for-dates: Refers to a baby whose birth weight is above the 90th percentile. Large-for-gestational-age.

larva (lar′-va): An embryo that is independent before it has assumed the characteristic features of its parents.—larvae, pl.; larval, adj.

larvicide (lar′-vi-sīd): Any agent that destroys larvae.—larvicidal, adj.

larvivorous (lar-viv′-ō-rus): Usually refers to fishes that are the natural enemy of mosquitoes; used in malarial control programs.

laryngeal (la-rin′-jē-al): Pertaining to the larynx. **L. STRIDOR,** a noisy crowing sound made on inspiration; in the infant may be congenital, due to immaturity of the larynx; see stridor.

laryngectomee (lar-in-jek′-tō-mē): A person who has had his larynx removed.— **L. SPEECH,** esophageal speech; see under esophageal.

laryngectomy (lar-in-jek′-to-mi): Excision of the larynx.

laryngismus stridulus (lar-in-jiz′-mus strīd′ ū-lus): Momentary attack of laryngeal spasm, inspiration producing a crowing sound and followed by a period of apnea caused by the spasmodic closure of the glottis. Associated with low blood calcium in infantile rickets.

laryngitis (lar-in-jī′tis): Inflammation of the mucous membrane lining of the larynx; may be acute or chronic; may be associated with a cold or be caused by heavy smoking, exposure to irritating fumes, overuse of the voice. Usual symptoms are dryness and soreness of the throat, difficulty in swallowing, pain. **ACUTE SPASMODIC L.,** croup; a mild inflammation of the larynx with spasm of the laryngeal muscles, causing partial obstruction; seen most often in young children; attacks often occur at night; symptoms dramatic with dyspnea, coughing, high-pitched rasp with inspiraton, cyanosis of lips and nails, rapid pulse, elevation of temperature.

laryngo-: Combining form denoting relationship to the larynx.

laryngocele (la-ring′gō-sēl): A congenital condition in which an air sac communicates with the laryngeal cavity; may appear as a tumor on the outside of the neck.

laryngofissure (la-ring′gō-fish′ūr): The operation of opening the larynx at midline.

laryngologist (lar′-ing-gol′o-jist): A specialist in laryngeal diseases and disorders.

laryngology (lar′-ing-gol′o-ji): The branch of medical practice that deals with diseases of the larynx.

laryngoparalysis (la-ring′gō-pa-ral′i-sis): Paralysis of the muscles of the larynx.

laryngopharyngectomy (la-ring′gō-far-in-jek′to-mi): Excision of the larynx and the lower part of the pharynx.

laryngopharyngitis (la-ring′gō-far-in-jī′tis): Inflammation of the larynx and the pharynx.

laryngopharynx (la-ring′gō-far′inks): The lower portion of the pharynx.—laryngopharyngeal, adj.

laryngoscope (la-ring′gō-skop): A lighted instrument for exposing and visualizing the larynx.—laryngoscopy, n.; laryngoscopic, adj.

laryngoscopy (lar-ing-gos′ko-pi): Examination of the interior of the larynx with a laryngoscope.

laryngospasm (la-ring′gō-spasm): Convulsive involuntary muscular contraction of the larynx, usually accompanied by spasmodic closure of the glottis.

laryngostenosis (la-ring′gō-ste-nō′sis): Narrowing of the glottic aperture, or of the lumen of the larynx.

laryngostomy (lar′ing-gos′to-mi): The surgical creation of an artificial opening from the neck into the larynx.

laryngotomy (lar′ing-got′o-mi): The operation of opening the larynx.

laryngotracheal (la-ring′gō-trā′kē-al): Pertaining to the larynx and the trachea.

laryngotracheitis (la-ring′gō-trā-kē-ī′tis): Inflammation of the mucous membrane lining of the larynx and the trachea.

laryngotracheobronchitis (la-ring′gō-trā′kē-ō-brong-kī′tis): Inflammation of the larynx, trachea, and bronchi. Usually refers to an acute respiratory condition in young children; attended by fever, toxemia, laryngeal obstruction, hoarseness, dyspnea, inspiratory stridor, barking cough. Syn., viral croup. See **croup**.

larynx (lar′inks): The organ of voice situated below and in front of the pharynx and at the upper end of the trachea. It is composed of muscular and cartilaginous tissue and is lined with mucous membrane. The vocal cords pass from front to back across the lumen of the structure. It also serves as a passageway for air entering the trachea.—laryngeal, adj.

lascivia (la-siv′i-a): Abnormal degree of sexual desire.

Lasègue (lah-sezh′): **LASEGUE'S SIGN,** pain in the hip when the knee is extended but no pain on flexion; it differentiates sciatica from hip disease.

laser (lā′zer): An acronym for *L*ight *a*mplification by *s*timulated *e*mission of *r*adiation. An electron device containing a gaseous, solid, or liquid substance in which atoms that are stimulated by focused light rays magnify and concentrate these waves which may then be emitted as a very narrow, concentrated, powerful beam of light. **LASER BEAM,** the precisely aimed, high-intensity beam of light emitted by a laser and which transmits energy as heat; it permits visual examination of body cavities and allows for greater precision in surgery; has been used in treatment of iridectomy, detached retina, and cataract surgery as well as in a variety of surgical procedures to destroy tissue, to fix tissue in place, or to divide or create adhesions.

laserbrasion (lā′-zer-brā-zhun): The bloodless removal of layers of sun-damaged skin utilizing a carbon dioxide laser; done under local anesthesia.

Lassa fever: Named for the Nigerian town in which several fatal cases occurred among American missionary nurses in 1969. Caused by the exceptionally virulent Arenavirus, of which the rat is the carrier; isolated and identified during the same year. Symptoms vary widely and include very high fever, skin rash with tiny hemorrhages, mouth ulcers, pharyngitis, dysphagia, edema, pneumonia, pleural effusion, kidney damage, infection of the heart leading to heart failure. Not limited to the tropics or Africa; the first cases in the U.S. occurred in scientists in research laboratories where the virus was being studied. No known cure; treatment consists of supportive measures and relief of symptoms.

Lassar's paste: A paste used in treating several skin conditions; composed of starch, salicylic acid, and zinc oxide in a white petrolatum base.

lassitude (las′i-tūd): Exhaustion; lack of energy.

latency (lā′ten-si): The period between the application of a stimulus and the reaction or response to the stimulus.

latent (lā′tent): Concealed, hidden, not active. **L. STAGE,** the period in development of the libido, from about the sixth to the thirteenth year, when the endocrine activity slows down and the child's need for sexual gratification is slight but the need for belonging and social acceptance by peers is increased.

lateral (lat′er-al): 1. Pertaining to a side. 2. Denoting a position away from the midline or the median plane, either to the right or left.

lateral geniculate body: A small flattened area of nerve cells in the thalamus that receive impulses from the optic tract and relay them to the occipital area of the cortex.

lateralization (lat′er-al-ī-zā′shun): Localization on one side of the body or one part of the body, as in one cerebral hemisphere.

lateroversion (lat′er-ō-ver′zhun): A turning to one side or the other; said especially of the uterus.

latex agglutination test: A widely used test to detect the presence of rheumatoid factor in verifying the diagnosis of rheumatoid arthritis; also used to test for presence of antibodies to Hashimoto's disease. Also called latex fixation test.

latissimus dorsi (la-tis′si-mus dor′si): A large, broad, flat muscle of the back; it arises from the spinous processes of the six lower thoracic vertebrae, the lumbar vertebrae, sacrum, and the posterior iliac crest (all via the lumbosacral fascia), and is inserted into a groove on the under side of the humerus. Its action is to adduct and medially rotate the arm.

Latrodectus (lat-rō-dek′tus): A genus of small poisonous spiders, including the widow spiders which have very poisonous neurotoxic bites. **L. MACTANS,** the "black widow" spider, found commonly in southern U.S.; the bite of the female causes severe, sometimes fatal, symptoms.

laughing gas: Nitrous oxide (*q.v.*).

Laurence-Moon-Beidl syndrome: A recessive hereditary disorder characterized by obesity, metal retardation, visual disturbances, genital atrophy, and polydactyly.

lavage (la-vazh′): The irrigation of or washing out of an organ such as the stomach or colon, or the instillation and withdrawal of a rinsing fluid from a body cavity such as the peritoneal or pleural cavity. In **BRONCHIAL L.,** small amounts of warm water or saline solution are injected into the airway to clear tenacious bronchial material. **ENDOMETRIAL L.,** see under **endome-**

trial. **GASTRIC L.**, **L.** of the stomach. **LUNG L.**, the instillation and draining out of isotonic saline solution via a catheter inserted into the bronchi, to assist in removing collected mucus; used primarily in cystic fibrosis patients. **PERITONEAL L.**, the rinsing out of the peritoneal cavity by instilling and then withdrawing a dialyzing solution.

laxative (laks'a-tiv): A mild cathartic (*q.v.*); an aperient.

layer: A sheet of substance lying upon another sheet of substance, but not connected or continuous with it, and differentiated by cellular structure, function, or some other characteristic, *e.g.*, one of the three primary layers of the early embryo—the ectoderm, entoderm, or mesoderm.

lazaret (laz'a-ret): A hospital for treatment of contagious diseases, usually for leprosy; also called lazaretto and leprosarium.

LBBB: Abbreviation for left bundle branch block. See under **block.**

lb: Abbreviation for *libra* [L.], meaning pound.

LD: Abbreviation for lethal dose. **LD_{50}**, the median **LD**; lethal to 50% of test animals.

LDH: Abbreviation for lactic acid dehydrogenase. (*q.v.*).

L-Dopa: Levodopa. A drug used to control the symptoms of Parkinson's disease.

L.E.: Abbreviation for: 1. Left eye. 2. Lupus erythematosis.

LE cells: Characteristic cells found in the bone marrow of patients with lupus erythematosus, together with a special globulin in the plasma.

lead (lēd): 1. A wire carrying electricity to or from a device. 2. A pair of electrodes that are placed in or on the body and are connected to an instrument that measures and records the difference in the electrical potential between them. 3. One of the electrical connections for the records made in electrocardiography; the pattern of the lead varies with the body site to which the electrode is attached.

lead (led): A metal, the salts of which are astringent when applied externally. **L. POISONING**, rarely occurs in the acute form, but, in children, may be the cause of acute encephalopathy; the chronic form, due to absorption of small amounts of lead over a period is fairly common; it can happen to children who suck on articles made of lead alloys or painted with lead paint. It may also be an occupational danger to painters, the usual symptoms being anemia that is due to interference with production of heme and to short life of red blood cells; loss of appetite; abdominal cramps; metallic taste; and the formation of a blue line around the gums.

leadpipe rigidity: An increase in the tone of the skeletal muscles, making the limb appear stiff due to pathology in the extrapyramidal tract. Also called plastic rigidity.

Leber's disease: 1. A hereditary form of optic atrophy, transmitted through the female; occurs chiefly in young men; progresses rapidly to blindness of central vision, with preservation of peripheral vision. 2. Leber's congenital amaurosis, a rare type of blindness occurring in early infancy characterized by diffuse pigmentation and optic atrophy.

Leboyer methodology: An approach to childbirth that emphasizes avoidance of trauma, pain, and fear in the transition from uterine to extrauterine life; includes dimming of lights, silence insofar as possible, patience, warmth, and loving tender handling of the infant.

lecithin (les'-i-thin): A nitrogenous, fatty substance in cell protoplasm; widely distributed throughout the body, being found in nerve tissue, semen, bile, and blood. Also found in egg yolk, soy beans, and other seeds.

leech (lēch): *Hirudo medicinalis*. A bloodsucking aquatic worm formerly much used for sucking blood from local areas. Its saliva contains hirudin, an anticoagulant.

left handedness: The use of the left hand in preference to the right in performing various tasks. Also called sinistrality.

leg: The lower leg from the knee to the ankle. **BANDY L.**, bowleg. **MILK L.**, thrombophlebitis of a femoral vein; phlegmasia alba dolens (*q.v.*). **PHANTOM L.**, the sensation of presence of a leg after it has been amputated. **SCISSOR L.**, a hyperadducted leg that crosses the midline of the body; see **scissor leg, scissoring.**

Legg-Calvé-Perthes disease: Osteochondritis (*q.v.*) of the head of the femur occurring in children. Also called Perthe's disease, Waldenstrom's disease, and coxa plana.

Legg's disease: Quiet hip disease; osteochondritis deformans juvenilis or arthritis of the hip.

Legionella pneumophilia: A virus thought to be one cause of atypical pneumonia; see **Legionnaire's disease.**

Legionnaire's disease: Term coined to describe a disease affecting many who attended a meeting in Philadelphia in 1976; thought to be contagious and caused by a bacterium-like organism isolated from lung tissues; many cases were fatal. Sporadic outbreaks have occurred elsewhere since that time with the causative organism being cited as a pneumonia-like virus called *Legionella pneumophilia*. Symptoms include acute onset, chills, fever, tachypnea, cough, pleuritic pain, bradycardia, abdominal pain, diarrhea. Also called legionellosis.

legume (leg'-ūm): A class of plant foods containing the protein legumin, *e.g.*, peas, beans, lentils, peanuts.

legumin (le-gū'-min): A protein resembling casein, found in plant foods classified as legumes (*q.v.*).

leiodermia (lī-ō-der′-mi-a): A skin disorder characterized by abnormal glossiness and atrophy.

leiomyoma (lī′ō-mī-ō′ma): A benign tumor originating in smooth muscle tissue. **L. UTERI.**, a benign tumor of the uterus; see fibroid.

leiomyosarcoma (lī′ō-mī-ō-sar-kō′ma): A malignant tumor derived from smooth muscle tissue.

Leishman-Donovan bodies: A species of intracellular flagellated parasite that causes visceral leishmaniasis (kala azar) (*q.v.*).

Leishmania (lēsh-mā′-ni-a): A flagellated protozoan that is responsible for several recognized types of leishmaniasis (*q.v.*).

leishmaniasis (lēsh′ma-nī′a-sis): Any of several communicable protozoan diseases caused by Leishmania (*q.v.*); spread by sand flies. Generalized (or visceral) manifestation is kala azar (*q.v.*). **CUTANEOUS L.**, **L.** caused by *Leishmania tropica;* also called Aleppo boil, Delhi boil, or oriental sore; characterized by nodules and ulcerating lesions on the skin. The nasopharyngeal manifestation causes ulceration of the nose and throat; espundia. The disease occurs in the Mediterranean and Near East areas, China, and some parts of Africa, and is occasionally brought to the U.S. by persons who have visited in these areas.

Lenegre's disease: Complete heart block caused by degeneration of the conduction system of the heart; due to small lesions in both the right and left bundle branch.

lenitive (len′-i-tiv): 1. Relieving discomfort or pain; soothing. 2. An agent that relieves discomfort or pain; a demulcent (*q.v.*).

lens (lenz): 1. The small, transparent, biconvex crystalline body that is supported in the suspensory ligament immediately behind the iris of the eye. On account of its elasticity, the lens can alter in shape, enabling light rays to focus exactly on the retina. 2. A piece of transparent material, usually glass, with a regular curvature of one or both surfaces, used for conveying or diffusing light rays, as in a camera, microscope or eyeglasses. **CONTACT L.**, a thin, usually plastic, curved lens that fits over the cornea and is used instead of an eyeglass. **L. IMPLANT**, a thin artificial lens to correct any visual abnormality such as myopia, following a cataract operation.

lentectomy (len-tek′-to-mi): Surgical removal of the lens of the eye.

lenticonus (len-ti-kō′-nus): A conical prominence on the anterior or posterior surface of the lens; may be congenital; see in Alport's syndrome (*q.v.*).

lenticular (len-tik′-ū-lar): 1. Pertaining to or shaped like a lens. 2. Shaped like a lentil. **L. NUCLEUS**, a mass of gray matter on the outer surface of the caudate nucleus, with which it unites to form the corpus striatum.

lentiform (len′-ti-form): Shaped like a lens. **L. NUCLEUS**, the globus pallidus and the putamen considered together.

lentigines (len-tij′-i-nēz): Plural of lentigo (*q.v.*). **L. LEPROSAE**, the pigmented lesions that occur in leprosy.

lentigo (len-tī′-gō): A smooth, brownish pigmented spot on the skin, usually seen on normally exposed areas and in people of middle age or older; caused by changes in the skin rather than sunlight; a freckle. **L. MALIGNA**, appears as a tan spot that becomes dark and nodular and often malignant; usually occurs on the face after age 60; also called Hutchinson's freckle. **L. SENILIS**, flat dark-colored spots that appear on exposed areas after middle age; usually benign; syn., liver spots.

lentil (len′-til): A widely cultivated European plant whose seeds and stalks furnish a cheap and nutritious legume containing a large amount of protein.

leontiasis (lē′on-tī′a-sis): Enlargement of face and head giving a lion-like appearance, in such diseases as elephantiasis and leprosy.

Leopold's maneuvers: A series of four maneuvers performed with the hands, for palpating the abdomen to determine the position and presentation of the fetus in utero.

leper (lep′-er): A person who has leprosy.

lepidosis (lep-i-dō′-sis): Any skin eruption accompanied by scaling or desquamation, *e.g.*, pityriasis.

leproma (lep-rō′-ma): A granulomatous nodule in the skin; seen in some patients with leprosy.—lepromata, pl.; lepromatous, adj.

leprosarium (lep-rō-sar′-i-um): A colony or hospital for persons with leprosy. Also leprosary.

leprosy (lep′-ro-si): A chronic, progressive, communicable disease; endemic in warmer climates; infrequently seen in the U.S. Caused by *Mycobacterium leprae* (Hansen's bacillus) and very resistant to treatment. One of the two types of the disease affects the peripheral nerves, resulting in anesthesia in areas of the skin; the other type affects the skin, causing the formation of nodules in skin and mucous membrane that become granulomatous. Transmission of the disease results only from prolonged and intimate contact with an infected person; the incubation period is estimated at two to four years. Also called Hansen's disease.—leprous, adj.

lept-, lepto-: Combining forms denoting small, thin, weak, fine.

leptocephaly (lep-tō-sef′-a-li): Abnormal height and narrowness of the skull.

leptocyte (lep′-tō-sīt): A red blood cell that is abnormally thin and flattened, has a central area of pigmented material surrounded by an area of clear unpigmented material, and is enclosed by an outer pigmented rim; sometimes referred to as a "target" or "Mexican hat" cell.

leptocytosis (lep'tō-sī-tō'sis): The presence of thin, flattened red cells circulating in the blood (leptocytes). Characteristic of Cooley's anemia (*q.v.*). Also seen in jaundice, hepatic disease, and sometimes after splenectomy.

leptodermic (lep'-tō-der'-mik): Having a thin skin.

leptomeninges (lep-tō-me-nin'-jēz): The pia mater and the arachnoid membranes considered together.—leptomeningeal, adj.

leptomeningitis (lep'tō-men-in-jī'tis): Inflammation of the two inner covering membranes of the brain or spinal cord. See leptomeninges.

Leptospira (lep-tō-spī'ra): A genus of bacteria. Very thin, coiled spirochetes. Common in water as saprophytes; many pathogenic species may infect both man and animals, producing leptospirosis. *L. icterohaemorrhagiae* causes Weil's disease in man. *L. canicola* causes "yellows" in dogs and pigs; transmissible to man. See canicola fever.

leptospirosis (lep-tō-spī-rō'sis): Infection by *Leptospira* organisms; transmitted to man by water in swamps or ponds, infected rats, dogs, and swine; usual symptoms include hepatitis, nephritis, lymphocytic meningitis; may occur in epidemics. See Leptospira, Weil's disease.

Leriche's syndrome: A syndrome occurring mostly in males; marked by fatigue and coldness of hips and lower extremities following exercise, by lack of femoral pulsation, and sometimes impotence; caused by an obstruction, usually atheromatous, at the bifurcation of the aorta.

Lermoyez's syndrome: Unexplained attacks of loss of hearing followed by dizziness, after which hearing returns to normal or near normal.

lesbian (lez'-bi-an): A female homosexual (*q.v.*).

lesbianism (lez'-bi-an-izm): Homosexuality between women.

Lesch-Nyhan syndrome: A rare inherited disorder of purine metabolism marked by severe mental and physical retardation, choreoathetosis, self-mutilation particularly of the fingers and lips by biting; also neurological problems similar to cerebral palsy, failure to thrive, and defective kidney function.

lesion (lē'-zhun): Any pathological change in the continuity or structure of a bodily tissue; may be caused by trauma or disease. SPACE-OCCUPYING L., a L. within a confined space, as the skull, that compresses the contents, interferes with blood supply, and may lead to loss of function; most often refers to tumors of the brain substance.

lethal (lē'thal): Deadly, fatal. L. DOSAGE, the amount of a drug or other agent that will cause death.—lethality, adj.

lethargy (leth'-ar-jē): Abnormal drowsiness; torpor; apathy. Characteristic of certain diseases, *e.g.*, encephalitis.—lethargic, adj.

lethe (lē'-thē): Loss of memory; amnesia.

lethologica (lēth-ō-loj'i-ka): Temporary inability to recall a proper name or noun.

Letterer-Siwe disease: A fatal disease of infancy and early childhood involving the reticuloendothelial system; cause unknown. Characterized by erythematous skin eruptions; a tendency to hemorrhage and purpura; enlarged spleen, liver, and lymph nodes; progressive anemia; osseous defects, especially of the skull; bone marrow involvement; anorexia and weight loss. Also called systemic aleukemic reticuloendotheliosis.

leuc-, leuco-: For words beginning thus and not found here, see words beginning leuk-, leuko-.

leucine (lū'-sēn): One of the essential amino acids that is obtained from protein; it is required for optimal growth and development in infants and for maintaining the nitrogen balance in adults. L. SENSITIVITY, seen more often in infants than adults; characterized by the occurrence of hypoglycemia following high protein intake; also occurs on fasting.

leuk-, leuk-: Combining forms denoting 1) white; 2) a type of blood cell; 3) white matter of the brain.

leukemia (lū-kē'-mi-a): A usually fatal disease of the blood-forming organs; many forms are recognized, both chronic and acute; of unknown cause. Chief symptom is an increase in the number of white blood cells, along with the presence of immature leukocytes. Other symptoms include poor appetite, lesions in the mouth, enlarged spleen and lymphatics, and bone marrow changes. Classified according to the kind of leukocyte found and whether the condition is acute or chronic. ACUTE L., characterized by rapid onset, anemia, susceptibility to infection and hemorrhage; blast forms of cells predominate in the bone marrow. ALEUKEMIC L., refers to a leukemic condition in which the white cell count in the blood remains normal or is below normal. CHRONIC LYMPHOCYTIC L., characterized by proliferation and enlargement of the lymphocytes in any lymphoid tissue such as the spleen, lymph nodes, bone marrow. MONOCYTIC L., L. in which the predominating cells are monocytes; in the Naegeli type, many of the cells closely resemble myelocytes; in the Schilling type they resemble monocytes. MYELOGENOUS L., L. involving the bone marrow, especially that of the ribs, sternum, and vertebrae.

leukemoid (lū-kē'-moyd): Resembling leukemia but due to some other cause; usually refers to a condition that is marked by the presence in the blood of immature cells but that is not leukemia.

leukoagglutinin (lū'kō-a-gloo'ti-nin): An antibody that acts against leukocytes; see agglutinin.

leukocidin (lū-kō-sī'-din): A substance produced by certain bacteria that is toxic to polymorphonuclear leukocytes.

leukocyte (lū'-kō-sīt): A white corpuscle of the blood; a spherical, colorless, nucleated mass that has ameboid movement; produced in lymph nodes and in the lymphatic tissue of the spleen, liver, and other organs; chief function is to produce antibodies and act as scavengers in protecting the body from invading organisms. May be classified into two categories, 1) granulocytes, including neutrophils, basophils, eosinophils; and 2) agranulocytes, including monocytes and lymphocytes. See basophil, eosinophil, lymphocyte, mononuclear, polymorphonuclear.—leukocytic, adj.

leukocythemia (lū'-kō-sī- thē'-mi-a): An increase in the number of white blood cells; leukemia.

leukocytolysis (lū'-kō-sī- tol'-i-sis): Destruction and disintegration of white blood cells.—leukocytolytic, adj.

leukocytometer (lū'-kō-sī- tom'-e-ter): An instrument for counting white blood cells.

leukocytosis (lū-kō-sī-tō'sis): Increased number of leukocytes in the blood. Often a physiological response to infection.—leukocytotic, adj.

leukocyturia (lū'-kō-sī-tū'-ri-a): Presence of leukocytes in the urine.

leukoderma (lū-kō-der'ma): Defective skin pigmentation, especially when it occurs in patches or bands.

leukodystrophy (lū'kō-dis'trō-fi): A neurologic condition characterized by abnormally formed or abnormally broken-down myelin; due to an inborn error of metabolism; appears in several forms with varying symptoms at different stages of life. METACHROMATIC L., a form of L. due to an enzyme deficiency that results in metachromasia in cerebral white matter, peripheral nerves, kidneys, and liver, and in progressive neurological disease; usually occurs in early childhood.

leukoedema (lū'kō-ē-dē'ma): A condition of the buccal mucosa, characterized by thickness and edema; resembles early leukoplakia (*q.v.*).

leukoencephalitis (lū'kō-en-sef-a-lī'tis): Inflammation of the white matter of the brain. SUBACUTE SCLEROSING L., subacute sclerosing panencephalitis; see under panencephalitis.

leukoencephalopathy (lū'-kō-en-sef'-a-lop'-a-thi): Any inflammatory or degenerative pathological condition involving chiefly the white matter; occurs most often in patients with leukemia, lymphoma, granulomatosis; usually fatal. PROGRESSIVE MULTIFOCAL L., usually occurs secondary to certain neoplastic diseases; probably caused by a virus; characterized by demyelination in the white matter but is also seen in the brain stem and cerebellum; usually fatal.

leukoerythroblastosis (lū'kō-ē-rith'rō-blastō'sis): A condition characterized by the presence of immature leukocytes and erythrocytes in the peripheral blood.

leukokoria (lū-kō-kor'-i-a): A condition in which a whitish mass appears in the area back of the lens. Also spelled leucocoria.

leukoma (lū-kō'-ma): White opaque spot on the cornea.—leukomata, pl.; leukomatous, adj.

leukonychia (lū-kō-nik'-i-a): White spots on the nails.

leukopenia (lū-kō-pē'ni-a): A white blood cell count that is below normal; less than 5000 per cu mm.—leukopenic, adj.

leukopheresis (lū-kō-fer-ē'-sis): A procedure by which leukocytes, particularly granulocytes, are collected from the blood of a healthy donor for transfusion to patients with severe granulocytopenia, which is sometimes due to leukemia, cancer chemotherapy, or toxic drugs.

leukoplakia (lū-kō-plā'ki-a): A disease characterized by the occurrence of white, thickened patches on mucous membrane, usually on the lips and inside of mouth; may also occur on genitalia. Often seen in smokers, but also due to bad fitting dentures, vitamin A deficiency, or uncleanliness. Sometimes becomes malignant. Often occurs in conjunction with kraurosis vulvae (*q.v.*).

leukopoieses (lū-kō-poy-ē'sis): The formation of white blood cells.—leukopoietic, adj.

leukorrhea (lū-kō-rē'-a): A sticky, whitish vaginal discharge containing mucus and pus cells.—leukorrheal, adj.

leukosarcoma (lū'kō-sar-kō'ma): A blood condition that may develop in patients originally diagnosed as having lymphocytic malignant lymphoma; characterized by the presence in the bloodsteam of lymphocytes that are morphologically different from those found in chronic lymphocytic leukemia.

leukotomy (lū-kot'-o-mi): PREFRONTAL L., an operation for the treatment of certain forms of chronic insanity by cutting the connection fibers in the white matter of the frontal lobe of the brain. May produce a state of irreversible apathy and inertia; it is usually reserved for chronic schizophrenics and patients in whom there is gross behavior disorder such as prolonged violence, self-mutilation, and extreme restlessness.

leukotoxic (lū-kō-tok'-sik): Pertaining to any substance that is toxic to leukocytes.

levator (le-vā′-tor): 1. A muscle that acts by raising a part. 2. An instrument for lifting a depressed part.—levatores, pl.

levatores ani (lev-a-tō′-rēz-ā′-ni):A pair of broad muscles extending from the back of the pubis to the sacrum and coccyx and to the lateral pelvic walls; forms the strongest part of the pelvic floor.

LeVeen shunt: See under shunt.

Levin tube: A rubber or plastic nasal gastroduodenal catheter; it is inserted through the nose into the upper alimentary tract for continuous gastric suction, especially after operations, for the purpose of decompression, for nasogastric feedings, or for obtaining material for tests. [Abraham Louis Levin, American physician. 1880-1940.]

Levine scale: A scale used to describe the intensity of a heart murmur, from Grades I through IV, from faint to extremely loud.

levitation (lev′-i-tā′- shun): 1. The sensation of rising or floating in the air. 2. The act of supporting a patient on a cushion of air.

levodopa (lev-ō-dō-pa): An antiparkinson drug. L-Dopa.

levoversion (lē′-vō-ver′-zhun): Turning to the left. In ophthalmology, the simultaneous movement of the eyes to the left.

levulose (lev′-ū-lōs): Fructose or fruit sugar. Sweeter and more easily digested than ordinary sugar; useful in treatment of diabetes.

Lev's disease: A condition in which lesions develop in the fibrous tissues of the heart and its valves and interfere with the functioning of the conduction system; may lead to complete heart block.

lewisite (lū′-i-sit): A lethal war gas resembling mustard gas. It causes blisters on the skin, tearing of the eyes, and is a systemic poison that enters the bloodstream through the skin or lungs. [W. Lee Lewis, American chemist. 1879-1943.]

Lewy bodies: Round bodies found in the cytoplasm of some of the neurons of the midbrain of patients with paralysis agitans.

-lexia: Combining form denoting 1) speech; 2) word; 3) a type of incapacity to read.

Leydig cell: One of the interstitial cells of the testis that produce the male sex hormone.

LFT: Abbreviation for liver function test.

LGA: Abbreviation for large for gestational age.

LH: Abbreviation for leutinizing hormone (*q.v.*).

Lhermitt's sign (ler′-mits): A condition seen in multiple sclerosis and certain diseases of the cervical cord; when the head is flexed a transient electric shock-like sensation spreads down the arms and legs; may persist for a few days or weeks and then disappears without treatment.

libidinous (li-bid′-i-nus): Pertaining to libido; erotic; lustful; lascivious.

libido (li-bē′-dō): The vital force or energy that results in purposeful actions. Freud's name for the urge to obtain sensual satisfaction which he believed to be the mainspring of human behavior. Sometimes more loosely associated with the meaning of sexual urge. Freud's meaning was satisfaction through all the senses. In Jungian psychology the term denotes psychic energy.—libidinal, adj.

lice (līs): See louse.

licensure (lī′-sen-shur): In health care, a process whereby a governmental agency grants permission to individuals, educational institutions, and health care facilities to function in a specified capacity after having met certain minimum qualifications and requirements. Licensure for professional nursing, which has the effect of law, is a function of the various states; it ensures a minimal level of nursing competence and has the effect of restricting entry into practice; candidates who meet the set requirements are required to take an examination to demonstrate competency; several states now require evidence of having taken continuing education courses before granting re-licensure. In 1986 North Dakota became the first state to require that applicants for licensure as registered nurse must have received the BSN degree.

lichen (lī′-ken): In medicine, aggregates of papular skin lesions. **L. AMYLOIDOSIS**, a form of localized cutaneous amyloidosis; seen most often on the shins. **L. NITIDUS**, characterized by minute, shiny, flat-topped, pink papules of pinhead size; most frequently seen on the abdomen, breasts, and on the genitalia of males. **L. PLANUS**, aggregates of small, persistent, polygonal papules, flat-topped with a characteristic sheen, and of reddish-purple color, occurring in well defined patches on the wrists, ankles, and abdomen; grayish patches on mucous membranes; and may involve hair follicles and nails. **L. SCLEROSIS ET ATROPHICUS**, a chronic skin condition in which flat papules appear and later coalesce into larger white areas, and the skin becomes thin, hyperpigmented, and telangiectasic; cause unknown; occurs most often in women as kraurosis vulvae; in men it is known as balanitis xerotica obliterans. **L. SCROFULOSSUS**, small flat-topped papules that may occur as an allergic phenomenon in tuberculosis. **L. SIMPLEX** or **L. SIMPLEX CHRONICUS**, a psychosomatic condition characterized by the development of localized areas of irritating, leathery, shiny papules (lichenification); skin abrasions and dry scaling are kept going by itching, rubbing, scratching; syn., chronic neurodermatitis. **L. SPINULOSIS**, characterized by small spines protruding from the openings of the hair follicles; seen especially around the anogenital area, dorsa of the hands and feet, bend of the elbow or knee, and back of the neck; appears to be a result of vitamin A deficiency. **L. TROPICUS**, characterized by redness and inflammation of the skin; also called malaria rubra and prickly heat. **L. URTICATUS**. papular urticaria; see urticaria.—lichenoid, adj.

lichenification (lī′-ken-i-fi-kā′-shun): Thickening and hardening of the skin; is usually secondary to pruritus, and due to scratching and excoriation of the skin.

lid lag: A condition in which a rim of sclera may be seen between the upper lid and the sclera when the patient gazes downward; usually a sign of hyperthyroidism.

lie detector: An apparatus that records changes in breathing rate, pulse rate, blood pressure, and sweating of the hands—symptoms thought to be indicative of emotional reactions to certain words or questions when one is not telling the truth. A polygraph.

Lieberkühn's crypts, glands, or follicles (lē′-ber-kēnz): Simple tubular glands in the mucous membrane of the small intestine. [Johann Nathaniel Lieberkühn, German physician and anatomist. 1711-1756.]

lien (lī′-en): The spleen.—lienal, adj.

lien-, lieno-: Combining forms denoting the spleen. See also splen- , spleno-.

lienculus (lī-en′-kū-lus): A small accessory spleen.

lienitis (lī-e-nī′-tis): Old term for inflammation of the spleen.

lienorenal (lī′-en-ō-rē′- nal): Pertaining to the spleen and kidney.

life expectancy: The number of years a person can expect to live, based on statistical averages.

life island: A plastic tent that encloses the patient, his bed, and immediate surroundings; used to protect him from infection. See also laminar air flow.

life style: The way an individual adapts to the social milieu or environment in which he is placed; or, the life style he has adopted for himself which may or may not conform with that of his contemporaries.

Lifeline: A support system for older people living alone; allows a person to request aid by pressing a button on a portable pocket-sized unit, which will ring a telephone in a central unit.

ligament (lig′-a-ment): A strong band of fibrous connective tissue serving to bind bones or other parts together, to support a structure or organ, and to strengthen joints.—ligamentous, adj.

ligate (lī′-gāt): 1. To constrict a blood vessel or a duct, or the pedicle of a tumor by tying a thread or like material very tightly around it. 2. To apply a ligature.—ligation, n.

ligation (lī-gā′-shun): The application of a ligature (*q.v.*). **TUBAL L.**, sterilization of the female by applying a ligature to the uterine tubes to constrict them; the tubes may or may not be severed or crushed; when performed through the vagina, it is referred to as **VAGINAL TUBAL LIGATION.**

ligature (lig′-a-chūr): The material used for tying tightly around a blood vessel to constrict blood flow, or around part of a body structure or a tumor to constrict it, or for sewing tissues. Silk thread, horsehair, catgut, silver wire, synthetic fibers, cotton, linen, kangaroo tendon, sheep intestine, or strips of the patient's own fascia are used. See suture.

light bath: Exposure of uncovered skin to light rays from the sun or from electric or other light sources.

light headedness: Dizziness, faintness, delirium.

lightening: Term used to denote the relief of pressure on the diaphragm by the abdominal viscera when the presenting part of the fetus descends into the pelvis in the last two to three weeks of pregnancy.

lightning (līt′-ning): Descriptive of paroxysmal, stabbing pains, as those that occur in the lower limbs in tabes dorsalis.

limb-girdle dystrophy: A form of muscular dystrophy most often seen in late childhood or early adulthood; first affects the shoulder girdle or the pelvic girdle, then spreads to other parts of the body.

limbic system: A term loosely applied to a group of structures in the rhinencephalon (*q.v.*) of the brain, including the hippocampus, amygdala, and hypothalamus, that have to do with various senses, emotions, and feelings, and certain automatic functions. Lesions in this system result in a wide range of abnormal behaviors.

limbus (lim′-bus): A border. In anatomy, a border or edge of certain structures, *e.g.*, the edge where the cornea joins the sclera.—limbic, adj.

lime water: Solution of calcium hydroxide (about 0.15 percent). It is used in a number of skin lotions, and with an equal volume of linseed or olive oil it forms a soothing application. It is also used in infant feeding as it hinders the formation of large curds.

limen (lī′-men): In physiology, a threshold, as of a stimulus.—limina, pl.; liminal, adj.

liminal (lim′-i-nal): The lowest intensity of a stimulus that can be perceived by the human sense. See subliminal.

limulus assay test: A rapid test for detecting the presence of clinical septicemia due to gram-negative organisms; utilizes an extract obtained from the king crab. Limulus gelatin test.

linctus (lingk′-tus): A sweet, syrupy liquid, made of a powdered drug combined with honey or other syrup; has a soothing effect on the mucous membrane of the pharynx; should be taken undiluted and sipped slowly.

Lindau's disease: von Hippel-Lindau disease (*q.v.*).

line: In anatomy, a mark, stripe, streak, or bony ridge; may be imaginary, referring to two anatomical points. **AXILLARY L.**, a vertical line passing through the center of the axilla, dividing the body into anterior and posterior halves. **MEDIAL L.**, a **L.** passing through the midline of the body from the crown of the head to the ground between the feet; it divides the body into right and left halves. **MIDCLAVICULAR L.**, a **L.** on the anterior surface of the body passing through the center of the nipple; also called linea mamillaris. **MIDSPINAL L.**, a perpendicular **L.** down the middle of the spinal column. **MIDSTERNAL L.**, a perpendicular **L.** passing from the cricoid cartilage down through the center of the sternum to the xiphoid process.

linea (lin′-ē-a): A line. **L. ALBA,** the white line between the two rectus muscles, visible after removal of skin from the center of the abdomen, stretching from the ensiform cartilage to the pubis, its position being indicated by a slight depression on the surface. The transversalis and parts of the oblique muscles are inserted into it. **L. ALBICANTES,** white lines that appear on the abdomen after reduction of tension caused by stretching such as occurs in tumors, pregnancy, edema, etc. **L. ASPERA,** roughened line on posterior aspect of the femur. **L. NIGRA,** a pigmented line from umbilicus to pubis that appears in pregnancy. **L. TERMINALIS PELVIS,** a line on the inner surface of either iliac bone; runs from the scaroiliac joint to the eminence of the symphysis pubis; it marks the division between the false and true pelves.—lineae, pl.

lingua (ling′-gwa): The tongue.—lingual, adj.

lingual (ling′-gwal): Pertaining to the tongue. **L. GOITER,** an enlargement at the back of the tongue.

lingula (ling′-gū-la): General term used to describe a small tongue-shaped structure extending from a body part or organ.

liniment (lin′-i-ment): A medicinal oily liquid to be applied to the skin by friction.

linin (lī′-nin): The substance that makes up the thread-like network in a cell and on which the granules of chromatin are situated.

linked (linkt): In genetics, descriptive of characters that are so united to each other that they are always inherited together.

linoleic acid (lin-ō-lē′-ik): An unsaturated, essential fatty acid. Found in the glycerides of linseed and vegetable oils.

lint: A soft, absorbent material used for surgical dressings. It is fluffy on one side and smooth on the other.

liothyronine (lī′ō-thī′rō-nēn): One of two thyroid hormones, normally present in the thyroid gland and the blood; it is important in tissue metabolism. Also prepared synthetically and used in treatment of hypothyroidism.

lip: labium (*q.v.*).

lip-, lipo-: Combining forms denoting 1) fat: 2) fatty tissue.

lipase (lī′-pās): Any fat-splitting enzyme. Lipoprotein l., an enzyme that promotes the storage of fat in the fat cells of the body; this activity seems to be reduced in cigarette smokers but becomes more active when the individual stops smoking. **PANCREATIC L.**, steapsin (*q.v.*).

lipemia (li-pē′-mi-a): Increased lipid (especially cholesterol) in the circulating blood.—lipemic, adj.

lipid (lip′-id): Any one of a widely varying group of fats and fat-like organic substances that are insoluble or only slightly so in water but are soluble in alcohol, ether, chloroform, and other such substances, and that can be metabolized and easily stored in the body; obtained from plants and animals. Along with carbohydrates and proteins, lipids are important constituents of living cells and an important source of fuel in the body.

lipidosis (lip-i-dō′-sis): Overall term for disorders of fat metabolism that result in the accumulation of abnormal amounts of lipids in the body tissues.

lipiduria (lip-i-dūr′-ri-a): The presence of lipids in the urine.

lipoatrophy (lip-ō-at′-rō-fi): Atrophy of subcutaneous body fat.

lipocardiac (lip-ō-kar′-di-ak): Pertaining to fatty degeneration of the heart muscle, or to a person affected with this condition.

lipochondrodystrophy (lip′-ō-kon′-drō-dis′-tro-fi): A congenital abnormality of fat metabolism involving the bones, skin, cartilage, brain, and other organs; characterized by short stature, kyphosis, and possibly mental deficiency. Syn., Hurler's syndrome.

lipocyte (lip′-ō-sīt): A fat or fat-storing cell.

lipodystrophy (lip-ō-dis′-trō-fi): Any disturbance of fat metabolism. **INTESTINAL L.**, a condition characterized by diarrhea, fatty stools, emaciation, arthritis, and deposits of fat in intestinal lymphatic tissue.

lipofibroma (lip′ō-fi-brō′ma): A fibrous fatty tumor.

lipofuscin (lip-ō-fūs′sin): A brown pigment that accumulates in neural cells and is found in many body tissues; may be a product of degenerated lysosomes; has been associated with senile confusion.

lipogenesis (lip′-ō-jen′-e-sis): 1. The production of fat. 2. The deposition of fat in the body. 3. The conversion of protein or carbohydrate into fat.

lipogenous (li-poj′-e-nus): Producing fat or fatness.

lipogranuloma (lip′ō-gran-ū-lō′-ma): A nodule made up of fatty tissue with a necrotic center; occurs in granulomatous inflammation.

lipogranulomatosis (lip′-ō-gran′-ū-lō-ma-tō′-sis): A condition characterized by the occurrence of several lipogranulomas.

lipoid (lip′-oyd): 1. Resembling fat. 2. A lipid.—lipoidal, adj.

lipoidosis (lip-oy-dō′-sis): Disease that is due to disorder of fat metabolism.

lipolysis (li-pol′-i-sis): The chemical breaking down of fat.

lipolytic (lip-ō-lit′-ik): Pertaining to or causing lipolysis.

lipoma (li-pō′-ma): A benign tumor containing fatty tissue, usually multiple but not metastatic.—lipomata, pl.; lipomatous, adj.

lipomatosis (lip′ō-ma-tō′sis): A condition marked by an abnormal accumulation of fat in a localized area.

lipophilic (lip-ō-fil′-ik): 1. Having an affinity for lipids. 2. Absorbing fat.

lipoprotein (lip′ō-prō′tē-in): A conjugated protein formed by the combination of a lipid and a protein, and having the general properties of proteins. ALPHA L., tiny particles, rich in protein and apparently not related to atherosclerosis. BETA-L., L. rich in cholesterol, therefore of significance in atherosclerosis.

liposarcoma (lip′-ō-sar-kō′-ma): A rare malignant tumor seen most often in the elderly; usually occurs in the retroperitoneal or mediastinal fat desposits.

lipotropic (lip′-ō-trō′-pik): Acting on fat metabolism by promoting the reduction of fat deposit in the liver, or an agent that has this effect.

Lippes loop: A once popular intrauterine contraceptive device.

lipuria (li-pū′-ri-a): The presence of lipids in the urine.—lipuric, adj.

Liq: Abbreviation for liquor.

liquefaction (lik-we-fak′-shun): The conversion of a solid or gas into a liquid.

liquid (lik′-wid): A substance that flows freely, is neither a solid nor a gas, has no definite shape, but takes the shape of its container.

liquor (lik′-er): A solution. In anatomy, refers to certain body fluids; in pharmacology, refers to an aqueous solution. L. AMNII, the fluid surrounding the fetus. L. FOLLICULI, the fluid surrounding a developing ovum in a graafian follicle. L. SANGUINIS, the fluid part of the blood (plasma).

lisp: To pronounce the letters s and z with the sound of th.

Lissauer's paralysis: A rapidly progressive general paralysis; characterized by seizures and by symptoms of unilateral frontal or temporal lobe disease. Also called **Lissauer's cerebral sclerosis.**

Lister, Lord Joseph: English surgeon 1827–1912. In 1867 Lister published *On the Antiseptic Principle in the Practice of Surgery* which, along with his own practice of surgery, laid the foundation for the development of modern surgery.

Listeria (lis-tēr′-i-a): A genus of coccoid and bacillary microorganisms that occur in lower animals as the cause of septicemia or encephalitis and in humans as the cause of septicemia, conjunctivitis, lymphadenitis, and upper respiratory infections. L. MONOCYTOGENES, a cause of sporadic cases of purulent meningitis, septicemia, and sometimes mononucleosis.

listeriosis (lis-tēr-′-i-ō′-sis): Infection caused by *Listeria* organisms. See **Listeria.**

liter (lē′-ter): A unit of liquid measurement in the metric system, being 1000 cc or 1000 ml. Equivalent to 1.0567 quarts U.S. liquid measure. Also litre.

lith-, litho-, -lith: Combining forms denoting calculi (stones).

lithagogue (lith′a-gog): An agent that promotes the expulsion of calculi, especially urinary calculi.

lithiasis (li-thī′-a-sis): Formation of calculi, or concretions. L. BILIARIS, gallstones. L. RENALIS, kidney stones.

lithicosis (lith-i-kō′-sis): Pneumoconiosis (*q.v.*).

lithium (lith′-i-um): A soft, silver-white metallic element, the salts of which are solvents of uric acid. Sometimes used in drug therapy for individuals with certain psychiatric disorders.

litholapaxy (li-thol′-a-pak-si): Crushing a stone within the urinary bladder and removing the fragments by irrigation. Syn., lithotripsy.

litholysis (li-thol′-i-sis): The dissolving of calculi, especially urinary calculi in the bladder.

lithonephrotomy (lith′ō-ne-frot′ō-mi): Surgical incision of the kidney for the removal of a calculus.

lithopedion (lith-ō-pē′-di-on): A fetus that has died and calcified in situ; often extrauterine.

lithosis (li-thō′-sis): Pneumoconiosis (*q.v.*).

lithotomy (lith-ot′-o-mi): An operation on a duct or organ for the removal of a calculus, especially from the urinary tract or bladder. L. POSITION, that in which the patient lies in the dorsal position with the thighs raised and the knees supported and widely separated.

lithotripsy (lith′-ō-trip-si): An operation for crushing calculi in the bladder or urethra.

lithotrite (lith′-ō-trīt): An instrument for crushing a stone in the urinary bladder, or in the urethra.

lithotrity (li-thot′-ri-ti): The operation of crushing a stone in the urinary bladder. Also called litholapaxy and lithotripsy.

lithous (lith′-us): Pertaining to or resembling a calculus.

lithuresis (lith′ū-rē′sis): Voiding of gravel in the urine.

lithuria (lith-ū′ri-a): The presence of small stones or uric acid crystals in the urine.

litmus (lit′-mus): A vegetable pigment, obtained from lichen, used as an indicator of acidity or alkalinity. Blue **L.** paper turns red when in contact with an acid. Red **L.** paper turns blue when in contact with an alkali.

litre (lē′-ter): See liter.

litter: A portable stretcher or couch used for transporting the sick or wounded.

Little's disease: Diplegia of spastic type causing scissor-leg deformity. Congenital disease in which there is cerebral atrophy or agenesis. [William John Little, English surgeon. 1810-1894.]

livedo (li-vē′-dō): A bluish discoloration of the skin; may occur in localized patches or generally. **L. RETICULARIS,** cutis marmorata; see under cutis. May indicate the presence of an acute disease or a serious failure of the circulation; characterized by reddish blue mottling of the skin, occurring particularly in the extremities.

liver: The largest gland in the body, lobular in structure, weighing from 3 to 4 pounds in the adult male, less in women. It is dark red in color and is situated in the upper right section of the abdomen; dome-shaped from fitting closely under the diaphragm. It produces bile, converts most sugars into glycogen, which it also stores, and is essential to life. The liver of some animals is used as food and as the source of pharmaceutical preparations used in treatment of certain anemias. **L. SPOTS,** yellowish-brown patches or spots on the skin. See also cirrhosis, hobnail.

livid (liv′-id): Ashen, cyanotic. Blue discoloration due to bruising, congestion of blood, or insufficient oxygenation; black and blue.—lividity, n.

living will: A written statement by a mentally competent adult that, should that person ever be in such a condition as to be unable to make decisions regarding his or her care and is clearly dying, that no extraordinary measures be used to prolong life.

LMP: Abbreviation for last menstrual period.

LOA: Abbreviation for left occipitoanterior position (of the fetus in utero).

Loa loa (lō′a lō′-a): A species of nematode found mostly in West Africa; it penetrates the subcutaneous tissues, particularly around the eye and under the conjunctiva; flies are the intermediate host. Also called the African eye worm. See loiasis.

loading dose: In pharmacotherapeutics, the administration of a drug in larger doses than the body can eliminate in order to bring the concentration of the drug to an effective level; usually by giving several doses close together; when this has been achieved the daily dose is reduced to the amount that equals the amount of drug that is eliminated each day.

lobar (lō′-bar): Pertinent to a lobe. **L. PNEUMONIA,** see pneumonia.

lobate (lō′-bāt): Divided into or made up of lobes.

lobe (lōb): 1. The lower part of the external ear. 2. A more or less well-defined section of an organ, separated from neighboring sections by a fissure, sulcus, or connective tissue. 3. A subdivision of the lung.—lobar, adj.

lobectomy (lō-bek′-to-mi): Excision of a lobe, as of the lung, brain, thyroid, or liver.

lobotomy (lō-bot′-o-mi): Incision into a lobe. **FRONTAL** or **PREFRONTAL L.,** cutting through the nerve fibers that pass from the frontal lobe of the cerebrum to the thalamus; done to relieve certain mental states or intractable pain.

lobster-claw hand: An inherited deformity in which the middle digits of the hand are missing and the structures are fused so as to form a hand that resembles a lobster's claw. When only the first and fifth fingers are present, the condition is referred to as bidactyly.

lobule (lob′-ūl): A small lobe or a subdivision of a lobe.—lobular, lobulated, adj.

local: Not general; restricted to one part or area of the body. **L. ANESTHETIC,** see anesthetic. **L. INFECTION,** one restricted to a relatively small area, *e.g.*, a boil.

localize (lō′-kal-īz): 1. To limit the spread. 2. To determine the site of a lesion.—localization, n.; localized, adj.

localized: Restricted to one area or spot; not spread throughout the body. Opp. to systemic.

lochia (lō′-ki-a): The vaginal discharge of blood and tissue debris that occurs during the puerperium. At first pure blood, it later becomes pale, diminishes in quantity, and finally ceases.—lochial, adj.

lochiometra (lō-ki-ō-mē′-tra): Retention of lochia in the uterus.

lockjaw: Tonic muscle spasm making it impossible to open the jaws. See trismus.

locomotion (lō-kō-mō′-shun): The act of or ability to move from place to place.

locomotor (lō-kō-mō′-tor): Can be applied to any tissue or system used in human movement. Most usually refers to nerves and muscles. Sometimes includes the bones and joints. **L. ATAXIA,** the disordered gait and loss of sense of position in the lower limbs that occurs in tabes dorsalis (*q.v.*). Tabes dorsalis is sometimes referred to, still, as locomotor ataxia.

loculated (lok′-ū-lā-ted): Divided into numerous cavities or pockets.

loculation (lok-ū-lā′-shun): The formation of loculi in the tissues. See loculus. **L. SYNDROME**, see Froin's syndrome.

loculus (lok′-ū-lus): A small depression, cavity, or space.—loculi, pl.; locular, adj.

locus (lo′-kus): A specific site or place.—loci, pl.

log-, logo-, -log, -logue: Combining form denoting 1) speech; 2) discourse.

logoclonia (lō-gō-klon′-i-a): The spasmodic repetition of the final syllables of words. Also logoclony.

logopathy (log-op′-ath-i): Any speech disorder of central nervous system origin.

logopedics (log′ō-pē′diks): The study and treatment of speech defects.

logorrhea (log′ō-rē′a): Excessive talkativeness; garrulousness.

-logy: Combining form denoting 1) science, theory, doctrine; 2) speaking, saying.

loiasis (lō-ī′-a-sis): A chronic disease caused by a nematode; transmitted by a fly of the genus *Chrysops;* found in central Africa. After as long as two or three years, the larvae of the organism *Loa loa* mature and move into the connective tissue, producing a creeping sensation, intense itching, and pain. Also spelled loaiasis.

loin: The lower part of the back, between the lower ribs and the iliac crest; the area immediately above the buttocks.

longevity (lon-jev′-i-ti): 1. Length of life. 2. Long individual life.

longsightedness: Hyperopia (*q.v.*).

long-term care: Medical and personal care that extends over a long period of time, often years, for patients who require some nursing care, who may or may not be bedridden, and whose chronic illnesses may improve somewhat or become controllable. **LONG-TERM CARE FACILITY**, essentially a chronic disease facility where patients who may be convalescing, incurably ill, or unable to care for themselves in some way, stay for longer than 30 days, and where medical care receives more emphasis than in a nursing home.

loop: 1. A curve or bend. **HENLE'S L.**, a loop in the uriniferous tubule of the kidney. 2. A heat-resisting wire set into a handle and used in the laboratory for transferring bacteriological material. 3. Lay term for a commonly used intrauterine contraceptive device; may be of metal or plastic.

Looser's zones: Narrow ribbon-like zones seen on an x-ray photograph of the tibia and other long bones in cases of deficient calcification or decalcification along the nutrient arteries; sometimes seen in rickets and in osteomalacia.

lophotrichous (lō-fot′-ri-kus): Having two or more flagella at one or both ends; said of bacteria.

Lorain's infantilism: Pituitary dwarfism; see under dwarfism.

lordosis (lor-dō′-sis): An exaggerated forward, convex curve of the lumbar spine; sometimes called hollow back or saddle back.

lotion (lō′-shun): A liquid preparation, usually medicated, used externally on the skin.

Lou Gehrig's disease: Popular name for amyotrophic lateral sclerosis (*q.v.*).

Louis-Bar syndrome: Ataxia-telangiectasia (*q.v.*).

loupe (loop): A magnifying lens worn on the eyeglasses or a headband by the surgeon when operating on very small structures or by the opthalmologist when examining the eye.

louse: A small parasitic insect; three varieties of which infest man.—lice, pl. See Pediculus.

low birth weight: A weight at birth that is below 2.5 Kg (5½ pounds); the baby may be either preterm or small-for-dates.

low salt diet: See under diet.

low salt syndrome: A syndrome caused by a drop in the salt concentration of the serum; occurs in heat exhaustion as well as in chronic heart and renal disorders; symptoms include nausea, vomiting, muscle cramps, hypotension, and tachycardia, possibly convulsions.

lower motor neuron: An efferent neuron with a nucleus either in the anterior horn of the spinal cord or in the corresponding gray matter of the brain stem, and an axon that terminates in a skeletal muscle. See upper motor neuron.

lower respiratory tract: Composed of the right and left bronchi and their subdivisions, and the right and left lungs; abbreviated LRT. **LRT INFECTION**, infection involving the bronchi and lungs; often an extension of an upper respiratory tract infection.

Lowe's syndrome: A hereditary condition characterized by mental retardation, decreased ammonia production by the kidneys, cataract, glaucoma, osteomalacia, rickets, retardation of growth, myotonia. Has been observed only in male infants.

Lown-Ganong-Levine syndrome: An electrocardiographic syndrome in which the P-R interval is short, but the QRS interval is normal; often associated with paroxysmal tachycardia.

loxoscelism (lok-sos′-sel-izm): A condition resulting from the bite of the brown recluse spider (*Loxosceles reclusa*), common in North and Central America, whose venom produces a painful red vesicle that progresses to a black gangrenous slough, accompanied by chills, fever, nausea, vomiting, weakness. The sometimes fatal viscerocutaneous form is characterized by high fever and hematuria.

lozenge (loz′-enj): A medicated, sweetened tablet that is held in the mouth until it is dissolved; a troche.

Löffler's syndrome: Löffler's eosinophilia, a condition characterized by an increase in the eosinophilic leukocytes in the blood, accompanied by transient infiltration of the lungs.

LP: Abbreviation for lumbar puncture.

L.P.N.: Abbreviation for licensed practical nurse; see under nurse.

LSD: Lysergic acid diethylamide. Derivative of an alkaloid found in ergot. Has potent hallucinogenic action and produces mind-changing experiences. Sometimes used in medicine to produce abreaction (*q.v.*).

LTC: Abbreviation for long-term care.

lubb-dupp (lubb-dupp′): The sounds heard through the stethoscope when listening to the normal heartbeat. *Lubb* is heard when the atrioventricular valves close and *dupp* when the semilunar valves close. The first sound is longer and of lower pitch than the second. Also called lupp-dupp.

lubricant (loo′-bri-kant): Any substance such as oil, that lessens or prevents friction when applied between two solid surfaces.

lucent (lū′-sent): Clear; transparent.

Lucey-Driscoll syndrome: A type of congenital jaundice occurring in infants as a result of defective conjugation of bilirubin.

lucid (lū′-sid): Clear, particularly in reference to the mind.—lucidity, n.; lucidly, adv.

Ludwig's angina: See angina.

Luer syringe: A glass syringe for injecting substances hypodermically or intravenously.

lues (lū′-ēz): Syphilis.—luetic, adj.

Luft's disease: A disorder of striated muscle, characterized by muscle weakness, profuse sweating, and increased rate of metabolism.

Lugol's solution: A deep brown, transparent solution consisting of iodine and potassium iodide, in purified water; used as a source of iodine in treating hyperthyroidism because it inhibits the release of thyroid hormone.

lumb-, lumbo-: Combining forms denoting 1) the loin; 2) the lumbar area.

lumbago (lum-bā′-gō): Incapacitating low back pain, usually of muscular origin.

lumbar: Pertaining to the loins. **L. NERVE,** one of five pairs of spinal nerves. **L. PUNCTURE,** puncture into the subarachnoid space of the spinal cord, usually between the fourth and fifth lumbar vertebrae, to remove an excess of fluid, to obtain fluid for examination, or to inject a medicament. **L. SYMPATHECTOMY,** surgical removal of the sympathetic chain in the lumbar region; used to improve the blood supply to the lower limbs by allowing the blood vessels to dilate.

lumbocostal (lum′-bō-kos′-tal): Pertaining to the loins and ribs.

lumbosacral (lum′-bō-sā′-kral): Pertaining to the loin or lumbar vertebrae and the sacrum.

lumen (loo′-men): The channel of a tubular structure.—lumina, pl.; luminal, adj.

lumpectomy (lum-pek′-to-mi): Removal of a tumor; usually refers to breast surgery for removal of a lump only, leaving the surrounding tissues and lymph glands largely intact.

lunacy (lū′-na-si): Insanity; so called because in olden times it was thought to be due to the moon's influence.

lunate (lū′-nāt): One of the bones of the wrist.

lunatic (lū′-na-tik): A term formerly much used to describe a mentally ill person.

Lund and Browder's chart: A chart for estimating the surface area involved in burns of children; it indicates percentages for four growth periods from age one to age 16. An adaptation of Wallace's rule of nines (*q.v.*).

lung: One of the two main organs of respiration which occupy the greater part of the thoracic cavity. They are made up of an arrangement of air tubes terminating in air vesicles; connect with the outside by the bronchi and the trachea; and are divided into lobes, the right lung being composed of the superior, middle, and inferior lobes and the left lung of the superior and inferior lobes. The lungs are separated from each other by the heart and other organs in the mediastinum. Together they weigh about 42 oz. and they are concerned with oxygenation of the blood.

lungmotor: A respiratory apparatus similar to a pulmotor (*q.v.*), used to force air into the lungs in cases of asphyxia.

lunula (lū′-nū-la): A small semicircular area, especially the semilunar pale area seen at the root of the nail.

lupoid (lū′-poyd): Pertinent to or resembling lupus. **L. HEPATITIS,** a chronic form of hepatitis in which the serologic reactions are similar to those occurring in lupus erythematosus.

lupus (lū′-pus): A destructive, chronic nodular skin condition with many manifestations. **L. ERYTHEMATOSUS;** see collagen, LE cells. The discoid variety is characterized by a superficial inflammation of the skin with disk-like patches that have reddish edges and depressed centers; commonest on the nose where the eruption appears in a butterfly pattern extending over the adjoining cheeks. The disseminated type is characterized by large areas of erythema on the skin, pyrexia, toxemia, enlargement of lymph nodes, involvement of serous membranes (pleurisy, pericarditis) and renal damage; may be an autoimmune process; often fatal. **L. PERNIO,** a form of sarcoidosis (*q.v.*); lesions of the hands and ears resembling those of frostbite; usually accompanied by a pulmonary disorder; granulomatous nodules may appear on the skin, especially in old scars. **L. VULGARIS,** the commonest form of skin tuberculosis; ulceration occurs over cartilage (nose or ear) with necrosis and facial disfigurement. **SYSTEMIC L. ERYTHEMATOSUS,** the disseminated variety of lupus.—lupiform, lupous, adj.

lutein (lū′-tē-in): Yellow pigment in the corpus luteum (*q.v.*): also in egg yolk and fat cells.

luteinizing hormone (lū′-tē-in-īz-ing hor′-mōn): A gonadotropic (*q.v.*) hormone of the anterior pituitary, which acts with the follicle stimulating hormone to cause ovulation and the secretion of sex hormones; is also involved in the formation of corpus luteum (*q.v.*). In males, it stimulates the interstitial cells of Leydig in the testes to produce testosterone.

Lutembacher's syndrome: A combination of atrial septal defect and mitral stenosis.

luteotrophin (lū′-tē-ō-trō′-fin): Hormone secreted by the anterior pituitary gland; it assists the formation of the corpus luteum in the ovary. Stimulates milk production after parturition. Previously called lactogenic hormone. Also luteotropin.

luxation (luk-sā′-shun): Dislocation.—luxated, adj.

L.V.N.: Abbreviation for licensed vocational nurse: see under nurse.

lying-in: **L. PERIOD,** the puerperium (*q.v.*). The term postnatal is now preferred. **L. HOSPITAL,** a maternity hospital.

Lyme disease or arthritis: An acute, transient disease thought to be caused by a virus transmitted by the bite of a tick; characterized by skin lesions, erythema, fever, headache, stiff neck, malaise; sequelae include cardiac and neurological disorders and acute arthritis affecting the knees and other large joints. So called because it was first identified in Lyme, Connecticut.

lymph (limf): The pale, colorless or slightly yellow fluid that exudes from the blood through the capillaries, bathes the cells, and passes into lymphatic ducts which return the fluid to the bloodstream. Its function is to serve as the medium of exchange of nutrients and wastes between the blood and the cells. It resembles plasma, but contains only one type of blood cell, the lymphocyte. **L. GLAND, L.** node. **L. NODE,** see under node.

lymph-, lympho-: Combining forms denoting 1) lymph; 2) lymphatic tissue; 3) lymphocytes.

lymphadenectasis (lim′-fad-e-nek′-ta- sis): Enlargement of one or more lymph nodes.

lymphadenectomy (lim-fad′-e-nek′-to- mi): Excision of one or more lymph nodes.

lymphadenitis (lim′-fad-e-nī′-tis): Inflammation of one or more lymph nodes; usually produced by bacteria or their products; may be acute or chronic. The gland swells and there may be suppuration; the surrounding area may be red, hot, and tender to the touch. **MESENTERIC L., L.** of the mesenteric lymph nodes. **TUBERCULOUS L.,** tuberculosis of the lymph glands, particularly those of the neck and mediastinum, by metastasis from the lungs; suppuration may occur and form draining sinuses; formerly called scrofula.

lymphadenogram (lim-fad′-e-nō-gram): Radiography of lymph glands; a radiopaque dye is inserted into the gland before x-ray films are made; the dye is retained for several months, making it possible to take follow-up films.

lymphadenoid (lim-fad′-e-noid): Pertaining to or having the characteristics of a lymph gland.

lymphadenoma (lim-fad′-e-nō′- ma): An old term for an enlarged lymph node. **MULTIPLE L.,** Hodgkin's disease.

lymphadenopathy (lim-fad′e-nop′a-thi): Any disease of the lymph glands.—lymphadenopathic, adj. **IMMUNOBLASTIC L.,** a serious progressive **L.,** marked by fever, sweats, splenomegaly, thrombocytopenia, pruritus, hemolytic anemia; proliferation of the smaller blood vessels; and generalized lymphadenopathy.

lymphangiectasis (lim-fan′-ji-ek′-ta-sis): Dilation of the lymph vessels, resulting from some obstruction in the flow of lymph. May cause formation of lymphangioma.—lymphangiectatic, adj.

lymphangiectomy (lim-fan′-ji-ek′to-mi): The surgical removal of a lymph vessel.

lymphangiogram (lim-fan′ji-ō-gram): Radiograph demonstrating the lymphatic system after injection of an opaque medium.—lymphangiography, n.; lymphangiographical, adj.; lymphangiographically, adv.

lymphangioma (lim-fan′ji-ō′ma): A fairly well circumscribed swelling or simple tumor consisting of lymph vessels; frequently associated with similar formation of blood vessels. May be present at birth or soon afterwards; occurs most commonly on the head, neck, axilla. **L. CAVERNOSUM,** usually appears before two years of age and disappears in late childhood; characterized by dilatation of lymph vessels, forming cavities that are filled with fluid; seen mostly in the neck, axilla and mediastinum. **L. CIRCUMSCRIPTUM, L.** present at birth or occurring in childhood; marked by appearance of one or more yellow to red patches. **L. SIMPLEX,** small **L.** due to dilation of a lymph vessel in a circumscribed area.

lymphangioplasty (lim-fan′-ji-ō-plas-ti): Replacement of lymphatics by artificial channels (buried silk or nylon threads) to drain the tissues. Relieves the "brawny arm" after radical mastectomy.—lymphangioplastic, adj.

lymphangiosarcoma (lim-fan′-ji-sō-sar-kō′-ma): A malignant tumor of lymphatic vessels, usually occurring in a limb that has been the site of chronic lymphedema following radical mastectomy.

lymphangitis (lim-fan-ji′-tis): Inflammation of lymph vessel or vessels. May be due to infection through the skin, usually by streptococci; in fingertip infections a red line may be seen running up the arm. The condition usually terminates at the lymph node into which the vessel empties, but may result in septicemia. Symptoms include headache, chills, fever, malaise, increased white blood cell count.

lymphatic (lim-fat′-ik): 1. Pertaining to, or conveying or containing lymph. 2. A vessel that conveys lymph. **L. SYSTEM,** the vessels and glands (nodes) through which the lymph passes as it returns to the blood stream.

lymphedema (lim-fē-dē′-ma): Swelling of the subcutaneous tissues with excess lymph fluid due to faulty lymph drainage. May be congenital or hereditary, or may result from trauma or excision of lymph nodes. **L. PRAECOX,** gradual enlargement of the lower extremities of girls, starting in the feet; begins between the age of 10 and 25. See elephantiasis. **L. SLEEVE,** a tight-fitting elastic sleeve that extends from the wrist to the shoulder, or a sleeve that alternately inflates and deflates, thus providing intermittent compression; enhances venous return, and improves circulation; used in treatment of lymphedema following mastectomy.

lymphoblast (lim′fō-blast): An immature lymphocyte (*q.v.*).

lymphoblastoma (lim-fō-blas-tō′ma): Any one of several types of malignant lymphoma in which single or multiple tumors arise from lymphoblasts in lymph nodes. Sometimes associated with acute lymphatic leukemia. Term is sometimes used synonymously with lymphosarcoma (*q.v.*). **L. MALIGNUM,** Hodgkin's disease (*q.v.*).

lymphocyte (lim′fō-sīt): A variety of white blood cell formed in the lymphoid tissues of the body; round, colorless, somewhat motile, with a single nucleus and no cytoplasmic granules. Classified as large and small. They make up 20 to 30 percent of the total white blood cells and serve as a defense mechanism for the body. Their function is to produce antibodies. **B-LYMPHOCYTES** are those that migrate directly into the tissues without passing through the thymus, while **T-LYMPHOCYTES** are preprocessed in the thymus, especially early in life; thus children in whom the thymus is congenitally absent are highly susceptible to infections.—lymphocytic, adj.

lymphocythemia (lim′-tō-sī-thē′-mi-a): Excess of lymphocytes in the blood. Seen in such infectious diseases as infectious mononucleosis, undulant fever, measles, mumps, whooping cough.

lymphocytic choriomeningitis (lim-fō-sit′ik kōr-i-ō-men-in-jī′tis): Acute meningitis due to a specific virus; benign; runs a short course with symptoms resembling those of aseptic meningitis; occurs chiefly in young adults.

lymphocytoma (lim′-fō-sī-tō′-ma): A malignant lymphoma characterized by the presence of cells that closely resemble mature lymphocytes. **L. CUTIS,** a benign collection of lymphocytes in the dermis.

lymphocytopenia (lim′fō-sī-tō-pē′ni-a): A reduction in the normal number of lymphocytes in the blood.

lymphocytopoiesis (lim′fō-sī-tō-poi-ē′sis): The formation of lymphocytes.

lymphocytosis (lim′fō-sī-tō′sis): An excess of normal lymphocytes in the blood. **ACUTE INFECTIOUS L.,** an acute communicable disease of children in which there is an excess of normal small lymphocytes in the blood without disorder of the lymph glands or spleen.

lymphoepithelioma (lim′fō-ep-i-thēl-i-ō′ma): A rapidly growing malignant tumor arising in the modified epithelial tissue in the area of the tonsil and nasopharynx; often metastasizes to the cervical lymph nodes.—lymphoepitheliomata, pl.

lymphogram (lim′-fō-gram): X-ray demonstration of the lymphatic system or part of it after the injection of a radiopaque medium into the lymph system of an arm or leg.

lymphogranuloma (lim′-fō-gran-ū-lō′-ma): Term descriptive of several diseases in which the chief pathological change is the development of lesions resembling granulomas (*q.v.*). **L. VENEREUM,** an important contagious venereal disease, transmitted by sexual contact; primary lesion on genitalia may go unnoticed; later, regional lymph nodes enlarge and typical buboes form followed by formation of draining sinuses that leave thick scars when they heal. General symptoms are fever, malaise, joint pains. May cause elephantiasis of genitalia, ischiorectal abscesses and rectal stricture, the latter particularly in women. Also called lymphogranuloma inguinale; Nicolas-Favre disease, sixth venereal disease, climatic or tropical bubo.

lymphography (lim-fog′-ra-fi): A diagnostic x-ray procedure used in diagnosis of Hodgkin's disease and lymphoma; consists of injecting a dye, usually between the toes, which makes the lymph vessels and nodes visible on x ray.—lymphographical, adj.

lymphoid (lim′-foyd): Pertaining to or resembling lymph or the tissues of the lymphatic system.

lymphokines (lim′-fo-kīns): Soluble chemical factors released by T-lymphocytes in response to an antigen; they are hormone-like substances produced by the thymus, the best known one being interferon (*q.v.*).

lymphokinesis (lim′-fō-kī-nē′-sis): 1. The circulation of lymph through the lymph channels and nodes. 2. The movement of endolymph in the semicircular canals of the internal ear.

lymphoma (lim-fō′-ma): Term includes several tumors of lymphatic tissue, the three main types being Hodgkin's disease, lymphosarcoma, and reticulum sarcoma. Of unknown cause, the tumor starts as an enlargement of lymph nodes, usually cervical or inguinal; later extends to adjacent lymphatic chains. liver, and spleen. May be transformed into one of the malignant types including Hodgkin's disease. The benign form remains localized and does not recur after surgical removal. BURKITT'S L., a type of malignant L. that occurs in children in certain parts of Africa. NODULAR L., a malignant L. that occurs chiefly in people over 40; asymptomatic at first followed by slowly progressive painless growth of nodules primarily in the axillary, inguinal, or femoral regions.—lymphomatous, lymphomatoid, adj.

lymphopenia (lim-fō-pē′-ni-a): A reduction in the proportion of lymphocytes in the circulating blood.

lymphoplasmia (lim-fō-plaz′-mi-a): A blood condition in which the red blood cells lack hemoglobin.

lymphoproliferative (lim′-fō-prō-lif′-e-rā-tiv): Referring to or characterized by proliferation of lymphoid tissue.

lymphoreticular (lim′-fō-re-tik′-ū-lar): Pertaining to the reticuloendothelial cells of the lymph nodes. L. SYSTEM, the reticuloendothelial system; see reticuloendothelial.

lymphorrhagia (lim-fō-rā′ji-a): An outpouring of lymph from a severed or ruptured lymphatic vessel.

lymphosarcoma (lim-fō-sar-kō′ma): A malignant tumor of unknown cause, arising in the lymphatic tissue and tending to metastasize freely.—lymphosarcomata, pl.; lymphosarcomatous, adj.

lymph-vascular (limf-vas′-kū-lar): Relating to lymphatic vessels.

lyophilization (lī-of′i-lī-zā′shun): The process of creating a stable preparation of a biological substance such as blood or plasma by first freezing it rapidly and then dehydrating it.—liophilize, v.

lys-, lysi-, lyso-, -lysis: Combining forms denoting 1) disintegration, decomposition, dissolution, lysis; 2) a loosening.

The Lysaught Report: Popular name for *An Abstract for Action,* the report of the National Commission for the Study of Nursing and Nursing Education, of which Jerome Lysaught was the Chairman. This intensive three-year study involved assessment of nursing education and the current practice of nursing, and recommendations for improvement in these areas. Published in 1970 and followed by a second volume of Appendices in 1971.

lyse, lyze: To produce, cause, or undergo lysis (*q.v.*).

lysergic acid: See LSD.

lysergide (lī-ser′-jīd): A hallucinogenic compound derived from lysergic acid; see LSD.

lysin (lī′sin): An antibody that has the capability of causing the dissolution of cells. See bacteriolysin, hemolysin.

lysine (lī′-sēn): An essential amino acid necessary for growth in infants and to maintain nitrogen balance in adults. Deficiency may cause nausea, dizziness, and anemia. It is destroyed by dry heating, *e.g.*, as in toasted bread and cereals such as puffed wheat.

lysinogen (lī-sin′-ō-jen): A substance that is capable of inducing the formation of lysins. Also spelled lysogen.

lysis (lī′-sis): 1. A gradual return to normal, used especially in relation to pyrexia. Opp., crisis. 2. Dissolution and disintegration of bacteria and cells by the action of a lysin. 3. Loosening of an organ from adhesions.—lytic, adj.

lysogen (lī′-sō-jen): See lysinogen.

lysogenicity (lī′sō-je-nis′i-ti): 1. The ability to produce lysins. 2. The ability of a bacterial organism to produce a phage (*q.v.*).

Lysol: Well-known disinfectant containing creosol in soap solution. It has a wide range of activity, but the preparation is toxic to humans and this limits its use to disinfection of excreta and inanimate objects.

lysosome (li′-sō-sōm): One of a group of minute, cytoplasmic, intracellular, digestive bodies having a single membrane and containing a large number of powerful enzymes; found in saliva, tears, egg white, and many animal tissues. Shock, sepsis, or trauma may cause lysosomes to break down and release the enzymes which may damage the cells and, consequently, are an important factor in such wasting diseases as muscular dystrophy.

lysozyme (lī′sō-zīm): A bacteriolytic enzyme present in tears, saliva, nasal mucus and many animal fluids; also found in egg white.

lyssic (lis′-ik): Pertaining to rabies.

lytic (lit′-ik): 1. Pertaining to lysis. 2. Producing lysis.

-lytic: A suffix denoting lysis. In pharmacology, it refers to the ability of a drug to block or inhibit the actions of the autonomic nervous system.

M

M: Abbreviation for: 1. Thousand. 2. Mixture. 3. Meter. 4. Molar. 5. Myopia.

m: Abbreviation for: 1. Minim (min. is preferred): 2. Meter (M is preferred).

μ: Symbol for micron; the Greek letter *mu*.

M.A.: Abbreviation for: 1. Mental age. 2. Master of Arts.

MAA: Medical Assistance to the Aged: The Kerr-Mills Bill, passed in 1960. Relates to federal assistance for care of the aged in nursing homes.

Macaca mulatta: The rhesus monkey; much used in physiologic experimentation.

maceration (mas-er-ā′-shun): The softening of a solid by moisture, *e.g.*, the softening of the horny layer of the skin by moisture around the toes in tinea pedis (*q.v.*). In obstetrics, term is applied to the changes in the tissues of a fetus that is retained in the uterus after it has died.—macerated, adj.; macerate, v.

Mackenrodt's ligament: The lateral cervical ligament of the uterus. [Alwin Karl Mackenrodt, German gynecologist. 1859–1925.]

macr-, macro-: Combining forms denoting 1) large size (opp. to micro-); 2) abnormally large, *e.g.*, macrocolon; 3) visible to the naked eye.

macrencephaly (mak′-ren-sef′-a-li): A condition in which the head and brain are abnormally large in relation to the rest of the body; a congenital anomaly. Also called macrencephalia.

macroaggregate (mak′rō-ag′rē-gāt): An unusually large accumulation of a substance.

macroamylase (mak′-rō-am′-i-lās): A blood serum amylase in which the molecules have a high molecular weight and a tendency to combine with molecules of other proteins in the blood serum, forming a complex too large for the kidney to excrete.

macroamylasemia (mak′rō-am′il-a-sē′mi-a): The presence of macroamylase in the blood.

macroangiopathy (mak′rō-an-ji-op′a-thi): Disease of the larger blood vessels.

macrobiosis (mak′rō-bī-ō′sis): Longevity.

macrobiotic (mak′rō-bī-ot′ik): 1. Having a long life. 2. Tending to prolong life. **M. DIET**, a diet that began to be popular in the 1960s that emphasizes whole grains and foods native to one's environment, with gradual elimination of highly refined foods, sugar, and dairy products; was thought to reduce blood pressure and cholesterol levels. Some nutritionists held that the diet was injurious to health. Also called Zen macrobiotic diet.

macroblast (mak′-rō-blast): An abnormally large nucleated red blood cell.

macroblepharia (mak′rō-ble-fā′ri-a): The condition of having unusually large eyelids.

macrocephalia (mak′rō-se-fā′li-a): The condition of having an excessively long or large head.—macrocephalic, macrocephalous, adj.

macrocheilia (mak-rō-kī′li-a): The condition of having abnormally large lips. Macrolabia.

macrocheiria (mak-rō-kī′ri-a): The condition of having unusually large hands. Also megalocheiria, chiromegaly, macrochiria.

macrocnemia (mak-rō-nē′-mi-a): Excessive development of the legs below the knees.

macrocyte (mak′-rō-sīt): A large red blood cell, found in the blood in some forms of anemia, especially pernicious anemia.—macrocytic, adj.

macrocythemia (mak′-ro-sī-thē′-mi-a): A condition characterized by the presence of unusually large numbers of macrocytes in the circulating blood. Macrocytosis.

macrodactyly (mak-rō-dak′-ti-li): Excessive development of the fingers or toes. Also called macrodactilia and megadactyly.

macrodrip (mak′rō-drip): An IV apparatus that delivers intravenous solutions, with the drops being larger than those in the microdrip, the drop size being regulated by the caliber of the delivery tubing.

macroencephaly (mak′rō-en-sef′a-li): See macrencephaly.

macroesthesia (mak′rō-es-thē′zi-a): A sensation that things seen or felt are larger than they really are.

macrogenesy (mak-rō-jen′-e-si): Gigantism.

macrogenitosomia (mak′-rō-jen-i-tō-sō′-mi-a): Excessive development of the body in general, and especially of the sex organs. When this occurs at an early age it is called **M. PRAECOX.**

macroglobulin (mak′ro-glob′ū-lin): A globulin (*q.v.*) of high molecular weight; found in blood in certain diseases, particularly those affecting the lymphoid plasma cells and the reticuloendothelial system. See reticuloendothelium.

macroglobulinemia (mak′rō-glob′ū-li-nē′mi-a): A condition characterized by an increase in macroglobulins in the blood. **WALDENSTRÖM'S M.**, a rare progressive syndrome involving the reticuloepithelial system; usually seen in elderly males; marked by an increase in macroglobulins and Bence-Jones proteins, adenopathy, splenomegaly, hepatomegaly, anemia, anorexia, plasmocytosis (*q.v.*) of the bone marrow, and neurological manifestations; in some patients it resembles cancer and may be fatal; cause unknown.

macroglossia (mak-rō-glos′-i- a): Abnormal enlargement of the tongue. Megaglossia.

macrognathia (mak-rō-nā′thi-a): Abnormal enlargement of the jaw. Megagnathia.

macrogyria (mak-rō-jī′-ri-a): A congenital anomaly in which the convolutions of the brain are greatly enlarged; often associated with mental retardation.

macrolides (mak′-rō-līdz): A class of antibiotics of the genus *Streptomyces;* erythromycin is one of them.

macromastia (mak-rō-mas′-ti-a): Abnormally large breasts.

macromolecule (mak′-rō-mol′-e-kūl): A molecule of very large size, as found in such substances as proteins, nucleic acids, and polysaccharides.

macrophage (mak′-rō-fāj): A large "wandering" phagocytic cell that ingests foreign matter; plays an important part in resisting infection and in the organization and repair of tissue.

macroplasia (mak-rō-plā′zi-a): Overgrowth of a tissue or part. Gigantism.

macropodia (mak-rō-pō′-di-a): Abnormally large feet.

macropsia (ma-krop′-si-a): A disorder of vision in which things appear larger than they really are.

macropthalmous (mak-rof-thal′mus): Having abnormally large eyes.

macroscopic (mak′rō-skop′-ik): Visible to the naked eye; gross. Opp. to microscopic.

macroscopy (ma-kros′-ko-pi): Examination with the naked eye.

macrosomia (mak-rō-sō′-mi-a): Abnormally large body size. Also megasomia.

macrosurgery (māk′-rō-ser′-jer-i): Surgery that can be performed without the use of a microscope or miniature instruments. Opp. of microsurgery (*q.v.*).

macrotia (mak-rō′-shi-a): Abnormal largeness of the external ear.

macula (mak′-ū-la): A spot or stain on a body tissue, not elevated but differentiated from surrounding tissue. **M. DENSA,** a dense collection of cells in the distal convoluted tubule of the nephron; its function is to regulate the reabsorption of sodium ions. **M. LUTEA,** the yellow spot on the retina, the area of clearest vision. **M. SOLARIS,** a sunspot; a freckle.—maculae, pl.; macular, adj.; maculation, n.

macular (mak′-ū-lar): 1. Of, or pertaining to the macula lutea of the retina. 2. Of, or pertaining to the presence of macules. **M. DEGENERATION,** irreversible loss of central vision due to pathological changes in the macula lutea causing a gradual loss of clear central vision; may occur early in life but usually starts at about age 60; may be due to trauma, atherosclerosis, or senility, in which case it increases with age and may lead to total blindness. Individuals at high risk appear to be those with blue eyes, farsightedness, cardiovascular disease, and lengthy exposure to sunlight. Early treatment is imperative; the laser beam has been used to seal off the affected area to prevent the spread of the disease.

macule (mak′-ūl): A small, circumscribed spot or stain on the skin, not raised above the skin surface; usually refers to an area up to 1 cm in diameter.—macular, adj.

maculopapular (mak′ū-lō-pap′ū-lar): The presence of macules and raised palpaple spots (papules) on the skin.

maculopathy (mak-ū-lop′-a-thi): Any disease or disorder of the macula lutea (*q.v.*).

mad hatter's disease: Mercurialism (*q.v.*).

madarosis (mad′-a-rō′-sis): Loss of eyelashes and/or eyebrows.

Madura foot: A fungus disease of the foot found in India and the tropics. Characterized by swelling and the development of nodules and sinuses from which there is a characteristic exudate containing granules that may be white, yellow, red, brown, orchid or black. See mycetoma.

maduromycosis (mad′ū-rō-mī-kō′sis): Madura foot (*q.v.*).

magic bullet: The term was first used in connection with the use of arsphenamine in treatment of syphilis; discovered by Ehrlich in 1909. Syn., salvarsan, Ehrlich's 606. **MAGIC BULLET METHOD,** the use of a specific drug in the study or treatment of a specific disease.

magma: 1. A substance made up of finely divided particles suspended in a small amount of fluid. 2. A paste-like substance or salve.

magnesium (mag-nē′-zi-um): A silvery metallic substance found in bone, muscle, and blood; considered essential to nutrition and growth. Present in many animal and vegetable foods; deficiency in the diet causes disturbance in bone development and irritability of the nervous system that may result in convulsions and tetany. Chemical symbol is Mg. **MAGNESIUM SULFATE,** small, colorless, bitter tasting crystals, soluble in water; used as a cathartic and anti-inflammatory; Epsom salt.

magnum (mag′-num): Large or great, as the foramen **M.** in the occipital bone.

Mahaim fibers: Fibrous connections between the atrioventricular node and the ventricular septum.

Mahoney, Mary: The first trained black nurse in America; an 1879 graduate of the New England Training School for Nurses, the first such school to be established in the U.S. A Mary

Mahoney medal is now granted by the American Nurses' Association.

maidenhead: The hymen.

maim (mām): To disable or wound by violence.

main (mān): Hand.

mainlining: Slang term used to describe the injection of a drug directly into a vein.

mal: Disease or disorder. **M. DE MER,** seasickness. **GRAND M.,** major epilepsy. **PETIT M.,** minor epilepsy.

mal-: Combining form denoting 1) ill, bad, badly, poor, poorly, inadequate; 2) abnormal, irregular.

mala (mā'-la): The cheek or cheek bone.—malar, adj.

malabsorption (mal'-ab-sorp'-shun): Inadequate or disordered absorption of nutrients from the intestinal canal. **M. SYNDROME,** refers to a group of disorders including giardiasis, Whipple's disease, cystic fibrosis of the pancreas, Hirschprung's disease, and adult onset sprue, which are characterized by malabsorption of essential nutrients including electrolytes, vitamins, iron, and calcium; symptoms include pallor, lassitude, anorexia, failure to gain weight, weakness, large foul-smelling stools, and diarrhea.

malac-, malaco-: Combining forms denoting a condition of abnormal softness or softening.

malacia (ma-lā'-shi-a): 1. Abnormal softening of a part. See keratomalacia, osteomalacia. 2. Abnormal craving for certain foods, especially spicy foods.

malacosteon (mal-a-kos'-tē-on): Old term for osteomalacia (*q.v.*).

maladaptation (mal'a-dap-tā'shun): The inability to make normal adjustments in personal relationships and in society, with resulting abnormal or antisocial behavior.

maladie de Roger: The murmur produced by ventricular septal defect; is most likely to be heard in children and disappears as the child matures and the defect corrects itself; Roger's disease.

maladjustment (mal'ad-just'ment): Bad or poor adjustment to environment socially, mentally, emotionally, or physically; often results in conflict-producing behavior.

malady (mal'-a-di): A disease, disorder or indisposition.

malaise (ma-lāz'): A feeling of discomfort and uneasiness; often a sign of developing disease or infection.

malalignment (mal'a-līn'ment): Faulty alignment, as of the teeth, or of a fracture.

malar (mā'-lar): Relating to the cheek. **M.** or **ZYGOMATIC BONE** forms the prominence of the cheek.

malaria (ma-lā'-ri-a): An infectious, febrile, tropical disease caused by one of the genus *Plasmodium,* and carried by mosquitoes of the genus *Anopheles.* Characterized by anemia, toxemia, splenomegaly, and intermittent paroxysms of fever, chills, and sweating that occur at intervals corresponding to the time it takes for a new generation of the parasites to develop in the blood. If the paroxysms occur every 24 hrs. the malaria is known as quotidian; if every 48 hrs. tertian; if every 72 hrs., quartan. Sometimes classified on the basis of occurrence as 1) unstable **M.,** in which the amount of transmission varies from year to year and epidemics are possible; and 2) stable, in which the amount of transmission is generally high and epidemics are likely. **ALGID M.,** a condition resembling surgical shock; the skin is pale, cold, clammy; the respirations are slow, pulse is weak, and blood pressure low; often fatal. **CEREBRAL M.,** falciparum **M.** caused by localization of the causative organism in the brain; symptoms include delirium and coma. **FALCIPARUM M.,** the most serious form of **M.,** caused by *Plasmodium falciparum;* often fatal. **THERAPEUTIC M.,** deliberately induced **M.,** a therapy formerly much used for its beneficial effects in treating other diseases, especially neurosyphilis; not commonly used since the advent of penicillin. **TRANSFUSION M.,** caused by transfusion of blood from a symptomless infected donor.

malariologist (ma-lā-ri-ol'o-jist): A person knowledgeable about or engaged in the study of malaria.

malariology (ma-lā-ri-ol'-ō-ji): The study of malaria.

malariotherapy (ma-lā-ri-ō-ther'a-pi): The introduction of hyperpyrexia by inoculation with a benign form of malaria. Formerly used in treatment of neurosyphilis and certain other affections. Pyretotherapy.

malassimilation (mal'a-sim-il-ā'shun): Poor or disordered assimilation.

malaxation (mal'-ak-sā'-shun): 1. A kneading maneuver in massage. 2. The act of kneading the materials to be made into pills or plasters.

maldigestion (mal'-dī-jes'-chun): Imperfect or disordered digestion.

maleness (māl'-nes): Anatomic and physiological characteristics that relate to a male person's procreative capacity.

malformation (mal'-fōr-mā'-shun): Abnormal or incorrect shape or structure; deformity.

malignancy (ma-lig'-nan-si): 1. Virulence. 2. A life-threatening disorder or neoplasm as opposed to a benign condition.

malignant (ma-lig'-nant): Virulent and dangerous; that which is likely to become progressively worse and to have a fatal termination. **M. GROWTH** or **TUMOR,** cancer or sarcoma. **M. HYPERTENISON,** see under hypertension. **M. PUSTULE,** anthrax.—malignancy, n.

malinger (ma-ling′er): To feign, induce, or deliberately prolong an illness or incapacitation to avoid work or a duty or to excite sympathy.—malingerer, n.; malingering, v.

malleolus (mal-lē′-ō-lus): A part or process of a bone shaped more or less like a hammer. **EXTERNAL M.**, the process at the lower end of the fibula. **INTERNAL M.**, the process at the lower end of the tibia.—malleoli, pl.; malleolar, adj.

malleus (mal′-ē-us): The hammer-shaped lateral bone of the middle ear.

Mallory-Weiss syndrome: The vomiting of blood or melena following prolonged vomiting, hiccups, or coughing; due to small lacerations in the gastric mucosa or submucosa, most often near the junction of the esophagus and the stomach. Also called Mallory-Weiss tear.

Mallory's bodies: 1. Round or ovoid hyalin inclusion bodies found in the cytoplasm of some of the degenerated cells of the liver in certain nutritional disorders of the liver. 2. Bodies found in the lymph spaces and epidermal cells in some cases of scarlet fever.

malnutrition (mal-nū-trish′-un): The state of being poorly nourished. May be caused by inadequate food or of one of the essential nutrients, by malassimilation, or by a metabolic defect that prevents the body from utilizing nutrients properly.

malocclusion (mal′o-kloo′zhun): Failure of the upper and lower teeth to meet properly when the jaws are closed.

malodorous (mal-ō′-dor-us): Having an offensive or unpleasant odor.

malpighian (mal-pig′-i-an): 1. **M. CORPUSCLES** or **CAPSULES**, the renal glomeruli with Bowman's capsule enclosing them (see glomerulus). 2. Name given to certain small lymphoid bodies or patches distributed throughout the spleen. [Marcello Malpighi, Italian anatomist, founder of microscopic anatomy. 1628–1694.]

malposition (mal-pō-zish′-un): Any abnormal position of a part.

malpractice (mal′-prak′-tis): In health care, the failure of a health care professional to meet the accepted standards of care for professionals licensed to practice in a specific area, or the committment by a health care professional of acts considered improper, negligent, or injurious to another; referred to as unethical **M.** when the misconduct involves actions or behavior that is considered improper or immoral, and criminal **M.** when the action or behavior involved is criminal in nature.

malpresentation (mal′-prē-zen-tā′-shun): 1. Any unusual presentation of the fetus in the pelvis. 2. Abnormal or faulty position of the body or any part of it.

malrotation (mal′-rō-tā′-shun): 1. Abnormal position of the child at birth, making natural delivery difficult or impossible. 2. A developmental anomaly in which the intestine becomes fixed to the mesentery in an abnormal way.

Malta fever: See Brucella, brucellosis.

maltase (mawl′-tās): A sugar-splitting (saccharolytic) enzyme found in the body, especially in intestinal juice.

malthusian (mal-thū′-zi-an): Refers to the theory that populations tend to increase faster than their means of subsistence, unless intentionally checked and controlled. [Thomas Malthus, English economist. 1766–1834.]—malthusianism, n.

maltose (mawl′-tōs): Malt sugar, a disaccharide; produced by the hydrolysis of starch during digestion.

malunion (mal-ūn′-yon): Union of a fracture in faulty position.

mamma (mam′-a): The breast; milk-secreting gland.—mammae, pl., mammary, adj.

mammal (mam′-al): An individual belonging to the highest class of vertebrates; including man; a warm-blooded animal, usually hairy, that suckles its young.—mammalian, adj.

mammary (mam′-e-ri): Pertaining to the breasts. **M. GLAND**, the specialized tuboalveolar glands of the female breast that secrete milk.

mammectomy (mam-mek′-to-mi): Surgical removal of one or both breasts; mastectomy.

mammilla (ma-mil′-a): 1. The nipple. 2. A small papilla or nipple-like structure.—mammillae, pl.; mammillated, mammillary, adj.

mammilliplasty (mam-mil′i-plas-ti): Plastic reconstruction of a nipple and areola.—Syn., theleplasty.

mammillitis (mam′il-ī′tis): Inflammation of the nipple.

mammitis (mam-ī′-tis): Mastitis (*q.v.*).

mammogenesis (mam-mō-jen′-e-sis): The development of the mammary glands of the breast to their functional state.

mammogram (mam′-ō-gram): A roentgenogram of the breast.

mammography (mam-og′-ra-fi): X-ray examination of the breast after injection of an opaque agent. **ULTRASOUND M.**, a technique used in breast examination that does not require the use of x ray; said to be 80 to 90 percent accurate in determining whether a lesion is present. Syn., mastography.—mammographic, adj., mammographically, adv.

mammoplasty (mam′-ō-plas-ti): An operation to correct pendulous or sagging breasts; skin and glandular tissue is removed and the glands are fixed in their ordinary position. **AUGMENTATION M.**, plastic surgery to increase the size and shape of the breast.

mammose (mam′ōs, ma′mōs): Having large breasts.

mammotropic (mam-ō-trōp′-ik): 1. Having an effect on the breast. 2. Having a stimulating effect on the mammary gland.

mammotropin (mam-o-trō-pin): The lactogenic hormone; old term for prolactin.

mandible (man′-dib′l): The lower jawbone.—mandibular, adj.

mandibulectomy (man-dib′-ū-lek′-tō-mi): Surgical removal of the mandible.

mandibulofacial (man-dib′-ū-lō-fā′-shul): Pertaining to the mandible and some other parts of the face. **M. DYSOSTOSIS,** a hereditary disorder characterized by underdevelopment of the mandible and zygoma, defects of the ear, abnormally large mouth, and downward slant of the angles of the eyelids, giving a person a peculiar, fish-like appearance. Also called Treacher-Collins syndrome.

maneuver (man-nū′-ver): 1. A skillful procedure or act. 2. Special movement or procedure, using the hand or an instrument for a specific purpose. See Heimlich maneuver, Leopold's maneuvers, and Valsalva's maneuver.

manganese (mang′-ga-nēs): A metallic element that resembles iron and is often associated with it in ores; some of its salts are used in medicine.

mania (mā′-ni-a): A mood disorder that occurs as one phase in major affective disorders, bipolar disorders in particular, and in certain organic mental disorders such as dementia and delirium; characterized by undue elation and excitement, pronounced psychomotor activity, flight of ideas, talkativeness, anger, and destructiveness. **M. Á POTU,** delirium tremens; a pathologic intoxication in which the patient has hallucinations following alcoholic intake, remains unconscious, and often attempts suicide; may lead to schizophrenia.

-mania: Formerly denoted any kind of madness. Currently used to denote a morbid preoccupation with some idea or activity, or a compulsive need to carry out a certain kind of behavior.

maniac (mā′-ni-ak): A person affected with mania (*q.v.*). A person who is insane or violently disturbed.—maniacal, adj.

manic (man′-ik): Pertaining to or affected with mania (*q.v.*).

manic-depressive: Refers to a serious mental illness characterized by a cyclic, recurring pattern of short periods of mania alternating with longer periods of depression.

manikin (man′-i-kin): A model of the human body, used in teaching anatomy and also for demonstrating and teaching nursing procedures.

manipulation (ma-nip′ū-lā′shun): 1. In medicine, using the hands skillfully, as in reducing a fracture, dislocation, or changing the fetal position. 2. In physical therapy, the movement of a joint beyond the limit to which the individual can move it voluntarily. 3. A means of influencing others' behavior; methods may be overt or covert.

manipulative (ma-nip′-ū-lā-tiv): Usually refers to an individual who tries to control the behavior of others in order to meet his or her own needs and desires regardless of the others' needs and desires; sometimes seen in psychiatric patients.

mannerism (man′-er-izm): A way of speaking, acting, or behaving that is unusual or peculiar, and characterizes a particular person.

mannitol (man′-i-tol): An alcohol derived from manna and other plant sources; has various uses in medicine, especially in kidney disorders, when it may be used in kidney-function testing and as an osmotic diuretic.

manometer (ma-nom′-e-ter): An instrument for measuring the pressure exerted by liquids or gases or the tension of blood vessels. See sphygmomanometer.

Mantoux test (man-too′): A test for tuberculosis; a minute amount of diluted tuberculin (PPD) (*q.v.*) is injected intradermally. If the person has, or has had tuberculosis, hyperemia and a wheal will develop at the site of the injection. See tuberculin.

manual (man′-ū-al): Related to or involving use of the hands. **M. EXPRESSION OF URINE,** pressure on the abdominal wall at regular intervals to assist the patient to void when the bladder is paralyzed because of an interruption in the spinal cord. **M. THERAPY,** treatment performed by the hands *e.g.*, massage, manipulation. **M. TRACTION,** see under traction.

manubrium (ma-nū′-bri-um): A handle-shaped structure; the upper part of the breast bone or sternum.

manus (mā′-nus): The hand, including the fingers.

MAO inhibitors: See under monoamine oxidase.

maple bark disease: A type of pneumonitis caused by the spores of a mold found under the bark of maple logs.

maple syrup urine disease: A familial metabolic disorder, of unknown origin, with urine smelling of maple syrup, and with involvement of the central nervous system, sometimes resulting in mental subnormality. Usually fatal within the first few months of life.

marantic (ma-ran′-tik): Pertaining to or resembling marasmus (*q.v.*).

marasmus (mar-az′-mus): Wasting away of the body, especially that of a baby, without apparent cause.—marasmic, adj.

marble bones: Osteopetrosis (*q.v.*).

marche à petits pas (marsh′ah-ptē′-′pa): A slow, uncertain gait with small steps, usually with a slightly flexed posture, seen mostly in the aged who are senile.

Marchiafava-Bignami disease: A degenerative disorder involving the corpus callosum; occurs chiefly in persons who drink excessive amounts of red wine.

Marchiafava-Micheli's syndrome: Paroxysmal nocturnal hemoglobinuria; see under hemoglobinuria.

Marcus Gunn phenomenon: An hereditary condition of the upper eyelids in which chewing motions or opening the mouth cause an exaggerated elevation of the upper lids, and ptosis when the mouth is closed. Also called jaw-winking syndrome.

Marfan's syndrome: Hereditary congenital disorder of unknown cause. There is dislocation of the optic lens, congenital heart disease, and arachnodactyly, with hypotonic musculature and lax ligaments, occasionally excessive height, and abnormalities of the iris. [B.J.A. Marfan, French physician. 1858–1942.]

margin: An edge or border, as of an organ or structure.—marginal, adj.

marihuana, marijuana (mar-i-wah′-na): Cannabis (*q.v.*).

marmorization (mar′mo-rī-zā′shun): A marble-like mottling of the skin. See cutis marmorata, under cutis.

marrow: See bone marrow.

Marshall-Marchetti operation: A procedure that fixes the urethra to the back of the pubic bone; one treatment for stress incontinence.

marsupialization (mar-sū′pi-a-lī-zā′shun): The surgical creation of a pouch by evacuating a cyst and exterioralizing it by suturing the cyst walls to the cut edges of the skin, which heals by granulation, thus creating a pouch.

masculine (mas′-kū-lin): The qualities and role behavior that are considered characteristic of a male person, *e.g.*, strength, manliness, vigor, virility.

masculinize (mas′-kū-lin-īz): To confer or produce so called male characteristics in a female.—masculinization, n.

MASH: Abbreviation for Mobile Army Surgical Hospital.

mask: 1. A covering for the nose and mouth, sometimes the entire face, used to protect either the wearer or a patient, to prevent the inhalation of toxic substances or pathogenic organisms, or to administer oxygen or other medications in gas form. 2. An expression characteristic of a certain disorder or condition. AEROSOL M., a M. similar to a face M. but which has a nebulizing attachment that humidifies the inspired air. PARKINSON'S MASK, a fixed expression with staring and infrequent winking; characteristic of patients with Parkinson's disease. M. OF PREGNANCY, a brownish patchy discoloration on the face and neck; occurs during pregnancy and disappears after delivery. SURGICAL M., a mouth and nose mask worn by operating room personnel to deflect the air from the nose and mouth and filter out any droplets that may contain pathogenic organisms; also worn for self-protection by those caring for patients with communicable disease. VENTURI M., a M. that delivers precise fixed concentrations of oxygen.

masochism (mas′-ō-kizm): A form of sexual perversion in which one has a pathological desire to inflict pain upon oneself or to suffer pain, abuse, or humiliation at the hands of another. Opp. of sadism. [Leopold von Sacher-Masoch, Austrian historian. 1836–1895.]

masochist (mas′-ō-kist): One who derives sexual pleasure from humiliation, pain, or abuse inflicted by another.

mass: 1. A lump. 2. A mixture so prepared that it can be made up into pills.

massage (mas-sahzh′): Physical therapy that consists of manipulating the tissues of the body by the use of friction, stroking, kneading, etc. CARDIAC M., see under cardiac. CAROTID ARTERY M., a procedure sometimes used for patients with paroxysmal atrial tachycardia; gentle pressure in small circular motion is applied to one carotid artery for a short period of time.

masseter (mas-sē′-ter): The chief muscle of mastication; situated at the side of the face. It raises the lower jaw.

masseur (ma-ser′): A man who gives massage.

masseuse (mas-sūz′): A woman who gives massage.

massotherapy (mas′-sō-ther′-a-pi): Treatment by massage.

MAST: Abbreviation for military antishock trousers (*q.v.*).

mast cell: A large, round or ovoid, plump, granulated cell normally found in connective tissues; specific function undetermined; thought to contain heparin, histamine, bradykinin, and serotonin.

mast-, masto-: Combining forms denoting: 1. The breast. 2. The mastoid process.

mastadenoma (mast-ad-e-nō′ma): A benign tumor of the breast.

mastalgia (mas-tal′-ji-a): Pain in the breast.

mastatrophia (mas-ta-trō′-fi-a): Atrophy or shrinking of the breasts.

mastectomy (mas-tek′-to-mi): Surgical removal of the breast. ADENOMASTECTOMY, subcutaneous M. MODIFIED RADICAL M., one in which part of the pectoralis major or minor is preserved. RADICAL M., removal of the breast with the overlying skin and underlying pectoral muscles, together with the axillary lymph nodes; combined with radiotherapy, this operation is a common type of therapy for carcinoma of the breast. SIMPLE M., removal of the breast only with the overlying skin. **SUBCUTANEOUS M.**, involves removing all of the breast tissue and usually some of the axilla but leaves the breast skin and sometimes the areola; a silicone prosthesis may be inserted during surgery or later. **SUPERRADICAL M.**, in addition to the procedure for a radical **M.** the sternum is split and the lymph nodes in the mediastinum are also removed. **TOTAL M.**, removal of the breast and axillary lymph nodes, leaving the pectoral muscles intact.

Master's two-step exercise test: A stress test for coronary insufficiency; the patient makes two steps, each 9 inches high, for a predetermined length of time while connected to a monitor that records heart rate and rhythm; useful in determining the patient's capacity for exercise.

mastication (mas-ti-kā'-shun): The act of chewing food.

masticatory (mas'-ti-ka-tō-ri): Pertaining to mastication. 1. A medication to be chewed. 2. An agent affecting the muscles of mastication. **M. SPASM OF THE FACE,** trismus (*q.v.*).

mastitis (mas-tī'-tis): Inflammation of the mammary gland, common in nursing women; characterized by fever, chills, lethargy, pain on palpation; usually caused by a staphylococcus. **CHRONIC CYSTIC M.**, the name formerly applied to nodular and cystic changes in the breast, now usually called fibrocystic disease of the breast. **M. NEONATORUM,** any of several abnormal conditions of the breast in the newborn, including hypertrophy, inflammation, engorgement with secretion, abscess formation.

mastocarcinoma (mas'-tō-kar-si-nō'-ma): Carcinoma of the breast.

mastocytoma (mas'-tō-sī-tō'-ma): A nodular, circumscribed accumulation of mast cells that resembles a neoplasm.

mastocytosis (mas'-tō-sī-tō'sis): Excessive local or systemic proliferation and accumulation of mast cells in the tissues. The systemic form is marked by urticaria pigmentosa (*q.v.*) and may involve the spleen, liver, lymph nodes, bones, digestive system.

mastodynia (mas-tō-din'-i-a): Pain in the breast.

mastography (mas-tog'-ra-fi): See mammography.—mastographic, adj.

mastoid (mas'-toyd): 1. Nipple-shaped. 2. Pertaining to the **M.** process, antrum, cells, etc. **M. CELLS,** small intercommunicating cavities in the mastoid process that empty into the mastoid antrum. **M. ANTRUM,** the air space within the mastoid process, lined by mucous membrane continuous with that of the tympanum and mastoid cells. **M. PROCESS,** the rounded prominence on the mastoid portion of the temporal bone just behind the ear.

mastoidectomy (mas-toy-dek'-to-mi): Drainage of the mastoid air cells and excision of diseased mastoid tissue.

mastoiditis (mas-toy-dī'-tis): Inflammation of any part of the mastoid process; usually the result of an extension of a middle ear infection.

mastoidotomy (mas-toy-dot'-o-mi): Incision into the mastoid process of the temporal bone.

mastoptosis (mas-to-tō'-sis): Sagging or ptosis of the breasts.

masturbation (mas-tur-bā'-shun): Self-stimulation of the genital organs, manually or by other contact, but not sexual intercourse, usually resulting in orgasm.

match test: A rough test of respiratory function. If a person is unable to blow out a lighted match held four inches from a fully open mouth, there is significant reduction of respiratory function.

mater (mā'-ter): The latin word for mother. **DURA M.**, the fibrous outer covering of the brain and spinal cord. **PIA M.**, the vascular delicate membrane that immediately invests the brain and spinal cord. Between it and the dura **M.** lies the arachnoid (*q.v.*).

materia medica (ma-tēr'i-a med'i-ka): The science dealing with the origin, preparation, action, and dosage of drugs.

maternal (ma-ter'-nal): Pertaining to the female parent.

maternity (ma-ter'-ni-ti): Motherhood.

Maternity Center Association: A nonprofit organization, founded in 1918; devoted to improved maternity care; conducts research and educational programs for nurses, childbirth educators, and expectant couples; conducts demonstration projects in home delivery; promotes family-centered care; publishes materials on childbirth education, including *A Baby is Born,* and *Briefs,* a monthly magazine. Address, 48 E. 92nd St., New York NY 10028.

mate' (ma-tā'): A medication prepared from the dried leaves of a South American tree; contains caffeine and tannins; used as a laxative, tonic, diuretic, and stimulant.

matriarchy (mā'-tri-ark-i): A social system in which inheritance is traced through the female line; often the family life is dominated by the wife, mother, or other significant female who also has priority in certain other areas such as inheritance of property.

matrix (mā'-triks): The foundation substance in which the tissue cells are embeded. The basic material from which a thing develops.

matter: 1. Any material substance that occupies space and has weight. 2. Pus; material discharged from a suppurative process. **GRAY M.**, found in the cortex of the brain; composed mainly of nerve cell bodies and unmyelinated nerve fibres. **INORGANIC M.**, substances that are not living and never have been. **ORGANIC M.**, substances that are or have been alive. **WHITE M., M.** composed mostly of myelinated nerve fibers; the conducting tissues of the brain and spinal cord.

maturation (mat ū-rā'shun): The process of attaining full development and maturity.—maturate, v.

mature (ma-tūr'): To be fully developed, or to reach full development; to ripen.

maturity (ma-tūr' -i-ti): The state of completed growth or ripeness.

Mauer's dots: Characteristic coarse reddish dots seen in erythrocytes infected with *Plasmodium falciparum*.

maxilla (mak-sil' -a): The jawbone; in particular the upper jaw.—maxillary, adj.; maxillae, pl.

maxillary (mak' -si-ler-i): Pertaining to the maxilla. **M. SINUS,** either of a pair of large air cells that form a pyramidal cavity in the maxilla; lined with mucous membrane that is continuous with that of the nasal cavity.

maxillectomee (mak-si-lek' -tō-mē): A person who has undergone a maxillectomy.

maxillectomy (mak-sil-ek' -tō-mi): Partial or complete removal of the upper jaw.

maxillofacial (mak-sil-ō-fā'shal): Pertaining to the maxilla and the face. A subdivision in plastic surgery.

maximum (mak' -si-mum): The largest; utmost; the greatest possible size, quantity, value or degree.—maximal, adj.

maze: A labyrinth consisting of blind alleys and one correct path, used in the study of animal and human learning processes.

mazoplasia (mā-zō-plā' -zi-a): Degenerative hyperplasia of the acini of the breast. See acini.

MBD: Abbreviation for: 1. Minimal brain damage. 2. Minimal brain dysfunction.

McArdle's disease: Glycogen storage disease, Type V; most commonly seen in adults; characterized by pain, fatigability, and stiffness of muscles following exertion.

McBurney's point: A point about one-third of the way between the anterior superior iliac spine and the umbilicus, the site of maximum tenderness in cases of acute appendicitis. [Charles McBurney, American surgeon. 1845–1913.]

MCCU: Mobile Coronary Care Unit: A specially equipped vehicle, available on an emergency basis; manned by personnel trained to detect heart failure, carry out cardiopulmonary resuscitation at the site of the attack, and to transfer the patient safely to a hospital.

McDowell's operation: The operation for removal of an ovarian cyst through an abdominal incision. Named for the surgeon who first performed it in 1809. [Ephraim McDowell, American surgeon. 1771–1830.]

mcg: Abbreviation for microgram.

MCH: Abbreviation for Maternal and Child Health.

McMurray's test: A test involving rotation of the tibia on the femur; diagnostic for tears in the meniscus of the knee joint.

M.D: Abbreviation for Doctor of Medicine.

Meals-on-Wheels: A community service often provided by churches and private agencies for those who cannot do their own food shopping or cooking.

measles (mē' -zlz): Rubeola. Morbilli. An acute, highly contagious, febrile, exanthematous viral disease; spread by droplets; characterized by fever, a blotchy rash, and catarrhal inflammation of the mucous membranes; associated with a high rate of complications. Endemic and worldwide in distribution. See Koplik's spots and German measles (rubella).

meatotomy (mē-a-tot' -o-mi): An operation for enlarging the external urethral opening; sometimes done on infants with hypospadias (*q.v.*)

meatus (mē-ā' -tus): An opening or channel, usually referring to the external opening of a passageway into or out of the body. **AUDITORY M.,** the external opening into the auditory canal; also called external acoustic **M. URINARY M.,** the external orifice of the urethra; situated at the end of the penis in the male and between the clitoris and the vagina in the female.—meati, pl.

mechanical lift: A device for moving heavy, disabled, or helpless persons from bed to chair, toilet, etc.; consists of a frame, a source of hydraulic power, various levers, and supportive straps. See Hoyer patient lifter.

mechanoreceptors (mek' -an-ō-rē-sep'tors): Receptors that are sensitive to differences in pressure, such as those experienced through the sense of touch or hearing.

mechanotherapy (mek' -an-ō-ther'-a-pi): The treatment of disease by the use of various kinds of mechanical apparatus, especially as in physiotherapeutics.

Meckel's diverticulum (mek'els dī-ver-tik'ū-lum): A blind, pouch-like sac sometimes arising from the free border of the ileum. It may be 2 to 3 in. in length and is a remnant of the duct which, in the embryo, connects the yolk sac with the primitive alimentary canal. [Johann Friedrich Meckel, German anatomist and gynecologist. 1781–1833.]

meconium (mē-kō'ni-um): The discharge from the bowel of a newly born baby. It is greenish-black, viscid, and contains epithelial cells, mucus, and bile. **M. ASPIRATION SYNDROME,** characterized by severe asphyxia resulting from failure of the lungs to expand at birth because of the presence of aspirated meconium in the trachea or lungs; aspiration of meconium in utero is thought to be due to hypoxia. **M. ILEUS,** obstruction in the ileum of the newborn caused by impaction of unusually thick tenacious meconium; may be the earliest sign of cystic fibrosis; also called meconium plug syndrome.

MED: Abbreviation for: 1. Minimal effective dose. 2. Minimal erythema dose.

Medex: Any one of the health care programs based on the one originally designed for military corpsmen. Three variations now exist; all require a certain amount of time spent in study of the care of the sick, and a preceptorship or internship.

media (mē′-di-a): 1. In anatomy, the middle coat of an artery. 2. Plural of medium (*q.v.*).

mediad (mē′-di-ad): Toward the middle; toward a median line or plane of the body.

medial (mē′-di-al): Pertaining to or near the middle.—medially, adv.

median (mē′-di-an): The middle. **M. LINE,** an imaginary line passing through the center of the body from a point between the eyes to between the closed feet. In statistics, the value midway in a distribution of frequencies, that is, half of the observations fall above and half below the median value. **M. NERVE,** runs down the inner side and middle of the arm; innervates the flexor muscles of the wrist and hand.

mediastinal (mē′-di-as-tī′-nal): Pertaining to the mediastinum. **M. SHIFT,** a complication of certain respiratory conditions and of sucking wounds of the chest; because inspired air cannot escape, the intrapleural pressure builds up, the lung collapses, and the heart and great vessels shift to the side of decreased pressure; may lead to shock.

mediastinitis (mē′-di-as-ti-nī′-tis): Inflammation of the mediastinum.

mediastinoperidarditis (mē′-di-as-tī′-nō-per′-i-kar-dī′-tis): Inflammation of the pericardium and its surrounding mediastinal tissues.

mediastinoscope (me′di-as-tī′-nō-skōp): An instrument used in direct visual examination of the tissues in the mediastinal area.

mediastinoscopy (mē′di-as-tī-nos′kō-pi): Examination of the mediastinum by means of a tubular instrument which makes it possible to directly view the tissues of the area and to take tissue for biopsy.

mediastinum (mē-di-as-tī′- num): The space between the lungs; bounded by the lungs on either side, the sternum in front, the vertebrae in back, and the diaphragm at the bottom; contains all the organs of the chest except the lungs, *i.e.*, the heart, great vessels, and the esophagus.—mediastinal, adj.

Medicaid: Essentially, a health care insurance program for the poor, inaugurated along with Medicare (*q.v.*). It is organized as a federal-state partnership and is funded by local, state, and federal tax revenues; each state designs and administers its own program, consequently there is considerable variation in services covered and benefits offered. In general, Medicaid pays the cost of hospitalization, outpatient hospital care, laboratory tests and x-ray studies, nursing home care for those over 21, and physicians' services; the various states also provide coverage for several other health care services.

medical (med′-i-kal): Pertinent to medicine or the treatment of disease. **M. JURISPRUDENCE,** the application of medical science and facts to legal problems. Forensic medicine.

Medical Center: A care facility that differs from a community hospital in that it is usually larger, has a house staff, sponsors and conducts research, and is usually connected with a medical school and thus is a teaching hospital.

medical examiner: A public officer who performs postmortem examinations of bodies to determine the cause of death.

medical laboratory technician: A person who works in a pathological laboratory testing and analyzing specimens of body tissue, fluids, or excretions. A medical technologist.

medical social worker: A health care professional who is concerned with social aspects of illness; assists patients with many practical problems that may influence their emotional states and affect the course of their illnesses, treatments, and recovery.

Medic-Alert: An identification bracelet or necklace worn by persons with specific medical problems; inscription includes telephone number of a central office that has pertinent information about the person. Available from Medic-Alert Foundation, Inc., Turlock CA 95308, or from some local drug-stores; costs $10-25 depending on the metal used.

medicalization (med′-i-kal-ī-zā′ shun): Refers to a health care system that emphasizes inpatient services and the sick role; patients may be hospitalized longer than necessary, and subjected to tests and procedures that may or may not be required for diagnosis or effective therapy.

medicament (med′-i-ka-ment): A remedy or medicine.

Medicare: A federal assistance program inaugurated in 1965 by amendment to the Social Security Act (1935) which provides insurance for hospitalization and certain other health care services for nearly all people over 65 who qualify for Social Security and for certain others under 65 who qualify as disabled. Part of the program is financed by the Social Security system and part by general tax revenues; it is administered by 50 Blue Cross/Blue Shield state organizations; they determine the benefits and make payments which are the same throughout the U.S. Part A provides insurance coverage for a portion of short-term hospital bills (not including private rooms or private duty nursing costs) and for skilled care at home if the patient is housebound. Not covered are housekeeping services or custodial care. Part B is elective and available to most individuals over 65 who qualify for Social Security in return for a specified monthly payment; it provides insurance coverage for necessary physicians' fees and a certain percentage of outpatient hospital service.

medicate (med'i-kāt): 1. To impregnate with a drug or medicine. 2. To treat disease by administering a drug or drugs.—medicated, adj.

medication (med-i-kā'-shun): 1. Administration of a medicine or remedy. 2. A medicinal substance or agent. **HYPODERMIC M.**, one given by hypodermic under the skin. **ORAL M.**, a **M.**, given by mouth. **SUBLINGUAL M.**, one placed under the tongue and allowed to dissolve before it is swallowed.

medicinal (me-dis'-i-nal): 1. Pertaining to a medicine. 2. Having healing or curing effects or properties.

medicine (med'-i-sin): 1. The science or art of treating or preventing disease. 2. That branch of the healing art that deals with the treatment of disease by the administration of internal remedies as distinguished from such specialties as surgery. 3. A drug. 4. A therapeutic agent.

medicolegal (med'-i-kō-lē'-gal): Term referring to legal problems arising in the practice of medicine; *e.g.*, problems that may be associated with such procedures as therapeutic abortion, or those that may arise in the treatment of minors or mentally incompetent persons.

medionecrosis (mē'-di-ō-nē-krō'-sis): Necrosis of the tunica media of an artery.

meditation: TRANSCENDENTAL M., an exercise in contemplative relaxation that induces changes in physiological functions including lowered metabolic rate, reduced oxygen consumption, decreased cardiac output, and altered brain wave activity, and resulting in a feeling of exaltation and well-being.

Mediterranean fever: See Brucella, brucellosis.

medium (mē'-di-um): A substance used in bacteriology for the growth of organisms.—media, pl.

MEDLARS: Medical Literature Analysis and Retrieval System; the computerized literature retrieval center of the National Library of Medicine which is part of the National Institutes of Health. Persons studying or working in the health sciences have access to the professional literature through any of eleven access centers in the U.S. or any of twelve located in other countries. MEDLARS contains approximately four and a half million references to books and journal articles in the health sciences that have been published since 1965. Information can be obtained for use of the service from the Office of Inquiries and Publications Management, National Library of Medicine, 8600 Rockville Pike, Bethesda, MD 20014.

MEDLINE: A telephone library service that is linked with a computer retrieval system that can furnish, in a short period of time, a printout of literature related to health; gives access to all medical and nursing journals in the National Library of Medicine in Bethesda, Maryland, and to biomedical articles published during a current year and contained in the monthly and annual editions of *Index Medicus*.

medulla (me-dul'a): 1. The marrow in the center of a long bone. 2. The soft, internal portion of glands, as distinguished from the outer part, as seen in the kidneys, adrenals, lymph nodes, etc. **M. OBLONGATA**, the upper part of the spinal cord between the foramen magnum of the occipital bone and the pons varolii; contains the automatic control centers for breathing, arterial blood pressure, and vomiting.—medullary, adj.

medullary (med'-ū-lar-i): Pertaining to 1) a medulla; 2) bone marrow; or 3) the medulla oblongata. **M. CANAL**, the central cavity of a long bone; contains yellow bone marrow.

medullated (med'-ū-lā-ted): Containing or surrounded by a covering or sheath, particularly referring to nerve fibers.

medulloblastoma (med'-u-lō-blas-tō'-ma): A malignant, rapidly growing tumor, seen mostly in children; usually appears in the midline of the cerebellum obstructing the flow of cerebrospinal fluid through the fourth ventricle and producing hydrocephalus.

meg-, mega-, megal-, megalo-: Combining forms denoting great size, powerful, enlarged. Mega denotes one million units (metric system).

megacephalic (meg'-a-se-fal'- ik): Large-headed. Syn., macrocephalic, megalocephalic.

megacolon (meg'-a-kō'-lon): A condition of dilated and elongated colon; most common in males. In an adult the cause is unknown. In a child, the parasympathetic ganglion cells are absent in the distal part of the colon; Hirschprung's disease (*q.v.*). Also called congenital **M.** and aganglionic **M.**

megacurie (meg-a-kū'-ri): A unit of radioactivity; 1,000,000 curies (*q.v.*). Abbreviated Mc.

megaesophagus (meg'-a-ē-sof'-a-gus): A markedly dilated or enlarged esophagus; see achalasia.

megakaryocyte (meg'-a-kar'-i-ō-sīt): Giant multinucleated cells in the bone marrow from which the mature blood platelets originate.

megalencephaly (meg′-a-len-sef′-a-li): Having an abnormally enlarged head.

megaloblast (meg′-a-lō-blast): A large, nucleated, primitive red blood cell.—megaloblastic, adj.

megalocardia (meg′-a-lō-kar′-di-a): Cardiomegally (*q.v.*).

megalocephalic (meg′al-ō-se-fal′ik): See megacephalic.

megalocornea (meg′a-lō-kor′nē-a): An unusually large cornea; a developmental anomaly which may be inherited. Usually bilateral; present at birth.

megalokaryocyte (meg′a-lō-kar′i-ō-sīt): Megakaryocyte (*q.v.*).

megalomania (meg′-a-lō-mā′ni-a): Delusions of grandeur or self-importance, characteristic of general paralysis of the insane. See general.

megalopsia (meg-a-lop′-si-a): Macropsia (*q.v.*).

megaloureter (meg′-a-lō-ū-rē′-ter): An enlarged dilated ureter. Also called megaureter.

megaphonia (meg-a-fō′-ni-a): Abnormal loudness of the voice.

megavitamin (meg-a-vī′-ta-min): Usually refers to a type of therapy characterized by the administration of massive doses of vitamins.

meibomian (mī-bō′-mi-an): **M. GLANDS,** sebaceous glands lying in grooves on the inner surface of the eyelids, their ducts opening on the free margins of the lids. **M. CYST,** chalazion (*q.v.*). [Heinrich Meibom, German anatomist. 1638-1700.]

Meig's syndrome (meg′-zes): Benign, solid ovarian tumor or other pelvic tumor, associated with hydroperitoneum and hydrothorax. [Joe V. Meigs, American surgeon. 1892–1963].

meiosis (mī-ō′-sis): 1. The division occurring in the last two stages of cell division in the maturation of sex cells when the cell bodies divide twice but the chromosomes separate from each other only once, thus halving the number in the mature cells. 2. Constriction of the pupil as a result of contraction of the ciliary muscle. Also spelled miosis.

Meissner's corpuscles: Important receptors for the sense of touch; consist of elongated bodies enclosing the terminal ends of several afferent nerve fibers; lie just beneath the epidermis. Most numerous on the finger tips, palms of the hands and soles of the feet, tip of the tongue, and in the skin around the mouth and nipples. Sensitive to light touch and pressure. Also called Wagner-Meissner corpuscles.

mel-; melo-: Combining forms denoting: 1. An extremity or limb. 2. Cheek.

melan-, menano-: Combining forms denoting 1) melanin; 2) black, dark.

melancholia (mel-an-kō′-li-a): Extremely unhappy state, usually accompanied by inhibition of mental and physical activity. In psychiatry the term is reserved to mean severe forms of depression.—melancholic, adj. **INVOLUTIONAL M.,** a major affective disorder, chiefly of the middle-aged and elderly; marked by anxiety, agitation, insomnia, feelings of guilt and hypochondria.

melanemesis (mel-a-nem′-e-sis): Black vomit.

melanin (mel′-a-nin): A dark brown or black pigment found normally in hair, skin, choroid and retina of the eye, pia mater, cardiac muscle, and in some tumors. Accounts for racial differences in skin color.

melanism (mel′-a-nizm): Excessive deposit of pigment in tissues or the skin.

melanization (mel-a-nī-zā′-shun): The formation and deposition of melanin in the body tissues or organs.

melanocarcinoma (mel′-a-nō-kar-si-nō′-ma): A malignant tumor believed to be of epithelial origin. A malignant melanoma (*q.v.*).

melanocyte (mel′a-nō-sit, me-lan′-): A pigment-containing cell located between the epidermis and dermis; is responsible for the synthesis of melanin and provides for different colors of the skin, as yellow, brown, black.

melanoderma (mel′-a-nō-der′-ma): 1. The appearance of pigmented spots on the skin resulting from deposition of an abnormal amount of melanin. 2. Discoloration of the skin due to the administration of metallic substances such as silver or iron. 3. **SENILE M.,** cutaneous pigmentation as occurs in the aged.

melanoglossia (mel′-a-nō-glos′-i-a): Black tongue. See under tongue.

melanoma (mel-a-nō′-ma): A deep-seated tumor occurring usually in individuals over 30; derived from cells that are capable of forming melanin. **MALIGNANT M.,** often starts from a pigmented mole on the skin; also arises in mucous membranes of the mouth, anus, genitalia; has a strong tendency to metastasize; can be fatal if not recognized and treated early. In people with deeply pigmented skin, the toes and soles of the feet are often affected. In older people, should be differentiated from senile lentigo (*q.v.*).

melanosarcoma (mel′-a-nō-sar-kō′-ma): One form of malignant melanoma.—melanosarcomata, pl.; melanosarcomatous, adj.

melanosis (mel-a-nō′-sis): A condition characterized by the appearance of dark brown or brownish-black pigmentation in tissues of the body, as in the skin in sunburn or Addison's disease, or around the nipples and elsewhere during pregnancy.—melanotic, adj.

melanous (mel′-a-nus): Dark-complexioned.

melanuria (mel′-a-nū′-ri-a): The presence of

melanin in the urine which causes it to be dark or to turn dark upon standing.

melasma (me-laz′-ma): Any dark discoloration of the skin, as in Addison's disease.

melatonin (mel′-a-tō′-nin): A hormonal secretion of the pineal gland; is thought to depress gonadal function, to affect the functioning of several other endocrine glands, and to decrease pigmentation of the skin.

melena (mel′-e-na, me-lē′-na): 1. Black vomit. 2. Dark, tarry stools resulting from the action of intestinal juices on free blood. **M. NEONATORUM,** melena of the newborn, resulting from the extravasation of blood into the alimentary canal during the first few hours after birth.

melenemesis (mel-e-nem′-e-sis): The vomiting of dark material that has been colored as a result of the action of gastric juices on blood.

meli-: Combining form denoting 1) sweetness; 2) honey.

-melia: Combining form denoting a condition of the limbs.

melioidosis (mē′-li-oy-dō′-sis): An often fatal disease with symptoms resembling those of glanders (*q.v.*); affects rats and transmissible to man by the rat flea; occurs in certain parts of Asia and the Far East. The causative organism is *Pseudomonas pseudomallei*.

melitis (me-lī′-tis): Inflammation of the cheek.

melodiotherapy (mel-ō′-di-ō-ther′-a-pi): Treatment by music. Syn., musicotherapy.

meloplasty (mel′-ō-plas-ti): 1. Plastic surgery of the cheek. 2. Plastic surgery of an extremity.

member: An organ or a part of the body, particularly a limb.

membrane (mem′-brā-n): A thin, soft, pliable sheet of tissue that lines a tube or cavity, covers an organ or structure, or divides a space or organ. There are four major types in the body: cutaneous, mucous, serous, synovial. All are protective in function and secrete a fluid.—membranous, adj. **BASEMENT M.,** a thin layer beneath the epithelium of mucous surfaces. **CELL M.,** the thin, semipermeable **M.** that surrounds the cytoplasm of cells. **CROUPOUS M.,** a yellow-white false **M.** that forms on the tracheal surfaces in laryngotracheobronchitis. **CUTANEOUS M.,** the skin. **DIPHTHERITIC M.,** a thick, tough fibrinous false **M.** that forms on mucous surfaces, characteristic of diphtheria. **HYALINE M.,** a thin sheet of material lining the alveoli, alveolar ducts and bronchioles, sometimes found in postmortem examination of infants whose death was due to idiopathic respiratory distress. **HYALOID M.,** that surrounding the vitreous humor of the eye. **MUCOUS M.,** contains glands that secrete mucus. Lines cavities and passages that communicate with the exterior of the body. **SEMIPERMEABLE M.,** one that allows the passage through it of a solvent such as water, but not any of the substances held in solution. **SEROUS M.,** a lubricating **M.,** lining closed cavities, and reflected over their enclosed organs. **SYNOVIAL M.,** that lining the intra-articular parts of bones and ligaments; secretes synovial fluid for lubrication. **TYMPANIC M.,** that which separates the middle ear from the external auditory canal; the ear drum.

membranous croup (mem′-bra-nus kroop): A lay term for diphtheria (*q.v.*).

memory: The mental faculty of being able to retain and consciously or unconsciously recall or relive that which has been learned or experienced in the past. **ANTEROGRADE M., M.** for things that occurred in the distant past but not for recent events. **PRIMARY M.,** short-term **M.** acquired by shallow processessing of information; does not last unless rehearsed. **RETROGRADE M., M.** for things that occurred recently but not for those that occurred in the distant past. **SECONDARY M.,** permanent **M.** acquired by deep processing of information; limitless amounts can be acquired and used, both in the present and the future. **SENILE M., M.** for events that occurred in the distant past, characteristic of the aged. **SHORT-TERM M.,** primary **M. VISUAL M.,** the ability to recall visual impressions that are unusually vivid and exact.

men-, meno-: Combining forms denoting menstruation; the menses.

menacme (me-nak′-mi): The period of a woman's life during which menstruation persists.

menadione (men-a-dī′-ōn): A yellow crystalline chemical substance, soluble in vegetable oils; promotes synthesis of prothombin in conditions characterized by hypoprothrombinemia; used as a supplement for vitamin K. Also called menapthone.

menarche (me-nar′-kē): 1. The first menstrual period. 2. When the menstrual periods commence and other bodily changes occur.—menarcheal, adj.

mendelian (men-dē′-li-an): Pertaining to Mendel's theory. See Mendel's law.

Mendelson's syndrome: Postoperative chemical pneumonitis due to inhalation of vomited or regurgitated gastric contents; marked by bronchospasm, dyspnea, cyanosis, pulmonary edema.

Mendel's law: A theory of heredity, evolved by an Austrian monk, which deals with the interaction of dominant and recessive characters in crossbreeding. Foundation of the present theory of heredity. [Gregor Johann Mendel. 1822-1884.]

Ménière's disease, syndrome (mān-ē-airz′): A disorder of the membranous labyrinth of the inner ear; occurs in adult life. May accompany such disorders as drug poisoning, blood dyscrasias, circulatory disorders, neuritis or tumor, although the exact cause of the symptoms may be unknown. The most characteristic and disturbing symptom is sudden dizziness; tinnitus, nausea, vomiting, and progressive deafness may also occur. [Prosper Ménière, French otologist. 1799–1862.]

mening-, meningi-, meningo-: Combining forms denoting membrane, particularly one of the membranes (meninges) that cover the brain and spinal cord.

meningeal (me-nin′-jē-al): Pertaining to or affecting the meninges. **M. CARCINOMATOSIS,** infiltration of the leptomeninges by a malignant tumor, *e.g.*, melanoma, medulloblastoma, or leukemia. **M. GLIOMATOSUS,** proliferation of a glioma into the subarachnoid space. **M. SARCOMA,** a sarcomatous tumor of the meninges, arising in the dura. **M. SPACES,** the space between the dura mater and the arachnoid and that between the arachnoid and the pia mater.

meninges (men-in′-jē-s): Membranes, specifically the three protective and nutritive membranes surrounding the brain and spinal cord: the dura mater (outer); the arachnoid (middle); the pia mater (inner).— meninx, sing.; meningeal, adj.

meningioma (me-nin′-ji-ō′-ma): A slowly growing benign extracerebral encapsulated tumor; arises from the dura but may also occur on the spinal cord; accounts for 15 percent of all brain tumors, usually occurring after age 30. Tends to remain localized; may cause damage by pressing on the brain and adjacent tissues. Symptoms include headache, seizures, and signs of optic nerve compression. Recurrence after surgical removal is rare.

meningism, meningismus (me-nin′jizm, men-in-jis′mus): Condition presenting with signs and symptoms of meningitis (*e.g.*, neck stiffness) but meningitis does not develop. It may be hysterical in origin; may also result from irritation of the meninges at the onset of acute febrile diseases, particularly in children.

meningitis (men-in-jī′-tis): Inflammation of the meninges. Inflammation of the dura mater is called pachymeningitis. The arachnoid and pia mater are most commonly affected and the condition is known as leptomeningitis. May be caused by any one of several microorganisms, the most common being meningococcus, pneumococcus, streptococcus, and the tubercle bacillus. Presence of the organism in the spinal fluid is diagnostic. Fever, malaise, stiff neck, vomiting, severe headache, stupor, confusion, delirium, convulsions, and unconsciousness are among the symptoms. Sometimes only the cerebral meninges are involved, sometimes only those of the spinal cord, and sometimes both. See leptomeningitis, pachymeningitis. An epidemic form of **M.** is often called cerebrospinal fever; the infecting organism is *Neisseria meningitidis* (meningococcus). **ASEPTIC M.,** most often caused by an enterococcus but also by the various herpes viruses, and by nonviral infections such as syphilis, leptospirosis, and lupus erythematosus; symptoms include headache, nausea, fever, malaise, stiff neck; course is short and usually uncomplicated. **BENIGN LYMPHOCYTIC M.,** viral **M. MENINGEAL M.,** the only type of bacterial **M.** that occurs in epidemic form. **PURULENT M., M.** that is suppurative. **RECURRENT BACTERIAL M.** recurring infections in the subarachnoid space; may be associated with a persistent suppurative focus in the skull, ears, or paranasal sinuses, or to lack of immunity to bacterial infections. **TUBERCULOUS M.,** a severe form caused by *Mycobacterium tuberculosis*. **VIRAL M.,** caused by various viruses, including the coxsackieviruses; characterized by fever, malaise, headache, stiff neck, increased number of lymphocytes. Also called aseptic **M.** and benign lymphocytic **M.**—meningitides, pl.; meningitic, adj.

meningocele (me-ning′-gō-sēl): Protrusion of the meninges through a bony defect in the skull or spinal column. It forms a cyst filled with cerebrospinal fluid. See spina bifida.

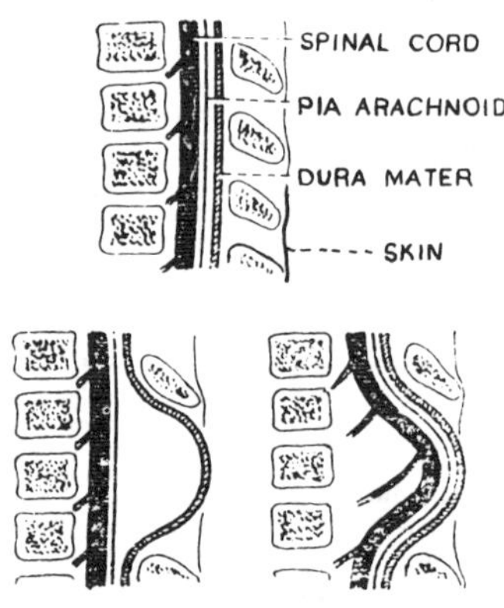

meningococcemia (me-ning′-gō-kok-sē′-mi-a): The presence of meningococci in the bloodstream; see Neisseria meningitidis. **ACUTE FULMINATING M.,** Waterhouse–Friderichsen syndrome (*q.v.*).

meningococcus (me-ning′-gō-kok′-us): An individual organism of the species *Neisseria meningitidis*.—meningococcal, adj.

meningoencephalitis (me-ning′-gō-en-sef′-a-lī′-tis): Inflammation of the brain and the meninges. May follow such infections as measles, mumps, tularemia, influenza, and some types of pneumonia.

meningomyelitis (me-ning′-gō-mī′-e-lī′-

tis): Inflammation of the spinal cord and its coverings.

meningomyelocele (me-ning-gō-mī′-e- lō-sēl): A malformation that results from failure of the bone and tissues over the dorsal aspect of the spine to develop, allowing a portion of the spinal cord and its enclosing membranes to protrude through the defect; usually occurs in the lumbar area—Syn., myelomeningocele.

meningopathy (men′-ing-gop′-a-thi): Any disease of the meninges of the brain or spinal cord.

meninx (mē′-ninks): 1. The singular of meninges. 2. Any membrane but particularly one of the coverings of the brain and spinal cord.

meniscectomy (men′-i-sek′-to- mi): The removal of a semilunar cartilage, especially from the knee joint, following injury and displacement. The medial cartilage is damaged most commonly.

meniscocytosis (me-nis-kō-sī-tō′-sis): Sickle cell anemia; see under anemia.

meniscus (me-nis′-kus): 1. A fibrocartilaginous structure found between the articulating surfaces of some joints. 2. The curved upper surface of a column of liquid; may be concave or convex. DISCOID M., swelling of the lateral M., of the knee joint observed when the knee is slightly fixed; more painful on pressure and during the night. LATERAL M., a crescent-shaped fibrocartilage attached to the lateral superior end of the tibia. MEDIAL M., a crescent-shaped fibrocartilage attached to the medial surface of the superior end of tibia.

Menke's disease or syndrome: An inherited disorder of unknown cause; onset in infancy; characterized by light kinky hair, failure to develop, degeneration of cerebrum and cerebellum, and early death. Also called kinky hair syndrome.

menometrorrhagia (men′-ō-met-rō-rā′-ji-a): Heavy bleeding from the uterus at irregular intervals as well as during regular menstrual periods.

menopause (men′-ō-pawz): The permanent cessation of menstruation, occurring normally between the ages of 45 and 50; involves hormonal changes, vascular phenomena, psychological disturbances; characterized by such symptoms as flushing, sweating, headache, dizziness, fatigue, irritability, palpitations, insomnia, vaginal pruritus. ARTIFICIAL M., an earlier menopause induced by surgery or radiotherapy for a pathologic condition. NATURAL M., that which occurs spontaneously without any medical or surgical treatment. PREMATURE M., that which occurs before the age of 35–40.—menopausal, adj.

menorrhagia (men-ō-rā′-ji-a): An excessive regular menstrual flow. Syn., menorrhea.

menostasis (me-nos′-ta-sis): Amenorrhea.

menses (men′-sēz): The sanguineous fluid discharged from the uterus during menstruation; menstrual flow.

menstrual (men′-stroo-al): Relating to the menses. M. CYCLE, the cyclical chain of uterine and ovarian changes that result from hormonal influence and that occur in the time from the beginning of one menstrual period to that of the next. M. EXTRACTION, extraction of the products of menstruation, utilizing a soft double-walled cannula that is inserted through the vagina; usually done to avoid the inconvenience of blood flow.

menstruation (men-stroo-a′-shun): The periodic physiologic shedding of blood, secretions, and the functional layer of endometrium from the non-pregnant uterus; occurs at approximately four-week intervals; lasts four-five days; commences at about age 13 and ceases at about age 45.—menstrual, menstrous, adj.

menstruum (men′-stroo-um): 1. Menstrual fluid. 2. A solvent; a solution that contains another solution.

mental: 1. Pertaining to the chin. 2. Pertaining to intellect or the mind. M. AGE, see under age. M. CONFUSION, a state characterized by mingling of ideas leading to disturbed comprehension; to be differentiated from senility. M. DEFICIENCY, feeblemindedness; failure of or incompetent mental development, usually considered to be of nervous system origin and not curable; classified according to degree of intellectual capacity. M. DISEASE, one that affects the mind or intellect. M. HYGIENE, the science of maintaining mental health and preventing development of mental disorders such as neuroses and psychoses. M. INCOMPETENCE, inability to manage one's own life or affairs. M. TELEPATHY, ESP; mind reading. M. TEST, one given to determine an individual's mental capacity.

mental disorder: Descriptive of an emotional or behavioral disturbance that is characterized by symptoms that may have their origin in genetic, organic, psychological or psychosocial factors. See Appendix VI for classification and categories of mental disorders.

mental health: A state of well-being characterized by the absence of mental or behavioral disorder; the condition existing when the individual has made an adjustment satisfactory to himself and the community in regard to his emotional, behavioral, and social reactions. MENTAL HEALTH NURSING, see psychiatric nursing.

Mental Health Association (MHA): A nonprofessional voluntary agency that works to improve mental health care, facilities, and services in the community, and promotes mental health legislation and research, and the education of mental health workers. Functions at national, state, and local levels. Formerly called National Association for Mental Health. Address: 1800 North Kent St., Arlington, VA 22209

mental retardation: Classified (in the Diagnostic and Statistical Manual of Mental Diseases III-R) as disorders usually first evident in infancy, childhood, or adolescence, and further categorized as mild, moderate, severe, profound, and unspecified. These disorders are characterized by subnormal intellectual and, usually, social functioning; may or may not be evident at birth; varies in degree with IQ's as low as 20 to 70–80; often accompanied by emotional and maturational disturbances.

mentality (men-tal′-i-ti): Mental power or learning ability.

mentation (men-tā′-shun): Mental activity; the process of thinking.

mentoplasty (men′-tō-plas-ti): Plastic surgery on the chin; often consists of an insertion of a Silastic implant for augmentation purposes.

mentovertical diameter (men-tō-ver′tik-al): The measurement from the point of the chin to above the posterior fontanelle; it is the presenting diameter in a brow presentation of the fetus.

mentum (men′-tum): The chin.

mephitic (mē-fit′-ik): Noxious; poisonous; foul.

Meq: Abbreviation for milliequivalent. Also written meq.

mer-, mero-: Combining forms denoting: 1. The thigh. 2. Part, partial, or division into segments.

meralgia (mer-al′-ji-a): Pain in the thigh. **M. PARESTHETICA,** a disorder marked by paresthesia, tingling, and burning pain over the outer lower aspect of the thigh; due to entrapment of the femoral cutaneous nerve by the inguinal ligament; common in obese women and those who wear tight belts or corsets.

mercurial (mer-kū′-ri-al): Pertaining to mercury. **M. DIURETICS,** potent diuretic drugs that contain mercury in organic combination.

mercurialism (mer-kū′-ri-al-izm): Chronic poisoning from misuse of mercury as a drug or from industrial exposure to the metal or its fumes. Symptoms include stomatitis with ulceration and sloughing of the mucous membrane of the mouth, salivation, loosening of the teeth, gastroenteritis with griping and diarrhea, sometimes bloody stools, skin eruptions. In severe cases prognosis is grave.

Mercurochrome (mer-kū′-ro-krōm): A red dye containing mercury in combination; formerly much used for its local antiseptic properties.

mercury (mer′-kū-ri): Quicksilver. A heavy metallic element, liquid at ordinary temperatures. **M.** and its salts formerly much used as purgatives, antisyphilitics, intestinal antiseptics, and astringents. An important medical use is in the manufacture of various types of manometers and thermometers. Symbol is Hg.—mercurial, adj.

mercy death: Euthanasia (*q.v.*).

merotomy (me-rot′-o-mi): 1. The sectioning of a cell for the purpose of studying its different segments. 2. Experimental division of unicellular organisms such as amoebas.

merozoite (mer′-ō-zō′-īte): Any one of the segments resulting from the splitting up of the schizont (*q.v.*) during the life cycle of the malarial parasite; it is released into the blood where it invades the erythrocytes.

mes-, meso-: Prefix denoting 1) in or toward the middle; 2) an intermediate connecting part; 3) the mesentery or a membrane that supports a specific part.

mesangium (mes-an′-ji-um): The thin suspensory membrane containing sponge fibers that helps to support the capillary loops in the glomerulus.

mesaortitis (mes-a-ōr-tī′-tis): Inflammation of the middle coat of the aorta.

mesarteritis (mes-ar-ter-ī′tis): Inflammation of the middle coat of an artery.

mescaline (mes′-ka-lēn): Peyote. A hallucinogenic agent derived from small tubercles on the mescal cactus, native to Mexico and southwestern U.S. Produces hallucinations similar to those produced by LSD; useful in experimental psychiatry.

mesencephalon (mes′en-sef′a-lon): The midbrain (*q.v.*).

mesenchyme (mes′-en-kīm): Embryonic connective tissue from which the connective tissue of the body and the vessels of the circulatory and lymphatic systems develop.

mesenteritis (mes′en-te-rī′tis): Inflammation of the mesentery (*q.v.*).

mesentery (mes′en-ter-i): A large fold of peritoneum that invests the intestines and attaches them to the posterior abdominal wall; it holds the organs in place and carries blood vessels, nerves and lymphatics to them. Usually refers specifically to the fan-shaped fold of peritoneum that encircles the small intestine (particularly the jejunum and the ileum) and attaches it to the posterior abdominal wall.

mesial (mē′-zi-al): Situated at the middle. Toward the midline of the body.

mesioclusion (mē-si-ō-klew′-zhun): A malrelation of the teeth in which the mandible is farther forward than normal, thus causing the lower teeth to be farther forward than in normal occlusion.

mesmerism (mes′-mer-izm): 1. The induction of hypnosis by the method practiced by Mesmer and believed to involve animal magnetism; broadly, hypnotism. 2. Intense fascination.—

mesmerize, v. [Franz A. Mesmer, Austrian physician. 1733-1815.]

mesoblast (mes′-ō-blast): The mesoderm, particularly during its early stage of development.

mesocephalic (mes′-ō-se-fal′-ik): Having a head of medium length or an individual with such a head. See microcephalic and macrocephalic.

mesocolon (mes′ō-kō′lon): The fold of peritoneum that attaches the colon to the posterior abdominal wall.—mesocolic, adj.

mesoderm (mes′-ō-derm): The middle one of the three primary germ layers of the embryo; from it are developed all connective tissues, bone, muscle, cartilage, circulatory and lymphatic tissues, the lining of serous cavities and of the organs of the genitourinary tract. It lies between the ectoderm and the entoderm (*q.v.*).—mesodermal, adj.

mesometrium (mes′-ō-mē′-tri-um): The part of the broad ligament that lies below the mesovarium (*q.v.*); it is made up of layers of peritoneum that separate to enclose the uterus, and extends to the lateral wall of the pelvis.

mesomorph (mes′-ō-mōrf): A person whose tissues are derived mostly from mesoderm, that is, the muscle, bone, and connective tissues predominate. A well-proportioned individual.

mesonephros (mes′-ō-nef′-rōs): The excretory organ of the fetus; consists of a long tube in the lower part of the body cavity, parallel to the spinal axis.

mesosalpinx (mes′-ō-sal′-pinks): The upper free part of the broad ligament that is above its attachment to the uterus; it encloses the fallopian tube.

mesothelioma (mes′-ō-thē-li-ō′-ma): A rare, painful, progressive tumor originating in the mesothelium (*q.v.*). One type is a rapidly fatal tumor that spreads over the pleural covering of the lung; of current interest because it has frequently occured in workers and others who had been exposed to asbestos particles.

mesothelium (mes′-ō-thē′-li-um): The squamous epithelium that develops from the mesoderm (*q.v.*) of the embryo and forms the epithelial layer of membranes that line serous cavities—peritoneal, pleural, pericardial, and scrotal.—mesothelial, adj.

mesovarium (mes′-ō-vā′-ri-um): The part of the broad ligament that encloses the ovary and holds it in place; it lies between the mesosalpinx (*q.v.*) and the mesometrium (*q.v.*).

mestranol (mes′-tra-nōl): A synthetic estrogen used in various combinations as an oral contraceptive.

meta-: Prefix denoting: 1. Change, transformation in. 2. Between, among, after, over, along with.

metabolic (met-a-bol′-ik): Pertaining to metabolism. **BASAL M. RATE** (BMR), the figure that expresses the amount of energy (heat) released in the body, based on the amount of oxygen utilized and carbon dioxide produced in a given period of time when the body is at complete rest in a warm atmosphere at least 12 hours after the ingestion of food. See metabolism. **M. ACIDOSIS,** see acidosis. **M. ALKALOSIS,** see alkalosis. **M. DISEASE,** any condition that interferes with metabolism.

metabolism (me-tab′-ō-lizm): The sum of physical and chemical changes in the body by which nutrition is effected, energy is provided for life processes, and life is maintained. The tissues are broken down by wear and tear (catabolism) and rebuilt (anabolism) continuously. **BASAL M.,** the energy used by the body at complete rest, being the minimum necessary to maintain life. **ERROR OF M.,** see inborn error of metabolism. —metabolic, adj.

metabolite (me-tab′-ō-līt): Any product of metabolism. **ESSENTIAL M.,** a substance necessary for proper metabolism, *e.g.*vitamins.

metacarpal (met′-a-kar′-pal): 1. Pertaining to that part of the hand called the metacarpus (*q.v.*). 2. Any one of the five bones of the metacarpus.

metacarpophalangeal (met′a-kar′pō-falan′jē-al): Pertaining to the metacarpus and the phalanges.

metacarpus (met-a-kar′-pus): The part of the hand between the wrist and the fingers.

metachromasia (met-a-krō-mā′-zi-a): 1. The taking on of different colors by different elements of a substance when treated with a given stain. 2. A change in color produced by application of a stain.

metachromatic (met-krō-mat′-ik): Refers to tissues of which different elements take on different colors when stained with the same dye. **M. GRANULES,** granules that take on a different color from that of the dye used to stain them. **M. LEUKODYSTROPHY,** see under leukodystrophy.

metal-fume fever: An occupational disorder due to breathing concentrated, freshly generated metallic oxide fumes from such metals as copper, brass, zinc, iron, lead, magnesium, cobalt, mercury, nickel, and tin; symptoms resemble those of influenza and include intense thirst, weakness, chills, and sweating.

metamorphopsia (met′a-mor-fop′si-a): A disturbance of vision in which the shapes of objects seen are distorted; caused by retinal edema or damage.

metamorphosis (met′-a-mor′-fō- sis): 1. A change in the shape, size, function or structure of a substance. 2. A transition from one stage of development to another.

metamyelocyte (met′-a-mī′-e-lō-sīt): An immature granular leukocyte.

metanephrine (met′-a-nef′-rin): A metabolite of epinephrine, found in urine and some tissues, along with normetanephrine.

metaphase (met′-a-fāz): The middle stage in mitotic cell division; it is the stage at which the chromosomes separate in a particular manner. See **mitosis**.

metaphyseal (met-a-fiz′-ē-al): Pertaining to a metaphysis. **M. CHONDRODYSPLASIA**, a rare condition in which x-ray photographs show the metaphyses to consist largely of cartilaginous material and to be unevenly calcified. **M. DYSOSTOSIS**, an abnormal condition characterized by defective mineralization of the metaphyseal area of bones, resulting in dwarfism; several types are recognized.

metaphysis (me-taf′-i-sis): That part of a long bone that lies between the shaft (diaphysis) and the extremity (epiphysis). During the growth period it consists of spongy bone; after growth is completed, it is continuous with the epiphysis.—metaphyses, pl.; metaphyseal, adj.

metaplasia (met-a-plā′-zi-a): Conversion of one type of tissue into another, *e.g.*, cartilage into bone. **MYELOID M.**, a condition characterized by splenomegaly, anemia, the formation of red blood cells outside of the bone marrow, and the presence of immature red and white blood cells in the peripheral blood.—metaplastic, adj.

metapsychology (met′a-sī-kol′ō-ji): That branch of speculative or theoretical psychology that deals with the purpose and structure of the mind, mental processes, the nature of the body-mind relationship, and other hypotheses that cannot be verified by experiment or observation.

metarterioles (met′-ar-tē′-ri-ols): Small peripheral blood vessels between the arterioles and capillaries.

metastasis (me-tas′-ta-sis): 1. The transference of bacteria or body cells, especially cancer cells, from the original site to another part of the body, usually by blood or lymph, and resulting in development of a similar lesion at the new site. 2. A secondary growth that results from the transference of disease to a site distant from the original lesion. Term is used particularly with reference to malignant growths. —metastases, pl.; metastatic, adj.; metastasize, v.

metatarsal (met′-a-tar′-sal): 1. Pertaining to that part of the foot called the metatarsus (*q.v.*). 2. Any one of the five bones of the metatarsus.

metatarsalgia (met′-a-tar-sal′-ji-a): Pain in the forefoot due to osteochondrosis of the heads of the metatarsal bones or to a structural abnormality of the foot; causes include arthritis, weakness of foot muscles, ill-fitting shoes; seen most often in older women. Also called Morton's metatarsalgia, Morton's toe, Morton's neuralgia.

metatarsophalangeal (met′a-tar′so-fa-lan′jē-al): Pertaining to the metatarsus and the phalanges.

metatarsus (met′-a-tar′-sus): The five bones that form the skeleton of the foot between the ankle and the toes. **M. ABDUCTUS, M.** valgus; a congenital deformity in which the forepart of the foot deviates away from the midline of the body. **M. ADDUCTUS**, a congenital deformity in which the front part of the foot deviates toward the midline of the body. **M. ATAVICUS**, a congenital abnormality in which the first metatarsal is shorter than normal so that it must bear more than the normal amount of weight. **M. LATUS**, a broad spread-out foot; widened forefoot. **M. VARUS**, a congenital deformity in which the sole of the foot turns inward and the person walks on the outer border of the foot.

Metchnikoff's theory: The theory that invading bacteria or other disease-producing agents are attacked and destroyed by the phagocytes (*q.v.*) and that this activity produces inflammation. [Elie Metchnikoff, Russian zoologist in Paris. 1845–1916.]

meteorism (mē′-tē-ō-rizm): Excessive accumulation of gas in the intestines. Tympanites.

-meter: Combining form denoting relationship to 1) a measurement; 2) an instrument for making a measurement.

meter, metre (mē′-ter): 1. Basic unit of length in the metric system; equivalent to approximately 39.37 inches. 2. An apparatus for measuring the quantity of anything passing through it.

methadone treatment: The treatment of a person addicted to a drug, usually heroin, with methadone, a narcotic that is also addicting but less socially disabling than heroin.

methane (meth′-ān): Marsh gas; the colorless, odorless, flammable gas that is given off by decomposing organic matter. It is the fire damp given off in coal mines. See **fire damp**.

methanol (meth′-a-nōl): Methyl alcohol; see under **alcohol**.

methemoglobin (met-hē-mō-glō′- bin): A form of hemoglobin consisting of a combination of globin with an oxidized heme, containing ferric iron. This pigment is unable to transport oxygen. **M.** may be formed following the administration of a wide variety of drugs, including the sulfonamides. **M.** may be present in blood as a result of a congenital abnormality.

methemoglobinemia (met-hē′-mō-glō-bi-nē′-mi-a): Methemoglobin in the blood. If large quantities are present, individuals may show cyanosis, but otherwise no abnormality except, in severe cases, breathlessness on exertion, because the methemoglobin cannot transport oxygen.—methemoglobinemic, adj.

methemoglobinuria (met-hē′-mō-glō-bi-nū′-ri-a): Methemoglobin in the urine.—methemoglobinuric, adj.

methionine (me-thī′-o-nēn): One of the sulphur-containing amino acids; essential for growth in infants and for maintenance of nitrogen equilibrium in adults. Occasionally used therapeutically in hepatitis and other conditions associated with liver damage.

method: The manner of performing any act; a procedure. **RHYTHM M.**, a method of contraception that involves abstinence from sexual intercourse during the period of the menstrual cycle when ovulation is most likely to occur.

methodology (meth-o-dol′-ō-ji): 1. A set of principles and methods that govern or regulate a discipline. 2. The principles and procedures involved in a study in a particular area.

methoxyflurane (mē-thok′si-flū′rān): A potent, non-flammable inhalation anesthetic; widely used in obstetrics.

methyl alcohol: Wood alcohol. See alcohol.

methylene blue (meth′-i-lēn): A basic dye used in histologic and microbiologic studies. Also used as an antidote for methemoglobinemia. **M. B. TEST**, may be 1) a test for renal function; 2) a test for the presence of vitamin C; or 3) a test for the presence of bilirubin in the urine. Used in medicine as a urinary antiseptic and as an antidote for cyanide poisoning.

methylprednisolone (meth′-il-pred-nis′-ō-lōn): An adrenocortical steroid that has the actions and uses of prednisolone (*q.v.*).

metopic (mē-top′ik): Pertaining to or relating to the forehead.

metra-, metro-: Combining forms denoting the uterus.

metralgia (mē-tral′-ji-a): Pain in the uterus; metrodynia.

metratonia (mē-tra-tō′-ni-a): Atony of the uterus.

metratrophia (mē-tra-trō′fi-a): Atrophy of the uterus.

-metria: A combining form denoting condition of the uterus.

metric system: A system of weights and measures, invented and first used in France in the late 18th century. Now used in most countries except most English-speaking ones but even in those it is now used in scientific research and increasingly in other areas. Employs a decimal scale. The unit of weight is the gram; of length is the meter; and of capacity is the liter.

metritis (mē-trī′-tis): Inflammation of the uterus.

metrocele (mē′-trō-sēl): Hernia of the uterus.

metrocolpocele (mē′trō-kol′pō-sēl): A hernia of the uterus into the vagina; prolapse of the uterus.

metrodynia (mē-trō-din′-i-a): Pain in the uterus.

metrofibroma (mē′-trō-fī-brō′-ma): A fibroma of the uterus.

metropathia hemorrhagica (mē-trō-path′-i-a hem-or-aj′-ik-a): Irregular episodes of uterine bleeding due to excessive and unopposed estrin in the bloodstream. Usually associated with a follicular cyst in the ovary.

metropathy (mē-trop′-a-thi): Any disorder of the uterus.

metroptosis (mē′trō-tō′sis): Prolapse of the uterus.

metrorrhagia (mē-trō-rā′ji-a): Uterine bleeding between the menstrual periods.

metrorrhexis (mē-tro-rek′-is): Rupture of the uterus.

Meyer-Betz disease: A rare familial disease characterized by attacks of myoglobinuria following strenuous exercise; the muscles become weak, tender, and swollen.

mg: Abbreviation for milligram.

MHA: Abbreviation for microhemagglutin. **MHA TEST**, a confirmatory test for *treponema pallidum*, the causative agent in syphilis.

MI: Abbreviation for: 1. Mitral insufficiency. 2. Myocardial infarction.

mi-, mio-: Combining forms denoting less, fewer, slightly.

micelles (mi-sel′lēz): Small, spherical, water soluble structures formed by the aggregation of bile salt molecules during digestion of lipids; they diffuse into the epithelial cells of the small intestine where they are concerned with the synthesis of phospholipids and protein and the absorption of fat and cholesterol.

Michel's clips (mi′-shels): Small metal clips used instead of sutures for the closure of a wound.

MICN: Mobile Intensive Care Nurse; a professional nurse with special training and accreditation in the specialty of mobile emergency care; is responsible to the Director of Emergency Medicine at the base station of the unit.

micr-, micro-: Combining forms denoting 1) small or minute size or amount; 2) abnormal smallness, *e.g.*,microcephalia; 3) instruments or objects used in dealing with minute objects, *e.g.*, microscope, microtome; 4) one millionth part (metric system).

micrencephaly (mī′kren-sef′a-li): Abnormal smallness of the brain.—micrencephalic, adj. Also micrencephalia, microencephaly.

microabscess (mī′krō-ab′ses): A very small abscess.

microaerophil (e) (mī′-krō-ā′-er-ō-fīl): An aerobic organism that grows best in an atmosphere with an oxygen content lower than that of the air.—microaerophilic, adj.

microanalysis (mī'krō-nal'i-sis): The analysis of minute quantities of material.

microanatomy (mī'krō-a-nat'o-mi): Histology (*q.v.*).

microaneurysm (mī'krō-an'ū-rizm): An aneurysm occurring in a capillary; often seen in diabetic retinopathy and in thrombotic purpura. See **retinopathy** and **purpura**.

microbe (mī'-krōb): A microscopic unicellular organism, especially one capable of causing disease. Syn., microorganism.—microbial, microbic, adj.

microbicide (mī-krō'-bi-sīd): An agent that destroys microbes.—microbicidal, adj.

microbiologist (mī'-krō-bī- ol'-o-jist): A person who specializes in the study of microbes.

microbiology (mī'krō-bī-ol'o-ji): The branch of biology that is concerned with the study and science of microbes. **DIAGNOSTIC M.**, is concerned with tests done to aid in diagnosis and in prescribing medications, and to check for freedom from pathogenic microorganisms.

microbiosis (mī'-krō-bī- ō'-sis): 1. Shortness of life. 2. The condition of being infected with microbes.

microbrachia (mī-krō-brā'ki-a): A congenital anomaly consisting of abnormal shortness of the arms.

microcephalic (mī-krō-sef-al'-ik): 1. Pertaining to an abnormally small head. 2. An individual with an abnormally small head.

microcephalus (mī-krō-sef'-a-lus): An individual with an abnormally small or imperfectly formed head.

microcephaly (mī-krō-sef'-a-li): Abnormal smallness of the head.—microcephalic, adj.

microcirculation (mī'-krō-sir-kū-lā'-shun): Circulation in the smallest of the blood vessels, that is, the arterioles, capillaries, and venules.

Micrococcus (mī'krō-kok'us): A genus of saprophytic gram-positive spherical bacteria occurring in irregular masses. They comprise saprophytes, parasites, and pathogens.

microcolorimeter (mī'-krō-kol-o- rim'-e-ter): A colorimeter used for examining small blood samples.

microcornea (mī'krō-kor'nē-a): An unusually thin flat cornea; usually bilateral and often associated with other inherited or developmental anomalies or disorders of the eye.

microcurie (mī'krō-kū'rē): A unit of radioactivity; one millionth of a curie.

microcyte (mī'-krō-sīt): An undersized red blood cell found in anemic blood.—microcytic, adj.

microcythemia (mī'krō-sī-thē'mi-a): The presence of abnormally small erythrocytes in the blood.

microcytosis (mī-krō-sī-tō'-sis): A blood condition characterized by the presence of large numbers of microcytes (*q.v.*).

microdactylia (mī'-krō-dak-til'-i-a): Abnormal smallness of the fingers and toes.

microdissection (mī'-krō-di-sek'-shun): Dissection of cells or tissues under the microscope.

microdrip (mī'-krō-drip): An apparatus for delivering intravenous solutions by small drops; refers particularly to the administration of small amounts of solution slowly. See **macrodrip**.

microembolus (mī-krō-em'bō-lus): An embolus of microscopic size.—microembolism, n.

microflora (mī-krō-flō'-ra): Plant life that is visible only under a microscope.

microgenitalia (mī'krō-jen-i-tā'li-a): The condition of having unusually small genitalia, particularly external genitalia.

microglossia (mī-krō-glos'i-a): An abnormally small tongue.

micrognathia (mī-krō-nā'thi-a): Small jaw, especially the lower one, which recedes due to a poorly developed mandible.

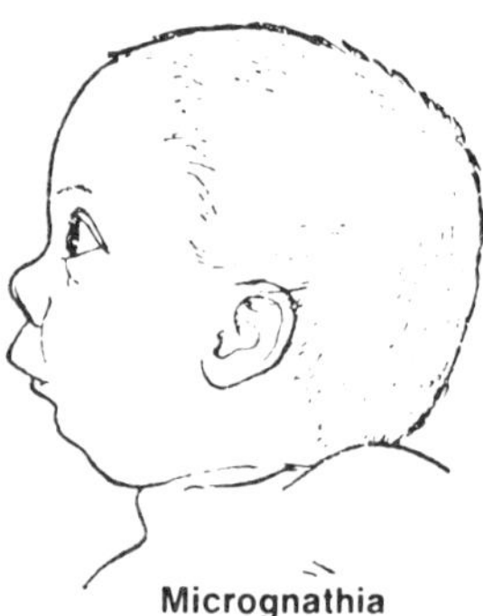

Micrognathia

microgram (mcg): One thousandth of a milligram; one millionth of a gram. Represented by the symbol μg.

microgyrus (mī-krō-jī'rus): An unusually small convolution of the brain.

microlens (mī'-krō-lens): A small thin corneal contact lens.

microlipoinjection (mī'-krō-lī'-pō-in-jek'-shun): A procedure whereby fat tissue is suctioned by needle from one part of the body and injected into the tissues of the face or other part of the body. **M.** corrects the deep skin furrows caused by aging; also used to raise depressed areas of scars caused by surgery or injury.

microliter (mī'-krō-lē-ter): One millionth of a liter, or one thousandth of a milliliter. Usually abbreviated μl.

microlithiasis (mī'-krō-li-thī'-a-sis): The formation of multiple small concretions or stones in an organ.

micrometer (mī-krom′-e-ter): An instrument for measuring objects being viewed under the microscope.

micron (mī′-kron): A unit of length in the metric system. One thousandth of a millimeter, or one millionth of a meter; approximately 1/25,000 of an inch. Used for measuring blood cell diameters and bacteria. Represented by the Greek letter μ(mu).

micronodular (mī-krō-nod′ū-lar): Marked by the presence of small nodules; often said of the liver.

micronystagmus (mī′krō-nī-stag′mus): Very fine movements of the eye, normally present at all times.

microorganism (mī′krō-or′gan-izm): A microscopic cell. (Often synonymous with bacterium but includes virus, protozoon, rickettsia, fungus, alga, and lichen.

microphage (mī′-krō-fāj): A very small phagocyte (*q.v.*).

microphallus (mī-krō-fal′-us): An abnormally small penis; also called micropenis.

microphobia (mī-krō-fō′-bi-a): 1. Morbid dread of microbes. 2. Morbid dread of small things.

microphotograph (mī-krō-fō′tō-graf): A small photograph of a microscopic object; usually magnified for viewing and interpreting.

microphthalmia (mī-krof-thal′-mi-a): Abnormal smallness of the eyeballs.

microphysics (mī-krō-fiz′iks): That branch of physics that deals with molecules, atoms, and elementary particles of matter.

microplasia (mī-krō-plā′zi-a): Dwarfism.

micropodia (mī-krō-pō′di-a): Abnormal smallness of the feet.

micropsia (mī-krop′-si-a): A pathological condition in which objects appear to be smaller than they actually are. Micropia. —microptic, adj.

microsaccades (mī′-krō-sa-ka′-dez): Imperceptible jerks of the eye that occur during fixation.

microscope (mī′-krō-skōp): An instrument consisting of a lens or an arrangement of lenses for making enlarged images of minute cells or objects. **BINOCULAR M.**, one that has two eyepieces. **COMPOUND M.**, one that has two lens systems. **DARK FIELD, M.**, a **M.** modified to permit lateral lighting. **ELECTRON M.**, one in which an electric beam causes an image to be projected on a fluorescent screen, where it may be viewed or photographed. **SIMPLE M.**, one that has only one lens; a magnifying glass. Many special types of microscopes are available including those that utilize infrared and ultraviolet radiation, x rays, ultrasound, laser beam, television, and scanning techniques. See also microsurgery.

microscopic (mī-krō-skop′ik): Extremely small; visible only with the aid of a microscope.

microscopy (mi-kros′-ko-pi): Examination by means of a microscope.

microsomia (mī-krō-sō′-mi-a): Abnormal smallness of the body.—microsomal, adj.

microspherocytosis (mī′-krō-sfē-rō-sī-tō′-sis): A condition in which most of the red blood cells are more round and smaller than usual; seen in hemolytic icterus.

Microsporum (mī-kros′-pō-rum): A genus of fungi that causes various superficial cutaneous infections; it is parasitic, living in the keratin-containing tissues of man and animals. **M. AUDOUINII**, the commonest cause of scalp ringworm (tinea tonsurans) in children. **M. CANIS**, the species of **M.** that causes dermatophytosis (*q.v.*) in children and adults; usually contracted from infected cats or dogs.

microsurgery (mi-kro-ser′-jer-i): Dissection, or the performance of surgery, under a high-powered microscope capable of magnifying nerves and blood vessels up to 40 times, using specially developed miniature instruments; the microscope is often hooked up to television screens so that other members of the operating team can see what the surgeon is doing.—microsurgical, adj.

microthrombus (mī-krō-throm′bus): A small thrombus located in a capillary or other small vessel.

microtia (mī-krō′-shi-a): The condition of having ears with exceptionally small pinnae but which are of normal shape.

microtome (mī′-krō-tōm): An instrument for making thin sections of tissue for microscopic study.

microvilli (mī-krō-vil′lī): Microscopic processes on the surface of a cell, which increase the area available for absorption of nutrients or for excretion; found particularly in the cells of the proximal renal tubule and the intestinal epithelium.

microwave (mī′-krō-wāv): An electromagnetic wave of very short length and high frequency.

micturate (mik′-tū-rāt): The act of voiding or passing urine.

micturating urethrogram: An x-ray photograph of the bladder after injection of a radiopaque substance; taken when the patient is at rest and while actually voiding.

micturition (mik-tū-rish′-un): The act of passing urine. **M. SYNCOPE**, syncope following rapid emptying of a distended bladder; results from sudden drop in blood pressure; may be associated with postural hypotension, but may also occur in otherwise healthy persons.

midaxillary line (mid-ak′-si-lar-i): An anatomical landmark consisting of an imaginary line drawn vertically on the surface of the body from the apex of the axilla, dividing the body into an anterior and a posterior portion.

midbrain: The mesencephalon, that short portion of the brain stem that lies just above the pons and just below the cerebrum; it connects the cerebrum with the pons and the cerebellum and is involved in motor coordination.

midclavicular line (mid-kla-vik′-ū-lar): An anatomical landmark consisting of an imaginary line drawn vertically on the surface of the body from the outer end of the clavicle through the center of the nipple.

middle age: Commonly considered to be the years between 40 or 45 and 60, but usually defined by psychosocial rather than physiological events and changes.

middle ear: The space on the medial side of the tympanic membrane; connects with the mastoid cells and the eustachian tube; contains the auditory ossicles. See ossicle.

middle ear disease: A condition common in the elderly; starts with a feeling of fullness in the ear and general discomfort; may be a sign of developing nasopharyngeal cancer, lymphoma, or leukemia.

midget (mij′-et): An individual who is smaller than normal, but whose organs and parts are perfectly formed.

midgut (mid′-gut): The region between the foregut and the hindgut in the developing embryo.

midline (mid′-līn): An imaginary line that divides the body into right and left halves.

midriff (mid′-rif): 1. The diaphragm (*q.v.*). 2. The middle region of the human torso, particularly the front external aspect.

midsternal line: An anatomical landmark consisting of a vertical line drawn from the cricoid cartilage through the sternum to the xiphoid process.

midstream specimen: See clean catch specimen.

midwife (mid′-wīf): A woman who attends women in childbirth. Accoucheuse (*q.v.*). NURSE-MIDWIFE, a professional nurse who has had advanced educational preparation for the independent management and care of normal newborns and their mothers before, during, and after delivery, according to standards defined by the Americal College of Nurse-Midwives. CERTIFIED NURSE-MIDWIFE (CNM); a professional nurse who has had advanced education in midwifery and who has passed the certification examination of the American College of Nurse-Midwives.

midwifery (mid′-wif′-ri): The practice of delivering babies or of assisting women in childbirth, by women who are not physicians but who are trained in obstetrical procedures. NURSE-MIDWIFERY, the practice of midwifery by a professional nurse who has had advanced education in the care of newborns and their mothers before, during, and following delivery.

migraine (mī′-grān): Hemicrania. A syndrome characterized by recurring throbbing headache, usually bilaterally initially; of unknown cause. Symptoms include photophobia, phonophobia, nausea, vomiting. More common in women than men; often there is a family history of M.; may result from unconscious emotional conflicts; when severe may result in incapactitation. CLASSIC M., of three types: 1) muscle contraction M., formerly called tension headache; differs from vascular M., in that the pain is occipital, dull, aching, and bilateral; 2) traction and inflammatory M., caused by some disease or disorder of the skull contents; and 3) vascular M.,the most common type of M., due to depression and conversion reactions; two classes are identified: a) hemiplegic M., in which there is slight paralysis of one side of the body; may occur two or three times a day and last for about 45 minutes; and b) ophthalmoplegic M., recurrent vascular headache that occurs periodically on one side only; characterized by transient oculomotor palsy (see under palsy).

migrainous (mī′-gran-us): Pertaining to or resembling migraine. M. NEURALGIA, characterized by attacks of severe pain over the eye and forehead, with fever, rhinorrhea, and lacrimation, tending to occur in clusters and lasting from 15 to 30 minutes; also called cluster headache, histamine cephalalgia, and Horton's headache. See headache.

migration (mī-grā′-shun): In physiology, the passage of leukocytes through the walls of vessels into tissue spaces in order to combat organisms that have invaded tissues.

Mikulicz's disease or syndrome: Chronic hypertrophic enlargement of the lacrimal and salivary glands; of unknown etiology, but sometimes occurs as a syndrome in association with certain other diseases such as leukemia or lymphosarcoma. [Mikulicz-Radecki, Rumanian surgeon. 1850-1905.]

milia (mil′i-a): Whiteheads. Tiny white epidermal cysts appearing usually over the face, nose, upper eyelids and neck, and sometimes over the chest; due to blocked pilosebaceous glands. M. NEONATORUM, M. occurring in the newborn, thought to be due to blocked hair follicles and sweat glands; the whiteheads are filled with keratinous material and disappear without specific treatment.

miliaria (mil-i-ār′i-a): An inflammatory skin condition characterized by vesicular and erythematous eruption caused by blocking of sweat ducts and their subsequent rupture, or their infection by bacteria or fungi. Often accompanied by burning, itching, prickling sensation. Common in the tropics. Also called heat rash, prickly heat, summer rash, wildfire rash, strophulus.

miliary (mil'i-er-i): Resembling a millet seed. **M. TUBERCULOSIS,** a form in which minute tuberculous nodules are widely disseminated throughout the organs and tissues of the body.

milieu (mil-yū'): Environment; surroundings. **M. THERAPY,** treatment, usually psychiatric, in a carefully structured environment in which all elements such as furnishings, equipment, staff, etc. enhance the medical therapy, encourage acceptable and responsible behavior, and help the patient toward rehabilitation.

military antishock trousers (MAST): A wraparound device with Velcro fasteners, consisting of three bladders, one for each leg and one for the abdomen, which are slowly inflated to 88–100 mmHg pressure after being applied, the effect being to shunt blood from the lower extremities and lower abdomen to the heart-brain-lung circulation. Used in treatment of trauma victims with hypovolemic shock, in congestive heart failure, and in cases of massive hemorrhage; also used for splinting fractures of the lower extremities and/or the pelvis. Also called medical antishock trousers, shock pants, compression pants.

milium (mil'i-um): A small pearly epidermal cyst, thought to be due to a blocked pilosebaceous gland. Usually referred to in the plural, milia. Whitehead.

milk leg: Phlegmasia alba dolens (*q.v.*).

milk line: In anatomy, an imaginary line extending from the axilla to the groin; so called because extra nipples sometimes develop at points along the line.

milk sugar: Lactose (*q.v.*).

milk teeth: The first set of teeth.

milk-alkali syndrome: A condition of hypercalcemia characterized by renal insufficiency, azotemia, calcinosis, conjunctivitis, and mild alkalosis, but without excess excretion of calcium in the urine; occurs in individuals on prolonged milk treatment for peptic ulcer and in infants on milk diets for long periods of time.

Miller-Abbott tube: A double-lumen rubber tube with an inflatable balloon at the distal end; used in diagnosis and treatment of obstructive lesions of the small intestine.

Miller-Kurzrok test: A test to determine the ability of the sperm to penetrate the mucous plug normally present in the cervix of the uterus.

milli-: Prefix denoting one thousandth part of the root to which it is affixed (metric system),

milliampere (ma) (mil'li-am'pēr): One thousandth of an ampere.

millicurie (mCi, mc) (mil'li-kū're): The unit of radioactivity used to determine dosage; one thousandth of a curie.

milliequivalent (mEq/L) (mil'li-ē-qwiv'a-lent): Term used to express the concentration of a substance in a liter of solution, that is, the number of grams of a solvent in one milliliter of normal solution.

milligram (mg) (mil'li-gram): One thousandth of a gram. Approximately 0.015 grains.

milligrams-percent (mg%): In biochemistry, milligrams of a substance in 100 milliliters of solution.

milliliter (ml) (mil'i-lē-ter): One thousandth of a liter; in liquid measure, equivalent to a cubic centimeter.

millimeter (mm) (mil-li-mē'ter): One thousandth of a meter; approximately 1/25th of an inch.

millimicron (mμ) (mil-li-mī'kron): One thousandth of a micron (*q.v.*).

millimole (mM) (mil'i-mōl): One thousandth of a mol.

millirad (mil' -li-rad): One thousandth of a rad. A measurement of a unit of absorbed radiation dose.

millisecond (ms, msec) (mil'li-sek-ond): One thousandth of a second.

millivolt (mV) (mil'li-volt): One thousandth of a volt.

Milroy's disease: Congenital lymphedema. Hereditary lymphedema of the legs caused by chronic obstruction of lymphatic vessels; may also affect other parts of the body.

Milwaukee brace: A splint commonly used for children; it extends from the back of the head to the hips and maintains extension of the spine from fixed points on the pelvis, chin, and occiput; longitudinal struts are utilized in such a way that they can be lengthened as the child grows; used in treatment of scoliosis, lordosis, and kyphosis, and requires careful fitting.

mimesis (mī-mē'sis): 1. Mimicry. 2. The appearance of symptoms of one disease in a person with another, different, disease.

-mimetic: Combining form denoting the ability of a drug to mimic the action of the autonomic nervous system.

min: Abbreviation for minim. Also m. (Should be written out because min may be confused with minute and m with meter.)

Minamata disease: Named for the town in Japan where it was first discovered in 1951; mercurial poisoning caused by eating fish or shellfish from waters contaminated by industrial chemical wastes. Characterized by ataxia, dysarthria, salivation, impaired hearing, speech, and sight; paralysis and brain damage. Fetuses in utero may be affected.

mine damp: See damp 2.

mineralocorticoid (min'er-al-ō-kor'ti-koyd): A secretion of the adrenal cortex that affects the fluid and electrolyte balance of the body, chiefly through its influence on sodium retention and potassium loss from the body. See **aldosterone.**

Minerva jacket or **brace:** A cast that covers the head, with cutouts for the face and ears, and reaching to the hips; used in cases of cervical and/or thoracic vertebral fracture.

miner's anemia: Ancylostomiasis (*q.v.*).

miner's elbow: Inflammation of the olecranon bursa over the point of the elbow; caused by leaning on the elbow; also called student's elbow.

minilaparotomy (min′i-lap-a-rot′o-mi): A sterilization procedure for women that can be done under local anesthesia; consists of ligation of the fallopian tubes through a small suprapubic incision.

minim (min′im): A unit of capacity in the apothecaries' system, being one-sixtieth of a fluid dram. Now largely replaced by metric measurement in milliliters, one minum being equal to 0.06 milliliters.

minimal brain dysfunction syndrome: Usually occurs in children with some functional disorder of the central nervous system; the child is of near average intelligence but may have difficulty with language and memory and controlling his emotions and impulses. Occurs more often in boys than girls; may be caused by perinatal or postnatal disease or injury, genetic factors, or pathologic biochemical conditions. Also called hyperkinesis, hyperkinetic syndrome, attention deficit disorder (*q.v.*).

minimum lethal dose (MLD): The smallest dose of a medication or drug that will cause death.

Minnesota Multiphasic Personality Inventory (MMPI): A frequently used device for self-rating; measures various aspects of personality; most often used to test patients over 16 years of age who have various kinds of psychological disorders. Abbreviated MMMP.

minor: In surgery, an operation that can be done under local anesthesia and in which the risk of death and the death rate are negligible.

minute respiratory volume (MRV): The total amount of air breathed in during one minute.

miosis (mī-ō′sis): Contraction of the pupil of the eye.

miotic (mī-ot′ik): 1. Pertaining to or producing miosis. 2. A medication that causes constriction of the pupil.

mirror writing: Backward writing that resembles ordinary writing as reflected in a mirror.

misalignment (mis-a-līn′ment): The condition of being out of line or improperly adjusted.

misanthropy (mis-an′thrō-pi): Hatred, distrust of, or contempt for mankind.—misanthrope, n.; misanthropic, adj.

miscarriage (mis-kar′ij): Expulsion of the fetus before it is viable, *i.e.*, before the 28th week.

misce: A term used in prescription writing; means to mix.

miscegenation (mis′e-je-nā′shun): Intermarriage or cohabitation between persons of different races.

misdiagnosis (mis′dīag-no′sis): An incorrect diagnosis.

miso-: Combining form denoting hatred of.

misogyny (mi-soj′e-ni): Hatred of women.

misopedia (mis-ō-pē′di-a): Hatred of children.

mit-, mito-: Combining forms denoting: 1. Thread or thread-like. 2. Mitosis.

mite (mīt): A minute arthropod, related to the spiders, that is parasitic on man and that produces various skin irritations. Some mites are intermediary hosts for certain pathogenic organisms, *e.g.*, that causing scrub typhus.

mitochondria (mī′tō-kon′dri-a): Organelles in the cytoplasm of cells, disclosed by differential staining; in the presence of oxygen they convert nutrients into energy and during this process adenosine triphosphate is formed.—mitochondrion, sing.

mitosis (mī-tō′sis): A complicated method of division occurring in specialized cells; usually consists of a series of stages—prophase, metaphase, anaphase, and telephase.—mitotic, adj.

mitral (mī′tral): 1. Mitre-shaped. 2. The biscuspid valve between the left atrium and left ventricle of the heart. **M. INCOMPETENCE,** a defect in the closure of the mitral valve, whereby blood tends to flow backward into the left atrium when the valve is closed. **M. MURMUR,** a murmur produced at the mitral valve orifice. **M. STENOSIS,** narrowing of the mitral orifice, usually due to the formation of fibrous tissue as a result of rheumatic fever. **M. VALVE,** a valve with two flaps, located in the septum between the left atrium and left ventricle; it allows blood to flow from the atrium into the ventricle and prevents backflow into the atrium. Also called bicuspid **V.,** and atrioventricular **V. M.VALVULOTOMY,** the operation of splitting the cusps of a stenosed mitral valve.

MITS: Medically Impaired Transportation Service, a community service that provides vans or other suitable means of transportation for patients in wheelchairs or who are otherwise unable to take themselves to health care facilities.

mittelschmerz (mit′el-schmertz): Pain or discomfort in the lower abdomen experienced by some women midway in the intermenstrual interval; thought to be the result of irritation of the pelvic peritoneum caused by the escaping fluid or blood from the ovarian follicle.

mixture (miks′tūr): A combination of two or

more substances, usually in liquid form, with each substance retaining its particular physical characteristics.

mmHg: Abbreviation for millimeters of mercury. Usually refers to the height of the mercury in the mercury manometer on the sphygmomanometer.

MMR: Abbreviation for the combination of measles (rubeola), mumps, and rubella (German measles) vaccines, given in one injection and producing lifetime immunity for these diseases.

mnemonics (nē-mon'iks): The science of improving the memory, or the techniques used for this purpose. **M. DEVICE,** a scheme for aiding the memory by establishing an artificial relationship between two things that are normally not related.

MNR: Nuclear Magnetic Resonance: A process that utilizes magnets to produce three-dimensional images of internal organs to locate tumors without using x rays or radioactive elements.

mobile intensive care system: An emergency care system designed to respond quickly and appropriately to medical emergencies in a designated jurisdiction. The care unit consists of an automotive vehicle with trained staff and with equipment and supplies needed to administer emergency care to individuals or groups of individuals. Paramedics on the staff have had special training in resuscitative procedures, administration of drugs and IV therapy, splinting, instituting cardiac monitoring, and maintaining an open airway; they receive instructions via radiophone from a base station facility, which is usually a local hospital.

mobility (mō-bil'i-ti): Being capable of moving one's self or of being moved.

mobilization (mō'bi-li-zā'shun): The process by which a fixed part is made movable, or motion is restored to an ankylosed joint. **STAPES M.,** surgery to correct immobility of the stapes; has been used in treating certain types of deafness.

Mobitz heart block, types I and II. See under block.

Möbius: [Paul Julius Möbius, German neurologist, 1853–1907.] **M's. DISEASE,** periodic migraine with oculomotor paralysis. **M's. SIGN,** impairment in the convergence of the eyes; seen in Graves' disease. **M's SYNDROME,** hereditary paralysis of facial muscles, due to imperfectly developed motor nuclei of some of the motor nerves; often associated with speech and hearing defects and mental deficiency.

modality (mō-dal'i-ti): A method of applying or using a therapeutic agent or procedure.

modiolus (mō-dī'ō-lus): The central, bony pillar of the cochlea, around which the spiral canal winds.

modus (mō'dus): Manner. **M. OPERANDI,** a way of performing an operation or of working.

moiety (moy'i-ti): 1. A portion or part of a molecule that has a characteristic pharmacological or chemical effect. 2. One or two equal parts into which something is divided.

mol: The molecular weight in grams of a compound or the atomic weight in grams of an element.

molality (mō-lal'i-ti): The concentration of a solution expressed as mols per 1000 grams of solvent.

molar (mō'lar): 1. The double teeth or grinders; three on either side of the jaw. 2. A solution containing one mole of solute per liter of solution.

molarity (mō-lar'i-ti): The concentration of a solution expressed in gram molecular weight of solute per liter of solution.

mold (mōld): 1. Multicellular fungus; a member of the plant kingdom with no differential into root, stem, or leaf, and without chloryphyll. Structurally consists of hyphae which aggregate into a mass of cobwebby filaments called mycelium. Propagation is by means of spores. Occurs in infinite variety, commonly as saprophytes contaminating foodstuffs, and more rarely as pathogens. 2. The process of changing the shape of something, referring particularly to the change in shape of the fetal head to acommodate to the birth canal. 3. A shaped receptacle into which a malleable substance is poured or placed in making a cast.

molding (mōl'ding): The shaping of the fetal head in adjustment to the shape and size of the birth canal during the passage of the fetus through the canal in labor.

mole: Term used to express molecular weight; see gram-molecule. Also mol.

mole (mōl): Lay term for a nevus; a circumscribed, pigmented, elevated area on the skin. **CARNEOUS M.,** the dead and organized remains of a fetus that has died in utero. **HYDATIDIFORM M.,** a condition in which the chorionic villi of the placenta undergo cystic degeneration and the fetus is absorbed; may be a harmless condition safely corrected, but a proportion of these moles are active and if remnants are left in the uterus after abortion of the mole, malignant changes may ensue, giving rise to a chorionepithelioma (*q.v.*).

molecular (mō-lek'ū-lar): Pertaining to a molecule. **M. BIOLOGY,** the branch of biology that deals with the function and structure of the molecular constituents of biological systems and their physical and chemical roles in living tissues. **M. CLOCK HYPOTHESIS,** the assumption that senescence and death are the final steps in a program that begins with the development of the embryo.

molecule (mol′e-kūl): The smallest particle into which matter can be divided and still retain its identity.—molecular, adj.

mollities (mol-ish′i-ēz): Softness. Malacia.

molluscum (mō-lus′kum): A soft tumor. **M. CONTAGIOSUM,** a mildly contagious type of wart that appears especially on the face, buttocks, and perineum as a waxy papule, often umbilicated; spread is by autoinoculation. **M. FIBROSUM,** the superficial tumors of Recklinghausen's disease (*q.v.*).

mon-, mono-: Combining forms denoting 1) involving, having, or affecting a single element or part; 2) restricted to one. In chemistry, denotes in combination with one atom.

Monafo regimen: A regimen of fluid replacement utilized in the care of burn patients; consists of 250 Meq/L of sodium, 150 Meq/L chloride, and 100 Meq/L of lactate, administered rapidly to maintain urine output (for adults) at 30 to 50 ml per hour.

monarticular (mon′ar-tik′ū-lar): Relating to or affecting only one joint.

monaural (mon-aw′al): 1. Pertaining to one ear. 2. One ear functioning alone. 3. Hearing with one ear.

mongol (mong′gol): A person affected with mongolism (*q.v.*).—mongoloid, adj.

mongolian (mon-gō′li-an): Pertaining to or resembling a Mongol. **M. BLUE SPOT,** or **M. SPOT,** discoloration on the lumbosacral area of the newborn; fades gradually; not a birth defect and probably of no real significance. **M. IDIOCY,** Down's syndrome (*q.v.*). **M. FOLD,** see epicanthus.

mongolism (mon′gol-izm): A congenital condition characterized by mental deficiency and physicial characteristics resembling those of mongoloid people; now usually called Down's syndrome.

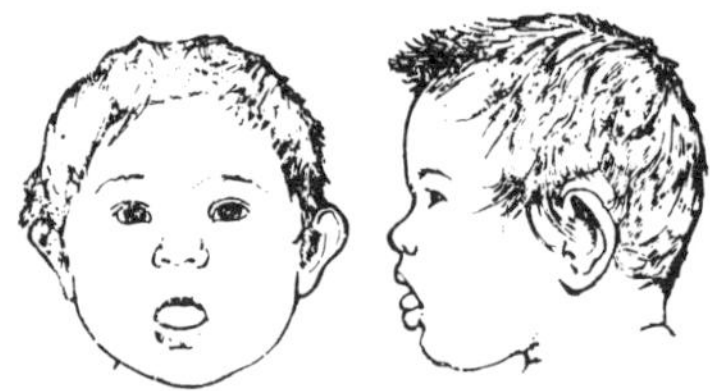

Mongolism

Monilia (mo-nil′i-a) The generic name for a large group of fungi or molds; those that are pathogenic are now more commonly called Candida (*q.v.*).

monilial vaginitis (mō-nil′i-al vaj-in-ī′tis): Candidiasis (*q.v.*).

moniliasis (mō-ni-lī′a-sis): Candidiasis (*q.v.*). **ORAL M.,** *Candida* infection of the mouth; seen in the very young and the very old; also called thrush (*q.v.*).

moniliform (mo-nil′i-form): Like a string of beads; beaded. Used to describe the arrangement of microorganisms, or such manifestations as skin rash.

monitor (mon′-i-tor): 1. To watch, observe, or check constantly on a state or condition. 2. An electronic apparatus that is attached to the patient and automatically records on a screen such physical signs as respiration, pulse, and blood pressure; may be employed in caring for an anesthetized person who is undergoing or recuperating from surgery or other procedure.

monitoring (mon′-i-tor-ing): The continuous or periodic observing, reporting and/or controlling of certain physiologic, biochemical, or bacterial processes, activities, or conditions. **INVASIVE M.,** involves instrumental penetration of the body, *e.g.*, central venous monitoring. **NONINVASIVE M.,** is based on observations, *e.g.*, blood pressure, pulse rate, respiratory rate.

monoamine (mon-ō-am′-ēn): An amine compound that contains only one amine group. See amines.

monoamine oxidase (MAO) (mon-ō-am′-en oks′-i-dās): An enzyme present in most tissue cells; its function is to act as a catalyst in the deamination of certain monoamines such as epinephrine and serotonin. **MAO INHIBITOR,** any drug or chemical that inhibits the action of monoamine oxidase with the result that the amines normally acted on by the enzyme accumulate in the body. Drugs in this class are sometimes used as psychic energizers in the treatment of fairly severe depression, but under close medical supervison because of their side effects and incompatibilities with certain other drugs and foods.

monoblast (mon′-ō-blast): A large immature monocyte.

monoblepsia (mon-ō-blep′-si-a): A condition of vision in which one is able to see better with only one eye than with two. The term is also applied to color blindness in which all colors appear to be the same.

monochromatic (mon′ō-krō-mat′ik): 1. Existing in one color only. 2. Staining with only one dye at a time. 3. A person who exhibits monochromatism (*q.v.*).

monochromatism (mon′ō-krō′ma-tizm): Complete color blindness; all colors appear as shades of gray. A rare disorder.

monoclonal (mon-ō-klō′-nal): Pertaining to a single group of cells, or a clone, involving an identical cell product.

monococcus (mon-ō-kok′-us): A coccus that occurs singly, not in pairs, chains, or groups.

monocular (mon-ok′-ū-lar): Pertaining to or affecting one eye only. See microscope.

monocyte (mon′-ō-sīt): A large mononuclear leukocyte. The monocytes are phagocytic; they make up about 5 percent of the total white blood cell count.

monocytopenia (mon′ō-sī-tō-pē′ni-a): Less than the normal number of monocytes in the circulating blood.

monocytosis (mon′-ō-sī-tō′-sis): An abnormal increase in the proportion of leukocytes in the circulating blood.

monogenesis (mon-ō-jen′-e-sis): Nonsexual reproduction.

monoideism (mon-ō-ī-dē′-izm): Inability to stop talking or thinking about a certain idea or group of ideas; a degree of monomania.

monomania (mon′ō-mā′ni-a): Obsessed with a single idea or group of ideas.

monomer (mon′-ō-mer): A simple molecule that is capable of combining with other similar or unlike molecules to form a polymer.

mononeuritis (mon′-ō-nū-rī′-tis): Neuritis affecting only one nerve. See **neuritis.**

mononeuropathy (mon′ō-nū-rop′a-thi): A condition in which pain and weakness develop suddenly in the areas of distribution of one or two nerves; usually occurs in the leg with the femoral or sciatic nerve being involved; may be seen in diabetics and in cases of herniated vertebral disk. **CRANIAL M.,** a disease involving one of the cranial nerves.

mononuclear (mon′ō-nū′klē-ar): With a single nucleus. Usually refers to the largest type of blood cell, characterized by a round or oval shape and indented nucleus. Monocyte.

mononucleosis (mon′-ō-nū-klē-ō′-sis): An increase in the number of circulating monocytes (mononuclear cells) in the blood. **INFECTIOUS M.,** is an acute infectious type of **M.** caused by a virus; characterized by sudden onset, fever, malaise, sore throat, enlargement of lymph nodes and spleen. Occurs most frequently between the ages of 20 and 30 and is usually self-limited and benign.

monoparesis (mon′-ō-par-ē′-sis): Weakness of the muscles of one arm or one leg.

monophasia (mon′ō-fā′zi-a): Aphasia in which the individual is able to utter only one word or phrase and repeats it constantly.

monoplegia (mon-ō-plē′-ji-a): Paralysis of only one limb, or of one muscle or group of muscles.—monoplegic, adj.

monorchidism (mon-or′-ki-dizm): Having only one testis, or the condition of only one testis having descended into the scrotum. Monorchism.

monosaccharide (mon-ō-sak′-a-rīd): A simple sugar ($C_6H_{12}O_6$). Examples are glucose, fructose, and galactose.

monosexual (mon-ō-seks′-ū-al): Having the characteristics of only one sex.

monosodium glutamate (mon-ō-sō′-di-um glū′-ta-māt): A salt of glutamic acid; used as a food additive for flavoring and also in the treatment of encephalopathy associated with liver disease.

monotrichous (mo-not′-ri-kus): Having a single flagellum at one end; said of a bacterial cell.

monovular (mon-ov′-ū-lar): Pertaining to a single ovum; or derived from a single ovum, as identical twins.

monoxide (mon-ok′-sīd): An oxide in which the molecules have only one atom of oxygen. Commonly used by the laity to mean carbon monoxide.

monozygotic (mon′ō-zī-got′ik): Referring to twins that develop from the same fertilized ovum, *i.e.,* identical twins.

mons veneris (mons ven′-er-is): The eminence formed by the pad of fat that lies over the symphysis pubis in the female. Also called mons pubis.

monster (mon′-ster): Term formerly much used to describe an infant grossly malformed at birth. Many are born dead or die soon after birth; in a few cases surgery can be performed to correct the anomaly.

Montgomery's tubercles: Name given to the sebaceous glands on the areola of the breast when they become enlarged during pregnancy.

mood: A prevailing attitude or state of mind. In psychiatry, a sustained emotional state such as melancholia or mania.

moon face: The rounded full face that is characteristic of hyperadrenocorticism (*q.v.*).

Moore pin: A metal pin used in hip surgery.

morbid (mor′-bid): Diseased. Pertaining to, affected by, or productive of disease. Grisly or gruesome. **M. ANATOMY,** that branch of anatomy that is concerned with the study of diseased tissues and organs.

morbidity (mor-bid′-i-ti): 1. The state of being sick or diseased. 2. The incidence of disease. 3. The sick rate; the ratio of sick persons or of cases of disease to the number of well persons in a specified geographic area during a specific period of time.

Morbidity and Mortality Weekly Report: A publication of the Centers for Disease Control. By law, all deaths must be reported, but the only category of illness that the physician is required to report is that of infectious diseases of which only ten are significant—chickenpox; gonorrhea; hepatitis A and B and unspecified; measles; mumps; German measles; salmonellosis; tuberculosis; syphilis; and acquired immunodeficiency syndrome.

morbific (mor-bif′-ik): Causing disease; pathogenic.

morbilli (mor-bil′lī): Measles (*q.v.*).

morbilliform (mor-bil′-i-form): Descriptive of a rash resembling that of measles.

morbus (mor′-bus): Disease.

mordant (mor′-dant): In microbiology, a substance used to fix a dye or stain.

mores (mō′-rēz): The fixed values and customs of a particular group. Habits; manners; moral code.

morgue (morg): A place where bodies of the deceased are placed temporarily until they are identified or claimed for burial.

moribund (mor′-i-bund): Dying; having no vital force left.

morning after pill: A contraceptive pill that is taken after sexual intercourse, usually the next morning. It blocks the formation of corpus luteum following ovulation and presumably prevents implantation of the fertilized ovum. Has been used after rape, or incest, or when there is undue anxiety about the possiblity of pregnancy.

morning sickness: Nausea and vomiting when arising in the morning, especially that which occurs during the first 4 to 16 weeks of pregnancy. Occurs in about 50 percent of pregnant women.

Moro reflex: See reflex, Moro.

moron (mō′-ron): An obsolete term for an individual with a potential mental age of 8 to 12 years with an IQ of 50 to 70, thus ranking below normal and highest in the group of mental defectives (the other two grades were formerly identified as imbecile and idiot).

morph-, morpho-: Combining forms denoting form, shape, type, structure.

-morph, -morphous: Combining forms denoting shape, form.

morphea (mor′-fē-a): Localized scleroderma; see under scleroderma.

morphine (mor′-fēn): The active principle of opium and a valuable narcotic, hypnotic, and analgesic. Habit-forming, thus its sale and distribution are controlled by federal law.

morphinism (mor′-fin-izm): Addiction to morphine.

morphogenesis (mor′-fō-jen′-e-sis): The morphological changes, including growth and cell differentiation, during human development.

morphology (mor-fol′-o-ji): The science that deals with the form and structure of living things, regarded as a whole, and apart from their function.—morphological, adj.; morphologically, adv.

morphometry (mor-fom′-e-tri): Measurement of the forms of organisms.—morphometric, adj.

Morquio's syndrome: A rare hereditary form of mucopolysaccharidosis (*q.v.*), marked by severe dwarfism, dorsolumbar kyphosis, waddling gait, flatfeet, deafness, and some facial abnormalities; often not noticeable until the child begins to walk; mentality is seldom affected.

mortal: 1. Fatal; causing or resulting in death. 2. Human.

mortality (mor-tal′-i-ti): 1. The quality of being mortal (*q.v.*). 2. The death rate; the number of deaths in a unit of population occurring within a prescribed time. Mortality rates for deaths from all causes are usually expressed as number of deaths per 1000 population. **INFANT M. RATE,** the number of deaths during the first year of life per 1000 live births for the year. **MATERNAL M. RATE,** the number of deaths due to pregnancy or childbearing per 1000 registered births per year. **PERINATAL M. RATE,** the number of stillbirths and babies that die during the first week of life per 1000 registered births in a year.

Mortenson's syndrome: Hemorrhagic thrombocythemia; a blood disorder characterized by increased thrombocytic count, prolonged bleeding time, hemoptysis, easy bruising, and enlarged spleen; may occur in association with leukemia or polycythemia, or following splenectomy.

mortician (mor-tish′-an): A funeral director. An undertaker; one who is trained to care for the dead, as regulated by law and custom.

mortification (mor′-ti-fi-kā′- shun): Local death of tissue. See gangrene.

Morton's syndrome or neuralgia: A painful condition in which congenital shortness of the first metatarsal causes hypertrophy and pain in the second metatarsal; the pain is caused by irritation of the nerve between the heads of the metatarsals. If the nerve becomes thickened and hypertrophied, the condition is referred to as **MORTON'S NEUROMA.** See metatarsalgia.

morula (mor′-ū-la): In embryonic development, the solid mass that results from cleavage of a fertilized ovum; consists of blastomeres.

mosaicism (mō-zā′-i-sizm): The presence of cells with differing genetic makeup in the same individual.

Mosenthal test: A kidney function test involving measuring the variability of the specific gravity of the urine over 24 hours.

mosquito (mō-skē′-tō): A large family of blood-sucking arthropods, several varieties of which are carriers or vectors of infectious disease.

mother complex: Oedipus complex (*q.v.*).

motile (mō′-til): Capable of spontaneous movement.—motility, n.

motion sickness: Nausea and usually vomiting due to stimulation of the semicircular canals caused by the irregular or rhythmic motion of an airplane, car or boat, or by swinging.

motivation (mō-ti-vā'-shun): Drive; incentive; need; attitude and expectation that results in action.

motor: Pertaining to 1) action or motion; or 2) a muscle, nerve, or center that is concerned with motion. See neuron. **M. APHASIA,** see under aphasia. **M. APRAXIA,** see under apraxia. **M. AREA,** the area in the cerebral cortex that controls the contraction of voluntary muscles.

motor end plate: A specilized structure at the terminus of a motor nerve fiber where it makes functional contact with a muscle fiber.

motor fibers: Nerve fibers that are responsible for voluntary movement; consist of 1) pyramidal fibers that originate in the cortex of the brain, cross in the medulla oblongata, descend in the pyramidal tract of the spinal cord and end in roots that enervate skeletal muscles; and 2) extrapyramidal fibers that orginate in the brain stem and descend in close association with the pyramidal fibers.

motor neuron, upper and lower. See under neuron.

motor point: A point on the skin over a muscle where the application of an electric current will cause the muscle to contract.

motor unit: An anatomical unit consisting of an anterior horn cell, its axon with all of its branches, the motor end plates, and the muscle fibers that are innervated.

mottling (mot'-ling): Spotty discoloration of the skin without a distinct pattern; patches have varying sizes, shapes, and depth of color.

mould (mōld) Mold (*q.v.*).

mountain: **M. SICKNESS,** symptoms of sickness, dyspnea, and tachycardia; due to low oxygen content of rarefied air at high altitudes. **M. FEVER,** see Rocky Mountain spotted fever.

mourning: See bereavement.

mouth: An aperture or opening into a cavity; specifically the opening through which food passes into the body.

mouth sticks: Sticks of varying lengths that are held in the mouth and can be manipulated by handicapped persons, *e.g.*, quadriplegics, to assist in such activities as typing, drawing, dialing telephone numbers, etc.

mouth-to-mouth resuscitation: See resuscitation.

movement: 1. Motion; the act of moving. 2. The act of emptying the colon; defecation. 3. The material evacuated from the rectum during one bowel movement; the stool.

moxa (mok'-sa): A small soft tuft of downy material used in moxibustion (*q.v.*).

moxibustion (mok'-si-bus'-chun): The burning of a moxa (*q.v.*) placed on the skin, to produce counterirritation or cauterization; a very old form of treatment formerly much used in China and Japan.

M.P.H.: Abbreviation for Master of Public Health.

MS: Abbreviation for 1. Multiple sclerosis. 2. Master of Science.

msec.: Abbreviation for millisecond.

M.S.N.: Abbreviation for Master of Science in Nursing.

MSU: Abbreviation for midstream specimen of urine. See clean-catch specimen.

M.T.: Abbreviation for medical technologist.

mu: The twenty-sixth letter of the Greek alphabet; written μ; used as a symbol for micron.

mucin (mū'-sin): A mixture of mucopolysaccharides found in or secreted by many cells and glands. The chief constituent of mucus.—mucinous, adj.

mucobuccal (mū-kō-buk'-al): Pertaining to the mucous lining of the mouth and cheek.

mucocele (mū'-kō-sēl): 1. Distention of a cavity with mucus. 2. A cyst or cyst-like structure that contains mucus.

mucocutaneous (mū'-kō-kū-tā'nē-us): Pertaining to mucous membrane and skin.

mucoid (mū'-koyd): Resembling mucus.

mucolysis (mū-kol'-i-sis): Dissolution or liquefaction of mucus.—mucolytic, adj.

mucolytic (mū-kō-lit'-ik): 1. Capable of destroying or dissolving mucus. 2. An agent that liquefies or dissolves mucus.

mucopolysaccharide (mū'-kō-pol-i-sak'-a-rīd): A polysaccharide widely distributed in nature; a complex material that makes up the amorphous substance in the intercellular material in the body.

mucopolysaccharidosis (mū'kō-pol-i-sak'a-ri-dō'sis): An inherited disorder of mucopolysaccharide metabolism; characterized by mental retardation, skeletal deformities, clouding of the cornea, and the secretion of mucopolysaccharides in the urine. Several types are identified on the basis of findings, including Hurler's syndrome, Hunter's syndrome, Morquio's syndrome, Sanfilippo's syndrome, and Scheie's syndrome.

mucoprotein (mū'kō-prō'tē-in): One of a group of complex protein compounds that occur in body tissues and fluids; has chemical characteristics of a protein but does not coagulate when heated.

mucopurulent (mū'kō-pū'roo-lent): Containing mucus and pus.

mucopus (mū'-kō-pus): Mucus containing pus.

Mucor (mū'-kor): A general name for a variety of molds that are frequently found on dead or decaying vegetable matter; some of them are pathogenic to man.

Mucorales (mū-kor-ā'-lez): An order of fungi, including the bread molds; the majority are saprophytic; the cause of mucormycosis, which is often a complication of debilitating disease, diabetes in particular. See mucormycosis.

mucormycosis (mū′-kor-mī-kō′-sis): An acute, usually fulminating, infection by a fungus of the *Mucorales* order; usually accompanies a systemic disorder such as diabetes, lymphoma, or leukemia; often starts in the respiratory tract and metastasizes to other parts of the body, including the skin, brain, and gastrointestinal tract.

mucorrhea (mū-kō-rē′-a): An increase in the discharge of mucus from the cervix at the time of ovulation; usually continues for three to four days and has the general appearance of egg white. See spinnbarkheit.

mucosa (mū-kō′sa): A mucous membrane (*q.v.*).—mucosal, adj.: mucosae, pl.

mucosanguineous (mū′-kō-sang-gwin′-ē-us): Composed of both mucus and blood.

mucositis (mū-kō-sī′-tis): Inflammation of a mucous membrane.

mucous (mū′-kus): Pertaining to, secreting, or containing mucus. See membrane. **M. COLITIS,** mucomembranous colitis; possibly a functional disorder, manifested by passage of mucus in the stool, obstinate constipation and occasional colic. **M. POLYPUS,** condition in which the mucous membrane becomes pedunculated and projects from the surface in polypoid masses.

mucoviscidosis (mū′kō-vis′i-dō′sis): A congenital hereditary disease with failure of development of normal mucus-secreting glands, sweat glands and pancreas. May be present in a newborn as meconium ileus; in infancy with septic bronchitis and steatorrhea. Stools contain excess fat; trypsin is absent from stool and duodenal juice. See cystic fibrosis.

mucus (mū′-kus): the viscid fluid secreted by the mucous glands. Contains mucin and such other substances as inorganic salts, epithelial cells, leukocytes, and water. Serves as a protective lubricant coating.

Müllerian ducts: Embryonic structures from which the urinary system develops; in the female, the origin also of the fallopian tubes, uterus, and most of the vaginal canal.

multi-: Combining form denoting 1) multiple, many, much; 2) affecting many parts.

multiarticular (mul′ti-ar-tik′ū-lar): Pertaining to or affecting several joints.

multicellular (mul-ti-sel′-ū-lar): Constructed of many cells.

multifocal (mul-ti-fō′-kal): Arising from, pertaining to, or having several foci.

multiform (mul′-ti-form): Having many forms or shapes.

multiglandular (mul-ti-glan′-dū-lar): Pertaining to or affecting several glands.

multigravida (mul-ti-grav′-id-a): A woman who has been pregnant more than once. —multigravidae, pl.

multilobar (mul-ti-lō′-bar): Possessing several lobes.

multilobular (mul-ti-lob′-ū-lar): Possessing many lobules.

multilocular (mul-ti-lok′-ū-lar): Possessing many small cysts, loculi or pockets.

multinuclear (mul-ti-nū′-klē-ar): Possessing many nuclei.—multinucleate, adj.

multipara (mul-tip′-a-ra): A woman who is having or has had two or more pregnancies resulting in viable children. Written Para II, III, etc. **GRANDE M.,** name given to a woman who has had seven or more children.—multiparae, pl.; multiparous, adj.

multiparity (mul-ti-par′-i-ti): 1. The production of more than one child in the same gestation. 2. The condition of being a multipara (*q.v.*).

multiple endocrine adenomatosis: See adenomatosis.

multiple sclerosis: See sclerosis.

multivalent (mul-ti-vā′-lent): 1. In chemistry, having the power of combining with three or more univalent atoms. 2. Pertaining to an agent that is effective against several varieties or strains of a certain microorganism.

multivitamin (mul-ti-vī′-ta-min): Pertaining to a preparation that contains several vitamins, especially those considered to be essential to life and health.

mummification (mum-i-fi-kā′-shun): 1. Dry gangrene. 2.The drying up of a dead fetus in the uterus. 3. Restraining a patient by wrapping him in a sheet; used to keep mental patients from injuring themselves and others and to restrain a restive child during an operation or other procedure.

mummy restraint: A type of physical restraint in which the entire body is wrapped in a sheet or blanket and only the head is exposed.

mumps: An acute, infectious disease, characterized by inflammation of one or both parotid (*q.v.*) glands; caused by a filterable virus. The chief symptom is a sensitive swelling below and in front of the ear and edema of the surrounding tissues, distorting the features. The most common complication in the adult male is orchitis; in the female, ovaritis and mastitis. Syn., epidemic parotitis.

Munchausen syndrome: A condition characterized by repeated presentations with fictitious symptoms and an untrue history; these individuals often produce symptoms by various means and willingly undergo any suggested treatment or tests to get attention or, sometimes, drugs.

mural (mū′-ral): Pertaining to or occurring in the wall of a cavity, organ or vessel.

muriatic acid (mū-ri-at′ik-as′id): Hydrochloric acid (*q.v.*).

murmur (mur′-mur): An abnormal, usually soft, blowing sound, but may be rasping, harsh, or musical; caused by vibration produced by the turbulent flow of blood between two pressure areas and/or within the heart or the adjacent great vessels; not necessarily significant. **AORTIC M.**, one heard at the aortic orifice of the heart; may be regurgitant or obstructive. **DIASTOLIC M.**, one that occurs during ventricular diastole and may be classified as 1) regurgitant, a high-pitched long **M.**, or 2) filling, a low-pitched rumbling **M.** **FUNCTIONAL OR INNOCENT M.**, one commonly heard in young children; not associated with a heart lesion. **MILL WHEEL M.**, a churning **M.** produced by air embolism to the heart. **MITRAL M.**, one heard at the mitral valve, due to obstruction or regurgitation. **ORGANIC M.**, a **M.** caused by an organic lesion. **PRESYSTOLIC M.**, one that occurs just before the systole and is usually due to stenosis of one of the atrioventricular orifices. **PULMONARY M.**, a **M.** heard at the pulmonary orifice of the heart; may be due to obstruction or regurgitation. **SYSTOLIC M.**, an abnormal quality of the first heart sound, usually related to the area of one of the heart valves, *e.g.*, systolic mitral murmur; may be classified as 1) **SYSTOLIC EJECTION M.**, produced by the blood moving over the pneumonic and aortic valves, heard early in systole at the base of the heart, and in older people without signs of heart disease; or 2) **REGURGITANT M.**, heard when there is backflow from ventricles to atria or through a septal defect. Systolic **M.**, may also be pansystolic or holosystolic, lasting throughout the entire phase of systole.

Murphy button: A device consisting of two hollow cylinders; one is inserted into each open end of the intestine, sutured in place, and then the intestinal ends are sutured together; formerly widely used in the operation for creating an intestinal anastomosis

Murphy drip: The continual slow drip of a fluid into the body, usually into the rectum, or the apparatus used for administering fluid in this way.

Murphy's sign: A sign of gallbladder disease when the patient cannot take a deep breath while the physician's fingers are pressed deeply beneath the right costal margin.

Musca domestica (mus′ka dom-es′ti-ka): The common house fly, capable of transmitting many organisms pathogenic to man.

muscae volitantes (mus′kē vol-i-tan′tēz): The sensation of moving spots before the eyes. Caused by the presence of cells or cell fragments in the vitreous humor. See floater.

muscarine (mus′ka-rēn): A deadly alkaloid found in certain mushrooms and certain rotten fish.

muscle (mus′el): Strong, contractile tissue that produces movement of the body. Depending on structure, muscle tissue is classified as striated (striped), nonstriated (smooth), and indistinctly striated. Also classified according to whether it is voluntary (under conscious control) or involuntary (under control of the autonomic nervous system). Characteristics of muscle tissue are contractility, excitability, extensibility, and elasticity. **CARDIAC M.** forms the walls of the heart, is indistinctly striated and involuntary. **SKELETAL M.**, surrounds the skeleton, is striated and voluntary. **VISCERAL M.** (internal) is nonstriated (except for the heart) and involuntary.—muscular, adj.

muscle cramp: A sudden, involuntary, painful contraction of a skeletal muscle.

muscle-bound: Having some of one's muscles enlarged, tense, and lacking in elasticity; usually due to overexercise.

muscul-, musculo-: Combining forms denoting muscle, muscular.

muscular (mus′kū-lar): 1. Pertaining to muscle or muscles. 2. Descriptive of an individual with well-developed muscles.

muscular dystrophy: See under dystrophy.

musculature (mus′kū-la-tūr): The muscular system of the body or part of it.

musculocutaneous (mus′kū-lō-kū-tā′nē-us): Pertaining to both muscle and skin.

musculomembranous (mus′kū-lō-mem′bra-nus): Pertaining to both muscle and membrane. Descriptive of such muscles as the occipitofrontalis, which is largely membranous.

musculoskeletal (mus′kū-lō-skel′e-tal): Pertaining to the muscular and skeletal systems.

musculotendinous (mus′kū-lō-ten′di-nus): Pertaining to or composed of muscle and tendon.

musculotrophia (mus′kū-lō-trō′fi-a): Having an affinity for or affecting chiefly muscular tissue.

mushroom worker's lung: See farmer's lung.

musicomania (mū′zi-kō-mā′ni-a): An insane preoccupation with music.

musicotherapy (mū′zi-kō-ther′a-pi): Music therapy. The use of music in treatment of disease, especially mental disorders.

Musset's sign: Subtle, rhythmic up and down movements of the head in synchronization with the heartbeat; seen in cases of aortic aneurysm and aortic insufficiency.

mussitation (mus-i-tā′shun): Movement of the lips without producing any sound; sometimes seen in delirious patients.

mustard: The powdered seed of a plant of the genus *Brassica;* has been used in medicine as an emetic and rubefacient. **M. GAS**, a poisonous gas used in warfare; it causes vesication and corrosion of the skin and mucous membranes; is particularly damaging to the membranes of the respiratory system. **NITROGEN MUSTARDS,** mustard compounds that have been used therapeutically in treatment of certain cancers.

mutagen (mū'ta-jen): A physical or chemical agent that is capable of causing a heritable alteration in the DNA (*q.v.*), which induces a genetic mutation, *e.g.*, drugs, ultraviolet light, ionizing radiation.

mutagenesis (mū'ta-jen'e-sis): The production of genetic change.

mutagenic (mū-ta-jen'ik): Capable of causing genetic mutations.—mutagenicity, n.

mutant (mū'tant): A cell that is the result of a genetic change. It has characteristics that are different from those of the parent cells and that can be passed on to the offspring. A sport.

mutation (mū-tā'shun): 1. A transformation or change in form, quality, or some other characteristic. 2. A genetic change in the germ plasm of a cell which results in a change of the characters of the cell. This change is heritable, remaining until further mutation occurs. **INDUCED M.,** a gene mutation produced by a known agent outside the cell, *e.g.*, ultraviolet radiation. **NATURAL M.,** a gene mutation taking place without apparent influence from outside the cell.

mute (mūt): 1. Unable to speak. 2. A person who is unable to speak. **DEAF-M.,** a person who is unable to speak or to hear. In psychiatry, a person who refuses to speak in order to keep others at a distance.

mutilate (mū'ti-lāt): To maim or disfigure the body by removing, destroying, or deforming some essential and conspicuous part.—mutilation, n.

mutilation (mū-ti-lā'shun): 1. The destruction or removal of a body part. 2. The loss of an important part of the body with consequent disfigurement.

mutism (mū'tizm): Dumbness; speechlessness. In psychiatry, refusal or inability to speak. May be conscious or unconscious, organic or functional. **AKINETIC M.,** a type of **M.** in which the person makes no bodily or other response to sound.

mutualism (mū'tū-a-lizm): Symbiosis. Equally beneficial interactions between organisms, *e.g.*, between humans and certain bacteria.

mV: Abbreviation for millivolt.

my-, myo-: Combining forms denoting relationship to muscle.

myalgia (mī-al'ji-a): Pain in the muscles.—myalgic, adj.

myasthenia (mī'as-thē'ni-a): Muscular weakness. **M. GRAVIS,** a progressive disorder, seen mostly in adults, chiefly women, 20 to 50 years of age; characterized by marked fatigability of voluntary muscles, especially those of the face, lip, tongue, throat and neck, and eye. The patient has a characteristic sleepy expression due to ptosis of the eyelids and weakness of the facial muscles. Results from lack of acetylcholine or excess of cholinesterase at the myoneural junction.

myasthenic syndrome (mī-as-then'ik): Weakness of the limb girdle muscles; often associated with cancer, particularly of the lung; to be distinguished from myasthenia gravis, which it resembles.

myatonia (mī-a-tō'ni-a): Absence of tone in muscle. **M. CONGENITA,** a form of congenital muscular dystrophy in infancy. Child is unable to bear the weight of the head on the shoulders.—myatonic, adj.

myatrophy (mī-at'rō-fi): Atrophy of muscle.

myc-, myceto-, myco-: Combining forms denoting fungus.

mycelium (mī-sē'li-um): The tangled mass of branching filaments (hyphae) that represents the body of a mold or fungus.—mycelial, mycelian, mycelioid, adj.

mycetoma (mī-sē-tō'ma): A fungus infection, usually of the feet, occurring in tropical and subtropical regions. Similar to actinomycosis and aspergillosis (*q.v.*). Syn., Madura foot, maduromycosis.

Mycobacterium (mī-kō-bak-tēr'i-um): Small slender rod bacteria, gram-positive and acid-fast, both to a varying degree. Saprophytic, commensal, and pathogenic species. **M. BALNEI,** the cause of "swimming-pool" granuloma; see granuloma. **M. BOVIS,** the bovine variety of the tubercle bacillus; causes bovine tuberculosis, which may be acquired by man, usually through infected milk. **M. TUBERCULOSIS,** the cause of tuberculosis. **M. LEPRAE,** the cause of leprosy.

mycology (mī-kol'o-ji): The study of fungi.—mycologist, n.; mycological, adj.; mycologically, adv.

Mycoplasma (mī'kō-plaz-ma): A genus of microorganisms intermediate in size between viruses and bacteria; includes the pleuropneumonia-like organisms (PPLO); important in respiratory diseases. One type is associated with acute leukemia. **M. HOMINIS,** found in genital and rectal mucosa; associated with nongonococcal urethritis. **M. ORALE,** found in human saliva. **M. PNEUMONIAE,** the cause of primary atypical pneumonia; also called Eaton agent. **M. SALIVARIUM,** found in human saliva and the upper respiratory tract.—mycoplasmal, mycoplasmic, adj.

mycoplasmosis (mī'kō-plaz-mō'sis): Infection with mycoplasma (*q.v.*).

mycoprotein (mī-kō-prō'te-in): The protein in fungi or bacteria.

mycopus (mī-kō'pus): Mucus that contains pus.

mycosis (mī-kō'sis): Any disease caused by a fungus; may be superficial, affecting only the skin, or systemic. **M. FUNGOIDES,** a rare, chronic, usually fatal skin malignancy; characterized by pruritus and psoriasis-like dermatitis, followed by skin abscesses; in the late stages it spreads to the lymph nodes and the viscera resulting in the development of large painful tumors that ulcerate; seen most often in adult males and the elderly.

mydriasis (mi-drī'a-sis): Abnormal dilatation of the pupil.

mydriatics (mid-ri-at'iks): Drugs that cause mydriasis (*q.v.*).

myectomy (mī-ek'to-mi): Surgical removal of part of a muscle.

myel-, myelo-: Combining forms denoting: 1. Bone marrow. 2. Spinal cord.

myelencephalitis (mī'el-en-sef-a-lī'tis): Inflammation of the brain and spinal cord.

myelencephalon (mī'el-en-sef'a-lon): The lower part of the embryonic hindbrain; it develops into the medulla oblongata.

myelic (mī-el'ik): Pertaining to: 1. Bone marrow. 2. The spinal cord.

myelin (mī'e-lin): The white, fatty substance constituting the medullary sheath of certain nerve fibers.

myelinization (mī'e-li-nī-zā'shun): The accumulation or supplying of myelin during the process of nerve development or repair.

myelinolysis (mī'e-lin-ol'i-sis): Disintegration of myelin.—myelinotic, adj.

myelinosis (mī'e-li-nō'sis): Necrosis or decomposition of fat, with the formation of myelin.

myelitis (mī-e-lī'tis): Inflammation of 1) the spinal cord; 2) bone marrow. **TRANSVERSE M., M.** that extends across the spinal cord.

myeloblast (mī'e-lō-blast): An immature cell in the bone marrow which develops into a granular leukocyte.

myeloblastoma (mī'e-lō-blas-tō'ma): A fairly well circumscribed malignant tumor consisting of a mass of myelobasts (*q.v.*).

myeloblastosis (mī'e-lō-blast-tō'sis): Abnormally large number of myeloblasts in the blood or in the tissues, sometimes seen in acute leukemia.

myelocele (mī'e-lō-sēl): A form of spina bifida (*q.v.*); the development of the spinal cord itself has been arrested, and the central canal of the cord opens on the skin surface, discharging cerebrospinal fluid. Incompatible with life.

myelocystomeningocele (mī'e-lō-sis'tō-mening'gō-sēl): A congenital anomaly in which a cystic tumor composed of spinal cord and meningeal tissues protrudes through a defect in the bony spinal column. Also called meningomyelocele.

myelocyte (mī'e-lō-sīt): 1. An immature bone marrow cell of the type from which leukocytes develop. Present in blood in some pathological conditions, *e.g.*, leukemia. 2. Any cell in the gray matter (*q.v.*).

myelodysplasia (mī'e-lō-dis-plā'zi-a): Defective development of the spinal cord; occurs most often in the lumbosacral region.—myelodysplastic, adj.

myeloencephalitis (mī'e-lō-en-sef-a-lī'tis): Acute inflammation of the brain and spinal cord. **EPIDEMIC M.,** acute anterior poliomyelitis (*q.v.*).

myelofibrosis (mī'e-lō-fī-brō'sis): Excessive growth of bone marrow.

myelogenesis (mī'e-lō-jen'e-sis): Myelinization (*q.v.*).

myelogenous (mī-e-loj'e-nus): 1. Produced in or by the bone marrow. 2. Myelogenic.

myelogram (mī'e-lō-gram): An x ray of the spine after injection of a radiopaque substance into the subarachnoid space. **AIR M.,** a **M.** in which air or oxygen is injected into the subarachnoid space instead of a radiopaque substance.

myelography (mī-e-log'ra-fi): Visualization of the spinal cord after the injection of a contrast medium into the subarachnoid space. **GAS M.,** radiographic examination of the spinal cord following the injection of gas into the subarachnoid space.—myelographic, adj.; myelographically, adv.

myeloid (mī'e-loyd): 1. Pertaining to or derived from bone marrow. 2. Pertaining to the spinal cord.

myeloma (mī-e-lō'ma): 1. A tumor of the medullary canal. 2. A tumor containing cells of the type normally found in bone marrow. **MULTIPLE M.,** a primary tumor of bone marrow; usually malignant; associated with hyperplasia of the bone marrow, Bence Jones protein in the urine, neuralgic pain, sometimes spontaneous fracture; bone pain in the back or hip is the usual complaint; occurs most often in the elderly.

myelomalacia (mī'e-lō-ma-lā'shi-a): Softening of the spinal cord.

myelomatosis (mī'e-lō-ma-tō'sis): Multiple myeloma (*q.v.*). See Bence Jones protein.

myelomeningocele (mī'e-lō-me-ning'gō-sēl): Meningomyelocele (*q.v.*).

myelopathy (mī-e-lop'a-thi): Any disease or pathological change in the spinal cord.

myelophthisis (mī-e-lof'thi-sis): 1. Atrophy or wasting of the spinal cord. 2. A pathological condition in which the blood-cell forming tissues of the bone marrow are displaced by fibrous or bony tissue, resulting in anemia that is characterized by the presence of immature granulocytes in the blood (myelopathic anemia).

myelopoiesis (mī′-e-lō-poy-ē′sis): The formation of bone marrow, or of the cells that arise in the bone marrow.

myeloproliferation (mī′e-lō-prō-lif-er-ā′shun): Proliferation of one or more elements of the bone marrow without other signs of neoplasia.—myeloproliferative, adj.

myelosclerosis (mī′e-lō-sklē-rō′sis): Multiple sclerosis of the spinal cord. See **sclerosis**.

myelosis (mī-e-lō′sis): 1. The development and presence of a tumor on the spinal cord. 2. A bone marrow condition characterized by proliferation of the tissue, or cellular elements resulting in changes in the blood, as seen in myelocytic leukemia. **ERYTHREMIC M.**, a malignant blood condition associated with anemia, enlarged liver and spleen, hemorrhagic tendencies, and the presence in the blood of erythrocytes in all stages of development, including megaloblasts.

myelotomy (mī′e-lot′o-mi): A surgical procedure in which nerve tracts in the spinal cord are severed.

myelotoxic (mī′e-lō-tok′sik): Depressing or destructive to the bone marrow or pertinent to diseased bone marrow.

myiasis (mī-ī′a-sis): Any infection that develops as a result of invasion of a body tissue or cavity by the larvae of dipterous insects (houseflies, mosquitoes, gnats, etc.); may involve the eye, ear, nasal passages, intestinal tract, or skin.

mylohyoid (mī′lō-hī′oyd): Pertinent to molar teeth or the lower part of the jaw and the hyoid bone; denotes various structures as nerves, muscles.

myoasthenia (mī-ō-as-thē′ni-a): Lack or loss of muscle strength.

myoblastoma (mī′ō-blas-tō′ma): A neoplasm occurring in striated muscle, often in the tongue; made up of immature muscle cells.

myobradia (mī-ō-brā′di-a): Sluggish reaction of muscle to electrical stimulation.

myocardia (mī-ō-kar′di-a): A noninflammatory disease of the myocardium. The term is often used to describe heart failure when the cause is unknown.

myocardial (mī-ō-kar′di-al): Pertaining to the myocardium. **M. INFARCTION**, the formation of an infarct (*q.v.*) in the myocardium.

myocarditis (mī-ō-kar-dī′tis): Inflammation of the myocardium.

myocardium (mī′ō-kar′di-um): The middle and thickest of the layers of the heart wall; composed of indistinctly striated, involuntary muscle tissue.—myocardial, adj.

myocele (mī′ō-sēl): Protrusion of a muscle through its ruptured sheath.

myocelialgia (mī′ō-sē-li-al′ji-a): Pain in the abdominal muscles.

myocelitis (mī-ō-sē-lī′tis): Inflammation of the abdominal muscles.

myoclonus (mi-ok′lo-nus): Clonic contractions of individual muscles or groups of muscles. Twitching. **M. MULTIPLEX**, a disorder characterized by rapid contractions of unrelated muscles, either simultaneously or consecutively; also called paraclonus and Friedreich's disease.

myocytoma (mī′-ō-sī-tō′ma): A benign muscle tumor usually involving nonstriated muscle.

myodegeneration (mī′ō-dē-jen-er-ā′shun): Degeneration of muscle tissue.

myodemia (mī-ō-dē′ mi-a): Fatty degeneration of muscle tissue.

myodynia (mī′ō-din′i-a): Pain in a muscle; myalgia.

myodystonia (mī′ -ō-dis-tō′ -ni- a): Any disorder of muscle tone.

myoelectric (mī′ -ō-ē-lek′ -trik): Pertaining to the electrical properties of muscle. **M. ARM.**, an artificial arm that is activated by amplifying the electric currents produced by the patient's own muscles.

myoendocarditis (mī′ -ō-en-dō- kar-dī′ -tis): Inflammation of the heart muscle and of the endocardium.

myofacial pain-dysfunction syndrome: Temporomandibular joint syndrome: see under **temporomandibular**.

myofascitis (mī′ -ō-fa-sī′ -tis): Musculoskeletal pain, probably due to inflammation of a muscle and its fascia.

myofibril (mī-ō-fī′ -bril): One of the long fibrils that make up a muscle fiber.

myofibroma (mī-ō-fī-brō′ -ma): A tumor of muscular and fibrous tissue.

myofibrosis (mī-ō-fī-brō′sis): Replacement of muscle with fibrous tissue; leads to inadequate functioning of the involved part.—myofibroses, pl.

myogenic (mī-ō-jen′ -ik): Originating in, or starting from, muscle.

myoglobin (mī-ō-glō′ - bin): Oxygen-transporting muscle protein. Syn., myohemoglobin.

myoglobinuria (mī′ō-glō-bin-ū′ri-a): Excretion of myoglobin in the urine as occurs in crush syndrome. Syn., myohemoglobinuria.

myogram (mī′ -ō-gram): A radiologic or graphic study of muscle activity.

myohemoglobin (mī′ō-hē-mō-glō′bin): A hemoglobin present in muscle, of much lower molecular weight than blood hemoglobin. It is liberated from muscle and appears in the urine in the crush syndrome.

myohemoglobinuria (mī′ō-hē-mō-glō-bin-ū′ri-a): The presence of myohemoglobin in the urine.

myohypertrophy (mī′ō-hī-per′trō-fi): Abnormal increase in muscle size.

myoid (mī'-oyd): Resembling muscle.

myoischemia (mī'-ō-is-kē'-mi-a): A deficiency of blood supply to a muscle.

myokymia (mī-ō-kim'-i-a): Twitching of a few isolated muscle bundles within a single muscle; may be transitory or persistent; may occur after exercise or chilling, or may be a sign of infection or tumor of the brain stem.

myolipoma (mī-ō-lī-pō'ma): A benign fatty tumor of smooth muscle tissue.

myolysis (mī-ol'-i-sis): Degeneration or disintegration of muscle tissue.

myoma (mī-ō'-ma): A benign tumor of muscle tissue; most often refers to tumor of uterine muscle. Also called fibroid or fibroids.—myomas, myomata, pl.

myomalacia (mī'ō-ma-lā'shi-a): Softening of muscle, as occurs in the myocardium after coronary occlusion.

myomatosis (mī-ō-ma-tō'-sis): The presence of multiple myomas, as often occurs in the uterus. See leiomyoma.

myomectomy (mī-ō-mek'to-mi): Surgical removal of a myoma, specifically a uterine myoma.

myomeningocele (mī'-ō-me-ning'-gō-sēl): A congenital anomaly in which there is a saclike protrusion of meningeal and spinal cord substance; usually occurs in the lumbosacral region; may be associated with other abnormalities including mental retardation. See meningocele.

myometer (mī-om'-e-ter): An instrument for measuring the strength of muscle contraction.

myometritis (mī-ō-me-trī'tis): Inflammation of the muscular wall of the uterus.

myometrium (mī'ō-mē'tri-um): The thick muscular wall of the uterus.

myonarcosis (mī'-ō-nar-kō'-sis): Numbness of muscles.

myonecrosis (mī'ō-ne-krō'sis): Death of individual muscle fibers. **CLOSTRIDIAL M.**, gas gangrene; caused by the anaerobic *Clostridium perfringens;* seen in deep wound infections; early signs and symptoms include pain, tenderness, fever, accumulation of gas in the muscle tissue, shock with tachycardia, and hypotension.

myoneural (mī-ō-nū'-ral): Pertaining to muscle and nerve. **M. JUNCTION**, the place where a nerve ending terminates in muscle tissue.

myoneuralgia (mī'ō-nū-ral'ji-a): Muscular pain.

myoneurasthenia (mī'ō-nū-ras-thē'ni-a): A relaxed state of muscles, seen in neurasthenia (*q.v.*).

myoneuroma (mī'ō-nū-rō'ma): A neuroma (*q.v.*) that contains muscle tissue.

myopachynsis (mī-ō-pa-kin'sis): Abnormal enlargement or thickening of muscle.

myopalmus (mī-ō-pal'mus): Twitching of a muscle or muscles.

myopathy (mī-op'a-thi): Any disease or abnormal condition of muscle tissue. **ALCOHOLIC M.**, **M.** occurring in alcoholics, marked by acute myoglobulinuria (*q.v.*) and weakness of the limbs. **OCULAR M.**, slowly progressive muscular dystrophy characterized by ptosis and immobility of the eye.

myope (mī'ōp): A nearsighted person.—myopic, adj.

myophosphorylase (mī-ō-fos-for'a-las): The phosphorylase of muscle. See phosphorylase.

myopia (mī-ō'pi-a): Nearsightedness. The light rays come to a focus in front of, instead of on, the retina.—myopic, adj.

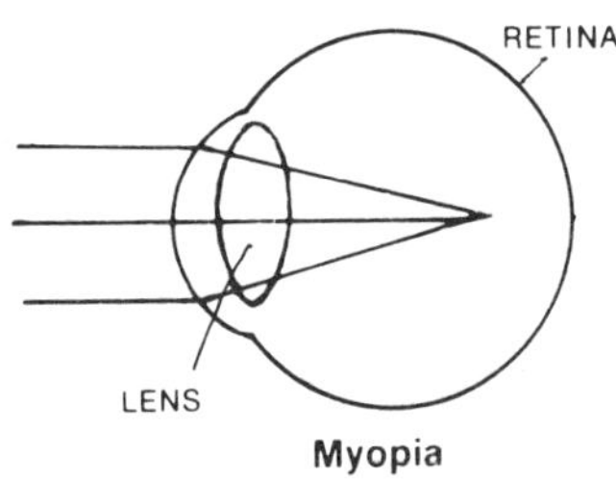

Myopia

myoplasty (mī'ō-plas-ti): Plastic surgery of muscles, or the use of muscle tissue in plastic surgery.—myoplastic, adj.

myorrhaphy (mī-or'a-fi): Suturing of a wound in muscle, or of a divided muscle.

myorrhexis (mī-ō-rek'sis): Rupture or tearing of a muscle.

myosarcoma (mī'ō-sar-kō'ma): A malignant tumor derived from muscle.—myosarcomata, pl.; myosarcomatous, adj.

myosclerosis (mī'ō-sklē-rō'sis): Fibrous myositis; see under myosis.—myosclerotic, adj.

myosin (mī'ō-sin): A globin that makes up about 68 percent of the muscle substance. Along with actin, it is responsible for contraction and relaxation of muscles.

myosis (mī-ō'sis): See miosis.

myositis (mī-ō-sī'tis): Inflammation of a voluntary muscle. **FIBROUS M.**, characterized by formation of fibrous tissue in muscle. **INTERSTITIAL M.**, usually of viral origin; characterized by fever, headache, aching limbs, sore throat; also called Bornholm disease. **M. OSSIFICANS**, deposition of active bone cells in muscle, resulting in hard swellings.

myospasm (mī'ō-spazm): Spasmodic contraction of a muscle.

myotenositis (mī'ō-ten-ō-sī'tis): Inflammation of a muscle and its tendon.

myotics (mī-ot'iks): Drugs that cause myosis (*q.v.*).

myotomy (mī-ot'om-i): Cutting, or dissection of, muscle tissue.

myotonia (mī-ō-tō'ni-a): A disorder characterized by increased muscular contractions and decreased relaxation; tonic muscle spasm. **M. CONGENITA,** an inherited disorder characterized by early onset and by stiffness of muscles, which is accented by cold weather; the skeletal muscles become hypertrophied. **M. DYSTROPHICA,** myotonic dystrophy; see under dystrophy.

myotonic (mī-ō-ton'ik): Pertaining to myotonia. **M. REACTION,** the delay in relaxation of a muscle after contraction.

myringa (mi-ring'ga): The eardrum or tympanic membrane.

myringitis (mir-in-jī'tis): Inflammation of the eardrum (tympanic membrane). **M. BULLOSA,** viral otitis media characterized by the formation of serous or hemorrhagic blisters on the tympanic membrane.

myringoplasty (mī-ring' -gō-plas-ti): A plastic operation on the eardrum (tympanic membrane).—myringoplastic, adj.

myringotome (mī-ring'gō-tōm): A delicate instrument for incising the eardrum (tympanic membrane).

myringotomy (mir-in-got'o-mi): Incision of the eardrum (tympanic membrane).

mysophobia (mī-sō-fō'bi-a): A morbid fear of dirt or germs, or of touching even familiar objects, *e.g.*, doorknobs.

myx-, myxo-: Combining forms denoting mucus, mucous.

myxadenitis (miks-ad-e-nī'tis): Inflammation of a mucous gland or glands.

myxadenoma (miks-ad-e-nō'ma): A benign tumor with the structure of a mucous gland, or one that contains mucous elements.

myxedema (mik-se-dē'ma): A syndrome resulting from hypofunction of the anterior pituitary, or deficiency of iodine in the diet, or to excessive use of antithyroid drugs; may also be secondary to removal of the thyroid gland. Symptoms include lethargy, mental dullness, bradycardia, subnormal temperature, dry skin, alopecia, edema of the face and extremities. The basal metabolic rate is low, and blood cholesterol is elevated, but there is no enlargement of the thyroid gland. **CONGENITAL M.,** see cretinism.—myxedematous, adj.

myxoma (mik-sō'ma): A connective tissue tumor composed largely of mucoid material.—myxomata, pl.; myxomatous, adj.

myxosarcoma (mik-sō-sar-kō'ma): A malignant tumor of connective tissue with a soft, mucoid consistency.—myxosarcomata, pl.; myxosarcomatous, adj.

myxovirus (mik-sō-vī'rus): Name proposed by the International Congress of Microbiology, 1953, for the influenza group of viruses. They infect mucus-secreting tissue and include the parainfluenza viruses, measles virus, respiratory syncytial virus.

N

N: 1. Chemical symbol for nitrogen. 2. Abbreviation for 1) nasal, 2) normal, 3) nerve.

NA: Abbreviation for: 1. Nomina Anatomica (*q.v.*). 2. Not applicable. 3. Nurses' aid.

Na: Chemical symbol for sodium (natrium).

NAACOG: Nurses Association of the American College of Obstetrics and Gynecology.

nabothian (nā-bō′-thi-an): **N. CYSTS,** tiny cysts that form in the cervical glands of the uterus when these become inflamed and their secretions are retained because of obstruction in the ducts. Also called Naboth's follicles. **N. GLAND,** any of several small mucous glands in the uterine cervix. [Martin Naboth, German anatomist. 1675–1721.]

NaCl: Chemical formula for sodium chloride.

nacreous (nā′-krē-us): Having a lustrous, mother-of-pearl appearance; said of bacterial colonies.

Naegele's rule: Used to estimate date of confinement; calculated by subtracting 90 days from the first day of the last menstrual period and adding seven days. [Franz K. Naegele, German obstetrician. 1777–1851.]

Naga sore (nah′-gah): One of several names for the chronic sloughing ulcer seen chiefly on the lower extremities of people living in tropical areas; thought to be due to a nutritional deficiency.

$NaHCO_3$: Chemical formula for sodium bicarbonate.

nail: 1. A rod of material (usually bone or metal) used to hold pieces of fractured bones together. 2. The horny cutaneous plate that covers the dorsal surface of the distal ends of fingers and toes; the root is that part embedded in a deep fold of skin at the base, and the body is the exposed part lying on a bed of matrix of the skin from which the new substance develops. The white crescent at the base of the nail is called the lunula. Discoloration of the nails may occur due to hemorrhage, trauma, certain pathologic conditions such as diabetes, anemia, or certain poisonings, or in persons receiving certain substances such as silver. **EGG SHELL N.,** a condition of thinning, softening and splitting of the nails; associated with several general pathological conditions. **HANG N.,** a bit of skin hanging loose at one side or root of a **N.** **INGROWN N.,** a painful aberrant growth, usually of a toenail, with the edges pressing into the soft tissues at the side. **KÜNTSCHER N.,** a stainless steel flanged nail used for intermedullary fixation of fractures. **NEUFELD N.,** a **N.** used for fixation of an intertrochanteric fracture of the femur. **REEDY N.,** a **N.** with lengthwise furrows. **SMITH-PETERSEN N.,** a trifid, cannulated metal **N.,** formerly much used to provide internal fixation of the head of the femur in fracture of the neck of the femur. **SPOON N.,** a **N.** that is depressed in its central portion. **TURTLE-BACK N.,** a distorted nail that is more convex than normal.

nailing: The operation of fastening the ends of a fractured bone together with a nail.

nail-patella syndrome: A congenital condition characterized by absence of the nails, various skeletal abnormalities, including absence of the patella, and abnormalities of the eyes and ears.

nalidixic acid: An antibacterial agent frequently used in treatment of urinary tract infections caused by gram-negative organisms.

nandrolone (nan′-drō-lōn): An anabolic steroid that promotes skeletal growth and protein metabolism.

nanism (nā′-nizm): Dwarfism; of much smaller size than normal.

nano-: 1. A combining form denoting small or dwarfish. 2. A prefix denoting one-billionth of a measure.

nanocephaly (nā-nō-sef′-a-li): Abnormal smallness of the head. Also nanocephalia, nanocephalism, nanocephalus.—nanocephalous, adj.

nanocurie (nā-nō-kū′-ri): A unit of radiation equal to one-billionth of a curie.

nanogram (nā′nō-gram): In the metric system, a unit of mass weight; one-billionth of a gram. Abbreviated ng.

nanomelus (na-nom′-e-lus): An individual with unusually short extremities; often refers to a fetus. Also nanomelia.—nanomelous, adj.

nanometer (nā-nom′-e-ter): The official International Standard Unit of Wavelength, 10 Angströms; equal to one-billionth of a meter; a millimicron.

nanophthalmus (nan-of-thal′-mus): The condition of having abnormally small eyeballs. Microphthalmus.

nanus (nā′-nus): A dwarf.—nanoid, nanous, adj.; nanism, n.

NaOH: Chemical formula for sodium hydroxide.

nape: The back of the neck; the nucha.

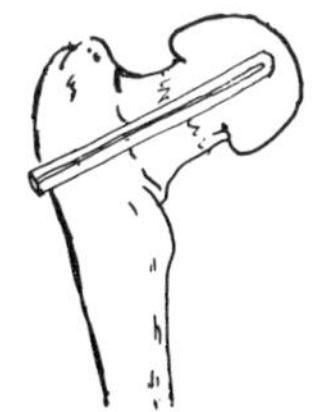

Smith-Petersen nail

napex (nā′-peks): The part of the scalp that is immediately below the occipital protuberance.

naphthol (naf′-thol): A substance obtained from coal tar; has antiseptic qualities.

NAP-NAP: Abbreviation for National Association of Pediatric Nurse Associates/Practitioners.

NAPNES: Abbreviation for National Association for Practical Nurse Education and Service.

naprapathy (na-prap′-a-thi): A school of folk medicine that utilizes diet, massage, and manipulation of muscles, ligaments, and joints of the spine, pelvis, and thorax.

NARA: National Addict and Rehabilitation Act (*q.v.*).

narcissism (nar-sis′-izm): Self-love; absorption with one's own perfections. In psychiatry, the narcissistic personality is one in which the sexual love-object is the self; named for a character in Greek mythology who fell in love with his own image reflected in a fountain.—narcissistic, adj.

narco-: Combining form denoting 1) stupor; 2) deep sleep; 3) numbness.

narcoanalysis (nar-kō-a-nal′-a-sis): Psychotherapy conducted while the individual is under light anesthesia produced by certain drugs, *e.g.*, sodium pentothal or sodium amytal. The purpose is to assist the person to recover repressed memories along with the emotion that accompanied the experience, with the idea of helping him to accept the memories and integrate them into his self-image.

narcoanesthesia (nar′-kō-an-es-thē′-zi-a): Anesthesia resulting from a subcutaneous injection of a narcotic such as morphine and scopolamine.

narcohypnia (nar-kō-hip′-ni-a): A sensation of general numbness felt upon awakening.

narcohypnosis (nar-kō-hip-nō′-sis): A hypnotic state produced by some drugs and used sometimes in psychotherapy.

narcolepsy (nar′kō-lep-si): An irresistible tendency to fall into deep sleep during the daytime, but from which the individual can be easily aroused; may occur several times a day and last for only a few minutes or for hours; seen in diverse clinical conditions.—narcoleptic, adj.

narcomania (nar-kō-mā′-ni-a): 1. Uncontrollable craving for narcotics. 2. Insanity resulting from alcoholism or from a narcotic drug habit.

narcose (nar′-kōs): Stuporous.

narcosis (nar-kō′-sis): Unconsciousness, stupor, or insensibility produced by a drug and from which recovery is possible. **BASAL N.**, a state of unconsciousness produced by drugs prior to giving an anesthetic. **NITROGEN N., N.** produced by 1) nitrogenous substances in the blood, as occurs in hepatic coma and uremia, or 2) increased nitrogen pressure in the blood, as occurs in deep sea divers; often called "rapture of the deep."

narcosynthesis (nar-kō-sin′-the-sis): The building up of a clearer mental picture of an incident involving the patient by reviving memories of it under semi-narcosis, so that both patient and therapist can examine the incident in clearer perspective.

narcotherapy (nar-kō-ther′-a-pi): Narcoanalysis (*q.v.*).

narcotic (nar-kot′-ik): 1. Pertinent to or producing narcosis. 2. Any substance that in moderate doses relieves pain and produces profound sleep, particularly substances derived from opium; most are habit-forming.

narcotic addict: A person who has become physiologically or psychologically dependent on a narcotic drug.

Narcotic Addict Rehabilitation Act: Passed in 1966; provides for treatment of addicts charged with violation of federal laws as well as those who are not involved in any criminal acts. This Act and significant legislation that followed it have resulted in the establishment of community-based programs for the treatment of drug addicts and drug abusers, and training centers for program personnel that are supported, at least in part, by the federal government.

narcotism (nar′-kō-tizm): 1. Addiction to narcotics. 2. A state of stupor produced by a narcotic drug.

narcotize (nar′-kō-tīz): To place under the influence of a narcotic drug.

nares (nā′-rēz): The nostrils. **ANTERIOR N.**, the pair of openings from the exterior into the nasal cavities. **POSTERIOR N.**, the pair of openings from the nasal cavities into the nasopharynx. Syn., choanae.—naris, sing.

narrative notes: A written record of a patient's progress or response to therapy; part of the patient's chart.

nasal (nā′-zal): Pertaining to the nose. **N. BONE**, either of two small oblong bones which together form the arch of the nose. **N. CANNULA**, a cannula inserted through the nasal cavity for administering oxygen. **N. CATHETER**, one inserted through the nose to deliver oxygen. **N. CAVITY**, that in the nose, separated into right and left halves by the **N.** septum. **N. CONCHAE**, three long thin projections from the lateral walls of the **N. CAVITY**; identified according to position as superior, medial, and inferior. **N. DECONGESTANT**, a drug that reduces local inflammation in nasal passages in ordinary rhinitis and sinusitis; many are antihistamines. **N. DRIP**, see postnasal drip. **N. FEEDING** or **GAVAGE**, see under feeding. **N. FOSSA**, one of the two parts of the **N.** cavity extending from the exterior to the nasopharynx. **N. INTUBATION**, an endotracheal tube is inserted through the nostril and advanced through the vocal cords during inspiration, to establish an airway. **N. MUCOSA,** the mucous membrane lining the nose. **N. POLYP,** focal hyperplasia of the submucous connective tissue of the nose with accumulation of edematous fluid. **N. SEPTUM,**, the thin bony cartilaginous structure that separates the nostrils. **N. SINUSES,** any of several cavities in the bones of the skull that communicate with the **N.** cavity; in particular, the frontal, ethmoid, sphenoid, and maxillary (also called the antrum of Highmore) sinuses; they are lined with mucous membrane that is continuous with that of the nasal cavity and are often irritated. **N. SOUNDS,** so called because to produce them air is resonated in the nasal cavity; they are the sounds of *m, n,* and *ng*.

nasalis (nā-zal'is): Relating to the nose.

nascent (nā'-sent): 1. At the moment of birth. 2. Coming into existence or in the process of emerging.

nas-,nasi-, naso-: Combining forms denoting 1) the nose; 2) nasal.

nasoantral (nā'-zō-an'-tral): Pertaining to the nose and the maxillary antrum.

nasoantritis (nā'-zō-an-trī'-tis): Inflammation of the nose and the antrum of Highmore (maxillary sinus).

nasobronchial (nā-zō-brong'-ki-al): Pertaining to the nose and bronchi.

nasoduodenal (nā'-zō-dū-ō-dē'-nal): Pertaining to the nose and the duodenum; usually refers to a tube used for enteral nutrition.

nasofrontal (nā'-zō-frun'-tal): Pertaining to the nasal and frontal bones or forehead.

nasogastric (nā'-zō-gas'-trik): Pertaining to the nose and stomach. **N. FEEDING,** see under feeding. **N. TUBE,** a soft rubber tube that is inserted through the nostril into the stomach; used for instilling liquids and foods and for withdrawing stomach contents.

nasojejunal feeding: See feeding, transpyloric.

nasolabial (nā'-zō-lā'-bi-al): Pertaining to the nose and the upper lip. **N. SEBORRHEA,** enlarged follicles at the sides of the nose; they contain plugs of sebaceous material.

nasolacrimal (nā'-zō-lak'-ri-mal): Pertaining to the nose and the lacrimal apparatus. **N. DUCT,** carries the tears from the **N.** sac to the inferior meatus of the nose; see under lacrimal.

naso-oral (nā'-zō-or'-al): Pertaining to the nose and the mouth.

nasopalatine (nā'-zō-pal'-a-tīn): Pertaining to the nose and the palate.

nasopharyngeal (nā'-zō-fa-rin'-jē-al): Pertaining to the nasopharynx. **N. ANGIOFIBROMA,** a relatively benign tumor of the nasopharynx, seen most often in teenage boys; characterized by nasal and auditory tube obstruction resulting in adenoidal speech.

nasopharyngitis (nā'zō-far-in-jī'tis): Inflammation of the nasal passages and the pharynx; caused by a virus or group of viruses. The common cold.

nasopharyngoscope (nā'-zō-far-ing'-gō-skōp): An endoscopic device for viewing the nasal passages and the postnasal space.—nasopharyngoscopic, adj.

nasopharynx (nā'-zō-far'-ingks): The portion of the pharynx above the soft palate and which opens anteriorally into the nasal cavity.—nasopharyngeal, adj.

nasoscope (nā'-zō-skōp): An instrument for examining the nasal cavity. Rhinoscope.

nasoseptal (nā'-zō-sep'-tal): Pertaining to the nasal septum.

nasosinusitis (nā'-zō-sī-nū-sī'-tis): Inflammation of the nasal cavities and adjacent sinuses.

nasotracheal (nā'-zō-trā'-kē-al): Pertaining to the nasal cavity and the trachea. **N. TUBE,** a tube that is inserted into the trachea via the nasal cavity and the pharynx.

nasus (nā'-sus): The nose.

natal (nā'-tal): Pertaining to: 1. Birth. 2. The buttocks.

natality (nā-tal'-i-ti): 1. The birth rate; the ratio of births to the population in a given area. 2. Birth.

nates (nā'-tēz): The buttocks.

natimortality (nā'-ti-mor-tal'-i-ti): The proportion of fetal deaths and stillbirths to the general birth rate.

National Association for Practical Nurse Education and Service (NAPNES): Maintains accreditation and consultation services for schools of practical nursing; promotes recruitment of students; concerned with both the education and practice performance of practical/vocational nurses. Address, 254 W. 31st St., New York, NY 10001

National Bureau of Standards: Established in 1901 as a federal agency within the Department of Commerce; conducts research on improved methods of measurement standards in physical, chemical, and materials measurement; collects data on, and sets measurement standards for, material needed and used by the government, industry, commerce, and educational institutions. Mailing address, Washington, D.C. 20234

National Center for Health Statistics: The major body dealing with health statistics in the U.S.; created in 1974 to develop a uniform system for collecting and analyzing statistics from the federal, state, and local health care agencies; functions within the U.S. Public Health Service.

National Center for Nursing Ethics: A non-profit organization for the study of nursing ethics. Conducts research; publishes *Journal of*

Nursing Ethics. Address, P.O. Box 2237, Cincinnati, OH 45201

National Centers for Disease Control: See Centers for Disease Control.

National Council Licensure Examination for Registered Nurses (NCLEX-RN): Beginning in 1982 this examination replaced the National League for Nursing's State Boards Test Pool Examination for Registered Nurses. It is administered by the National Council of State Boards of Nursing (NCSBN) which was established in 1980. Address, 303 E. Ohio St., Chicago, IL 60611

National Council of State Boards of Nursing (NCSBN): Founded in 1980; its predecessor was the American Nurses' Association's Council of State Boards of Nursing. Objectives are to establish policies and procedures concerning licensing examinations; to promote uniformity of standards in nursing; to promote nursing education programs for members, boards of nursing, and professional workers; to identify and take positions on trends affecting nursing and nursing education; to provide consultation services for national council members, governmental and voluntary agencies, and individuals concerned with health and welfare of the public; to define a legal code of conduct and unprofessional conduct.

National Death Index: A national computer file started in 1979; collates and stores information from state offices of vital statistics regarding deaths of U.S. citizens and their causes.

National Federation of Licensed Practical Nurses: Founded in 1949. Membership confined to licensed practical nurses. Aim is to preserve and foster the ideal of comprehensive nursing care for the ill and aged, to improve standards of practice, and to conduct continuing education programs for practical nurses; cooperates with other professional groups concerned with better patient care. Address, P.O. Box 11038, 214 S. Driver St., Durham, N.C. 27703

National Federation of Nursing Specialties and the American Nurses' Association: A voluntary organization, founded in 1973, with the purpose of working toward communication and coordination among participating nursing organizations in matters that relate to nursing practice, nursing education, and other matters of mutual concern. Among the Federation's functions are 1) supporting collective efforts to improve nursing practice; 2) developing statements on matters of concern to nurses nationally; 3) facilitating cooperation among member organizations; and 4) emphasizing the nurse's role as patient advocate. Meets twice yearly; membership includes 28 ± specialty organizations and the American Nurses' Association.

National Formulary: An official drug compendium, published by the United States Pharmacopeia Convention (formerly issued by the American Pharmaceutical Association), and revised frequently; provides standards and specifications for use in evaluating the quality of pharmacologic agents. Contains some drugs not listed in the U.S. Pharmacopeia and, along with it, is recognized by the courts as an official source.

National Institutes of Health (NIH): The principal research division of the United States Public Health Service. Sponsors, conducts, and supports biomedical research and scientific investigation of causes, prevention, and cure of disease. Aim is to improve the health of the American people through modern methods of communicating medical information. Composed of the National Cancer Institute; National Heart, Lung, and Blood Institute; the National Library of Medicine; National Institute of Arthritic, Metabolic, and Digestive Diseases; National Institute of Allergy and Infectious Diseases; National Institute of Child Health and Human Development; National Institute of Dental Research; National Institute of Environmental Health Science; National Institute of Medical Sciences; National Institute of Neurological and Communicative Disorders and Stroke; National Eye Institute; National Institute on Aging; and a Clinical Center in addition to divisions on international health affairs and on various aspects of research. Address, 9000 Rockville Pike, Bethesda, MD 20205

National League for Nursing (NLN): A national organization formed in 1952 by the fusion of seven groups: The National League for Nursing Education; The National Organization for Public Health Nursing; The Association of Collegiate Schools of Nursing; The Joint Committee on Careers in Nursing; The National Committee for Improvement of Nursing Services; The National Accrediting Service; and The Joint Committee on Practical Nurses and Auxiliary Workers in Nursing Services. Its objective is to foster the development of hospital, industrial, public health, and other organized nursing services and of nursing education through the coordinated action of nurses, allied professional groups, citizens, agencies, and schools to the end that the nursing needs of the people will be met. Its functions in the furtherance of these objectives are: 1) to identify the nursing needs of society and to foster programs designed to meet these needs; 2) to develop and support services for the improvement of nursing service and nursing education through consultation, continuing education, testing, evaluation, and other activities; 3) to work with voluntary, governmental, and other agencies, groups, and organizations for the advancement of nursing and toward the achievement of comprehensive health care; 4) to respond in appropriate ways to universal nursing needs. There are constituent Leagues in almost all states and in many local communities. Membership includes individuals, nursing and other health professionals, and agencies such as hospitals, community health agencies, and nursing education facilities. The official journal is *Nursing and Health Care*. National office is at 10 Columbus Circle, New York, NY 10019

National Library of Medicine: Established in 1836 as the Library of the Surgeon General's Office; in 1956 was transferred to the Department of Health, Education and Welfare and upgraded to be the National Library of Medicine. Holdings include over 2,500,000 books, journals, technical papers, theses, microfilms, and audiovisual materials, with some items dating from the 11th century. Provides medical library services to public and private institutions and to individuals; operates a computer-based toxicology system; acquires and distributes audio-visual instructional material in addition to many other services. Address, 8600 Rockville Pike, Bethesda, MD 20209

National Safety Council (NSC): A nonprofit organization of local and state safety agencies, institutions, and industries concerned with accident prevention. The purpose is to reduce all kinds of occupational illnesses and injuries by gathering and disseminating material regarding their causes and prevention. Collects statistics and conducts courses in safety training. Address, 444 N. Michigan Ave., Chicago IL 60611.

National Second Step Project (in nursing education): A project for studying the people who study for the BSN degree after becoming registered nurses.

National Student Nurses Association (NSNA): Membership composed of undergraduate students in state approved schools of nursing. Purpose is to aid in the professional development of individual student nurses. Encourages programs and activities in affiliated state groups concerned with nursing and health; holds career workshops and annual conventions; awards scholarships; participates in community health programs; works closely with the ANA, NLN, and the ICN. Publishes the journal, *Imprint*. Address, 10 Columbus Circle, New York, NY 10019.

natremia (nā-trē'-mi-a): The presence of more than the normal amount of sodium in the blood.

natrium (nā'-tri-um): Sodium.

natriuresis (nā'-tri-ū-rē'-sis): A condition in which there is an unusually large amount of sodium in the urine; occurs in certain diseases and following the administration of diuretic drugs.

natriuretic (nā'-tri-ū-ret'-ik): 1. Pertaining to natriuresis. 2. An agent that promotes natriuresis by inhibiting the reabsorption of sodium ions by the glomerulus.

natural: 1. Neither artificial nor pathological. 2. Inborn. 3. Normal. **N. CHILDBIRTH,** a system of management for childbirth in which anesthesia, sedation, and surgical intervention are replaced by prenatal education and psychological preparation for delivery and continuous support of the mother during delivery. **N. DEFENSES OF THE BODY,** include the skin, lymphatic tissue, white blood cells, and antibodies in the blood. **N. HEALING PROCESSES,** processess such as blood clot formation, scar tissue formation, bone repair after fracture, and cell division. **N. IMMUNITY,** immunity resulting from the genetic composition of the host; may be manifested in individuals, families, or races.

naturopathy (nā'-tūr-op'-a-thi): A system of treatment that makes use of such physical agents as light, heat, water, massage, exercise, and diet; no surgical procedures are used and only such medications as are derived from herbs vitamins, etc.

Nauheim bath: A bath of all or part of the body in naturally hot carbonated water, followed by exercise; originated at the spas in Bad-Nauheim, Germany for use in treating cardiac conditions.

naupathia (naw-path'-i-a): Seasickness.

nausea (naw'-zē-a): 1. A sensation of discomfort or sickness in the area of the stomach; usually precedes vomiting but not always. 2. Extreme disgust; loathing.—nauseating, adj.; nauseate, v.

nauseant (naw' zē-ent): A drug that produces nausea.

nauseous (naw'-zē-us): Producing nausea, disgust, or loathing.

navel (nā'-vel): The umbilicus. The depression in the center of the abdomen marking the place where the umbilical cord is attached to the fetus.

navicular (nav-ik'-ū-lar): 1. Shaped like a boat or canoe. 2. Pertaining to a bone in the wrist or one in the ankle.

N-CAP: Abbreviation for Nurses' Coalition for Action in Politics (*q.v.*).

NCLEX-RN: Abbreviation for National Council Licensure Examination for Registered Nurses (*q.v.*).

NCSBN: Abbreviation for National Council of State Boards of Nursing (*q.v.*).

nearsightedness: Lay term for myopia (*q.v.*).

nebula (neb'-ū-la): 1. A grayish, corneal opacity. 2. An oily mixture for use in a nebulizer (*q.v.*). 3. A cloudiness of the urine.

nebulization (neb'-ū-lī-zā'-shun): 1. Conversion into a spray. 2. Treatment of an area by spraying.

nebulize (neb′-ū-līz): To convert into a fine spray or vapor.

nebulizer (neb′-ū-līz-er): An apparatus for converting a liquid into a fine spray. Syn., atomizer.

Necator (nē-kā′-tor): A genus of nematodes (see Nematoda); **N. AMERICANUS,** the hookworm found in the U.S. and Central and South America. See hookworm.

neck: 1. The part between the head and the shoulders. 2. The constricted portion of bone or an organ, *e.g.*, the neck of the femur, the neck of the uterus.

necr-, necro-: Combining forms denoting 1) death; 2) a dead body; 3) dead tissue.

necrectomy (nek-rek′-to-mi): Surgical removal of necrosed tissue.

necrobiosis (nek′-rō-bī-ō′-sis): The degeneration or death of cells followed by replacement; may be normal as in red blood cells and epithelial cells, or abnormal as in a pathological process. **N. LIPOIDICA,** a skin disease characterized by the formation of reddish yellow plaques, mostly on the legs; occurs most often in older women, epecially those with diabetes; also called necrobiosis lipoidica diabeticorum.

necrocytosis (nek′-rō-sī-tō′-sis): The death of cells.

necrogenic (nek′-rō-jen′-ik): Caused by or productive of necrosis.

necrology (nek-rol′-ō-ji): 1. The study of death statistics. 2. The science of collecting, classifying, and interpreting death statistics.—necrologic, adj.

necrolysis (nek-rol′-i-sis): The dissolution or breaking down of dead tissue.

necromania (nek′rō-mā′ni-a): 1. Morbid interest in death or in corpses. 2. A form of mania in which one wishes to die.

necrophile (nek′-rō-fīl): A person who derives pleasure from dead bodies, who is sexually aroused by thoughts of death, or who derives pleasure from sexual activity with a dead body.

necrophilia (nek′-rō-fil′-i-a): 1. A morbid preoccupation with death and a liking for being in the presence of dead bodies. 2. A morbid desire to have sexual intercourse with a corpse.—necrophiliac, adj.

necrophobia (nek′-rō-fō′-bi-a): A morbid dread of dead bodies.

necropsy (nek′-rop-si): The examination of the internal organs of a dead body; autopsy.

necrose (ne′-krōz): 1. To become necrotic. 2. To be necrotic.

necrosis (ne-krō′-sis): Localized death of tissue or bone. When **N.** occurs in bone the dead part is referred to as a sequestrum; when it occurs in soft tissue it is referred to as slough; when large areas are affected the condition is referred to as gangrene. May be caused by lack of normal circulation to a part, trauma, radiant energy such as x rays or radium, or bacterial invasion; and may be described according to cause, location, extent, and consistency of the dead tissue. **AVASCULAR N., N.** due to lack of normal circulation to a part; also called **ANEMIC N. CASEOUS N., N.** in which the dead tissue has a cheesy consistency. **DRY N., N.** in which the dead material is dry, as compared with that which is termed **MOIST. EPIPHYSIAL ASEPTIC N.,** usually occurs in the head of the femur, medial condyle, head of the humerus, or the tibial tubercle; associated with sickle cell anemia and alcoholism. **PUTREFACTIVE N., N.** caused by bacterial invasion of tissue. **TOTAL N., N.** that destroys all or most of an organ or part. **TUBULAR N., N.** of the epithelial tissue along the kidney tubules.—necroses, pl., necrotic, adj.

necrotic (nē-krot′-ik): Pertaining to or characterized by necrosis.

necrotize (nek′-rō-tīz): 1. To undergo necrosis. 2. To produce or cause necrosis.—necrotizing, adj.

necrotomy (nek-rot′-o-mi): An operation for the removal of a sequestrum (*q.v.*) or other necrotic tissue.

needle: 1. A slender, sharp, pointed instrument used for suturing wounds or for puncturing. Needles may be straight or curved, and have a cutting or rounded edge. 2. A hollow pointed instrument used to deliver medication into the body or to withdraw fluid from a tissue, blood vessel, or hollow organ. **ASPIRATING N.,** a long hollow **N.** used for removing fluid from a cavity. **HYPODERMIC N.,** a short hollow **N.** used for administering medications through the skin. **SCALP VEIN N.,** a **N.** originally designed for use in administering intravenous fluids to infants, now often used for prolonged intravenous therapy for patients of all ages; is made in various lengths and gauges and fitted with plastic wings that fold flat on the skin to help to anchor the **N.** in place. **SWAGED N.,** has no eye; the suture material is fused to the needle. See needle biopsy under biopsy.

needling (nēd′- ling): Puncturing with a needle as in discission of the lens capsule in surgical treatment of cataract. Discission.

negation (nē-gā′-shun): Denial.

negative: 1. Not affirmative; the opposite of positive. 2. Denoting that a substance or microorganism tested for is not present in the material examined.

negativism (neg′-a-tiv-izm): 1. Habitual skepticism. 2. Tendency to do the opposite of what one is asked or expected to do. Occurs commonly in children at the age of two, but not usual in adults. Often associated with schizophrenia.

negatron (neg′-a-tron): A negatively charged electron.

negligence (neg′-li-jens): In the health sciences, the basis for many lawsuits for malpractice. Includes actions of both commission and omission, *e.g.*, failure to provide care that a reasonably prudent health care professional would provide in the given circumstances, failure to provide care that meets the accepted standards of care, or giving care that results in harm or injury to the patient.

Negri bodies: Microscopic bodies found in the cytoplasm of certain nerve cells of animals or persons with rabies; of diagnostic importance.

neighborhood health centers: Federally funded outpatient facilities that began to develop in the 1960s to provide comprehensive ambulatory services to the sick poor.

Neisseria (nīs-ēr′-i-a): A genus of coccus microorganisms; gram-negative, nonmotile, usually found in pairs with their adjacent sides slightly flattened. *N. catarrhalis,* found in sputum normally and also in the respiratory tract during infections. *N. gonorrhea,* the causative agent of gonorrhea and ophthalmia neonatorum. *N. meningitidis,* also called *N. intracellularis,* the causative agent of epidemic cerebrospinal meningitis.

Nélaton's line: A line that demonstrates the normal level of the greater trochanter of the femur, that is, the tip of the trochanter should lie just below or on a line from the anterior spine of the ilium to the tuberosity of the ischim; in dislocation of the hip the tip of the trochanter lies above this line.

Nemathelminthes (nem-a-thel-min′-thēz): The roundworms.

nemathelminthiasis (nem′-a-thel-min-thī′-a-sis): Infestation with roundworms of the phylum *Nemathelminthes*.

nematocide (nem′a-tō-sīd): An agent that destroys nematode worms.

Nematoda (nem-a-tō′-da): A class of *Nemathelminthes* (*q.v.*) that includes the true roundworms; many are parasitic in man.—nematode, sing.

nematode (nem′-a-tōd): Any member of the class *Nematoda*.

nematodiasis (nem′-a-tō-dī′-a-sis): Infestation with a nematode parasite.

nematoid (nem′-a-toid): Threadlike; refers to a nematode parasite.

nematosis (nem-a-tō′-sis): The condition of being infested with nematode parasites (roundworms).

neo-: Combining form denoting new, newness, strange.

neoarthrosis (nē′-ō-ar-thrō′-sis): Abnormal articulation; a false joint as at the site of a fracture. Also refers to a joint created in an operation for total joint replacement.

neocerebellum (nē′-ō-ser-e-bel′-um): The more recently evolved part of the cerebellum; is concerned with voluntary movement.

neocortex (nē-ō-kor′-teks): The more recently evolved part of the cerebral cortex, which is most highly developed in man; contains a larger number of nerve cells than the allocortex(*q.v.*). Also called isocortex and neopallium.

neocyte (nē′-ō-sīt): An immature leukocyte.

neocytosis (nē′-ō-sī-tō′-sis) The presence of neocytes in the blood.

neofetus (nē-ō-fē′-tus): The embryo at about the eighth week of gestation.

neoformation (nē-ō-for-mā′-shun): 1. A neoplasm (*q.v.*). 2. Regeneration, as of tissue or bone.

neogenesis (nē-ō-jen′-e-sis): The regeneration of tissue.—neogenicity, adj.

neoglottis (nē-ō-glot′-is): Name given to an artificial larynx, a prosthetic device for persons who have had the larynx removed.

neoglycogenesis (nē′-ō-glī-kō-jen′-e-sis): See glyconeogenesis.

neohymen (nē-ō-hī′-men): A new or false membrane.

neokinetic (nē′-ō-kī-net′-ik): Referring to movement, particularly to the nervous mechanism that regulates voluntary muscle activity.

neolalia (nē-ō-lal′-i-a): Speech in which neologisms are used freely, a common habit among schizophrenics.

neologism (nē-ol′-o-jizm): A specially coined word, phrase, or usage, often meaningless to everyone except the person who invented it.

neon (nē′-on): A colorless, odorless, tasteless, inert gas; found in minute quantities in the air; used in electric lamps.

neonatal (nē-ō-nā′-tal): Pertaining to the period immediatey following birth and continuing through the first month of life. **N. MORTALITY,** the death rate of babies in the first month of life. **N. PERIOD,** the first 28 days of life.

neonate (nē′-ō-nāt): A newborn baby up to one month old.

neonatologist (nē′-ō-nā-tol′-o-jist): A physician who specializes in the care and treatment of the newborn.

neonatology (nē′-ō-nā-tol′-o-ji): That branch of medicine that is concerned with the care and treatment of the newborn.

neonatorum (nē′-ō-nā-tor′-um): Pertaining to the newborn.

neopallium (nē-ō-pal′-i-um): All of the cerebral cortex except the rhinencephalon. (*q.v.*).

neopathy (nē-op′-a-thi): 1. A new disease or condition arising in a patient who already has another disease. 2. A newly recognized disease.

neopenthic (nē-ō-pen′-thik): Having the effect of inducing peace and forgetfulness.

neophobia (nē-ō-fō′-bi-a): A morbid dread of newness or new things.

neoplasia (nē-ō-plā′-zi-a): Literally the formation of new tissue. By custom refers to the pathological process in tumor formation.—neoplastic, adj.

neoplasm (nē′-ō-plazm): Any abnormal, progressive, uncontrolled growth of cells or tissues that serves no useful purpose; a tumor. May be benign, malignant, or potentially malignant.—neoplastic, adj.

neostomy (nē-os′-to-mi): The creation of an artificial opening into an organ or between two organs.

neovascularization (nē′ō-vas′kū-lar-ī-zā′shun): Formation of new blood vessels as occurs in tumors or in abnormal places, as in the retinae of patients with diabetic retinopathy.

nephalism (nef′-a-lizm): Total abstinence from alcohol or alcoholic liquors.

nephelopia (nef-e-lō′-pi-a): Visual defect due to cloudiness of the cornea.

nephr-; nephro-: Combining forms denoting relationship to the kidney.

nephradenoma (nef′-rad-e-nō′-ma): Adenoma (*q.v.*) of the kidney.

nephralgia (ne-fral′-ji-a): Pain in the kidney.—nephralgic, adj.

nephrectasia (nef-rek-tā′-zi-a): Distention of the pelvis of the kidney. Also nephrectasis.

nephrectomy (ne-frek′-to-mi): Removal of a kidney.

nephredema (nef′-re-dē′ma): Edema caused by disease of the kidney. Rarely, edema of the kidney.

nephric (nef′-rik): Pertaining to the kidney.

nephridium (ne-frid′-i-um): The embryonic tube that is the excretory organ of the fetus and from which the kidney develops.

nephrism (nef′-rizm): Cachexia due to kidney disease or disorder.

nephritic (ne-frit′-ik): 1. Pertaining to a) nephritis; b) the kidney. 2. A person with nephritis.

nephritides (ne-frit′-i-dēz): Plural of nephritis; the term is used collectively to refer to all types of nephritis.

nephritis (ne-frī′-tis): A term embracing a group of conditions in which there is either an inflammatory or an inflammatory-like condition, focal or diffused, in the kidneys. **ACUTE N.**, Bright's disease. A diffuse inflammatory reaction of both kidneys, usually following a streptococcal infection, and classically manifest by puffiness of the face and scanty blood-stained urine. **CHRONIC N.**, a chronic condition in which there is widespread fibrous replacement of functioning kidney tissue, resulting in progressive renal failure and arterial hypertension, and terminating ultimately in death. **INTERSTITIAL N.**, nephritis affecting the interstitial tissue of the kidney. **LUPUS N.**, diffuse glomerulonephritis occurring in patients with lupus erythematosus or systemic lupus; characterized by hematuria and progressing to renal failure. **NEPHROTIC N.**, a chronic condition of unknown cause, characterized by massive edema and heavy proteinuria.

nephritogenic (ne-frit′-ō-jen′-ik): Giving rise to nephritis.

nephroangiosclerosis (nef′-rō-an′-ji-ō-sklē-rō′-sis): Necrosis of the renal arterioles; usually associated with high blood pressure; symptoms include headache, blurred vision, enlarged heart, retinal hemorrhage, and papilledema; when untreated, progresses to heart and kidney failure.

nephroblastoma (nef′-rō-blas-tō′-ma): A malignant tumor of the kidney; occurs almost exclusively in children. Thought to develop from embryonic structures. Also called embryoma and Wilms' tumor.

nephrocalcinosis (nef′-rō-kal-sin-ō′-sis): A form of renal lithiasis (*q.v.*); characterized by calcium deposits in many areas of the kidney, resulting in renal insufficiency.

nephrocapsectomy (nef′-rō-kap-sek′-to-mi): Surgical removal of the kidney capsule. Usually done for chronic nephritis. Also nephrocapsulectomy.

nephrocardiac (nef′-rō-kar′-di-ak): Pertaining to the kidney and the heart.—Also nephritocardiac.

nephrocele (nef′-rō-sēl): A hernia of the kidney.

nephrocolic (nef-rō-kol′-ik): Pertaining to the kidney and the colon.

nephrocoloptosis (nef′-rō-kō-lop-tō′-sis): The downward displacement of both the kidney and the colon.

nephrocystanastomosis (nef′-rō-sist-an-as-to-mō′-sis): The surgical creation of a communicating passageway between the kidney and the urinary bladder to correct an irremovable obstruction in the urethra.

nephrocystitis (nef′rō-sis-tī′tis): Inflammation of the kidney and the urinary bladder.

nephrocystosis (nef′-rō-sis-tō′-sis): The development of cysts in the kidney substance.

nephrogenic (nef′-rō-jen′-ik): 1. Arising in a kidney. 2. Produced by the kidneys. 3. Capable of generating kidney tissue.

nephrogenous (nef-roj′-e-nus): Arising in a kidney.

nephrogram (nef′-rō-gram): X ray of renal shadow following injection of opaque medium.—nephrography, n.; nephrographical, adj.; nephrographically, adv.

nephrography (ne-frog′-ra-fi): Roentgenography of the kidney.

nephrohemia (nef-rō-hē′-mi-a): Congestion of the kidney.

nephrohydrosis (nef′-rō-hī-drō′-sis): Hydronephrosis (*q.v.*).

nephrohypertrophy (nef′-rō-hī-per′-tro-fi): Hypertrophy of the kidney.

nephrolith (nef′-rō-lith): A kidney stone.

nephrolithiasis (nef′-rō-lith-ī′-a-sis): The presence of stones in the kidney.

nephrolithotomy (nef′-rō-lith-ot′-o-mi): Removal of a stone from the kidney by an incision through the kidney substance.

nephrologist (ne-frol′-o-jist): A physician who specializes in diseases and disorders of the kidney.

nephrology (ne-frol′-o-ji): Scientific study of the kidneys and the diseases that affect them.—nephrologic, adj.

nephrolysis (ne-frol′-i-sis): 1. Destruction of kidney substance. 2. The operation of freeing a kidney from adhesions.—nephrolytic, adj.

nephroma (ne-frō′-ma): A tumor that arises in the kidney.

nephromalacia (nef′rō-ma-lā′shi-a): Softening of the kidney substance.

nephromegaly (nef-rō-meg′-a-li): Enlargement of one or both kidneys.

nephron (nef′-ron): The basic structural and functional unit of the kidney, comprising a glomerulus (*q.v.*) within Bowman's capsule, proximal and distal convoluted tubules with the nephronic loop (loop of Henle) connecting them, and a straight collecting tubule via which urine is conveyed to the renal pelvis. There are more than a million nephrons in each kidney.

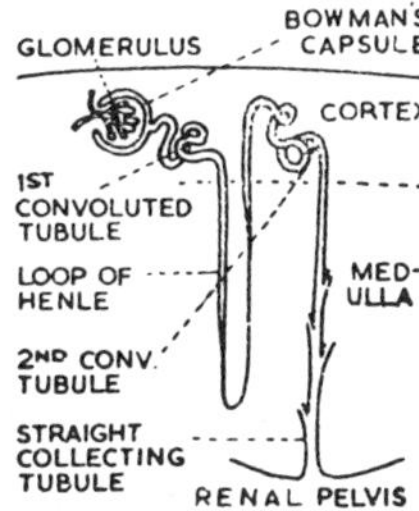

Diagram of nephron

nephropathy (ne-frop′-a-thi): Any disease of the kidney(s).—nephropathic, adj.

nephropexy (nef′-rō-pek-si): Surgical fixation of a floating kidney.

nephrophthisis (ne-frof′-thi-sis): Tuberculosis of the kidney.

nephroptosis (nef-rop-tō′-sis): Downward displacement of the kidney; also called floating kidney.

nephropyelitis (nef′-rō-pī-e-lī′-tis): Inflammation of the pelvis and the parenchyma of the kidney.

nephropyelography (nef′rō-pī′e-log′ra-fi): Roentgenography of the kidney including its pelvis.

nephropyelolithotomy (nef′-rō-pī′-e-lō-lith-ot′-o-mi): The surgical removal of a stone from the pelvic area of the kidney.

nephropyeloplasty (nef′-rō-pī′-e-lō-plas-ti): A plastic operation on the pelvis of the kidney.

nephropyosis (nef′-rō-pī′-ō′-sis): Pus formation in the kidney.

nephrorrhagia (nef′-rō-rā′-ji-a): Hemorrhage from a kidney or into the pelvis of the kidney.

nephrorrhaphy (nef-ror′-a-fi): Suturing a kidney or fixing a kidney in place by suturing. Nephropexy.

nephrosclerosis (nef′-rō-sklē-ro′-sis): Hardening or sclerosis of the kidney. Seen in cardiovascular-renal disease. May be benign or malignant. **ARTERIOLAR N.,** sclerosis of the small arteries of the kidney.—nephrosclerotic, adj.

nephrosis (ne-frō′-sis): A term descriptive of any degenerative change in the kidney, the tubules in particular, that is not associated with inflammation as occurs in nephritis, or with vascular involvement which may occur. **ACUTE N., N.** caused by certain chemical poisons, toxemia of pregnancy, or obstructive jaundice; characterized by low urine output, and little or no edema or proteinuria. **HYPOXIC N.,** acute renal failure caused by hypovolemia resulting from such conditions as burns, hemorrhage, or shock. **LIPOID N., N.** characterized by edema and albuminuria, and increased blood cholesterol; occurs most often in children. **TOXIC N.,** acute renal failure caused by ingestion of such poisons as mercuric chloride or by septicemia.—Syn., nephropathy; nephrodystrophy.

nephrostomy (ne-fros′to-mi): A surgically established fistula from the pelvis of the kidney to the body surface. **N. TUBE,** a tube inserted through the abdominal wall into the pelvis of the kidney to provide for drainage of urine.

nephrotic (ne-frot′ik): Pertinent to, resembling, or caused by nephrosis. **N. SYNDROME,** a protein-wasting kidney condition; may be primary or secondary to some systemic disease; caused by damage to the glomerular membrane; characterized by fatigue, severe generalized edema, ascites, proteinuria, hypoproteinemia, hyperlipidemia, lipiduria, hypoalbuminemia, pleural effusion, lowered resistance to intercurrent infections. May be associated with diabetes mellitus, hypovolemia, sickle cell disease, allergic reactions. Also called nephrosis.

nephrotomography (nef′rō-tō-mog′ra-fi): An x-ray procedure for obtaining sectional views of the kidney.

nephrotomy (ne-frot′o-mi): An incision into the kidney.

nephrotoxic (nef-rō-tok′sik): Toxic or destructive to cells of the kidney.—nephrotoxicity, n.

nephrotoxin (nef-rō-tok′sin): A cytotoxin that is destructive to kidney cells.—nephrotoxic, adj.

nephroureterectomy (nef′rō-ū-rē′ter-ek′to-mi): Removal of a kidney along with a part or the whole of the ureter.

nephroureterocystectomy (nef′rō-ū-rē′ter-ō-sis-tek′to-mi): Surgical excision of a kidney, ureter, and part or all of the urinary bladder.

nerve: An elongated bundle of fibers that may or may not be myelinated, along with blood vessels and connective tissue. The individual fibers are covered with a sheath called endoneurium; the individual bundles are covered with a sheath called perineurium; and the nerve is covered with a sheath called epineurium. **AFFERENT N.**, a **N.** conveying impulses from the tissues to a nerve center; also known as receptor and sensory **N. EFFERENT N.**, one that conveys impulses outward from a nerve center. **MIXED N.**, one that consists of both motor and sensory fibers. Nerves are also known as effector, motor, secretory, trophic, vasoconstrictor, vasodilator, etc., according to function and location—nervi, pl.

nerve block: Regional anesthesia produced by interruption of the passage of impulses over a nerve, usually by injection of an anesthetic close to the nerve supplying the area to be anesthetized.

nerve gas: A chemical compound in gaseous form which, following inhalation, ingestion, or application to the skin, is absorbed by the body, with serious effects on the nervous system and various body functions.

nervous (ner′vus): 1. Relating to nerves or nerve tissue. 2. Referring to a state of restlessness or timidity. 3. Easily excited or agitated. 4. Exhibiting undue irritation or excitability of the nervous system. **N. BREAKDOWN,** a common nonmedical term for an emotional illness or psychosis.

nervous system: The structures that control the actions and functions of the body, which allow the individual to react and adjust to varying internal and external conditions. It comprises the central nervous system and the peripheral nervous system with its subsystems, the somatic and the autonomic systems. **AUTONOMIC NERVOUS SYSTEM,** is concerned with regulating the activities of cardiac muscle, smooth muscle, and the glands of internal secretion. The autonomic system has two subsystems, 1) the parasympathetic nervous system, which consists of some of the cranial and sacral nerves that are concerned with the innervation of smooth and cardiac muscle and glands; and 2) the sympathetic nervous system, which comprises a chain of ganglia on either side of the vertebral column in the thoracolumbar region; it sends fibers to all involuntary muscle tissue and glands. **CENTRAL NERVOUS SYSTEM,** includes the brain and spinal cord; it is the integrative and control center of the entire nervous system. **PERIPHERAL NERVOUS SYSTEM,** consists of all parts of the nervous system outside of the pia arachnoid membrane of the brain and spinal cord; it includes the 12 pairs of cranial nerves and 31 pairs of spinal nerves and their many ganglia, branches, and fibers that reach out to the periphery of the body. **SOMATIC NERVOUS SYSTEM,** consists of motor and sensory nerves that supply skeletal muscles and somatic tissues; it initiates voluntary actions.

nervousness (nerv′us-nes): A state of unrest, jitteriness, and irritability.

nesidiectomy (nē-sid′i-ek′to-mi): Surgical removal of the pancreatic islands of Langerhans.

nesidioblastoma (nē-sid′i-ō-blas-tō′ma): A tumor of islet tissue of the pancreas.

nesidioblastosis (nē-sid′ -ē-ō-blas-tō′sis): Excessive proliferation of the islet cells and tissue of the pancreas.

nestia (nes′ti-a): Abstinence from food; starvation.

nestiostomy (nes-tē-os′tō-mi): The surgical creation of a permanent opening into the jejunum through the abdominal wall; jejunostomy.

nestis (nes′tis): The jejunum.

nettle rash (net′t′l): 1. Popular term for urticaria; wheals of the skin; see **urticaria.** 2. A fine intensely itchy rash caused by contact with nettles; self-limited and of short duration.

network: In anatomy, a structure resembling a net; formed by intertwining fibers.

Neufeld nail: A nail used in orthopedic surgery for fixation of an intertrochantic fracture of the femur.

neur-, neuro-: Combining forms denoting 1) nerve; 2) neural tissue; 3) nervous system.

neural (nū′ral): Pertaining to a nerve or nerves. **N. TUBE,** the embryonic epithelial tube from which the brain and spinal cord develop.

neuralgia (nū-ral′ji-a): Severe, paroxysmal pain occurring along the course of one or more nerves. Many varieties are distinguished and named according to the part affected or the nerve that supplies the part affected. **GENICULATE N.,** severe pain in the middle ear and auditory canal, facial paralysis, lack of tearing and salivation, and loss of taste; due to a lesion of the facial nerve at the geniculate ganglion; often associated with herpes zoster. MIGRAINOUS N., characterized by severe burning pain over the eye and part of the face, with fever, rhinorrhea, lacrimation; usually occurs in the morning and characteristically in clusters. POSTHERPETIC N., often follows herpes zoster in which the trigeminal nerve is involved; marked by burning, unrelenting pain. TRIGEMINAL N., may affect all or only one branch of the nerve; marked by excruciating episodic pain along the distribution of the nerve; also called tic douloureux, cluster headache, and Horton's headache, facial neuralgia and Fothergill's neuralgia.

neuralgic (nū-ral′jik): Pertaining to or resembling neuralgia.

neuranagenesis (nūr′an-a-jen′e-sis): The regeneration of a nerve following injury or destruction of part of the nerve.

neurapraxia (nū′ra-prak′si-a): Temporary loss of function in peripheral nerve fibers without interruption of the nerve. Most commonly due to crushing or prolonged pressure; recovery is usually rapid and complete.

neurasthenia (nū′ras-thē′ni-a): A condition of nervous exhaustion characterized by lassitude, inertia, fatigue, loss of initiative, oversensitivity, and undue irritability; may be a sequela of psychiatric illness.

neurasthenic (nū-ras-then′ik): 1. One suffering from neurasthenia (*q.v.*). 2. Pertaining to neurasthenia.

neuraxis (nū-rak′sis): 1. An axon. Also called neuraxon. 2. The central nervous system.

neurectasis (nū-rek′ta-sis): The stretching of, or an operation for, the stretching of a nerve.

neurectomy (nū-rek′to-mi): The surgical division of a nerve or excision of part of a nerve to relieve pain.

neurectopia (nū′rek-tō′pi-a): A condition in which a nerve follows an abnormal course.

neurergic (nūr-er′jik): Pertaining to the action or activity of a nerve.

neuriatry (nū-rī′a-tri): The medical practice concerned with the treatment of the diseases and disorders of the nervous system.

neuricity (nū-ris′i-ti): The energy inherent in nervous tissue.

neurilemma, neurilema (nū-ri-lem′ma): The thin membranous layer of cells that covers the myelinated sheaths of the fibers of peripheral nerves or the axon of a nonmyelinated nerve. See also endoneurium and sheath of Schwann.

neurilemmitis, neurilemitis (nū′ri-lem-ī′tis): Inflammation of the neurilemma of one or more nerves.

neurilemmoma, neurilemoma (nū′-ri-lem-mō′ma): A benign slow-growing tumor that arises from the neurilemma of certain cranial or spinal nerves. Also called neurolemmoma and schwannoma.

neurinoma (nū-ri-nō′ma): A benign encapsulated fibroma (*q.v.*) which arises in the endoneurium of the sheath of Schwann of peripheral, autonomic, or cranial nerves. ACOUSTIC N., acoustic neuroma (*q.v.*).

neurinomatosis (nū′ri-nō-ma-tō′sis): A condition marked by the appearance of numerous neuromas.

neurite (nū′rīt): An old term for axon.

neuritis (nū-rī′tis): Inflammation of a nerve, accompanied by pain and tenderness over the nerve, sometimes by paresthesias and loss of reflexes. DISSEMINATED N., polyneuritis; also called multiple N. NUTRITIONAL N., beri-beri (*q.v.*). OPTIC N. Inflammation of the optic nerve. PERIPHERAL N., N. of nerve endings or of terminal nerves. RETROBULBAR N., acute impairment of vision, especially of central visual acuity, in one or both eyes; due to demyelination or other pathology of the orbital part of the optic nerve. SCIATIC N., inflammation of the sciatic nerve; sciatica. VESTIBULAR N., irritation of the vestibular part of the 8th cranial nerve; characterized by vertigo, vomiting, imbalance; to be differentiated from Ménière's disease.

neuroanastomosis (nū′rō-an-as-to-mō′sis): The operation of joining or making a junction between nerves.

neuroanatomy (nū′rō-a-nat′o-mi): The anatomy of the nervous system.—neuroanatomic, adj.

neuroarthropathy (nū′rō-ar-throp′a-thi): A pathological joint condition occurring simultaneously with a disease of the nervous system.

neuroastrocytoma (nū′rō-as-trō-sī-tō′ma): A glioma (*q.v.*) made up chiefly of astrocytes; may arise in almost any part of the nervous system but most often occurs in the third ventricle of the brain.

neurobiology (nū′rō-bī-ol′o-ji): The biology of the nervous system.

neuroblast (nū′rō-blast): A primitive nerve cell.

neuroblastoma (nū-rō-blas-tō′ma): A malignant tumor seen mostly in infants and young children; composed of immature cells resembling neuroblasts; usually occurs in the retroperitoneal area, the adrenal medulla especially, and metastasizes to other organs and bones.

neurocanal (nū′-rō-kan-al): The vertebral column, which contains the spinal cord.

neuroceptor (nū′rō-sep-tor): A terminal branch of a dendrite that receives a stimulus from an adjoining neuron.

neurochemistry (nū′rō-kem′is-tri): The branch of neurology that deals with the chemistry of nerve substance.

neurochorioretinitis (nū-rō-kō′ri-ō-ret-i-nī'tis): Inflammation of the optic nerve, choroid, and retina.

neurocirculatory (nū-rō-sir'kū-la-tō-ri): Pertaining to both the nervous and circulatory systems. **N. ASTHENIA,** see under **asthenia.**

neurocladism (nū-rok'la-dizm): The formation of new branches by a process of a neuron; said especially of the formation of a bridge between the two ends of a divided nerve.

neuroclonic (nū-rō-klon'ik): Pertaining to or characterized by nervous spasm.

neurocranium (nū'rō-krā'ni-um): The part of the cranium that contains the brain.

neurocutaneous (nū'rō-kū-tā'nē-us): Pertaining to 1) the nervous system and the skin; or 2) the nerves of the skin.

neurocyte (nū'rō-sīt): A nerve cell. Neuron.

neurocytoma (nū-rō-sī-tō'ma): A tumor made up of nervous system cells, usually ganglionic. See **ganglion.**

neurodeatrophia (nū'rō-dē-a-trō'fi-a): Atrophy of the retina.

neurodendrite (nū'rō-den'drīt): A dendrite (*q.v.*).

neurodermatitis (nū'rō-der-ma-tī'tis): Lichen simplex (*q.v.*). Leathery, thickened patches of skin secondary to pruritus or anything that causes habitual scratching, *e.g.*, insect bites, psoriasis, contact with chemicals. As the skin thickens, irritation increases, scratching causes further thickening and thus a vicious circle is set up.

neurodiagnosis (nū'rō-dī-ag-nō'sis): The diagnosis of nervous disorders.—neurodiagnostic, adj.

neurodynia (nū'rō-din'i-a): Pain in one or more nerves. Neuralgia.

neuroelectricity (nū'rō-ē-lek-tris'i-ti): The electrical currents generated by the nervous system.

neuroencephalomyelopathy (nū'rō-en-sef'a-lō-mī-e-lop'a-thi): Pathology involving the nerves, brain, and spinal cord.

neuroendocrine (nū'rō-en'dō-krēn): 1. Pertaining to the relationship between the nervous and endocrine systems. 2. Pertaining to cells that release a hormone into the bloodstream following a neural stimulus, *e.g.*, the beta cells of the islets of Langerhans in the pancreas.

neuroendocrinology (nū'rō-en'dō-krin-ol'ō-ji): The study of the relationships between the nervous and the endocrine systems and their interactions.

neuroepithelium (nū'rō-ep-i-thē'li-um): Simple columnar epithelium made up of cells that act as receptors for external stimuli, as in the nose, tongue, and cochlea.—neuroepithelial, adj.

neurofibril (nū-rō-fī'bril): One of the many fine fibrils that run through the cytoplasm and the axons and dendrites of a nerve cell. It is thought that they may form the conducting element of the neuron.—neurofibrillary, adj.

neurofibrillary (nū-rō-fib'ri-lar-i): Pertaining to neurofibrils. **N. TANGLE,** bundles of fibrillary material within the cytoplasm of neurons and projecting into the axon and dendrites, particularly those of the hippocampus; commonly seen in cerebral cortex of persons over 65 years of age.

neurofibroma (nū'rō-fī-brō'ma): A somewhat firm benign tumor occurring on a peripheral nerve sheath and including portions of nerve fibers; often multiple; due to disorderly proliferation of Schwann cells. Also called Schwann's tumor.

neurofibromatosis (nū'rō-fī-brō-ma-tō'sis): A condition characterized by the formation of multiple neurofibromata and possible neuromas. See Recklinghausen's disease.

neurogangliitis (nū'rō-gang-gli-ī'tis): Old term for inflammation of a neuroganglion.

neuroganglion (nū-rō-gang'gli-on): A mass of nerve cell bodies in either the central or peripheral nervous system.

neurogastric (nū-rō-gas'trik): Pertaining to the nerves of the stomach.

neurogenesis (nū-rō-jen'e-sis): The development of nerve tissue.

neurogenic (nū-rō-jen'ik): 1. Originating within or forming nervous tissue. 2. Stimulating nervous energy. **N. BLADDER,** a condition resulting from any defect in the functioning of the urinary bladder that is the result of damage to the nerve supply of that organ. **N. SHOCK,** see under **shock.**

neurogenous (nū-roj'e-nus): Arising from nervous tissue.

neuroglia (nū-rog'li-a): The tissue that supports elements of the central nervous system, especially the brain, spinal cord, and ganglia; of ectodermal origin; consists of a network of fine fibrils, stellate cells, and many radiating fibrillar processes.—neuroglial, adj.

neurogliacyte (nū-rog'li-a-sīt): A neuroglial cell.

neurogliocytoma (nū-rog'li-ō-sī-tō'ma): A tumor composed of neuroglial cells.

neuroglioma (nū-rōg'lī-ō'ma): A tumor composed of neuroglial tissue. Glioma.

neurogliosis (nū-rog'li-ō-sis): A condition characterized by formation of multiple foci of glioma in the brain and spinal cord.

neurogram (nū'rō-gram): The imprint that a mental experience makes on the brain; important in the development of memory and of personality.

neurohistology (nū'rō-his-tol'o-ji): The histology (*q.v.*) of the nervous system.

neurohormone (nū'rō-hor-mōn): A hormone

that stimulates neuronal activity, *e.g.*, adrenaline.

neurohumor (nū'rō-hū'mor): A chemical substance that is formed in the neuron and liberated at the nerve endings; participates in the transmission of nerve impulses from one neuron to another or to a muscle or gland.—neurohumoral, adj.

neurohypophyseal (nū'rō-hīpō-fiz'ē-al): Pertaining to the neurohypophysis (*q.v.*).

neurohypophysis (nū'rō-hī-pō-f'i-sis): The posterior lobe of the pituitary gland. See also pituitary.

neuroid (nū'royd): Resembling a nerve.

neurolemma (nū-rō-lem'ma): Neurilemma (*q.v.*).

neurolemmoma, neurolemoma (nū'rō-lem-mō'ma): Neurilemmoma (*q.v.*).

neurolepsis (nū-rō-lep'sis): A state of consciousness in which anxiety and psychomotor activity are reduced and the individual is unresponsive to elements in the environment; sleep may occur but the individual responds to commands; may be induced by administration of analeptic (antipsychotic) drugs.

neuroleptanalgesia (nū'rō-lept-an-al-jē'zi-a): A state produced by the administration of a major tranquilizer and a narcotic analgesic together, most often after minor surgery, to produce somnolence and lessen the stress on the central nervous system that results from anesthesia.

neuroleptic (nū-rō-lep'tik): 1. An agent that acts to produce symptoms resembling those of certain disorders of the nervous system. 2. An agent that acts on the nervous system to reduce anxiety and psychomotor activity; includes the tranquilizers and antipsychotics; used in psychotherapy for treating acute and chronic psychoses and the psychoses associated with old age.

neurologic (nū-rō-log'ik): Pertaining to neurology or to the nervous system.

neurologist (nū-rol'o-jist): A physician who specializes in diseases of the brain, spinal cord, and nerves.

neurology (nū-rol'o-ji): The branch of medical science that deals with the nerves, their structure, function, and pathology, and with the diseases and disorders of the nervous system.

neurolymph (nū'rō-limf): Cerebrospinal fluid.

neurolysis (nū-rol'i-sis): 1. The breaking down of nerve substance. 2. The operation of freeing a nerve from adhesions. 3. Exhaustion of nerve from overstimulation.—neurolytic, adj.

neuroma (nū'rō'ma): A tumor made up of nerve cells and nerve tissue. An old general term for many neoplasms of the nervous system. **ACOUSTIC N.**, a **N.** arising in the vestibular portion of the 8th cranial nerve; lies in the auditory canal and enlarges progressively, causing headache, dizziness, staggering gait, diplopia, and eventual hearing loss; may be unilateral or bilateral; is usually benign. **N. CUTIS**, a **N.** arising in the skin; nerve tissue may be involved, making the neoplasm extremely sensitive to painful stimuli. **JOPLIN'S N.**, perineural fibrosis of the plantar proper digital nerve; may result from bunionectomy or trauma to the first metatarsal joint; characterized by pain and paresthesia on the plantar aspect of the joint.

neuromalacia (nū'rō-ma-lā'shi-a): Pathological softening of the nerves.

neuromatosis (nū'rō-ma-tō'sis): A condition characterized by the presence of numerous neuromas.

neuromuscular (nū' -rō-mus'kū-lar): Pertaining to nerves and muscles.

neuromyasthenia (nū'rō-mī-as-thē'ni-a): Muscular weakness associated with emotional lability. Cause unknown; symptoms usually include sore throat, headache, slight fever, malaise.

neuromyelitis (nū'rō-mī-e-lī'tis): Myelitis (*q.v.*) occurring in conjunction with neuritis. **N. OPTICA**, demyelination of the optic nerve and spinal cord, marked by dimming of vision and possible blindness, flaccid paralysis of extremities, disturbances of sensation; more common in children than adults. Also called Devic's disease.

neuromyopathic (nū'rō-mī-op'a-thik): Pertaining to a pathologic condition of muscle and of the nerves supplying the muscles.

neuromyositis (nū'rō-mī-ō-sī'tis): Inflammation of both the nerves and muscles of a part.

neuron (nū'ron): The structural and functional unit of the nervous system comprising the fibers (dendrites) that convey impulses to the nerve cell, the nerve cell itself, and the fibers (axons) that convey impulses from the cell. May be classified according to function as 1) afferent, which carry impulses from receptors in all parts of the body to the central nervous system; 2) efferent, which carry impulses from the central nervous system to muscles and glands of the body; and 3) interneurons, which connect neurons within the nervous system. **BIPOLAR N.**, one with two processes arising from opposite poles of the cell body. **CONNECTOR N.**, one that serves as a link between a receptor and an effector neuron. **INTERNUNCIAL N.**, an **N.** between two other **N.'s** connecting them. **LOWER MOTOR N.**, an **N.** with the cell in the gray matter of the anterior horn of the spinal cord and the axon passing to skeletal muscle. **UPPER MOTOR N.**, an **N.** with the cell in the cerebral cortex and the axon passing down the spinal cord to arborize with a lower motor **N.**—neural, adj.

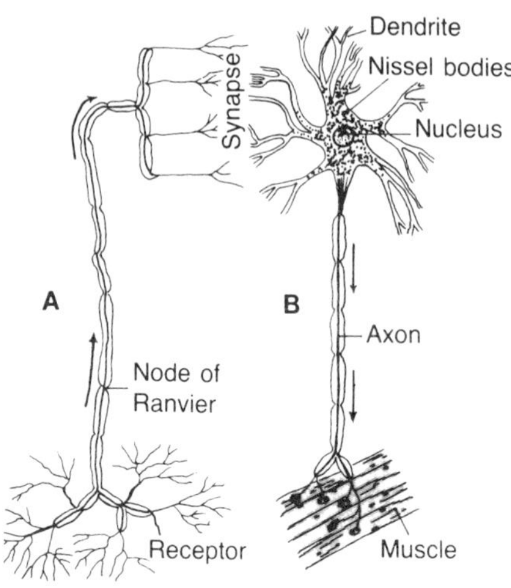

neuron

neuronitis (nū-rō-nī'tis): Term applied to a disorder of the more proximal part of the peripheral nervous system; it involves breakdown of the fibers due to inflammation. **VESTIBULAR N.,** may follow a viral infection; the patient feels dizzy when lying down and tends to fall or deviate to one side when walking; may persist for a few days or weeks; to be differentiated from Ménière's disease.

neuronophage (nū-ron'ō-fāj): A phagocyte that destroys nerve cells.

neuro-ophthalmology (nū'rō-of-thal-mol'o-ji): The study of, or branch of medicine that deals with the diseases of the eye as related to the nervous system.

neuroparalysis (nū' -rō-pa-ral'i-sis): Paralysis caused by disease of the nerve(s) supplying the affected part.—neuroparalytic, adj.

neuropathic (nū-rō-path'ik): 1. Relating to disease of the nervous system. 2. Having a nervous disease.

neuropathology (nū' -rō-path-ol'oj-i): A branch of medicine dealing with diseases of the nervous system.—neuropathologic, adj.

neuropathy (nū-rop' -a-thi): A general term for any disease of the nerves, of known or unknown cause, in which there is functional disturbance in the peripheral nervous system. **ASCENDING N., N.** that progresses from the feet upward. **DESCENDING N., N.** that starts at the shoulders and progresses downward. **DIABETIC N., N.** that arises as a complication in diabetic patients; characterized by leg pain, abnormal burning sensation, tingling, and numbness. **ENTRAPMENT N., N.** due to compression of a nerve in a confined space such as the carpal tunnel in the wrist; characterized by pain, weakness; seen more often in women.

neuropharmacology (nū'rō-far-ma-kol'o-ji): The branch of pharmacology dealing with the drugs that affect the nervous system.

neurophonia (nū-rō-fō'ni-a): The involuntary uttering of peculiar cries or sounds often resembling the sounds produced by animals; characteristic of certain nervous disorders.

neurophysiology (nū'rō-fiz-ē-ol'o-ji): The physiology of the nervous system.—neurophysiologic, adj.

neuroplasm (nū'rō-plazm): The cytoplasm of a nerve cell.

neuroplasty (nū'rō-plas-ti): Surgical repair of nerves.—neuroplastic, adj.

neuropraxia (nū-rō-prak'si-a): Contusion or trauma to a nerve that results in temporary disruption of its function by blocking conduction of the nerve impulse.

neuropsychiatry (nū'rō-si-kī'a-tri): The combination of neurology and psychiatry; a specialty dealing with organic and functional diseases of the nervous system and utilizing the results of psychological tests in the diagnosis of neuropathology.

neuropsychology (nū'rō-sī-kol'o-ji): A system in psychology that is based on neurology; it is the study of the relationships between the brain and behavior.

neuropsychopathy (nū' -rō-sī-kop'a-thi): Emotional illness that involves disease or disorder of the nervous system.

neuropsychosis (nū'rō-sī-kō'sis): Psychosis of neurologic origin.

neuroradiology (nū'rō-rādi-ol'o-ji): Radiology of the central nervous system. Neuroroentgenology.

neuroretinitis (nū'rō-ret-in-ī'tis): Inflammation of the optic nerve and the retina.

neuroroentgenography (nū'rō-rent-ge-nog'ra-fi): Neuroradiology (*q.v.*).

neurorrhaphy (nū-ror'a-fi): Suturing the ends of a divided nerve.

neurosarcoma (nū' -rō-sar-kō'ma): A sarcoma made up of nerve, connective, and vascular tissue.

neurosciences (nū'rō-sī'en-sis): The disciplines that are concerned with the anatomy, structure, function, development, and pathology of the various elements that make up the nervous system.

neurosclerosis (nū'rō-sklē-rō'sis): The hardening of a nerve or of nerve tissue.

neurosecretory (nū'rō-sē'kre-to-ri): Pertaining to the secretory activity of nerves.

neurosensory (nū-rō-sen'so-ri): Pertaining to sensory nerves.

neurosis (nū-rō'sis): A functional emotional disorder, the commonest types being anxiety state, reactive depression, hysteria, and obsessional **N.** To be differentiated from psychosis by the fact that it arises from stresses and anxieties in the environment and that the individual usually retains his relation to reality. **ANXIETY STATE N.**, an apprehensive state and feeling of uncertainty and helplessness without sufficient cause; occurs as a result of a threat to the person's self-esteem or identity; marked by recurrent anxiety attacks (panics) with symptoms that include all the signs of fear, leading up to fear of impending collapse and sometimes of death. **CHARACTER N.**, a personality disorder in which the individual's character and life-style are abnormal but whose interpersonal relationships may or may not be normal. **COMPULSIVE N., N.** characterized by compulsion to perform certain acts against one's will to the extent that this interferes with living and functioning. **DEPERSONALIZATION N., N.** in which the individual has strong feelings of unreality and estrangement from himself as well as from his environment. **DEPRESSIVE N., N.** characterized by severe depression due to internal conflict; often follows the loss of a loved one or object. **HYPOCHONDRIACAL N.**, a condition in which the individual is certain he has a physical illness although none can be detected. **HYSTERICAL N., CONVERSION TYPE,** a form of psychoneurosis characterized by signs and manifestations that have no organic basis but arise from anxiety caused by some emotional conflict and which involve the special senses and the voluntary nervous system, *e.g.*, blindness, deafness, anesthesia, pain, paralysis. **INSTITUTIONAL N.**, apathy, nonparticipation, and withdrawal occurring in long-term patients in reaction to institutionalization. **OBSESSIONAL N.**, of two types: 1) The patient has obsessive-compulsive thoughts, *i.e.*, he is preoccupied with constantly recurring thoughts that he may wish to eliminate but cannot; the thoughts are always painful and out of keeping with his normal personality. 2) The patient has obsessive-compulsive thoughts and also engages in actions that are both obsessional and compulsive, such as handwashing, not touching doorknobs, etc., which he does not choose to do but cannot stop doing. The ideas are often concerned with feelings of guilt. **PHOBIC N., N.** characterized by intense anxiety and unwanted fears that interfere with the person's adjustment to his environment. **SOMATIC N., N.** in which the patient's anxiety is fixed on his body. **SYMBOLIC N., N.** in which the patient's anxiety is transformed into bizarre behavior. **TRAUMATIC N., N.** that results from injury. **WAR N.**, shell shock; see under shock.

neuroskeletal (nū'rō-skel'e-tal): Pertaining to the nervous system and the skeletal muscles.

neurospasm (nū'rō-spazm): Twitching of a muscle due to a disorder of the nerve supplying the muscle.

neurospongioma (nū' -rō-spon-ji-ō'ma): Medulloblastoma (*q.v.*).

neurostatus (nū-rō-stā'tus): The state of the patient's nervous system as shown in the case history.

neurosurgeon (nū-rō-sur'jun): A surgeon who specializes in surgery on nerves and other parts of the nervous system.

neurosurgery (nū-rō-ser'jer-i): Surgery involving any part of the nervous system.—neurosurgical, adj.

neurosyphilis (nū-rō-sif'i-lis): Infection of the brain or spinal cord, or both, by *Treponema pallidum*. The variety of clinical pictures produced is large, but the two common syndromes encountered are tabes dorsalis and dementia paralytica. The basic pathology is disease of the blood vessels, with later development of pathological changes in the meninges and the underlying nervous tissue. Very often symptoms of the disease do not arise until 20 years or more after the date of primary infection. See Argyll Robertson pupil.—neurosyphilitic, adj.

neurotendinous (nū'rō-ten'din-us): Pertaining to both a nerve and a tendon.

neurotension (nū'rō-ten'shun): See neurectasis.

neurothecitis (nū'rō-thē-sī'tis): Inflammation of the sheath of a nerve.

neurotherapy (nū-rō-ther'a-pi): The treatment of nervous diseases and disorders.

neurothlipsis (nū-rō-thlip'sis): Irritation or pressure on one or more nerves.

neurotic (nū-rot'ik): 1. Pertaining to neurosis. 2. Nervous. 3. A person suffering from a neurosis or from instability of the nervous system; usually characterized by over-reaction to stresses, but without loss of contact with reality.

neurotic disorders: Mental disorders in which there is no demonstrable organic disorder, and that are relatively enduring and/or recurring unless treated; the symptoms are not acceptable to the patient; anxiety states and panic states characterized by fear and apprehension may interfere with the person's social functioning. Many neurotic disorders were formerly classified as neuroses.

neuroticism (nū-rot'i-sizm): The condition of being neurotic or suffering from abnormal nervousness.

neurotization (nū-rot'ī-zā'shun): 1. The regeneration of a nerve. 2. The implantation of a nerve into a paralyzed muscle.

neurotmesis (nū-rot-mē'sis): Complete destruction of the connective tissue of a nerve causing interruption of the nerve; may be caused by scarring or cutting.

neurotomy (nū-rot'o-mi): Surgical cutting or division of a nerve.

neurotony (nū-rot′o-ni): The stretching of a nerve; sometimes done to relieve intractable pain. Neurectasia.

neurotoxic (nū-rō-toks′ik): Harmful or destructive to nerve tissue.—neurotoxicity, n.

neurotoxin (nū-rō-toks′in): Any toxic substance that acts directly on the nervous system and is destructive to nerve tissue, *e.g.*, the venom of certain snakes.

neurotransmission (nū′rō-trans-mish′un): The process by which a presynaptic cell releases a specific chemical agent to cross the synapse and stimulate or inhibit a postsynaptic cell.

neurotransmitter (nū′rō-trans-mit′ter): Any of several chemical substances that make possible the transmission of nerve impulses within the brain and from one nerve cell to another.

neurotrauma (nū-rō-traw′ma): Injury to a nerve or nerves.

neurotripsy (nū-rō-trip′si): The surgical crushing of a nerve.

neurotrophia (nū-rō-trō′fi-a): Impaired nutrition of the nervous system.

neurotrophic (nū-rō-trō′fik): 1. Pertaining to the influence of nervous impulses on the nutrition and normal condition of nerves. 2. Having a predilection for the nervous system, said especially of *Treponema pallidum,* some forms of which seem always to produce neurosyphilitic complications. **N. VIRUSES** (rabies, poliomyelitis, etc.) make their major attack on the cells of the nervous system.

neurovascular (nū-rō-vas′kū-lar): Pertaining to 1) both nerve and vascular tissues, or 2) the nerves that supply the walls of the blood vessels.

neurula (nū′roo-la): The period in the development of an embryo when the nervous system tissues begin to differentiate; occurs about 20 to 26 days after fertilization.

neutral (nū′tral): Having no positive properties or characteristics. In chemistry, neither acid nor basic in reaction.

neutralization (nū′tral-ī-zā′shun): 1. The conversion of an acid or basic substance into a neutral one. 2. The process of rendering any action or process ineffective. 3. In bacteriology, the action of an antibody in coating the membrane of a host cell, thus preventing a virus from attaching to it and invading the body.

neutralize (nū′tra-līz): 1. To render something neutral. 2. To render ineffective.

neutroclusion (nū′trō-klū′zhun): Irregularities in occulsion of some of the teeth, although the jaws are in normal position.

neutron (nū′tron): One of the basic particles of the nucleus of the atom; it breaks down into a proton and an electron.

neutropenia (nū-trō-pē′ni-a): The condition in which there is a much lower percentage of neutrophils in the blood than normal.

neutrophil (nū′trō-fil): One form of polymorphonuclear leukocyte (*q.v.*); its nucleus has two or more lobes that are connected by strands of chromatin; stains readily with neutral dyes with the nucleus staining a dark blue and the cytoplasm pink. **N.'S** constitute from 50 to 65 percent of the leukocytes in the blood and are essential for phagocytosis of bacteria and cellular debris. The number of **N.'S** in the blood increase in certain pathological conditions and hemorrhage.

neutrophilia (nū-trō-fil′i-a): An increase in the percentage of neutrophils in a differential white blood cell count.

neutrophilic (nū-trō-fil′ik): Refers to cells that take up both acidic and basic stains.

nevoid (nē′voyd): Pertaining to or resembling a nevus.

nevolipoma (nē′vō-lī-pō′ma): A nevus that contains fibrofatty tissue; rare.

nevosarcoma (nē′vō-sar-kō′ma): A malignant melanoma presumed to have developed from a nevus.

nevus (nē′vus): 1. A general term used to describe any congenital circumscribed pigmented lesion on the skin; may be epidermal, connective tissue, or vascular in origin. 2. A mole. 3. A birthmark. **N. FLAMMEUS,** a diffuse, poorly defined area of skin varying in color from pink to deep purple; a port-wine **N. N. MATERNUS,** a birthmark. **N. PILOSUS,** a hairy nevus. **SPIDER N.,** a congenital or acquired lesion composed of lines radiating from a center, due to capillary dilatation. **STRAWBERRY N.,** a raised, bright red skin lesion; cavernous hemangioma; see hemangioma.—nevi, pl.; nevoid, adj.

newborn (nū′born): 1. A recently born infant. 2. Recently born.

Newcastle disease: A highly contagious viral disease of fowl, transmissible to man; symptoms include those of severe follicular conjunctivitis and lymphangiitis.

New England Training School for Nurses: Credited with being the first school of nursing in the U.S.; established in 1872 in association with the New England Hospital for Women and Children in Roxbury, Massachusetts. Requirements for graduation were one year of service to the hospital and attendance at twelve lectures. Melinda Ann Richards is credited with being the first graduate.

NHO: National Hospice Organization. Incorporated in 1978. Has established guiding principles for hospice organizations and developed standards of care for hospice patients.

NIAAA: Abbreviation for National Institute on Alcohol Abuse and Alcoholism.

niacin (nī'a-sin): Nicotinic acid; a member of the vitamin B complex; essential for glycolysis, fat synthesis, and prevention of pellagra. Found in high protein diets that include meats, fish, poultry, organ meats, eggs, certain legumes, yeast, wheat germ, enriched or whole grain flour and cereals, nuts, peanuts, milk. Deficiency results in rough skin, loss of strength, gastrointestinal disturbances, pellagra, and depression. Niacin is not stored in the body and must be supplied daily.

niche (nēsh): A depression or defect in an otherwise smooth surface, as in the wall of a hollow organ; is detected by x ray.

Nicholas-Favre disease (nē'kō-la-fav'ri): A venereal disease involving the inguinal lymph glands; see lymphogranuloma venereum under lymphogranuloma.

nicking (nik'ing): Localized constriction of blood vessels in the retina; sometimes occurs in patients with arterial hypertension.

nicotinamide (nik-ō-tin'a-mīd): Nicotinic acid amide; it has the same vitamin action as nicotinic acid, but is not a vasodilator. Deficiency occurs in alcoholics and is associated with the severe vomiting seen in cancer of the stomach, pancreas, and colon, and in intestinal obstruction. Also called niacinamide.

nicotine (nik'ō-tēn): A poisonous alkaloid (*q.v.*) derived from tobacco.

nicotinic acid (nik-ō-tin'ik): Niacin (*q.v.*); vitamin B_3. Occurs as a white crystalline powder; essential for metabolism of carbohydrate; used as a vasodilator and in the prevention and treatment of pellagra. Occurs naturally in milk, cheese, liver, yeast, and cereals.

nicotinism (nik'ō-tin-izm): Poisoning caused by excessive use of tobacco or nicotine; characterized by stimulation of the central and autonomic nervous systems, followed by depression. Symptoms incude nausea, vomiting, diarrhea, salivation, weakness, mental confusion, sometimes shock and respiratory depression.

nictitation (nik-ti-tā'shun): Rapid and involuntary blinking of the eyelids.—nictitate, v.

NIDA: National Institute on Drug Abuse. Gives support and emphasis to treatment facilities for drug addicts, particularly heroin addicts.

nidal (nī'dal: Pertaining to a nidus (*q.v.*).

nidation (nī-dā'shun): Implantation of the early embryo in the uterine mucosa.

nidus (nī'dus): 1. The focus of an infection. Septic focus. 2. A group of cells within the central nervous system.

Niemann-Pick disease: A hereditary disease of lipid metabolism, occurring chiefly in female Jewish infants. There is enlargement of the liver, spleen, and lymph nodes and mental subnormality. There is no effective treatment and the affected children die early. [Albert Niemann, German pediatrician. 1880–1921. Ludwig Pick, German pediatrician. 1868–1935.]

night: **N. BLINDNESS,** nyctalopia (*q.v.*); reduced visual adaptation to darkness; may be associated with vitamin A deficiency. **N. CRY,** a shrill cry uttered by children during sleep; may signify beginning hip joint disease when pain occurs in the relaxed joint. **N. SWEAT,** sweating during sleep; often a symptom of tuberculosis; in debilitated children, a sign of rickets. **N. TERRORS,** a disorder similar to nightmare; occurs most often in children who waken from sound sleep screaming in fright; the episode may last for some time, with the child remaining unconscious. **N. VISION,** the ability to see at night or in a dim light.

night guard: A dental device worn at night to prevent and correct the effects of bruxism (*q.v.*).

Nightingale, Florence: British woman, considered the founder of modern nursing; in 1860, established the first organized school of nursing at St. Thomas' Hospital, London, which set the pattern for nursing education throughout the world. [1820–1910]

nightmare: A terrifying dream occurring during REM sleep (*q.v.*) in which the person is unable to help himself or get out of a frightening situation; often accompanied by a feeling of suffocation.

nightshade: A plant of the genus *Solanum*. **DEADLY N.,** belladonna, the active principle in atropine, a drug used in medicine as a mydriatic, sedative, antispasmodic, antisudorific, and narcotic.

nightwalking: Walking during sleep. Somnambulism.

nigral (nī'gral): Pertaining to the substantia nigra: see under substantia.

nigrities (nī-grish'i-ēz): Blackness. **N. LINGUAE,** black tongue; see under tongue.

nigrostriatal (nī'grō-strī-ā'tal): Pertaining to the substantia nigra and the corpus striatum, or to the efferent connection between them. See substantia and corpus.

NIH: Abbreviation for National Institutes of Health (*q.v.*).

nihilism (nī'hil-izm): 1. In psychiatry, a form of delusion in which the patient denies the reality of everything, including that of himself, in whole or in part. 2. In medicine, **THERAPEUTIC N.,** disbelief in the therapeutic value of drugs. 3. The performance of acts that are self-destructive to the world at large as well as to one's self.

Nikolsky's sign: A condition in which the external layer of skin "slips" or rubs off with slight friction or injury; seen in pemphigus vulgaris (*q.v.*). [Pyotr V. Nikolsky, Russian dermatologist. 1858–1940.]

niphablepsia (nif-a-blep′si-a): Snow blindness. Also niphotyphlosis.

nipple (nip′l): 1. The conical eminence in the center of each breast, containing the outlets of the milk ducts; a teat. 2. An artificial substitute for the human nipple used on an infant's nursing bottle. **ACCESSORY N.**, a structure resembling a nipple occurring in an abnormal location; see milk line.

nirvana (nir-vah′na): A state of bliss, with freedom from worry and the cares of the world; a Buddhist concept.

Nissl('s) bodies: Granular, stainable protein bodies within the cytoplasm of nerve cells and dendrites; they contain ribonucleoprotein, and are concerned with protein synthesis and metabolism.

nit: The egg of a louse. The nits of head lice are found firmly attached to the hair shaft.

niter, nitre (nī′ter): Saltpeter (*q.v.*).

nitrate (nī′trāt): Any salt of nitric acid.

nitric acid (nī′trik as′id): A colorless, corrosive inorganic acid that gives off choking fumes. It is exceedingly caustic; sometimes used for removing warts. Also used in certain tests for albumin in the urine.

nitrite (nītrīt): Any salt of a nitrous acid. Organic nitrites are used in treatment of certain heart diseases; they cause the blood vessels to dilate and thus lower blood pressure.

nitrituria (nī-tri-tū′ri-a): The presence of nitrites in the urine.

nitrogen (nī′trō-jen): A colorless, tasteless, odorless gaseous element; constitutes about four-fifths of the atmosphere and is an essential constituent of protein foods. **N.** is excreted mainly in the urine as urea; ammonia, creatine, and uric acid account for a further small amount; less than 10 percent total nitrogen is excreted in feces. **N. BALANCE**, the difference between the intake and output of **N.** by the body; a person is in positive **N.** balance when the intake exceeds the output, in negative balance when the intake of **n.** is less than the output. **N. EQUILIBRIUM**, the condition that exists when the amount of **N.** excreted equals the amount taken into the body in foods. **NONPROTEIN N.**, (NPN), nitrogenous constitutents in the blood that are not protein, *i.e.*, urea, uric acid, creatine, creatinine, amino acids, ammonia. See blood urea nitrogen.

nitrogen mustard: A warfare agent (mechlorethamine hydrochloride) from which a series of therapeutic compounds are derived; have been used in medicine as antineoplastic agents in treatment of Hodgkin's disease, certain leukemias, lymphosarcoma, and lymphoblastoma.

nitrogenous (nī-troj′en-us): Relating to or containing nitrogen.

nitroglycerin (nī′trō-glis′er-in): A vasodilating drug used in the prophylaxis and treatment of pain, particularly that of angina pectoris.

nitrosamines (nī-trōs-am′ēns): A group of derivatives of secondary amines, some of which appear to have carcinogenic properties.

nitrosurea (nī′trō-sū-rē′a): Any of a certain group of antineoplastic compounds that have severe toxic effects due to their alkylating properties; have been used in treatment of brain tumors, Hodgkin's disease, certain leukemias, lymphomas, myelomas, and cancer of the breast and ovaries. See alkylation.

nitrus (nī′trus): Pertaining to or containing nitrogen in its lowest valency. **N. OXIDE**, a colorless, sweet-tasting gas with a not unpleasant odor; widely used in obstetrics, dental surgery, and for induction anesthesia. Laughing gas.

N_2O: Chemical formula for nitrous oxide (*q.v.*). See under nitrous.

Nocardia (nō-kar′di-a): A genus of branching aerobic microorganisms of the same family as *Actinomyces* (*q.v.*); a few are pathogenic to man. **N. ASTEROIDES**, cause of a pulmonary infection resembling tuberculosis. **N. BRASILIENSIS**, cause of mycetoma and nocardiosis. **N. MADURAE**, widely distributed in soil; causes maduromycosis.

nocardiosis (nō′kar-di-ō′sis): Infection caused by certain species of *Nocardia;* characterized by chills, sweating, anorexia, weight loss, dyspnea.

nociassociation (nō′si-a-sō-si-ā′shun): The unconscious discharge of nervous energy following overstimulation of nociceptors (*q.v.*), as occurs in surgical shock, trauma, and some diseases.

nociceptive (nō-si-sep′tiv): 1. Pertaining to a neuron that is receptive to painful sensations. 2. Painful; injurious.

nociceptor (nō-si-sep′tor): A receptor that is stimulated by injuries that cause pain.

noci-influence: A traumatic or harmful influence.

no-code: Sometimes written on a patient's chart when the patient is so seriously ill that death is inevitable; it means "do not attempt resuscitation."

noct-, nocti-, nocto-: Combining forms denoting night or during the night.

noctalbuminuria (nok′-tal-bū-min-ū′ri-a): The presence of large amounts of albumin in urine secreted during the night.

noctambulation (nok-tam′bū-lā′shun): Sleepwalking.

noctiphobia (nok-ti-fō′bi-a): Morbid fear or dread of the night or darkness.

nocturia (nok-tū′ri-a): Excessive urination during the night. May or may not be a sign of kidney disease. Also nycturia.

nocturnal (nok-tur'nal): 1. Pertaining to the hours of darkness. 2. Nightly; during the night. 3. Descriptive of an individual or animal that is awake and active during the night and sleeps during the day. **N. EMISSION,** "wet dreams," expulsion of semen resulting from erotic dreams that culminate in orgasm; a common occurrence in males.

nodal (nō'dal): Pertaining to a node, often the atrioventricular node. **N. RHYTHM,** see under rhythm.

node (nōd): 1. A small rounded protruberance, mass, or swelling. 2. A constriction. **ATRIOVENTRICULAR N.,** a small mass of neuromuscular fibers in the septa between the atria and the ventricles; conducts impulses from the atria to the bundle of His. **HEBERDEN'S N.,** see HEBERDEN. **LYMPH N.,** a mass of lymphoid tissue resembling a gland, found along the course of lymph vessels. **N. OF RANVIER,** a constriction in the neurilemma of a nerve fiber. [Louis Antoine Ranvier, French pathologist. 1835–1922.] **SINOATRIAL N.,** situated at the opening of the superior vena cava into the right atrium; the wave of contraction begins here, then spreads over the heart; called the pacemaker of the heart. **SINGER'S N.,** a small node that develops on the vocal cord(s) of singers as a result of over-use or improper use of the voice. **SINUS N.,** sinoatrial **N.**

nodose (nō'dōs): Characterized by the presence of nodes; protuberances, or knotty swellings.

nodosity (nō-dos'i-ti): A node or protuberance.

nodular (nod'ū-lar): 1. Resembling or like a node or nodule. 2. Having nodules.

nodule (nod'ūl): A small, solid, palpable, elevated area, extending deeper into the dermis than a papule, and which moves when the skin is palpated.

noematachometer (nō-ē'ma-tak-om'e-ter): A device that measures the time it takes for a simple perception to occur.

noesis (nō-e'sis): Cognition; intellectual apprehension.—noetic, adj.

Nofnagel's syndrome: Unilateral third cranial nerve paralysis combined with ipsilateral cerebellar ataxia.

noli me tangere (nō'li-mē-tan'jer-ē): Literally, "touch me not." An old term applied to destructive skin lesions; now used chiefly in referring to basal cell carcinoma (rodent ulcer).

noma (nō'ma): Gangrenous stomatitis; usually observed in malnourished children and debilitated adults. Starts with ulcers of the mucous membrane at the corners of the mouth and spreads to lips and cheeks, sometimes to the genitalia, and progesses with necrosis, sloughing of tissues and destruction of bone; marked by a foul odor. Also called water canker, stomatonecrosis, and cancrum oris.

nomenclature (nō'men-klā'chur): A system of words and terms used in a particular science or discipline.

Nomina Anatomica: An international system of nomenclature for anatomy; approved by the Sixth International Congress of Anatomists in 1950 and amended several times since. Abbreviated NA.

nomogram (nō'mō-gram): A diagram, chart, or graph on which several variables can be plotted; usually consists of three parallel scales graduated for different variables, so placed that when a straight line is drawn between any two scales, the related value may be read directly from the third at the point where the line intersects the scale. Such graphs may be constructed to show the relation between quantities, values, numbers, and so on.

nomothetic (nō-mō-thet'ik): 1. In research, refers to a study in which a relatively small amount of data is collected from many people. Opp. of idiographic (*q.v.*). 2. Refers to general or universal laws concerned with the behavior of people in groups rather than as individuals.

non-: Prefix denoting not, without, absence of.

non compos mentis (non kom'pos men'tis): Of unsound mind.

non repetat: Do not repeat. Term used in ordering medications.

nona-; noni-: Combining forms denoting nine or ninth.

nonan (nō'nan): Occuring every ninth day, as a symptom.

nonapeptide (non-a-pep'tīd): A peptide that contains nine amino acids.

noncompliance (non-kom-plī'ans): In health care, refers to the actions of a person who deviates from a prescribed therapeutic regimen because of some personal belief and who claims the right to some control over his treatment. In 1976 noncompliance was accepted as a nursing diagnosis by the North American Nursing Diagnosis Association and is based on evidence that the patient is not complying as shown by his failure to keep appointments or the lack of change in his pathologic condition.

nonconductor (non-kon-duk'tor): A substance that does not readily conduct heat, light, sound, or electricity.

nonelectrolyte (non-ē lek'trō-līt): A substance that in solution will not conduct electricity because the molecules do not dissociate into ions.

nongranulocyte (non-gran'ū-lō-sīt): A nongranular leukocyte.

nonigravida (nō-ni-grav'i-da): A woman pregnant for the ninth time.

noninfectious (non-in-fek'shus): Not communicable; not spread by contact.

noninvasive (non-in-vā'siv): 1. Referring to a test or a type of therapy that does not involve penetrating the skin or going into a body cavity. 2. Referring to a tumor that has not spread.

nonipara (nō-nip′a-ra): A woman who has given birth to nine viable offspring.

nonmyelinated (non-mī′-e-lin-ā-ted): Referring to 1) a substance that contains no myelin, or 2) a nerve process that has no myelin sheath.

non-nucleated (non-nū′klē-ā-ted): Not having a nucleus.

nonpathogenic (non-path-ō-jen′ik): Not productive of or causing disease.

nonprescription (non-pre-skrip′shun): Referring to drugs that may be purchased over the counter, *i.e.,* without a doctor's prescription.

nonproprietary (non-prō-prī′-e-tar-i): Refers to the name of a drug other than the trade name; may or may not be the same as the generic name.

nonpurulent (non-pū′roo-lent): Nonpyogenic (*q.v.*).

nonpyogenic (non-pī-ō-jen′ik): 1. Not containing or associated with pus. 2. Not promoting the formation of pus.

nonrapid eye movements (NREM): Eye movements that occur during the early stages of sleep and which are not rapid as are those that occur during the later stage of deep sleep. See also rapid eye movements and sleep.

nonseptate (non-sep′tāt): Without a septum or dividing wall.

nonspecific (non-spē-sif′-ik): 1. Not caused by a specific agent. 2. Referring to a disease for which the specific causative agent or organism has not been identified.

nontoxic (non-toks′ik): 1. Not poisonous. 2. Not capable of producing disease or injury. **N. GOITER,** simple or colloid **G.**; see under goiter.

nontropical sprue: See celiac disease.

nonunion (non-ūn′yun): Failure of the ends of a fractured bone to unite or knit together.

nonurgent (non-ur′jent): In emergency department management or in triage, refers to a patient who presents for care but who does not require emergency service, and who is usually referred for appropriate routine medical attention.

nonviable (non-vī′a-b′l): Not capable of life, or of living independently. Often said of a fetus that is born before it is capable of living outside the uterus.

Noonan's syndrome: A condition of unknown cause occuring only in males; the individual is of low stature with webbed neck, low-set ears, antimongoloid-slanted eyes, valvular pulmonic stenosis. See also Turner's syndrome.

noradrenaline (nor-ad-ren′a-len): Norepinephrine (*q.v.*).

norepinephrine (nor′ep-i-nef′rin): A hormone secreted by the adrenal medulla; it acts to increase blood pressure by constricting the blood vessels; also available as an agent used in treatment of acute hypotension.

norethindrone (nor-eth′in-drōn): A steroid hormone with action similar to that of progesterone; used in treatment of certain uterine conditions and, in combination with estrogen or mestranol, as an oral contraceptive.

norm: A fixed standard or model.

norm-, normo-: Combining forms denoting normal.

normal: Natural, average, or healthy. **N. SALINE** or **SALT SOLUTION;** see under solution.

normalcy (nor′mal-si): The state of being normal.

normergic (nor-mer′jik): Reacting or behaving in a normal manner.

normetanephrine (nor-met-a-nef′rin): A catabolite of epinephrine, found in some tissues and in urine, along with metanephrine.

normoblast (nor′mō-blast): A normal sized nucleated red blood cell, the precursor of the erythrocyte. Normally present in the bone marrow, but appears in the blood in certain types of anemia.

normocalcemia (nor-mō-kal-sē′mi-a): The presence of a normal amount of calcium in the blood.

normocapnia (nor-mō-kap′ni-a): The condition in which the carbon dioxide tension in the blood is normal.—normocapnic, adj.

normocephalic (norm′ō-sef-al′ik): Mesocephalic (*q.v.*).

normochromia (norm-ō-krō′mi-a): Normal color and hemoglobin content of the red blood cells.—normochromic, adj.

normocyte (nor′mō-sīt): A nucleated red blood cell of normal size and hemoglobin content.—normocytic, adj.

normoglycemia (nor-mō-glī-sē′mi -a): The condition of having the normal amount of glucose in the blood.—normoglycemic, adj.

normokalemia (nor-mō-kal-ē′mi-a): The presence of the normal amount of potassium in the blood.—normokalemic, adj.

normoproteinemia (nor-mō-prō′te-in-ē′mi-a): The presence of the normal protein content in the blood.

normoskeocytosis (nor-mō-skē′ō-sī-tō′sis): The presence of the normal number of leukocytes in the blood, many of which, however, are immature.

normotension (nor-mō-ten′shun): Normal tension, by current custom alluding to blood pressure.—normotensive, adj.

normotensive (nor-mō-ten′siv): 1. Pertaining to normal tone, tension, or pressure, by custom referring to blood pressure. 2. An individual with normal blood pressure.

normothermia (nor-mō-ther'mi-a): Normal body temperature, as opposed to hyperthermia and hypothermia.—normothermic, adj.

normotonia (nor-mō-tō'ni-a): Normal strength, tension, or tone, by current custom referring to muscle tissue.—normotonic, adj.; normotonicity, n.

normotopia (nor-mō-tō'pi-a): In anatomy, normal location.

normotrophic (nor-mō-trō'fik): Of normal size and development.

normouricuria (nor'mō-ū-ri-kū'ri-a): The presence of the normal amount of uric acid in the urine.

normovolemia (nor-mō-vō-lē'mi-a): Having the normal volume of blood.—normovolemic, adj.

North American Nursing Diagnosis Association: Formerly called the National Conference Group on Classification of Nursing Diagnoses. Has met at regular intervals since 1973 to develop a classification system for nursing diagnoses that are concerned with the alterations or potential alterations in individuals' health status and the human responses to these alterations to the extent that they involve the nursing process. At each meeting of the Association the list of previously approved nursing diagnoses is reviewed and corrected as necessary and the newly approved diagnoses are added. See nursing diagnosis and Appendix V.

Norton scale: A scoring chart (devised in England) that lists five characteristics of geriatric patients who are at risk of developing decubitus ulcers and rates them on a scale of 1 to 4, from good (4) to very bad (1); the characteristics are physical condition, mental condition, activity, mobility, and incontinence.

nos-, noso-: Combining forms denoting disease, pathology.

nose: The prominent structure in the middle of the face; the organ of smell and the beginning of the respiratory tract; it warms and filters the inspired air.

nosebleed: Hemorrhage from the nose. Syn., epistaxis.

Nosema: A group of several spore-forming protozoan species that cause infections in invertebrates and, rarely, in humans.

nosematosis (nō-sēm-a-to'sis): Infection with a *Nosema* organism which, in humans, causes necrotizing keratosis of the cornea and painful inflammation of the conjunctiva; may also be associated with meningoencephalitis and meningitis.

nosetiology (nōs'ē-ti-ol'o-ji): The study of the causes of disease.

nosh: To eat or snack between meals, or the food taken as snacks between meals.

nosocomial (nōs'ō-kō'mi-al): Pertaining to a hospital. **N. DISEASE,** a new disorder, not related to the original disease, that is caused or aggravated by hospital life. **N. INFECTION,** an infection acquired during hospitalization; organisms commonly involved include *Staphylococcus, Pseudomonas, Escherichia coli, Candida albicans, Streptococcus,* and the viruses of herpes and hepatitis.

nosocomium (nōs'ō-kō'mi-um): A hospital or infirmary. Also nosocomion.

nosogenesis (nōs'ō-jen'e-sis): Pathogenesis (*q.v.*).

nosology (nō-sol'o-je): The science of the systematic classfication of diseases.

nosomania (nos-ō-mā'ni-a): The unfounded and irrational belief that one is afflicted with a particular disease.

nosophilia (nōs'ō-fil'i-a): A morbid desire to be ill. —nosophiliac, adj.; n.

nosophobia (nōs'ō-fō'bi-a): A morbid dread or fear of disease, or of contracting a certain disease.

Nosopsyllus fasciatus (nōs'ō-sil'us fas-si-ā'tus): A species of the rat flea that transmits murine typhus and possibly plague.

nosotaxy (nōs-ō-tak'si): The classification of diseases.

nosotherapy (nōs-ō-ther'-a-pi): Treatment that involves the introduction of another agent or organism into the body in addition to the one being treated.

nostrils (nos'trils): The anterior openings in the nose; the anterior nares.

nostrum (nos'trum): A quack or patent remedy; or a secret remedy that is recommended by its maker.

notalgia (nō-tal'ji-a): An old term for pain in the back. Dorsalgia.

notch: A rather deep impression or indentation; usually refers to such an indentation on the surface of a bone or organ. **INFRASTERNAL N.,** a landmark depression in the anterior abdominal wall just above the xiphoid cartilage. **SUPRASTERNAL** or **JUGULAR N.,** the depression in the center of the upper part of the sternum; an anatomical landmark.

notencephalocele (nō-ten-sef'a-lō-sēl): A hernial protrusion of brain substance through a malformed occiput.

Notes on Nursing: What It Is and What It Is Not: A treatise on nursing by Florence Nightingale, published in 1859. The first book on nursing written by a nurse; points out the author's ideas concerning hospital construction, ventilation, cleanliness, diets for patients, the nurse's functions, and the need for careful observation of the patient in order to plan for prevention of disease and for care of the sick.

notifiable (nō-ti-fī'a-b'l): In health care, referring to a disease that is required to be reported to the local board of health.

notochord (nō'tō-kord): The long rod of cells that forms the longitudinal supportive structure in an embryo. Traces of it remain in the adult in the central portion of the intervertebral disks.

notomelus (nō-tom'e-lus): A congenital anomaly in which supernumerary limbs are attached to the back.

notomyelitis (nō'-tō-mī-e-lī'tis): Inflammation of the spinal cord.

nourish (nur'ish): To provide the foods and other substances that are essential for maintaining and supporting growth and life.

nourishment (nur'-ish-ment): Food, vitamins, minerals, and other substances needed to maintain and support growth and life.

NOW: National Organization for Women. Supports full equality for women and acts to end prejudice against them in government, church, industry, professions, and many other areas. Seeks passage of an equal rights amendment to the Constitution through research, litigation, and political processes. Address, 425 13th St., NW, Washington D.C. 20004

noxious (nok'shus): Harmful; not wholesome; injurious to health.

NPN: Abbreviation for nonprotein nitrogen.

NPO: Abbreviation for *nil per os* [L.], meaning nothing by mouth.

NREM: Nonrapid eye movement. **NREM SLEEP,** that which begins as the person passes from wakefulness to deep sleep and no rapid eye movements occur; represents about three-fourths to four-fifths of one's total sleeping time. See sleep and REM.

NSR: Abbreviation for normal sinus rhythm; see sinus rhythm under rhythm.

nubecula (nū-bek'ū-la): Cloudiness, especially that of the cornea or of urine. See nebula, I.

nubile (nu-b'l): Marriageable; said of a girl or young woman, especially in regard to physical development or age.

nucha (nū'ka): The nape of the neck.—nuchal, adj.

nuchal (nū'kal): Pertaining to the nucha (*q.v.*). **N. CORD,** an umbilical cord that is looped around the baby's neck as it is being born; occurs most often with long cords and can usually be slipped over the baby's head. **N. RIGIDITY,** stiffness of the neck; may be associated with spasm and pain on movement; a common sign of meningeal irritation.

Nuck: Canal of Nuck, a diverticulum of the peritoneal membrane extending into the inguinal canal; in the female, the round ligament passes along it to the pubic region; in the male, it accompanies the testes into the scrotum; may be the seat of inguinal hernia or the development of cysts. [Anton Nuck, Dutch anatomist. 1650–1692.]

nuclear (nū'klē-ar): 1. Pertaining to or containing a nucleus. 2. Forming, or like, a nucleus. 3. Characterized by the use of atomic energy. 4. Relating to atomic nuclei. **N. CHEMISTRY,** The branch of chemistry that deals with changes in the nucleus of the atom. **N. ENERGY,** energy that is released in reactions involving the nuclei of atoms. **N. FISSION,** the splitting of certain heavy atomic nuclei into large fractions, accompanied by conversion of part of the mass into energy; the principle of the atomic bomb. **N. PHYSICS,** that branch of physics that deals with the structure and properties of the nuclei of atoms.

nuclear family: A family consisting only of a father, mother, and their children.

nuclear magnetic resonance imaging: A process that utilizes magnets to produce three-dimensional images of internal organs to locate tumors without using x rays or radioactive elements.

nuclear medicine: That branch of medicine which deals with the use of radionuclides (*q.v.*) in diagnosis, therapy, and research.

nucleated (nū'klē-āt-ed): Possessing one or more nuclei.

nucleic acid (nū-klē'ik): Any of a large group of important chemical substances containing phosphoric acid, sugar, and purine and pyrimidine bases; found in the nuclei and cytoplasm of the cells of all living organisms; are concerned with the storage and release of energy and with genetic characteristics and their transmission. Two important types are ribonucleic acid and deoxyribonucleic acid.

nucleocapsid (nū'klē-ō-kap'sid): Part of the structure of certain viruses; consists of a protein coat called a capsid, which encloses the viral nucleic acid.

nucleolus (nū-klē'ō-lus): A small, rounded, basophilic body within the cell nucleus; usually single but there may be several; rich in ribonucleic acid (RNA) and protein; essential in the formation of ribosomes (*q.v.*). Also called plasmosome.—nucleoli, pl.; nucleolar, adj.

nucleoplasm (nū'klē-ō-plazm): The protoplasm that makes up the nucleus of the cell. Also called karyoplasm.

nucleoproteins (nū'klē-ō-prō'tē-inz): The form in which nucleic acids are found in the nuclei of plant and animal cells; consist of conjugated proteins in which the protein molecules are closely associated with those of nucleic acid; are broken down during digestion, producing purine and pyrimidine bases. An end product of nucleoprotein metabolism is urea which is excreted in the urine.

nucleoside (nū'klē-ō-sīd): A compound

formed by the combination of a purine or pyrimidine base with a pentose sugar.

nucleotide (nū'klē-ō-tīd): The structural unit of a nucleic acid; consists of an ester of a nucleoside and phosphoric acid.

nucleotoxin (nū'klē-ō-tok'sin): Any agent that is toxic to cell nuclei, including drugs, toxins, and viruses.—nucleotoxic, adj.

nucleus (nū'klē-us): 1. The inner essential part of a tissue cell, being necessary for the growth, nourishment, and reproduction of the cell, and for the transmission of hereditary characteristics. 2. A circumscribed accumulation of nerve cells of the central nervous system having a particular function. 3. The central core of an atom. **N. PULPOSIS**, the soft core of an intervertebral disk which can prolapse (*q.v.*) into the spinal cord and/or nerve roots. Most common in the lumbar region where it causes low back pain and/or sciatica.—nuclei, pl.; nuclear, adj.

nuclide (nū'klīd): A specific type of atom characterized by the number of its protons and neutrons and the energy content state of its nucleus, and with the capability of existing for a measureable length of time.

nudomania (nū-dō-mā'ni-a): Obsessive desire to be naked.

nudophobia (nū-dō-fō'bi-a): Abnormal aversion to being nude or unclothed.

null hypothesis: A hypothesis indicating that, in a research study, there is no significant relationship between an independent variable and a dependent variable; the concept is related to the statistical method to be used. Rejection of the null hypothesis indicates that there is no significant difference between the groups examined. See also **variable**.

nulligravida (nul-i-grav'i-da): A woman who has never been pregnant.

nullipara (nul-lip'a-ra): A woman who has not had a pregnancy that lasted to the stage of viability.

nulliparity (nul-li-par'i-ti): The condition of not having borne any children.

numb (num): 1. Lacking sensation, especially when caused by anesthesia or cold. 2. Lacking emotion; indifferent.

numbness (num'nes): Lack or diminution of sensation in a part.

nummular (num'ū-lar): Coin-shaped; resembling rolls of coins, as seen in the sputum in pulmonary tuberculosis.

nummulation (num'ū-lā'shun): An aggregation of red blood cells in a row resembling a roll of coins; rouleaux (*q.v.*).

nurse: 1. To care for the sick, wounded, or helpless. 2. To feed an infant at the breast. 3. A person who is specially prepared and licensed to provide care for the sick, wounded, or helpless, as well as those with potential health problems, usually in collaboration with a physician. **A.D. NURSE**, a graduate of an Associate Degree Program (*q.v.*). **CERTIFIED NURSE**, one who has met predetermined qualifications and can prove recency of nursing knowledge and skills. **CERTIFIED NURSE SPECIALIST**, must meet the same specifications as for Certified Nurse but must also have a Masters degree. **CHARGE NURSE**, one who is in charge of a unit when the head nurse is off duty. **CIRCULATING NURSE**, one who does not "scrub" but who is responsible for many functions in preparing the operating room before surgery and following surgery, for providing various materials and services that may be required during surgery, and for seeing that sterility in the surgical field is maintained. **CLINICAL NURSE SPECIALIST**, a professional nurse who has had special training and experience in a particular clinical specialty, holds a Masters degree, and is prepared to give expert care to the acutely or chronically ill and to assist clients to maintain health; may be certified by American Nurses' Association. **COMMUNITY HEALTH NURSE**, a professional nurse who provides nursing service to families and communities, with special emphasis on preventing disease and promoting wellness. **CRITICAL CARE NURSE**, a professional nurse who has the qualifications required by the policies of the critical care unit and has had a basic course in acute care nursing. **GENERAL DUTY NURSE**, a professional nurse who does not specialize in any particular field of nursing but is available for service in any area of nursing. **GRADUATE NURSE**, one who has graduated from a professional school of nursing. **HEAD NURSE**, a professional nurse who is in charge of a unit or ward in a health care facility and who is responsible for providing or supervising nursing services to patients. **HIGH-RISK PERINATAL NURSE**, a registered professional nurse who is prepared through advanced study and experience to provide perinatal care to infants and families at risk during the child-bearing period and through the fourth trimester. **INDEPENDENT NURSE GENERALIST**, an independent nurse practitioner; see under **nurse practitioner**. **INDUSTRIAL NURSE**, an occupational health nurse. **LICENSED PRACTICAL/VOCATIONAL NURSE**, one who has had appropriate education and experience to qualify for meeting the basic needs of patients and to give care under the supervision of a registered nurse, physician, or dentist. **NURSE ADMINISTRATOR**, a registered professional nurse who is accountable for the administration, management, and nursing services provided in a health agency or a unit of such agency. **NURSE ANESTHETIST**, a professional nurse who has had one or two years of training in the administration of anesthetics and is prepared to function as an anesthetist under the direction of a physician. **NURSE CLINICIAN**, a professional nurse with a Masters degree and experience in a particular field of nursing practice, who has received certification and is qualified to provide primary care to families, adult medical/surgical patients, gerontologic patients, obstetric patients and their infants, normal high-risk mothers and infants, psychiatric patients, or patients with mental health problems. The nurse clinician may practice independently, but also collaborates with physicians and other health care personnel when the patient or the situation make this desirable. **NURSE EDUCATOR,** a professional nurse who is involved with classroom and clinical teaching of student nurses. **NURSE GENERALIST,** a registered nurse who has graduated from an associate degree, diploma, or baccalaureate program in nursing and who provides nursing care in hospitals and nursing homes. **NURSE PSYCHOTHERAPIST,** a nurse practitioner who has at least a Masters degree and experience in psychiatric and mental health nursing and who practices in the field of psychotherapy. **NURSE SPECIALIST,** a registered nurse who has graduated from a Masters program in nursing or who holds a doctoral degree and is certified through a professional society; may hold positions in administration, education, a clinical specialty, or research. **OCCUPATIONAL HEALTH NURSE,** one employed in industry who gives immediate care to ill or injured workers, follows up on the sick and injured, and helps develop accident prevention and health programs for workers. **OFFICE NURSE,** a registered nurse employed by a physician or group of physicians and whose varied functions include working with other personnel involved in the patients' care, giving required nursing care to office patients, counselling patients regarding preventive health care, keeping an appointment book and carrying out any other required procedures which may or may not involve nursing. **PRACTICAL NURSE,** see Licensed Practical/Vocational N. **PRIMARY CARE NURSE,** consistently represents the nursing staff to assigned patients and their families throughout their contact with the health care agency; is responsible for providing comprehensive nursing care while on duty and for directing others who give such care when the primary care nurse is off duty; is accountable to both the patient and the institutional administration for all outcomes of nursing activities on behalf of the patient. The primary care nurse is prepared, as a professional nurse to provide prenatal, postnatal, and well-child care; to give guidance regarding nutrition and immunization; to assist patients and families to cope with illness and adapt to disability and old age, to supervise treatment; to give physical and psychological comfort from birth to death; and to coordinate health care services for the patient. **PRIVATE DUTY NURSE,** one who cares for a single patient in his home or hospital. **PROFESSIONAL NURSE,** one who has graduated from a professional school of nursing and has passed a qualifying examination to practice as an R.N.; in addition to providing traditional patient care, is prepared to make independent judgments in the areas of nursing education, counseling, supervision, and administration. **PSYCHIATRIC NURSE,** a professional nurse, usually with a bachelors degree in nursing and experience in working with mentally disturbed patients. **PSYCHIATRIC NURSE THERAPIST,** a professional nurse with a minimum of a bachelors degree and advanced education and experience in psychiatric-mental health nursing. **PUBLIC HEALTH NURSE,** an R.N. who performs nursing services for patients in their homes, at school, at work, or in an outpatient clinic; is employed by a health care agency and collaborates with other medical and paramedical workers and citizens groups on community health programs; is concerned with keeping people in the community physically and mentally healthy. Also called community health nurse. **REGISTERED NURSE,** one who is licensed by a State Board of Examiners to practice nursing in the state in which she lives and/or works. **SCHOOL NURSE,** one employed by a school to participate in health programs for children. **"SCRUB" NURSE,** a nurse who assists a surgeon by handing him things he needs during an operation, holding retractors, etc.; she scrubs hands and arms thoroughly and dons sterile gown, mask, and gloves before the operation begins. **STAFF NURSE,** a professional nurse who gives bedside care to patients in a hospital or other health care facility. **TECHNICAL NURSE,** a graduate of an Associate Degree program or a Diploma program; is qualified to provide direct nursing care requiring a high degree of technical skill to carry out treatment plans. **TRAINED NURSE,** one who has graduated from an accredited program in nursing education. **VISITING NURSE,** a trained nurse who cares for the ill in their homes; is usually employed by a community agency, either private or governmental. **WET NURSE;** any woman who suckles someone else's child. See also nurse practitioner.

Nurse Corps: Consists of nurses in the various armed services. They now are eligible for the same rank, title, advancement, and benefits as other officers in these services.

nurse educator: A registered professional nurse who has also had education in the discipline of teaching and who specializes in the teaching of nursing and in planning and implementing nursing education programs at both the undergraduate and graduate level.

nurse examiners: Usually refers to a State Board of Nursing, or the agency that approves nursing programs, to assure that the graduates of the programs in each of the 50 States are eligible to take the licensing examination.

nurse practitioner: A registered professional nurse who has completed an advanced course that leads to certification as a primary nurse practitioner and is qualified to give care beyond that provided in the traditional setting for nursing care, to take histories, do physical examination's, and carry out selected aspects of clinical medicine; the title applies to clinical nurse specialists and nurse clinicians. Nurse practitioners are trained to exercise initiative and clinical judgment in the health care of adult patients; geriatric patients; psychiatric patients; pediatric patients; perinatal patients; children in the school setting; and families. **ADULT N.P.**, a registered professional nurse who has had advanced education and is prepared to assume expanded roles in the care of adults (except pregnant women). **COLLEGE N.P.**, a professional nurse who has had educational preparation for primary care nursing and is capable of assessing the health and illness status of college students, and of providing preventive as well as restorative care of students with physical and/or emotional problems. **COMMUNITY HEALTH N.P.**, a professional nurse who has completed a pertinent formal education program, or has included this content in a Masters program, and who is highly skilled in history taking, physical assessment, and interviewing. **EMERGENCY N.P.**, a professional nurse who has had an advanced course in emergency care, has received certification, and preferably, has had wide experience in critical care nursing. **FAMILY N.P.**, a professional nurse who holds a Masters degree, provides primary care for families, including counseling, guidance, and referral to physicians when necessary, and is qualified to direct the management of stable conditions and common self-limiting acute conditions. **GERONTOLOGIC N.P.**, a professional nurse who has completed an advanced course in the care of older people and their families, and is qualified to provide primary health care for the sick elderly. **INDEPENDENT N.P.**, a **N.P.** who is not on the regular staff of a health care facility but works alone, maintains an office, establishes a fee for service, and provides primary health care for patients that she is educationally and experientially qualified and licensed to treat; collaborates with physicians, and/or makes referrals to other health care professionals when this is necessary. The Independent Nurse Practitioner's objective is to supply nursing care that is complete, comprehensive, and health-focused rather than illness-focused. **PEDIATRIC N.P.**, a professional nurse who has had advanced education and experience in pediatric nursing and who is qualified to provide primary care for infants and children. **SCHOOL N.P.**, a professional nurse who has a background in pediatric and community health nursing, and is capable of doing physical examinations and assessments, diagnosing and treating students who are ill or injured at school, giving screening tests, administering first aid, and doing immunizations.

nurse psychotherapist: A nurse practitioner with a minimum of a Masters degree in nursing and experience in psychiatric-mental health nursing.

Nurse Training Act: A federal act of 1964, aimed at increasing the number of nurses prepared to give quality care; provided funds for student support, and for construction of educational facilities, and allowed schools of nursing to expand and reorganize their curriculums. The Nurse Training Act of 1971 expanded the Act of 1964, and resolutions through 1975 added capitation grants to schools of nursing to increase enrollments and to aid those in financial distress.

nurse-midwife: A registered nurse who has been educated in the two disciplines of nursing and midwifery, has experience in the care of mothers and babies throughout the maternity cycle, and has received certification from the American College of Nurse-Midwives.

nurse-midwifery: The management and care of women during normal pregnancy and delivery and the care of the normal newborn, by a professional nurse who has completed a special education program in midwifery and is licensed to practice in that field.

nursery: A unit or department in a hospital where the newborn are cared for. **DAY N.**, a place where children of preschool age are cared for during the daytime.

nurses' aide: A person who assists nurses to care for the sick, wounded, or helpless; may be a paid employee or a volunteer; may have a brief period of instruction before starting work or may be given on-the-job instruction in tasks that are less technical than those performed by nurses; works under the direct supervision of a professional nurse. Also called nursing assistant.

Nurses Coalition for Action in Politics (N-CAP): The political arm of the American Nurses' Association. Purpose: to promote improvement of health care of the people by encouraging nurses to take an active interest in the political process and in organizing themselves for more effective political action.

nurses' code: See Code for Nurses in Appendix XI.

Nurses Educational Funds: An independent organization established in 1954 to honor nursing pioneers; functions under a Board of Directors with administrative assistance from the American Journal of Nursing Company; grants and administers scholarships and fellowships to registered nurses for post-R.N. study.

Nurses House, Inc.: A national nonprofit organization of professional nurses, the chief objective of which is to provide emergency financial assistance to registered nurses in need, whether they are or are not members of the organization. Funds for this purpose are contributed by members and obtained through various fund-raising projects. Address, 10 Columbus Circle, New York, NY 10019

Nurses, Patients, and Pocketbooks: The report (1928) of an important study of the status of nurses and nursing; economic as well as professional issues of the time were reported.

nurses' registry: An office or listing service where nurses can register their availability for employment, usually private duty nursing or "specialing" a patient.

nurses' station: A centrally located administrative office in a health care facility, or a unit of such facility, where nurses meet to give and receive reports and assignments, where patients' charts and the Kardex file are kept, where the ward clerk or secretary handles the necessary paper work and answers the telephones, and where, in some instances, the computer terminals for centralized monitoring of patients are located.

nursigenic (nurs-i-jen'ik): A recently coined word used to identify a state or condition thought to have been induced by nursing action.

nursing: 1. Strictly, the activities involved in giving physical care and emotional support to the sick, wounded, and helpless. 2. Broadly, all activities performed by nurses and concerned with restoration or maintenance of individual and community health, both physical and mental. BARRIER NURSING, a nursing technique involving keeping the infectious person isolated in a private room or other personal space; everything used in this space is disinfected before removal; paper and other disposable products are used when available. Called reverse barrier nursing when the techniques involved protect the patient from acquiring infections from others. CLINICAL NURSING, direct interventions by a nurse on behalf of a client; involves observing, evaluating, diagnosing, treating, teaching, counseling, serving as a clinical advocate. COMMUNITY HEALTH NURSING, nursing practice aimed at promoting and preserving the health of populations, and extending continuous comprehensive nursing care to individuals, families, and groups; includes the work of visiting nurses, public health nurses, and independent nurse practitioners. FUNCTIONAL NURSING, a system of care wherein nurses perform only certain special duties, *e.g.*, one nurse gives all medications to all patients on a certain unit while others perform other specialized functions. GERIATRIC NURSING, is concerned with the assessment of nursing needs of elderly patients and with planning and implementing nursing care to meet these needs. GERIATRIC CLINICAL NURSING, is concerned with health maintenance of the older individual, prevention of illness and disability, and care of the ill in the older age group. GEROPSYCHIATRIC NURSING, is concerned with the care of older persons with emotional or psychiatric problems; includes assisting such persons to identify events that are stressful to them and helping them to find mechanisms for coping with these events. INTERNATIONAL NURSING, nursing in foreign countries, often under the auspices of some agency established for giving aid to countries with limited health care facilities, *e.g.*, a church, the Peace Corps, Project Hope. MENTAL HEALTH NURSING, usually spoken of as psychiatric and mental health nursing. MILITARY NURSING, usually refers to professional nursing within the Nurse Corps of the various armed services, the initial obligation being a three-year enlistment. Nurses now receive the same rank, privileges, and educational and retirement benefits as regular officers in these services. OCCUPATIONAL HEALTH NURSING, the application of nursing principles to the conservation and maintenance of workers' health; usually carried out at the place of employment. PRIMARY NURSING, continuous comprehensive nursing care by a professional nurse who is assigned complete responsibility for planning, implementing, coordinating, and delivering care to the patient from the time he enters the hospital until he leaves, for seeing that the patient's needs are met when the primary nurse is off duty, and for providing the teaching needed by the patient and his family. PRIVATE DUTY NURSING, caring for a single patient, either at the hospital or in his own home. PSYCHIATRIC NURSING, the branch of nursing that is concerned with the care of patients with mental disorders and with the prevention of such disorders; often involves working with families and others associated with the patient, and in many situations outside of institutions; often referred to as psychiatric and mental health nursing. SPECIALTY NURSING, a type of nursing in which the nurse works with patients in one of the specialty care units, *e.g.*, geriatrics, gynecology, obstetrics, pediatrics, psychiatry, etc. or in critical care units. TEAM NURSING, a system of nursing care in which a group of health care personnel, led by an R.N. who is appointed by the head nurse on a unit, is assigned specific patients for whom the various team members provide comprehensive nursing care services. TRANSCULTURAL NURSING, cross-cultural nursing, *i.e.*, working with people from varying cultural backgrounds; some U.S. universities offer masters and doctoral degrees in this field.

nursing action: An activity, stated in the nursing care plan, that is to be carried out by the nurse during a nursing intervention to meet a specific physical, psychologic, or socioeconomic need of the patient and which is expected to have a salutary effect on the patient's behavior and/or health status. An action to be taken by the nurse may be stated in the form of a nursing prescription or a nursing order.

Nursing and Health Care: The official magazine of the National League for Nursing. Published monthly by the Health Science Division of Technomic Publishing Company, 851 New Holland Ave., Bos 3535, Lancaster PA 17603

Nursing and Nursing Education in the United States: Published in 1923, the report of an extensive study of nurses and nurses' training schools; conducted by the Committee for the Study of Nursing Education, which had been appointed by the Rockefeller Foundation (1919) to study the proper education for public health nurses; often referred to as the Goldmark Report, so called because Josephine Goldmark, who was secretary for the Committee, prepared the report for publication. The report covered all aspects of nursing education in the United States, and made recommendations for improvement and change in the education programs; it became important in the development of university schools of nursing.

nursing assessment: The systematic collection and analysis of data pertaining to a patient's current health or illness problem; the first step in the nursing process. In addition to a physical inspection and the nurse's close observations as to how the patient is responding to his health problem, data is collected from the patient, his family, and significant others, usually through structured interviews. Data collected concern not only the patient's current or potential health problem but also his social, economic, emotional, and spiritual status, and his own view of his illness. All of this data is entered on the patient's permanent record, and may be added to or amended as the patient responds to various nursing interventions. The nursing assessment furnishes part of the data base on which nursing diagnoses and nursing care plans are formulated.

nursing assistant: A nonprofessional health care worker who assists professional nurses and who has had training in performing such basic procedures as bathing and taking temperature, pulse, and respirations; works under the direct supervision of a registered nurse; the term may be applied to nurses aides, orderlies, and certain other attendants.

nursing audit: A means of monitoring the results of the nursing process through a systematic, written appraisal of the formally constructed patient care plan and the nurses' notes on the patient's record; done for the purpose of implementing and maintaining a quality assurance program. The findings are compared to a set of standards of nursing care, which may be set by the specific hospital or facility, or they may be the *Standards of Practice* of the American Nurses' Association. The audit may be done concurrently, that is, while the patient is receiving nursing care, or retrospectively after the patient has been discharged; in the latter case the patient's chart is used to obtain the data for the audit. **EXTERNAL NURSING A.**, one done by a group of peers who were not involved in the patient's care. **CONCURRENT NURSING A.**, one done during the time that care is being given. **INTERNAL NURSING A.**, one done by the caregivers who were involved in the patient's care. **OUTCOME NURSING A.**, one in which the focus is on the patient and the end results of his care. **PEER NURSING A.**, evaluation of one's performance by a group of one's peers. **PROCESS NURSING A.**, an examination of the nature and sequence of the events that took place during the time the patient was receiving care. **RETROSPECTIVE NURSING A.**, one done after the care has been given. **STRUCTURAL NURSING A.**, an **A.** of the organizational and physical elements of a health care system.

nursing care plan: A written protocol for nursing care prepared by a professional nurse at the beginning of the nurse–patient relationship; it is kept updated and modified as the patient responds to treatment and it becomes part of the patient's permanent record. The plan identifies the patient's nursing care problems as they are revealed by the nursing assessment and nursing diagnosis, states the nursing actions and interventions to be undertaken to correct or ameliorate those problems, sets patient-centered goals and outcomes to be achieved by the nursing actions, and states the nurse's evaluation of the patient's responses to the nursing actions.

nursing conference: A group discussion involving a particular nursing or patient care problem or situation; may include only members of nursing staff from a particular unit or may include those from other units, depending on the topic for discussion; a teaching strategy.

nursing diagnosis: The statement of a judgment made by a professional nurse regarding an actual or potential health problem that occurs in association with a patient's current health status (whether the problem is acute, chronic, physical, emotional, sociologic, or spiritual) that requires nursing intervention that professional nurses are qualified to make and for which they are held accountable; is made early in the nurse–patient relationship as the first step in the nursing process, and amended and updated as the status of the patient changes; thus it becomes a structure for nursing practice and differs from a medical diagnosis which tends to remain the same throughout the course of an illness. There may be only one nursing diagnosis for a specific event or as many as four, or more, depending on the particular patient and the particular circumstances that affect the patient's behavior and responses to his illness. The elements or factors that enter into the formulation of a nursing diagnosis include: 1) determining the etiology of the problem and making a nursing assessment that utilizes the objective and subjective data obtained from the patient, his family, and other significant others, usually through structured interviews, which are kept updated as new data are collected; 2) identifying the signs and symptoms characteristic of the problem; 3) defining the health care problem involved; 4) determining the nursing actions and interventions to be performed by the nurse who is qualified and licensed to perform them and for which nurses are held accountable, along with the rationale for these actions; 5) making a nursing care plan including nursing orders and prescriptions; 6) stating patient-centered goals to be achieved; 7) stating expected outcomes of the nursing interventions; and 8) evaluating the outcomes of the nursing interventions. A differential diagnosis is also sometimes called for. At each biennial meeting of the North American Nursing Diagnosis Association the previously approved list of nursing diagnoses is reviewed and additions, deletions, or changes in diagnoses may be made; the newly approved list is published in the *National Conference Proceedings*. Some states have included nursing diagnosis in the State Practice Act or Education Law; for example, Section 6901 of the Education Law of the State of New York (1972) defines nursing diagnosis as follows: "Diagnosing in the context of nursing practice means that identification of and discrimination between physical and psychological signs and symptoms which is essential to effective execution and management of the nursing regimen. Such diagnostic privilege is distinct from a medical diagnosis." See also North American Nursing Diagnosis Association and Appendix V.

nursing education: Education for the practice of nursing. Several types of programs are available: ASSOCIATE DEGREE PROGRAMS—two years in length, often conducted in community colleges, prepare students to take the state board examination for licensure as professional nurses. In states that recognize only two levels of professional nursing practice the ADN degree represents graduates from all professional nursing programs other than the Bachelor of Nursing programs. BACCALAUREATE PROGRAMS—usually four years in length, granting the B.S.N. degree; course includes study of the arts, sciences, and humanities, and learning experiences in selected hospitals and community agencies; graduates are eligible to sit for state board examinations for licensure as professional nurses, and are prepared for general nursing practice in a variety of settings. CONTINUING EDUCATION PROGRAMS—aimed at updating, maintaining, and extending practicing nurses' knowledge and skills. DIPLOMA PROGRAMS—from two to three years in length, usually organized and sponsored by a hospital where students receive their clinical experience; graduates are eligible to sit for state board examinations for licensure as professional nurses. DOCTORAL PROGRAMS—prepare nurses for careers in research, teaching, and advanced clinical practice; the doctorate in nursing science is a professionally oriented degree while the Ph.D. for nurses is research oriented. EXTERNAL DEGREE PROGRAMS in nursing, education programs in which the student takes self-study courses at home with visits to concentrated classroom study during vacations or other free time, and may take examinations at home. These programs usually offer the associate degree or the bachelaureate degree in nursing. MASTERS PROGRAMS in nursing—prepare R.N.s for practice as clinical nurse specialists, primary nurse practitioners, nursing administrators, nurse educators. PRACTICAL NURSE PROGRAMS—one or two years in length; prepare graduates to sit for examination for licensure as Licensed Practical Nurses or Licensed Vocational Nurses.

nursing goal: A general goal that the nurse hopes to achieve through her interventions and activities in connection with the patient's treatment for a specific condition or disorder, *e.g.*, the development of the individual's ability to care for himself in regard to personal hygiene, nutrition, and compliance with a prescribed medical or health promotion regimen.

nursing history: Data obtained from the patient and his family, regarding the patient's present illness, previous illnesses and hospitalizations, any handicaps, marital status, religion, general life activities and interests, allergies, food preferences, sleeping habits, medicines taken regularly, use of habituating drugs including alcohol and tobacco, type of work engaged in and any hazardous conditions in the workplace, etc. Data is usually obtained at the time the nursing assessment is made and is useful in making nursing care plans and in understanding the patient and his reactions to his current situation.

nursing home: A small private hospital or convalescent home, particularly one designed for providing skilled long-term care by a range of health care professionals including physicians, nurses, social workers, physical therapists, etc.

nursing intervention: The nursing action selected and implemented by the nurse to meet or resolve a patient's current or potential health need or problem. The action is based on analysis of the need or problem as revealed in the first step of the nursing process, *i.e.*, the nursing assessment. (J. Fonseca)

nursing orders: Written instructions for the nurse who makes nursing interventions and carries out nursing activities called for by the nursing care plan; they are written and signed by a professional nurse and are not to be confused with medical orders.

Nursing Outlook: A bi-monthly magazine devoted to issues and trends in nursing. Published by the American Journal of Nursing Company.

nursing practice: 1. For registered, professional nurses, nursing practice is defined as "diagnosing and treating human responses to actual or potential health problems through such services as case finding, health teaching, health counseling, and provision of care supportive to or restorative of life and well-being, and executing medical regimens prescribed by a licensed or otherwise legally authorized physician or dentist. A nursing regimen shall be consistent with and shall not vary from any existing medical regimen."—[Section 6902, Education Law of the State of New York.] 2. For licensed practical nurses, nursing practice is defined as "performing tasks and responsibilities within the framework of case finding, health teaching, health counseling, and provision of supportive and restortive care under the direction of a registered, professional nurse or a licensed or otherwise legally authorized physician or dentist."—[Section 6902, Education Law of the State of New York.] INDEPENDENT N. P., nursing practice in which the nurse gives primary health care directly to the patient rather than assisting in giving medical care, the focus of care being the maintenance of health, rather than the patient's health deficits.

nursing practice acts: State laws enacted by each of the 50 states to 1) protect the public by establishing minimum standards for the safe practice of nursing; and 2) protect the titles of professional nurse and licensed practical nurse. These acts, in effect, control nursing education and practice in the various states; they are all quite similar and are amended from time to time to keep pace with developments in both nursing education and practice. They provide for the creation of State Boards of Nursing and identify the functions of these Boards; identify the requirements for licensure, for the revocation of licenses, and for reprocity of licensure among the states. The Acts also define nursing in the broad sense and identify the kinds of activities the nurse may legally engage in.

nursing prescription: A written recommendation prepared and signed by a professional nurse, for an action to be taken by 1) the nurse to assist her in implementing a nursing care plan, or 2) the patient to engage in some self-health-care activity. See also nursing orders.

nursing process: The scientific system of assessing, planning, organizing, implementing, delivering, and evaluating nursing care that progresses in orderly steps taken by the nurse. These steps begin with the collection of data obtained through a physical examination and interviews with the patient and significant others, progresses to the assessment and analysis of the patient's nursing care needs, the establishment of a nursing diagnosis and the making of a nursing care plan, the determination of priorities in carrying out the nuring interventions for which professional nurses are qualified and licensed to perform, the setting of goals for the outcome of the interventions and, finally, to the evaluation of the patient's responses to the nursing care and to his treatment. Thus, a structural framework for the nurse–patient relationship is formulated. At each step the nurse works closely with the patient, and, whenever possible, with his family and other involved persons in collecting significant data relative to the patient's health history, his current health status, and to his response to treatment. See also nursing action, nursing assessment, nursing audit, nursing care plan, nursing diagnosis, nursing intervention, nursing order, nursing prescription.

Nursing Research: A scholarly bimonthly refereed journal, published since 1952 by the American Journal of Nursing Company. It is devoted to the publication of research and scientific papers and reports, the objectives being to stimulate interest in nursing research and to keep members of the nursing profession informed about ongoing or completed projects in nursing research.

nursing research: A systematic inquiry to discover facts or to test theories for the purpose of obtaining valid answers to questions raised or hypotheses made regarding some aspect of nursing. Three types of research commonly identified are descriptive or survey, experimental or explanatory, and historical. Research in nursing may also be categorized as nursing practice research or clinical research, or as research related to nursing practice, *e.g.*, research in the field of nursing education or nursing service administration. The eventual goal of nursing research is improved nursing practice and better patient care. (L. Notter)

nursing rounds: Teaching conferences or meetings of members of the nursing staff, usually conducted at the beginning of a work shift; may or may not include visits to patients' bedside.

nursing-bottle-mouth syndrome: Extensive cavities and discoloration of the teeth in young children, particularly those who have prolonged bottle feedings and who take their bottles of milk or sweetened juice to bed, thus exposing the teeth to contact with the milk or juice for many hours. Also referred to as nursing-bottle caries.

nursling (nurs′ling): An infant that is still being breast-fed; one that has not been weaned.

nurturance (nur′chur-ans): Affectionate care and attention.—nurturant, adj.

nutation (nū-tā′shun): Nodding; applied especially to uncontrollable head shaking.

nutmeg (nut′meg): The dried ripe seed of the *Myristica fragrans* tree; a carminative, stimulant, and condiment; source of **N.** oil which, if taken in large quantities, produces narcosis and delirium, headache, restlessness, visual hallucinations, palpitation, flushing, and numbness of extremities; overuse may be accidental or intentional.

nutrient (nū′tri-ent): 1. Food that supplies the elements necessary to nourish the body. 2. Nourishing. 3. Serving as or providing nourishment. **N. ARTERY,** one that enters a long bone. **N. FORAMEN,** hole in a long bone that admits the **N.** artery.

nutriment (nū′tri-ment): Nourishment.

nutrition (nū-tri′shun): 1. The sum total of the processes by which the living organism receives and utilizes the materials necessary for survival, growth and repair of tissues, the creation and liberation of energy, and the elimination of waste products and of unusable portions of the materials. 2. The science that deals with the food requirements of the body.—nutritious, nutritive, adj.

nutrition, alteration in: less than body requirements: A nursing diagnosis accepted by the Fourth National Conference on Nursing Diagnoses.

nutritionist (nū-trish′un-ist): A health-care professional with special education in the field of human nutrition; usually holds a bachelors or higher degree; may function as a dietitian, a supervisor of food service in a health-care facility, a teacher, or a researcher in nutrition.

nutritious (nū-trish′us): Containing elements needed for growth, development, and health. Syn., nutritive.

nutritive (nū′tri-tiv): Pertaining to or supplying nutrition to the body.

nyct-, nycti-, nycto-: Combining forms denoting 1) night; 2) darkness.

nyctalgia (nik-tal′ji-a): Pain that occurs only during sleep.

nyctalopia (nik′ta-lō′pi-a): Imperfect or defective vision in a dim light or at night; may be caused by retinitis pigmentosum (see under **retinitis**), or other eye disorder, or by vitamin A deficiency. Night blindness.

nyctamblyopia (nik-tam-bli-ō′pi-a): Poor night vision that does not seem to be due to any change in the eyes.

nyctophilia (nik′tō-fil′i-a): An abnormal preference for nighttime over daytime.

nyctophobia (nik′tō-fō′bi-a): Abnormal fear of the night and darkness.

nycturia (nik-tū′ri-a): Nocturia (*q.v.*).

NYD: Abbreviation for not yet diagnosed.

nymphae (nim′fē): The labia minora—Sing., nympha.

nymphectomy (nim-fek′to-mi): Excision of the labia minora.

nymphitis (min-fī′tis): Inflammation of the labia minora.

nymphohymeneal (nim-fō-hī′me-nē-al): Pertaining to the labia minora and the hymen.

nymphomania (nim-fō-mā′ni-a): Excessive sexual desire in a female.—nymphomaniac, adj., n.

nymphomaniac (nim-fō-mā′ni-ak): 1. A woman who exhibits nymphomania. 2. Pertaining to nymphomania.

nystagmogram (nis-tag′mō-gram): The tracing of movements of the eyeball, produced by a nystagmograph.

nystagmograph (nis-tag′mō-graf): An instrument similar to the cardiograph for measuring the involuntary movements of the eyeball and recording them graphically.—nystagmography, n.

nystagmus (nis-tag′mus): Constant, rhythmic, involuntary, rapid movements of the eyeball, a neurological sign useful in diagnosing certain nervous conditions and drug toxicity, particularly that resulting from anticonvulsants and barbituates. **JERKING N., N.** marked by movements that are faster in one direction than the other; this is normal when watching a moving object but may indicate drug toxicity or neurologic or vestibular disorder. **MINERS' N.,** caused by working many years in the dark or in poor light. **OPTOKINETIC N.,** jerking movements of the eyes normally caused by watching moving objects or in situations like watching things from a moving train. **PENDULAR N.,** characterized by oscillations that are equal in length in both directions; occurs in miners' **N.,** albinism, and retinal pathology. **POSITIONAL N.,** occurs when the head is placed in an abnormal plane. **ROTARY N., N.** in which the eyes move about the visual axis.

O

O: 1. In chemistry, the symbol for oxygen (0_2). 2. In optics, the abbreviation for *oculus,* meaning eye; *e.g.*, oculus sinister (O.S.), left eye. 3. In hematology, the symbol for a particular blood type.

o- or **oo-:** Combining forms denoting 1) egg; 2) ovum.

oak poisoning: A condition resembling ivy poisoning (*q.v.*); caused by exposure to a climbing vine which is closely related to poison ivy.

OARS: Older Americans Resources and Services. An information system developed at the Duke University Center for the Study of Aging and Human Development; concerned with the health care process.

oat cell carcinoma: Carcinoma in which the cells are elongated and blunted at the ends and have long oval nuclei and very little protoplasm. The tumor is not formed into a mass, but the tightly packed cells spread along the lymphatics; most often affects the lung; the prognosis is usually poor. Also called small cell lung cancer.

ob-: A prefix denoting toward, against, over; inward; completely; in reverse order; in the way of (something).

OB, OBS: Abbreviation for obstetric, obstetrical.

OBD: Abbreviation for organic brain disturbance or disease.

obdormition (ob-dor-mish'un): Numbness and tingling in an extremity due to pressure on a sensory nerve; commonly referred to as being asleep.

obese (ō-bēs'): Excessively fat. Syn.—corpulent, fat.

obesity (ō-bē'si-ti): The condition of excessive accumulation and storage of fat in the body; occurs when more calories are consumed than are expended in the form of energy, and is evidenced when one's weight is greater than 20 percent of the expected weight for males and 25 percent for females. **ENDOGENOUS O.**, that due to certain endocrine or metabolic disorders with the fat being distributed in certain body areas, *e.g.*, the girdle area. **EXOGENOUS O.**, that due to excessive caloric intake. **HYPERPLASTIC O.**, that due to an increase in the number of fat cells in the body. **HYPERTROPHIC O.**, that due to increase in the size of fat cells in the body. **MORBID O.**, increase in body weight of at least 70 percent more than the ideal weight for that individual, or over 100 pounds over that weight.

obfuscate (ob'fus-kāt): To becloud, dim, confuse; to make obscure or unnecessarily complicated.—obfuscated, adj.; obfuscation, n.

obfuscation (ob-fus-kā'shun): 1. Clouding, as of the cornea. 2. Mental confusion.

obicularis oculi (ō-bik-ū-lar'is ok'ū-li): The circular, sphincter-like muscle that surrounds the orbit of the eye; its function is to allow the eyelids to close tightly.

objective (ob-jek'tiv): 1. An aim or purpose. 2. A lens or series of lenses in a microscope. 3. Pertaining to things external to one's self. Opp. of subjective (*q.v.*). **O. SIGNS**, signs of disease which the observer notes, as distinct from the symptoms of which the patient complains.

obligate (ob'li-gāt): 1. Compulsory; required; bound; of necessity. 2. To make necessary or require. In bacteriology, refers to an organism that can survive and thrive in only one particular environment; said particularly of certain bacteria; opp. of facultative.

oblique (ō-blēk'): Slanting. **EXTERNAL O. MUSCLE**, forms the outer side of the side wall of the abdomen. **INTERNAL O. MUSCLE**, forms the second layer of the side wall of the abdomen.—obliquity, n.

obliteration (ob-lit'er-ā'shun): 1. The complete closure of a lumen, as of a blood vessel. 2. The complete removal of a part by a pathological process or by surgery. 3. Complete loss of memory for certain events.—obliterative, adj.

oblongata (ob-long-ga'ta): The medulla oblongata (*q.v.*).

OBS: Abbreviation for: 1. Organic brain syndrome. 2. Obstetrics, obstetrical.

observation: The act or faculty of noticing or paying attention. In nursing, the active process of utilizing all of one's senses to note things about the patient for the purpose of collecting data needed for formulating a nursing diagnosis and making a nursing care plan.

obsession (ob-sesh'un): A persistent, recurring pathological concern with an overvalued idea or set of ideas that dominate the mind, often leading to irrational actions and/or compulsive performance of certain acts, *e.g.*, frequent handwashing; the person may wish to banish these ideas from the mind but cannot. A characteristic symptom of patients with a diagnosis of obsessive–compulsive disorder.

obsessive-compulsive: In psychiatry, a type of neurosis marked by insistent compulsion to repeatedly perform certain acts or rituals or to entertain unwanted ideas, which often interfere with performance of normal daily activities; the obsessional ideas usually have to do with dirt. Likely to occur in children whose parents stress cleanliness and neatness.

obstetrician (ob-ste-trish'un): A qualified physician who practices the science and art of obstetrics.

obstetrics (ob-stet'riks): The branch of medicine dealing with the care of the pregnant woman during the antenatal; parturient and puerperal stages; midwifery.—obstetric, obstetrical, adj.

obstipation (ob-sti-pā'shun): Obstinate constipation, sometimes due to intestinal obstruction.

obstruction (ob-struk'shun): 1. The blockage, clogging, or closing of a natural passageway. 2. An obstacle that blocks a passageway. 3. The condition of being blocked or clogged; may occur in any tubular structure including the colon, common bile duct, larynx, intestine, pancreatic duct.—obstructive, adj.

obstructive (ob-struk'tive): Obstructing or tending to obstruct. **O. ANOSMIA,** loss of the sense of smell, which may be due to an obstruction in the nasal cavity or to disorder of the olfactory nerve. **O. ANURIA,** a urologic condition in which an obstruction in the urinary tract results in scanty or almost complete lack of urination. **O. GLAUCOMA,** glaucoma in which the outflow of aqueous humor from the anterior chamber is obstructed; see glaucoma, narrow-angle. **O. JAUNDICE,** a condition in which there is interference with the flow of bile in some part of the biliary system; may be due to the presence of gallstones or tumor, hepatitis, alcoholism, or use of certain drugs. **O. PULMONARY DISEASE,** any condition or disorder in which an obstruction interferes with air flow through the respiratory tract; may be due to a structural change, spasm, or excess secretions as occur in such disorders as bronchiectasis, bronchiolitis, bronchitis, bronchial stenosis, asthma, emphysema, cystic fibrosis. The term is also sometimes used to describe cor pulmonale (*q.v.*), pulmonary emboli, and adult respiratory disease syndrome in which pulmonary ventilation is compromised. **O. SHOCK,** a state of shock resulting from obstruction in some part of the mainstream of blood flow; may be due to cardiac tamponade, compression on the vena cava, or pulmonary embolism.

obstruent (ob'stroo-ent): 1. Obstructing or blocking a passageway. 2. An agent that blocks or obstructs the passage of a discharge; usually refers to a discharge from the bowels.

obtund (ob-tund'): To blunt or to dull, said especially of pain or of sensation.—obtundent, adj.; n.

obtundent (ob-tun'dent): Having the action of dulling the sensation of pain.

obturation (ob-tū-rā'shun): Closure; occlusion. Usually said of an opening or a passageway.—obturate, v.

obturator (ob'tū-rā-tor): Any natural or artificial thing that closes an aperture or opening. **ESOPHAGEAL O.,** a single-lumen tube with a balloon attached; used as an airway in unconscious non-breathing patients; it occludes the esophagus and prevents gastric regurgitation. **O. FORAMEN,** the opening in the innominate bone, largely filled in by the **O. MEMBRANE** which is made up of muscle and fascia. **O. MUSCLES,** two muscles at each side of the pelvic area, the **O. INTERNUS** and the **O EXTERNUS;** they rotate the thigh laterally.

obtuse (ob-tūs'): Dense, stupid, dull, blunted; lacking awareness of perception or sensation.—obtuseness, adj.; obtusely, adv.

obtusion (ob-tū'zhun): A blunting or the condition of being blunted; usually said of sensation.

OC: Abbreviation for oral contraceptive.

occipital (ok-sip'it-al): Pertaining to the back part of the head. **O. BONE,** the bone at the back of the head, characterized by the large hole (foramen magnum) through which the cranial cavity communicates with the spinal canal. **O. LOBE,** the portion of the cerebral hemisphere that lies behind the parietal and temporal lobes.

occipitoanterior (ok-sip'it-ō-an-tē'ri-or): Denoting the position of the fetus when the occiput lies in the anterior half of the maternal pelvis.

occipitofrontal (ok-sip'i-tō-fron'tal): Pertaining to the occiput and forehead. **O. DIAMETER,** the measurement from the root of the nose to the occipital protuberance; it is the engaging diameter when the fetus is in the occipitofrontal position.

occipitomental (ok-sip'i-tō-men'tal): Pertaining to the occiput and the chin.

occipitoposterior (ok-sip'it-ō-pos-tē'ri-or): Denoting the position of the fetus when the occiput is in the posterior half of the maternal pelvis.

occiput (ok'si-put): The posterior region of the head.

occlude (o-klood'): 1. To shut, close, or stop up so as to prevent the normal passage of something. 2. To bring together, as the upper and lower teeth.

occlusion (o-kloo'zhun): The closure of an opening, especially of ducts or blood vessels, due to obstruction. In dentistry, the fit of the teeth as the two jaws meet.

occlusive (o-kloo'siv): Serving to cover or close; often refers to a dressing or bandage that closes a wound or prevents its exposure to air.

occult (o-kult'): 1. Hidden, concealed, obscure. 2. In medicine, not detectable except by microscopic or chemical means; used especially to describe conditions such as blood in the urine or feces, but also to describe certain infections, lesions or neoplasms. **O. BLOOD,**, see blood.

occupational: **O. DELIRIUM,** psychiatric term for a condition occurring in dementia and consisting of purposeless over-activity relating to a patient's occupation. **O. DERMATITIS,** see dermatitis. **O. DISEASE,** one contracted by reason of occupational exposure to an agent known to be hazardous to health, *e.g.*, dust, fumes, chemicals, radiation, etc. Also called industrial disease. **O. HEALTH NURSE,** see under nurse. **O. NEUROSIS,** a functional disorder of a part of the body caused by occupational activity, *e.g.*, writer's cramp. **O. THERAPIST,** a person who practices occupational therapy. **O. THERAPY,** see under therapy.

Occupational Safety and Health Act: A Federal Act, passed in 1970; purpose is to ensure safe and healthful on-the-job working conditions for working men and women and to reduce work-related injuries and illnesses. Abbreviation OSHA.

Occupational Safety and Health Administration (OSHA): A unit in the Department of Labor whose functions consist of preventive activities in the workplace; uses criteria developed by NIOSH (*q.v.*) to set national standards for occupational safety and health.

ochlophobia (ōk-lō-fō'bi-a): Abnormal dread of crowds.

ochrodermatosis (ō'krō-der-ma-tō'sis): Yellowness of the skin.

ochronosis (o-krōn-ō'sis): Bluish and/or brownish discoloration of the skin and of the cartilage and connective tissue, especially around joints; often associated with alkaptonuria and the long-time application of phenol compounds to the skin and mucous membrane.

octa-, octo-: Combining forms denoting eight.

octan (ok'tan): Occurring every eighth day, counting both the first and last day of the episode; said of certain fevers.

octipara (ok-tip'a-ra): A woman who has borne eight viable children.

octogenarian (ok'tō-je-ner'i-an): A person who is in his or her eighties.

ocul-, oculo-: Combining forms denoting 1) the eye; 2) ocular.

ocular (ok'ū-lar): 1. Pertaining to the eye, or the sense of sight. 2. The eyepiece of a microscope. **O. BOBBING,** sudden downward jerking of the eyes at irregular intervals followed by slow return to normal position; seen infrequently in otherwise normal newborns.

ocularist (ok'ū-lar-ist): A licensed optician who designs and fits artificial eyes.

oculentum (ok-ū-len'tum): An eye ointment.

oculisics (ok-ū-lis'iks): Eye movements that convey nonverbal communication.

oculist (ok'ū-list): Older term for ophthalmologist (*q.v.*).

oculocephalogyric (ok'ū-lō-sef-a-lō-jī'rik): Pertaining to rotary movements of the head and eyes.

oculocutaneous (ok'ū-lō-kū-tā'nē-us): Pertaining to or affecting both eyes and the skin.

oculofacial (ok'ū-lō-fā'shi-al): Pertaining to the eye and the face.

oculography (ok'ū-log'ra-fi): A technique for recording eye movements and eye position.

oculogyration (ok'ū-lō-jī-rā'shun): Circular movement of the eyeball.

oculogyric (ok-ū-lō-jī'rik): Referring to rotary movements of the eyeball. **O. CRISIS,** a spasm of eye muscles that occurs in some neurological disorders; the eyeballs become fixed in one position, usually upwards; seen sometimes in parkinsonism.

oculomotor (ok'ū-lō-mō'tor): Pertaining to or causing movements of the eyeball. **O. NERVE,** one of the third pair of cranial nerves that control eye movement and also supply the eyelid; fibers of this nerve also go to the pupil to control pupillary dilatation and contraction.

oculonasal (ok'ū-lō-nā'zal): Pertaining to the eye and the nose.

oculus (ok'ū-lus): The organ of vision; the eye. **O. DEXTER,** right eye. **O. SINISTER,** left eye.—oculi, pl.; ocular, adj.

O.D.: Abbreviation for: 1. *Oculus dexter* [L.], meaning right eye. 2. Overdose. 3. Doctor of optometry.

o.d.: Abbreviation for *omni die* [L.], meaning every day.

Oddi (ō'dī): Sphincter of **O.**, see under sphincter.

odditis (ō'dī'tis): Inflammation of the sphincter of Oddi at the junction of the duodenum and the common bile duct.

odont-, odonto-: Combining forms denoting a tooth or teeth.

odontalgia (ō' -don-tal'ji-a): Toothache.

odontectomy (ō'don-tek'to-mi): Surgical removal of a tooth or teeth.

odonterism (ō-don'ter-izm): Chattering of the teeth.

odontiasis (ō-don-tī'a-sis): The eruption of teeth; dentition.

odontitis (ō-don-tī'tis): Inflammation of the pulp of a tooth.

odontoclasis (ō-don-tok'la-sis): The fracture or breaking of a tooth.

odontodynia (ō-don'tō-din'i-a): Toothache.

odontogenesis (ō-don'tō-jen'e-sis): The formation and development of teeth.—odontogenic, adj.

odontoid (ō-don'toid): Resembling a tooth. **O. PEG** or **PROCESS,** the toothlike projection from the upper surface of the body of the second cervical vertebra or axis.

odontolith (ō-don′to-lith): Tartar; the concretions which are deposited around teeth.

odontology (ō-don-tol′o-ji): Dentistry.

odontoma (ō-don-tō′ma): A tumor developing from or containing tooth structures.—odontomata, pl.; odontomatous, adj.

odontonoid (ō-don′tō-noyd): Pertaining to a tumor that contains tooth substance.

odontopathy (ō′don-top′a-thi): Any disease of the teeth.

odontoprisis (ō′don-top′ri-sis): Grinding of the teeth. Bruxism (*q.v.*).

odontorrhagia (ō-don-tō-rā′ji-a): Hemorrhage following extraction of a tooth or other dental surgery.

odontotherapy (ō-don-tō-ther′a-pi): The treatment given for diseases of the teeth.

odor (ō′-der): A quality of a substance that affects the sense of smell. Odors are described as pure when only one sensation is produced, or mixed when more than one sensation is produced. One system of classifying odors lists six fundamental sensations—spicy, fruity, flowery, resinous, foul, and burnt.

-odynia: Combining form denoting pain in a specific location.

odynophagia (ō-din′ō-fā′ji-a): Painful swallowing; dysphagia.

oedipal (ed′i-p′l): Pertaining to the oedipus complex. **O. STAGE,** the stage in a child's development when there is a feeling of strong attachment for the parent of the opposite sex and envious and aggressive feelings toward the parent of the child's own sex. See **O. COMPLEX.**

oedipism (ed′i-pizm): 1. Infliction of injury to one's own eyes. 2. Manifestation of the Oedipus complex (*q.v.*).

Oedipus complex (ed′i-pus kom′pleks.): [Oedipus, King of Thebes, unwittingly killed his father and married his own mother. When he discovered the true relationship he tore out his own eyes.] A strong attachment of a child for the parent of the opposite sex resulting in a feeling of jealousy toward the parent of the same sex, and guilt, producing emotional conflict; usually said of a male offspring. This process was described by Freud as part of his theory of infantile sexuality and considered to be normal in male infants.

oes-: For words beginning thus and not found here, see words beginning with es.

oestrus (es′trus): Estrus (*q.v.*).

OH: The symbol that represents the hydroxyl ion in solution. When one or more OH groups unite with a metallic element, a base is formed.

o.h.: Abbreviation for *omni hora* [L.], meaning every hour.

ohm (ōm): A unit of electrical resistance; the resistance through which a potential difference of one volt can produce a current of one ampere.

Ohm's law: States that for a given resistance the current flowing through it will be proportional to the voltage across it.

-oid: A suffix denoting having the quality, form, or appearance of; resembling the item designated in the first part of the word, *e.g.*, epitheloid.

oil: A liquid of fatty consistency and greasy feel, insoluble in water but soluble in ether and some alcohols; classified as animal, vegetable, or mineral according to source, and as volatile or fixed according to its action on exposure to air or heat.

oil immersion objective: An objective for the microscope that is equipped for a special lens to be used when oil replaces the air between the objective and the object being studied.

ointment (oynt′ment): A semisolid fatty mixture that is applied externally as a protective covering or as a vehicle for a medicinal substance that is to be absorbed.

O.L.: Abbreviation for *oculus laevus* [L.], meaning left eye.

old: In statistics, one who has lived for a long time; often refers to the years between about 65 and 75. *Old age,* usually refers to the final years of one's life, most often any age over 75. The World Health Seminar on Aging (Kiev, 1965) developed the following definitions: *elderly,* persons 60–74 years old; *old,* those between 75–89; *very old,* those over 90. Another classification lists those 55–75 as *young old,* and those 75–89 as *old,* and still another classifies those 75 and older as *old-old.* The term old-old has also been used to identify elderly persons who have survived major debilitating illnesses or mental disorders and who require a range of health and social services.

Old Age Survivors Health and Disability Insurance Program: A federal program inaugurated in 1935, commonly referred to as Social Security; administered by the Social Security Administration; provides monthly cash payments to retired persons over 65, and to certain disabled persons and their dependents. Medicaid (*q.v.*) is part of this program.

old tuberculin: The first type of tuberculin; made by the German bacteriologist, Koch (*q.v.*); used as a skin test for tuberculosis. Currently, Protein Purified Derivative (PPD) is often preferred for this use. See tuberculin.

Older Americans Act: Important legislation passed in 1965; established a national policy on aging and provided grants to states and local governments for conducting programs for the aging. Amended in 1973 to change the focus from state to regional offices on aging. Revised in 1978 and again in 1987 to consolidate some of the services. Sections deal with income, food service, housing, mental and physical health, retirement, and many types of community services for dealing with other life activities and problems. Projects are carried out under the Administration on Aging.

ole-, olei-, oleo-: Combining forms denoting oil.

oleaginous (ō-lē-aj'i-nus): Greasy, oily.

oleate (ō'lē-āt): A combination of an alkaloid or a metallic base in oleic acid; used as an ointment.

olecranarthritis (ō-lek'ran-ar-thrī'tis): Inflammation of the elbow joint.

olecranon (ō-lek'ra-non): The large process at the upper end of the ulna; it forms the tip of the elbow when the arm is flexed and fits into the olecranon fossa when the forearm is extended.

oleic acid (o-lē'ik): An acid prepared from fats; occurs as a yellow liquid used in the preparation of lotions.

oleoresin (ō'lē-ō-rez'in): A natural compound extracted from certain plants, consisting of resin and an essential oil, having a pungent odor and taste, and used in pharmaceutical preparations such as balsams, stimulants, and expectorants. See balsam of Peru and balsam of Tolu.

oleum (ōl'ē-um): Oil. **O. RICINI**, castor oil, a purgative. **O. MORRHUAE**, cod liver oil (*q.v.*).

olfaction (ol-fak'shun): 1. The act of smelling. 2. The sense of smell.

olfactology (ol'fak-tol'o-ji): The science or study of the sense of smell.

olfactometer (ol'fak-tom'e-ter): A device for determining the keenness of an individual's sense of smell.

olfactorium (ol-fak-tor'-i-um): An air-conditioned temperature-controlled room into which a known concentration of an odor is introduced; the subject reports when he or she first detects the odor and when he or she recognizes it. Used to test a person's sense of smell.

olfactory (ol-fak'to-ri): Pertaining to the sense of smell. **O. NERVE**, one of the first pair of cranial nerves; some of the processes of the **O.** nerve are embedded in the mucosal lining of the nasal cavity, and others penetrate the cribriform plate of the ethmoid bone and join others in the **O. BULB** that lies just above the ethmoid bone from which they leave as olfactory tracts that travel to the cerebral cortex on the medial sides of the temporal lobes. **O. ORGAN**, the nose.—olfaction, n.

olig-, oligo-: Combining forms denoting 1) deficiency; 2) insufficiency; 3) little, few.

oligemia (ol-i-gē'mi-a): Diminished total quantity of blood in the body.—oligemic, adj. Also olighemia and oligohemia.

olighydria (ol'-ig-hid'ri-a): Scanty perspiration. Also oligidria.

oligocholia (ol'i-gō-kō'li-a): A deficiency in the secretion of bile.

oligochylia (ol'i-gō-kī'li-a): A deficiency of chyle or of gastric juice.

oligocythemia (ol'i-gō-sī-thē'mi-a): Deficiency in the cellular elements in the blood.

oligodactylia, oligodactyly (ol'i-gō-dak-til'i-a, ol-i-gō-dak'ti-li): Fewer than the normal number of fingers or toes.—oligodactylic, adj.

oligodendrocyte (ol'i-gō-den'drō-sīt): One of the non-neural cells that form part of the structure of the neuroglia of the central nervous system. See neuroglia.

oligodendroglioma (ol'i-gō-den-drō-glī-ō'ma): An intracerebral malignant tumor; arises from the oligodendrocytes; usually occurs in the frontal lobe; characterized by calcification, which gives a honeycomb appearance on x-ray.

oligodipsia (ol'i-gō-dip'si-a): Abnormally diminished sensation of thirst.

oligodontia (ol'i-gō-don'shi-a): Congenital absence of one or more of the teeth.

oligoerythrocythemia (ol'i-gō-e-rith'rō-sī-thē'mi-a): A deficiency of red blood cells or of coloring matter in these cells.

oligogalactia (ol'i-gō-ga-lak'shi-a): Diminished or deficient secretion of milk.

oligohydramnios (ol'i-gō-hī-dram'ni-ōs): Deficient amount of amniotic fluid in the pregnant uterus. Oligamnios.

oligohydruria (ol'i-gō-hī-drū'ri-a): Excretion of small amount of highly concentrated urine.

oligohypermenorrhea (ol'i-gō-hī-per-men-ō-rē'a): Infrequent menstruation but with excessive flow.

oligohypomenorrhea (ol'i-gō-hī-pō-men-ō-rē'a): Infrequent menstruation with less than normal flow.

oligoleukocythemia (ol'i-gō-lū'kō-sī-thē'mi-a): A reduction in the number of leukocytes in the circulating blood. Leukopenia.

oligomenorrhea (ol'i-gō-men-ō-rē'a): Scanty or infrequent menstruation.

oligophosphaturia (ol'i-gō-fos-fa-tū'ri-a): An abnormally small amount of phosphates in the urine.

oligophrenia (ol'i-gō-frē'ni-a): Mental deficiency due to faulty development. **PHENYLPYRUVIC O., O.** characterized by excretion of phenylpyruvic acid in the urine; see phenylketonuria.

oligopnea (ol-i-gop'nē-a): Abnormally slow or infrequent respirations.

oligoptyalism (ol'i-gō-tī'a-lizm): Diminished or deficient secretion of ptyalin.

oligosaccharide (ol'i-gō-sak'a-rīde): A carbohydrate that, on hydrolysis, yields ten monosaccharides.

oligospermia (ol'i-gō-sper'mi-a): Deficiency in the number of spermatozoa in the semen.

oligotrichia (ol′-i-gō-trik′-i-a): Congenital thinness of the hair.

oligotrophia (ol′-i-gō-trō′-fi-a): Lack of nourishment. Also oligotrophy.

oliguria (ol-i-gū′-ri-a): Deficient urine secretion in relation to amount of fluid intake; a condition frequently seen in persons with low cardiac output or renal failure.—oliguric, adj. Also oliguresia and oliguresis.

olivary (ol′-i-var-i): Olive shaped.

olive oil: The oil of the olive; used externally as an emollient and lubricant, internally as a lubricant, and as a food.

Ollier's disease: Dyschondroplasia (*q.v.*).

o.m.: Abbreviation for *omni mane* [L.] meaning every morning.

-oma: A suffix denoting a tumor or neoplasm of the part named in the stem.

omagra (ō-mag′-ra): Gout in the shoulder joint.

omalgia (ō-mal′-ji-a): Pain in the shoulder.

omarthritis (ō′-mar-thrī′-tis): Arthritic pain and inflammation of the shoulder joint.

ombudsman (om′-buds-man): In health care, an agent or representative of the client who receives his complaints, investigates reported problems, and strives to achieve an equitable solution for the client.

omentectomy (ō-men-tek′-to-mi): Excision of all or part of the omentum.

omentitis (o-men-tī′-tis): Inflammation of the omentum.

omentopexy (ō-men′tō-pek-si): A surgical procedure in which the omentum is fastened to the abdominal wall or some other tissues in the abdominal cavity.

omentorrhaphy (ō-men-tor′a-fi): Suturing of the omentum.

omentum (ō-men′tum): A double layer of peritoneum that covers the stomach and hangs down like an apron covering the anterior surface of the abdominal organs. The functions of the **O.** are protection, repair and fat storage. **GREATER O.**, the fold which hangs from the lower border of the stomach and covers the front of the intestines. **LESSER O.**, a smaller fold, passing between the transverse fissure of the liver and the lesser curvature of the stomach.—omental, adj.

omitis (ō-mī-tis): Inflammation of the shoulder.

Ommaya reservoir: A device used to avoid repeated spinal puncture for delivering drugs intrathecally to patients being treated with antibiotics, analgesics, and/or anticancer drugs. Consists of a catheter with a dome shaped reservoir attached, which is threaded through a burr hole in the skull and through the frontal lobe of the brain into the lateral ventricle; the reservoir remains under the skin flap and over the burr hole. When drugs are to be administered, the scalp is punctured with a hypodermic needle and a specific amount of cerebrospinal fluid is withdrawn from the reservoir before the medication is injected into it. The procedure, which is performed under strict aseptic technique, is usually carried out by the physician.

omo-: Combining form denoting shoulder.

omodynia (ō-mō-din′i-a): Pain in the shoulder.

omohyoid (ō-mō-hī′oyd): 1. Pertaining to the shoulder and the hyoid bone. 2. Refers to a digastric muscle that is attached to the scapula and the hyoid bone.

omphal-, omphalo-: Combining forms denoting the umbilicus.

omphalectomy (om-fa-lek′to-mi): Excision of the umbilicus.

omphalitis (om-fa-lī′tis): Inflammation of the umbilicus.

omphalocele (om-fal′-ō-sēl): Congenital umbilical hernia.

omphaloncus (om-fa-long′-kus): A swelling or tumor of the umbilicus.

omphaloproptosis (om′-fal-ō-prop-tō′-sis): Abnormal protrusion of the umbilicus.

omphalorrhagia (om′-fa-lō-rā′-ji-a): Hemorrhage from the umbilicus.

omphalotomy (om-fa-lot′-ō-mi): The severing or cutting of the umbilical cord.

omphalus (om′-fa-lus): The umbilicus.

o.n.: Abbreviation for *omni nocte* [L.], meaning every night.

onanism (ō′-nan-izm): Incomplete sexual intercourse with withdrawal before the emission of semen.

onc-, onco-: Combining forms denoting 1) tumor; 2) swelling or mass; 3) barb or hook.

Onchocerca (ong-ko-ser′-ka): A genus of filarial nematodes; parasitic to man as well as animals; inhabit the connective tissues with formation of nodules that contain the parasite.

onchocerciasis (ong′-kō-ser-kī′-a-sis): Infestation of man with worms of the genus *Onchocerca;* the adult worms are encapsulated in subcutaneous connective tissue; may migrate to the eye causing ophthalmic problems including cataract and blindness.

oncogene hypothesis: The theory that cancer may be caused by certain DNA viruses that insert themselves within the genetic material; ordinarily they are held in suppression.

oncogenesis (ong′-kō-jen′-e-sis): The production of tumors.

oncogenic (ong-kō-jen′-ik): 1. Capable of tumor production. 2. Pertaining to the origin and growth of a neoplasm: often used to describe the carcinogenic viruses.

oncogenous (ong-koj′-e-nus): Arising in, originating in, or inducing the development of a tumor.

oncologist (ong-kol′-o-jist): A physician who specializes in oncology (*q.v.*)

oncology (ong-kol′-o-ji): The scientific study of tumors.—oncological, adj.

Oncology Nursing Society (ONS): A national organization established in 1975, for professional nurses specializing in cancer care. Sponsors education and research programs; promotes high standards in cancer care; publishes *Oncology Forum*. Address, 701 Washington Road, Pittsburgh, PA 15228

oncolysis (ong-kol′-i-sis): The destruction of a neoplasm. Sometimes used to describe reduction in size of a tumor.—oncolytic, adj.

oncometer (ong-kom′e-ter): An instrument for measuring the variations in size or delineating the form of certain viscera such as the kidney.

oncosis (ong-kō′-sis): 1. Any condition characterized by the formation of a neoplasm. 2. Any swelling or tumor. 3. The formation of multiple tumors.

oncothlipsis (ong′-kō-thlip′-sis): Pressure caused by a pathological growth or a tumor.

oncotomy (ong-kot′o-mi): An incision into a tumor, an abscess, or a cyst.

Ondine's curse: Term sometimes used to describe a syndrome wherein the individual is apneic although the respiratory organs are able to function normally; due to a defect in the breathing control centers in the central nervous system which are sensitive to excess carbon dioxide. May occur following infections such as poliomyelitis or encephalitis, certain types of brain or spinal cord surgery, or overdose of certain drugs; may also be the condition causing infant apnea syndrome. [Ondine, a water nymph in fable, caused the human male who loved her to sleep continuously.]

oneiric (ō-nī′rik): Pertaining to dreams or dreaming.

oneiroanalysis (ō-nī′rō-a-nal′a-sis): Psychoanalysis that involves the exploration of the personality through the interpretation of drug-induced dreams.

oneirophrenia (ō-nī′rō-frē′ni-a): A form of schizophrenia marked by hallucinations, amnesia, confusion and disorientation, stupor, prolonged sleeplessness.

onomatopoiesis (on′-ō-ma-tō-poy-ē′-sis): In psychiatry, the creation by the patient of meaningless words, phrases, or sounds.

ontic (on′tik): Relating to or having real being or existence.

ontogenic, ontogenetic (on-tō-jen′ik, on-tō-je-net′ik): Referring to the development of an individual or organism as distinguished from the evolutionary development of a species.

ontogeny (on-toj′e-ni): The life history of an individual from a one-celled ovum to birth.

onych-, onycho-: Combining forms denoting the nails.

onychatrophia (on′i-ka-trō′fi-a): Atrophy of the finger- and toenails.

onychauxis (on-i-kawk′sis): Hypertrophy of a nail or nails.

onychectomy (on-i-kek′to-mi): Surgical removal of a nail.

onychia (ō-nik′i-a): Acute inflammation of the nail bed; may become suppurative and result in loss of the nail.

onychocryptosis (on′ik-ō-krip-tō′sis): Ingrowing of a nail.

onychogryphosis (on′-ik-ō-grī-fō′sis): A deformed overgrowth of the nails in which they become ridged, thickened, and elongated, sometimes with an inward curvature.

onycholysis (on-i-kol′i-sis): Loosening of toe- or fingernail.—onycholytic, adj.

onychomadesis (on′i-kō-ma-dē′sis): The separation or loosening of the nails, beginning at the base and continuing until the nails fall off.

onychomalacia (on′ik-ō-ma-lā′shi-a): Softening of the nails.

onychomycosis (on′ik-ō-mi-kō′sis): A fungal infection of the nails causing thickening and splitting. Also called ringworm of the nails.

onychophagia, onychophagy (on-i-ki-ō-fā′ji-a, on-i-kof′a-ji): Nailbiting.

onychorrhexis (on′i-kō-rek′sis): Spontaneous splitting of the nails at the free edge.

onychosis (on-i-kō′sis): Any disease or deformity of the nails.

onychotillomania (on-i-kot′-i-lō-mā′ni-a): A neurotic habit of picking or tearing at the nails.

onychotomy (on-i-kot′o-mi): Surgical incision of a fingernail or toenail, usually to remove a mass under the nail.

onyx (on′iks): 1. A finger- or toenail. 2. A collection of pus that resembles a nail, located between the layers of the cornea.

onyxis (ō-nik′sis): Ingrowing of a nail or nails.

OOB: Abbreviation for out of bed.

ooblast (ō′ō-blast): A cell from which an ovum develops.

oocyst (ō′ō-sist): The encysted zygote in the life of some sporozoa. See **ookinete.**

oocyte (ō′ō-sīt): An immature ovum.

oogenesis (ō-ō-jen′e-sis): The production and formation of ova in the ovary.—oogenetic, adj.

ookinete (ō′ō-kī-nēt): The zygote in the life cycle of some protozoan parasites, as that of the malarial parasite; it bores into the female mosquito's intestinal wall where it develops into an oocyst (*q.v.*).

oophor-, oophoro-: Combining forms denoting 1) ovary; 2) ovarian.

oophoralgia (ō-of′or-al′ji-a): Pain in an ovary.

oophorectomy (ō-of′ō-rek′to-mi): Excision of an ovary; ovariectomy.

oophoritis (ō-of-or-ī'tis): Inflammation of one or both ovaries.

oophorocystectomy (ō-of'or-ō-sis-tek'to-mi): Removal of an ovarian cyst.

oophorocystosis (ō-of'ō-rō-sis-tō'sis): The formation of an ovarian cyst.

oophorohysterectomy (o-of'ō-rō-his-ter-ek'to-mi): The surgical removal of the ovaries and the uterus.

oophoroma (ō-of-or-ō'ma): A malignant tumor of the ovary.

oophoron (ō-of'or-on): The ovary.

oophoropexy (ō-of'o-rō-pek-si): See ovariopexy.

oophorosalpingectomy (ō-of' -or-ō-sal-pin-jek'to-mi): Excision of an ovary and its associated fallopian tube.

oosperm (ō'ō-sperm): A fertilized ovum.

opacification (ō-pas'i-fi-kā'shun): The process of becoming opaque.

opacity (ō-pas'i-ty): Non-transparency; cloudiness; an opaque spot, as on the cornea or lens.

opaque (ō-pāk'): Not transparent.

OPD: Abbreviation for Outpatient Department.

open: 1. Exposed to the air. 2. Not covered by skin. 3. To puncture, as a boil or abscess. 4. To make an opening into a wound or cavity. **O. CARE,** care given to a patient in a community where programs aimed at supporting living in one's home are available. **O. FRACTURE,** one in which an external wound leads to the fractured bone. **O. HOSPITAL,** see under hospital. **O. REDUCTION,** reduction of a fracture after incision into the site of the fracture. **OPEN-HEART SURGERY,** performed on the opened heart; involves incision into one or more of the chambers of the heart. The term is often loosely used to refer to all heart surgery, whether or not the heart itself is opened. **O. WOUND,** one that opens to the surface of the body.

operable (op'er-a-b'l): Descriptive of a condition that it is thought can be cured or improved by surgery which will not endanger the patient's life or general health.

operant (op'er-ant): In behavioral experimentation, refers to the desired response or behavior chosen by the experimenter; hopefully, pairing the behavior with a reinforcer will either increase or decrease its occurrence whichever is desired. **O. BEHAVIOR,** behavior that operates on the environment. **O. CONDITIONING,** see under conditioning. **OPERANT LEARNING THEORY,** the theory that behavior is solely the result of environmental cues and rewards.

operation (op-er-ā'shun): A procedure in which a surgeon uses his hands or instruments to correct or alter a pathological condition or state, or for removing a tumor, limb, etc. **ELECTIVE O.,** one for which haste is not required; can be performed at the patient's and surgeon's convenience. **EMERGENCY O.,** one that must be done immediately in order to save the patient's life. **EXPLORATORY O.,** one done for diagnostic purposes. **MAJOR O.,** one involving risk to the patient's life. **MINOR O.,** a relatively simple one that usually does not involve risk to the patient's life. **RADICAL O.,** one done in an effort to effect a complete cure. **SUBTOTAL O.,** one in which not all of the involved organ is removed.

operculum (ō-per'kū-lum): 1. A lid or covering. 2. Obstructive tissue or substance. In obstetrics, the plug of mucus and mucoid material that fills the cervical canal during pregnancy and helps to prevent infection of the genital tract.

ophiasis (ō-fī'a-sis): A type of baldness in which hair is lost in one or more winding streaks around the hair margin.

ophidiophilia (ō-fid-i-ō-fil'i-a): Abnormal fondness for snakes.

ophidiophobia (ō-fid-i-ō-fō'bi-a): A morbid dread of snakes.

ophidism (ō'fi-dizm): Poisoning caused by snake venom.

ophiotoxemia (ō'fi-ō-tok-sē'mi-a): Poisoning by snake venom.

ophthal-, ophthalmo-: Combining forms denoting 1) the eyes; 2) the eyeball.

ophthalmacrosis (of-thal-ma-krō'sis): Abnormal enlargement of the eyeball.

ophthalmagra (of'thal-mag'ra): Sudden pain in the eye.

ophthalmalgia (of'thal-mal'ji-a): Pain in the eye.

ophthalmatrophia (of' -thal-ma-trō'fi-a): Atrophy of the eye.

ophthalmectomy (of-thal-mek'to-mi): Surgical removal of the eyeball by enucleation.

ophthalmia (of-thal'mi-a): Inflammation of the eye involving especially the conjunctiva. **O. NEONATORUM,** purulent infection of the eyes of an infant at birth as it passes through the genital tract; may be caused by the gonococcus. **PURULENT O., O.** neonatorum. **SYMPATHETIC O.,** inflammation of one eye secondary to injury or disease of the other.

ophthalmic (of-thal'mik): Pertaining to the eye.

ophthalmitis (of-thal-mī'tis): 1. Any inflammation of the eye. 2. Ophthalmia (*q.v.*).

ophthalmoblenorrhea (of-thal'mō-blen-ō-rē'a): Purulent ophthalmia (*q.v.*); often due to a gonococcal infection.

ophthalmocele (of-thal'mō-sēl): Exophthalmos (*q.v.*).

ophthalmocentesis (of-thal'mō-sen-tē'sis): Surgical puncture of the eye.

ophthalmocopia (of-thal-mō-kō'pi-a): Eyestrain or eye fatigue.

ophthalmodonesis (of-thal'mō-dō-nē'sis): Trembling movement of the eye or eyes.

ophthalmodynamometer (of-thal'mō-dī-na-mom'e-ter): An instrument for measuring 1) the arterial pressure in the retinal vessels, or 2) the power of convergence of the eyes.

ophthalmodynamometery (of-thal'mō-dī-na-mom'e-tri): Use of the ophthalmodynamometer for making indirect measurements of 1) the blood pressure in the retinal arteries, or 2) the power of the extraocular muscles.

ophthalmodynia (of-thal'mō-dī'ni-a): Pain in the eye.

ophthalmofundoscope (of-thal' -mō-fun'dū-skōp): An instrument for examining the fundus of the eye.

ophthalmograph (of-thal'-mō-graf): An instrument for photographing eye movements during reading.

ophthalmogyric (of-thal-mō-jī'rik): See **oculogyric.**

ophthalmolith (of-thal'mō-lith): A calculus in the eye or lacrimal duct. See also **dacryolith.**

ophthalmologist (of-thal-mol'o-jist): A physician who specializes in the diseases and refractive errors of the eye; may also do eye surgery, examine eyes, and prescribe corrective lenses.

ophthalmology (of-thal-mol'o-ji): The science that deals with the structure, function and diseases of the eye, and with the diagnoses and treatment of the diseases and disorders of the eye.

ophthalmomalacia (of-thal'mō-ma-lā'shi-a): Abnormal softness of the eyeball.

ophthalmometer (of'thal-mom'e-ter): An instrument for measuring the eye, particularly its refractive powers. See **keratometer.**

ophthalmometry (of'thal-mom'e-tri): Measurement of the acuity of vision and of the eye's refractive power.

ophthalmomyositis (of-thal'mō-mī-ō-sī'tis): Inflammation of the muscles that move the eyeball.

ophthalmomyotomy (of-thal'mō-mī-ot'o-mi): The surgical division of one or more muscles of the eye.

ophthalmoneuritis (of-thal'mō-nū-ri'tis): Inflammation of the ophthalmic nerve.

ophthalmopathy (of-thal-mop'a-thi): Any disease or disorder of the eye.

ophthalmoplegia (of-thal'mō-plē'ji-a): Paralysis of either or both certain extrinsic or intrinsic muscles of the eye.—ophthalmoplegic, adj.

ophthalmoptosis (of-thal' -mop-tō'sis): Protrusion of the eyeball; exophthalmos (*q.v.*).

ophthalmorrhagia (of-thal-mō-rā'ji-a): Hemorrhage from the eye.

ophthalmorrhexis (of-thal-mō-rek'sis): Rupture of the eyeball.

ophthalmoscope (of-thal'-mō-skōp): An instrument fitted with a lens and illumination for examining the posterior portion of the interior of the eye.—ophthalmoscopic, adj.

ophthalmoscopy (of-thal-mos'ko-pi): Examination of the interior of fundus of the eyeball with an ophthalmoscope.

ophthalmosteresis (of-thal'mō-ste-rē'sis): Loss of an eye.

ophthalmotomy (of-thal-mot'o-mi): Incision into the eyeball.

ophthalmotonometer (of-thal'mō-tō-nom'et-er): Instrument for determining the intraocular tension.

-opia: Combining form denoting sightedness, or visual condition, *e.g.*, myopia.

opiate (ō'pi-āt): 1. Any drug derived from opium. 2. In a broad sense, sometimes used to describe any drug that produces sleep.

opioids (ō'pi-oyds): 1. Substances produced in the body which have actions similar to those of the opiate, morphine. 2. Synthetic substances that have actions similar to those of opium but are not derived from it.

opisthotonos (op-is-thot'on-ōs): Extreme extension of the body, occurring in tetanic spasm. The spine is bent forward to such a degree that the patient may be supported on his head and heels alone. The symptom may be present in meningitis and strichnine poisoning as well as tetanus.—opisthotonic, adj.

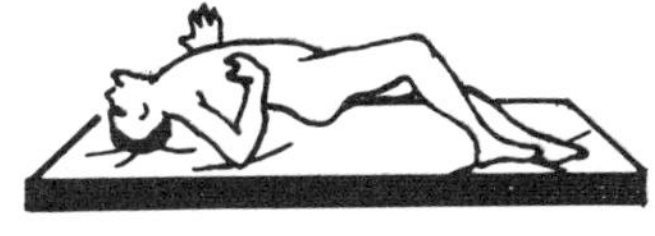

opisthotonos

opium (ō'pi-um): The dried juice of the unripe **o.** poppy capsules; long used as a narcotic, analgesic, astringent, and diaphoretic. Contains valuable alkaloids such as morphine, codeine, and papaverine.

opiumism (ō'pi-um-izm): The habit of using opium or the physiological condition resulting from the habitual use of opium.

opodidymus (op-o-did' -i-mus): Conjoined twins with a single body but two heads that are partly fused.

opotherapy (ō-pō-ther'a-pi): The use of animals' organs, or the products of such organs, in treatment of disease.

oppilation (op'i-lā'shun): 1. Constipation. 2. An obstruction.

opponens (ō-pō'nenz): 1. Opposing. 2. The name given to several small muscles of the hand or foot that act to draw the lateral digits across the palm or sole to oppose each other.

opportunistic (op′por-tū-nis′tik): 1. Said of infections that are capable of adapting to a host or environment other than the normal one for the particular organism. 2. Pertains to a serious infection with a microorganism that normally has little or no pathogenic activity but which has been activated by a serious disease or a modern method of treatment, or lowered resistance of the host.

opsin (op′sin): A protein in the rods and cones of the retina that is involved in the formation of the light-sensitive visual pigments.

opsinogen (op-sin′o-jen): A substance that induces the formation of opsonins (*q.v.*).

opsoclonia (op′sō-klō′ni-a): A condition characterized by irregular, jerking horizontal and vertical movements of the eyeball. Opsoclonus.

opsonic (op-son′ik): Pertaining to opsonins. **O. ACTION,** the effect produced by opsonins on susceptible microorganisms and other cells. **O. INDEX,** the numerical measure of opsonic activity of the blood serum; indicates the ability of phagocytes to ingest foreign bodies such as bacteria.

opsonin (op′ son-in) Any of several substances including antibody that unite with antigen and render bacteria and other cells more susceptible to phagocytosis. See antibodies.—opsonic, opsoniferous, adj.; opsonification, n.

opsonization (op-son-ī-zā′shun): In bacteriology, the rendering of bacteria and other cells susceptible to phagocytosis (*q.v.*).

-opsy: Combining form denoting examination of.

opthalmiatrics (of-thal-mi-at′riks): Treatment of diseases and disorders of the eye.

optic (op′tik): Pertaining to sight or to the eye. **O. ATROPHY,** refers to atrophy of the optic nerve. **LEBER'S O. ATROPHY,** a hereditary form of **O.** atrophy in which central vision is completely lost while peripheral vision is partially retained; is transmitted by the female and occurs in males. **O. CHIASM** or **CHIASMA,** the X-shaped crossing on the ventral surface of the brain where some of the fibers of the two optic nerves cross to the opposite sides and continue in the optic tracts of those sides; see chiasm. **O. DISK,** the point at the back of the retina where the **O.** nerve fibers converge to form the **O.** nerve. **O. GLIOMA,** a glioma of the optic nerve or the optic chiasm, characterized by slow growth, visual loss, protrusion of the eyeball, and strabismus. **O. NERVE,** one of the second pair of cranial nerves; they conduct visual stimuli from the retina to the brain. **O. NEURITIS,** involvement of any part of the optic nerve in a disease process that impairs nerve conduction; may be an inflammatory, vascular, or degenerative disease.

optical (op′ti-kal): Related to vision or the science of optics.

optician (op-tish′an): One who grinds lenses to prescription and dispenses spectacles to correct refractive errors in vision.

optics (op′tiks): That branch of physics that deals with light, its sources, transmission, refraction, absorption, etc., particularly as these phenomena relate to vision.

optimum (op′ti-mum): The quality of being the best or most favorable; conducive to the most favorable activity or result. In bacteriology, the temperature at which bacteria grow best. **O. POSITION,** that which will be the least awkward and most useful should a limb remain permanently paralyzed.

opto-: Combining form denoting: 1. Vision. 2. The eye. 3. Optic.

optokinetic (op-tō-kī-net′ik): Pertaining to or involving movements of the eyeball, particularly those that occur while the subject is watching moving objects.

optometer (op-tom′et-er): An instrument used for measuring the power and range of vision.

optometrist (op-tom′e-trist): One who holds an O.D. degree and is licensed to practice optometry.

optometry (op-tom′e-tri): 1. Measurement of visual acuity with an optometer. 2. An occupation consisting of examining the eye for refractive errors and prescribing lenses or any other means except drugs for the correction of these errors; non-medical visual care.—optometric, adj.

OPV: Abbreviation for oral poliovaccine. Also called Sabin's vaccine.

OR: Abbreviation for Operating Room.

orad (ō′rad): Toward the mouth, or situated near the mouth.

oral: Pertaining to the mouth. **O. CONTRACEPTIVE,** pills taken orally to block the possibility of impregnation during sexual intercourse. **O. HERPES,** herpes simplex (*q.v.*). **O. HYGIENE,** care of the mouth tissues and structures including brushing of the teeth, use of dental floss, massaging the gums, and ensuring that dentures are properly fitted. **O. HYPOGLYCEMIC AGENTS,** chemicals used in treating certain types of diabetes. **O. PHASE,** the earliest phase of psychosocial development (*q.v.*) in which the child derives pleasure from sucking or biting; persists in adult life in sublimated form.

oral personality type: In psychiatry, refers to a person who seeks gratification by eating, drinking, smoking; usually is also very talkative, envious, nagging, insecure.

orb: A sphere. In medicine, the eyeball.

orbicular (or-bik′ū-lar): Resembling a globe; spherical or circular.

orbicularis (or-bik-ū-lar′ is): Descriptive of a muscle that encircles an opening of the body. **O. OCULI,** the muscle that surrounds the eye. **O. ORIS,** the muscle that surrounds the mouth.

orbit (or′bit): In anatomy, the bony socket that encloses and protects the eyeball and its appendages.—orbital, adj. Also eye socket.

orchi-, orchid-, orchio-: Combining forms denoting the testes.

orchialgia (or-ki-al′ji-a): Pain in a testis. Also orchidalgia.

orchiatrophy (or-ki-at′rō-fi): Atrophy or shrinkage of the testes.

orchiauxe (or-ki-awk′sē): Enlargement of a testis.

orchidectomy (or-ki-dek′to-mi): Excision of one or both testes; castration. Also orchectomy, orchiectomy.

orchidic (or-kid′ik): Pertaining to the testes.

orchidopexy (or′ -ki-dō-pek′si): The operation of bringing an undescended testis into the scrotum, and fixing in in this position. Also orchiopexy, orchiorrhaphy.

orchidoptosis (or′ -ki-dop-tō′sis): Ptosis of the testes.

orchidotherapy (or′ -ki-dō-ther′a-pi): Treatment of disease with testicular extract. Orchiotherapy.

orchiepididymitis (or′ki-ep-i-did-i-mī′tis): Inflammation of a testis and an epididymis.

orchiocatabasis (or′ -ki-ō-ka-tab′a-sis): The descent of the testes into the scrotum.

orchioncus (or-ki-ong′ kus): A tumor of the testis.

orchiopathy (or-ki-op′a-thi): Any disease of the testis.

orchiotomy (or-ki-ot′o-mi): Incision and drainage of a testis. Also orchotomy.

orchis (or′kis): The testis.—orchitic, adj.

orchitis (or-kī′tis): Inflammation of a testis. **GRANULOMATOUS O.,** a hard painful testicular mass; develops suddenly or insidiously; seen mostly in older men.

Order of Deaconesses: A church order that existed as early as the 4th century but which fell into abeyance by the Middle Ages; it was revived by Pastor Theodore Fliedner at Kaiserswerth, Germany in 1833 with the aim of training women in the care of the sick; it was here that Florence Nightingale received her instruction in nursing.

orderly: An attendant in a hospital or other institution.

ordure (or′dūr): Excrement.

orexia (ō-rek′sē-a): Appetite.

orexigenic (ō-rek-si-jen′ik): 1. Stimulating the appetite. 2. An agent that stimulates the appetite.

orf: A disease of sheep, transmissible to man, but rare in humans; caused by a filterable virus; characterized by dark red papules that become indurated, but most often confined to a single self-limited lesion of the finger.

organ: A differentiated part of the body that may or may not be grouped with other parts to perform a specific function. **O. OF CORTI,** see Corti.

organ transplant: The replacement of a diseased or malfunctioning organ or part with one from another individual, either living or recently deceased. Organs that have been transplanted include kidney, heart, liver, lung, pancreas, spleen, and an entire human eye. The principal problem in transplants is the rejection of the organ by the immunological defenses of the donee which treat the transplanted organ as foreign and try to destroy it. Corneal transplants are frequently successful.

organelle (or′ga-nel): A specialized part of structure within the cytoplasm of a cell that is presumed to have a special function in the cell's overall activities in the life process.

organic (or-gan′ik): 1. Pertaining to an organ. 2. Associated with life. 3. Pertinent to or derived from animal or vegetable life. 4. In nutrition, refers to foods grown without use of manmade fertilizers, pesticides or herbicides. **O. ACID,** an acid containing one or more -COOH (carboxyl) groups, *e.g.*, acetic acid, formic acid, and fatty acids. **O. CHEMISTRY,** the study of substances that contain carbon. **O. CONFUSIONAL STATE,** in psychiatry, refers to a state of disturbed orientation to time, place, or person which sometimes appears to be of organic origin. **O. DISEASE,** one in which there is structural change in organs or tissues.

organic brain syndromes: A group of mental disorders caused by local or widespread cognitive impairment. Categories listed in Diagnostic and Statistical Manual of Mental Disorders III-R include 1) delirium and dementia in which the impairment is widespread; 2) amnestic syndrome and organic (or substance) hallucinosis in which selected areas of cognition are affected; 3) organic (or substance) delusional syndrome and organic (or substance) affective syndrome, which resemble schizophrenic or affective disorders; 4) organic (or substance) personality syndrome, in which the person's personality is affected; 5) intoxication and withdrawal, in which the disorder is associated with the ingestion or withdrawal of a substance, or which does not fit into any of the first four categories; 6) atypical or mixed organic brain syndrome, a category which includes any organic brain syndrome not included in the other five categories.

organic mental disorders: A large heterogeneous group of disorders that are characterized by behavioral and psychological abnormalities and which are associated with brain dysfunction. See Appendix VI for a listing of these disorders.

organism (or′gan-izm): A living cell or group of cells differentiated into functionally distinct parts that are interdependent. Any living individual, either plant or animal.

organization (or-gan-ī-zā′shun): 1. The process of providing or assuming a structure. 2. The change in the structure of a blood clot in a vein whereby it becomes fibrous.

organogenesis (or′gan-ō-jen′e-sis): The formation and development of the organs and organ systems of the body.

organology (or-ga-nol′ō-ji): The special study of the history and formation of organs of the body, including their anatomy, physiology, and functions.

organomegaly (or′gan-ō-meg′a-li): Abnormal enlargement of a viscus or of viscera. Also called splanchnomegaly and visceromegaly.

organopathy (or-ga-nop′a-thi): Organic disease. See organ.

organopexy (or′ga-nō-pek′si): The surgical fixation of an organ; refers often to the uterus after removal of a tumor.

organotherapy (or′ga-nō-ther′a -pi): Treatment of disease by administration of animal organs or the extracts of these organs.

organs of Zuckerlandl: Glandular cells of sympathetic origin found along the aorta in the abdominal cavity; they are chemoreceptors for oxygen, carbon dioxide, and hydrogen ion concentration; they help control and regulate respiration.

orgasm (or′gazm): The climax of sexual excitement.

oriental sore (o-ri-en′tal sōr′): Delhi boil. A form of cutaneous leishmaniasis producing papular, crusted, granulomatous eruptions of the skin. A disease of the tropics and subtropics. Also called Aleppo boil.

orientation (or-i-en-tā′shun): Clear awareness of one's position relative to time and the environment. In mental conditions **o.** in space and time means that the patient knows where he is and recognizes the passage of time, *i.e.*, can give the correct date. Disorientation means the reverse.

orifice (or′i-fis): 1. A mouth or opening. 2. The outlet or entrance of the body cavity or aperture, *e.g.*, the urethral meatus, vagina, anus, ducts of glands, and the mouth.

origin (or′i-jin): The commencement or source of anything. **O. OF A MUSCLE,** the end that remains relatively fixed during contraction of the muscle.

ornithine (or′ni-thēn): An amino acid formed when arginine is hydrolyzed; an important intermediate product in the urea cycle.

Ornithodoros (or-ni-thod′o-rōs): A genus of ticks which are the vectors of the organisms causing such diseases as spotted fever, Q fever, tick fever, tularemia, relapsing fever, and certain types of encephalitis.

ornithosis (or-ni-thō′sis): A contagious virus disease of wild birds and some domestic fowl, sometimes transmitted to man. Disease closely resembles psittacosis but is usually less severe.

orofacial (o-rō-fā′shi-al): Pertaining to the mouth and the face.

orolingual (or-ō-ling′gwal): Pertaining to the mouth and tongue.

oronasal (or-ō-nā′zal): Pertaining to the mouth and nose.

oropharyngeal (o′rō-far-in′jē-al): Pertaining to the mouth and the pharynx.

oropharynx (ō-rō-far′ingks): 1. That portion of the pharynx that is below the level of the hyoid bone. 2. Pertaining to the mouth and pharynx.—oropharyngeal, adj.

orotic acid (ō-rot′ik): An acid found in milk.

orphan: O. DRUGS, drugs that have been found useful in treating relatively rare diseases but which are not manufactured commercially. **O. VIRUSES,** viruses that have been isolated from tissue culture in the laboratory but which do not appear to be associated with any particular disease.

orrho-: Combining form denoting serum.

orrhology (or-rol′o-ji): Serology (*q.v.*).

orrhorrhea (or-ō-rē′a): A copious serous or watery discharge.

orrhos (or′ōs): Serum.

orris root: A powder derived from the rhizome of certain iris plants; used in cosmetics, dentrifices, perfumes, etc.

ORT: Abbreviation for operating room technician.

orth-, ortho-: Combining forms denoting 1) straight or normal; 2) correct or corrective.

orthesis (or-thē′sis): An orthopedic brace, splint, or other device used by patients with physical disability or impairment, but not a prosthesis.—orthetic, adj.

orthetics (or-thet′iks): Orthotics (*q.v.*).

orthobiosis (or-thō-bī-ō′sis): A lifestyle that is based on hygienic and moral principles and other factors that make for physical and mental well-being and longevity.

orthocephalic (or-thō-se-fal′ik): Having a well proportioned head.

orthodontics (or-thō-don′tiks): A branch of dentistry dealing with prevention and correction of irregularities and malocclusion of the teeth. Also orthodontia.

orthodontist (or-thō-don′tist): A dentist who specilizes in orthodontics (*q.v.*).

orthodromic (or-thō-drō′mik): Descriptive of

fibers that conduct impulses over an axon in a normal direction.

orthograde (or'thō-grād): The upright position of the body in standing or walking.

orthokeratology (or'thō-ker-a-tol'o-ji): A method of improving vision by utilizing a contact lens to mold the cornea.

orthomolecular (or-thō-mō-lek'ū-lar): Referring to the chemical makeup of the body, both the substances formed endogenously and those taken into the body through diet and administration, including vitamins.

orthopantograph (or-thō-pan'-tō-graf): A radiographic device that makes possible the visualization of all of the teeth, the alveolar bone, and the surrounding tissues on a single film.

orthopedics (or-thō-pē'diks): A branch of medicine dealing with deformities and diseases of the skeleton and its associated structures and their correction, whether by apparatus, manipulation, or surgery.

orthopedist (or-tho-pē'dist): A physician who specializes in diseases and disorders of the bones and joints.

orthopnea (or-thop-nē'a): Inability to breathe except in an upright, sitting position.—orthopneic, adj.

orthopsychiatry (or-thō-sī-kī'a-tri): That branch of psychiatry that deals with the amelioration of disorders of personality and behavior in normal or near-normal persons, particularly in children and young adults.

orthoptic (or-thop'tik): Relating to orthoptics (*q.v.*). **O. EXERCISES,** a system of eye exercises designed to strengthen the eye muscles and prescribed to help correct such conditions as strabismus (*q.v.*) or squint.

orthoptics (or-thop'tiks): The study and treatment of muscle imbalances of the eye, especially the treatment of strabismus by exercise of the ocular muscles.

orthosis (or-thō'sis): General term for an external device applied to a patient for supportive, preventive, or corrective purposes.—orthoses, pl.; orthotic, adj.

orthostatic (or-thō-stat'ik): Caused by or related to the upright stance. **O. ALBUMINURIA,** occurs in some healthy subjects only when they take the upright position; when lying in bed the urine is normal. **O. HYPOTENSION,** see **hypotension, orthostatic.**

orthotics (or-thot'iks): The science of orthopedic appliances and their use.

orthotist (or'thō-tist): One who makes and fits orthopedic appliances.

Ortoloni's sign: A positive click heard on abduction and external rotation of the hip; a sign of dislocated hip.

O.S.: Abbreviation for *oculus sinister* [L.], meaning left eye.

os: A mouth. **EXTERNAL O.,** the opening of the cervix into the vagina. **INTERNAL O.,** the opening of the cervix into the uterine cavity.—ora, pl.

os: A bone.—ossa, pl. **O. CALCIS,** the heel bone; the calcaneus. **O. COXAE,** the hip bone. **O. INNOMINATUM,** os coxae.

osche-, oscheo-: Combining forms denoting the scrotum.

oscheal (os'kē-al): Pertaining to the scrotum.

oscheitis (os-kē-ī'tis): Inflammation of the scrotum.

oschelephantiasis (osk'el-e-fan-tī'a-sis): Enlargement of the scrotum.

oscheocele (os'kē-ō-sēl): Swelling, tumor, or hernia of the scrotum.

oscheoma (os-kē-ō'ma): A tumor of the scrotum.

oscheoncus (os-kē-ong'kus): Tumor of the scrotum; oscheoma.

oscillating bed (os'il-āt-ing): A mechanical bed so designed that it may be tilted at regular intervals, thus changing the patient's posture and allowing for the alternate filling and draining of the blood vessels of the lower extremities.

oscillation (os-il-ā'shun): A swinging or moving to and fro; a vibration.

oscillograph (o-sil'ō-graf): An instrument that records alternating current waves or other types of electrical oscillation (*q.v.*) that are used in recording heart action.

oscillometry (os-i-lom'-e-tri): Measurement of vibration, using a special apparatus (oscillometer, oscilloscope). Measures the magnitude of the pulse wave more precisely than palpation.

oscillopsia (os'i-lop'si-a): The sensation that stationary objects one is viewing are swaying back and forth.

oscilloscope (o-sil'ō-skōp): An instrument that displays temporarily on a fluorescent screen the fluctuations in an electric quantity; used in monitoring various body functions, primarily heart function.

oscitation (os'i-tā'shun): Yawning.

-oscopy: Combining form denoting a looking into.

osculum (os'kū-lum): A small opening or aperture; a pore.

-ose: Combining form denoting 1) full of, or having the quality of; 2) a carbohydrate substance.

Osgood-Schlatter disease: Osteochondrosis of the tuberosity of the tibia. See **osteochondrosis.** Also called epiphyseal aseptic necrosis.

OSHA: Occupational Safety and Health Administration (*q.v.*). Also often refers to the Occupational Safety and Health Act (*q.v.*).

Osler, Sir William: Canadian teacher and medical historian (1849–1919); taught at

McGill University and in the United States, particularly the University of Pennsylvania and Johns Hopkins University; made important contributions to medical literature; considered the outstanding physician of his time. **O.'S DISEASE**, see polycythemia. **O.'S NODES**, small painful erythematous areas, due to emboli, in the pulp of fingers or toes, or palms and soles, occurring in subacute bacterial endocarditis. **O.'S SYNDROME**, a familial condition characterized by the development of many telangiectal lesions appearing chiefly on the skin of the cheeks, scalp, ears, fingers, toes, and on the nail beds and mucosa of the gastrointestinal organs, bladder, and genitalia. Known by many other names including Rendu-Osler syndrome, Rendu-Weber-Osler syndrome, and hereditary hemorrhagic telangiectasia.

osmatic (oz-mat'ik): Relating to the sense of smell.

osmesis (oz-mē'sis): The sense of smell; the act of smelling.

osmics (oz'miks): The science dealing with the sense and organs of smell.

osmidrosis (oz'mi-drō'sis): Bromhidrosis (*q.v.*).

osmolality (oz'mō-lal'i-ti): Osmotic pressure expressed in terms of osmoles or milliosmoles per kilogram of fluid; it reflects the concentration of a solute in a solution.

osmolarity (os'mō-lar'i-ti): The osmotic pressure exerted by a substance in aqueous solution, defined in terms of the number of active particles per unit of volume.

osmole (oz'mōl): The standard unit of osmotic pressure; based on the concentration of an ion in solution.

osmology (oz-mol'-o-ji): 1. The science that deals with odors and the sense of smell. 2. The study of osmosis.

osmophilic (oz-mō-fil'ik): Readily stained with osmic acid.

osmoreceptor (oz'mō-re-sep'tor): 1. A sensory nerve ending that is responsive to stimulation by odors. 2. A sensory nerve ending that is responsive to changes in the osmotic pressure of the surrounding medium.

osmose (oz-mōs'): To pass through a membrane by osmosis.

osmosis (os-mō'sis): The passage of fluid across a membrane under the influence of osmotic pressure (*q.v.*).—osmotic, adj.

osmotic fragility test: A laboratory test for determining the fragility of red blood cells.

osmotic pressure (os-mot'ik): The force with which the fluid part of a solution is drawn across a semipermeable membrane that separates two solutions of different concentrations and that permits passage of the fluid but not of the solutes, the direction of flow being from the solution of lesser to the solution of greater concentration. When the pressure is due to the movement of protein molecules over a semipermeable membrane it is called colloidal osmotic pressure or oncotic pressure.

osphresiolagnia (os-frē'zi-ō-lag'ni-a): Sexual stimulation or excitement produced by odors.

osphresiology (os-frē'zi-ol'o-ji): The science of odors and the sense of smell; osmology.

osphresis (os-frē'sis): Olfaction.—osphretic, adj.

osphyalgia (os-fi-al'ji-a): Pain in the lumbar region; see lumbago.

osphyarthrosis (os'-fi-ar-thrō'sis): Inflammation of the hip or loins area.

ossein (os'ē-in): The organic matter in bone.

osseous (os'ē-us): Pertaining to, composed of, or resembling bone; bony.

ossi-: Combining form denoting relationship to bone.

ossicle (os'ik'l): A small bone, particularly one of those contained in the middle ear: the malleus, incus, and stapes.—ossicular, adj.

ossiculectomy (os-ik'-ū-lek'to-mi): Removal of one or all the ossicles of the middle ear.

ossiferous (o-sif'er-us): Producing or containing bone tissue.

ossification (os'i-fi-kā'shun): The formation of bone; the conversion of cartilage, etc. into bone. **INTRACARTILAGINOUS O.**, the replacement of cartilaginous structures by bone; many bones are formed this way. **INTRAMEMBRANOUS O.**, the replacement of dense connective tissue by deposits of calcium salts, forming bone; the skull bones are formed this way.

ossify (os'i-fī): To change or develop into bone.

ost-, oste-, osteo-, osti-: Combining forms denoting bone.

ostealgia (os-tē-al'ji-a): Pain in a bone or bones.

osteanabrosis (os'tē-an-a-brō'sis): See osteoanabrosis.

ostearthritis (os'-tē-ar-thrī'tis): Osteoarthritis (*q.v.*).

ostectomy (os-tek'to-mi): Surgical removal of a bone or part of a bone. Osteectomy.

osteectopia (os'-tē-ek-tō'pi-a): Displacement of bone.

osteitis (os-tē-ī'tis): Inflammation of a bone. **ALVEOLAR O.**, alveoalgia (*q.v.*). **O. CONDENSANS ILII**, dense sclerosis on the iliac side of the sacroiliac joint, often leading to fibrositis syndrome or sciatica. **O. DEFORMANS**, Paget's disease; rarefaction leading to bowing of long bones and deformity of flat bones. **O. FIBROSA CYSTICA**, softening and resorption of bone and replacement of calcified bone with fibrous tissue; usually the result of excessive secretion of parathyroid hormone; Recklinghausen's disease. **O. FRAGILITANS**, osteogenesis imperfecta;

see under osteogenesis. **O. OSSIFICANS,** condensing **O.** in which an entire bone eventually becomes more or less cancellated. **O. PUBIS,** sclerosis of the pubic bones at the symphysis with pain radiating downward in the thigh, tenderness, and eventual widening of the symphysis.

ostemia (os-tē′mi-a): Abnormal congestion of blood in a bone.

ostempyesis (os′-tem-pī-ē′sis): Suppuration of or within a bone.

osteoanabrosis (os′tē-ō-an-a-brō′sis): Atrophy of bone.

osteoarthritis (os′-te-ō-ar-thrī′tis): Degenerative arthritis. A chronic disease of weight-bearing joints and interphalangeal joints of the fingers particularly; occurring mostly in middle or old age, characterized by degenerative changes in the bone and cartilage of all of the joints. The articular cartilage becomes worn and osteophytes may form at the periphery of the joint and loose bodies result. Apparently no specific cause; may be primary, or follow disease or injury involving the articular surfaces of synovial joints; other factors may be heredity, occupation, obesity, faulty posture.—osteoarthritic, adj.

osteoarthropathy (os′tē-ō-ar-throp′a-thi): 1. Increased bone formation at joints. 2. Any disease involving bones, or joints, accompanied by pain. 3. Osteoarthritis. **PULMONARY O.,** osteitis of the legs and arms, chiefly in the terminal epiphyses of long bones and in the phalanges; associated with dorsal kyphosis and joint abnormalities; often secondary to chronic pulmonary or cardiac disorders. Also called hypertrophic pulmonary osteoarthropathy.

osteoarthrosis (os′tē-ō-ar-thrō′sis): 1. Chronic arthritis. 2. Degenerative joint disease. 3. Osteoarthritis.

osteoarthrotomy (os′-tē-ō-ar-throt′o-mi): Surgical removal of the articular end of a bone.

osteoarticular (os′tē-ō-ar-tik′ū-lar): Pertaining to or affecting bones and joints.

osteoblast (os′tē-ō-blast): A bone-forming cell.

osteoblastoma (os′tē-ō-blas-tō′ma): An uncommon tumor of osteoblasts; occurs chiefly in the spine in young people.

osteocachexia (os′tē-ō-ka-kek′si-a): Chronic disease of the bone that results in malnutrition. See cachexia.

osteocarcinoma (os′-tē-ō-kar-sin-ō′ma): Carcinoma of a bone or bones.

osteocartilaginous (os′tē-ō-kar-til-aj′i-nus): Composed of both bone and cartilage.

osteocele (os′tē-ō-sēl): The presence in the scrotum of a mass that contains bony deposits.

osteochondral (os-tē-ō-kon′dral): Pertaining to or composed of both bone and cartilage.

osteochondritis (os′-tē-ō-kon-drī′tis): Inflammation of both bone and cartilage. Term most often applied to non-septic conditions, especially avascular necrosis involving a joint surface. **O. DEFORMANS JUVENILIS,** a form of **O.** occurring most often in boys 5–10 years of age; disturbance of growth at the epiphyseal cartilage results in flattening of the head of the femur causing muscle spasm, limitation of movement, limping and sometimes shortening of the leg. Syn., Legg's disease, Legg-Calvé-Perthes disease. **O. DISSECANS,** a form of **O.** in which small pieces of an articular joint may separate to form loose bodies in the joint; seen most often in the knee and shoulder.

osteochondrodystrophia (os′tē-ō-kon′drō-dis′trō-fi-a): Dysplasia of bone and cartilage with atrophy and abnormal development. See dysplasia.

osteochondrofibroma (os′tē-ō-kon′-drō-fī-brō′ma): A tumor containing elements of osteoma, chondroma, and fibroma.

osteochondroma (os′-tē-ō-kon-drō′ma): A benign tumor made up of osseous and cartilaginous tissue.

osteochondromatosis (os′tē-ō-kon-drō-ma-tō′sis): Multiple cartilaginous tumors that form on the surface of bones.

osteochondropathy (os′-tē-ō-kon-drop′a-thi): A pathologic condition of bone and cartilage.

osteochondrosarcoma (os′tē-ō-kon′drō-sar-kō′ma): A sarcomatous tumor of bone and cartilage.

osteochondrosis (os′-tē-ō-kon-drō′sis): A disease of the ossification centers in the bones of children. Usually begins with a degeneration that is followed by regeneration and calcification. May affect the femur, tibia, vertebrae, bones of the wrist or hand and result in deformity. See Scheuermann's disease.

osteoclasia (os′tē-ō-klā′zi-a): The destruction and absorption of bony tissue by osteoclasts.

osteoclasis (os-te-ok′la-sis): The intentional therapeutic fracture of a deformed or misshapen bone to correct the condition. Also osteoclasia, osteoclasty.—osteoclastic, adj.

osteoclast (os′tē-ō-klast): A large multinucleated cell that is formed in the bone marrow; its function is to dissolve or remove unwanted or dead bone.

osteoclastoma (os′-tē-ō-klas-tō′ma): A tumor made up of cells resembling osteoclasts. May be benign, recurrent, or frankly malignant. The usual site is near the end of a long bone. See myeloma.

osteocope (os′tē-ō-kōp): Extreme pain in bone; usually related to syphilitic bone disease.

osteocystoma (os′tē-ō-sis-tō′ma): A cystic tumor of bone usually occurring in childhood or early adolescence. Site is most often the shaft of a long bone, particularly the upper part of the humerus.

osteocyte (os′tē-ō-sīt): A bone cell.

osteodermia (os-tē-ō-der′mi-a): A condition characterized by bony deposits in the skin.

osteodiastasis (os′tē-ō-dī-as′ta-sis): Separation of two adjacent bones.

osteodynia (os-tē-ō-din′i-a): Pain in a bone.

osteodystrophy (os-tē-ō-dis′tro-fil): Faulty formation or growth of bone. Osteodystrophia. **RENAL O.**, renal rickets; see under **rickets**.

osteoempyesis (os′tē-ō-em-pī-ē′sis): Suppuration within a bone.

osteofibroma (os′tē-ō-fi-brō′ma): A tumor made up mostly of fibrous tissue but which has small foci of bony tissue.

osteogenesis (os′tē-ō-jen′e-sis): Formation of bone; development of bones. **O. IMPERFECTA,** an inherited condition in which the bones are brittle and subject to repeated fractures, often resulting in such deformities as pigeon breast and curvature of the spine. The sclera has a blue color and the person may be subject to bruising, hernias, constipation, deafness. Sometimes fractures occur in intrauterine life and sometimes not until the child is old enough to walk. Worldwide; affects both sexes. Also called brittle bones; fagilitas ossium.

osteogenic (os-tē-ō-jen′ik): Bone producing. **O. SARCOMA,** a general term for a malignant tumor arising in cells whose normal function is the production of bone; usually occurring in children and young adults; characterized by pain, swelling, and early metastases especially to the lung.

osteohalisteresis (os′tē-ō-hal-is-ter-ē′sis): Softening of bone due to loss or deficiency of mineral elements.

osteoid (os′tēoid): Resembling bone.

osteolipochondroma (os′tē-ō-līp′ -ō-kon-drō′ma): A chondroma that contains bony and fatty elements.

osteolipoma (os′tē-ō-lī-pō′ma): A lipoma that contains bony tissue.

osteology (os-tē-ol′o-ji): The branch of medicine that is concerned with the scientific study of bones.

osteolysis (os-tē-ol′i-sis): Softening or dissolution of bone, especially that caused by loss of calcium.

osteolytic (os-tē-ō-lit′ik): Relating to osteolysis. Destructive of bone.

osteoma (os-tē-ō′ma): A bony tumor; usually developing on a bone, but may also be on some other organ, *e.g.*, lung or pleura; may be single or multiple. **OSTEOID O.**, a circumscribed tumor, usually benign, seen mostly in the cortex of long bones, occasionally in the cancellous portion; occurs most often in younger persons.

osteomalacia (os′tē-ō-ma-lā′shi -a): A condition of adult life in which there is a softening of bone due to deficiency of vitamin D, calcium, and phosphate, or excessive absorption of calcium and phosphorus from the bones. May occur in malnutrition or pregnancy; often referred to as adult rickets.

osteomyelitis (os′ -tē-ō-mī-e-lī′tis): Inflammation of bone caused by infection with a pyogenic organism such as staphylococcus, streptococcus, pneumococcus, gonococcus, or meningococcus. Usually begins in the bone marrow; may remain localized or spread to other parts of the bone. May be acute, chronic, or iatrogenic, or may follow injury to the bone, a skin infection, or an abscess in another part of the body. **SCLEROSING NONSUPPURATIVE O.**, chronic iatrogenic osteomyelitis involving especially the tibia and the femur, characterized by diffuse inflammation without suppuration, and pain, especially at night; affects mostly young adults. **SUPPURATIVE O.**, may occur as a complication or sequela of typhoid fever or paratyphoid fever, other salmonella infections, or in association with sickle cell anemia. Usually involves the long bones and occurs most often in children under 12 years of age.

osteomyelodysplasia (os′tē-ō-mī′e-lō-dis-plā′zi-a): A condition characterized by thinning of the osseous tissue of bones and accompanying increase in size of the marrow cavity, leukopenia, and fever.

osteoncus (os-tē-ong′kus): A bone tumor. Osteoma.

osteonecrosis (os′tē-ō-nē-krō′sis): Death (necrosis) of bone when it occurs in areas considered large as compared with such small foci of necrosis as occur in dental caries.

osteonosus (os-tē-on′o-sus): Any disease of bone.

osteopath (os′tē-ō-path): One who practices osteopathy.

osteopathy (os-tē-op′a-thi): 1. Any disease of bone. 2. A theory that attributes a wide range of disorders to mechanical derangements of the skeletal system, which it claims can be rectified by suitable manipulations along with adequate nutrition and favorable environment.—osteopathic, adj.

osteopenia (os-tē-ō-pē′ni-a): Loss of bone mass which occurs when bone synthesis is not sufficient to compensate for bone lysis. The bones become less dense and there is a thinning of the cortex of the long bones. Seen in the elderly and in women more than men.

osteoperiostitis (os′tē-ō-per′i-os-tī′tis): Inflammation of periosteum and the bone under it.

osteopetrosis (os′ -tē-ō-pē-trō′sis): A condition in which progressive sclerosis causes a generalized increase in the density of the bones and eventual obliteration of the marrow; may be fatal due to bone marrow failure. Characteristics are clubbing of the ends of long bones, retarded growth, anemia, and a strong tendency to spontaneous fractures. Called also "marble bones" and Albers-Schonberg disease (*q.v.*).

osteophage (os′tē-ō-fāj): Syn., osteoclast (*q.v.*).

osteophlebitis (os′tē-ō-flē-bī′tis): Inflammation of veins in a bone.

osteophone (os′tē-ō-fōn): A device for helping the deaf to hear. An audiophone.

osteophony (os′tē-of′on-i): The conduction of sound waves to the inner ear by bone.

osteophyma (os-tē-ō-fī′ma): A tumor or outgrowth on a bone.

osteophyte (os′tē-ō-fīt): A bony outgrowth or spur, usually at the margins of joint surfaces, *e.g.*, in osteoarthritis.—osteophytic, adj.

osteophytosis (os′tē-ō-fī-tō′ -sis): A condition characterized by the formation of osteocytes. See osteophyte.

osteoplasty (os′tē-ō-plas-ti): Any plastic operation on bone.—osteoplastic, adj.

osteopoikilosis (os′tē-ō-poi-ki-lō′sis): A rare, probably congenital, condition of the bones in which there are multiple areas of sclerosis throughout the bones; usually asymptomatic but the bones are subject to easy fracture; usually discovered by accident on x-ray examination.

osteoporosis (os′tē-ō-po-rō′sis): Loss of density of bone and enlargement of the bone spaces due to disturbance of mineral metabolism, inadequate absorption of calcium into bone, and failure of the osteoclasts to lay down sufficient matrix; characterized by abnormal porousness, fragility, and reduction in quantity of bone. Cause is unknown; begins in the spine, causing compression of the vertebrae which results in low back pain, development of a "dowager's hump," and loss of weight; progresses to the bones of the pelvis, ribs, arms, and legs. Spontaneous fractures may occur. Most often seen in women after menopause; may also accompany pathologic conditions, *e.g.*, parathyroid tumor. **ALVEOLAR O.**, involves the alveolar part of bone which serves as a reservoir for minerals needed to maintain vital functions; seen most often in the alveolar processes of older people following the extraction of teeth and resorption of the processes.—osteoporotic, adj.

osteoradionecrosis (os′tē-ō-rā′di-ō-nē-krō′sis): Necrosis of bone following irradiation.

osteorrhaphy (os-tē-or′a-fi): The suturing or wiring of bone.

osteosarcoma (os′tē-ō-sar-kō′ma): A malignant tumor originating in bone cells or containing bony tissue. See under sarcoma.

osteosclerosis (os′tē-ō-skler-ō′sis): Abnormal density or hardness of bone.—osteosclerotic, adj.

osteosis (os-tē-ō′sis): Metaplastic formation of bone. See metaplasia.

osteospongioma (os′tē-ō-spon′ji-ō′ma): A spongy tumor of bone.

osteosynovitis (os′tē-ō-sin-ō-vī′tis): Inflammation of the synovial membrane covering a joint, along with osteitis of adjacent bone.

osteosynthesis (os-tē-ō-sin′the-sis): Bringing the ends of a fractured bone into close apposition by means of a metal plate or other mechanical means.

osteotabes (os′ -tē-ō-tā′bēz): Degeneration of bone; begins with destruction of bone marrow cells, progresses to spongy bone, then to compact bone.

osteothrombosis (os′tē-ō-throm-bō′sis): Thrombosis of the veins of a bone.

osteotome (os′tē-ō-tōm): An instrument for cutting bone; it is similar to a chisel, but bevelled on both sides of its cutting edge.

osteotomy (os-tē-ot′o-mi): The surgical division, cutting, or repositioning of bones in treatment of diseased or deformed joints or bones.

osteotropic (os′tē-ō-trō′pik): Pertaining to the nutrition of bone.

ostitis (os-tī′tis): Osteitis (*q.v.*).

ostium (os′ti-um): A mouth or opening; often refers to an opening between two cavities, *e.g.*, the entrance to the oviduct or fallopian tube.—ostia, pl.; ostial, adj.

ostomate (os′tō-māt): One who has an artificial opening or stoma into the gastrointestinal canal.

Ostomies Anonymous: A national organization of persons who have had mutilating surgery for treatment of gastrointestinal cancer. Its purpose is to assist such persons to express their fears and anxieties and to adjust to their condition.

ostomy (os′ -to-mi): An informal term referring to a surgical procedure that involves making an artificial opening between two organs or between an organ and the surface of the body. Also used in referring to a patient who has had such an operation.

Ostomy Clubs: Composed of people who are ostomates themselves and who are available to visit patients before and after surgery to answer questions and help in the adjustment to life with a colostomy or ileostomy.

OT: Abbreviation for: 1. Old tuberculin. 2. Occupational therapy.

ot-, oto-: Combining forms denoting the ear.

otalgia (ō-tal′ji-a): Earache.

OTC: Over the counter. Refers to drugs that can be purchased without a prescription.

otiatrics (ō-ti-at'riks): The branch of medicine that deals with the science and treatment of ear diseases.

otic (ō'tik): Pertaining to the ear.

otitis (ō-tī'tis): Inflammation of the ear. **O. EXTERNA,** inflammation of the external auditory canal. **O. INTERNA, O.** of the inner ear, usually caused by extension of inflammation from the middle ear; main symptoms are dizziness, nausea, nystagmus, headache and possibly deafness. **O. MEDIA, O.** of the middle ear; may be acute or chronic; may follow infectious disease such as measles or scarlet fever; chief symptoms are pain, fever, tinnitis, bulging of the tympanic membrane, possibly deafness. **SEROUS O. MEDIA,** a common disorder of the middle ear; usually occurs in children; not pyogenic; may be due to a virus or allergy. Marked by a serious discharge; when chronic may lead to conductive deafness.

otoantritis (ō-tō-an-trī'tis): Inflammation of the mastoid antrum.

otoblennorrhea (ō'tō-blen-ō-rē'a): A mucous discharge from the ear.

otocleisis (ō-tō-klī'sis): Closure of the eustachian tube or of the external auditory canal; may be caused by a new growth or by collection of cerumen in the external canal.

otodynia (ō-tō-din'i-a): Earache. Otalgia.

otoencephalitis (ō'tō-en-sef-a-lī'tis): Inflammation of the brain resulting from an extention of inflammation of the middle ear.

otogenic (ō'tō-jen'ik): Originating within the ear, inflammation of the ear in particular.

otolaryngologist (ō'tō-lar-in-gol'o-jist): A physician who specializes in otolaryngology.

otolaryngology (ō'tō-lar-in-gol'o-ji): Strictly speaking, the branch of medical science that deals with the structure, function, and diseases of the ear, larynx, and laryngeal area; sometimes includes diseases of the upper respiratory tract and some diseases of the head and neck.

otoliths (ō'tō-līths): Tiny dustlike deposits of calcium carbonate within the membranous labyrinth of the inner ear.

otologist (ō-tol'ō-jist): One specializing in the functions and diseases of the ear.

otology (ō-tol'o-ji): The branch of medical science that deals with the structure, functions, and diseases of the ear.—otologic, adj.

-otomy: Refers to a surgical incision.

otomycosis (ō' -tō-mī-kō'sis): A fungal (Aspergillus, Candida) infection of the external auditory meatus and canal, accompanied by itching, pain, and scaling; usually bilateral—otomycotic, adj.

otopathy (ō-top'a-thi): Any disease of the ear.

otopharyngeal (ō'tō-fa-rin'jē-al): Pertaining to the ear and pharynx.

otophone (ō'tō-fōn): An ear trumpet.

otoplasty (ō'tō-plas-ti): Plastic surgery for the correction of deformed, flattened, or protruding ears; done preferably during childhood.

otopyorrhea (ō' -tō-pī-o-rē'a): Flow of purulent discharge from the ear; often results from chronic otitis media with perforation of the ear drum.

otopyosis (ō-tō-pī-ō'sis): Suppuration occurring in the external auditory canal; often associated with suppuration in the middle ear.

otorhinolaryngology (ō'tō-rī'nō-lar-in-gol'o-ji): The branch of medical science that deals with the structure, function, and diseases of the ear, nose and larynx.

otorhinology (ō'tō-rī-nol'o-ji): The branch of medicine that deals with the ear and nose.

otorrhagia (ō-tō-rā' -ji-a): A bloody or purulent discharge from the external auditory canal due to inflammation of the ear.

otorrhea (ō-tō-rē'a): A discharge from the external auditory meatus, especially one that is mucopurulent.

otosalpinx (ō-tō-sal'pinks): The eustachian tube.

otosclerosis (ō'tō-skle-rō'sis): A condition of progressive deafness marked by new bone formation affecting primarily the labyrinth of the inner ear and causing ankylosis of the stapes to the margin of the round window. Of unknown origin; heredity may be a factor.—otosclerotic, adj.

otoscope (ō'tō-skōp): An instrument for examining the ear; auriscope (*q.v.*).—otoscopic, adj.

otoscopy (ō-tos'kō-pi): Visualization of the external auditory canal and the tympanic membrane by means of an otoscope.

otosis (ō-tō'sis): Mishearing spoken words.

otosteal (ō-tos'tē-al): Pertaining to the small bones of the middle ear.

ototomy (ō-tot'o-mi): 1. Incision of the drum membrane; myringotomy. 2. The anatomy of the ear.

ototoxic (ō-tō-tok'sik): Refers to a substance that has a toxic effect on the organs of balance and hearing, or on the eighth cranial nerve.

ototoxicity (ō-tō-tok-sis'i-ti): The quality of being toxic or damaging to the eighth cranial nerve or to the organs of equilibrium and hearing.

O.U.: Abbreviation for 1) *oculi unitas* [L.] meaning both eyes together; 2) *oculi uterque* [L.] meaning each eye.

ounce: A measure of weight. In the avoirdupois system it is 1/16 of a pound, or 437.5 grains. In the apothecaries' system it is 1/12 of a pound, or 480 grains. A fluid ounce is equal to

8 fluidrams in the apothecaries' system, 29.57 ml in the metric system. Abbreviation oz.

outlet: An opening, usually in the nature of a passageway, by means of which something escapes.

outpatient: An ambulatory patient who does not require admission to a hospital bed, but who comes to the hospital outpatient department for treatment; these patients may also be given attention at doctors' offices, emergency rooms, and hospital clinics.

output: 1. The quantity of waste substance produced by a process such as metabolism and excreted from the body, *e.g.*, the amount of urine voided in a given time. Opp. of intake. 2. The amount of a substance ejected from a given place, *e.g.*, the cardiac output of blood.

outreach: In health care, refers to a system or program that functions to help those in need of various services to learn what services are available to them and how to obtain them. O. WORKER, in health care, one who goes into the community to seek those in need of help.

ov-, ovi-, ovo-: Combining forms denoting ovum.

oval window: Fenestra ovalis: see under fenestra.

ovar-, ovari-, ovario-: Combining forms denoting 1) ovary; 2) ovarian.

ovarialgia (ō-var-i-al'ji-a): Pain in an ovary.

ovarian (ō-var'i-an): Pertaining to the ovaries. O. CYST, a tumor that forms on the surface of the ovary; may be benign or malignant. O. CYSTECTOMY, the removal of cystic tissue from an ovary without disturbing the remaining tissue.

ovariectomy (ō-var-i-ek'to-mi): Excision of an ovary. Oophorectomy.

ovariocele (ō-var'-i-ō-sēl): A hernia of an ovary.

ovariocentesis (ō-var'i-ō-sen-tē'sis): Surgical puncture of an ovary usually for the drainage of an ovarian cyst.

ovariocyesis (ō-var'i-ō-sī-ē'sis): Ovarian pregnancy.

ovarioncus (ō-var-i-ong'kus): Tumor of the ovary.

ovariopexy (ō-var'i-ō-pek'-si): The surgical procedure of elevating and fixing an ovary to the abdominal wall.

ovariorrhexis (ō-var'i-ō-rek'sis): Rupture of an ovary.

ovariosalpingectomy (ō-var'i-ō-sal-pin-jek'to-mi): The surgical removal of an ovary and uterine tube.

ovariotomy (ō-var-i-ot'om-i): Literally means incision of an ovary, but it is the term usually applied to the removal of an ovary. Also oophorectomy.

ovaritis (ō'var-ī'tis): Oophoritis (*q.v.*).

ovary (ō'va-ri): One of the paired sex glands of the female; an oval, flattened gland, about 1½ inches long, suspended on the posterior surface of the broad ligament, one on either side of the uterus. The substance is vascular and fibrous and contains the egg cells, one of which matures and is expelled periodically. Function of the gland is to develop the egg cells and also to produce the female sex hormones. CYSTIC O., retention cysts in the ovarian follicles. POLYCYSTIC O., the ovary is enlarged and the cortex contains multiple small follicular cysts; associated with an endocrine disturbance.

over the counter: In pharmacology, refers to drugs sold without a physician's prescription but within the law.

overcompensation (ō'ver-kom-pen-sā'shun): Name given any type of behavior a person adopts in order to cover up a deficiency in his personality, of which he is aware. Thus a person who is afraid may react by becoming arrogant or boastful or quarrelsome.

overdosage: The administration or taking of an excessive dose of a drug; the amount considered overdose varies with the individual and the degree of tolerance he may have built up for the drug.

overextension (ō-ver-eks-ten'shun): Extension beyond the usual normal limit, said of a joint or muscle.

overflow: Continuous escape of fluid such as tears or urine.

overhydration (ō-ver-hī-drā'shun): The presence of excess fluids in the body tissues; often associated with congestive heart failure and renal pathology; signs and symptoms include edema, puffy eyelids, tachypnea, oversecretion of antidiuretic hormone.

overriding: 1. The slipping of one end of a fractured bone past the other end. 2. The molding of the fetus's head during delivery.

overt (ō-vert'): Obvious, manifest; open to view.

overtoe: A condition in which the great toe lies over the adjacent toes. Hallux varus.

overventilation: See hyperventilation.

oviduct (ō'vi-dukt): Syn., fallopian tube (*q.v.*). Also called uterine tube.

ovotestis (ō-vō-tes'tis): A gonad that contains both ovarian and testicular tissue.

ovotherapy (ō-vō-ther'a-pi): Therapeutic use of ovarian secretion, particularly that from the corpus luteum.

ovulation (ov-ū-lā'shun): The process of maturation and rupture of a graafian follicle, with the discharge of the ovum; should occur 14 days before the next menstrual flow is expected. O. method, see Billings ovulation method.

ovule (ō′vūl): The ovum before it has been expelled from the ovary.

ovum (ō′vum): The female reproductive cell; a round cell about 0.1 mm in diameter that develops in the graafian follicle and, when mature, is expelled by the follicle into the abdominal cavity whence it enters the fallopian tube; unless fertilized is cast off; this occurs approximately every 28 days during a female's life, from puberty to menopause.—ova, pl.; ovarian, adj.

oxalate (ok′sa-lāt): Any salt of oxalic acid.

oxalemia (ok-sa-lē′mi-a): Presence of abnormally large amounts of oxalates in the blood.

oxalic acid (ok-sal′ik): An organic acid found in many plants that are used as foods.

oxalosis (oks-a-lo′-sis): A genetic disorder characterized by excessive urinary excretion of oxalate, nephrolithiasis, renal failure.

oxaluria (ok-sa-lū′ri-a): The excretion of urine containing calcium oxalate crystals; often associated with dyspepsia (*q.v.*).

oxidant (oks′i-dant): An oxidizing agent. See oxidize.

oxidase (ok′si-dās): Any enzyme which promotes oxidation.

oxidation (ok-si-dā′shun): The process of converting a substance into an oxide by the addition of oxygen. The carbon in organic compounds undergoes **O.** with the formation of carbon dioxide when they are combusted in air, or when they are metabolized in living material in the presence of oxygen. Also used in biochemistry in the process of removing hydrogen from a molecule (*e.g.*, in the presence of air, ascorbic acid undergoes **O.** with the formation of dehydroascorbic acid). The loss of an electron with an increase in valency (*e.g.*, the conversion of ferrous to ferric iron) is also an **O.** The greater part of the energy present in foods is made available to the body by the process of **O.** in the tissues.

oxide (ok′sīd): Any compound of oxygen with another element or radical, usually a metal.

oxidize (ok′si-dīz): To combine oxygen with an element or a radical, or to cause such combination to take place.

oxidosis (ok-si-dō′sis): Acidosis (*q.v.*).

oximeter (ok-sim′i-ter): A photoelectric device for measuring the level of oxygen saturation of the circulating blood.

oximetry (ok-sim′e-tri): The use of an oximeter to determine the oxygen saturation level in the arterial blood.

oxy-: Combining form denoting: 1. The presence of oxygen in a substance. 2. Pointed. 3. Sharp, 4. Sour. 5. Quick.

oxyblepsia (ok-sē-blep′si-a): Unusual acuteness of vision.

oxycephaly (ok-sē-sef′a-li): A congenital deformity in which the head is more pointed than rounded.

oxygen (ok′si-jen): A colorless, odorless gaseous element, necessary for life and combustion. The most abundant element on earth; constitutes 20 percent by weight of air. Used medicinally as an inhalation, supplied in cylinders in which the gas is at a high pressure. See hyperbaric. **O. MASK,** used mainly for administering oxygen when the patient requires it for only a short time, or intermittently. **O. TENT,** transparent plastic tent which encloses the patient and part or all of the bed; used to provide a constantly oxygenated environment. **O. THERAPY,** administration of oxygen in conditions resulting from oxygen deficiency, for example, pneumonia, congestive heart failure, coronary thrombosis; may be administered by mask, nasal catheter, tent, or special oxygen chamber.

oxygen dissociation curve: The release of oxygen from the red blood cells in the capillaries into the interstitial fluid from which it can enter the cells, as demonstrated on a plotted curve.

oxygenation (ok′si-je-nā′shun): The saturation of a substance (particularly blood) with oxygen.—oxygenated, adj.

oxygenator (ok′si-je-nā′tor): A device for oxygenating the blood outside of the body. The artificial lung as used in heart surgery.

oxygeusia (ok′si-gū′si-a): Abnormally keen sense of taste.

oxyhemoglobin (ok′ -si-hē-mō-glō′bin): Oxygenated hemoglobin, an unstable compound.

oxyhemoglobinometer (ok′si-hē′mō-glō-bin-om′e-ter): An instrument for measuring the oxygen level in the blood.

oxylalia (ok-si-lā′li-a): Abnormally fast speech.

oxymyoglobin (ok′ -si-mī-ō-glō′bin): Oxygen combined with myoglobin.

oxyntic (ok-sin′tik): Producing acid. **O. CELLS,** the cells in the gastric mucosa which produce hydrochloric acid.

oxyopia (ok-si-ō′pi-a): Abnormally acute vision.

oxyosmia (ok-si-os′mi-a): Abnormally acute sense of smell.

oxyphonia (ok-si-fō′ni-a): An unusually sharp quality of the voice.

oxytocic (ok-si-tō′sik): 1. Hastening parturition. 2. An agent promoting uterine contractions.

oxytocin (ok-si-tō′sin): One of two hormones formed in the posterior pituitary gland, the other being vasopressin (*q.v.*). Stimulates contraction of the uterine muscles.

oxyuriasis (ok-si-ū-rī'a-sis): Infestation with pinworms or threadworms.

oz: Abbreviation for ounce.

ozena (ō-zē'na): An atrophic condition of the nasal mucous membrane with associated crusting and an offensive-smelling discharge.

ozone (ō'zōn): 1. A modified and condensed form of oxygen; a slightly blue irritating gas, generated naturally by the action of ultraviolet light rays on oxygen; also made commercially; O_3. Has stronger oxidizing properties than oxygen; is used as an antiseptic and disinfectant, *e.g.*, in the purification of water. 2. May be descriptive of air that contains a perceptible amount of O_3, seaside air, *e.g.*

ozostomia (ō' -zō-stō'mi-a): Foul breath; halitosis.

P

P: Chemical symbol for phosphorus. P^{32} radioactive phosphorus.

P wave: In the electrocardiogram it represents the contraction of the ventricles during the heartbeat.

PA: Abbreviation for: 1. Paralysis agitans. 2. Pathology. 3. Percussion and auscultation. 4. Pernicious anemia. 5. Physicians' assistant. 6. Posterior-anterior. 7. Psychoanalyst. 8. Pulmonary artery.

PAS: Abbreviation for para-aminosalicylic acid. PASA is also used.

Pablum: Trade name for a precooked cereal food for infants; contains wheat, oat, and corn meals in addition to iron, sodium chloride, wheat embryo, alfalfa leaves.

pabulum (pab'ū-lum): Food or nourishment.

PAC: Abbreviation for: 1. Premature atrial contraction. 2. Phenacetin, aspirin, and caffeine.

Pacchioni's bodies (pak-ē-ō'nēz): Projections of the arachnoid membrane through the dura mater into the superior sagittal sinus. Also called arachnoid granulations.

PACE: Patient Appraisal and Care Evaluation; a system for assessing nursing home patients' needs; developed by the Department of Health, Education and Welfare in 1978.

pacemaker: In anatomy, a body part that initiates and maintains a rhythmic activity, the sinoatrial node in particular. **ARTIFICIAL P.**, an electrical device used to reestablish the muscular contractions of an arrested heart or to steady the heartbeat; consists of an electrode introduced into the right atrium or ventricle and attached to an electrical source that is either implanted within the body or located externally; it initiates an increase in the rate of contraction of the ventricle resulting in output adequate to allow the patient to participate in his usual activities. **ASYNCHRONOUS P.**, a device that paces the heartbeat when the heart beats too slowly or not at all without help; also called fixed-rate **P.** **ATRIAL P.**, used to stimulate atrial contraction when the conduction system between the atria and ventricles is intact. **DEMAND P.**, a **P.** that will provide or withhold stimulation depending on how the heart is functioning on its own. **EXTERNAL P.**, a temporary **P.** placed outside the body until a permanent **P.** can be implanted. **MONITORING P.**, allows the patient to lead a fairly normal life. **TEMPORARY P.**, used in certain emergency situations to correct severe cardiac arrhythmias; usually inserted into the subclavian, jugular, basilic, or femoral vein. **WANDERING P.**, a condition in which the origin of the heartbeat is shifted from the head of the sinoatrial node to the lower or other part of the atrium.

pachy-: Combining form denoting thick.

pachyblepharon (pak'i-blef'a-ron): Thickening of an eyelid, especially near the edge.

pachycephalia (pak'i-se-fā'li-a): Abnormal thickness of the skull bones.—pachycephalic, pachycephalous, adj.

pachycheilia (pak-i-kī'li-a): Abnormal thickness of the lips. Also pachycheilia.

pachydactyly (pak'i-dak'ti-li): Enlargement or thickening of the fingers or toes, especially at their ends.

pachyderma (pak-i-der'ma): Abnormal thickness of the skin. See **elephantiasis**. Also pachydermia.—pachydermatous, adj.

pachydermoperiostosis (pak-i-der'mō-per'i-os-tō'sis): A condition characterized by thickening of the skin over bones, especially those of the face and distal parts of the extremities, with clubbing of the fingers; may be hereditary or due to underlying pulmonary disease.

pachyglossia (pak-i-glos'i-a): Abnormal thickness of the tongue.

pachymeningitis (pak-i-men-in-jī'tis): Inflammation of the dura mater (or pachymeninx).

pachymeter (pa-kim'i-ter): An instrument for measuring thickness, especially of thin objects or tissues, *e.g.*, a membrane.

pachyonychia (pak'-i-ō-nik'i-a): Abnormal thickening of the fingernails or toenails, often congenital.

pachypleuritis (pak-i-ploo-rī'tis): Inflammation of the pleura accompanied by thickening of the membrane. Productive pleurisy.

pachysomia (pak-i-sō'mi-a): Abnormal thickening of parts of the body, especially of the soft parts, as seen in acromegaly.

pacifier (pas'i-fī-er): 1. A rubber nipple-shaped device for babies to suck or bite upon. 2. A tranquilizer.

pacing (pās'ing): The application of an electric stimulus to the heart to initiate contractions.

Pacini's corpuscles (pa-chē'nēz): Oval bodies in the deep parts of the corium of the skin that act as end organs for the sense of pressure; found especially in the skin of the hands and feet, but also in tendon and some internal structures. [Filippo Pacini, Italian anatomist. 1812–1883.]

pack: 1. A collection of instruments or equipment needed for a certain medical or surgical procedure. 2. To fill a cavity or tubular structure. 3. A hot or cold, wet or dry dressing applied to the body or part of it.

packed cells: Refers to whole blood from which the plasma has been removed by centrifugation or sedimentation; the cells then have a hematocrit of about 80 percent and are used in certain blood transfusions; also called packed red cells. **P. CELL VOLUME,** the volume of cells in 100 ml of a blood sample after it has been centrifuged.

$PaCO_2$: Abbreviation for partial pressure of carbon dioxide in the arterial blood; it is inversely proportional to alveolar ventilation; low concentrations indicate hyperventilation; high or elevated concentrations indicate hypoventilation.

paed-, paedo-: See words beginning ped- and pedo-.

Paget-Schroeffer syndrome: Axillary or subclavian vein thrombosis, often associated with effort, in fit young persons.

Paget's disease: 1. Osteitis deformans. A chronic disease of the bone that resembles arthritis; of unknown cause. Characterized by softening and thickening of the bones of the spine, skull, pelvis, thigh, and lower legs, and by degeneration of the joints, with consequent distortion and bowing deformity of the long bones. Occurs most often in people of Western European heritage, particularly those from the British Isles, France and Germany and who are in the 60 to 70 year age group. 2. A progressive, inflammatory, eczematous dermatosis of the nipple and surrounding area, seen most often in older women. There is itching, soreness, ulceration and retraction of the nipple. May be precancerous or associated with cancer of the breast. 3. Paget's disease of the vulva, a rare condition seen mostly in postmenopausal women; usually malignant and occurring in association with carcinoma in some other part of the vulvorectal area; symptoms include pain, pruritus, and burning; treatment is usually vulvectomy. [Sir James Paget, English surgeon. 1814–1899.]

pagophagia (pā′gō-fā′ji-a): Ice eating; thought to be a sign of iron deficiency.

pagoplexia (pā′gō-plek′si-a): Frostbite.

PAH: 1. Para-amminohippuric acid, a white crystalline powder the salts of which are used in various kidney function tests. 2. Polycystic aromatic hydrocarbon, found in automobile exhaust; said to be a possible cause of cancer.

pain: Physical or mental suffering. A state of localized or generalized discomfort that ranges from mild distress to acute agony; usually caused by injury to a part or disturbance of the normal condition or functioning of a part of the body. In the plural usually refers to the pains experienced during childbirth. **AFTERPAINS,** those due to contraction of the uterus following the birth of a child. **FALSE P'S,** occur late in pregnancy and resemble labor pains but do not result in labor. **GROWING P'S.,** those that sometimes occur in muscles and joints of adolescents and children; may be manifestation of rheumatic fever. **HUNGER P'S.,** those that occur in the stomach when it is time for a meal; sometimes a sign of gastric disorder. **INTERMENSTRUAL P.,** see mittleschmertz. **LABOR P'S.,** the progressively severe, involuntary, rhythmic pains that occur during childbirth. **PHANTOM LIMB P.,** that which is felt as being in a limb although the limb has been amputated. **PSYCHOGENIC P.,** imaginary **P. REFERRED P.,** that which is felt in a part other than where it is produced. **VASCULAR P.,** results from dilatation of blood vessels, particularly those around the brain; most common in migraine headache. See gate control theory,

painter's colic: Lead colic (*q.v.*). See lead poisoning.

palatable (pal′a-tab′l): Pleasant or agreeable to the taste; savory.

palate (pal′at): The roof of the mouth, consisting of the structures that separate the mouth from the nasal cavity, with its upper surface forming the floor of the nasal cavity; formed by parts of the palatine bones and the maxillae. **ARTIFICIAL P.,** prosthesis for use in correcting cleft palate. **CLEFT P.,** a congenital cleft between the palatal bones which leaves a gap in the roof of the mouth; usually associated with harelip. **HARD P.,** the anterior part of the **P.,** formed by parts of the palatine and maxillary bones. **SOFT P.,** situated at the posterior end of the palate and consisting of muscle covered with mucous membrane; forms the pillars of the fauces and the uvula.—palatal, palatine, adj.

palatine (pal′a-tīn): Pertaining to the palate. **P. ARCHES,** the bilateral double pillars or arch-like folds formed by the descent of the soft palate as it meets the pharynx. **P. BONE,** one of two irregular bones that form the back part of the palate, the lateral walls of the nasal cavity, and the floor of the orbit. **P. PROCESS OF THE MAXILLA,** a horizontal plate of bone extending from each side of the maxilla to form the hard palate. **P. TONSIL,** see tonsil.

palatitis (pal-a-tī′tis): Inflammation of the hard palate.

palatomaxillary (pal′a-tō-mak′si-lar-i): Pertaining to the palate and the maxilla.

palatonasal (pal-a-tō-nā′zal): Pertaining to the palate and the nasal cavity.

palatopharyngoplasty (pal′a-tō-făr-ing′-ō-plas-ti): The surgical removal of excess tissue in the upper throat which vibrates like a reed in a musical instrument, causing snoring.

palatoplasty (pal′a-tō-plas-ti): Plastic surgery of the palate, including operations to correct cleft palate. Uraniscoplasty.

palatoplegia (pal′at-ō-plē′ji-a): Paralysis of the muscles of the soft palate.—palatoplegic, adj.

palatorrhaphy (pal′a-tor′a-fi): An operation for the repair of a cleft palate. Syn., staphylorrhaphy, uraniscoplasty.

paleogenetic (pā′lē-ō-je-net′ik): Having originated in the past; not newly acquired. Said of traits, structures, abnormalities, etc.

paleopathology (pā′ -lē-ō-pa-thol′o-ji): The study of diseases in bodies preserved from ancient times, *e.g.*, mummies.

pali-, palin-: Combining forms denoting again.

palikinesia (pal-i-kī-nē′si-a): Pathological, involuntary repetition of certain movements.

palilalia (pal-i-lā′li-a): The constant repetition of a word or phrase with increasing rapidity and with the speech becoming less and less audible. May occur in persons with parkinsonism following encephalitis, or those with Pick's disease (*q.v.*).

palindromia (pal-in-drō′mi-a): The worsening or recurrence of a disease.—palindromic, adj.

palingenesis (pal′in-jen′e-sis): 1. The restoration or regeneration of a body part that has been lost or removed. 2. The appearance of ancestral characteristics particularly abnormal ones, in successive generations.

palliate (pal′ē-āt): To reduce the severity of; allay; abate; mitigate; lessen. To ease pain or symptoms without curing the condition.

palliative (pal′-ē-ā-tive): 1. Anything which serves to alleviate but cannot cure a disease. 2. Providing relief but not cure.

pallid (pal′id): Lacking the normal amount of color; wan.

pallidectomy (pal-i-dek′to-mi): Destruction of a predetermined section of globus pallidus. See chemopallidectomy and sterotactic surgery.

pallidotomy (pal-i-dot′o-mi): Surgical severance of the fibers from the cerebral cortex to the corpus striatum. Done to relieve the tremor in Parkinson's disease.

pallor (pal′lor): Absence of normal color in the skin, especially of the face; paleness.

palm: The anterior, somewhat concave, flexor surface of the human hand; extends from the wrist to the bases of the fingers. The flat of the hand.

palmar (pal′mar): Pertaining to the palm of the hand. **P. ARCHES**, superficial and deep, formed by the anastomosis of the radial and ulnar arteries.

palmaris (pal-mā′ris): Referring or related to the palm of the hand. **P. LONGUS** and **P. BREVIS**, two of the muscles of the palm of the hand.

palpable (pal′pa-b'l): 1. Evident, plain. 2. Capable of being felt or touched.

palpate (pal′pāt): To examine by touching with the fingers or palms of the hands.

palpation (pal-pā′shun): The act of feeling or touching the external surface of the body in order to determine the condition of a part or organ lying underneath; a procedure used in making physical diagnoses, and involving the ability to interpret the significance of what is being sensed by touch.

palpebra (pal′pe-bra): The eyelid. **INFERIOR P.**, the lower eyelid. **SUPERIOR P.**, the upper eyelid.—palpebral, adj.; palpebrae, pl.

palpebral (pal′pe-bral): Pertaining to the eyelids. **P. CARTILAGES**, the thin, cartilage-like plates of tissue that make up the framework of the eyelids. **P. COMMISSURE**, the union of the upper and lower eyelid, either medial or lateral. **P. FISSURE**, the opening between the two eyelids.

palpebration (pal′pe-brā′shun): 1. Winking. 2. Abnormally frequent winking.

palpebritis (pal′pe-bri′tis): Old term for blepharitis.

palpitation (pal-pi-tā′shun): The sensation that accompanies a condition in which the heart beats very rapidly or there is a change in rhythm of which the person is aware; flutter.

palsy (pawl′zi): Paralysis, temporary or permanent. Term most often used in combination. **BELL'S P.**, facial hemiparesis from a lesion in the seventh (facial) nerve, resulting in distortion of the facial features; cause unknown. [Charles Bell, Scottish physician. 1774–1842.] **BIRTH P.**, **P.** due to injury at birth. **BRACHIAL P.**, cause may be unknown, but may be due to birth trauma or may follow administration of antitoxin, or an influenzal infection; marked by pain across the shoulder and upper arm, weakness and focal paralysis; often bilateral. **BULBAR P.**, a chronic, usually fatal disease caused by degeneration of motor nuclei in the medulla oblongata; characterized by progressive paralysis of muscles of the mouth, pharynx, and larynx. **CEREBRAL P.**, progressive persistent disorder of motor power and coordination, due to damage to the brain. **CREEPING P.**, progressive muscular dystrophy (*q.v.*). **CRUTCH P.**, paralysis of the extensor muscles of the wrist, thumb, and fingers, due to pressure of the crutch crosspiece on the radial nerve in the axilla. **DUCHENNE'S P.**, bulbar **P.** **DYSKINETIC P.**, cerebral **P.**, characterized by uncontrolled movements that disappear during sleep. **ERB'S P.**, paralysis of a group of shoulder and arm muscles; caused by an injury to the brachial plexus or to the lower cervical nerve roots; the arm hangs loosely with the forearm pronated (waiter's tip position); also called Erb-Duchenne paralysis, Duchenne-Erb paralysis. [William Erb, German neurologist. 1840–1921.] **FACIAL P.**, unilateral paralysis of muscles supplied by the seventh cranial nerve. **OCULOMOTOR P.**, paralysis of the oculomotor nerve; accompanied usually by ptosis, dilatation of the pupil, and external deviation of the eye. **PERONEAL P.**, due to compression of the peroneal nerve by tight garters or by sitting with legs crossed; weakness of the peroneal muscles results in dorsiflexion, eversion of the foot, and foot drop. **PROGRESSIVE SUPRANUCLEAR P.**, characterized by staring facial expression, ocular dysfunction, dementia, and progressive spasticity. **PSEUDOBULBAR P.**, resembles bulbar **P.**, but not of bulbar origin; seen in arteriosclerotic parkinsonism when it is associated with emotional instability, dysphagia, dysarthria; marked by spastic weakness of facial muscles, tongue, and pharynx. **"SATURDAY NIGHT" P.**, temporary paralysis of the arm caused by compression of the radial nerve when a drunken person's arm hangs over the back of a chair for several hours; recovery is usually spontaneous within a few weeks. **SCRIVENER'S P.**, an occupational neurosis characterized by painful spasmodic cramps of the fingers, hand, and forearm whenever an attempt is made to write; often called writer's cramp. **SHAKING P.**, paralysis agitans (*q.v.*). **ULNAR P.**, due to injury of the ulnar nerve; usually bilateral; may occur as a result of activities which involve leaning on the elbows for long periods of time; marked by weakness, wasting, and sensory loss in the ulnar area of the hand. **WASTING P.**, progressive muscular dystrophy; see under muscular.

pan-, pant-, panta-, pano-, panto-: Combining forms denoting 1) all, completely whole; 2) general.

panacea (pan-a-sē'a): A universal remedy; a cure-all. Term derived from Panacea, the daughter of Aesculapius, who, along with her sister Hygiea, assisted in caring for the sacred serpents and in carrying out rites in early Greek temples of healing.

panarteritis (pan'ar-ter-ī'tis): Periarteritis nodosa (*q.v.*).

panarthritis (pan-ar-thrī'tis): Inflammation of all the structures of a joint, or of all of the joints.

pancarditis (pan-kar-dī'tis): Inflammation of all the structures of the heart.

Pancoast's tumor: A malignant tumor of the apex of a lung; characterized by neuritic pain in the arm and atrophy of the muscles of the arm and hand, due to involvement of the brachial plexus. Syn., Pancoast's syndrome.

pancreas (pan'krē-as): A long, narrow, tongue-shaped glandular organ lying below and behind the stomach. Its head or right end is encircled by the duodenum and its tail often touches the spleen. It is about 7 in. long and weighs about 3.5 oz. It secretes pancreatic juice which passes into the duodenum via the pancreatic duct and the common bile duct, and acts on all classes of foods. An internal secretion, insulin, produced in the islands of Langerhans (*q.v.*) is required for the regulation of carbohydrate metabolism. **ANNULAR P.**, an anomaly in which the **P.** forms a ring that completely surrounds the duodenum.

pancreatalgia (pan'krē-a-tal'ji-a): Pain in the pancreas or in the area of the pancreas.

pancreatectomy (pan'krē-a-tek'to-mi): Excision of part or the whole of the pancreas.

pancreatic (pan-krē-at'ik): Of or pertaining to the pancreas. **P. DUCT**, begins with the junction of small ducts from lobules in the tail of the pancreas and runs from right to left through the gland, receives other ducts along the way, and finally empties into the common bile duct. **P. JUICE.**, an external secretion of the pancreas; consists of clear alkaline fluid containing trypsinogen, which converts proteins to amino acids; amylase, which converts all starches to maltose and dextrin; and lipase, which converts fats to fatty acids and glycerol.

pancreatic function test: A test involving analysis of aspirated material from the stomach and second part of the duodenum to determine the response of the pancreas to various hormonal stimuli.

pancreatico-: Combining form denoting relationship to the pancreatic duct.

pancreaticojejunostomy (pan-krē-at'i-kō-jē-ju-nos'to-mi): The surgical anastomosis of the pancreatic duct, or of the divided end of the pancreas, with the jejunum.

pancreatin (pan'krē-a-tin): A mixture of pancreatic enzymes obtained from cattle or hogs; used as a digestive or in the preparation of predigested foods.

pancreatitis (pan'krē-a-tī'tis): Inflammation of the pancreas, acute or chronic; may be symptomless or characterized by pain and tenderness of the abdomen, nausea, vomiting, and tympanites. **ACUTE HEMORRHAGIC P.**, characterized by autolysis of pancreatic tissue by enzymatic action, which causes hemorrhage into surrounding tissues, often staining them. **CHRONIC P.** is of two types, 1) painless attacks progressing to loss of pancreatic function, and 2) recurring attacks of progressive severity with destruction of pancreatic tissues.

pancreato-: Combining form denoting relationship to the pancreas.

pancreatoduodenectomy (pan-krē-at'ō-dū-ō-dē-nek'to-mi): Surgical removal of the head of the pancreas and the adjoining loop of duodenum; most often a treatment for certain forms of biliary tract cancer.

pancreatography (pan'krē-a-tog'ra-fi): X-ray examination of the pancreas during surgical exploration, after a contrast medium has been injected into the pancreatic duct.

pancreatolith (pan-krē-at'ō-lith): A pancreatic calculus.

pancreozymin (pan'krē-ō-zī'min): A hormone of the duodenal mucosa that stimulates the secretion of pancreatic enzymes, amylase in particular.

pancytopenia (pan-sī-tō-pē'ni-a): A deficiency of all three types of blood cells—erythrocytes, lymphocytes, and platelets. Aplastic anemia.

pandemic (pan-dem'ik): 1. An infection spreading over a whole country or the world. 2. Widely epidemic.

panencephalitis (pan'en-sef-a-lī'tis): Inflammation of all or most of the brain. **SUBACUTE SCLEROSING P.**, a rare, progressive, often fatal form of **P.**, characterized by lesions in the white matter, demyelination, and pathologic changes in the nerve cells; probably caused by a virus, the measles virus in particular; symptoms include ataxia, seizures, blindness, progressive dementia; occurs most often in children and adolescents. Also called Dawson's encephalitis.

pang: A sudden piercing physical pain or feeling of mental anguish.

panhypopituitarism (pan'hī-pō-pi-tū'i-tar-izm): The condition of complete absence of pituitary secretion; results in pituitary dwarfism, absence of gonadal function, weight loss, hypotension, insufficient thyroid and adrenal function. See Simmon's disease.

panhysterectomy (pan'his-ter-ek'to-mi): Removal of the entire uterus, including the cervix.

panhysterosalpingo-oophorectomy (pan-his'ter-ō-sal-ping'ō-ō-of-ō-rek'tō-mi): Surgical removal of the uterus, cervix, fallopian tubes, and ovaries.

panic (pan'ik): Sudden overwhelming and unreasoning fear resulting in hysteria and irrational behavior. May be brought on by a trifling cause or a situation perceived to be of extreme danger; usually accompanied by frantic efforts to escape. In psychiatry, an attack of intense anxiety with distorted perceptions, loss of rational thought and often considerable disintegration of the personality. **HOMOSEXUAL P.**, an anxiety state that usually climaxes a prolonged period of tension from unconscious conflicts regarding the individual's imagined or real homosexual or bisexual tendencies; characterized by fear, paranoia, and personality disorganization; may herald the onset of schizophrenia.

panmyelopathy (pan-mī-a-lop'a-thi): A condition in which there is a proliferation of the bone marrow elements without visible evidence of neoplasm, along with extramedullary production of blood cells and the presence of immature cells in the circulating blood.

panniculectomy (pa-nik'ū-lek'tō-mi): Surgical removal of the abdominal panniculus adiposus; may be required after an obese person has had a significant weight loss. See panniculus.

panniculitis (pa-nik'ū-lī'tis): Inflammation of the thin sheet of fatty subcutaneous connective tissue of the anterior abdominal wall. **SYSTEMIC NODULAR P.**, recurrent crops of tender movable subcutaneous nodules, most commonly seen on the legs, thighs, buttocks, abdomen, breasts, arms; accompanied by chills, fever, malaise, musculoskeletal aching, splenomegaly, sometimes leukopenia.

panniculus (pa-nik'ū-lus): A layer or sheet of tissue. **P. ADIPOSUS**, a sheet of superficial fascia that contains deposits of fat.

pannus (pan'us): Vascularization of the cornea, usually the upper half, resulting in thickening and opacity and causing dimness of vision; often caused by conjunctival irritation; frequently also a complication of trachoma.

panophthalmitis (pan'of-thal-mī'tis): Inflammation and infection, usually purulent, in all parts of the eye.

panoptosis (pan-op-tō'sis): General prolapse or ptosis of all of the abdominal organs.

panosteitis (pan'os-tē-ī'tis): Inflammation of all constituents of a bone, *i.e.*, medulla, bony tissue, and periosteum.

panotitis (pan-ō-tī'tis): Inflammation of all the parts of the ear.

panphobia (pan-fō'bi-a): Morbid fear of everything.

panproctocolectomy (pan-prok'tō-kō-lek'tō-mi): The surgical excision of all of the rectum and the colon, and the creation of an ileostomy for the elimination of feces.

pansystolic (pan'sis-tol'ik): Holosystolic (*q.v.*).

pant: 1. A short, quick, labored breath. 2. To breathe quickly or with difficulty; to gasp for breath.

pantothenic acid (pan-tō-then'ik as'id): A constituent of the vitamin B complex. Widely distributed in plant and animal tissues; found in yeast, liver, heart, salmon eggs, various grains; also produced synthetically. Is essential for nutrition of certain animal species but its importance to human nutrition is not fully understood. Also known as vitamin B_3.

pantropic (pan-trōp'ik): 1. Having affinity for many body tissues, often said of viruses. 2. Having affinity for many body organs or parts.

panty-girdle syndrome: May occur in women of sedentary occupation when they wear a panty-girdle type of foundation garment; by the end of the day the ankles have become swollen.

PaO_2: Abbreviation for partial pressure of oxygen in arterial blood; it measures the state of oxygenation of the blood, and varies with the patient's age and the ambient air.

PAP: Abbreviation for pulmonary artery pressure.

Pap: **PAP SMEAR,** a vaginal smear prepared for microscopic examination of exfoliated cells. Can also be prepared from many other body secretions including sputum, gastric contents, mammary secretions, washings from a bronchoscope. **P. TEST,** Papanicolaou test; see Papanicolaou.

pap: Any soft, pulpy food for infants or invalids.

papain (pa-pā'in): An enzyme derived from the papaw; it acts as a catalyst in hydrolysis of proteins and polypeptides to amino acids; also has several uses in medicine.

Papanicolaou (pap-a-nik-ō-la'ow): **P. TEST,** a cytologic test for early detection of the presence of cancer cells utilizing cells scraped from the surface of a membrane, or from body secretions or fluids; most often done as a screen for cancer of the cervix. [George N. Papanicolaou, Greek physician and anatomist. 1883–1962.]

papilla (pa-pil'a): A small, nipple-shaped eminence. **CIRCUMVALLATE P.,** the large papillae found at the base of the tongue; arranged in a V shape; contain taste buds. **FILIFORM P.,** fine hairlike papillae at the tip of the tongue. **FUNGIFORM P.,** fungus-shaped papillae found chiefly on the dorsocentral area of the tongue. **MAMMARY P.,** the pigmented projection on the anterior aspect of the mammary gland into which the milk ducts open. **OPTIC P.,** the terminus of the optic nerve at the point where it enters the eyeball. **RENAL P.,** the summit of one of the renal pyramids. **TACTILE P.,** one that projects into the true skin and contains an end organ for touch. **VALLATE P.,** a circumvallate **P.**—papillae, pl; papillary, adj.

papillary (pap'i-ler-i): Pertaining to or resembling a papilla or nipple. **P. MUSCLES,** small cone-shaped muscles that project from the walls of the ventricles and attach to the chordae tendinae (*q.v.*); when the ventricles fill with blood and contract, these muscles also contract and tighten the chordae, pressing the valves shut but preventing them from being pushed back into the atria by the surging blood.

papilledema (pap-il-ē-dē'ma): Edema of the optic disk; indicative of increased intracranial pressure. Choked disk (*q.v.*).

papilliferous (pap'i-lif'er-us): Containing or provided with papillae.

papillitis (pap'i-lī'tis): 1. Inflammation of a papilla. 2. Inflammation and edema of the optic disk. **CHRONIC LINGUAL P.,** painful glossitis that often extends to the palate and cheeks; characterized by redness, burning, and desquamation of the stratum corneum; most often seen in middle-aged women; Moeller's glossitis. **NECRETIZING P.,** necrosis of the renal papillae; seen in the most severe forms of pyelonephritis (*q.v.*).

papilloma (pap-i-lō'ma): A branching or lobulated, circumscribed epithelial neoplasm, usually benign, arising in the skin or mucous membrane; may appear as a wart, condyloma, or polyp. **DUCTAL P.,** a benign tumor of the mammary duct system of the breast; characterized by atypical papillary structures. **VILLOUS P., P.** characterized by long slender processes; usually seen in the urinary bladder.

papillomatosis (pap'i-lō-ma-tō'sis): The simultaneous widespread development of several papillomata.

papillomavirus (pap'i-lō-ma-vī'rus): Any of a group of small viruses that cause papillomata in humans.

papovavirus (pa-po'-va-vī'rus): Any of a group of small viruses, many of which are thought to be the cause or potential cause of tumors, and some of which cause warts.

Pappenheimer's bodies: Granules containing iron that are sometimes found in the cytoplasm of normoblasts and erythrocytes after splenectomy.

papule (pap'ūl): A small, solid, usually round or conical, circumscribed elevation on the skin. A pimple.—papular, adj.; papulation, n.

papulopustular (pap'-ū-lō-pus'-tū-lar): Pertaining to an eruption composed of both papules and pustules.

papulosis (pap-ū-lō'sis): A condition marked by the presence of multiple papules on the skin. **LYMPHOMATOID P.,** a form of **P.** characterized by ulcerative lesions, with new lesions occurring as others recede.

papulosquamous (pap'ū-lō-skwā'mus): Both papular and scaly; pertains to certain dermatoses, including psoriasis, pityriasis rosea, and lichen planus.

papyraceous (pap-i-rā'shus): Like paper or parchment. **P. FETUS,** a dead twin fetus that has been compressed by the other growing twin and which has a mummy-like, parchment appearance.

par-, para-: Prefixes denoting 1) beside, alongside, parallel; 2) closely resembling a true form, *e.g.*, paratyphoid; 3) faulty, irregular, abnormal, perverted.

Para: A word used to designate the number of pregnancies a woman has had that have resulted in viable births. It is usually capitalized and combined with the proper numeral, *e.g.*, Para I, II, etc.

para-aminobenzoic acid (par-a-am'i-nō-ben-zō'ik as'id): Often occurs as a member of the vitamin B complex. Found in certain meats, cereal grains, milk products, and eggs; also occurs in small amounts in body fluids, particularly cerebrospinal fluid, blood, urine, and sweat; also known as vitamin H_1. Sometimes used as an antirickettsial drug, and in treatment of certain dermatoses. Abbreviated PABA.

para-aminosalicylic acid (par-a-am′i-nō-sal-i-sil′ik): A synthetic drug that acts as a tuberculostatic. Abbreviated PAS or PASA.

para-arthria (par-a-ar′-thri-a): The imperfect utterance of words.

Paracelsus (par-a-sel′sus): [Philippus Aureolus Theophrastus Bombastus Hohenheim Paracelsus, Swiss physician and alchemist. 1493–1541.] Introduced such substances as lead, iron, sulfur, and arsenic into medicine.

paracentesis (par′a-sen-tē′sis): Puncture, particularly the puncture of a fluid-filled body cavity by a needle or trocar for the purpose of drawing off fluid; designated according to the particular cavity that is punctured, *e.g.*, abdominal, thoracic, etc.

paracervical block: A form of regional anesthesia used during labor; consists of the injection of an anesthetic into the area on each side of the uterus.

paracholia (par-a-kō′li-a): A condition characterized by disordered secretion of bile.

parachroma (par-a-krō′ma): Abnormal or unusual coloration of the skin.

parachromatopsia (par′a-krō′ma-top′si-a): Partial color blindness. Dichromatopsia.

paracoccidioidomycosis (par′a-kok-sid-i-oy′dō-mī-kō′sis): South American blastomycosis, caused by the *Paracoccicioides brasiliensis;* see blastomycosis. Chronic mycosis, characterized by painful ulceration of mucocutaneous areas of the mouth and nose and disseminated to the lung, liver, spleen, pancreas, kidney, and possibly the brain. Symptoms include anorexia, abdominal pain, diarrhea. Fatal if untreated.

paracolpitis (par-a-kōl-pī′tis): Inflammation of the tissues surrounding the vagina.

paracusia (par-a-kū′si-a): Impaired or disordered hearing. Paracusis.

paracyesis (par-a-sī-ē′sis): Extrauterine pregnancy.

paradigm (par′a-dim): An example or pattern.

paradipsia (par-a-dip′si-a): A perverted and exaggerated appetite for fluids out of proportion to the needs of the body.

paradoxical (par-a-dok′si-kal): Occurring in a manner that is inconsistent with or contrary to the normal or usual. **P. BREATHING,** occurs in patients whose chest is opened by severe injury; during inspiration the affected part is sucked in as the lung fills and during expiration the affected part bulges out. **P. BLOOD PRESSURE,** a diminution in systemic arterial pressure on inspiration and a strengthening on expiration; this is normal in deep breathing; otherwise it may indicate cardiac tamponade. **P. PULSE,** see pulsus paradoxus.

paraesophageal (par′a-ē-sof-a-jē′al): Situated alongside the esophagus. **P. CYST,** a cyst that has its origin in a bronchus and ultimately connects with the esophageal wall. **P. HERNIA,** a hiatal hernia in which part of the stomach herniates into the thorax.

paraffin (par′a-fin): A colorless, odorless, tasteless, white or somewhat translucent substance obtained from petroleum. **P. BATH,** a physical therapy treatment in which part or all of an extremity is dipped into or brushed with liquid paraffin repeatedly to form a thick coating.

parafollicular (par-a-fo-lik′ū-lar): Associated with or in the vicinity of a follicular structure. **P. CELLS,** argyrophil cells, cells found between or among the follicles in the thyroid epithelium; they are thought to be the source of thyrocalcitonin and are rich in mitochondria.

paragammacism (par-a-gam′a-sizm): Faulty pronunciation of the letters *g* and *k* and of *ch*.

paraganglioma (par-a-gang-gli-ō′ma): A benign neoplasm that occurs in the medullary portion of the adrenal gland.

paraganglion (par-a-gang′gli-on): Any of the small chromaffin cells (*q.v.*) or group of them. They secrete epinephrine and norepinephrine.—paraganglia, pl.

parageusia (par-a-gū′si-a): 1. A disorder or perversion of the sense of taste. 2. An unpleasant taste in the mouth.

paraglossia (par-a-glos′i-a): Swelling of the tongue.

paragnathus (par′ag-nath′us): A fetus with a supernumerary or malformed jaw.

paragonimiasis (par′a-gon-i-mī′a-sis): The condition of being infected with one of the lung flukes of the genus *Paragonimus,* a fairly common human and animal parasite, occurring endemically in the Orient and frequently in western U.S.; occurs through eating raw fresh water shellfish; symptoms include hemoptysis, bronchitis, anorexia, cough, chest pain, diarrhea, possibly hemiplegia, brain involvement, seizures.

paragraphia (par-a-graf′i-a): A psychological condition in which a person understands words and their meanings but is unable to write correctly from dictation, or uses the wrong word in writing, or makes mistakes in writing.

parahemophilia (par′a-hē-mō-fil′i-a): An inherited tendency to hemorrhage due to absence of coagulation factor V.

parahormone (par-a-hor′mōn): A substance that acts to control the function of a distant part or organ but is not a true hormone. A common example is carbon dioxide which acts on the respiratory center in the brain.

parainfluenza virus: Several serotypes are recognized. Infection in adults is associated with pharyngitis, hoarseness, and tracheitis; in children the virus is associated with croup.

parakeratosis (par′a-ker-a-tō′sis): Any disorder of the horny layer of the skin, particularly if it interferes with keratinization.

paralalia (par-a-lā′li-a): A disorder of speech in which sounds are distorted or one letter is substituted for another.

paralambdacism (par-a-lam′da-sizm): Inability to pronounce the letter *l* (ell), or the substitution of another letter for it.

paralanguage (par-a-lang′waj): Nonverbal aspects of speech, *i.e.*, voice quality, intonation, pitch, rhythm, loudness, silence, head nodding, position, body movements, facial expression, etc.; important in studies of personality. Also called paralinguistics.

paralepsy (par′a-lep-si): Psycholepsy (*q.v.*).

paralexia (par-a-lek′si-a): An impairment of reading ability, characterized by the transposition of words and syllables so that the resulting combinations are meaningless.

parallagma (par-a-lag′ma): The displacement of the ends or the fragments of a fractured bone.

parallax (par′-a-laks): The apparent displacement of an object when viewed from different points not on a straight line with the object. Noted in cylinders or measuring glasses in which a reading taken at the lower line of the meniscus will differ from that at the upper line.

parallergy (par-al′er-ji):A condition in which sensitization of the body with a specific allergen predisposes the individual to susceptibility to nonspecific allergens.

paralogia (par′a-lō′ji-a): Inability to reason, marked by illogical speech and self-deception.

Paralympics (par-a-lim′piks): An international sports contest, organized in 1952 for paraplegic patients; since 1976 non-wheelchair contestants have been admitted, including the blind and amputees. Events are held in conjunction with the regular Olympic Games.

paralysis (pa-ral′i-sis): Complete or incomplete, temporary or permanent loss of motor function or of sensation in a part of the body; may be caused by damage to the central or peripheral nervous system by injury, disease, or certain chemical poisonings or drugs. Many types are described, usually according to etiology, the part or parts affected or the extent to which they are affected, or muscle tone, *i.e.*, whether the muscles are flaccid or spastic. See also palsy; paresis. **P. AGITANS**, see Parkinson's disease. **ASCENDING P.**, **P.** that begins in the legs and ascends toward the head. **BRACHIAL P.**, **P.** of the arm due to a lesion in the brachial plexus; see under palsy. **BULBAR P.**, involves the labioglossopharyngeal region; see under palsy. **DIPHTHERITIC P.**, affects the uvula and usually some other muscles; appears two or three weeks after an attack of diphtheria; due to toxic neuritis. **DIVER'S P.**, see caisson disease. **EMOTIONAL P.**, occurs in hysterical subjects. **ERB'S P.**, Erb's palsy; see under palsy. **ERB-DUCHENNE P.**, upper brachial plexus paralysis; due to birth injury of the upper cervical nerve roots; affects chiefly the muscles controlling abduction and external rotation of the arm and flexion and supination of the forearm; see under palsy. **FACIAL P.**, Bell's palsy, see under palsy. **FAMILIAL PERIODIC P.**, a condition characterized by episodes of weakness caused by a hereditary tendency to fluctuation in potassium balance; treated by correcting electrolyte balance. **FLACCID P.**, results mainly from lower motor neuron lesions; tendon reflexes are diminished or absent. **INFANTILE P.**, anterior poliomyelitis; see poliomyelitis. **KLUMPKE'S P.**, **P.** and atrophy of forearm and hand muscles, along with sensory and pupillary disturbances; due to injury of the lower part of the brachial plexus, often a birth injury; see Erb's palsy. **LANDRY'S P.**, acute ascending **P.** beginning in the feet and rapidly progressing; characterized by fever; may terminate in respiratory stasis and death. **PERIODIC P.**, a group of disorders characterized by attacks of muscular weakness beginning when the individual is exposed to cold or is at rest after exercise; there are no other symptoms and recovery between attacks is complete. **PROGRESSIVE BULBAR P.**, bulbar **P.** that begins in later life; due to the atrophic degeneration that is characteristic of aging. **PSEUDOBULBAR P.**, affects chiefly the facial muscles; there is gross disturbance in control of the tongue, bilateral hemiplegia, and mental changes following a succession of "strokes"; resembles bulbar **P.** **SPASTIC P.**, results mainly from upper motor neuron lesions; there are exaggerated tendon reflexes, rigidity of muscles of the extremities with atrophy. **TICK P.**, caused by the bite of a tick found in certain parts of the world; affects both animals and children; a flaccid ascending motor paralysis is the principal symptom, which usually disappears when the tick is removed; see Dermacenter.

paralytic (par-a-lit′ik): 1. A person afflicted with paralysis. 2. Pertaining to paralysis. **P. ILEUS**, paralysis of the intestinal muscle, so that the bowel content cannot pass onward even though there is no mechanical obstruction; may be a complication of abdominal surgery.—See also aperistalsis.

paralytogenic (par′a-lit-ō-jen′ik): Causing paralysis.

paralyze (par′a-līz): To produce a state of paralysis (*q.v.*).

paramania (par-a-mā′ni-a): A condition characterized by enjoyment of complaining.

Paramecium (par′a-mē′shi-um): A genus of ciliated protozoa.

paramedian (par-a-mē′di-an): Situated near the midline.

paramedic (par-a-med′ik): 1. A person who is not a physician who works in a paramedical field; may be a pharmacist; technician; physical, occupational, or speech therapist; or a medical social worker. 2. A person who has had training in emergency intensive care; often utilized to staff ambulances and rescue squads; fire fighters and police officers often receive this training.

paramedical (par-a-med′i-kal): Having an indirect or secondary relationship to the practice of medicine. **P. WORKERS,** include nurses; pharmacists; technicians; physical, occupational, and speech therapists; social workers; dentists; podiatrists.

paramenia (par-a-mē′ni-a): Disordered menstruation.

parametrial (par-a-mē′tri-al): Pertaining to the parametrium (*q.v.*).

parametric (par-a-met′rik): Around the uterus.

parametritis (par-a-mē-trī′tis): Inflammation of the parametrium (*q.v.*).

parametrium (par-a-mē′tri-um): The connective tissues and smooth muscle of the pelvic floor and immediately surrounding the lower part of the uterus and extending laterally between the layers of the broad ligament.—parametrial, adj.

paramimia (par-a-mim′i-a): Faulty or incorrect use of muscles and gestures in the verbal expression of thoughts.

paramnesia (par-am-nē′zi-a): A disorder of memory characterized by the belief that certain events that never took place actually occurred; it is involuntary falsification. Also sometimes denotes a person who remembers words but forgets their meanings so that use of them results in incomprehensible speech.

paramorphia (par-a-mor′fi-a): Any abnormality of structure or form.

paramyoclonus (par′a-mī-ok′lo-nus): A condition in which various unrelated muscles go into myoclonic contraction. See **myoclonus.**

paramyotonia (par′a-mī-ō-tō′ni-a): A condition in which impaired muscle tone results in tonic muscle spasms. **P. CONGENITA,** a congenital **P.** that is induced by exposure to cold, which causes intermittent flaccid paralysis but does not permanently affect the muscles.

paramyxovirus (par′a-mik-sō-vī′rus): A subgroup of the myxovirus group; includes the viruses that cause mumps, measles, parainfluenza, possibly syncytial virus disease. Infection with **P.,** may have serious complications involving the breast, seminal vesicles, prostate gland, or pancreas.

paranasal (par-a-nā′zal): Near the nasal cavities, as the various sinuses. **P. SINUSES,** air cavities in the skull bones which are lined with mucous membrane and communicate with the nasal cavity.

paranephric (par-a-nef′rik): 1. Near the kidney. 2. Referring to the adrenal gland.

paranoia (par-a-noy′a): A chronic, slowly progressive psychiatric disorder characterized by well organized delusions of grandeur or of persecution, or attitudes of suspicion. Mental powers, including clear, orderly thinking are preserved. True paranoia occurs rarely but many other psychotic conditions resemble it.—paranoid, paranoiac, adj.

paranoiac (par-a-noy′ak): 1. Resembling, pertaining to, or suffering from paranoia. 2. A person suffering from paranoia. **P. BEHAVIOR,** characterized by extreme suspicion of others, delusions of persecution, megalomania.

paranoid (par′a-noyd): Resembling paranoia. Term often used to describe people who are overly suspicious or jealous. **P. DISORDERS,** disorders characterized by the development of a delusional system in which one considers oneself endowed with superior and unique abilities, while one's thinking remains orderly and clear. **P. SCHIZOPHRENIA,** see under **schizophrenia.**

paranomia (par-a-nō′mi-a): A type of aphasia characterized by inability to properly name objects seen or touched.

paraparesis (par-a-par′e-sis): Partial paralysis affecting particularly the legs and lower part of the back.

parapertussis (par-a-per-tus′sis): A disease that resembles pertussis but is much less severe in nature.

paraphasia (par-a-fā′zi-a): A speech disorder characterized by inability to use the right words, or to arrange words correctly in sentences; the result is unintelligible speech.

paraphemia (par-a-fē′mi-a): A type of aphasia in which the person consistently uses the wrong words.

paraphia (pa-rā′fi-a): A disorder of the sense of touch.

paraphilia (par-a-fil′i-a): An emotional disorder characterized by unusual sexual behavior, including the practice of fetishism and sexual activities with unconsenting humans, or involving suffering or humiliation.

paraphiliac (par-a-fil′i-ak): 1. Pertaining to paraphilia. 2. A person who practices paraphilia (*q.v.*).

paraphimosis (par′a-fī-mō′sis): A painful condition in which the prepuce has been retracted behind the glans penis and cannot be replaced; the tight ring of skin interferes with the flow of blood in the glans. Surgical correction is possible.

paraphonia (par-a-fō′ni-a): Partial loss of the voice or any change in its quality. **P. PUBERUM,** the harsh, deep, irregular quality that develops in boys' voices at puberty.

paraphrasia (par-a-frā'zi-a): A type of aphasia in which incorrect words or senseless combinations of words are used.

paraphrenia (par-a-frē'ni-a): A paranoid state characterized by delusions of grandeur but in which the person's thinking processes are not disturbed.

paraplasm (par'a-plazm): 1. The fluid part of the protoplasm. 2. Any malformed substance or growth.

paraplegia (par-a-plē'ji-a): Paralysis of the lower half of the body, including the lower trunk and both legs; usually due to disease or injury of the spinal cord. **SENILE P., P.** in the elderly which involves changes in gait; may be associated with cervical spondylitis or vascular disease.—paraplegic, paraplectic, adj.

paraplegic (par-a-plē'jik): Pertaining to paraplegia. Also sometimes used to denote a person suffering from paraplegia.

parapraxia (par-a-prak'si-a): A term used to describe such minor aberations of behavior as forgetfulness, a tendency to misplace things, or slips of the tongue or pen.

paraprofessional (par'a-prō-fesh'un-n'l): In health care, a worker who assists a professionally trained personnel in caring for clients but who is not trained or licensed to practice as a professional, *e.g.*, a nurses' aide.

paraprotein (par-a-prō'tē-in): 1. Any plasma protein that differs in one or more characteristics from normal plasma protein, usually refers to a globulin. 2. A protein that has been modified so that it is slightly different from the native protein.

paraproteinemia (par'a-prō-tē-in-ē'mi-a): The presence of abnormal amounts of a paraprotein in the blood plasma.

parapsoriasis (par-a-sō-rī'a-sis): Name given to a group of rare skin diseases that are characterized by red scaly patches or papules that resemble those of psoriasis and are resistant to treatment.

parapsychology (par'a-sī-kol'o-ji): A term used to describe the branch of psychology dealing with motor and psychic phenomena that occur without the apparent mediation of sensory or motor organs and that cannot be accounted for by currently known scientific methods, *e.g.*, clairvoyance and extrasensory perception.

pararectal (par-a-rek'tal): Near the rectum.

parasellar (par-a-sel'lar): Adjacent to or near the sella turcica.

parasigmatism (par-a-sig'ma-tizm): Imperfect pronunciation of the letter *s*, resulting in a lisp.

parasinusoidal (par'a-sī-nū-soy'dal): Near or around a sinus; usually refers to a cerebral sinus, the superior sagittal sinus in particular.

parasite (par'a-sīt): Any organism that lives in or on another organism and obtains all or part of its nourishment from its host without giving anything in return.—parasitic, adj. **FACULTATIVE P.**, an organism that is parasitic on another but is also capable of existing independently. **OBLIGATORY P.**, an organism that cannot live independently of its host.

parasitemia (par'a-sī-tē'mi-a): The presence of parasites in the blood; usually refers to malarial parasites.—parasitemic, adj.

parasiticide (par-a-sit'-i-sīd): Any agent that destroys parasites.

parasitogenic (par'a-sī-tō-jen'ik): Caused by or due to parasites.

parasitology (par'a-sī-tol'o-ji): The science that treats of parasites and their effects on other living organisms, especially the human body.

parasitophobia (par'a-sī-tō-fō'bi-a): Morbid dread of parasites.

parasitosis (par'a-sī-tō'sis): The condition of being infested or infected with parasites.

paraspadias (par-a-spā'-di-as): A condition in which the urethra opens on one side of the penis.

paraspasm (par'a-spazm): 1. Spasm of corresponding muscles on both sides of the body. 2. Spasm or paralysis of the muscles of the lower extremities.

parasympathetic (par-a-sim-pa-thet'ik): **P. NERVOUS SYSTEM**, a division of the autonomic nervous system; see under **nervous system**.

parasympatholytic (par-a-sim'pa-thō-lit'ik): Opposing or blocking the action of parasympathetic nerve fibers, or an agent that has this physiological effect.

parasympathomimetic (par-a-sim' -pa-thō-mī-met'ik): Producing effects similar to those produced by stimulation of parasympathetic nerve fibers, or an agent that has this physiological action.

parasystole (par-a-sis'to-li): An irregular cardiac rhythm in which the heartbeat is paced at different rates by two pacemakers that function independently of each other.

parataxia (par-a-taks'i-a): 1. An emotional state in which one views all events, persons, and objects as entirely separate without any relationship to other aspects of one's personal experience. 2. Behavior that demonstrates lack of adjustment to emotions and desires.

paratendinitis (par' -a-ten-di-nī'tis): A rather common condition in young adults whose occupation involves repetitive movements of the hand and wrist which causes friction between the tendons; marked by swelling, local edema, fine crepitation, and pain at the back of the wrist and in the forearm. Syn., acute frictional tenosynovitis.

paratherapeutic (par' -a-ther-a-pū'tik): Refers

to a condition caused by treatment for another condition or disease; iatrogenic.

parathormone (par-a-thor'mōn): A hormone secreted by the parathyroid glands; controls the metabolism of calcium and phosphorus. Excess hormone causes mobilization of calcium from the bones, which become rarefied.

parathyroid (par-a-thī'royd): Any one of several, usually four, small endocrine glands lying close to or embedded in the posterior surface of the thyroid gland. They secrete a hormone, parathormone (*q.v.*). **P OSTEODYSTROPHY,** a condition in which an excess of parathyroid secretion causes generalized osteoporosis and cystic changes in some bones, usually the clavicle, long bones, hands, and skull; seen in adults.

parathyroidectomy (par'a-thī-roy-dek'to-mi): Excision of one or more parathyroid glands.

paratonia (par-a-tō'ni-a): A disorder of tension or tone, particularly of muscle, manifested in uneven resistance of limbs to passive movement; seen most often in stuporous patients or those with dementia. Syn., gegenhalten.

paratrigeminal syndrome (par'a-trī-jem'i-nal): A rare condition characterized by paroxysmal pain in the face, sensory loss on the affected side, ptosis of the upper eyelid, and weakness of the muscles of mastication. One cause is thought to be an aneurysm of the internal carotid artery.

paratrooper fracture: See under fracture.

paratyphoid fever (par-a-tī-foyd fē'ver): Descriptive of a variety of enteric fevers that closely resemble typhoid fever but which are less prolonged and severe. Usually contracted by eating food that has become contaminated with bacteria of the genus *Salmonella*. See TAB.

paraurethral (par'a-ūrē'thral): Near the urethra. **P. DUCTS.,** the ducts from two small glands that open into the posterior wall of the female urethra at the orifice; Skene's ducts. **P. GLANDS,** see Skene's glands.

paravaginal (par-a-vaj'in-al): Near or alongside the vagina.

paravertebral (par-a-ver'te-bral): Alongside or near the vertebral column. **P. BLOCK ANESTHESIA,** induced by infiltration of local anesthetic around the spinal nerve roots as they emerge from the intervertebral foramina. **P. INJECTION,** of local anesthetic into sympathetic chain; can be used as a test in ischemic limbs to see if sympathectomy will be of value.

paregoric (par-e-gor'ik): Camphorated tincture of opium, frequently used in cough syrups and mixtures; also used in treatment of diarrhea.

parencephalia (par'en-se-fā'li-a): Imperfect development of the brain.

parencephalitis (par'en-sef-a-lī'tis): Inflammation of the cerebellum.

parencephalocele (par-en-sef'al-ō-sēl): Protrusion of part of the cerebellum through a defect in the structure of the cranium.

parencephalon (par-en-sef'a-lon): The cerebellum.

parenchyma (pa-reng'ki-ma): The specialized tissue of an organ that, in contradistinction to its interstitial tissue, is concerned with its function.—parenchymal, parenchymatous, adj.

parenteral (pa-ren'ter-al): 1. Located or occurring outside of the intestine. 2. Refers to the administration of a substance by some manner other than via the alimentary tract, *i.e.*, subcutaneously or intravenously.—parenterally, adj.

Parents Anonymous: A self-help group for parents who are inclined to be abusive to their children or who have abused or maltreated them. Like Alcoholics Anonymous, it furnishes a forum where such parents can discuss their problems with other members.

paresis (pa-rē'sis), (par'e-sis): 1. Slight or partial paralysis. 2. General paralysis, a condition due to neurosyphilis, with late and insidious onset, beginning with headache and fatigability with slowly progressive deterioration, involving personality changes, tremor, speech disturbances, Argyll Robertson pupil (*q.v.*), increasing muscular weakness. Also called dementia paralytica.

paresthesia (par-es-thē'zi-a): Abnormal tactile sensation such as burning, tingling, prickling, creeping; may be a symptom of psychosis or neurological disease.

paretic (pa-ret'ik): 1. Pertaining to paresis. 2. A person afflicted with paresis.

pareunia (par-ū'ni-a): Sexual intercourse; coitus.

paries (pā'ri-ēz): A wall; by common usage refers to the wall of a hollow organ or cavity.—parietes, pl.; parietal, adj.

parietal (pa-rī'e-tal): Pertaining to a wall. **P. BONES,** the two bones that form the sides and vault of the skull. **P. LOBE,** one of the five lobes of each hemisphere of the cerebrum; lies over the parietal bone. **P. PLEURA,** see under pleura.

parietofrontal (pa-rī'ē-tō-fron'tal): Pertaining to the parietal and frontal bones or the part of the cerebral cortex that lies under them.

parietooccipital (pa-rī'e-tō-ok-sip'i-tal): Pertaining to the parietal and occipital bones or regions.

parity (par'i-ti): Status of a woman with regard to the number of children she has borne. See para.

parkinsonian (par-kin-sōn'i-an): 1. Of, like, or referring to Parkinson's disease. 2. A person afflicted with Parkinson's disease. **P. MASK,** a fixed, staring expression with eyebrows raised, infrequent winking, and immobility of facial muscles, the characteristic feature of parkinsonism. **P. TREMOR,** a fine, slowly spreading, rhythmic tremor of three or four per second; most prominent in repose; paralysis agitans (*q.v.*).

parkinsonism: See **paralysis agitans** under **paralysis,** and **postencephalitic.**

Parkinson's disease: Paralysis agitans (shaking palsy); a slowly progressive degenerative disease of the nervous system affecting especially the brain centers that control movement; seen more often in men than in women; cause unknown, but may follow encephalitis, various infections, head trauma, or use of psychotropic drugs. Disturbance in the production of dopamine in the brain results in the characteristic signs and symptoms, including onset in middle age, slowing of spontaneous movements, rigidity, peculiar shuffling gait with short steps, "pill-rolling" tremor of the hands, mask-like facial expression, diminished blinking, narrowing of the palpebral fissures, slow and monotonous speech, difficulty in swallowing, salivation, weakness, and inability to initiate movements. [James Parkinson, English physician. 1755–1824.]

parodynia (par-ō-din'i-a): Abnormal or difficult labor.

paronychia (par-ō-nik'i-a): Suppurative inflammation around a fingernail. A whitlow (*q.v.*).

paroophoron (par-ō-off'ō-ron): A group of vestigal tubular structures in the broad ligament of the uterus; usually disappear in the adult but may give origin to cysts.

parorexia (par'ō-rek'si-a): Morbid craving for certain foods or for substances that are not fit for food.

parosmia (par-oz'mi-a): Perverted or distorted sense of smell, usually of an hallucinatory nature.

parotic (pa-rot'ik): Situated or occurring near or about the ear.

parotid (pa-rot'id): Situated near the ear. **P. GLAND,** the largest of the three salivary glands, located on either side of the face just in front of and below the ear; empties into the mouth via Stenson's duct which opens opposite the second upper molar tooth.

parotidectomy (pa-rot'-i-dek'to-mi): Excision of the parotid salivary gland.

parotitis (par-ō-tī'tis): Inflammation of one or both parotid glands. **INFECTIOUS (SPECIFIC) P.,** mumps (*q.v.*). **SEPTIC P.** refers to ascending infection from the mouth via the parotid duct, when a parotid abscess may result. Also spelled parotiditis.

parous (par'us): Having borne a child or children.

paroxysm (par'ok-sizm): 1. A sudden, temporary attack or convulsive seizure. 2. A sudden exacerbation or intensification of the symptoms of a disease.

paroxysmal (par-ok-siz'mal): Coming on in attacks or paroxysms. **P. DYSPNEA,** occurs mostly at night in patients with cardiac disease. **P. FIBRILLATION,** occurs in the atrium of the heart and is associated with a ventricular tachycardia and total irregularity of the pulse rhythm. **P. TACHYCARDIA,** may result from ectopic impulses arising in the atrium or in the ventricle itself; of sudden onset and abrupt ending.

parrot disease or fever: Psittacosis (*q.v.*).

pars: A part or portion. In anatomy, a part of a structure that differs from the main part. **P. FLACCIDA MEMBRANAE TYMPANI,** the small, thin, lax, triangular portion of the upper part of the tympanic membrane. **P. TENSA MEMBRANAE TYMPANI,** the main portion of the tympanic membrane.

partial pressure: The pressure of any one gas in a mixture of gasses or in a liquid; it relates to the concentration of that gas and to the total pressure of all gasses in the liquid.

partial prothrombin time: a test for detecting coagulation defects and the presence of hemophilia. Abbreviated PPT.

partimute (par'ti-mūt): A deaf-mute.

partograph (part'ō-graf): A graphic device for recording the salient features of labor.

parturient (par-tū'ri-ent): Pertaining to childbirth.

parturition (par-tū-rish'un): The act of bearing a child; labor.

PAS: Abbreviation for para-aminosalicylic acid. PASA is also used.

Pascal's law: States that when pressure is exerted on one part of a fluid in an enclosed space, the increased pressure will be transmitted throughout the whole fluid. Also called Pascal's principle. [Blaise Pascal, French mathematician and scientist. 1623–1662.]

Paschen bodies (pash'en): Minute particles once thought to contain the virus of smallpox, found in great numbers in skin exanthemas. [E. Paschen, German bacteriologist. 1860–1936.]

passive (pas'iv): Neither active nor spontaneous. **P. CARRIER,** one who harbors the causative organism of a disease without having had the disease. **P. IMMUNITY,** see under **immunity. P. LEARNING,** incidental learning; learning without intention to learn. **P. MOVEMENT OR EXERCISE,** performed by the physiotherapist, the patient being relaxed. **P. RANGE OF MOTION,** the limits of motion through which a joint can be put without use of the muscles that cross the joint. **P. SMOKING,** inhaling smoke produced by someone else.

passivism (pas'i-vizm): Sexual act in which the individual submits to the will of another.

passivity (pas-iv'i-ti): The absence of activity or initiative; submissiveness; inertia. In psychiatry, a state of dependency on others and failure to take the initiative or personal responsibility for making decisions.

Pasteur, Louis: Noted French chemist (1822–1895); developed the germ theory of disease; discovered a treatment for rabies; and invented the process of pasteurization. With Robert Koch, considered to be a founder of modern bacteriology.

Pasteurella (pas-tur-el'a): A genus of bacteria. Short, gram-negative rods, staining more deeply at the poles (bipolar staining); pathogenic to man and animals. **P. TULARENSIS,** an obsolete name for **FRANCISELLA TULARENSIS;** see under Francisella. **P. PESTIS,** an obsolete name for **YERSINIA PESTIS,** the causative organism of classical plague.

pasteurization (pas'tur-ī-zā'shun): A process whereby nonsporebearing pathogenic organisms in fluid (especially milk) are killed by heat without affecting the food properties or flavor of the fluid. Flash method of **P.** (H.T.,S.T.—High temperature, short time), the fluid is heated to 161.5°F., maintained at this temperature for 30 minutes, then rapidly cooled; a useful procedure when the materials to be treated might be altered or damaged by excessive heat.

Pasteur's method or treatment: The method devised by Pasteur for preventing the development of rabies by injecting repeated doses of attenuated virus of the disease, gradually increasing the strength of the virus.

Pastia's sign: Transverse lines of small petechiae on the skin surfaces of the antecubital area; seen in scarlet fever.

pastille (pas-tēl'): A medicated disk or lozenge intended to be held in the mouth until dissolved; used for local action on mucous membrane of mouth and throat.

PAT: Abbreviation for paroxysmal atrial tachycardia.

Patau's syndrome: Trisomy 13. See trisomy.

patch: An area larger than a macule that differs in appearance from the surrounding surface. **PEYER'S P'S.,** small oval masses of typhoid tissue found on the mucous membrane of the small intestine. **P. TEST,** a test for hypersensitiveness to certain foods, pollens, or other substances; a small amount of the suspected substance is applied to an adhesive patch that is placed on the skin along with a plain patch which acts as a control; after about two days the patches are removed and if the skin under the one with the substance on it has reddened, it indicates that the individual is probably sensitive to that substance.

patella (pa-tel'a): The kneecap; a triangular, sesamoid bone.—patellar, adj., patellae, pl.

patellectomy (pat'e-lek'to-mi): Excision of the patella.

patent (pā'tent): Open; apparent; evident; not closed or occluded. **P. DUCTUS ARTERIOSUS,** failure of the ductus arteriosus to close soon after birth, so that the fetal shunt between the pulmonary artery and the aorta is preserved. **P. FORAMEN OVALE,** a congenital heart defect; the oval hole between the left and right atria of the fetal heart fails to close at or soon after birth. **P. INTERVENTRICULAR SEPTUM,** a congenital defect in the dividing wall between the right and left ventricles of the heart.

patent medicine (pat'ent): A medicine that has been patented and can be sold without a prescription; must be labeled as to content and dosage.

paternity (pa-ter'ni-ti): The state of being a father. **P. TEST,** a blood test in which the blood groups of the child, its mother and a certain man are compared to determine whether the man could be the father of the child; it does not always prove paternity.

Paterson-Kelly syndrome: Plummer-Vinson syndrome (*q.v.*).

-path: Combining form denoting: 1. One suffering from a specific ailment. 2. A physician who practices a specific kind of medicine, *e.g.*, a homeopath.

path-, patho-: Combining forms denoting: 1. Pathology; disease. 2. Emotion.

pathogen (path'ō-jen): A disease producing agent, usually restricted to a living agent, as a microorganism or a virus.—pathogenic, adj.; pathogenicity, n.

pathogenesis (path'ō-jen'e-sis): The origin and development of disease.—pathogenetic, adj.

pathogenicity (path'ō-jen-is'i-ti): The capacity to produce disease.

pathognomonic (pa-thog'no-mon'ik): Characteristic of or peculiar to a disease or pathologic condition.

pathologist (path-ol'ō-jist): A physician who is specially trained in the study of disease by laboratory examination of tissues and other body substances, for changes in structure or function caused by a disease process.

pathology (path-ol'ō-ji): The branch of medical science that deals with the cause and nature of disease and the changes in structure and function that result from disease processes.—pathological, adj.; pathologically, adv.

pathomimesis (path'ō-mim-ē'sis): Intentional or unconscious mimicry of disease; malingering. See Munchausen's syndrome.

pathophobia (path-ō-fō'bi-a): A morbid dread of disease.

pathophysiology (path'ō-fiz-i-ol'o-ji): The physiology of disordered function or of functions altered by disease, as distinguished from structural defects.—pathophysiologic, adj.

pathopsychology (path-ō-sī-kol′o-ji): The study of causes and processes in the development of mental diseases and disorders.

pathway: In neurology and neurophysiology, usually refers to a structure that carries impulses to or from the central nervous system. **MOTOR P.**, consists of afferent neurons that carry impulses from the brain to nerves that supply muscles or glands. **REFLEX P.**, bypasses the brain in transmitting impulses between efferent and afferent neurons. **SENSORY P.**, consists of efferent neurons that transmit impulses from the body to the brain via the spinal cord.

-pathy-: Word termination denoting: 1. Disease of a specific part. 2. A system of therapy. 3. A feeling *e.g.*, empathy.

patient (pā′shent): A person who is physically or mentally ill or who is undergoing treatment for physical or mental illness.

patient advocate: A knowledgeable person appointed by a health care agency to counsel a patient in regard to the law and his or her legal rights and obligations, or to act for the person who is incompetent to make his or her own decisions regarding health care.

Patients' Bill of Rights: Proposed by the American Hospital Association in 1973; includes what and when information should be given to patients about their diseases, treatments, and prognoses. The 12 points of the Bill recognize the patient's dignity as a human being and right to respectful care, to privacy, and to receive information necessary for giving informed consent, as well as to know whether the hospital proposes to engage in human experimentation. This bill of rights served as an example and an incentive for the formation of many similar bills including the Bill of Rights for Disabled Persons, passed by the U.S. Congress in 1972, which lists 16 rights that apply to health education, employment, housing, transportation, and civil rights of disabled persons; the Bill of Rights for the Handicapped drawn up by the Cerebral Palsy Association; the Bill of Rights for the Mentally Ill and Retarded; the Dying Person's Bill of Rights; the Pregnant Patient's Bill of Rights; New Jersey's Mental Patients' Bill of Rights; the Nursing Home Residents' Bill of Rights; the Indian Patients' Bill of Rights; the Rights of Hospital Patients.

patriarch (pā′tri-ark): The male head of a family, tribe, or other social organization.

patriarchy (pā′tri-ar-ki): A form of social organization in which the father is the supreme authority in the family or group and descent is traced through the male line with the children belonging to the father's group; or a society based on this type of social organization.

patulous (pat′ū-lus): Opened out; expanded.

pavor (pā′vor): Dread; terror. **P. NOCTURNUS**, night terrors during sleep.

PAWP: Abbreviation for pulmonary artery wedge pressure.

Pb: Chemical symbol for lead.

PBI: Abbreviation for protein-bound iodine.

p.c.: Abbreviation for *post cibum* [L.] meaning after meals.

PCN: Abbreviation for penicillin.

PCO_2: Chemical formula for partial pressure of carbon dioxide. The normal for arterial blood is about 40 mmHg; it is elevated in acidosis.

PCWP: Abbreviation for pulmonary capillary wedge pressure.

PD: Abbreviation for: 1. Pediatrics. 2. Pulmonary disease.

P.D. (s): Abbreviation for patient day(s).

peak flowmeter: An instrument used to determine how rapidly a person who has had or is recovering from a respiratory disorder can expel air from the lungs.

pearl: Perle (*q.v.*).

peccant (pek′ant): Unhealthy; causing disease.

pecten (pek′ten): 1. Any body structure with comb-like projections or processes. 2. The middle third of the anal canal.

pectin (pek′tin): A gelatinous substance found in fruits; used in preparing jams, jellies, and similar foods. In medicine, used as a plasma expander and, in conjunction with other agents, to control diarrhea.

pectinate line (pek′tin-āt): A sinuous or jagged line at the level of the anal valves that marks the junction of columnar epithelium and stratified epithelium that line the anal canal.

pectineus (pek-tin′ē-us): An anterior muscle of the femur; it acts to flex and adduct the thigh and to rotate it medially.

pectoral (pek′tor-al): Pertaining to the breast or chest.

pectoralgia (pek′to-ral′ji-a): Pain in the chest or breast.

pectoralis (pek-to-rā′lis): 1. Pertaining to the breast or chest. 2. Any one of the four muscles of the chest. **P. MAJOR**, the large, fan-shaped muscle that covers the upper anterior chest. **P. MINOR**, the thin, triangular muscle underlying the **P. MAJOR.**

pectoriloquy (pek-tō-ril′ō-kwī): The transmission of voice sound through the chest wall; can be heard on auscultation; indicates the presence of a large cavity in the chest or, when combined with bronchophony, consolidation of the lung. **WHISPERED OR WHISPERING P.**, the transmission of whispered sounds through the chest wall.

pectus (pek′tus): The chest. **P. CARINATUM**, pigeon chest. **P. EXCAVATUM**, funnel chest.

ped-, pedi-, pedio-, pedo-: Combining forms

denoting 1. The foot; or having foot-like projections. 2. Child; children.

pedal (ped'al): Pertaining to the foot.

pedatrophia (ped-a-trō'fi-a): Marasmus (*q.v.*); any wasting condition in children.

pederasty (ped'er-as-ti): Homosexual anal intercourse between men and boys.

pederosis (ped-er-ō'sis): A sexual interest in children; sexual abuse of children by adults.

Pediatric Bill of Rights: Formulated in 1974 by the Board of Trustees of the National Association of Childrens Hospitals and Related Institutions.

pediatric nurse practitioner: See nurse practitioner under nurse. Abbreviated PNP.

pediatrician (pē-di-a-trish'un): A physician who specializes in the health supervision and treatment of children.

pediatrics (pē-di-at'riks): The branch of medicine that deals with the development and care of the child and with the diseases of children and their treatment.

pedicellate (ped' -is-e-lāt): Resembling a pedicle; pedunculated. See peduncle.

pedicle (ped'ik-l): 1. A stalk, *e.g.*, the narrow part by which a tumor is attached to the surrounding structures. 2. The two processes that extend backward from the body of a vertebra and connect the laminae with the body of the vertebra.

pedicterus (pē-dik'ter-us): Jaundice of the newborn; icterus neonatorum.

pediculicide (pē-dik'ū-li-sīd): An agent that destroys lice (pediculi).

pediculosis (pē-dik'ū-lō'sis): Infestation with lice (pediculi).

pediculous (pē-dik'ū-lus): Infested with pediculi; lousy.

Pediculus (pē-dik'ū-lus): A genus of wingless, blood-sucking insects (lice) important as vectors of disease. **P. CAPITIS,** the head louse. **P. CORPORIS,** the body louse. **P. PUBIS** (more correctly, Phthirus), the pubic louse; also called the crab louse.

Pediculus capitis and "nit" attached to hair

pediluvium (ped-i-lū'vi-um): Footbath.

pedodontics (pē' -dō-don'tiks): The branch of dentistry that deals with the diagnosis and treatment of conditions of the teeth and surrounding tissues in children.

pedodontist (pē'dō-don'tist): A dentist who specializes in pediatric dentistry.

pedogomy (ped-og'o-mi): Fertilization by the union of two cells with the same chromatin inheritance; inbreeding. Also called endogomy.

pedograph (ped'ō-graf): 1. An imprint of the weight-bearing surface of the foot. 2. A device for taking footprints.

pedojet (ped-ō-jet'): Apparatus for introducing vaccine under pressure into the skin. Avoids use of the needle with consequent danger of spreading serum hepatitis.

pedologist (pē-dol'o-jist): A physician who specializes in pedology.

pedology (pē-dol'o-ji): The study of the life and development of children.

pedophilia (pē-dō-fil'i-a): Abnormal fondness for children. **P. EROTICA,** sexual perversion in which children are the preferred objects.

pedophobia (pē-dō-fō'bi-a): An abnormal fear or dread of children.

peduncle (pē-dung'kl): 1. A stalk-like narrow structure that serves as a support. 2. Any of several structures consisting of bands of nerve fibers that connect various parts of the central nervous system.

pedunculated (pē-dung'ū-lāt-ed): Having a peduncle or stem. Opp. of sessile.

pedunculus (pē dung'kū-lus): Peduncle (*q.v.*).

peeling: Desquamation (*q.v.*).

PEEP: Abbreviation for positive end expiratory pressure.

peer review: In nursing, nurses of equal status review nursing care given by each other; accepted standards of care are used as the measuring tool.

Peer Review Organization (PRO): A group of physicians and other health care personnel who review Medicare patients' hospital records to assure that treatment given was adequate and medically appropriate; may also review records, when requested, of patients under DRG system of admission if the patient thinks he is being discharged too soon.

PEFR: Abbreviation for peak expiratory flow rate.

PEG: Abbreviation for pneumoencephalogram.

pejorative (pe-jor'a-tiv): Changing for the worse; unfavorable.

Pel-Ebstein's fever: Recurring bouts of pyrexia in regular sequence found in lymphadenoma (Hodgkin's disease). [Pieter Klazes Pel, Dutch physician. 1852–1919. Wilhelm Ebstein, German physician. 1836–1912.]

pellagra (pel-ag'ra): A deficiency disease caused by lack of vitamin B complex (nicotinic acid) and protein. Syndrome includes glossitis, dermatitis, peripheral neuritis and spinal cord changes (even producing ataxia), anemia and mental confusion.

Pellegrini-Stieda's disease: A condition characterized by the formation of a semilunar bony deposit in the upper part of the medial lateral knee ligament; due to trauma; results in limitation of flexion.

pellet (pel'et): A small pill; may contain medication and be taken by mouth, or may contain pure steroid hormones and be implanted under the skin from which location it is slowly absorbed by the body.

pellicle (pel'i-kl): 1. A thin skin or membrane. A film on the surface of a liquid.

pelmatogram (pel-mat'o-gram): A footprint; an imprint of the sole of the foot made by pressing the inked sole on a piece of paper.

pelotherapy (pē'lō-ther'a-pi): The use of mud in the treatment of disease.

pelvic (pel'vik): Pertaining to the pelvis. **P. CAVITY,** the cavity within the bony pelvis; see pelvis. **P. ENDOSCOPY,** laparoscopy (*q.v.*). **PELVIC EXAMINATION,** see under examination. **P. EXENTERATION,** see under exenteration. **P. INFLAMMATORY DISEASE,** inflammation of the internal female genital tract, caused by any of several microorganisms, including the Neisseria gonorrhoeae; marked by abdominal pain, fever, and tenderness of the uterine cervix. **P. FLOOR,** the muscular lower part of the pelvis; includes the levator ani and coccygeus muscles, and fascia. **P. GIRDLE,** the bony framework of the pelvis; consists of two innominate bones and the sacrum. **P. ROLL,** an exercise involving motion of the pelvis around its transverse axis. **P. SLING,** a sling that encloses the hips and is suspended from an overhead bar; used in treatment of pelvic injuries. **P. TILT,** an exercise in which the patient lies flat on the back with the knees flexed and feet on the bed, and then contracts the abdominal and gluteal muscles firmly, thus flattening the lumbar back.

pelvimeter (pel-vim'e-ter): An instrument specially designed to measure the pelvic diameters.

pelvimetry (pel-vim'e-tri): The measurement of the dimensions of the pelvis by means of a pelvimeter. Four measurements are taken: the distances between (1) the anterior superior spines of the ilia; (2) between the crests of the ilia; (3) between the greater trochanters of the femurs; (4) between the spinous process of the 5th lumbar vertebra and the anterior surface of the symphysis pubis.

pelvis (pel'vis): 1. A basin-shaped cavity, *e.g.*, pelvis of the kidney. 2. The large bony basin-shaped cavity formed by the innominate bones and sacrum, containing and protecting the bladder, rectum, and organs of generation. **ANDROID P.,** a male type **P.** with heavy bones and a heart-shaped brim; the cavity has a poor curve and the outlet has less space than the normal female pelvis, thus presenting difficulties in delivery. **ANTHROPOID P.,** a female type pelvis characterized by an anterior-posterior diameter at the outlet that is as great or greater than the transverse diameter; most often seen in tall, long-legged women. **CONTRACTED P.,** one in which one or more diameters are smaller than normal and this may result in difficulties in childbirth. **FALSE P.,** the wide expanded part of the pelvis above the brim. **GYNECOID P.,** the normal female pelvis; rounded oval shape with rounded brim, and a well rounded anterior and posterior segment. **PLATYPELLOID P.,** has a short anterior-posterior diameter, lengthened transverse diameter, and a capacious outlet; seen as a sequela of rickets. **TRUE P.,** that part of the pelvis that lies below the pelvic brim.

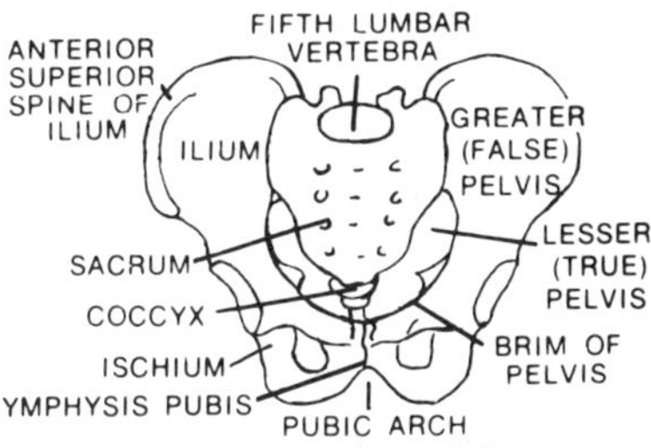

The bony pelvis

pemphigoid (pem'fi-goyd): 1. Allied to pemphigus. 2. A bullous eruption occurring chiefly in older women, marked by the formation of large lesions on the lower abdomen, groin, and inner thighs; of unknown cause; histological examination of the base of a lesion differentiates it from pemphigus.

pemphigus (pem'fi-gus): Name applied to a group of skin conditions marked by bullous eruptions that are absorbed and leave pigmented spots, but more correctly applied to a group of serious diseases called **P. VULGARIS, P. VEGETANS,** and **P. ERYTHEMATOSUS;** the latter two are rare. **P. NEONATORUM;** 1) a dangerous form of impetigo occurring as an epidemic in hospital nurseries; usually caused by *Staphylococcus aureus;* 2) bullous eruption seen in congenital syphilis in the newborn. **P. VULGARIS,** a bullous disease of middle age and later, of unknown etiology; edema of the skin results in blister formation in the epidermis, with resulting secondary infection and rupture, so that large raw areas develop; bullae also develop on mucous membranes; when death occurs it is usually due to intercurrent disease or malnutrition.

pen-, pent-, penta-: Combining forms denoting 1) five; 2) containing five atoms.

pendular (pen'dū-lar): 1. The movement of a

pendulum. 2. Resembling a swinging pendulum.

pendulous (pen′dū-lus): Hanging down.

-penia: A combining form used in a suffix to denote deficiency.

penicillin (pen-i-sil′in): The first antibiotic; derived from cultures of certain molds of the genus *Penicillium;* it is the parent substance of a large group widely used in treating diseases caused by most gram-positive and some gram-negative bacteria, some cocci and some spirochetes. Administered orally, topically, and intravenously.

penicillinase (pen-i-sil′in-āse): An enzyme produced in several strains of staphylococci that are resistant to penicillin; it inactivates penicillin and thus promotes resistance to it.

Penicillium (pen-i-sil′i-um): A genus of fungi comprising the blue molds, the hyphae of which bear spores characteristically arranged like a brush. Common contaminant of food. Found chiefly on decaying nonliving organic matter such as fruit. **P. CHRYSOGENUM,** is now used for the commercial production of penicillin, along with **P. NOTATUM.**

penile (pē′nīl): Pertaining to or affecting the penis. **P. PROSTHESIS,** an inflatable device inserted into the penis; consists of a pump and a reservoir; used in cases of impotence.

penis (pē′nis): The male organ of copulation; in mammals the penis is also the organ of urination. **P. ENVY,** in psychoanalytic theory, the desire of a female child to possess a penis.—penile, adj.

penitis (pē-nī′tis): Inflammation of the penis. Also phallitis, priapitis.

pennate (pen′āt): Shaped like a feather or looking like a feather. Penniform.

Penrose drain: A cigarette type of drain consisting of a piece of rubber tubing containing a length of absorbent gauze. [Charles B. Penrose, American gynecologist. 1862–1925.]

pentagastrin (pen-ta-gas′trin): A synthetic pentapeptide (*q.v.*) which has the same amino acids as the human gastrin; used therapeutically to stimulate production of hydrochloric acid in the stomach.

pentose (pen′tōs): A class of monosaccharides with five carbon atoms in their molecule; abundant in some fruits.

pentosuria (pen-tō-sū′ri-a): The occurrence of one or more pentoses in the urine. The alimentary type is temporary and due to ingestion of large amounts of certain foods, *e.g.*, plums, cherries, or grapes. May be caused by a hereditary error of metabolism. Not significant except that it may be mistaken for diabetes.

peotomy (pe-ot′o-mi): Surgical amputation of the penis.

pepsin (pep′sin): A proteolytic enzyme of the gastric juice; converts the native proteins of foods into proteoses and peptones. Along with dilute hydrochloric acid, it is the chief active ingredient of gastric juice.

pepsinogen (pep-sin′ō-jen): A pre-enzyme secreted by the peptic cells in the gastric mucosa and converted into pepsin by contact with hydrochloric acid.

peptase (pep′tās): An enzyme that splits peptides into amino acid.

peptic (pep′tik): Pertaining to the stomach, to pepsin or to digestion generally. **P. ULCER,** a nonmalignant ulcer in those parts of the digestive tract that are exposed to the gastric secretions; hence it usually occurs in the stomach or duodenum.

peptide (pep′tīd): A chemical combination of two or more amino acids; *e.g.*, dipeptide, tripeptide, polypeptide.

Peptococcus (pep′tō-kok′us): A genus of bacteria of the family *Pepococcaceae* (*q.v.*); an anaerobic, spherical, gram-positive organism; some species are found in the upper respiratory, gastrointestinal, and urinary tracts as nonpathogenic parasites.

peptone (pep′tōn): Substance produced when the enzyme pepsin acts upon the acid metaproteins produced in the first stage of digestion of proteins.

peptonuria (pep-tō-nū′ri-a): The excretion of peptones in the urine.

Peptostreptococcus (pep′tō-strep-tō-kok′us): One of a large group of anaerobic microorganisms of the tribe *Streptococceae* that occur in the intestinal tract of man and as secondary invaders in necrotic and gangrenous wounds.

per-: Prefix denoting 1) by means of; through; 2) completely, throughout, extremely. In chemistry, it denotes the highest member of a series.

per anum (per ā′num): By way of or through the anus.

per os: By or through the mouth.

peracidity (per-a-sid′i-ti): Excessive acidity.

peracute (per-a-kūt′): Extremely acute.

percentile (per-sen′tīl): A point on a frequency scale above and below which a certain percentage of observations fall.

percept (per′sept): 1. An object perceived; the impression of an object obtained through the senses. 2. The mental product of a sensation; a sensation plus memories of similar sensations and their relationships.

perception (per-sep′shun): The reception of a conscious impression through the senses by which we distinguish objects one from another and recognize their qualities according to the different sensations they produce. Intelligent discernment; insight.—perceptual, adj.

perceptive hearing loss: Sensorineural (*q.v.*) type of hearing loss.

percolation (per'kō-lā'shun): The process by which fluid slowly passes through a hard but porous substance.

percussible (per-kus'i-b'l): Detectable on percussion.

percussion (per-kush'un): 1. A diagnostic procedure consisting of tapping or striking the surface of the body to produce sounds that reflect the size, position, and density of the underlying organs and tissues in order to determine the condition of these organs or tissues. Normally a finger of the left hand is laid on the patient's skin and the middle finger of the right hand is used to strike the left finger. Useful in detecting consolidation, fluid, or pus in a cavity, change in the size of an organ, etc; used especially over the chest and abdomen. 2. A movement in massage consisting of taps of varying force. 3. Striking the hand on the chest wall to produce vibration that loosens secretions retained in the lung. **P. HAMMER**, see under **hammer**.—percuss, v.

percussor (per-kus'er): An instrument used in percussion, usually a hammer with a rubber or metal head.

percutaneous (per'kū-tā'nē-us): Through unbroken skin, as by absorption of substances applied by inunction. Also denotes procedures that are performed by needle puncture, *e.g.*, intravenous injection or intra-arterial catheterization.

perflation (per-flā'shun): The blowing of air into a cavity or canal to force its walls apart or to force out any secretions or other substances.

perforate (per'fō-rāt): To pierce through. May be applied to the fibers of a tendon, ligament, or muscle or to a nerve or blood vessel.

perforating ulcer: One that erodes through the wall of an organ such as the stomach or intestine; a serious development requiring immediate surgery.

perforation (per-fo-rā'shun): A hole in an intact sheet of tissue, or the act of making such a hole; may be pathogenic or intentional. Used especially in reference to the tympanic membrane or the wall of the stomach or intestine.

perforator (per'fō-rāt-er): 1. An instrument used to perforate a body tissue or structure. 2. A nerve, blood vessel, or tissue fiber that perforates a tissue or body structure.

perfusate (per'-fūz-āt): The fluid that is introduced during perfusion (*q.v.*).

perfuse (per-fūz'): To spread or pour over or through.

perfusion (per-fū'zhun): 1. The act of spreading or pouring over or through, specifically the artificial passage of fluid through an organ or tissue by way of the blood vessels. 2. The process whereby oxygen is carried from the lungs to body tissues and carbon dioxide is carried from tissues to the lungs.

peri-: Prefix denoting 1) all around, about; 2) near; 3) enclosing, surrounding.

periadenitis (per-i-ad-en-ī'tis): Inflammation in soft tissues surrounding a gland or glands.

perianal (per-i-ān'al): Around or surrounding the anus.

periapical (per-i-ap'i-kal): Relating to the tissues that enclose the apex of a tooth. **P. ABSCESS**, one that forms at or near the apex of a tooth.

periarterial (per'i-ar-tē'ri-al): Around or surrounding an artery.

periarteriolar (per'i-ar-tē-ri-ō'lar): Around an arteriole.

periarteritis (per-i-ar-tē-rī'tis): Inflammation of the outer sheath of an artery and the periarterial tissue. **P. NODOSA**, a widespread disease of the arteries; frequently produces renal damage and hypertension; see **collagen**, **polyarteritis**.

periarthritis (per-i-ar-thrī'tis): Inflammation of the structures surrounding a joint. Sometimes applied to frozen shoulder (*q.v.*).

periarticular (per'i-ar-tik'ū-lar): Around or surrounding a joint. **P. FIBROSITIS**, an inflammation of the fibrous tissues around a joint. **P. OSSIFICATION**, deposits of calcium around a joint.

periauricular (per'i-aw-rik'ū-lar): Around the external ear.

periblepsis (per-i-blep'sis): The characteristic staring expression of an insane or emotionally disturbed person.

peribronchial (per-i-brong'ki-al): Surrounding or occurring about a bronchus.

pericardectomy (per-i-kard-ek-to-mi): Surgical removal of a portion of the pericardium which has thickened from chronic inflammation and is embarrassing the heart's action. Also pericardiectomy

pericardial (per-i-kar'di-al): Pertaining to or affecting the pericardium. **P. EFFUSION**, see under **effusion**. **P. FRICTION RUB**, see under **rub**. **P. TAMPONADE**, see under **tamponade**.

pericardiocentesis (per-i-kar' -di-ō-sen-tē'sis): The withdrawal of fluid from the pericardial sac by insertion of a hollow needle or cannula.

pericarditis (per-i-kar-dī'tis): An acute or chronic inflammation of the outer, serous covering of the heart; caused by many agents; it may or may not be accompanied by an effusion and formation of adhesions between the two layers. **ACUTE IDIOPATHIC P.**, causes interference with the filling of the ventricles which results in dyspnea, ascites, fatigue, hepatomegaly, pain, peripheral edema. **ACUTE FIBRINOUS P.**, marked by a fibrinous exudate. **ADHESIVE P.**, **P.** characterized by adhesions that form between the two layers of pericardium. **P. CALCULOSA**, **P.** marked by deposits of calcium in the pericardium. **CONSTRICTIVE P.**, thickening, fibrosis, and sometimes calcification of the pericardium and constriction of the heart chambers; may follow inflammation or tuberculosis. **DRY P.**, inflammation and roughening of the pericardium without formation of effusion; interferes with cardiac functioning. **P. OBLITERANS, P.** marked by adhesions between the two layers of pericardium and obliteration of the pericardial cavity. **PYOGENIC P.**, inflammation of the pericardium by pyogenic bacteria such as staphylococcus, or by septicemia or pneumonia. **RHEUMATIC P.**, inflammation of the pericardium associated with rheumatic fever. **TUBERCULAR P.**, **P.** caused by *Mycobacterium tuberculosis*. **UREMIC P.**, occurs in patients with renal failure and high blood urea levels. See also Broadbent's sign and pericardectomy.

pericardium (per-i-kard'i-um): The double fibroserous membranous sac which envelops the heart. The layer in contact with the heart is called visceral; that reflected to form the sac is called parietal. Between the two is the pericardial cavity, which normally contains a small amount of serous fluid.—pericardial, adj.

pericholangitis (per-i-kō-lan-jī'tis): Inflammation of the tissues around the bile ducts.

pericholycystitis (per-i-kōl-ē-sis-tī'tis): Cholecystitis extending to the tissues around the gallbladder.

perichondrial (per'i-kon'dri-al): Composed of or pertaining to the perichondrium.

perichondritis (per-i-kon-dri'tis): Inflammation of the perichondrium.

perichondrium (per-i-kond'ri-um): The membranous covering of cartilage.—perichondrial, adj.

pericolic (per'i-kō'lik): Around the colon.

pericolitis (per'i-kō-lī'tis): Inflammation of the tissues around the colon, especially of the peritoneal coat.

pericolpitis (per-i-kōl-pī'tis): Inflammation of the tissues around the vagina.

pericoronitis (per-i-kor-o-nī'tis): Pain and inflammation around the crown of a tooth, especially around an erupting third molar (wisdom tooth).

pericranium (per'i-krān'i-um): The periosteal covering of the cranium.—pericranial, adj.

pericystitis (per-i-sis-tī'tis): Inflammation of the tissues around the urinary bladder.

pericyte (per'i-sīt): One of the peculiarly shaped elongated cells found outside the basement membrane of capillaries, usually having the power of contraction.

peridontoclasia (per'i-don-tō-klā'zi-a): 1. The loosening of one or more permanent teeth. 2. Any destructive disease of the periodontium.

peridural (per-i-dū'ral): Around or external to the dura mater.

perifollicular (per-i-fol-ik'ū-lar): Around a follicle.

perifolliculitis (per'i-fol-ik-ū-lī'tis): Inflammation around the root of a hair follicle.

perihepatic (per-i-hē-pat'ik): Situated or occurring around or near the liver.

perihilar (per-i-hī'lar): Around a hilus (*q.v.*).

perikaryon (per-i-kar'i-on): The protoplasmic part of the cell body, exclusive of the nucleus and processes.

perilymph (per'i-limf): The fluid contained in the internal ear, between the bony and membranous labyrinth.

perimeter (pe-rim'e-ter): 1. An outer border or edge. 2. A device used to determine the characteristics and extent of one's visual field.

perimetritis (per'i-mē-trī'tis): Inflammation of the perimetrium (*q.v.*).

perimetrium (per'i-mē'tri-um): The peritoneal (serous) covering of the uterus.—perimetrial, adj.

perimetry (per-im'e-tri): The determination of the extent of an individual's peripheral visual field.

perimyocarditis (per-i-mī'-ō-kar-dī'tis): A condition in which the patient has symptoms of both pericarditis and myocarditis.

perimysium (per-i-mis'i-um): The delicate connective tissue sheath that envelops and separates the bundles of voluntary muscle fibers.

perinatal (per-i-nā'tal): Occurring at, or pertaining to, the time of birth. **P. PERIOD.**, usually considered to be the period between the 28th week of gestation and four weeks after delivery.

perinate (per'i-nāt): An infant in the perinatal (*q.v.*) period.

perineal (per-i-nē'al): Pertaining to or involving the perineum. **P. BODY**, a wedge-shaped mass of tissue that lies between the anal canal and vagina in the female and between the anal canal and the corpus spongiosum of the penis in the male.

perineometer (per'i-nē-om'e-ter): An instrument for measuring the strength of the perivaginal muscles.

perineoplasty (per-i-nē'-ō-plas-ti): Reparative or plastic surgery of the perineum.

perineorrhaphy (per-i-ne-or'a-fi): The operation for the repair of a torn perineum. Perineoplasty.

perineotomy (per-i-nē-ot'o-mi): A surgical incision into the perineum. See also episiotomy.

perinephric (per'ī-nef'rik): Around or surrounding the kidney.

perinephritis (per'-i-nef-rī'tis): Inflammation of the peritoneal covering of the kidney and of the surrounding tissues.—perinephritic, adj.

perineum (per-i-nē'um): The area that lies between the vulva and the anus in the female and between the scrotum and the anus in the male. Often referred to as the pelvic floor (*q.v.*).—perineal, adj.

perineurium (per-i-nū'ri-um): The connective tissue sheath that surrounds the separate bundles of fibers of peripheral nerves.

period: An interval or extent of time. **GESTATION P.,** the period of pregnancy; in the human it is approximately 270 days. **INCUBATION P.,** the time between the entrance of a pathogenic organism into the body and appearance of first symptoms of disease.

periodic table: A table in which the elements are arranged according to their atomic numbers.

periodontal (per'i-ō-don'tal): Refers to the area surrounding a tooth or the teeth. **P. DISEASE,** a chronic inflammatory condition that attacks the supporting structures of the teeth, including the ligaments, and destroys the bone.

periodontitis (per'i-ō-don-tī'tis): Inflammation of the tissues surrounding a tooth; may be due to gingivitis, faulty dental restoration, oral sepsis, malnutrition, diabetes, scurvy, or pellagra; when untreated usually leads to loss of the tooth.

periodontium (per'i-ō-don'shi-um): The tissues surrounding and supporting the teeth, including the cementum, bone, and gingivae; strictly speaking, the tissue between the teeth and their bony sockets.

periodontologist (per'i-ō-don-tol'ō-jist): A dentist who practices in the field of periodontology.

periodontology (per'i-ō-don-tol'o-ji): The study of the tissues that surround and support the teeth, *i.e.*, the periodontium.

periomphalic (per'i-om-fal'ik): Around the umbilicus.

perionychia (per'i-ō-nik'i-a): Inflammation around a nail.

perioral (pe-ri-or'al): Around or surrounding the mouth.

periorbital (per-i-ōr'bi-tal): 1. The periosteum within the orbit of the eye. 2. Situated around or near the eye socket.

periosteal (per-i-os'tē-al): Pertaining to the periosteum.

periosteitis (per-i-os-tē-ī'tis): Periostitis (*q.v.*).

periosteoma (per'i-os-tē-ō'ma): A neoplasm on the surface of a bone.

periosteomyelitis (per-i-os' -tē-ō-mī-e-lī'tis): Inflammation of the bone including the marrow and the periosteum.

periosteum (per'i-os'tē-um): The thick, fibrous membrane that covers bones except at their articulations; it is protective and essential for regeneration of bone. Consists of two layers, the inner one being concerned with formation of bone tissue and the outer one serving to convey nerves and blood vessels to the bone.—periosteal, adj.

periostitis (per'i-os-tī'tis): Inflammation of the periosteum. **P. DIFFUSE,** that involving the periosteum of long bones. **P. HEMORRHAGIC,** that accompanied by bleeding between the periosteum and the bone.

periotic (per'i-ō'tik): Around the internal ear.

peripartum (per'i-par'tum): Pertaining to or occurring at or near the time of parturition.

peripatetic (per'i-pa-tet'ik): Walking around. Descriptive of certain illnesses, in which the patient does not remain in bed.

peripatologist (per'i-pat-ol'o-jist): A mobility instructor for the blind.

peripheral (per-if'er-al): Pertaining to the periphery (*q.v.*): situated away from the center of a structure. **P. LESION,** one in the periphery of the body, a peripheral nerve in particular. **P. NERVE,** any of the nerves in the peripheral nervous system. **P. NEUROPATHY,** pathology affecting any part of the peripheral nervous system. **P. RESISTANCE,** opposition to the flow of blood through the small vessels and capillaries. **P. VASCULAR DISEASE,** refers broadly to pathology of the blood vessels outside the heart, specifically to atherosclerosis affecting the legs, causing insufficient supply of blood to the feet; characterized by numbness, tingling, and cramplike pain in calf muscles; may lead to gangrene; see intermittent claudication. **P. VISION,** vision in that area of the retina which is outside of the macula lutea; less distinct than central vision but important to functioning in and adapting to the environment.

peripheral circulatory assist: A device for preventing decubiti; consists of an electrically monitored pad that creates pressure differentials in selected areas by introducing air into tubes in the pad.

periphery (per-if'er-i): The outward part or surface of the body; the parts away from the center or midline.

periportal (per-i-por'tal): Surrounding the portal vein and its branches.

periproctitis (per'i-prok-tī'tis): Inflammation of the tissues around the rectum and anus.

perirectal (per'i-rek'tal): Around the rectum.

perirenal (per'i-rē'nal): Around the kidney.

perisalpingitis (per' -i-sal-pin-jī'tis): Inflammation of the peritoneum and tissues around the fallopian tubes.

perisinusitis (per'i-sī-nū-sī'tis): Inflammation of the tissues around a sinus; often refers to a sinus of the dura mater.

perisplenitis (per-i-sple-nī'tis): Inflammation of the peritoneal coat of the spleen and of the adjacent structures.

perispondylitis (per' -i-spon-di-lī'tis): Inflammation of tissues around a vertebra.

peristalsis (per'i-stal'sis): The characteristic movements of the intestine consisting of a wave of contraction preceded by a wave of relaxation; begins with swallowing and continues throughout the digestive tube until the contents are moved forward into the rectum. **MASS P.**, strong peristaltic waves occurring several times a day in the large intestine and which move the contents from one division of the intestine to the next. **REVERSED P., P.** in which the wave is in a direction opposite to normal and the contents of the lumen are forced backward; may occur in malrotation of the bowel, duodenal ulcer or stenosis, gastrointestinal allergy, urinary tract infections.—peristaltic, adj.

peritectomy (per'i-tek'to-mi): Excision of a strip of conjunctiva at the edge of the cornea, a surgical treatment for pannus (*q.v.*).

peritendinitis (per' -i-ten-di-nī'tis): Inflammation of the sheath enclosing a tendon.

peritomy (per-it'o-mi): 1. Surgical incision of the conjunctiva around the entire circumference of the cornea; peritectomy. 2. Circumcision.

peritoneal (per'i-tō-nē'al): Referring or pertaining to the peritoneum. **P. CAVITY**, the potential space between the parietal and visceral layers of the peritoneum. **P. DIALYSIS**, the separating of particles from the blood by using the peritoneum as a semi-permeable membrane through which a fluid is repeatedly introduced into and removed from the peritoneal cavity.

peritoneocentesis (per'i-tō-nē'ō-sen-tē'sis): Paracentesis of the abdominal cavity. Abdominocentesis.

peritoneoscopy (per'i-tō-nē-os'ko-pi): Inspection of the peritoneal cavity by means of an electrically lighted, tubular optical instrument (peritoneoscope) introduced through the abdominal wall.—peritoneoscopic, adj.; peritoneoscopically, adv.

peritoneum (per'i-tō-nē'um): The delicate, smooth, transparent, serous membrane that lines the abdominal and pelvic cavities and is reflected over the organs contained in them, thus forming a sac. **PARIETAL P.**, the layer of **P.** that lines the abdominal walls. **VISCERAL P.**, the layer of **P.** that invests the abdominal organs.

peritonitis (per'i-tōn-ī'tis): Inflammation of the peritoneum, usually secondary to disease of one of the abdominal organs.

peritonsillar (per'i-ton'si-lar): Around the tonsil or tonsils, **P. ABSCESS**, caused by a streptococcal organism, characterized by pain, fever, malaise, and bulging of the tonsillar fauces; mediastinitis is a possible complication; see quinsy.

perityphlitis (per'i-tif-lī'tis): Inflammation of the peritoneum around the cecum and the appendix; appendicitis.

periumbilical (per'i-um-bil'ik-al): Around or surrounding the umbilicus.

periungual (per'i-un'gwal): Around a finger or toenail.

periurethral (per'i-ū-rē'thral): Surrounding the urethra, as a **P.** abscess.

periuterine (per'i-ū'ter-in): Around the uterus.

perivascular (per'i-vas'kū-lar): Around a blood vessel.

perkinism (per'kin-izm): A formerly popular type of quackery in which the patient was treated by the application of certain metals that were supposed to have magic power to cure or alleviate a disease. [Elisha Perkins, New England physician. 1741–1799.]

perle (purl): A very small, thin glass ampule containing one dose of a volatile drug; it is to be crushed in a handkerchief or sponge and the contents inhaled.

perléhe (per-lesh'): An inflammation at the angles of the mouth, sometimes with maceration, fissuring, or crust formation; causes lip licking and results in thickening and desquamation of the skin. Occurs mostly in malnourished children as a result of vitamin deficiency, thrush, bacterial infection, drooling or thumbsucking. In adults may result from poorly fitted dentures or from overclosure of the mouth in adentulous persons.

permeability (per'mē-a-bil'it-i): In physiology, the ability of cell membranes to allow salts, glucose, urea and other soluble substances to pass into and out of the cells from the body fluids.

permeable (per-mē-a-b'l): Capable of being traversed; pervious.

permissiveness (per-mis'siv-nes): The habitual or characteristic allowance or tolerance of behavior that others might disapprove or forbid.

permit (per'mit, per-mit'): 1. Permission. 2. To allow. **OPERATIVE P.**, a statement signed by the patient, or his or her parent or guardian, permitting an operative procedure to be performed on his or her body. The signature must be witnessed and the patient (or other signer) must receive an explanation of what will be done during surgery.

pernicious (per-nish'us): Deadly, noxious, destructive. In medicine, usually denotes a disease of severe character and tending to a fatal outcome. **P. ANEMIA.**, see anemia. **P. VOMITING**, see vomiting.

pernio (per'ni-ō): Chilblain. Congestion of the skin due to exposure to cold; may cause swelling, itching, burning, or even ulceration of the skin.

perniosis (per-ni-ō'sis): Chronic chilblains. The smaller arterioles go into spasm readily from exposure to cold.

pero-: Combining form denoting deformed.

peromelia (per-ō-mē'li-a): Severe congenital deformity of the limbs, including absence of hand or foot.

perone (per-ō'nē): Fibula.—peroneal, adj.

peroneal (per-ō-nē'al): Pertaining to the fibula or to the outer side of the leg, or to the muscles or tissues on the outer side of the leg. **P. MUSCULAR ATROPHY,** a chronic familial condition characterized by wasting of the muscles of the foot and lower leg, with footdrop; also called Charcot-Marie-Tooth disease. **P. NERVE,** a branch of the sciatic nerve; innervates the front of the leg and foot.

peroneotibial (per'o-nē' -ō-tib'i-al): Pertaining to both the fibula and the tibia.

peroral (per-ō'ral): By or through the mouth.

peroxide: See hydrogen peroxide under hydrogen.

PERRLA: Abbreviation for *p*upils *e*qual, *r*ound, *r*eact to *l*ight and *a*ccommodation.

persecution complex: The belief that others have harmful designs against one's person or well-being.

perseveration (per-sev-er-ā'shun): The continuation of an activity after the causative stimulus has been removed, or of a response that is no longer correct. In psychiatry, a mental symptom consisting of an apparent inability of the patient's mind to detach itself from one idea to another with normal speed. Thus, shown a picture of a cow, the patient repeats "cow" when shown further pictures of different objects. Common in senile dementia and schizophrenia.

persona (per-sō'na): In psychiatry, the mask or assumed personality that a person presents to the outside world as opposed to the anima (*q.v.*) which is his or her inner personality or true character.

personality (per'son-al'i-ti): The total complex of individual mental attitudes, characteristics, and ways of behaving and reacting to the environment that distinguish a person. **P.** is sometimes classified as Type A, which includes competitive impatient persons with excessive drive; believed to be associated with high incidence of coronary disease; and Type B., which describes persons who are relaxed, easy-going and less competitive than those in Type A.

personality disorder: Any deeply ingrained maladaptive way of thinking, believing, or perceiving that causes distress or inability to function normally; usually becomes apparent during childhood or adolescence and persists into adulthood, often identified according to the behavior characteristics of the individual. **ANAKASTIC P.,** see compulsive p. **ANAL P.,** descriptive of a person who is excessively orderly, miserly, obstinate; thought to originate during the anal phase of psychosocial development. **ASTHENIC P.,** characterized by emotional and intellectual sluggishness, lack of vigor in meeting the demands of ordinary life, susceptibility to stress. **ANTISOCIAL P.,** characterized by coldness, aggressiveness, disregard for social obligations. **AUTHORITARIAN P.,** characterized by dogmatism and fascistic tendencies, distortion of reality, holding to rigid beliefs and standards. **COMPULSIVE P.,** characterized by meticulous attention to detail, devotion to work, inability to express warm and tender emotions, and exclusion of pleasure. **CORONARY P.,** characterized by predisposition to coronary disease, specifically by aggressiveness, competitiveness, sense of urgency, and strong ambition. **CYCLOTHYMIC P.,** characterized by recurring alternating periods of depression and elation that have no apparent external cause. **DEPENDENT P.,** characterized by lack of self-confidence, avoidance of independence, and placing responsibility for one's life on others. **DISORDERED P.,** the person thinks of *self* as applying to someone else. **DUAL P.,** the person leads two lives, each independent of the other and not fully aware of the other. **EXPLOSIVE P.,** characterized by uncontrollable outbursts of anger, affection, and hate, expressed in aggressive physical violence in otherwise normally behaving persons. **HISTRIONIC P.,** characterized by excitability, overactivity, emotional instability, self-dramatization to attract attention, self-centeredness, immaturity, dependency. Also called hysterical **P. INADEQUATE P.,** term applied to a group of personality disorders that are characterized by fixed patterns of maladaptive behavior and lack of stamina; usually lifelong; to be differentiated from neuroses and psychoses. **MULTIPLE P.,** a **P.** that is capable of dissociating into several different personalities at the same time; the individual believes that one's personality consists of all of them; often a symptom of schizophrenia. **NARCISSISTIC P.,** the person has a grandiose sense of self-importance; needs constant attention and admiration. **PARANOID P.,** characterized by mistrust of others, suspiciousness, hypersensitivity. **PASSIVE-AGGRESSIVE P.,** characterized by aggressive behavior expressed passively as in pouting, exaggerated self-importance, obstinancy, obstructionism. **PSYCHOPATHIC P.,** a persistent pattern of conduct leading to aggressive, antisocial, or irresponsible behavior such as lying, cheating, criminalism, or sexual perversion; usually there is little evidence of guilt or concern about the effects of such behavior on others. **SCHIZOID P.,** characterized by eccentricity, oversensitivity, seclusiveness, daydreaming, avoidance of competitive relationships, detachment. **SPLIT P.,** one composed of two or more groups of behavior tendencies, each acting independently and apparently dissociated from the other.

perspiration (per-spi-rā'shun): 1. The excretion of sweat through the skin pores. **INSENSIBLE P.**, invisible **P.**; the **P.** evaporates immediately upon reaching the skin surface. **SENSIBLE P.**, visible drops of sweat on the skin. 2. Sweat, the fluid secreted by the sweat glands.

perspire (per-spīr'): To sweat.

Perthes' disease (Legg-Perthes-Calvé's disease): Syn., pseudocoxalgia. A vascular degeneration of the upper femoral epiphysis; revascularization occurs, but residual deformity of the femoral head may subsequently lead to arthritic changes. Occurs chiefly in male adolescents. [Georg Clemens Perthes, German surgeon. 1869–1927.]

Perthes' test: A test to determine whether the collateral circulation in the deep veins of the legs is adequate when the individual has varicose veins. A tourniquet or tight bandage is applied just below the knee and the person walks around with it on for a set period of time; when the bandage is removed the varicose veins will have been cleared if the collateral circulation is adequate.

pertussis (per-tus'is): Whooping cough. A highly communicable infectious disease of children with paroxysms of coughing that reach a peak of violence ending in a long-drawn inspiration that produces a characteristic "whoop." The basis of the condition is respiratory catarrh and the organism responsible is *Hemophilus pertussis*. Prophylactic vaccination is responsible for the decrease in case incidence.

pertussoid (per-tus'soid): Resembling whooping cough or a cough resembling that of whooping cough.

Peruvian bark: The dried bark of a South American tree of the Cinchona genus; discovered in the 17th century to be therapeutic for malaria and used widely throughout the world. Also called Jesuits' bark, Jesuits' powder.

perversion (per-vur'shun): A turning away from what is normal or right. In medicine, a pathological alteration of function. **SEXUAL P.**, indulgence in what is traditionally regarded as unnatural sexual practices.

pervert (per-vurt', per'vurt): 1. To turn aside, or cause to be turned aside from what is considered right or normal; to lead astray. 2. A person who has turned aside from what is considered proper and normal behavior; applied especially to one who exhibits any traditionally regarded unnatural sexual behavior.

pes: A foot or foot-like structure. **P. CAVUS**, "hollow" foot, when the longitudinal arch of the foot is accented; clawfoot. **P. PLANUS** or **P. PLANOVALGUS**, flatfoot, when the longitudinal arch of the foot is lowered.

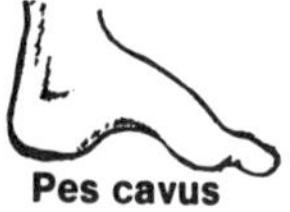
Pes cavus

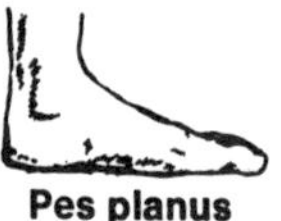
Pes planus

pessary (pes'a-ri): 1. An article inserted into the vagina to support the uterus or to correct uterine displacements. 2. A medicated suppository used to treat vaginal infections or as a contraceptive.

pest: 1. An epidemic disease usually associated with high mortality, specifically the plague. 2. A destructive or annoying plant or animal.

pesthouse: An old term for a shelter, retreat, or hospital where persons with epidemic or communicable diseases were cared for.

pesticide (pes'ti-sīd): A poisonous agent used to destroy a pest, *e.g.*, insect, rodent, fungus.

pestilence (pes'ti-lens): 1. A virulent, communicable, devastating disease, specifically the plague. 2. Something that is pernicious or extremely destructive.—pestilential, adj.

pestis (pes'tis): Plague.

PET: Abbreviation for positron emission tomography (*q.v.*).

petechia (pe-tē'ki-a): A pinpoint, reddish to brown spot of hemorrhage into the skin or a membrane.—petechiae, pl.; petechial, adj.

petit mal (pet'ē mal): Minor epilepsy (*q.v.*). The convulsions are mild and the seizures transient; may be clouding or momentary loss of consciousness.

Petri dish: A round glass dish with a cover; used in the laboratory for growing bacterial cultures.

pétrissage (pā-tri-shazh'): A movement in massage that resembles kneading.

petrolatum (pet'rō-lah'-tum): A yellowish, semisolid substance obtained from petroleum; used as an emollient and as a base for many ointments. Petroleum jelly.

petroleum distillates: Gasoline, kerosene, charcoal igniting fluids, paint thinners, and other like substances; a frequent cause of poisoning.

petroleum jelly: Petrolatum (*q.v.*).

petrosa (pē-trō'sa): The hardened cone-shaped part of the temporal bone; it contains the structures of the inner ear.

petrositis (pē-trō-sī'tis): Inflammation of the petrous part of the temporal bone; usually associated with inflammation of the middle ear or with mastoiditis. Also spelled petrousitis.

petrous (pē'trus): 1. Resembling stone. 2. Pertaining to the petrosa.

Peutz-Jeghers syndrome: An inherited condition, thought to be transmitted by a dominant trait, characterized by the development of multiple cysts in the ileum, colon, or stomach, and excessive pigmentation, usually involving skin, lips, oral mucosa, fingers, palms, toes, and umbilical area; complications include colic, anemia, intussusception.

pexis (pek′sis): The surgical fixation of a tissue or a part.

-pexy: Suffix denoting fixation; a making fast.

Peyer's patches (pī′ers): Flat patches of lymphatic tissue situated in the small intestine but mainly in the ileum; they are the seat of infection in typhoid fever. [Johann Conrad Peyer, Swiss anatomist. 1653–1712.]

peyote (pā-yō′-tē): Mescaline (*q.v.*).

Peyronie's disease: A chronic condition, of unknown cause, in which dense fibrous strands develop in the corpus cavernosum of the penis causing deformity of the penis and painful erections.

Pfannenstiel's incision: A transverse incision above the pubes; used in operations on the pelvic organs. [Emil Pfannenstiel, German gynecologist. 1862–1909.]

pH: The expression used to designate the concentration of hydrogen ions as a logarithm. A neutral solution has a pH of 7.0. With increasing acidity the pH falls and with increasing alkalinity it rises, in a range of 1 to 14.

phac-, phaco-: Combining forms denoting: 1. A lentil or a thing shaped like a lentil. 2. A lens. 3. The crystalline lens of the eye.

phacoanaphylaxis (fak′ō-an-a-fi-laks′is): Hypersensitivity of the crystalline lens to protein.

phacoemulsification (fak′ō-ē-mul-si-fi-kā′shun): A surgical procedure for dissolution of a cataract utilizing ultrasound waves.

phacolysis (fak-ol′i-sis): 1. The operation of breaking down the lens of the eye and then removing it. 2. The dissolution of the crystalline lens by some means other than surgery.

phacomalacia (fak′ō-ma-lā′shi-a): A soft cataract, or a softening of the crystalline lens.

phacomatosis (fak′ō-ma-tō′sis): Name given to several types of hereditary neurocutaneous syndrome which later develop into tuberous sclerosis, neurofibromatosis, and angiomatosis, involving particularly the brain, skin, and eye.

phacosclerosis (fak′o-skler-ō′sis): A hard cataract, or a hardening of the crystalline lens.

phag-, phago-: Combining form denoting something that eats, ingests, or devours.

phage (fāj): A substance of viral origin that has a lytic effect on bacteria. See bacteriophage.

-phagia: Combining form denoting a desire to eat a certain substance or food.

phagocyte (fag′ō-sīt): A cell capable of engulfing, sometimes digesting, bacteria, foreign particles, cells, and other debris in the tissues.—phagocytic, adj.

phagocytose (fag-ō-sī′tōs): To engulf and possibly destroy bacteria or other foreign material.

phagocytosis (fag-ō-sī-tō′sis): The engulfment, and usually the isolation or destruction by phagocytes, of foreign or other particles or cells harmful to the body.

phagomania (fag-ō-mā′ni-a): Abnormal craving for or obsession with food. Morbid desire to eat continually.

phak-, phako-: See phac-, phaco-.

phakitis (fa-kī′tis): Inflammation of the crystalline lens.

phakoma (fa-kō′ma): A microscopic grayish-white tumor occasionally seen on the retina in patients with tuberous sclerosis. Also spelled phacoma.

phalangeal (fa-lan′jē-al): Pertaining to a phalanx or phalanges.

phalangectomy (fal-an-jek′to-mi): Removal of one or more of the phalanges.

phalanges (fal-an′jēz): Plural of phalanx (*q.v.*).

phalanx (fā′lanks): Any one of the small bones of the fingers or toes; 14 in each appendage, two in the thumb and great toe, and three in each of the other digits.—phalanges, pl.; phalangeal, adj.

phall-, phallo-: Combining forms denoting the penis.

phallectomy (fal-ek′to-mi): Amputation of the penis.

phallic (fal′ik): Pertaining to the penis. **P. PHASE,** in psychoanalytic theory, the period in psychosocial development when a boy's interest is centered in the penis and a girl's, to a lesser extent, in the clitoris.

phallitis (fal-ī′tis): Inflammation of the penis.

phallodynia (fal-ō-din′i-a): Pain in the penis. Phallalgia.

phalloncus (fal-ong′-kus): An abnormal swelling or tumor of the penis.

phallorrhea (fal-o-rē′a): 1. A discharge from the penis. 2. Gonorrhea in the male.

phallus (fal′us): The penis.—phallic, adj.

phantasm (fan′tazm): A delusion or illusion. An impression not caused by an actual physical stimulus. Phantom.

phantasmatomoria (fan-taz′mat-ō-mō′ri-a): Silly phantasies, delusions, or childishness; seen in demented persons.

phantasy: See fantasy.

phantom (fan′tom): 1. A model of a part of the body, *e.g.*, a model of the pelvis, used in teaching obstetrics. 2. An apparition; something that a person sees but which does not actually exist. **P. LIMB,** term applied to a sensation that a patient has a limb although the limb has been amputated. **P. PAIN,** pain felt as though it were in a limb that has been amputated.

pharmaceutical (far-ma-sū'tik-al): 1. Relating to drugs. 2. A medicinal drug.

pharmacist (far'ma-sist): One who is qualified and licensed to prepare and dispense drugs; a druggist.

pharmaco-: Combining form denoting drug(s), medicine(s).

pharmacodynamics (far'ma-kō-dī-nam'iks): The study of the action of drugs on the human body.

pharmacogenetics (far'ma-kō-jen-et'iks): The study of genetically determined reactions of individuals to drugs.

pharmacogenic (far'ma-kō-jen'ik): Produced by drugs, usually referring to side-effects.

pharmacognosy (far-ma-kog'nō-si): The branch of pharmacology dealing with the economic, biological, and chemical aspects of natural drugs and their constituents.

pharmacokinetics (farm'a-kō-kī-net'iks): The study of the action of a drugs in the body and their movement through the body systems during absorption, distribution, biotransformation, and elimination, and including the time required for therapeutic or pharmacological responses to them.

pharmacologist (far-ma-kol'o-jist): One who studies drugs, their sources, uses, and actions.

pharmacology (far-ma-kol'o-ji): The science that deals with drugs in all their aspects and relations. **CLINICAL P.**, the study of the action of drugs in man.

pharmacomania (far'ma-kō-mā'ni-a): A morbid desire to give or take medicines.

pharmacopeia (far'-ma-kō-pē'a): A book in which accepted drugs and their preparations are listed and described, including dosages and other pertinent information. Prepared by an official authority of the government or of a medical group and accepted as a legal standard. See United States Pharmacopeia.

pharmacopsychosis (far'ma-kō-sī-kō'sis): Psychosis due to addiction to alcohol, a drug, or a poison.

pharmacotherapeutics (farm'a-kō-ther-a-pū'tiks): The study of the uses of drugs in the treatment of disease.

pharmacotherapy (far'ma-kō-ther'a-pi): Treatment of disease with drugs.

pharmacothymia (farm'a-kō-thī'mi-a): Drug addiction.

pharmacy (far'ma-si): 1. The practice of preparing and dispensing medications. 2. A place where medications are prepared and dispensed; a drugstore.

pharyng-, pharyngo-: Combining forms denoting the pharynx.

pharyngeal (fa-rin'jē-al): Pertaining to the pharynx.

pharyngectomy (far'in-jek'to-mi): Removal of part of the pharynx.

pharyngismus (far'in-jis'mus): Spasm of the muscles of the pharynx.

pharyngitis (far'in-jī'tis): Inflammation of the pharynx or tonsils, or both.

pharyngoconjunctival (fa-ring'gō-kon-junk-tī'val): Pertaining to the pharynx and the conjunctiva. **P. FEVER**, a disease of children, characterized by pharyngitis, conjunctivitis, rhinitis, fever, and inflammation of cervical lymph nodes; caused by an adenovirus. Also called "swimming-pool" conjunctivitis; see under conjunctivitis.

pharyngolaryngeal (far-ing'gō-la-rin'jē-al): Pertaining to the pharynx and larynx.

pharyngolaryngectomy (far-ing'gō-lar-in-jek'to-mi): Surgical removal of the pharynx and larynx.

pharyngolaryngitis (far-ing'gō-lar-in-jī'tis): Inflammation of both the pharynx and larynx.

pharyngoplasty (far-ing'gō-plas-ti): Any plastic operation on the pharynx.

pharyngoplegia (far-ing'gō-plē'ji-a): Paralysis of the muscles of the wall of the pharynx.

pharyngospasm (far-ing'gō-spazm): Pharyngismus (*q.v.*).

pharyngotomy (far'-ing-got'o-mi): The operation of making an opening into the pharynx, done from either the outside or the inside.

pharyngotonsillitis (fa-ring'gō-ton-sil-lī'tis): Inflammation of the pharynx and the tonsils.

pharyngotympanic (fa-ring'gō-tim-pan'ik): Pertaining to the pharynx and the tympanic cavity. **P. TUBE**, see eustachian tube under tube.

pharynx (far'ingks): The upper expanded portion of the digestive tube that forms the cavity at the back of the mouth. It is cone-shaped, 3 to 4 in. long, and is lined with mucous membrane; at the lower end it opens into the esophagus. The eustachian tubes pierce its lateral walls and the posterior nares pierce its anterior wall. The larynx lies immediately below it and in front of the esophagus. For descriptive purposes it is divided into the nasopharynx, that part above the level of the soft palate; the oropharynx, that part between the soft palate and the epiglottis; and the laryngopharynx, that part between the upper edge of the epiglottis and the larynx. It functions as a passageway for both food and air.—pharyngeal, adj.

-phasia, -phasy: Combining forms denoting a speech disorder, especially related to the symbolic use of language.

phen-, pheno-: Combining forms denoting: 1. Appearance; showing. 2. Derivation from benzene.

phencyclidine (fen-sī'kli-dēn): A white powder, colorless in solution; smoked, inhaled, or swallowed, it has a psychedelic action. A street drug, called "angel dust," "hog," and "crystal."

phenocopy (fē'nō-kop-i): An effect produced experimentally that resembles an effect that is normally produced genetically.

phenol (fē'nol): Carbolic acid. Formerly widely used as a disinfecting agent. Strong solutions are caustic.—phenolic, adj. **P. COEFFICIENT,** the disinfecting power of a chemical as compared with phenol.

phenolic (fē-nol'ik): **1.** Pertaining to or derived from a phenol (*q.v.*). **2.** Resembling phenol in action.

phenolsulfonphthalein (fē'nol-sul-fōn-thāl'ē-in): A bright red crystalline powder used in diagnostic tests. **P. TEST,** a kidney function test; **P.** is administered intravenously and the rate and amount of excretion of the **P.** in the urine is a measure of the functional ability of the kidney; normally 50 to 70% is eliminated within 2 hours. Abbreviated PSP.

phenomenology (fē-nom'-en-ol'o-ji): The scientific study of events and happenings as they occur in human experience, rather than from the viewpoint of their causes.

phenomenon (fe-nom'e-non): **1.** Any unusual occurrence or fact. **2.** In medicine, a symptom or any occurrence in relation to disease, whether or not it is unusual or extraordinary.—phenomena, pl.

phenothiazines (fē'-nō-thī'a-zēns): A group of drugs in the major tranquilizer category; administered orally or intramuscularly. They act as mood stabilizers and are used in both excited assaultive patients and those who are withdrawn and apathetic.

phenotype (fē'nō-tīp): **1.** The outward observable expression of one's hereditary physical makeup. **2.** Term applied to a group of persons who resemble each other but who have different genetic makeups.

phenylalanine (fen-il-al'a-nēn): One of the essential amino acids; found in all natural protein foods.

phenylalanine 4-hydroxylase (fen-il-al'a-nēn hī-droks'-i-lās): An enzyme that converts phenylalanine to tyrosine (*q.v.*), a reaction requiring oxygen; a deficiency of this enzyme occurs in phenylketonuria, a hereditary metabolic disorder. See also **phenylketonuria.**

phenylketonuria (fen'il-kē'tō-nū'ri-a): An inherited disorder caused by a deficit of phenylalanine 4-hydroxylase, an enzyme that causes conversion of phenylalanine into tryosine; this results in an inborn error of metabolism of amino acids and an increase in the phenylalanine level in the blood which, if untreated, leads to severe mental deficiency. Marked by the presence of phenylpyruvic acid in the urine. Other symptoms include tremor, convulsions, mental deficiency, hyperactivity, eczema, offensive odor to feces and urine. Early dietary therapy may help prevent mental retardation. Appears most often in families of Irish or Mediterranean descent. Abbreviated PKU. Syn., phenylpyruvic oligophrenia. See also **Guthrie test.**

phenylpyruvic acid (fen'il-pī-rū'vik as'id): A product of the metabolism of phenylalanine (*q.v.*): its appearance in the urine is indicative of phenylketonuria.

pheochromocytoma (fē'ō-krō-mō- sī-tō'ma): A tumor derived from the cells of the adrenal medulla; secretes epinephrine and norepinephrine; usually benign. Produces hypertension with palpitation, nausea, vomiting, pounding headache, sweating, tingling sensations in the extremities.

pheresis (fe-rē'sis): **1.** The separation of blood into its individual components and the removal of one or more selected components. **2.** The removal of one or more selected components from a donor's blood, followed by return of the blood to the donor.

pheromone (fer'ō-mōn): Any substance that is elaborated in the body, secreted to the exterior, and has a characteristic odor that serves as a means of communication with other individuals of the same species and arouses certain behaviors.

phi phenomenon: The sensation of motion when viewing a row of stationary lights that flash alternately.

phial (fī'al): A small glass bottle for medicine; a vial.

-phil, -phile, -philia, -phillic: Combining forms used in the suffix position to denote 1) loving, having a fondness for; 2) one who loves or has an affinity for.

Philadelphia collar: A two-piece molded plastic collar used to provide support and to maintain neck alignment following spinal cord injuries.

-philia: Suffix denoting 1) love or craving for; 2) tendency toward.

philtrum (fil'trum): Anatomical term for the vertical groove in the midline of the upper lip.

phimosis (fī-mō'sis): Tightness of the prepuce so that it cannot be retracted over the glans penis.

phleb-, phlebo-: Combining forms denoting vein(s).

phlebangioma (flēb-an-ji-ō'ma): An aneurysm in a vein.

phlebarterectasia (fleb'ar-te-rek-tā'-zi-a): A general dilatation of both veins and arteries.

phlebectasia (fleb-ek-tā'zi-a): The dilatation of a vein or veins; syn., varicosity. **P. LARYNGITIS, P.** affecting veins of the larynx, particularly the vocal cords; usually a permanent condition.

phlebectomy (fle-bek′to-mi): Excision of a portion of a vein, sometimes done to relieve varicose veins. **MULTIPLE COSMETIC P.**, removal of varicose veins through little stab incisions that heal without scarring.

phlebitis (fle-bī′tis): Inflammation of a vein, often one in the leg. **P. MIGRANS**, recurrent attacks of thrombophlebitis, usually in the leg, characterized by pain, tenderness, and swelling of a segment of a superficial vein; occurs most often in men and may be an early sign of Buerger's disease (*q.v.*).

phleboclysis (fle-bok′li-sis): The intravenous injection of a medicinal solution.

phlebogram (fleb′ō-gram): An x-ray picture of a vein, or the recording of the venous pulse, usually jugular, utilizing a contrast medium.

phlebolith (fleb′ō-lith): A concretion that forms in a vein.

phlebology (fle-bol′o-ji): The branch of medical science that deals with the anatomy and physiology of veins and their disorders and diseases.

phlebomanometer (fleb′ō-man-om′e-ter): An instrument for measuring blood pressure within the veins.

phlebophlebostomy (fleb′ō-flēb-os′to-mi): The surgical procedure of anastomosing vein to vein.

phleborrhagia (fleb-ō-rā′ji-a): Hemorrhage from a vein.

phleborrhaphy (fle-bor′a-fi): The procedure of suturing a vein; venisuture.

phleborrhexis (fleb-ō-rek′sis): Rupture of a vein.

phlebosclerosis (fleb′ō-sklē-rō′sis): Loss of elasticity of the walls of a vein; due to fibrous hardening.

phlebostasis (fle-bos′ta-sis): 1. Retardation of blood flow in a vein. 2. The temporary shutting off of venous circulation in a part by compression on the veins; also called bloodless phlebotomy.

phlebostenosis (fleb′ō-ste-nō′sis): Narrowing or constriction of the caliber of a vein.

phlebothrombosis (fleb′ō-throm-bō′sis): Thrombosis in a vein due to sluggish flow, accompanied by relatively slight inflammation, occurring chiefly in bedridden patients and affecting the deep veins of the lower limbs or pelvis; may also occur as a complication of intravenous therapy. The loosely attached thrombus is likely to break off and lodge in the lungs as an embolus.

phlebotomize (flē-bot′o-mīz): To perform phlebotomy (incision into a vein) for the purpose of drawing blood.

Phlebotomus (fle-bot′o-mus): A genus of bloodsucking sandflies that transmit various forms of leishmaniasis, sandfly fever, Oroyo fever, kala-azar, and bartonellosis; found chiefly in China, the Middle East, and India.

phlebotomy (fle-bot′o-mi): Venesection. A bleeding of 400 to 500 ml of blood; a therapeutic measure in pulmonary congestion to relieve the work load of the heart, to reduce the red cell volume in polycythemia vera, or to reduce the total body iron in hemochromatosis. May also be done to obtain blood for a blood bank or for autotransfusion. **BLOODLESS P.**, the temporary production of phlebostasis in the extremities by compression of the veins.

phlegm (flem): Thick, viscid mucus that is secreted in abnormal quantities in the respiratory tract and expectorated.

phlegmasia (fleg-mā′zi-a): Inflammation. **P. ALBA DOLENS**, inflammation of the femoral vein; sometimes follows childbirth; marked by swelling of the leg, usually without redness; also called milk leg and white leg. **P. CERULEA DOLENS**, acute fulminating thrombophlebitis involving both deep and superficial veins of the leg, characterized by severe pain, cyanosis, edema, purpura; possibly circulatory collapse.

phlegmatic (fleg-mat′ik): 1. Emotionally stolid; not easily excited; apathetic. 2. Resembling phlegm.

phlegmon (fleg′mon): Inflammation of subcutaneous connective tissue, often terminating in ulceration or abscess formation. Cellulitis (*q.v.*).

phlogistic (flo-jis′tik): Pertaining to or inducing fever or inflammation.

phlyctena (flik′te-na): A small vesicle, such as occurs following a first-degree burn.—phlyctenae, pl.

phlyctenulae (flik-ten′ū-lē): Small vesicles, usually occurring on the conjunctiva or cornea, most often in debilitated or tubercular children.—phlyctenula, sing.; phlyctenular, adj.

phob-, phobo-: Prefix denoting: 1. Fear. 2. Avoidance of.

-phobe: Suffix denoting a person with a phobia.

phobia (fō′bi-a): A persistent, unreasonable, exaggerated, irrational fear or dread that focuses on a definite subject. The term is often used as the termination of a word in which the main stem indicates the object of the person's fear.—phobic, adj.

-phobia: Combining form used as a suffix denoting fear, hatred, or aversion to a subject.

-phobic: Combining form denoting morbid fear of, or aversion to, something.

phocomelia (fō-kō-mē′li-a): 1. A developmental anomaly in which the hands and feet are attached directly to the trunk, giving a seal-like appearance. 2. Congenital absence of part of a limb.

phon-, phono-: Combining forms denoting sound, voice, speech, tone.

phonal (fō'nal): Pertaining to speech or the voice.

phonasthenia (fō-nas-thē'ni-a): Weakness or hoarseness of the voice due to fatigue.

phonation (fō-nā'shun): The utterance of sounds produced by vibration of the vocal cord.—phonate, v.

phonetic (fō-net'ik): Relating to the voice and pronunciation of speech. Phonic.

phonetics (fō-net'iks): The science of speech and of pronunciation. Syn., phonology.

phoniatrics (fō-ni-at'riks): The study and treatment of the voice and speech defects.

phonoangiography (fō'nō-an-ji-og'ra-fi): The process of recording and then analyzing the sound produced by the blood passing through an artery; often used to measure the extent to which the vessel's lumen has been narrowed by atherosclerosis.

phonocardiogram (fō-nō-kar'di-ō-gram): A graphic record of heart sounds and murmurs.

phonocardiography (fō'nō-kar-di-og'ra-fi): The electronic recording of heart sounds, utilizing a highly sensitive stethoscope and microphone that detects sounds not otherwise available, displays the patterns on an oscilloscope screen, and makes a permanent record by photography.

phonopathy (fō-nop'a-thi): Any disease or disorder of the voice.

phonophobia (fōn-ō-fō'bi-a): 1. Abnormal fear of speaking or of one's own voice. 2. Abnormal fear of any sound.

phonophoresis (fō'nō-fō-rē'sis): The introduction of a medication through the skin by use of ultrasonic energy.

phonopsia (fō-nop'si-a): A sensation of seeing certain colors when one hears certain sounds.

-phoria: A combining form meaning: 1. A turning; in ophthalmology, a turning of the visual axis. 2. An emotional state.

phosgene (fos'jēn): A suffocating, extremely poisonous gas, which was used extensively in World War I; now used in the production of several chemical and pharmaceutical products.

phosphatase (fos'fa-tās): One of a group of enzymes that hastens the hydrolysis and synthesis of organic esters of phosphoric acid; essential in the absorption and metabolism of carbohydrates, phospholipids, and nucleotides, and in the calcification of bones.

phosphate (fos'fāt): A salt or ester of phosphoric acid; has a minor buffering action in the blood; important in maintaining the acid-base balance in the blood. Phosphates eliminated in the urine are decreased in nephritis and hypoparathyroidism, and increased in starvation, extreme prolonged muscular exercise, and in those on high protein diets.

phosphatemia (fos-fa-tē'mi-a): The presence of a higher than normal concentration of phosphates in the blood.

phosphaturia (fos-fa-tū'ri-a): The presence of an excess of phosphates in the urine; may be the cause of renal calculi. Also called phosphoruria and hyperphosphaturia.

phosphene (fos'fēn): The subjective sensation of light due to stimulation of the retina by pressure on the eyeballs or any stimulus other than light.

phosphofructokinase (fos'fō-fruk-tō-kī'nas): An enzyme of importance in glycolysis (*q.v.*).

phospholipase (fos-fō-lī'pās): Any one of four enzymes that act as catalysts in the splitting of a phospholipid (*q.v.*). Formerly called lecithinase.

phospholipid (fos-fō-lip'id): A class of greasy or waxy compounds widely distributed in plants and animals, particularly in membranes such as red blood cell membranes and in the myelin sheaths of nerve cells; on hydrolysis they yield phosphoric acid and several carbon compounds, including lecithin, cephalin, and sphingomyelin.

phosphonecrosis (fos-fō-nē-krō'sis): "Fossy-jaw," necrosis of the jaw with loosening of the teeth, occurring in workers engaged in the manufacture of products made with white phosphorus, *e.g.*, matches.

phosphorus (fos'fō-rus): A non-metallic constituent of bones, teeth, and nerve tissue, not found in the pure form in the body but in combination with alkalies. Important in conversion of glucogen to glucose, in the metabolism of proteins and calcium, and as a source of energy in muscle contraction. Vitamin D is required for its absorption and metabolism. Phosphorus compounds are found in the protein in many foods such as dairy products, eggs, legumes and many other vegetables, some nuts, liver, many cereals, figs, pineapple, and prunes. Deficiency in the diet results in perverted appetite, weight loss, retarded growth, rickets, anemia, and imperfect development of teeth and bones. **RADIOACTIVE PHOSPHORUS** (P^{32}) is used in treating certain pathological conditions, *e.g.*, leukemia and polycythemia vera, and as a tracer substance in certain physiological studies.

phosphorylase (fos-for'i-las): An enzyme that acts as a catalyst in the formation of glucose from glycogen; found in many plants, animals, and microorganisms.

phot-, photo-: Combining forms denoting: 1. Light. 2. Photograph or photographic.

photalgia (fō-tal'ji-a): Pain in the eyes from exposure to intense light.

photic (fō'tik): Of, related to, or caused by light.

photoallergy (fō'tō-al'er-ji): Hypersensitization to sunlight following ingestion of certain plant foods or certain drugs. See hypersensitivity.

photobiology (fō'tō-bī-ol'o-ji): The branch of biology that deals with the effects of light and other forms of radiant energy on living organisms.

photobiotic (fō'tō-bī-ot'ik): Capable of living and growing only in the presence of light; said of certain microorganisms.

photochemical (fō-tō-kem'ik-al): Related to or produced by the chemical properties of light.

photocoagulation (fō'tō-kō-ag-ūlā'shun): The use of controlled light rays to treat such conditions as intraocular tumor or detached retina, or to destroy abnormal retinal blood vessels. See laser.

photodermatitis (fō'tō-der-ma-tī'tis): Skin lesions due to exposure to sunlight or ultraviolet rays.

photodissociation (fō'tō-dis-sō-si-ā'shun): The chemical decomposition of a substance due to exposure to light.

photodynia (fō-tō-din' -i-a): Pain in the eyes caused by too great intensity of light; see photophobia.

photoelectricity (fō'tō-ē-lek-tris'i-ti): Electricity produced by the action of light.

photoerythema (fō'tō-er-i-thē'ma): Erythema (*q.v.*) caused by exposure to light.

photofluorography (fō'tō-flū-o-rog'ra-fi): Photography of fluoroscopic images on film; a procedure utilized in mass x-ray photography of the chest.

photokeratosis (fō'tō-ker-a-tō'sis): Mild corneal irritation due to overexposure to the ultraviolet rays of the sun.

photomania (fō'tō-mā'ni-a): 1. A morbid desire for light. 2. Insanity or maniacal symptoms induced by prolonged exposure to bright light.

photometer (fō-tom'e-ter): A device for determining 1) the intensity of light, or 2) the degree of sensitivity of the eye to light.

photomicrograph (fō'tō-mī'krō-graf): An enlarged photograph of a minute object or particle as viewed under the light microscope; syn., microphotograph.—photomicrography, n.

photomidriasis (fō'tō-mid-ri-ā'sis): A technique for enlarging a miotic pupil, utilizing the laser beam.

photophobia (fō-tō-fō'bi-a): 1. Profound intolerance for light; may be a significant symptom of a central nervous system disorder, *e.g.*, meningitis. 2. Dread or avoidance of light places.—photophobic, adj.

photopsia (fō-top'si-a): The subjective sensation of seeing sparks or flashes of light before the eyes; may be due to irritation of the retina, or certain diseases of the brain or optic nerve. Also photopsy.

photo-pulse sensor: An apparatus for detecting and measuring pulse rate, usually at the earlobe or finger tip. See plethysmograph.

photoreceptor (fō'tō-rēsep'tor): A sensory end organ capable of receiving stimuli caused by light, *i.e.*, the rods and cones of the retina.

photoscan (fō'tō-skan): A two-dimensional photograph showing the distribution and concentration of a radioactive isotope that has been administered internally.

photosensitive (fō-tō-sen'si-tiv): 1. Sensitive to light, as the retina of the eye. 2. Exhibiting an increased reactivity of the skin to sunlight.—photosensitivity, n.

photosensitization (fō'tō-sens-i-tī-zā'shun): Hypersensitivity of the skin to light, sunlight or ultraviolet rays in particular; due to the presence in the body of certain drugs, hormones, or heavy metals that have been used, either internally or externally; may occur immediately after ingestion (or use) of such substances for weeks, even months, afterward.

photosynthesis (fō-tō-sin'the-sis): The process by which plants, utilizing light energy, formulate carbohydrate (glucose) from carbon dioxide and water in the presence of chlorophyll.

phototaxis (fō'tō-taks'is): The response of an organ to a stimulus of light, involving movement toward or away from the source of the stimulus.

phototherapy (fō-tō-ther'a-pi): Therapeutic treatment by exposure to sunlight or artificial light, ultraviolet in particular; often used in treatment of skin disorders such as acne, psoriasis, and decubitus ulcer.

phototoxic (fō-tō-tok'sik): Pertaining to the harmful reaction caused by exposure to light, particularly the reaction of the skin to exposure to the ultraviolet rays in sunlight.

phototoxis (fō-tō-tok'sis): A disorder caused by over-exposure to ultraviolet light or from exposure to light in combination with a phototoxic substance. See photosensitization.

phren (fren): 1. The diaphragm. 2. The mind.—phrenic, adj.

phren-, phreni-, phreno-: Combining forms denoting: 1. The mind. 2. The diaphragm. 3. The phrenic nerve.

phrenasthenia (fren-as-thē'ni-a): 1. Loss of muscle tone of the diaphragm. 2. Feeblemindedness; mental deficiency.

phrenemphraxis (fren'em-frak'sis): Crushing of the phrenic nerve for the purpose of temporarily paralyzing the diaphragm.

phrenetic (fren-et'ik): 1. Frenzied. 2. A person who is maniacal or frenzied.

-phrenia: Combining form denoting a disordered condition of mental functioning.

phrenic (fren'ik): 1. Pertaining to the diaphragm. 2. Relating to the mind. **P. AVULSION,** see avulsion. **P. NERVE,** a general motor and sensory nerve originating in the cervical plexus and distributed to the pleura, pericardium, diaphragm, and peritoneum.

phrenicectomy (fren-i-sek'to-mi): Resection of all or part of the phrenic nerve.

phrenicotomy (fren-i-kot'o-mi): Division of the phrenic nerve to paralyze one half of the diaphragm, done to produce compression of a diseased lung.

phrenitis (fren-ī'tis): 1. Inflammation of the diaphragm. 2. Inflammation of the brain. 3. Frenzy; delirium.

phrenology (fre-nol'o-ji): A pseudoscience based on the belief that the external configurations of the skull indicate areas of development in the brain of certain mental faculties, and that therefore one's mental characteristics can be determined by examination of the various prominences of the skull.

phrenoplegia (fren'ō-plē'ji-a): 1. Paralysis of the diaphragm. 2. Paralysis or sudden loss of mental faculties.

phrynoderma (frin'ō-der'ma): A dry eruption of the skin; possibly due to vitamin A deficiency. Follicular keratosis.

PHS: Public Health Service. See United States Public Health Service.

phthiriasis (thi-rī'a-sis): Infestation with the crab or pubic louse.

Phthirus (thir'us): A louse. **P. PUBIS,** the crab louse; infests the pubic area primarily but also the axillae, eyebrows, and beard on occasion.

phthisis (tī'sis): 1. Progressive, general or local atrophy and wasting. 2. Old term for pulmonary tuberculosis. **FIBROID P.,** 1) interstitial pneumonia; 2) chronic fibrotuberculosis in which fibrous tissue develops around a cavity in the lung. **P. BULBI,** shrinkage of the eyeball.—phthisic, adj.

Phycomycetes (fī'kō-mī-sē'tēz): A class of fungi, including black bread mold and water mold; may be pathogenic to humans, particularly diabetics and debilitated individuals.

phycomycosis (fī'kō-mī-kō'sis): An acute or chronic systemic infection caused by one of the *Phycomycetes,* often *Mucor*. The central nervous system, blood vessels, or lungs may be affected; usually occurs in debilitated individuals.

phylaxis (fī-laks'is): The body's action in protecting or defending itself against infection.

physiatrics (fiz-i-at'riks): The branch of medicine that utilizes physical agents such as heat, cold, light, water, and electricity in the prevention, diagnosis and treatment of disease. Physical medicine.

physiatrist (fiz-i-at'rist): A physician who specilizes in physical medicine (physiatrics).

physic (fiz'ik): 1. Old term for the art and science of medicine. 2. A purgative or laxative drug.

physical (fiz'i-kal): Pertaining to: 1) the body; 2) natural science; 3) material things; 4) physical science. **P. ASSESSMENT,** the process of evaluating a client's health status utilizing data obtained from the client and the findings of a physical examination. **P. MEDICINE,** a medical specialty that utilzes physical and occupational therapy and physical reconditioning in the management of the sick and injured. **P. THERAPY,** see under therapy.

physical therapist: A person skilled in the therapeutic use of physical agents rather than drugs in carrying out treatments prescribed by a physician.

physician (fi-zish'un): A person fitted by knowledge and training, and licensed by the proper authorities, to care for the sick; a doctor. **ATTENDING P.,** one who visits his or her patients in the hospital and gives orders for their care. **HOUSE P.,** one who lives in the hospital and is responsible for patients' care during the absence of attending physicians.

physician's assistant: A fairly new category of health care worker who works under the direction of a physician in performing certain functions traditionally performed by physicians and professional nurses. Many serve as primary health care givers to low income populations in both urban and rural areas where there is a scarcity of physicians and professional nurses.

Physicians' Desk Reference: A reference book of information about many drug products; this information is much the same as that in the package inserts. Revised annually. Published by Medical Economics, Inc., Oradell, N.J. 07649

physicochemical (fiz' -i-kō-kem'ik-al): Pertaining to physics and chemistry.

physics (fiz'iks): A fundamental science that deals with the phenomena and laws of nature; it treats particularly of the properties of matter and energy.

physiognomy (fiz-i-og'-no-mi): The facial appearance, facial features, and expression that are thought by some to reveal inner character and quality.

physiologic (fiz-i-ō-loj'ik): 1. Of or related to physiology. 2. Denoting the action of a drug in a healthy person as distinguished from its therapeutic action. 3. Normal as opposed to pathologic; in accordance with natural processes of the body. Adjective often used to describe a normal process or structure, to distinguish it from an abnormal or pathological feature. **P. SALINE,** a solution consisting of 0.9 gram sodium chloride per 100 ml distilled water; it has the same osmotic pressure as plasma; also called physiologic salt solution, normal saline, and normal salt solution.—physiological, adj.

physiology (fiz-i-ol'ō-ji): The branch of biology that deals with the normal vital processes, activities, and functions of living organisms.

physiopathology (fiz' -i-ō-pa-thol'o-ji): The science of body functions in disease or as modified by disease.

physiopsychic (fiz-i-ō-sī'kik): Pertinent to or involving both the body and the mind.

physiotherapist (fiz'i-ōther'a-pist): A person specially skilled and trained in the use of physical agents to assist patients to overcome or adjust to physical disabilities. See physiotherapy.

physiotherapy (fiz'i-ō-ther'a-pi): Treatment of disease, injury, or disability by physical means, *e.g.*, light, heat, electricity, water, massage, regulated exercises. Physiatrics. Physical therapy.

physique (fi-zēk'): The general bodily structure or type. Syn., body build.

pia (pī'a, pē'a): Soft, tender. **P. MATER**, the innermost of the three meninges (*q.v.*); the vascular membrane that lies in close contact with the substance of the brain and spinal cord. See mater; meninges.

pia-arachnitis (pī'a-ar-ak-nī'tis): Leptomeningitis (*q.v.*).

pia-arachnoid (pī' -a-ar-ak'noid): Pertaining to the pia mater and the arachnoid membrane.

pica (pī'ka): 1. The habit of eating non-food substances such as plaster, chalk, ashes, etc., after the age when it might be considered natural behavior. Often indicates a nutritional deficiency. 2. The desire for extraordinary articles of food. See geophagia.

Pick's disease: A progressive type of presenile dementia in which atrophy of the cerebral cortex occurs, especially in the frontal and temporal lobes; a hereditary condition with onset in the 4th to 6th decade, characterized by apathy, mutism and altered speech pattern, personality changes; patients are often bedridden. [Arnold Pick, Czechoslovakian physician. 1851–1924.]

Pickwickian syndrome: A condition characterized by obesity, sleepiness, hypoventilation, cyanosis, erythrocytosis, hypoxia. Named for an obese character in Charles Dickens' writings.

picogram (pī'kō-gram): Micromicrogram. One trillionth of a gram.

picornavirus (pi-kor-na-vī'rus): Any one of a large group of RNA viruses that includes the enterovirus of poliomyelitis as well as the Coxsacki groups, echovirus, and many rhinovirus types.

PID: Abbreviation of pelvic inflammatory disease; see under pelvic.

piebaldism (pī'bawl-dizm): An inherited condition in which some areas of the skin, and sometimes of the hair, are white, due to hypomelanosis; partial albinism.—piebald, adj.

Pierre Robin syndrome: A congential condition in which micrognathia (*q.v.*), with a high arched palate and glossoptosis (*q.v.*), occurs; congenital glaucoma and retinal detachment are often present.

piesesthesia (pī-es-es-thē'zi-a): Sensivity to pressure.

piezocardiogram (pī-e-zō-kar'di-ō-gram): A graphic tracing of pressure changes caused by pulsations of the heart, often recorded through the esophagus.

pigeon breast: A deformity in which a narrow chest causes the sternum to bulge anteriorally resulting in an increased anterior-posterior diameter; occurs especially in rickets. Pectus carinatum.

pigeon toe: A condition in which the toes permanently turn inward toward the median line.—pigeon-toed, adj.

piggy-back: Refers to the simultaneous administration of two or more intravenous solutions.

pigment (pig'ment): In anatomy, any coloring matter in the body.

pigmentation (pig'men-tā'shun): The deposit of pigment in any of the body tissues, especially when abnormal or excessive.

pigmentum nigrum (pig-men'tum nī'grum): The black pigment that lines the choroid coat of the eye.

piitis (pī-ī'tis): Inflammation of the pia mater.

pil-, pili, pilo-: Combining forms denoting hair(s).

pilar (pī'-lar): Related to hair. Covered with hair. **P. CYST**, an epidermal cyst of the scalp; a wen.

piles: See hemorrhoids.

pili (pī'lī): Plural of pilus (*q.v.*).

pill: 1. A small, usually rounded mass of some cohesive substance containing a medication; may or may not be coated; to be swallowed whole. **BREAD P.**, one made of bread crumbs pressed into a ball; usually a placebo. **ENTERIC COATED P.**, one coated with a substance that will not dissolve until the pill reaches the intestine. **PEP P.**, one that contains a drug with a stimulating effect, especially benzedrine. 2. A contraceptive substance taken orally.

pillar: In anatomy, a supporting structure or part that resembles a column, usually in pairs, *e.g.*, the pillars of the fauces.

Pills Anonymous: A self-help group fellowship which derives its principles from Alcohol Anonymous; for those who have become chemically dependent on mood-altering drugs. Pill-

Anon is the co-existing group for family and friends of chemically dependent persons.

pilocarpine (pī-lō-kar′pēn): An alkaloid obtained from the leaves of the pilocarpus, a shrub native to Central America; it stimulates perspiration, the flow of saliva, and intestinal motility when given internally; used externally as a miotic and for treatment of glaucoma.

pilocystic (pī-lō-sis′tik): Denoting a cyst that contains hair.

piloerection (pī′lō-ē-rek′shun): Raising up of the hair accompanying chilling of the body; "goose pimples."

pilomotor (pī-lō-mō′tor): Causing the hair to move. **P. MUSCLES,** the arrectores pili of the skin. **P. NERVES,** tiny nerves attached to the hair follicle; innervation causes the hair to stand upright and give the appearance of "goose flesh."

pilonidal (pī-lō-nī′dal): Hair-containing. **P. CYST,** see under cyst. **P. SINUS,** see under sinus.

pilose (pī′los): Covered with hair, especially that of a soft texture; hairy.

pilosebaceous (pī′lō-sē-bā′shus): Pertaining to the hair follicle and the sebaceous gland opening into it.

pilosis (pī-lō′sis): An abnormal growth of hair.

pilula (pi-loo′la): A pill.

pilus (pī′lus): A hair.—pili, pl.

pimple: A small, circumscribed, usually pointed, erythematous elevation on the skin; often suppurated. See pustule; papule.

pin: A slender metal rod used in the surgical fixation of the ends of fractured bones.

pinch gauge: An instrument for measuring the strength of a finger pinch. Pinch meter.

pineal (pin′ē-al): 1. Having a shape like a pine cone. 2. Pertaining to the pineal body (*q.v.*).

pineal body (pin′ē-al): The small reddish-gray conical structure extending from the posterior part of the third ventricle of the brain; it apparently secretes the hormone melatonin which is thought to influence the metabolic actions of several hormones. Also called pineal gland and epiphysis cerebri.

pinealoma (pin′ē-a-lō′ma): A tumor of the pineal gland; usually occurs in young people in association with obesity and early puberty.

pinguecula (ping-gwek′ū-la): A small slightly elevated fat pad on the conjunctiva near the junction of the cornea and the inner canthus, or sometimes the outer canthus; usually does no harm but may disturb the individual who fears loss of vision.—pingueculae, pl.

pink disease: See acrodynia.

"pink puffer": Term applied to patients with pure emphysema; the patient is thin, breathless, has an enlarged heart, produces little sputum, and has a pink color.

pinkeye: Popular name for acute contagious conjunctivitis.

pinna (pin′a): That part of the ear which is external to the head; the auricle.—pinnae, pl.

pinocytosis (pīn′ō-sī-tō′sis): The absorption of liquids by cells with phagocytic properties such as the macrophage.

pint: A unit of capacity in the apothecaries' system; 16 fluid ounces, ½ quart. Equivalent to 473.167 ml in the metric system.

pinta (pin′ta): A chronic, nonvenereal disease caused by a spirochete; characterized by the eruption of patches of varying color that finally become white. Occurs mostly in children. Is endemic among dark-skinned peoples of the tropics and sub-tropics.

pinworm: Enterobius vermicularis (*q.v.*).

pipette (pī-pet′): A glass tube with a small lumen used in the laboratory for transferring and measuring small amounts of fluid.

piriform (pir′i-form): Having the shape of a pear.

Pirquet's reaction (pir′kāz): A local inflammatory reaction in response to the application of tuberculin to scarified skin to determine the presence of tuberculosis; used especially with children. [Baron Clemens von Pirquet, Austrian pediatrician. 1874–1929.]

pisiform (pis′i-form): 1. Having the shape or size of a pea. 2. One of the bones of the carpus.

pit: 1. Any hollow or depression on the surface of the body or of an organ. 2. A dimple or pockmark. 3. A depression in the enamel of a tooth. 4. To make an indentation, as occurs when a finger is pressed against edematous tissue.

pitchblende (pitsh′blend): A brown to black lustrous mineral that contains a large amount of uranite; it is the principal source of uranium and the elements produced from its breakdown, chiefly radium.

pith: 1. The spinal cord and medulla oblongata. 2. The center of a hair shaft. 3. To destroy the spinal cord or the entire central nervous system of an animal by introducing a sharp pointed instrument at the base of the skull or passing it down the spinal canal; done to destroy sensibility in animals to be used for experimental or teaching purposes.

pitting: 1. Depressed scars left on the skin, especially after smallpox. 2. Indentations remaining temporarily in edematous tissue after pressure with a finger.

pituitarism (pi-tū′ -i-tar-izm): Any dysfunction of the pituitary gland.

pituitary (pit-ū′i-tar-i): Pertaining to the hypophysis cerebri or the pituitary gland. **P. GLAND,** a small, two-lobed, oval endocrine gland located at the base of the brain in the sella turcica of the sphenoid bone; often called the master gland because it influences the secretory activity of all the endocrine glands except the adrenals. The larger anterior part (adenohypophysis) secretes several hormones that have an effect on other endocrine glands—the follicle stimulating hormone, adrenocorticotropic hormone, growth hormone, prolactin, thyroid stimulating hormone, luteinizing hormone. The smaller posterior lobe (neurohypophysis) furnishes a secretion that stimulates lactation, and vasopressin (antidiuretic hormone) which has an effect on the fluid and electrolyte balance in the body; it also acts to regulate and stimulate smooth muscle tissue, thus affecting blood pressure and the activity of intestinal and uterine musculature. **P. DWARFISM,** dwarfism due to hypofunctioning of the anterior lobe of the pituitary gland.

pituitectomy (pi-tū-i-tek′to-mi): Surgical removal of the pituitary gland.

pituitrin (pi-tū′i-trin): 1. A secretion of the posterior lobe of the pituitary gland; it acts specifically on the smooth muscle of the uterus increasing tone and contraction. 2. Trademark for a prepararation of pituitary extract made from the pituitary gland of certain animals.

pityriasis (pit-i-rī′a-sis): Name given to a group of skin diseases characterized by scaly (branny) eruption of the skin. **P. ALBA,** a very common skin disorder of children; characterized by the appearance of one or many round or oval finely scaling macules; may last for several years and apt to recur if untreated; also called impetigo sicca. **P. CAPITIS,** dandruff. **P. ROSEA,** a slightly scaly eruption of ovoid erythematous lesions widespread over the trunk and proximal parts of the limbs. There may be mild itching. It is a self-limiting condition. **P. RUBRA,** a form of exfoliative dermatitis. **P. RUBRA PILARIS,** a chronic skin disease characterized by tiny red papules of perifollicular distribution. **P. VERSICOLOR,** called also tinea versicolor, is a fungus infection which causes the appearance of buff-colored patches on the chest.

Pityrosporum (pit-i-ros′pōr-um): A fungus associated with dandruff and seborrheic dermatitis.

PKU: Abbreviation for phenylketonuria.

placebo (pla-sē′bō): An inactive substance given for its psychologic or suggestive effect. In experimental research, an inert substance, identical in appearance with the material being tested; neither the physician nor the patient knows which is which.

placenta (pla-sen′ta): Afterbirth. A plate-shaped spongy, vascular structure that develops about the third month of pregnancy and attaches to the upper part of the inner wall of the uterus; the umbilical cord usually arises from a place near its center, and is the means by which the fetus is supplied with oxygen and gets rid of its waste products; it also produces several hormones including estrogen and progesterone, which are responsible for many of the physical changes that occur in the mother during pregnancy. The **P.** is expelled within an hour after the birth of an infant; it usually weighs approximately 500 grams. **P. ACCRETA,** a **P.** that is embedded in uterine muscle; treatment is usually hysterectomy. **BATTLEDORE P.,** a **P.** that develops in the shape of a battledore when the umbilical cord arises in the periphery instead of the center. **P. PREVIA,** a **P.** that is attached to the lower part of the uterus so that it covers all or part of the internal os; usually causes antepartal hemorrhage. **RETAINED P.,** one that is not expelled within the normal time after childbirth. **P. SUCCENTURIATA,** a **P.** in which one or more accessory lobules form at some distance from the placenta but still within the membranes and connected with it by vascular channels.

placental (pla-sen′tal): Pertaining to the placenta. **P. ABRUPTION,** premature separation of a normally affixed placenta from the wall of the uterus; abruptio placentae. **P. BARRIER,** the tissues between the maternal and fetal blood of the placenta which prevent certain substances from passing from the mother to the fetus. **P. INSUFFICIENCY,** inefficiency of the **P.,** may be due to maternal disease or postmaturity of the fetus. **P. TRANSFUSION SYNDROME,** occurs in twin pregnancies; one twin is anemic at birth and the other is plethoric resulting from the forcing of placental blood into its circulation from that of the other twin.

placentography (plas-en-tog′ra-fi): X-ray examination of the placenta after delivery, using a contrast medium.

plagiocephaly (plā′ji-ō-sef′a-li): A lopsided or unsymmetrically shaped head, due to abnormal closure of the cranial sutures.

plague (plāg): Any disease of wide prevalence and high mortality, but particularly the very contagious epidemic disease caused by *Pasteurella pestis,* and spread by infected rats that transfer the infection to humans through the agency of fleas. It is characterized by high fever, prostration, a petechial eruption, glandular swellings. The main clinical types are bubonic, pneumonic, septicemic, and sylvatic. Also called pest, black death, oriental plague. See **bubo, bubonic plague.**

plane (plān): A flat smooth surface. In anatomy, an assumed or imaginary surface extending from certain landmarks through an axis of the body, *e.g.,* the **SAGITTAL P.** extends from the sagittal suture downward and divides the body into right and left portions, the **FRONTAL P.** runs (often referred to as the **CORONAL P.**) at right angles to the sagittal **P.** and divides the body into anterior and posterior portions; the **TRANSVERSE P.** divides the body into superior and inferior portions.

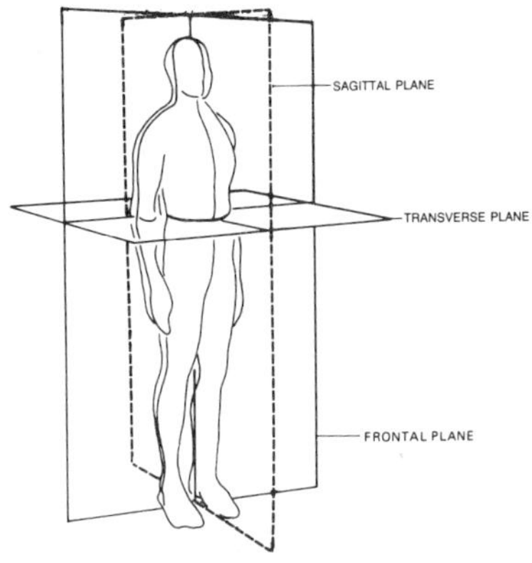

Planes of the Body

planigraphy (pla-nig′ra-fi): Tomography (*q.v.*).

planned parenthood: 1. The practice of measures (including contraception) that limit the number of offspring and determine the time interval between pregnancies. 2. An organization that promotes and distributes information regarding the number and spacing of children in families, *e.g.*, Planned Parenthood Federation of America.

planta (plan′ta): The sole of the foot.—plantae, pl.

plantar (plan′tar): Pertaining to the sole of the foot. **P. ARCH**, the union of the **P.** and dorsalis pedis arteries in the sole of the foot. **P. FLEXION**, downward movement of the big toe; opp. of dorsiflexion. **P. WART**, one that occurs on the sole of the foot; usually very painful and difficult to cure; thought to be caused by a specific virus that attacks irritated tissue.

planus (plan′us): Flat. Refers to a foot having a low arch; flatfoot.

plaque (plak): 1. A small flattened localized abnormal area or patch on a body surface or part. 2. A blood platelet. **ARGYROPHILIC P.**, microscopic areas of degeneration in the cerebral cortex which stain readily with silver; a diagnostic sign of Alzheimer's disease. **ATHEROMATOUS P.**, a deposit of fatty or fibrous material in the walls of a blood vessel, as occurs in atherosclerosis. **DENTAL P.**, deposit of material which may or may not contain colonies of bacteria on the surface of a tooth; it causes fermentation of carbohydrates with the formation of acids which demineralize the tooth enamel, then the dentin, resulting in a cavity. **SENILE P.**, areas of incomplete necrosis in the cerebral cortex of persons with senile dementia.

-plasia: Combining form denoting formation, development.

plasm: 1. Plasma. 2. That part of the germ cell that contains the substance by which individual characteristics are transmitted from generation to generation.

plasm-, plasmo-: Combining forms denoting; 1. The blood plasma. 2. The substance of a cell.

plasma: 1. Cytoplasm or protoplasm. 2. The liquid fraction of lymph. 3. The liquid fraction of the circulating blood; to be differentiated from serum (*q.v.*). It is clear, straw-colored and 90 percent water. Suspended or dissolved substances in it include the blood corpuscles, fibrinogen, electrolytes, proteins, hormones, vitamins, various waste products, and gases.—plasmic, adj.

plasma cell: See B lymphocyte.

plasmacyte (plaz′ma-sit): Plasma cell.

plasmacytoma (plaz′ma-sī-tō′ma): A focal neoplasm consisting of plasma cells. See also multiple myeloma.

plasmacytosis (plaz′ma-sī-tō′sis): An abnormal number of plasmacytes in 1) the peripheral blood, or 2) in the lymph nodes, spleen, liver, kidney, or bone marrow.

plasmapheresis (plaz′ma-fer-ē′sis): A complex technique using a large quantity of blood from which the cells are separated by centrifugation and are then added to a nonprotein fluid and reinjected into the body; done for both experimental and therapeutic reasons.

plasmin (plaz′min): The active substance in fibrinolysin that has the particular ability to dissolve fibrin clots.

plasminogen (plaz-min′ō-jen): The inactive precursor of plasmin; found in many body fluids and tissues; the release of inactivators from damaged tissues promotes its conversion into plasmin.

Plasmodium (plaz-mō′di-um): A genus of protozoa; parasitic in the red blood cells of warm-blooded animals; they complete their sexual cycle in blood-sucking arthropods. Four species cause malaria in man—**P. FALCIPARUM**, **P. MALARIAE**, **P. OVALE**, and **P. VIVAX**.

plasmolysis (plaz-mol′i-sis): Contraction or shrinking of a cell due to loss of water by osmosis; occurs when the cell is suspended in a hypertonic solution.

plasmoptysis (plaz-mop′ti-sis): The swelling of a cell and bursting of its wall with the escape of protoplasm; occurs when the cell is suspended in a hypotonic solution.

plaster: A fabric or similar material, spread with a mixture or substance that may or may not contain a medication, to be applied externally. **ADHESIVE P.**, fabric coated with a gummy substance; used to hold dressings in place, to protect wounds, sometimes for immobilization of a part. **COURT P., P.** made of isinglass spread on fine fabric; used for covering small lesions. **MUSTARD P.**, made of mustard and flour mixed with water and spread on a cloth; a counterirritant. See also **plaster of Paris.**

plaster of Paris: Gypsum cement (calcium sulfate), which forms a quick setting paste when mixed with water; used for casts and stiff bandages to immobilize a part.

plastic (plas′tik): 1. Tending to build up or regenerate tissue. 2. Capable of taking the form of a mold. 3. A substance that has been produced chemically. **P. SURGERY,** a surgical procedure in which healthy tissue is transferred, or tissues are reconstructed or repaired in order to correct deformities or abnormalities present at birth or caused by injuries, burns, etc.

plasticizer (plas′ti-sīz′er): Any of a group of agents that can be combined with other organic or synthetic substances to make them softer and more pliable.

-plasty: Combining form denoting 1) molding or shaping; 2) repair, reconstruction, plastic surgery.

plate: 1. In anatomy, a thin, flat structure, especially a bone. 2. A narrow, flat piece of metal that is screwed to the ends of fractured bones to keep them in alignment. 3. Common term for a denture.

plateau level: In drug administration, refers to the time when the amount of drug eliminated remains at the same level regardless of the amount of the drug that is in the body.

platelet (plāt′let): Small, oval, disk-like colorless cell found in the blood plasma; does not contain hemoglobin; is essential for clotting. A thrombocyte. **P. PHERESIS,** the removal of platelets from whole blood and immediate return of the red cells, white cells, and plasma to the donor.

plating (plāt′ing): The cultivation of bacteria on solid medium in a Petri dish.

platy-: Combining form denoting broad or flat.

platybasia (plat′i-bāz′i-a): A developmental anomaly in which the cervical spine appears to have pushed the floor of the occipital bone upward, producing a short neck, torticollis, and features of Arnold-Chiari deformity (*q.v.*).

platycephalic (plat′i-se-fal′ik): Having a skull that is flattened on top. Also platycephalous.

Platyhelminthes (plat′i-hel-min′thēz): Flatworm; fluke. See **schistosomiasis.**

platymorphic (plat′i-mor′fik): Having a flattened shape; used especially in reference to the eyeball.

platyopic (plat′i-op′ik): Having a broad face.

platypnea (pla-tip′nē-a): Dyspnea occurring when one is in the upright position and which is relieved when the person assumes a recumbent or semi-recumbent position; the opposite of orthopnea.

platypodia (plat-i-pō′di-a): Flatfootedness.

platysma (pla-tiz′-ma): The broad, thin sheet of muscle on each side of the neck; it acts to depress the lower jaw and draw down the corners of the mouth.

play therapy: See under **therapy.**

pleasure principle: The tendency to direct one's behavior toward immediate satisfaction of innate drives and immediate relief from any pain or discomforting situation.

pledget (plej′et): A small compress of gauze or a tuft of wool or cotton.

-plegia: Combining form denoting paralysis.

pleio-, pleo-, plio-: Combining forms denoting more.

pleocytosis (plē′ō-sī-tō′sis): 1. An increase of cells any place in the body. 2. An increase in the number of lymphocytes in the cerebrospinal fluid.

pleomastia (plē-ō-mas′ti-a): The condition of having supernumerary breasts or nipples.

pleomorphism (plē′ō-mor′fizm): Denotes a wide range in shape and size of individuals within a species or group of organisms.—pleomorphic, pleomorphous, adj.

pleonexia (plē-ō-nek′si-a): Greediness.

pleoptics (plē-op′tiks): A system of eye exercises to improve vision of a poorly functioning eye.

plethora (pleth′o-ra): Fullness; overloading. Used especially to describe a condition of overfullness of the blood vessels accompanied by congestion of tissues, a feeling of tension in the head, flushed complexion, bounding pulse.—plethoric, adj.

plethysmograph (pleth-iz′mō-graf): A device for measuring the volume variations in an organ, an extremity, or other body part. **OCULAR P.**, a device for measuring the systolic pressure in the ophthalmic artery.

plethysmography (pleth′iz-mog′ra-fi): 1. The determination of variations in the size of an organ or part by measuring change in its volume. 2. Determination of the variation in size of a body part by measuring the volume of blood contained in it or passing through it.

pleura (ploo′ra): A thin serous membrane covering the surface of the lung and reflecting, at the root of the lung, on to the chest wall. **PARIETAL P.**, that portion of the pleura that lines the inner surface of the chest wall and covers the top of the diaphragm. **VICERAL P.**, that portion of the pleura that is closely adherent to the lung surface. It is separated from the parietal **P.** by a very thin layer of fluid.—pleurae, pl.; pleural, adj.

pleuracentesis (ploor′a-sen-tē′sis): Surgical puncture of the chest wall for drainage of fluid. Pleurocentesis. Thoracocentesis.

pleural (ploor′al): Of or pertaining to the pleura. **P. CAVITY,** the potential space between the parietal and visceral pleura. **P. EFFUSION,** the presence of fluid in the pleural space; heard on auscultation as a crackling, grating sound during both inspiration and expiration. **P. FRICTION RUB,** see under rub. **P. SPACE,** the potential space between the parietal and visceral layers of pleura; it contains a very small amount of serous fluid which prevents friction on breathing. **P. TAP,** thoracentesis (*q.v.*).

pleuralgia (ploo-ral'ji-a): Pain in the pleura or in the side of the chest.—pleuralgic, adj.

pleurisy (ploor'-i-si): Inflammation of the pleura. Pleuritis. May be fibrinous (dry), associated with an effusion (wet), or complicated by empyema. **DIAPHRAGMATIC P.,** inflammation of the pleura of the diaphragm. **DRY P.,** a painful type of **P.** in which the two pleural surfaces are covered with a fibrinous exudate resulting in acute pain, especially when coughing. **PURULENT P., P.** marked by high fever, chills, and sweating; aspirated fluid is purulent.—pleuritic, adj.

pleuritic (ploo-rit'ik): Pertaining to the pleura or to one suffering from pleurisy.

pleuritis (ploo-rī'tis): Pleurisy (*q.v.*).

pleurocele (ploo'rō-sēl): A hernia of the lungs or of the pleura.

pleurodynia (ploo'rō-dın'ē-a): Intercostal myalgia; muscular rheumatism, with pain and fever; symptoms are increased by movement and coughing; may appear in epidemic form. See Bornholm's disease.

pleurolysis (ploo-rol'i-sis): Loosening of the pleura from the thoracic wall to allow for collapse of the lung in treatment for pulmonary tuberculosis.

pleuropericardial (ploo'rō-per-i-kar'di-al): Pertaining to or affecting both the pleura and pericardium.

pleuropericarditis (ploo'rō-per-i-kar-dī'tis): Inflammation of the pleura and the pericardium.

pleuropneumonia-like organisms: A widely distributed group of minute organisms that cause atypical pneumonia (Mycoplasma); abbreviated PPLO.

pleuropulmonary (ploo'rō-pul'mo-nar-i): Pertaining to the pleura and lungs.

pleurothotonos (ploo'rō-thot'o-nos): A bending of the body to one side, due to tetany of the muscles.

pleurotomy (ploo-rot'o-mi): An incision into the pleural cavity to allow escape of effused fluid. Thoracotomy.

pleximeter (plek-sim'e-ter): A finger or small, thin oblong plate of hard material, that is held against the skin to receive the stroke of a finger or percussion hammer in indirect percussion; also called plessimeter. See percussion.

plexor (plek'sor): 1. A percussion hammer; see hammer. 2. The finger that applies the tap in the indirect method of percussion, usually the third right finger.

plexus (pleks'us): A network of vessels or nerves. **AUERBACH'S P.,** a network of nerves and ganglia located between the circular and longtitudinal muscle fibers of the esophagus, stomach, and intestine. **BRACHIAL P.,** one located at the side of the neck and extending into the axilla; made up of branches of three of the cervical nerves and the first two thoracic nerves; supplies the upper arm. **CELIAC P.,** one located in the peritoneal cavity at the level of the first lumbar vertebra; consists of a large mass of sympathetic nerves and ganglia which supply nerves to the abdominal viscera. **CERVICAL P.,** one made up of branches of the upper four cervical nerves; supplies nerves to the muscles of the neck and shoulders. **CHOROID P.,** projections of tufts of blood vessels from the pia mater into each of the ventricles of the brain; concerned with the secretion of cerebrospinal fluid. **ESOPHAGEAL P.,** one surrounding the esophagus; formed by branches of the vagus nerve and sympathetic trunks. **LUMBAR P.,** one located in the posterior part of the psoas major muscle; made up of branches of the 4th and 5th lumbar nerves. **LUMBOSACRAL P.,** the lumbar and sacral plexuses considered together because of their contiguity. **MEISSNER'S P.,** one in the submucosal coat of the intestine; consists of nerves and ganglia that supply the muscles and submucous membrane of the intestine. **SACRAL P.,** one made up of sacral nerves and parts of the 4th and 5th lumbar nerves; supplies nerves to the pelvic structures, buttocks, and lower limbs; gives off the sciatic nerve. **SOLAR P.,** the celiac **P.**

-plexy: Combining form denoting seizure or stroke.

plica (plī'ka): A fold.—plicate, adj.; plication, n.

plica syndrome (plī'ka): Inflammation of the folds in the synovium of the knee joint; marked by pain and effusion; caused by a blunt or twisting injury.

plication (plī-kā'shun): The taking of tucks in a structure to shorten it or in the walls of a hollow organ to make it smaller.

plinth: In health care, a bed or couch upon which the patient lies while being examined, receiving treatment, or performing therapeutic exercises.

-ploid: Suffix denoting: 1. Multiple in form. 2 Number of chromosomes.

plombage (plom-bazh'): The use of an inert material to fill the space between the lung and the chest wall in order to compress the lung in treatment for pulmonary tuberculosis.

plosive (plō'siv): The speech sound heard when the air stream is blocked for a moment and then suddenly released, as in pronouncing the letters *p* and *t*.

plumbism (plum′bizm): Chronic lead poisoning (*q.v.*).

plumbum (plum′bum): Lead.

Plummer-Vinson syndrome: Combination of severe glossitis with dysphagia caused by degeneration of the muscle of the esophagus, atrophy of the papillae of the tongue, and secondary (nutritional) anemia. [Henry Stanley Plummer, American physician. 1874–1937. Porter Paisley Vinson, American surgeon. 1890–1959.]

Plummer's disease: Hyperthyroidism occurring in patients having a toxic adenoma of the thyroid gland.

pluri-: Prefix denoting 1) several; 2) more.

pluriglandular (plū′ri-gland′ū-lar): Pertaining to or affecting several glands, as mucoviscidosis (*q.v.*)

pluripara (plū-rip′ara): Multipara; a woman who has had two or more pregnancies resulting in viable offspring.

pluripotent (plū-rip′o-tent): Having the potential for affecting more than one organ or tissue. **P. CELLS**, immature cells in the bone marrow that have the potential for developing into any of several types of tissue cells.

plutomania (plū′tō-mā′ni-a): The obsessional delusion that one possesses great wealth.

plutonium (plū-tō′ni-um): A radioactive metallic element (chemical symbol Pu), similar to uranium; used in nuclear weapons and as nuclear fuel. ^{238}Pu has been used as an energy source in pacemakers.

P.M.: Abbreviation for *post meridian* [L.] meaning after noon.

PNC: Abbreviation for premature nodal contraction.

-pnea, -pnoea-: Combining forms denoting 1) breath; 2) breathing.

pneum-, pneumo-: Combining forms denoting: 1. Lungs. 2. Air or gas. 3. Respiration.

pneumat-, pneumato-: Combining forms denoting: 1. Air or gas. 2. Breathing.

pneumathemia (nū-ma-thē′mi-a): Air embolism (*q.v.*); the presence of bubbles of air or gas in the blood.

pneumatic (nū-mat′ik): Pertaining to air or gas. **P. BOOT** or **SLEEVE**, a boot or sleeve of varying lengths which is applied to a limb and rhythmically compressed by inflation with air; used to decrease swelling and to prevent postoperative thrombophlebitis. **P. TOURNIQUET**, a narrow rubber band that is wrapped around a limb and then inflated with air to furnish pressure on the limb. **P. TROUSERS**, see military antishock trousers.

pneumatocele (nū′mat-ō-sēl): 1. A thin-walled cavity that forms within the lung. 2. A hernial protuberance of lung tissue. 3. A tumor that contains gas, especially one occurring in the scrotum.

pneumatograph (nū-mat′-ō-graf): An instrument for recording the movements of the chest wall during breathing. Pneumograph.

pneumatosis (nū-ma-tō′sis): The presence of air or gas in an abnormal place in the body. **P. CESTOIDES INTESTINALIS**, the presence of subserosal or submucosal gas-containing cysts in the wall of the intestine.

pneumatotherapy (nū′-mat-ō-ther′a-pi): Treatment with rarefied or condensed air. **CEREBRAL P.**, treatment of certain psychoses by introducing oxygen into the subarachnoid space.

pneumaturia (nū-ma-tū′ri-a): The passage of flatus during or after urination; usually the result of a bladder-bowel fistula but may also be due to decomposition of bladder urine. Pneumatinuria.

pneumobacillus (nū′mō-ba-sil′us): See Friedländer's bacillus and Klebsiella pneumoniae.

pneumocele (nū′mo-sēl): Pneumatocele (*q.v.*).

pneumocentesis (nū′mō-sen-tē′sis): Surgical puncture of a lung to allow drainage of accumulated fluid or pus, to evacuate a cavity, or to obtain material for diagnostic study.

pneumocephalus (nū-mō-sef′a-lus): The presence of air or gas within the cerebral ventricles.

pneumococcus (nū-mō-kok′us): *Diplococcus pneumoniae*. A gram-positive, encapsulated coccal bacterium, characterically arranged in pairs; the common cause of lobar pneumonia; also causal agent for otitis media, mastoiditis, and leptomeningitis as well as many other infections.—pneumococcal, adj.

pneumonoconiosis (nū′mō-nō-kō-ni-ō′sis): Dust disease. Fibrosis of the lung caused by long continued inhalation of dust in industrial occupations, such as coal mining, stone cutting, etc. The most important complication is the occasional superinfection with tuberculosis. Examples are silicosis, coal worker's **P.**, asbestosis, siderosis, grinder's lung and byssinosis, described elsewhere.—pneumonoconioses, pl.

Pneumocystis (nū′mō-sis′tis): A genus of microorganisms considered to be protozoa. **P. CARINII**, causative agent of a type of pneumonia in patients receiving immunosuppressive therapy for cancer or who have had an organ transplant, in premature infants, and in debilitated persons; may be called interstitial cell pneumonia or pneumocystosis.

pneumocyte (nū′mō-sīt): Any of the epithelial cells of the alveoli of the lungs. Also called pneumonocyte.

pneumoderma (nū-mō-der′ma): Subcutaneous emphysema; the presence of air or gas under the skin.

pneumodynamics (nū'mō-dī-nam'iks): The study of the mechanism and forces involved in breathing.

pneumoencephalogram (nū'-mō-en-sef'a-lō-gram): X-ray picture of the brain after replacement of the cerebrospinal fluid with gas or air.

pneumoencephalography (nū'mō-en-sef-a-log'ra-fi): The making of an x-ray film of the brain after replacing the cerebrospinal fluid of the subarachnoid space with a gas, accomplished through spinal puncture; will reveal any distortion that may be caused by the presence of a tumor or a degenerative disease; may be done under local or general anesthesia.

pneumogastric (nū-mō-gas'trik): Pertaining to the lungs and stomach. See **vagus**.

pneumography (nū-mog'ra-fi): 1. Roentgenology of the lungs. 2. The x-ray recording of the respiratory movements in breathing. 3. Roentgenology of a body organ or part after injection of a gas.

pneumohydrothorax (nū'mō-hī-drō-thō'raks): The presence of either gas or air and fluid in the pleural cavity.

pneumolysis (nū-mol'i-sis): Separation of the two pleural layers, or the outer pleural layer, from the chest wall to collapse the lung. Also pneumonolysis.

pneumomediastinogram (nū'mō-mē'-di-a-stī'no-gram): X-ray photograph of the mediastinum after rendering it opaque with air.

pneumomediastinum (nū'mō-mē-di-a-stī'num): The presence of air or gas in the mediastinal tissues; may result from emphysema or other pulmonary pathology such as respiratory distress syndrome in infants, cystic fibrosis, or asthma, or be introduced during certain diagnostic procedures.

pneumomelanosis (nū'mō-mel-a-nō'sis): A condition in which lung tissue becomes discolored or black due to inhalation of such substances as coal dust.

pneumomycosis (nū'-mō-mī-kō'sis): Fungus infection of the lung such as aspergillosis, actinomycosis, moniliasis.—pneumomycotic, adj.

pneumon-, pneumono-: Combining forms denoting lung(s).

pneumonectomy (nū'mo-nek'to-mi): Excision of a lung or of lung tissue.

pneumonia (nū-mō'ni-a): Inflammation of the lung with the production of alveolar exudate, which consolidates, resulting in symptoms of fever, cough, lethargy, dyspnea and/or apnea, anorexia, and fine crackling rales. Traditionally two main types were recognized on an anatomical or radiological basis, viz., lobar **P.** and broncho-**P.** The tendency now is to classify according to the specific bacterium or virus causing the infection (specific pneumonias) on the one hand, and the aspiration or secondary pneumonias on the other. **ASPIRATION P., P.** caused by inhalation by unconscious patients of foreign particles such as vomitus. **ATYPICAL P.,** primary atypical **P.** caused by bacteria, most commonly diplococcus, staphylococcus, streptococcus, tuberculosis bacillus. **ATYPICAL VIRAL P., P.** caused by a virus. **BRONCHIAL P.,** an inflammation of the lungs that begins in the bronchioles. **FRIEDLÄNDER'S P.,** acute **P.** characterized by massive exudation of mucoid material; caused by *Klebsiella pneumoniae*. **HYPOSTATIC P.,** the result of stasis; occurs in debilitated patients from lack of movement in the dependent part of the lung. **INFLUENZAL P.,** severe, often fatal **P.** caused by the influenza virus; characterized by high fever, prostration, sore throat, dyspnea; may be complicated by bacterial pneumonia. **INHALATION P.,** aspiration **P.** LOBAR P., an acute febrile disease caused by the *Diplococcus pneumoniae;* characterized by inflammation and consolidation of one or more lobes of the lung, chills, dyspnea, pain in the chest, cough, bloody expectoration. **PNEUMOCOCCAL P.,** lobar **P. PRIMARY ATYPICAL P.,** an acute **P.** caused by *Mycoplasma pneumoniae* and various viruses; marked by fever, myalgia, sore throat, unproductive cough which later becomes productive; also called viral **P. TERMINAL P., P.** that develops during the course of another disease and often hastens death. **VIRAL P., P.** caused by a virus, most commonly adenoviruses, influenza virus, or varicella virus.

pneumonitis (nū-mō-nī'tis): Acute inflammation of lung tissue. **ASPIRATION P.,** caused by inhalation of foreign matter into the lung; may be an extremely serious complication of anesthesia. **CHEMICAL P.,** caused by inhalation of an irritating chemical. **GRANULOMATOUS P.,** farmer's lung (*q.v.*). **HYPERSENSITIVITY P.,** occurs in individuals whose occupations expose them to dusts containing animal or vegetable products or fungal spores, and who develop diseases such as farmer's lung or bagassosis.

pneumopericardium (nū'mō-per-i-kar'di-um): The presence of air in the pericardial sac.

pneumoperitoneum (nū'mō-per-it-o-nē'um): Air or gas in the peritoneal cavity. May follow perforated gastric ulcer, peritonitis, other pathologic conditions, or may be introduced for diagnostic or therapeutic reasons.

pneumoradiography (nū'mō-rā-di-og'ra-fi): Radiographic examination of a region after injection of air, oxygen or other gas.

pneumoresection (nū'mō-rē-sek'shun): Surgical removal of part of a lung.

pneumorrhagia (nū-mō-rā'ji-a): Hemorrhage from the lungs.

pneumotachograph (nū-mō-tak'ō-graf): A device for measuring the flow of air going to and from the lungs. Some models also measure several other parameters of respiration, *e.g.*, tidal volume, inspired oxygen fraction, expired carbon dioxide.

pneumotaxic (nū-mō-tak′sik): Pertaining to pneumotaxis. **P. CENTER,** the center in the pons that stimulates the expiratory center in the medulla.

pneumotaxis (nū-mō-tak′sis): The control of the rate of respiration.—pneumotaxic, adj.

pneumothorax (nū-mō-thō′raks): Air or gas in the pleural cavity; causes severe pain, dyspnea, absence of breath sounds, abnormal distention of the chest. **ARTIFICIAL P.,** induced in the treatment of pulmonary tuberculosis. **OPEN P., P.** caused by an injury to the chest wall that exposes the pleural cavity to the atmosphere. **SPONTANEOUS P.,** occurs when an overdilated pulmonary air sac ruptures, permitting communication between the respiratory passages and pleural cavity. **TENSION P.,** occurs when a valve-like wound allows air to enter the pleural cavity at each inspiration but not to escape on expiration, thus progressively increasing intrathoracic pressure.

pneumotoxin (nū-mō-tok′sin): An endotoxin produced by the pneumococcus and believed to be responsible for the systemic symptoms of lobar pneumonia.

pneumoventriculography (nū′mō-ven-trik′ū-log′ra-fi): Examination of cerebral ventricles by x ray after removal of the fluid content and direct injection of air.

PNP: Abbreviation for Pediatric Nurse Practitioner.

PO_2: The symbol for the partial pressure of oxygen; in arterial blood normally about 100 mgHg; lower than 70 mmHg denotes a serious oxygen lack.

p.o.: Abbreviation for *per os* [L.], meaning per mouth. Also written P.O.

pock: A pustule, specifically the pustular lesion characteristic of smallpox.

pockmark: The small, depressed mark, scar, or pit left after the pustular lesion of smallpox heals.

pod-, podo-: Combining forms denoting foot or foot-like.

podagra (pō-dag′ra): Gout in the foot, especially that in the metatarsophalangeal joint of the big toe.

podalgia (pō-dal′ji-a): Pain in the foot or feet.

podalic (pōdal′ik): Pertains to accomplishment by means of the feet. **P. VERSION,** see under version.

podarthritis (pod-ar-thrī′tis): Arthritis of the joints of the feet.

podiatrist (po-dī′a-trist): One who specializes in the diagnosis and treatment of diseases and defects of the feet. Syn., chiropodist.—podiatry, n.

podobromidrosis (pōd′ō-brō-mid-rō′sis): Offensive perspiration of the feet.

pododynia (pōd-ō-din′i-a): Pain in the foot or feet. Syn., podalgia.

podogeriatric (pōd-ō-jer-i-at′ric): Refers to foot care for the elderly.

-poiesis: Combining form denoting production or the formation of.

poikilocyte (poy′kil-ō-sīt): A large irregularly shaped red blood cell; frequently found in severe hemolytic anemias.

poikilocytosis (poy′kil-ō-sī-tō′sis): 1. Variation in the shape of red blood corpuscles, *e.g.*, the pear-shaped cells found in the blood in pernicious anemia. 2. The presence of poikilocytes in the circulating blood.

poikiloderma (poy′kil-o-der′ma): A skin disorder characterized by dryness, pigmentation, purpura, mottling, and atrophy. **P. CONGENITALE,** a hereditary disorder characterized by erythema and pigmentation of the skin, telangectasia, skeletal defects, baldness, hypogonadism, and juvenile cataracts.

poikilotherm (poy′kil-ō-therm): An organism whose body temperature varies with that of the environment; a so-called cold-blooded animal.

poikilothermy (poy′kil-ō-ther′mi): 1. A characteristic of certain animals in which the temperature changes in accordance with the changes in temperature of the environment. 2. Having a body temperature that changes with that of the environment.—poikilothermism, n.; poikilothermal, poikilothermic, adj.

poison (poy′z′n): Any substance that is harmful or lethal when applied to or taken into the body. **P. IVY,** see ivy poisoning.

poison control center: A facility equipped with personnel and reference works adequate to answer questions of the public about poisons and treatments for poisoning. Often associated with hospitals, medical schools or health departments. There are over 400 such centers in the U.S.; most of them are open 24 hours a day.

poisoning (poy′z′n-ing): A state produced by the introduction of a poisonous substance into the body or by exposure to such substance. **ACID P.,** causes erosion of the tissues and skin. **ALKALI P.,** corrosive **P.;** most often due to ingestion or contact with lye, or with sodium or potassium hydroxide. **CARBON MONOXIDE P., P.** due to inhalation of carbon monoxide gas which is contained in automobile exhaust, illuminating gas, sewer gas, and in mines.

poker back: Ankylosing spondylitis. See under spondylitis.

polarity (po-lar′i-ti): 1. In physics, the property of having two opposite poles, as in a magnet or storage battery. 2. The presence of manifestation of opposing or contrasting principles, tendencies, or emotions, as love and hate, or femininity and masculinity.

polarization (pō'lar-ī-zā'shun): 1. The separation of the positive and negative charges in a molecule. 2. The production or acquisition of polarity. 3. A condition in which substances of opposite electrical charges are separated by a membrane, as in the cells of the body.—polarize, v.

poli-, polio-: Combining forms denoting relationship to the gray matter of the nervous system.

polio: Colloquial term for poliomyelitis (*q.v.*).

polio vaccine: Vaccine given for the purpose of conferring immunity to poliomyelitis.

polioencephalitis (pō'li-ō-en-sef-a-lī'tis): Inflammation of the gray matter of the brain. Caused by poliomyelitis virus; marked by fever, headache, anxiety, confusion, trembling, twitching of facial muscles, insommnia, sometimes convulsions, lethargy; often fatal.—polioencephalitic, adj.

polioencephalomyelitis (pō'li-ō-en-sef'a-lō-mī-e-lī'tis): Inflammation of the gray matter of the brain and the spinal cord; caused by poliovirus.

poliomyelitis (pō'li-ō-mī'e-lī'tis): Inflammation of the gray matter of the spinal cord; an acute epidemic viral disease affecting children especially; marked by fever, headache, sore throat, stiff neck, gastrointestinal symptoms. May lead to paralysis and atrophy of one or more groups of skeletal muscles with resulting permanent deformity and disability. It is estimated (1987) that 20 to 25 percent of the people who had the disease in the epidemic of 1940–1950 have had late effects, with symptoms that resemble those of the disease including pain in muscles along with weakness of muscles that had not been affected earlier, joint pain, fatigue, and general weakness; may require the use of braces and portable respirators; seldom fatal. **ACUTE ANTERIOR P., P.**, in which the virus attacks the anterior horns of the gray matter of the spinal cord. **ASCENDING P., P.** that is first manifested in the legs and progresses upward. **BULBAR P.**, a serious form of **P.** in which the virus attacks the medulla oblongata; there may be inability to swallow, paralysis, respiratory distress leading to respiratory failure. **CEREBRAL P., P.** that involves the brain stem and areas of the motor cortex; polioencephalitis. **POSTINOCULATION P.**, symptoms of **P.** that appear, usually within three weeks, following some types of inoculation. **SPINAL PARALYTIC P.**, the classic form of **P.** with flaccid paralysis of one or more limbs.

poliosis (pōl-i-ō'sis): Premature graying of the hair.

poliovirus (pō'li-ōvī'rus): The causative agent of poliomyelitis. Three types are recognized serologically, of which Type One is the most frequent cause of paralytic poliomyelitis.

Politzer's bag: A soft, rubber, pear-shaped bag with a long tube and nozzle; used to inflate the inner ear via the nose and eustachian tube.—politzerization, n.

pollex (pol'eks): The thumb. **P. PEDIS**, the great toe.—pollices, pl.

pollinosis (pol-i-nō'sis): Allergic condition characterized by catarrh affecting the mucous membranes of eyes, nose, and respiratory tract; caused by sensitivity to pollen and recurs annually, usually in the spring or late summer. Hay fever and rose fever are examples of **P.** Also pollenosis.

pollutant (pō-lū'tant): Anything that acts to contaminate, befoul, dirty, or render impure the atmosphere or any other necessity for life; usually refers to agents that contaminate the human environment.

pollute (pol-lūt'): To render the environment or some substance impure, unclean, or unhealthful; to defile.

pollution (po-lū'shun): 1. Defilement; uncleanness; impurity. 2. Emission of semen at times other than during coitus, *e.g.*, nocturnal emission.

poly: Abbreviation and colloquial term often used to designate polymorphonuclear leukocyte.

poly-: Combining form denoting many, several, diverse, excessive, multiple.

polyadenitis (pol'i-ad-e-nī'tis): Inflammation of several lymph nodes at the same time; refers especially to the cervical nodes.

polyandry (pol-i-an'-dri): A social setting in which a woman may be legally married to more than one man at the same time.—polyandrous, adj.

polyarteritis (pol-i-ar-te-rī'tis): Simultaneous inflammation of several arteries. **P. NODOSA**, inflammation of the coats of the arteries in multiple circumscribed areas resulting in the formation of nodules; see **periarteritis nodosa**.

polyarthritis (pol'i-ar-thrī'tis): Inflammation of several joints at the same time. See **Still's disease**. Occasionally occurs in epidemic form, thought to be due to a virus; characterized by slight fever, rash, pain in joints of hands and feet.

polyarticular (pol-i-ar-tik'ū-lar): Pertaining to or affecting several joints simultaneously.

polyavitaminosis (pol'i-a'vī-ta-min-ō'sis): A pathological condition in which there is a deficiency of more than one vitamin in the diet.

polyblennia (pol-i-blen'i-a): Excess production of mucus.

polycholia (pol-i-kō'li-a): Excessive secretion of bile.

polychondritis (pol′i-kon-drī′tis): Inflammation of cartilage in several parts of the body. **RELAPSING P.**, an idiopathic condition in which recurring bouts of **P.** are accompanied by fever and malaise and may eventually result in deformities; affects chiefly the ears, nose, larynx, trachea, bronchi.

polychromasia (pol′i-krō-mā′zi-a): 1. In physiology, variation in the amount of hemoglobin in the red blood cells. 2. Polychromatophilia (*q.v.*).

polychromatic (pol′i-kro-mat′ik): Having various or changing colors.

polychromatophilia (pol-i-krō′ma-tō-fil′i-a): 1. The presence in blood of red blood cells that are susceptible to staining with more than one dye. 2. The tendency of cells to stain with both basic and acid stains.

polychromia (pol-i-krō′mi-a): Increased pigmentation or coloration in any part of the body.

polyclinic (pol-i-klin′ik): A clinic or hospital that cares for several types of diseases and injuries.

polycrotic (pol-i-krot′ik): Descriptive of a pulse that has several secondary waves following each pulse beat.

polycyesis (pol-i-sī-ē′sis): Multiple pregnancy.

polycystic (pol-i-sis′tik): Containing or composed of many cysts. **P. KIDNEY DISEASE,** may be 1) congenital and slowly fatal, or 2) familial, with cysts forming in the medulla of the kidney, and usually seen in children. **P. OVARY SYNDROME,** See Stein-Leventhal syndrome.

polycystoma (pol-i-sis-tō′ma): A condition in which a part of the body has many cysts; said especially of the breast.

polycythemia (pol′i-sī-thē′mi-a): Excess in the number of circulating red blood cells. This may result from dehydration or be a compensatory phenomenon to increase the oxygen carrying capacity, as in congenital heart disease. **P. VERA,** an idiopathic condition in which the red cell count is very high. The white cell count, platelets, volume and viscosity of the blood are also increased; there is hyperemia of all organs and enlargement of the spleen. The patient complains of headache and lassitude and there is danger of thrombosis and hemorrhage. **RELATIVE P.,** a relative increase in red blood cell count, due to loss of fluid from the blood.—polycythemic, adj.

polycytosis (pol′i-sī-tō′sis): An increase in the red and white cells of the blood with a reduction in blood volume.

polydactly (pol-i-dak′ti-li): A congenital anomaly consisting of the presence of more than the normal number of fingers or toes. Also called polydactilia and polydactylism.

polydipsia (pol-i-dip′si-a): Frequent drinking because of excessive thirst, a characteristic of diabetes; may also be of psychogenic origin, due to a personality disorder.

polyemia (pol-i-ē′mi-a): Excess amount of blood in the body.

polyethylene (pol-i-eth′i-lēn): A synthetic plastic material, highly resistant to chemicals; frequently utilized in making materials used in surgical procedures and in making tubing used in medicine.

polygalactia (pol′i-ga-lak′shi-a): Excessive secretion of milk.

polygene (pol′i-jēn): Any of a group of genes which, acting together, tend to influence the same character traits in the same way, resulting in a cumulative effect in the individual.

polyglandular (pol-i-glan′dū-lar): Pertaining to or affecting several glands and/or their secretions.

polygraph (pol′i-graf): An instrument that records several impulses or pulsations simultaneously; *e.g.*, pulse beat, blood pressure, and respiratory movements, any or all of which may be affected by emotional reactions, and thus is useful in detecting lying or deception. Commonly called a lie detector.

polyhidrosis (pol′i-hīd-rō′sis): Excessive secretion of sweat; hyperhydrosis.

polyhydramnios (pol′i-hī-dram′ni-ōs): The presence of more than the normal amount of amniotic fluid in the uterus at term; appears to be associated with a high percentage of congenital anomalies, especially anencephaly and esophageal atresia.

polyhydruria (pol-i-hi-drū′ri-a): The presence of an abnormally large fluid content of the urine.

polyhypermenorrhea (pol′i-hī′per-men-ō-rē′a): Frequent profuse menstruation.

polyhypomenorrhea (pol′i-hī′pō-men-ō-rē′a): Frequent scanty menstruation.

polyinfection (pol-i-in-fek′shun): Mixed infection; infection with two or more organisms at the same time.

polyleptic (pol-i-lep′tik): Descriptive of diseases that have many remissions and exacerbations, *e.g.*, malaria.

polymastia (pol-i-mas′ti-a): The condition of having more than two breasts.

polymenorrhagia (pol′i-men-ō-rāj′i-a): Menstrual periods that are both too heavy and too frequent.

polymenorrhea (pol′i-men-ō-rē′a): Menstrual periods that are normal in amount but occur too frequently.

polymer (pol′i-mer): A natural or synthetic chemical compound that results when two or more molecules of the same substance are combined to form a larger molecule.

polymerization (pol'i-mer-ī-zā'shun): The building up of large molecules, usually of high molecular weight, by combining identical smaller ones.

polymicrogyria (pol'i-mī-krō-jī'ri-a): A condition of the cerebral cortex, characterized by many small convolutions; caused by faulty brain development.

polymorphic (pol-i-mor' -fik): Multiform; existing or occurring in several forms.

polymorphonuclear (pol'i-mor-fō-nū'klē-ar): Having a many-shaped or lobulated nucleus; usually applied to the neutrophil leukocytes which constitute about 75 percent of the total white blood cell count and which function as phagocytes. See eosinophil; basophil.

polymorphous (pol-i-mor'fus): Occurring in many different morphologic forms; polymorphic.

polymyalgia (pol'i-mī-al'ji-a): Myalgia affecting several muscles at the same time. **P. RHEUMATICA,** a syndrome affecting older people; marked by pain and stiffness in the proximal muscles and joints in the neck, and in the shoulder and pelvic girdles, accompanied by a high sedimentation rate; responds to corticosteroid therapy.

polymyositis (pol-i-mī-ō-sī'tis): Inflammation of several muscles at the same time. Often refers to a group of disorders characterized by slowly developing muscle pain and weakness, especially of the shoulder and pelvic girdles, dysphagia, arthralgia, fever, erythematous rash and purplish discoloration of the skin of the face, neck, chest, hands and elbows; seen most often in females. In older people often associated with malignancy.

polyneuritis (pol-i-nū-rī'tis): Inflammation of many peripheral nerves at the same time. Some of the causes are alcoholism; poisoning, particularly from metals; vitamin deficiency, especially of thiamine. **ACUTE IDIOPATHIC P.,** may follow a febrile illness; characterized by sensory disturbances, muscular weakness, impaired reflexes; see also Guillain-Barré syndrome and Landry's disease.

polyneuropathy (pol'i-nū-rop'a-thi): Disease involving several nerves simultaneously, usually peripheral and/or cranial nerves; characterized by aching, burning, numbing, and tingling of the lower legs and feet; symptoms may extend to the arm; may be associated with such systemic disorders as diabetes, uremia, carcinoma, alcoholism, poisonings.

polyopia (pol'i-ō'pi-a): Seeing many images of a single object simultaneously; multiple vision.

polyorchidism (pol-i-or'ki-dizm): The condition of having more than two testes.

polyp or polypus (pol'ip-us): A small, smooth, finger-like growth arising from skin or a mucous surface (in the cervix, uterus, nose, rectum), usually attached by a stem. Most often benign but may become malignant.—polypi, pl.; polypous, adj.

polypectomy (pol-i-pek'to-mi): Surgical removal of a polyp.

polypeptides (pol-i-pep'tīdz): Proteins with long chains of amino acids linked together by peptide bonds.

polyphagia (pol-i-fā'ji-a): Pathological overeating; excessive appetite. See bulimia.

polyphobia (pol-i-fō'bi-a): Morbid fear of many things.

polyphrasia (pol-i-frā'zi-a): Excessive or insane talkativeness. Syn. verbigeration.

polyplegia (pol-i-plē'ji-a): Paralysis of several muscles at the same time.

polypnea (pol-ip-nē'a): Very rapid breathing; panting.

polypoid (pol'i-poyd): Resembling a polyp.

polyposis (pol'i-pō'sis): A condition in which there are numerous polypi in an organ. **P. COLI,** a hereditary condition in which polypi occur throughout the large intestine, starting in childhood and increasing progressively with symptoms of colitis; it almost always leads to carcinoma of the colon when untreated. Also called familial intestinal **P.**

polysaccharide (pol-i-sak'a-rid): Any one of a class of carbohydrates containing a large number of monosaccharide groups $(C_6H_{12}O_6)_x$. Starch, inulin, glycogen, and cellulose are examples.

polyserositis (pol'i-sē-rō-sī'tis): Widespread, chronic inflammation of serous membranes, particularly those of the upper abdomen, with serous effusion.

polysinusitis (pol'i-sīn-ūsī'tis): Inflammation of several sinuses at the same time.

polysomnography (pol' -i-sōm-nog'ra-fi): The continuous recording of such physical parameters as eye movements, heart rate, brain waves, muscle tonus, etc.; used in diagnosing sleep disorders.

polythelia (pol-i-thē'li-a): The condition of having supernumerary nipples; may be on the breast or elsewhere on the body.

polytrichia (pol-i-trik'i-a): Excessive hairiness.

polyunsaturated (pol'i-un-sat'ū-rā-ted): A chemical term referring to fatty acids that have two or more unsaturated bonds; they tend to be liquid at room temperature; found in soybeans; fish oil; corn, sunflower, safflower, and cottonseed oils. These oils, and foods made from them, are less likely to form plaque than saturated fats.

polyuria (pol-i-ū'ri-a): Excretion of excessive amounts of urine; may be due to intake of excess solute that has to be excreted, failure of the kidney to concentrate the urine, inadequate secretion of antidiuretic hormone, or renal pathology including atherosclerosis of renal arteries, congestive heart failure, hypertension, diabetes insipidus.—polyuric, adj.

polyvalent (pol'i-vā-lent, po-liv'a-lent): Usually refers to a serum or vaccine that is effective against several strains of a particular organism.

Pompe's disease: Glycogen storage disease, Type II; a hereditary condition characterized by excessive storage of glycogen in the heart, liver, and skeletal muscles; severe weakness and enlarged heart. Prognosis for life is poor.

pompholyx (pom'fol-iks): Vesicular skin eruption on the palms of the hands or soles of the feet. See cheiropompholyx.

pomphus (pom'fus): A blister or wheal on the skin.—pomphoid, adj.

POMR: Abbreviation for problem-oriented medical records.

PONS: Abbreviation for problem-oriented nursing service. See problem-oriented medical records.

pons: A bridge; a process of tissue joining two sections of an organ.—pontine, adj. **PONS VAROLII**, the white convex mass of nerve tissue at the base of the brain which serves to connect the cerebrum, cerebellum, and medulla oblongata.

pontine (pon'tēn): Pertaining to the pons varolii.

popliteal (pop-li-tē'al, pop-lit'e-al): Pertaining to the posterior surface of the knee. **P. CYST**, see Baker's cyst. **P. SPACE**, the diamond shaped depression at the back of the knee joint, bounded by the muscles and containing the popliteal nerve and vessels.

popliteus (pop-li-tē'us): A muscle at the back part of the knee joint; it assists in flexing the leg at the knee and in rotating the leg.

POR: Abbreviation for problem-oriented records.

poradenitis (por'ad-e-nī'tis): A condition characterized by the formation of small abscesses in the iliac glands; occurs in lymphogranuloma inguinale (*q.v.*).

pore: A small opening. One of the minute openings of the ducts that lead from the sweat glands to the surface of the skin; they are controlled by fine papillary muscles that contract in the cold, and dilate in the presence of heat.

porencephalia, porencephaly (por'en-sefā'li-a, sef'a-li): A condition in which there is inflammation of the brain in early infancy with the formation of cavities in the brain substance; may be congenital, or due to imperfect development, infection, or injury following birth.

pores of Kohn: Small holes in the walls of the alveoli that allow communication between parts of the lung lobules that are supplied by different bronchioles.

pornography (por-nog'ra-fi): 1. The depiction of erotic behavior in books or other media with the objective of arousing sexual excitement. 2. Devices such as pictures and books intended to arouse sexual excitement through depiction of erotic behavior.

porosis (pō-rō'sis): The formation of cavities or holes in tissue, *e.g.*, osteoporosis (*q.v.*).

porosity (pō-ros'i-ti): 1. A pore, as in the skin. 2. The condition of being porous.

porphobilinogen (por'fō-bī-lin'ō-jen): A chromogen involved in the biosynthesis of heme and porphyrin; found in the urine of some patients with acute intermittent porphyria.

porphyria (por-fī'ri-a, por-fir'i-a): A pathological state due to an inborn error of metabolism of blood pigments, resulting in the production of excess porphyrins in the blood, feces, and urine. Symptoms include abdominal pain, profound neuritis, weakness that may progress to total paralysis, pathological changes in nervous and muscular tissue, a variety of mental symptoms, and excessive amounts of porphyrin precursors in the urine. **ACUTE INTERMITTENT P.**, a rare form of **P.** that may be precipitated by certain drugs, infection, or pregnancy; seen mostly in young and middle-aged persons; characterized by extreme sensitivity to light along with other symptoms of **P. CONGENITAL ERYTHROPOIETIC P.**, a rare form of **P.** seen in infants and young children; due to a defect in the synthesis of hemoglobin; characterized by cutaneous photosensitivity that leads to formation of multilating lesions, enlarged spleen, hemolytic anemia, and the presence of porphyrins in the blood; often causes early death. **P. CUNEA TARDA**, a form of **P.** marked by photosensitivity, skin lesions, liver disease, and the presence of porphyrins in the urine; may be caused by the ingestion of certain drugs or alcohol. **P. HEPATICA**, includes several types of **P.** including those that occur following hepatitis or heavy metal poisoning.

porphyrin (por-fī'rin, por'fi-rin): Any one of a group of organic pigments that are widely distributed in nature and also exist in small amounts in the human body.

porphyrinuria (por'fi-rin-ū'ri-a): Excretion of porphyrins in the urine. Such pigments are produced as a result of an inborn error of metabolism. The urine becomes red or dark brown in color. See porphyria.

porrigo (po-rī'gō): Any disease condition of the scalp in which there is scaling or loss of hair and a tendency to spread.

porta: The depression (hilum) of an organ at which the vessels and nerves enter and, in some organs, excretory ducts leave.—portal, adj. **P. HEPATIS**, the transverse fissure through which the portal vein, hepatic artery and bile ducts pass on the under surface of the liver.

portacaval (por′ta-kā′val): Pertaining to the portal vein and inferior vena cava. **P. ANASTOMOSIS,** a fistula made between the portal vein and the inferior vena cava with the object of reducing the pressure within the portal vein in cases of cirrhosis of the liver. **P. SHUNT, P.** anastomosis.

portahepatitis (por′ta-hep-a-tī′tis): Inflammation around the transverse fissure of the liver.

portal (por′tal): 1. Pertaining to any porta or hilum, especially to the porta hepatis (*q.v.*). 2. The point of entrance of a pathogenic organism into the body: the most common **P.'S OF ENTRY** are 1) through the mouth and/or nose to the respiratory tract, by inhalation; 2) through the mouth to the alimentary tract, by ingestion; and 3) through the skin to the deeper tissues, by inoculation. **P. VEIN,** that conveying blood into the liver; about three inches long, it is formed by the union of the superior mesenteric and splenic veins.

Porter-Silber test: A laboratory test for the amount of 17-corticosteroids excreted in the urine as a means of evaluating adrenocortical function.

portogram (por′tō-gram): X-ray film of the portal vein after injection of radiopaque liquid.

portosystemic (por′tō-sis-tem′ik): Pertaining to the portal system. **P. ENCEPHALOPATHY,** see **hepatic encephalopathy** under **encephalopathy.**

port-wine stain or mark: A purplish-red superficial hemangioma of the skin occurring as a birthmark; a nevus (*q.v.*).

position: Posture; attitude. An arrangement of the parts of the body considered desirable or necessary for some medical or surgical procedure or for an examination. In obstetrics, the situation of the fetus in the pelvis as determined by the relation of an arbitrary point (occiput, chin, sacrum) to the right or left side of the mother. **ANATOMICAL P.,** the person stands erect with the arms at the sides and palms facing forward. **DORSAL P.,** the person lies flat on the back. **DORSAL RECUMBENT P.,** the person lies flat on the back with the knees slightly flexed and rotated outward. **FOWLER'S P.,** the person's head or the head of the bed is elevated to 18 or 20 inches above bed level; the knees are flexed and supported by a pillow; variations are specified as high, low, and semi-Fowler's. **FROG P., P.** sometimes assumed by premature infants or those with central nervous system disorders; the child lies prone with the thighs held in external rotation at the hips and abducted to about 90°. **GENUPECTORAL P.,** the person kneels on the table with the head and upper part of the chest also resting on the table; the arms are raised and crossed over the head. **GYNECOLOGICAL P.,** the lithotomy **P. JACKNIFE P.,** the person lies on the back with the legs flexed and the thighs at right angles to the torso. **KNEE-CHEST P.,** the genupectoral **P. LATERAL P.,** the person lies on the side with the knees slightly flexed. **LITHOTOMY P.,** the person lies on the back with the thighs flexed and abducted; the feet may be supported in stirrups. **PRONE P.,** the person lies flat and face downward. **RECUMBENT P.,** the person lies on the back with knees slightly flexed and the arms crossed over the abdomen. **SHOCK P.,** the patient is kept lying down in full Trendelenberg **P.** (*q.v.*), with the head of the bed

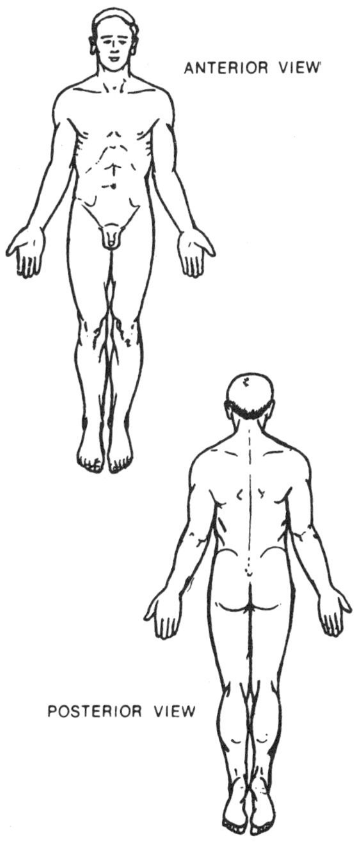

Anatomical position

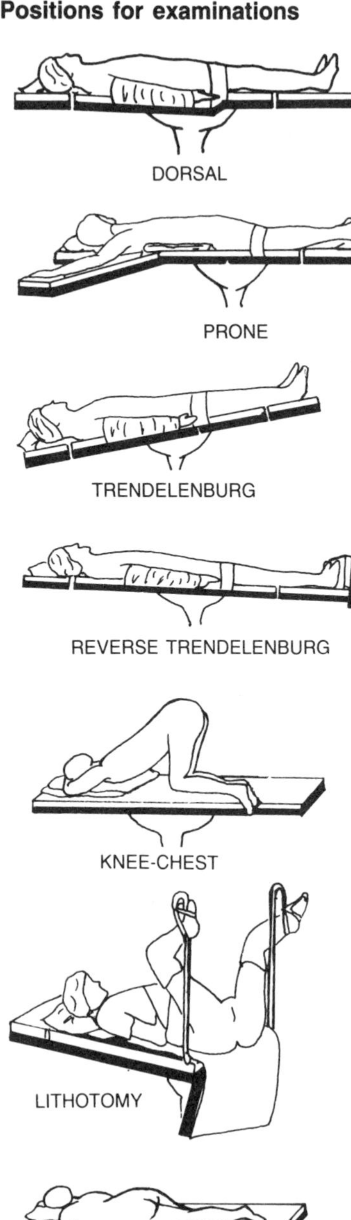

Positions for various examinations

lowered, or in a modified Trendelenberg **P.** in which only the legs are elevated. **SIM'S P.**, the person lies on the left side, with the right knee and thigh drawn up well above the left, the left arm behind the person and hanging over the edge of the table, and the chest inclined forward so the person rests on it. **SUPINE P.**, the dorsal **P. TRENDELENBERG P.**, the person lies on the back, with the body elevated at an angle of 45°, the head down, and the lower legs and feet hanging over the edge of the table; the hands are crossed over the chest.

Position Paper: The first position paper on education for nurses, published by the American Nurses Association in 1965. States the ANA position that the minimum level for beginning professional nursing practice should be baccalaureate degree education.

positioning: Placing a patient in a bed or chair in a position that corrects postural faults, minimizes dangers of faulty posture, and helps correct impaired breathing.

positive: 1. Definite as opposed to negative. 2. Indicates that a substance, microorganism, or condition tested or examined for is present in the material or individual examined.

positive end expiratory pressure: The pressure that is held at some pre-set level at the end of expiration, to keep the lungs partially inflated and to prevent collapse of the alveoli. Abbreviated PEEP.

positive pressure breathing: Inflation of the lungs with air (or oxygen) under pressure to produce inspiration. Exhaled air, hand bellows, or more sophisticated apparatus can be used. Elastic recoil of lungs produces expiration. Abbreviated PPB.

positron (pōz'i-tron): A subatomic particle that has the same mass and magnitude of charge as an electron but the charge is positive. **POSITRON EMISSION TOMOGRAPHY**, see under **tomography**.

posology (pō-sol'o-ji): That branch of materia medica that is concerned with dosage.

posset (pos'set): In infant feeding, refers to regurgitation of clotted milk.

post-: Prefix denoting 1) behind, after, posterior; 2) subsequent to, later.

post mortem: After death.

postanesthetic (pōst-an-es-thet'ik): Occurring after anesthesia.

postauditory (post-aw'di-tō-ri): Situated posterior to the external auditory meatus.

postcibal (pōst-sī'bal): Occurring after a meal or after taking food. Abbreviated p.c.

postclimacteric (pōst-klī-mak'ter-ik): Occurring after the end of the reproductive period.

postcoital (post-kō'i-tal): After sexual intercourse. **P. CONTRACEPTION,** the application or administration of a contraceptive after the act of coitus. **P. PILL,** a high-dose estrogen pill taken after coitus; it prevents implantation of the fertilized ovum; sometimes called the "morning after" pill. **P. TEST,** a test for human fertility, done as soon as possible after intercourse, one or two days before ovulation; involves microscopic examination of the cervical mucus for active and motile sperm. Also called Huhner's test.

postconcussional syndrome (pōst-kon-kush'on-al sin'drōm): The headache, dizziness, and feeling of faintness that may follow a head injury and persist for a cosiderable length of time.

postdiphtheritic (pōst-dif'-ther-it'ik): Following an attack of diptheria. Refers especially to paralysis of the limbs and palate.

postencephalitic (pōst-en-sef'-a-lit'ik): Following encephalitis lethargica. The adjective is commonly used to describe the syndrome of the parkinsonism which often results from an attack of this kind of encephalitis.

postepileptic (pōst-ep-i-lep'tik): Following or occurring as a consequence of an epileptic seizure. **P. AUTOMATISM.,** a fugue state, following a fit, when the patient may undertake a course of action, even involving violence, without having any memory of this; see **fugue**.

posterior (pos-tēr'-i-or): 1. Situated toward the rear or behind a structure; opp. of anterior. 2. Situated at or relating to the back of the body; dorsal. **P. CHAMBER OF THE EYE,** the space between the anterior surface of the lens and the posterior surface of the iris. See **aqueous**.

postero-: Combining form denoting posterior, behind, at the back of.

posteroanterior (post'er-ō-an-tē'ri-or): From the back to the front.

posteroinferior (pōs'ter-ō-in-fē'ri-or): Situated behind and below a part of the body.

posterolateral (pos-ter-ō-lat'er-al): Situated behind and to one side of the body, specifically the outer side.

posteromedian (pōs-ter-ō-mē'di-an): Situated at the back and/or near the midline.

posterosuperior (pōs'-ter-ō-sū-pēr'i-or): Situated behind and above a part of the body.

postganglionic (pōst'gang-gli-on'ik): Situated distal to a collection of nerve cells (ganglion) as a **P.** nerve fiber.

postherpetic (po'st-her-pet'ik): Occurring after an attack of herpes or as a sequel.

posthetomy (pos-thet'o-mi): Circumcision (*q.v.*).

posthitis (pos-thī'tis): Inflammation of the prepuce.

posthumous (pos'tū-mus): 1. After death. 2. Born after the father's death. 3. In obstetrics, born by cesarean section after the mother's death.

posthypnotic (post-hip-nōt'ik): After hypnosis. **P. SUGGESTION,** one made while the person is under hypnosis but carried out after returning to a normal state, without being aware of the origin of the suggestion.

postictal (post-ik'tal): Following a sudden fall, attack, stroke, or seizure such as an epileptic seizure.

postmature (pōst-ma-tūr'): 1. Overly developed. 2. Past the expected date of delivery. A baby is postmature when labor is delayed beyond 40 weeks.—postmaturity, n.

postmenopausal (pōst'-men-ō-paw'zal): Pertaining to or occurring in the period following menopause.

postmortal (pōst-mor'tal): Occurring after death.

postmortem (pōst-mor'tem): 1. Related or pertaining to the period after death. 2. Pertaining to an examination of the body after death. **P. EXAMINATION,** an examination of the dead body to determine the cause of death or the pathological changes produced by the disease; autopsy.

postmyocardial infarction syndrome (post'mī-ō-kar'di-al in-fark'shun sin'drōm): Pyrexia and chest pain associated with inflammation of the pleura, lung, or pericardium; due to sensitivity to products released from affected muscle. Also called Dressler's syndrome.

postnasal (pōst-nā'zal): Situated behind the nose and in the nasopharynx.—postnasally, adv. **P. DRIP,** the continual dripping of nasal mucus down the back of the throat instead of out of the nostrils; often more annoying than significant. Causes include allergies, low-grade infections, cold or foggy climate, polluted air, excessive smoking.

postnatal (pōst-nā'tal): Occurring after birth.

postocular (pōst-ok'ū-lar): Situated behind the eyeball.

postoperative (pōst-op'er-at-iv): Occurring or following soon after surgery.—postoperatively, adv.

postoral (pōst-ō'ral): Situated behind or in the back part of the mouth.

postpartum (pōst-par'tum): Occurring soon after childbirth. **P. HEMORRHAGE,** that occurring soon after childbirth and as a result of it. **P. DEPRESSION,** see under **depression**. **P. PSYCHOSIS,** a psychosis arising soon after childbirth, usually referring to one arising within three months of childbirth; often schizophrenic in nature; cause may be organic or emotional, or due to endocrine imbalance; symptoms include insomnia, instability of mood, hallucinations, withdrawal, restlessness, elation, suspiciousness.

postphlebitic syndrome (pōst-flē-bit'ik): A condition following thrombosis of a vein, especially a leg vein; the valves are destroyed and the thrombosed vein is obliterated resulting in chronic venous insufficiency.

postprandial (pōst-pran′di-al): Following a meal.

post-term (post-term): Refers to an infant born after more than 42 weeks of gestation.

post-transfusion syndrome (post-trans-fū′zhun sin′drōm): A condition that may occur several weeks or months after blood transfusion or sometimes after heart surgery; symptoms resemble those of mononucleosis, including fever, hepatomegaly, splenomegaly, and the presence of atypical lymphocytes in the blood; thought to be caused by cytomegalovirus. Also called postperfusion syndrome.

postulate (pos′tū-lat): A self-evident claim, demand, requirement, or basic principle, assumed without proof. **KOCH'S POSTULATES**, a list of four experimental conditions that an organism must meet before it can be declared to be the cause of a disease.

postural (pos′tū-ral): Pertaining to or affected by posture. **P. DRAINAGE**, usually infers drainage from the respiratory tract, by elevation of the foot of the bed, positioning the patient, or using a special frame. **P. HYPOTENSION**, see hypotension, orthostatic.

posture (pos′tūr): Active or passive arrangement of the whole body, or a part, in a definite manner.

postvaccinal (pōst-vak′sin-al): Following, or resulting from vaccination.

pot: A street term for marijuana.

potable (pō′ta-b'l): Drinkable; suitable for drinking.

potassemia (pot-a-sē′mi-a): The presence of more than the normal amount of potassium in the blood.

potassium (pō-tas′i-um): A soft, silvery-white alkaline, metallic element, occurring widely in nature but always in combination. Present in all animal cells and important for normal growth and development, in maintenance of acid-base balance, and in normal muscle activity, especially cardiac muscle. It is poorly conserved by the body but because it is present in many foods the daily requirement is easily met: symptoms of deficiency include changes in the electrocardiogram, weakness of muscles, thirst; see hypokalemia. Its salts have long been used in medicine. **P. ACETATE**, white powder or crystalline flakes; used as an alkaline diuretic, diaphoretic, and systemic and urinary alkalizer. **P. BICARBONATE**, white crystals or powder; used as a diuretic, to acidify urine, and to correct electrolyte imbalance. **P. CHLORIDE**, used to correct potassium deficiency. **P. GLUCONATE**, used to correct hypokalemia and as a replentisher of potassium. **P. IODIDE**, white crystalline substance used in expectorants. **P. PERMANGANATE**, odorless purple prisms, used as an antiseptic and deodorizer, and as an antidote in certain poisonings.

potbelly: A large, protruding belly, a fairly common condition in middle-aged males of sedentary occupations; due to a collection of fat in the omentum and weakening of the abdominal muscles. In children, often a symptom of disease conditions such as congenital megacolon, or the result of improper diet.

potency (pō′ten-si): 1. Inherent strength; force; or power. 2. The ability of a male to carry out sexual intercourse; often refers specifically to penile erection. See impotence. 3. The strength of a drug.

potent (pō′tent): 1. Possessing inherent strength, force. 2. Describing a medicinal preparation that is highly effective. 3. Capable of producing powerful mental or physical effects. 4. The ability of a male to engage in sexual intercourse.

potential (pō-ten′shal): Latent: existing as a possibility and having the power to eventually become an actuality. **P. ENERGY**, energy that is stored in the body but not in actual use. See also action potential.

potentiation (pō-ten-shē-ā′shun): 1. The synergistic effect of a substance which, when added to another, increases the potency of that substance. 2. The effect of combining two or more drugs which together produce an action greater than when the drugs are given separately.—potentiate, v.

potion (pō′shun): A large draught of liquid medicine or other liquid mixture.

potomania (pō-tō-mā′ni-a): 1. An abnormal desire to imbibe liquids; said especially of alcoholics. 2. Delirium tremens.

Pott: [Percival Pott, English physician. 1714–1788.] **P'S. DISEASE**, spondylitis: occurs primarily in children and young adults. Usually of tuberculous origin affecting one or more vertebrae; necrosis of the bone causes compression of the vertebrae and results in stiff spine, pain on motion, and kyphosis. **P'S. FRACTURE**, a fracture at the lower end of the fibula and of the medial malleolus of the tibia with lateral and backward displacement of the foot. **P'S PUFFY TUMOR:** osteomyelitis of the skull following injury without laceration; accompanied by edema.

Potter's syndrome: A rare congenital anomaly marked by skeletal and renal abnormalities; pulmonary hypoplasia; characteristic facies with widely spaced eyes, furrowed forehead, large low-set, floppy ears; and small jaw; clubbed feet. Often associated with oligohydramnios (*q.v.*). Affected infants are often stillborn or die soon after death.

Potts' operation: A direct side-to-side anastomosis between the aorta and the pulmonary artery; used in cases of tetralogy of Fallot. [Willis J. Potts, American surgeon. 1895–1968.] Also called Potts-Smith-Gibson operation.

pouch: A pocket, recess, or cul-de-sac. **RECTOUTERINE P.**, a cul-de-sac that lies between the posterior surface of the uterus and the anterior surface of the rectum; also called Douglas' pouch. **RECTOVESICLE P.**, the fold of peritoneum that in the male extends downward between the urinary bladder and the rectum. **UTEROVESICLE P.**, the fold of peritoneum that in the female lies between the anterior surface of the uterus and the urinary bladder.

poultice (pōl'tis): A soft, moist, pulpy mass spread between two layers of material and applied, usually hot, to an external surface to relieve pain and congestion and improve circulation in the area, or to hasten suppuration. Materials used include bread, mustard, flaxseed, linseed.

pound: A unit of weight; in the avoirdupois system the pound contains 16 ounces; in the apothecaries' system it contains 12 ounces; in the metric system it is the equivalent of 0.4536 kilograms.

Poupart's ligament: Inguinal ligament; see under **ligament**.

powder: 1. A mass of dry substance separated into minute particles; 2. A single dose of a drug in powdered form, usually contained in a paper. 3. To reduce a solid mass of a substance to fine particles.

pox: 1. Any disease characterized by an eruption, especially a pustular eruption. 2. An eruption. 3. Colloquial term for syphilis. See **smallpox, chickenpox**.

poxvirus (poks'vī'rus): Any of a group of relatively large viruses, including those that cause vaccinia and variola in man.

PPC: Abbreviation for progressive patient care.

PPD: Abbreviation for Purified Protein Derivative (*q.v.*).

PPLO: Abbreviation for pleuropneumonia-like organisms.

ppm: Abbreviation for parts per million.

PPMH: Abbreviation for pertinent past medical history.

PPT: Abbreviation for partial prothrombin time.

PQRST: A commonly used device for assessing emergency room problems and nursing needs of emergency room patients; P for provokes, *i.e.*, the cause of the pain or injury; Q for quality of the pain; R for whether the pain radiates; S for severity of the pain or injury; T for time, *i.e.*, when the pain started and how long it has persisted.

P-R interval: One of the segments of the ECG; it is a measure of the time between the beginning of the atrial depolarization and the beginning of the ventricular depolarization.

P-R segment: On the electrocardiogram, the interval between the end of the P wave and the beginning of the QRS complex.

practical nurse: See under **nurse**.

practitioner (prak-tish'un-er): 1. A person engaged in practice in any profession. 2. A person who practices medicine. **NURSE P.**, see under **nurse**.

Prader-Willi syndrome: A congenital condition characterized by mental retardation, various skeletal and facial abnormalities, obesity, hypogonadism.

prae-: See words beginning pre-.

pragmatic (prag-mat'ik): Practical; matter-of-fact; concerned with practical aspects.

praxiology (prak'si-ol'o-ji): The science or study of behavior.

praxis (prak'sis): The performance of a purposeful act or skilled movement.

pre-: Prefix denoting 1) anterior, before, in front of; 2) preparatory, beforehand.

preanesthesia (prē'an-es-thē'zi-a): Preliminary or light anesthesia; usually produced by medication and induced prior to general anesthesia.

preanesthetic (prē'an-es-thet'ik): Pertaining to preanesthesia, the period preceding anesthesia, or to a drug given prior to general anesthesia.

preauricular (prē'aw-rik'ū-lar): Situated in front of the auricle of the ear; used especially with reference to the lymphatic nodes in this area.

precancer (prē'kan-ser): A condition that is expected eventually to become malignant.

precancerous (prē-kan'ser-us): 1. Occurring before cancer, with special reference to nonmalignant pathological changes which are believed to lead on to, or to be followed by, cancer. 2. Tending to become malignant.

preceptor (prē'sep-tor): In nursing, an experienced professional nurse who works on a one-to-one basis with a recent graduate of a nursing school, and who serves as a role model and clinical instructor thus helping to reduce the reality shock often experienced by the new nurse on entering professional nursing practice. A preceptor may also be appointed to work with an experienced professional nurse during the orientation period when the nurse has moved into a new position or institution. Some schools of nursing use preceptors for students just prior to graduation to help students gain confidence and learn how to integrate the theoretical instruction they have had into their nursing practice.

precipitate (pre-sip'i-tāt): 1. To separate out or cause a substance in a solution or suspension to separate out. 2. A solid that is separated out from a solution or suspension. 3. Hasty or unduly rapid, as labor.—precipitation, n.

precipitin (prē-sip'i-tin): An antibody which forms a specific complex with precipitinogen (antigen); under certain physiochemical conditions this results in the formation of a precipitate. This reaction forms the basis of many delicate diagnostic serological tests for the identification of minute traces of material and bacteria. See antibodies.

preclinical (prē-klin'i-kal): 1. Referring to the period before symptoms of a disease are recognizable. 2. The period in the education of a physician or nurse before there is contact with patients.

precocious (prē-kō'shus): Exhibiting unusually early physical or mental development.

precomatose (prē-kō'ma-tōs): Pertaining to the state of consciousness which precedes the state of coma.

preconscious (prē-kon'shus): In psychoanalysis, thoughts that are submerged in the consciousness but which one can recall to mind when one wishes to do so.

precordial (prē-kor'di-al): Pertaining to the precordium. **P. SHOCK,** a brief, high-voltage electric shock applied to the precordial area to convert abnormal arrhythmias to normal, or to correct ventricular fibrillation. **P. THUMP,** a single sharp blow with the fist delivered over the midsternum from a distance of 8 to 12 inches above the sternum; an emergency measure that may be utilized by qualified personnel when a patient on a monitor develops ventricular fibrillation.

precordialgia (prē-kōr-di-al'ji-a): Pain in the precordium (*q.v.*).

precordium (prē-kōr'di-um): The area on the ventral surface of the body that lies immediately over the heart and stomach; comprises the epigastrium and lower, middle part of the thorax.—precordial, adj.

precursor (pre-kur'sor): Forerunner.

prediabetes (prē-dī-a-bē'tēz): Refers to potential predisposition to diabetes mellitus. Urine testing can detect the condition and it can sometimes be controlled by diet alone.—prediabetic, adj.; n.

predigestion (prē-di-jest'chun): Partial artificial digestion of foods before they are ingested.

predisposing (prē-dis-pōz'ing): Rendering one more vulnerable or susceptible to a disease condition.

predisposition (prē-dis-pō-zish'un): A latent or increased susceptibility to develop or contract certain diseases.

prednisolone (pred-nis'ō-lōn): A synthetic glutocorticoid having anti-inflammatory and antiallergic effects.

preeclampsia (prē'ē-klamp'si-a): A condition characterized by albuminuria, proteinuria, edema, azotemia, hypertension, headache, confusion, irritability, and visual disturbances; arises usually after the 30th week of pregnancy; varies from mild to fatal; occurs most often in teenagers and women over 35; cause unknown.—preeclamptic, adj.

prefrontal (prē-fron'tal): Situated in the anterior portion of the frontal lobe of the cerebrum. See leukotomy.

preganglionic (prē'gang-gli-on'ik): Preceding or in front of a collection of nerve cells (ganglion) as a **P.** nerve fiber.

pregnancy (preg'nan-si): Being with child, *i.e.*, from conception to parturition, normally 40 weeks or 280 days. **ABDOMINAL P.,** development of the ovum in the peritoneal cavity; usually follows rupture of tubal **P.,** primary abdominal implantation seldom occurs. **EXTRAUTERINE P., P.** developing outside the uterus. **MULTIPLE P.,** more than one fetus in the uterus. **PHANTOM P.,** see pseudocyesis. **TOXEMIA OF P.,** see under toxemia.

pregnancy test: Any procedure used to diagnose pregnancy. See human chorionic gonadotropin under gonadotropin.

pregnanediol (preg-nān-dī'ōl): A metabolite of progesterone found in the urine during pregnancy and during the progestational phase of the menstrual cycle; determinations during pregnancy indicate status of the placental function.

pregnant: Gravid; being with child; containing unborn young within the body.

prehensile (prē-hen'sil): Equipped or adapted for grasping or seizing.

prehension (prē-hen'shun): The act of grasping or taking hold of.

prehypophysis (prē-hī-pof'i-sis): The anterior lobe of the pituitary body.

preictal (prē-ik'-tal): Occurring before a stroke or a seizure, such as an epileptic seizure.

preinvasive (prē-in-vā'siv): Usually refers to malignant growths in which the cells are confined to their normal location and have not invaded surrounding tissues.

preload (prē'lōd): Refers to the volume of blood the heart has to pump out at each contraction *i.e.*, the amount of blood that returns to the heart via the veins.

premature (prē-ma-tūr'): Occurring before the usual or proper time. **P. BABY,** one whose weight at birth is less than 5.5 pounds (2.5 kg); and therefore requires special treatment. Current synonyms are low-weight or dysmature baby. Not all low birth weight babies are premature, but are included in the category "small for dates." See placental insufficiency. **P. BEAT,** extrasystole (*q.v.*). **P. LABOR,** expulsion of the fetus before the 280th day of pregnancy.

premature ventricular contraction: A contraction that is out of regular sequence in the rhythm of the heartbeat; may or may not indicate the presence of heart disease. Abbreviated PVC.

premedication (prē-med-i-kā'shun): Drugs given before the administration of another drug, *e.g.*, those given before an anesthetic for the purposes of allaying apprehension, producing sedation, inhibiting secretion of saliva and mucus from the upper respiratory tract, or to facilitate the administration of the anesthetic.

premenarchal (prē-me-nar'kal): Pertaining to or occurring before menstruation has become established.

premenopausal (prē-men'ō-paw-zal): Before the menopause. **P. AMENORRHEA,** variation in the intermenstrual periods occurring before cessation of the menses.

premenstrual (prē-men'strōō-al): Preceding menstruation. **P. TENSION,** see under tension.

premenstrual syndrome: A cluster of symptoms that occur a few days prior to the appearance of the menses and subside with the onset of menstruation; most common in women over 30; exact cause unknown, but may be due to hormonal activity during the menstrual cycle. Symptoms include edema of the hands and feet, breast tenderness, emotional instability, depression, anxiety, irritability. Mild analgesics are sometimes prescribed. Also called premenstrual tension.

premolar (prē-mō'lar): One of 8 bicuspid teeth. There are two on each side of each jaw, between the canine and first molar.

premonitory (prē-mon'i-tōr-i): Pertaining to a warning experienced in advance of an event or a recognizable pathologic condition. See prodromal.

premunition (prē-mu-nish'un): A state of immunity that develops after an actue infection has become chronic and lasts as long as the causative organism remains in the body.

prenaris (prē-nā'rēz): One of the anterior nares; nostril.—prenares, pl.

prenatal (prē-nā'tal): Occurring or existing before birth. Antenatal.—prenatally, adv.

preoperative (prē-op'er-at-iv): Before operation.—preoperatively, adv.

prep: Colloquial term meaning the preparation of an area (cleansing, shaving, etc.) for surgery, delivery, or other procedure.

preparalytic (prē-par-a-lit'ik): Before the onset of paralysis, often referring to the early stage of poliomyelitis.

prepartal (prē-par'tal): Before labor.

prepatellar (prē-pa-tel'ar): Situated in front of the kneecap. **P. BURSITIS,** see under bursitis.

preprandial (prē-pran'di-al): Before a meal.

prepuberty (prē-pū'ber-ti): The age preceding puberty.—prepubertal, adj.

prepuce (prē'pūs): When used alone it designates the foreskin; the free fold of skin that covers the glans penis. In the female, a fold of tissue formed by the union of the labia minora anteriorally, the lower folds are attached under the surface of the clitoris.

preputium (prē-pū'shi-um): The prepuce (*q.v.*).—preputial, adj.

prerectal (prē-rek'tal): Situated in front of the rectum.

presacral (prē-sā'kral): Situated in front of the sacrum.

presacral air insufflation: Injection of air into retroperitoneal interstitial tissues, mainly used for x-ray demonstration of renal and adrenal outlines.

presby-, presbyo-: Combining forms denoting 1) old; 2) old age.

presbycardia (pres-bi-kar'di-a): Changes in the myocardium due to the aging process along with pigmentation of the cardiac tissues; the heart reserve is decreased, but heart failure does not usually follow. Also called senile heart disease.

presbycusis (pres-bi-kū'sis): A sensorineural hearing loss which occurs typically in older persons; there is loss of sensitivity to sound, particularly those of high frequencies, and/or of the ability to distinguish words in speech; in addition to the aging process, may be caused by long exposure to noise, certain drugs, or previous attacks of otitis media; usually bilateral and progressive. Also called presbycusia, presbyacusia, presbyacusis.

presbyesophagus (pres-bi-ē-sof'a-gus): Diffuse spasm of esophageal muscles due to loss of peristalsis (*q.v.*) or to "corkscrew" esophagus; usually seen in the elderly.

presbyope (pres'bi-ōp): A farsighted person.

presbyophrenia (pres-bi-ō-frē'ni-a): A mental disorder most often seen in the elderly; characterized by memory loss; disorentation, and confabulation. Often judgment remains relatively unimpaired. Wernicke's syndrome.

presbyopia (pres-bi-ō'pi-a): Farsightedness due to loss of elasticity of the crystalline lens of the eye with consequent failure of accommodation; seen mostly in persons 45 and more years of age.—presbyopic, adj.; presbyope, n.

prescribe (prē-skrīb'): To give directions orally or in writing for the administration of a remedy in the treatment of any disease condition.

prescription (prē-skrip'shun): A written formula, signed by a physician, directing the preparation and administration of a remedy. Also refers to instructions for grinding corrective lenses for eyeglasses. **P. DRUG,** one that may be dispensed only on order of a physician. **SHOTGUN P.,** one containing many ingredients, some of which may be inert.

presenile dementia: See dementia.

presenility (prē'sē-nil'i-ti): 1. Before senility is established. 2. Premature old age.—presenile, adj.

present (prē-sent'): 1. To precede or appear first, as the part of the fetus that appears first at the os uteri. 2. To come forward as a patient.

presentation (prē'zen-ta'shun): In obstetrics, the part of the fetus that is felt through the cervix at the start of labor and which first enters the brim of the pelvis. May be vertex, face, brow, shoulder or breech.

presenting symptoms: The symptoms or complaint for which a person seeks health care service.

pressor (pres'or): 1. A substance that tends to raise blood pressure. 2. Involving or stimulating the vasomotor center in the brain. **P. DRUGS,** drugs that cause blood pressure to rise through increasing peripheral vasoconstriction.

pressoreceptor (pres'ō-rē-sep'tor): Baroreceptor (*q.v.*).

pressure: (presh'ur): 1. A force or compression exerted against an area of the body. 2. The sensation of touch aroused by compression against the skin. **P. AREAS,** bony prominences of the body, over which the flesh of bedridden patients is compressed between the bone and an external source of pressure; the latter is usually the bed, but may be a splint, plaster, upper bedclothes, etc. **ARTERIAL P.**, the **P.** of blood

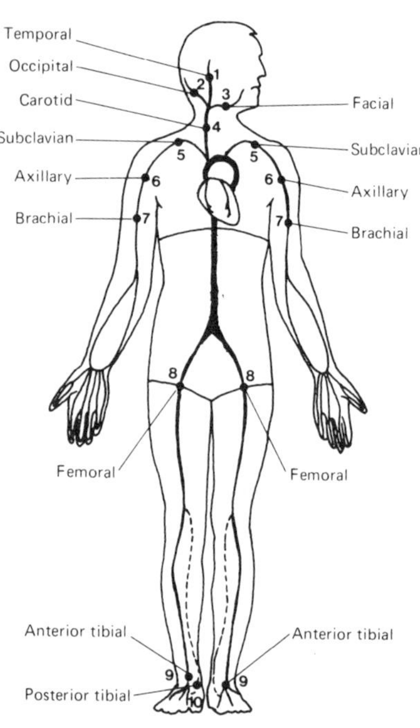

Arterial pressure points

within the arteries. **P. BANDAGE,** one applied so as to produce pressure; used to stop bleeding, prevent swelling, or to compress varicose veins. **BLOOD P.,** see under blood. **CENTRAL VENOUS P., P.** of the blood within the heart and great vessels of the thorax; can be measured accurately and automatically recorded. **DIASTOLIC P.,** arterial blood pressure during the period of dilatation of the chambers of the heart. **INTRACRANIAL P.,** the **P.** of the cerebrospinal fluid in the space between the brain and the skull. **INTRAOCULAR PRESSURE,** see under intraocular. **MEAN ARTERIAL PRESSURE** measured by means of an intraarterial catheter; it is determined by averaging the systolic and diastolic pressure according to the formula:

$$\frac{\text{diastolic p.} + 2 + \text{systolic p.}}{3}$$

NEGATIVE P., P. that is less than that of the atmosphere. **P. POINT,** a place at which an artery

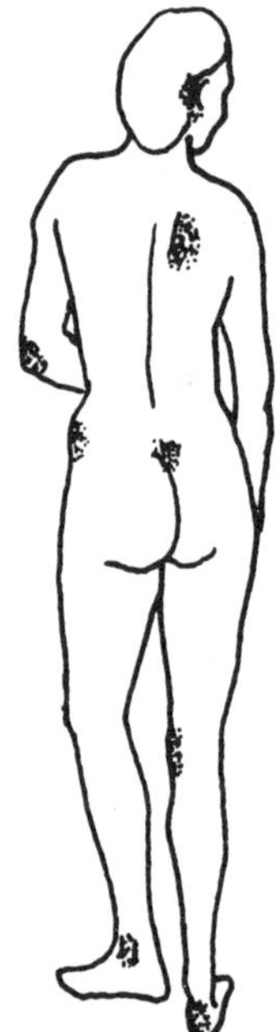

Pressure areas where decubitus ulcers are likely to develop.

passes over a bone, against which it can be compressed, to stop bleeding. **P. SORE,** decubitus ulcer; see under ulcer. **PULMONARY ARTERY P.,** pressure exerted on the pulmonary artery walls by blood being pumped out of the right ventricle. **PULMONARY CAPILLARY WEDGE P.,** the blood pressure in the most distal peripheral capillaries of the pulmonary artery; measured by use of the Swan-Ganz catheter, which is wedged into such a capillary; it is identical with left atrial pressure. **PULSE P.,** the difference between the systolic and diastolic blood pressure. **VENOUS P.,** may be either 1) peripheral, the constant pressure exerted by blood on venous walls, or 2) central, which is the venous blood pressure just before it enters the right atrium; read in centimeters of water and involving an invasive procedure utilizing either the cephalic or basilic vein; useful as a guide for treatment or for monitoring fluid replacement in patients with burns, shock, cardiac failure, or other critical condition.

presynaptic (pre′si-nap′tik): Located near or occurring before a synapse.

presystole (prē-sis′to-li): The interval just preceding the systole or contraction of the heart muscle.—presystolic, adj.

pre-term: Refers to the birth of a child before the end of 37 weeks gestation; approximately 7 percent of all live births fall in this category.

pretibial (prē-tib′i-al): In front of or on the front of the tibia.

prevalence (prev′-a-lens): In statistics, the total number of new cases of a specific disease at a particular point in time or during a specific period of time. **P. RATE,** the number of cases present in a given geographical area or community at one time divided by the population of the area at the same time.

preventive (prē-ven′tiv): Acting to prevent the occurrence of. **P. MEDICINE,** that branch of medicine that deals with preventing the occurrence of disease in individuals or in the community at large.

preventorium (prē-ven-tō′ri-um): An institution for the care of persons (usually children) who are believed to be in danger of contracting some disease; formerly much used for individuals who had been exposed to tuberculosis or who were in poor physical condition and likely to contract tuberculosis.

prevesical (prē-ves′ik-al): Situated anteriorally to a bladder, especially the urinary bladder.

priapism (prī′a-pizm): [*Priapus,* the god of procreation.] Persistent and painful erection of the penis in the absence of sexual stimulation; usually due to disease; sometimes seen in sickle cell crisis and cord lesions.

priapitis (prī-a-pī′tis): Inflammation of the penis.

prickle cells: Cells of the stratum spinosum layer of the epidermis; so-called because of the rod shaped processes that form intercellular bridges.

prickly heat: A noncontagious eruption that often occurs in hot humid weather; consists of small red pimples that itch, burn and tingle. See miliaria.

primary (prī′ma-ri): 1. First or most important in order of time or development. 2. First in rank or importance. **PRIMARY COMPLEX, GOHN'S FOCUS,** (*q.v.*) **P. UNION,** see under union.

primary care nurse: See under nurse.

primary care physician: A physician who provides the first contact care with a patient and is the primary medical resource and advisor to a patient or to an entire family; is responsible for medical care and for integrating it with that delegated to other specialists and care givers.

primary degenerative dementia, senile onset (before age 65 and at or after age 65): See Dementias Arising in the Senium or Presenium in Appendix VI.

primary health care: Refers to either or both of two kinds of care: 1) care the person receives at his first point of contact with the health care system; 2) continued care of a health care consumer by the same individual or team; it stresses holistic care and includes identification, management, and/or referral of health problems, integration of health care services, restoration and maintenance of the consumer's health by preventive actions, which may be performed in the patient's home, a health care facility, or a community institution; the emphasis is on a close, long-term relationship between the patient, his or her family, and the practitioner.

primary health care system: Refers to the system or the context in which primary health care is given, *e.g.,* occupational health unit, school health unit, public health service, clinic.

primary system of nursing: A system for providing nursing care for well clients or those who are not in an acute stage of an illness, usually in an outpatient or community setting.

primigravida (prīm-i-grav′i-da): A woman who is pregnant for the first time.—primigravidae, pl.

primigravidy (prī-mi-grav′i-di): The condition of being pregnant for the first time.

primipara (prī-mip′a-ra): A woman who is giving birth to her first child or who has just had her first viable infant.—primiparous, adj.

primordial (prī-mor′di-al): Primitive, original; applied to the ovarian follicles present at birth.

primordium (prī-mor′di-um): The origin or earliest form of something, *e.g.,* the earliest recognizable part of an organ or part in an embryo.

principle (prin'si-p'l): 1. A fundamental truth, doctrine, or law. 2. A scientific law that explains the method of a natural action. 3. A rule of conduct, especially right conduct. 4. In pharmacology, the constituent of a drug or compound that is chiefly responsible for its action.

Printzmetal's angina: See under angina.

privates: The external organs of generation. Colloq.

privileged communication: Confidential information given by a patient to health care personnel during physical examination or other procedures in connection with his diagnosis and treatment; some states have laws making it illegal for personnel to divulge this information. See confidentiality.

p.r.n.: Abbreviation for *pro re nata* [L.], meaning whenever necessary.

pro-: Prefix denoting 1) earlier than, prior to, before; 2) anterior to, located in front of; 3) projecting.

pro re nata: Whenever necessary; as the occasion arises. Sometimes used in prescription writing to indicate that the medicine is to be given according to the patient's need for it. Abbreviated p.r.n.

proaccelerin (prō-ak-sel'er-in): A factor in the blood (Factor V) that is required for the formation of a blood clot. Also called the labile factor.

proband (prō'band): Propositus (*q.v.*).

probe (prōb): 1. A slender, somewhat flexible rod-like metal instrument with a blunt tip, used typically for exploring body cavities or wounds. 2. To use a probe for exploration purposes.

problem list: See problem oriented records.

problem oriented medical information system: A medical record system that records, manipulates, and retrieves, the entire health and health care data on individual patients over time. It provides a framework for health care professionals to analyze and improve health care actions including nursing. Abbreviated PROMIS.

problem oriented medical records: A system of record keeping in which an individual's health problems are listed in order of need for care at his entrance into the health care system; all team members record care given and plan their care according to priorities implied by the list, which also becomes a checklist for the nursing audit. Consists of four logically sequenced parts: the data base, the problem list, plans for care, and follow-up.

procedure (prō-sē'jur): In health care, a series of orderly steps followed in carrying out a treatment or operation.

procephalic (prō-se-fal'ik): Related to or situated on or near the anterior part of the head.

process (pros'es): 1. A projection or outgrowth from the mass of an organism or part, especially from a bone. 2. A method, system, or mode of action utilized in doing something. ACROMIAL P., the acromion (*q.v.*). ALVEOLAR P., the parts of the mandible and maxilla that surround the teeth. ARTICULAR P., any of the four articulating processes of the vertebrae (two superior and two inferior). CAUDATE P., a P. on the caudate lobe of the liver. DENDRITIC P., the branching processes of a nerve cell; a dendrite. ENISFORM P., see under xiphoid. ODONTOID P., the toothlike process extending upward from the body of the axis; it articulates with the atlas. OLECRANON P., the olecranon (*q.v.*). TRANSVERSE P., a p. that projects laterally on either side of a vertebra. See also coracoid, ciliary, coronoid, mastoid, palatine, pterygoid, styloid, xiphoid.

procidentia (prō-si-den'shi-a): Complete prolapse of an organ or part, especially the uterus so that it lies within the vaginal sac but outside the contour of the body.

procoagulant (prō-kō-ag'ū-lant): 1. Favoring coagulation. 2. A precursor to a natural substance that is required for coagulation of the blood.

proconvertin (prō-kon-vert'in): A blood factor required for the formation of a blood clot (Factor VII). Also called the stable factor.

procreate (prō'krē-āt): To beget; produce offspring. Term applied usually to the male parent.—procreation, n.

proct-, procti-, procto-: Combining forms denoting anus or rectum, or both.

proctalgia (prok-tal'ji-a): The occurrence of pain in the anal region or the rectum.

proctatresia (prok-ta-trē'zi-a): Imperforation of the anus. Anal atresia. See atresia.

proctectomy (prok-tek'to-mi): Surgical removal of the rectum, usually because of the presence of a malignancy.

proctitis (prok-tī'tis): Inflammation of the mucous membrane of the rectum.

proctocele (prok'tō-sēl): Prolapse of the mucous coat of the rectum. Rectocele (*q.v.*).

proctoclysis (prok-tok'li-sis): The slow continuous injection of large quantities of fluid into the rectum. Murphy drip. (*q.v.*).

proctocolectomy (prok'tō-kōl-ek'to-mi): Surgical removal of the rectum and colon.

proctocolitis (prok'tō-kō-lī'tis): Inflammation of the rectum and colon; usually a type of ulcerative colitis.

proctologist (prok-tol'o-jist): A physician who specializes in proctology.

proctology (prok-tol'o-ji): That branch of medicine that deals with the study of the anus, rectum, and sigmoid and the treatment of their diseases.

proctoperineoplasty (prok'tō-per-i-ne'ō-plas-ti): An operation for repair of the anus and perineum. Also proctoperineorrhapy.

proctopexy (prok'to-pek-si): Operation for surgical fixation of the rectum to some other part.

proctoplasty (prok'to-plast-ti): Plastic surgery of the anus and rectum.

proctoptosis (prok-top-tō'sis): Prolapse of the anus and rectum.

proctorrhagia (prok-to-rā'ji-a): Bleeding from the anus.

proctorrhaphy (prok-tor'a-fi): Suturing of a lacerated anus or rectum.

proctorrhea (prok-to-rē'a): Discharge of mucus from the rectum.

proctoscope (prok'tō-skōp): An instrument with a light at the distal end, used for dilating and visually examining the rectum. See endoscope.—proctoscopic, adj.; proctoscopy, n.

proctoscopy (prok-tos'kō-pē): Examination of the rectum by means of a proctoscope (*q.v.*).

proctosigmoidectomy (prok'tō-sig-moi-dek'to-mi): Surgical removal of the anus, rectum, and sigmoid flexure.

proctosigmoiditis (prok'tō-sig-moy-dī'tis): Inflammation of the rectum and sigmoid colon.

proctosigmoidoscopy (prok'tō-sig-moy-dos'kō-pi): Direct inspection of the rectum and the sigmoid colon with a sigmoidoscope.—proctosigmoidoscopic, adj.

proctostasis (prok-tos'ta-sis): Constipation with retention of feces in the colon due to the inability of the rectum to respond to the stimulus for defecation.

proctostenosis (prok' -tō-ste-nō'sis): Narrowing or stricture of the rectum or anus.

proctotomy (prō-tok' -tō-mi): Incision of the rectum to relieve a stricture.

prodromal (prō-drō'mal): Preceding, as the transitory rash before the true rash of an infectious disease.

prodrome (prō'drōm): 1. An aura. 2. An early manifestation of a disease condition before signs and symptoms develop. Also prodroma.—prodromata, pl.

proenzyme (prō-en'zīm): A precursor of an enzyme which requires some change to render it active, *e.g.*, pepsinogen. Zymogen.

professional nurse: See under nurse.

Professional Standards Review Organization: A local organization, authorized by an amendment to the Social Security Act of 1972, which states that physicians are responsible for carrying out peer review of all health care institutions and the services and practices of all professionals delivering these services to patients whose care is supported by federal funds. The purpose is to assure that these services are needed and are of high quality. Abbreviated PSRO.

profundus (prō-fun'dus): Deep; deep-seated; profound. Term usually applies to certain deep-seated muscles or nerves. Also profunda.

progeria (prō-jer'i-a): Premature senility, particularly that occurring in childhood.

progestational (prō'jes-tā'shun-ul): 1. Before pregnancy; favoring pregnancy. 2. Term applied to a phase of the menstrual cycle that immediately precedes menstruation. 3. Pertaining to a class of drugs that have similar effects to those of progesterone. **P. AGENTS,** a group of hormones produced by the corpus luteum and placenta and in small amounts by the adrenal cortex, including progesterone; also produced synthetically, *e.g.*, progestin.

progesterone (prō-jes'te-rōn): A hormone produced by the corpus luteum, placenta, and adrenal cortex; plays an important part in regulation of the menstrual cycle and in pregnancy. Also prepared synthetically for use in certain gynecological disorders.

progestin (prō-jes'tin): Name used for certain synthetic progestational agents. See progestational, progesterone.

proglottis (prō-glot'is): A sexually mature segment of tapeworm.—proglottides, pl.

prognathic (prog-nath'ik): Having projecting jaws.

prognathism (prog'na-thizm): Protrusion or abnormal enlargement of the lower jaw.

prognosis (prog-nō'sis): A forecast of the probable course, duration, and termination of a disease.—prognostic, adj.

programmed instruction: Medium for self-instruction that is individualized so that the student can progress at his or her own speed by a technique that enables self-pacing. The unit of instruction is an individual frame in which a question is asked, a response is requested, and knowledge of the correct response is available through feedback. May be presented on paper or by a teaching machine, film, recording or flip chart. Sometimes used in teaching certain subjects in nursing school curriculums.

progressive bulbar palsy or paralysis: Progressive degeneration of the motor nuclei of the medulla and pons with atrophy and paralysis of the denervated muscles; onset usually late in life; associated with amyotrophic lateral sclerosis; may be hereditary.

progressive patient care: A system of caring for patients whereby the facilities are adapted to the needs of various types of patients. Acutely ill patients are cared for in an intensive care unit; those who are moderately ill are cared for in an intermediate care unit; those who need very little assistance with their physical care but who must remain in the hospital, are cared for in a self-care unit. The objective is to allow patients to live as nearly normal lives as possible and to make the best use of the available nursing staff.

proinsulin (prō-in′sū-lin): A percursor of insulin, elaborated in the beta cells of the pancreas.

Project HOPE: An experiment in international health and nursing care education, sponsored by the People to People Health Foundation, begun in 1958 with the outfitting and staffing of a hospital ship that visited various countries of the world to bring American medical and nursing skills and techniques to people in other countries and to help them adapt these skills to their own environment. The first visit was to Viet Nam in 1960. The nurses and physicians on the staff were highly-trained competent specialists who worked with their foreign counterparts on a one-to-one basis. The ship was retired in 1973 and has been replaced with land-based programs in both the United States and other countries. Address: 2233 Wisconsin Ave., N.W., Washington, D.C. 20007

Project ORBIS: A U.S. based international flying teaching eye hospital housed in a DC 8 jet aircraft; established in 1982. ORBIS' objective is to combat the high rate of preventable blindness around the world through the exchange of surgical skills and worldwide teaching of opthalmologists, and other medical personnel, the latest techniques in eye surgery.

projectile vomiting: Sudden vomiting, usually without preceding nausea, so forcibly that the vomitus is projected for some distance.

projection (prō-jek′shun): A prominence or extending process of a bone. In psychology, a defense mechanism occurring in normal people unconsciously, and in an exaggerated form in mental illness, especially paranoia, whereby the person fails to recognize certain emotionally unacceptable motives, feelings, and behaviors in himself but attributes them to others, thus imparting his own faults to another.

prolactin (prō-lak′tin): A hormone produced by the anterior lobe of the pituitary gland; stimulates and sustains the production of milk by the mammary glands.

prolactinoma (prō-lak-tin-ō′ma): A large tumor of the pituitary gland which secretes prolactin as does the gland itself.

prolapse (prō-laps′): 1. Descent; downward displacement of an organ or body structure from its usual position. 2. A falling forward or down. **P. OF THE CORD,** premature expulsion of the cord during labor. **P. OF THE IRIS,** part of the iris bulges forward through a corneal wound. **P. OF THE RECTUM,** the lower part of the intestinal tract extends downward in varying degrees, sometimes protruding through the external anal sphincter. **P. OF THE UTERUS,** the uterus descends into the vagina and may be visible at the vaginal orifice. See **procidentia.** **P. OF AN INTERVERTEBRAL DISK** (PID), nucleus pulposis; see **nucleus.**

proliferate (prō-lif′er-āt): To increase by cell division.—proliferation, n.; proliferative, adj.

proliferation (prō-lif-er-ā′shun): Rapid and increasing production, especially of cells and morbid growths.

prolific (prō-lif′ik): Fruitful, multiplying abundantly.

proline (prō′lēn): One of the amino acids.

prominence (prom′i-nens): A protrusion or projection. **LARYNGEAL P.,** that in the front of the neck, formed by the thyroid cartilage of the larynx; Adam's apple.

PROMIS: Abbreviation for problem oriented medical information system (*q.v.*).

promontory (prom′on-tō-ri): A projection; a prominent part.

promyelocyte (prō-mī′e-lō-sīt): A cell in the intermediate stage between a myeloblast and a myelocyte.

pronate (prō′nāt): To turn the ventral surface downward, *e.g.*, to lie on the face; or to turn the palm of the hand downward.—pronation, n. Opp., supinate.

pronation (prō-nā′shun): The position of the forearm and hand when the palm is turned down, or of the foot when the sole is turned downward.

pronator (prō-nā′tor): That which pronates, usually applied to a muscle, Opp., supinator.

prone (prōn): Lying with the face downward. Opp., supine.

pronormoblast (prō-nor′mō-blast): A precursor and the earliest recognizable form of the erythrocyte.

propagation (prop-a-gā′shun): 1. Growth. 2. Reproduction.

properdin (prō-per′din): A macroglobulin found in normal blood plasma that is capable of destroying certain bacteria and viruses under certain conditions.

prophase (prō′faz): The first stage in cell mitosis (*q.v.*) in which the centrosome divides and the two parts move away from each other although still attached by a thread-like structure.

prophylactic (prō-fi-lak′tik): 1. Acting to defend against something, particularly infection or disease. 2. An agent that acts to protect or defend (as a condom) against infection or disease.

prophylaxis (prō-fi-lak′sis): Prevention.—prophylactic, adj.; prophylactically, adv.

propositus (prō-poz′i-tus): In studies in human genetics, the person whose particular mental or physical characteristics served as a stimulus for the study. Also called proband.

proprietary (prō-prī'e-ta-ri): Refers to any medicine that is protected from competition by secrecy as to its composition or manufacture, or by trademark, copyright, or patent. **P. DRUGS** are sold over the counter without prescription and are advertised to the general public. **P. HOSPITAL,** a hospital that is organized and operated for profit.

proprioception (prō'pri-ō-sep'shun): The awareness of one's balance and position in space, and of the position of one's body parts without looking at them.

proprioceptive (prō'pri-ō-sep'tiv): Refers to neural stimuli arising from receptors in internal tissues.

proprioceptor (prō-pri-ō-sep'tor): One of the sensory nerve terminals of the afferent nerves in the deeper structures of the body, *e.g.*, muscles, tendons, joints. They are responsible for the sensation of position of the body and its parts and of changes in position.—proprioception, n., proprioceptive, adj.

proptosis (prop-tō'sis): Forward protrusion of any organ, especially of the eyeball. **OCULAR P.,** exophthalmos (*q.v.*).

prosencephalon (pros-en-sef'a-lon): The part of the brain that includes the diencephalon and the telencephalon (*q.v.*). Also called the forebrain.

proso-: Combining form denoting forward or anterior.

prosopagnosia (pros' -ō-pag-nō'si-a): Inability to recognize faces, usually associated with other forms of agnosia (*q.v.*).

prosopo-: Combining form denoting 1) the face; 2) a person.

prosopoplegia (pros-ō-pō-plē'ji-a): Facial paralysis.

prospective medicine: Preventive medicine. Involves intervention before signs or symptoms of disease appear, and regulating life patterns to prevent disease through periodic appraisals of health hazards.

Prospective Payment System (PPS): A system under Medicare in which the hospital patient pays in advance of treatment. Charges are based on the average cost of one day's hospitalization and the average length of stay of patients assigned to the particular category under the Diagnosis Related Group to which the patient is assigned. In many cases this results in shorter hospitalization.

prostaglandins (pros-ta-glan'dins): A group of several hormone-like, physiologically active substances of similar chemical structure, formerly thought to be produced only in the prostate but now believed to be produced by most body tissues; found in high concentrations in seminal fluid, menstrual blood, amniotic fluid, and in maternal blood during labor. Apparently involved in normal body functioning and in certain pathological conditions. Four types have been recognized, some of which have been synthesized and may be administered by mouth, intravenously, or by nebulizer for use in certain endocrine, nervous system, and blood and blood vessel disorders, although the therapeutic usefulness of prostaglandins has not been fully established. Prostaglandin F_{24} has been approved by the Food and Drug Administration for use in interruption of pregnancy when it is administered by intra-amniotic instillation.

prostate (pros'tāt): A small conical gland at the base of the male bladder and surrounding the first part of the urethra. It secretes a milky fluid that is discharged into the urethra and mixes with the semen at the time of emission.—prostatic, adj.

prostatectomy (pros-ta-tek'to-mi): Surgical removal of part or all of the prostate gland. **RADICAL P.,** removal of the entire prostate gland and its capsule, the seminal vesicle and rim of the bladder neck; may be indicated in cancer. **RETROPUBIC P.,** removal of a mass from the prostate via an incision into the prostatic bladder. **SUPRAPUBIC P., P.** through an abdominal incision into the urinary bladder. **TRANSURETHRAL P., P.** by means of an operating cystoscope.

prostatic (pros-tat'ik): Pertaining to the prostate gland. **BENIGN P. HYPERTROPHY,** a common disorder of middle-aged men; the glandular and cellular tissue of the prostate enlarge putting pressure on the urethra and causing urinary problems; the usual treatment is surgical.

prostaticovesical (pros-tat'i-kō-ves'i-kal): Pertaining to both the prostate gland and the urinary bladder.

prostatism (pros'ta-tizm): The condition of chronic disorders of the prostate, particularly enlargement of the prostate gland, which obstructs the flow of urine.

prostatitis (pros-ta-tī'tis): Inflammation of the prostate gland.

prostatocystitis (pros'-ta-tō-sis-tī'tis): Inflammation of the prostatic urethra and the male urinary bladder.

prostatodynia (pros'ta-tō-din'i-a): Pain in the prostate.

prostatolithotomy (pros'tat-ō-li-thot'o-mi): Removal of a stone from the prostate gland.

prostatomegaly (pros'ta-tō-meg'a-li): Enlargement or hypertrophy of the prostate gland.

prostatorrhea (pros'ta-tō-rē'a): A thin catarrhal discharge from the prostate gland; often occurs in prostatitis.

prostatoseminovesicular (pros'ta-tō-sem'i-nō-ve-sik'ū-lar): Pertaining to the prostate and seminal vesicles.

prostatoseminovesiculectomy (pros′ta-tō-sem′i-nō-ve-sik-ū-lek′tō-mi): Surgical removal of the prostate and the seminal vesicles.

prostatovesiculitis (pros′ta-tō-ve-sik′ū-lī′tis): Inflammation of the prostate and the seminal vesicles.

prosthesis (pros-thē′sis): An artificial substitute for a body part, *e.g.*, eye, tooth, heart valve, blood vessel, limb, breast. **MYOELECTRIC P.**, a device that enables an amputee to carry out ordinary tasks such as picking up things.—prostheses, pl.; prosthetic, adj.

prosthetics (pros-thet′iks): The art and science of making and adjusting artificial parts of the body (prostheses).

prosthetist (pros′the-tist): One skilled in making and adjusting prostheses.

prosthodontics (pros′thō-don′tiks): The branch of dentistry that deals with the construction of prostheses to replace missing teeth, or other oral structures.

prosthodontist (pros′thō-don′tist): A dentist who specializes in prosthodontics.

prosthokeratoplasty (pros′thō-ker′a-tō-plas-ti): Keratoplasty (*q.v.*) in which the corneal implant is of some material other than human or animal tissue.

prostitution (pros-ti-tū′shun): 1. The soliciting of or engaging in sexual intercourse for money. 2. The act of debasing one's self or one's abilities, especially when it is done for money.

prostration (pros-trā′shun): Complete exhaustion; extreme loss of strength. **NERVOUS P.**, neurasthenia (*q.v.*). See heat exhaustion.

prot-, proto-: Combining forms denoting; 1. First in time, formation, rank, status, or importance. 2. Giving rise to.

protanomaly (prō′ta-nom′a-li): A defect of vision in which the response of the retina to the color red is diminished.

protanopia (prō′ta-nō′pi-a): Red-green color blindness. Also called protanopsia.

protease (prō′tē-ās): Any protein-splitting enzyme. **GASTRIC P.**, pepsin.

protein (prō′tē-in): A highly complex, nitrogenous compound, found in all animal and vegetable tissues; the principal constituent of cell protoplasm. Proteins are built up of amino acids and are essential for growth and repair of the body. Those from animal sources are of high biological value since they contain the essential amino acids. Those from vegetable sources contain some but not all of the essential amino acids. **P.** is hydrolyzed in the body to produce amino acids which are then used to build up new body tissues. **COMPLETE P., P.** that contains all of the essential amino acids. **INCOMPLETE P., P.** that lacks one or more of the essential amino acids. **SECOND CLASS P., P.** that contains only slight amounts of some of the amino acids.

proteinaceous (prō′-tē-in-ā′shus): Pertaining to protein or being protein in nature.

protein-bound iodine: Iodine combined with protein as part of the thyroid hormone. It is low in thyroid deficiency.

proteinemia (prō′-tē-in-ē′mi-a): More than the normal amount of protein in the blood.

proteinosis (prō′tē-in-ō′sis): Accumulation or increase of protein in the tissues. **ALVEOLAR P.**, a chronic disorder of the lung characterized by the accumulation of eosinophilic proteinaceous material in the distal alevoli; symptoms include chest pain, dyspnea, productive cough, hemoptysis, and weakness.

proteinuria (prō′tē-in-ū′ri-a): The presence of protein in the urine. May be an isolated finding or indicate some abnormality or pathology of the kidney. Syn., albuminuria; nephrotic syndrome. **ORTHOSTATIC P.**, occurs when individuals with lumbar lordosis are in the upright position; usually no renal pathology is present.

proteolysis (prō-tē-ol′i-sis): The breaking down of proteins into simpler substances.—proteolytic, adj.

proteolytic (prō-tē-ō-lit′ik): Pertaining to or promoting proteolysis. **P. ENZYME**, an enzyme that acts as a catalyst in the digestion of protein.

proteose (prō′tē-ōs): The first cleavage product in the breakdown of proteins, intermediate between protein and peptone.

Proteus (prō′tē-us): A genus of gram-negative, flagellated, motile, rod-shaped microorganisms; found in damp surroundings and other putrefying material. May be pathogenic, especially in wound or urinary tract infections as a secondary invader. **P. MIRABILIS**, usually saprophytic and found in putrefying materials; may be pathogenic and associated with prostatitis, cystitis, infections of the uterus, and wounds. **P. MORGANI**, a normal inhabitant of the gastrointestinal tract. **P. RETTGERI**, cause of chicken cholera and often gastroenteritis in humans. **P. VULGARIS**, found in dirty wounds, particularly those soiled with animal dung or mud.

prothrombin (prō-throm′bin): A factor in the plasma of the blood; a precursor of thrombin. It is synthesized in the liver when the supply of vitamin K is adequate. In the presence of thromboplastin and calcium it is converted into thrombin. **P. TIME** is 1) widely used one-stage test for clotting time (normal time is 12–18 seconds), or 2) the time it takes for clot formation after tissue prothrombin and calcium have been added to blood plasma; it is increased in certain hemorrhagic conditions.

prothymia (prō-thim′i-a): Mental alertness.

protocol (prō′tō-kol): 1. A written statement or report that includes a statement of the patient's condition in medical terms, diagnostic procedures to be followed, and the important elements of therapeutic management; often includes instructions for continued care needed after the patient leaves the hospital. 2. An outline of the steps taken in performing a procedure.

protocoproporphria (prō′-tō-kop′-rō-por-fir′-i-ah): Increased secretions of coproporphyrins.

protodiastolic (prō′tō-dī-a- stol′ik): Refers to the period immediately following the second heart sound; the initial one-third of the diastole.

protogyny (prō-toj′i-ni): A form of hermaphrodism in which the female gonad matures before the male gonad.

proton (prō′ton): One of the basic parts of the nucleus of the atom, around which the electrons revolve; it carries a positive charge.

protopathic (prō-tō-path′ik): Primary; primitive. **P. SENSIBILITY,** term applied to peripheral sensory fibers that are of low sensibility for degree and location of the sensations of pain and heat. Opp. to epicritic (*q.v.*).

protoplasm (prō′tō-plazm): The thick, viscid, complex chemical compound constituting the main part of tissue cells; it may be clear or granulated and is surrounded by an invisible membrane. **P.** is the physical basis of all living cells.

protoporphyria (prō′tō-por-fir′i-a): A condition in which there is an abnormal amount of protoporphyrin (*q.v.*) in the feces. **ERYTHROPOIETIC P.,** an inherited disorder characterized by increased fecal excretion of protoporphyrin, increased protoporphyrin in the red blood cells, and development of acute urticaria or eczema soon after exposure to sunlight.

protoporphyrin (prō-tō-por′fir-in): A porphyrin (*q.v.*) which is linked with iron to form the heme of hemoglobin.

protopsis (prō-top′sis): Protrusion of the eyeball; exophthalmos.

protosyphilis (prō-tō-sif′i-lis): Primary syphilis.

prototype (prō′tō-tīp): 1. The primitive or original member of a class or species on which subsequent members are modeled. 2. An individual or quality that exemplifies the standard for members of a particular class or species.

protozoa (prō-tō-zō′a): The smallest type of animal life; single-celled organisms, capable of asexual reproduction. Diseases produced by them include malaria, amebic dysentery, leishmaniasis.—protozoon, sing.; protozoal, adj. See **ameba.**

protozoiasis (prō′tō-zō-ī′a-sis): Any disease caused by protozoa.

protozoology (prō-tō-zō-ol′o -ji): The science that treats of protozoa.

protraction (prō-trak′shun): An extension forward or outward. **FACIAL P.,** a facial anomaly in which some facial structure such as the jaw stands farther forward than usual. In dentistry, the extension of the teeth or other part of the upper or lower jaw to a position farther forward than usual.

protuberance (prō-tū′ber-ans): A projecting part, outgrowth, swelling, knob.

proud flesh: Excessive growth of granulation tissue in a wound or ulcer with little tendency toward scar formation.

provitamin (prō-vī′ta-min): A principle in certain foods which the body is able to convert into a vitamin, *e.g.*, carotene is converted into vitamin A.

proxemics (prok-sem′-miks): The study of the personal and cultural needs of people and of their interactions with various aspects of their environment; including urban overcrowding.

proximal (prok′si-mal): Nearest the head or source. In anatomy, the part of an extremity, nerve, vessel, etc. that is nearest the trunk or point of origin of the part.—proximally, adv.

proximate (prok′si-māt): Nearest, immediate. **P. CAUSE,** the particular cause, among several, which is the immediate cause of disease. **P.PRINCIPLE,** the active part of a drug substance.

prudent (proo′-dent): Refers to a person who exhibits knowledge, judiciousness, and cautiousness in activities or behavior. **REASONABLY PRUDENT,** in nursing, a legal term used in connection with some disputed nursing action or procedure that resulted in injury or harm to a patient, but which would not have occurred had the nurse acted with reasonable prudency.

prurigo (prū-rī′gō): A chronic skin disease marked by formation of papules that itch intensely, occurring most frequently in children. **BESNIER'S P.,** a common skin condition usually called infantile eczema when it occurs in infants and atopic dermatitis when it occurs in adults. **P. ESTIVALE,** hydroa aestivale (*q.v.*). **P. FEROX,** a severe form. **P. MITIS,** a mild form. **P. NODULARIS,** a rare disease of the adult female in which intensely pruritic pea-sized nodules occur on the arms and legs.

pruritus (prū-ri′tus): An unpleasant sensation that produces itching and the desire to scratch; caused by drugs, bites, or disease, including allergy. **P. ANI** and **P. VULVAE** are considered to be psychosomatic conditions (neurodermatitis) except in a few cases where a local cause can be found, *e.g.*, worm infestation, vaginitis. Generalized **P.** may be a symptom of systemic disease as in diabetes, icterus, Hodgkin's disease, carcinoma, etc. It may be psychogenic, *e.g.*, widow's itch which occurs shortly after bereavement. **P. ANI,** itching of the skin around the anus. **P. ESTIVALIS,** occurs during the summer; associated with prickly heat; syn., summer itch. **P. HIEMALIS,** occurs in cold weather; appears mostly on the legs. **P. SENILIS,** common in the aged; probably due to lack of oil in the skin; worse in cold weather; may be associated with diabetes, gout, myxedema, atherosclerosis, neurosis, liver disease. P. VULVAE, irritative condition of the vulva with intolerable itching; causes are poor hygiene, vaginitis, allergies, carcinoma, skin disorders, jaundice, glycosuria, nutritional deficiencies, psychological factors, tissue changes following menopause.

prussic acid (prus'ik as'id): A 4 percent solution of hydrogen cyanide; hydrocyanic acid. Both the solution and its vapor are poisonous, with death occurring very rapidly from respiratory paralysis.

psammotherapy (sam-ō-ther'a-pi): Treatment by the use of sand baths.

psellism (sel'izm): Stammering; stuttering; mispronunciation or substitution of letter sounds.

pseud-, pseudo-: Combining forms denoting: 1. False, counterfeit, faked, feigned, or illusory. 2. A deceptive resemblance. 3. Abnormal, aberrant.

pseudacusis (sū-da-kū'sis): A defect in hearing in which sounds are heard as altered in pitch or quality. Syn., pseudacousma.

pseudaphia (sū-daf'i-a): A defect in the perception of touch.

pseudarthrosis (sū-dar-thrō'sis): A false joint, *e.g.*, due to ununited fracture; also congenital. Occurs primarily in the long bones. Also pseudoarthrosis. GIRDLESTONE P., the creation of a false joint by removing the head and neck of the femur and upper half of the wall of the acetabulum and suturing a mass of soft tissue in the gap to form a cushion between the bones.

pseudoaneurysm (sū' -dō-an'ū-riz-em): False aneurysm. May be a rupture of all of the arterial coats, with the blood being retained by the tissues surrounding the vessel, or it may be due to a hematoma that does not involve the walls but which presents the appearance of an aneurysm.

pseudoangina (sū-dō-an-jī'na): False angina. Sometimes referred to as left mammary pain, it occurs in anxious individuals. Usually there is no cardiac disease present. May be part of effort syndrome (*q.v.*).

pseudoarthritis (sū'dō-ar-thrī'tis): A condition resembling or mimicking arthritis.

pseudoblepsis (sū-dō-blep'sis): A condition in which a person sees objects as different from what they really are; visual hallucinations.

pseudobulbar palsy (sū-dō-bul'bar): See under palsy.

pseudocide (sū'dō-sīd): Consciously acting to harm oneself in such a way as to attract attention or gain sympathy, without intending to take one's life.

pseudocoxalgia (sū'dō-kok-sal'ji-a): Legg-Calve-Perthes' disease (*q.v.*).

pseudocrisis (sū-dō-krī'sis): A rapid reduction of body temperature resembling a crisis, followed by further fever.

pseudocroup (sū-dō-kroop'): Laryngismus stridulus (*q.v.*).

pseudocryptorchism (sū'dō-krip'tor-kizm): A fairly common condition in which both testes are in the inguinal canal but can be brought down into the scrotum without surgery.

pseudocyesis (sū-dō-sī-ē'sis): The existence of signs and symptoms simulating those of early pregnancy occurring in a childless person with an overwhelming desire to have a child and who believes she is pregnant when, in fact, this is not so.

pseudocyst (sū'dō-sist): A dilated space in an organ that resembles a cyst but which does not have the epithelial lining found in a true cyst. PANCREATIC P., the accumulation of pancreatic secretion in a space behind the peritoneum; occurs in chronic pancreatitis following the rupture of a pancreatic duct.

pseudodementia (sū'dō-dē-men'shi-a): Extreme apathy and indifference to environment and general behavior that simulates dementia but without impairment of the mental faculties; usually reversible; often refers to the masked expression frequently seen in the elderly. HYSTERICAL P., see Ganser's syndrome.

pseudodiabetes (sū'ō-dī-a-bē'tēz): Subclinical diabetes; a condition marked by abnormal glucose tolerance test findings but no other signs of diabetes.

pseudoepilepsy (sū-dō-ep'i-lep-si): See hysteroepilepsy.

pseudoexophthalmos (sū'dō-eks-of-thal'mos): Abnormal protrusion of the eyeball for any reason other than exophthalmos, *e.g.*, shallow orbits or extreme myopia.

pseudogeusia (sū-dō-gū'si-a): A sensation of taste arising without any external stimulus to produce it.

pseudogout (sū'dō-gowt): A condition in which there is deposit of calcium crystals rather than urate crystals in and around small joints but especially the cartilage of the knee; occurs mostly in older people; pyrophosphate arthropathy.

pseudogynecomastia (sū'dō-jīn-ē-kō-mas'ti-a): Increase in size of the male breast by deposit of adipose tissue rather than breast tissue.

pseudohallucination (sū'dō-ha-lū-si-nā'shun): The appearance to an individual of geometric forms and figures which the person recognizes as hallucinatory, not real.

pseudohematuria (sū' -dō-hem-a-tū'ri-a): False hematuria; reddish discoloration of the urine due to ingestion of certain drugs or foods, not to the presence of blood.

pseudohemophilia (sū'dō-hē-mō-fil'i-a): A non-hereditary disease of both men and women in which the clotting time is normal but the bleeding time is prolonged. False hemophilia.

pseudohemoptysis (sū'dō-hē-mop'ti-sis): The spitting of blood that does not come from the bronchial tubes or the lungs.

pseudohermaphrodite (sū'dō-her-maf'rō-dīt): A person with the gonads of one sex but with external genitalia that resemble those of the opposite sex.

pseudohermaphroditism (sū'dō-her-maf'rō-dit-izm): A condition in which the gonads are definitely of one sex but there are morphologic contradictions in the individual's makeup. **FEMALE P.**, pertaining to a genetic female with female gonads but with some masculine characteristics. **MALE P.**, pertaining to a genetic male with male gonads but with some feminine characteristics.

pseudohypertrophic muscular dystrophy: A type of muscular dystrophy, occurring most often in young boys; probably hereditary. Marked by hypertrophy of the muscles, especially those of the calf and shoulder, difficulty in walking, and later dystrophy of the muscles.

pseudohypertrophy (sū'dō-hī-per'trō-fi): Increase in size, of some part of the body, that is not true enlargement, *e.g.*, in muscular **P.** in which the increase in size is due to infiltration of the muscle tissue by other tissues, not to enlargement of the muscle fibers.

pseudohyponatremia (sū'dō-hī-pō-na-trē'mi-a): Low serum concentration of sodium that is the result of hyperglycemia or hyperlipemia; it does not indicate a diminution in serum osmotic pressure.

pseudohypoparathyroidism (sū'dō-hī'pō-par-a-thī'royd-izm): A condition in which the symptoms are the same as in hypoparathyroidism, but which is due to the body's inability to respond to the parathyroid hormone rather than to lack of the hormone. See hypoparathyroidism.

pseudologia (sū-dō-lō'ji-a): Pathological lying, manifested in either speech or writing. **P. FANTASTICA,** a constitutional tendency to tell and defend fanastic lies plausibly; seen in some individuals with hysteria.

pseudolymphoma (sū'dō-lim-fō'ma): Lymphocytoma cutis; see under lymphocytoma.

pseudomembrane (sū'dō-mem'brān): A false membrane such as that which forms on the mucous membrane of the throat in diphtheria.

pseudomembranous (sū'dō-mem'bra-nus): Pertaining to a pseudomembrane. **P. ENTEROCOLITIS,** a serious, often fatal disease involving the mucosa of the small bowel thought to be caused by a staplylococcus organism; a pseudomembrane forms over the mucosa causing the latter to become inflamed and necrotic; symptoms include vomiting and severe bloody diarrhea; may occur in persons receiving antibiotics.

pseudomnesia (sū-dom-nē'zi-a): False memory. Memory of events that have never occurred.

Pseudomonas (sū-dō-mōn'as): A bacterial genus. Gram-negative motile rods, found commonly in water, soil, and decomposing vegetable matter. Several species are recognized. Some are pathogenic to plants and animals and occasionally to man, *e.g., P. pyocyanea (Bacillus pyocyaneus),* found commonly in intestinal dejecta, sinuses and suppurating wounds; a secondary invader in some urinary tract infections and wound infections; produces a blue or blue-green pigment which colors the exudate or pus; also called *P. aeruginosa.*

pseudomyxoma peritonei (sū'dō-mik-sō'ma per-i-tō-nē'ī): The accumulation of large amounts of mucoid material in the peritoneal cavity; may result from a ruptured ovarian neoplasm or a ruptured appendiceal mucocele.

pseudonystagmus (sū'dō-nis-tag'mus): Rhythmic jerking movements of the eyeball occurring as a symptom in various diseases of the central nervous system.

pseudoparalysis (sū'dō-pa-ral'i-sis): See pseudoplegia.

pseudopelade (sū'dō-pē'lahd): A form of alopecia characterized by small patches of folliculitis that are followed by a scarring type of alopecia.

pseudophakia (sū'dō-fā'ki-a):An eye condition in which mesodermal tissue replaces a degenerated crystalline lens. **P. ADIPOSA,** the lens is replaced by fatty tissue. **P. FIBROSA,** the lens is replaced by extension of the connective tissue that surrounds it.

pseudoplegia (sū'dō-plē'ji-a): Paralysis mimicking that of organic nervous disorders but usually hysterical in origin.

pseudopodia (sū'dō-pō'di-a): False legs. The temporary projection of protoplasmic processes of an ameba or of ameboid cells (leukocytes) for the purposes of locomotion or for the ingestion of food or other particles.—pseudopodium, sing.

pseudopolyposis (sū'dō-pol-i-pō'sis): Widely scattered polypi, usually the result of previous inflammation—sometimes ulcerative colitis.

pseudopsia (su-dop'si-a): False vision; visual hallucinations; See pseudoblepsia.

pseudoptosis (su-dō-tō'sis): The apparent ptosis of the eyelid resulting in a decrease in the palpebral fissure size.

pseudopuberty (sū'dō-pū'ber-ti): A condition characterized by varying bodily and functional changes typical of puberty before the natural chronological age of puberty; may be due to the hormonal secretions of a tumor.

pseudosmia (sū-doz′mi-a): The subjective sensation of perceiving an odor that is not present.

pseudostrabismus (sū′dō-stra-biz′mus): The false appearance of convergent strabismus seen particularly in infants and Orientals in whom the nasal bridges are flat, the interpupillary distances are narrow, and there is less sclera showing at the nasal side of the eyes. See strabismus and epicanthus.

pseudotumor (sū′dō-tū′mor): The appearance of signs and symptoms of tumor in the absence of a tumor; spontaneous recovery usually ensues. **P. CEREBRI,** a condition marked by signs of an intracranial tumor in the absence of any neoplasm; sometimes seen in hypervitaminosis or prolonged use of steroids; recovery is usually spontaneous but the optic nerve may be affected and cause blindness unless treated.

pseudoxanthoma elasticum (sū-dō-zan-thō′ma ē-las′ti-kum): An inherited form of dermatosis in which elastic fibers become calcified; the skin becomes lax with yellow, slightly elevated plaques; may also be associated with changes in the elasticity of blood vessels. Also called Grönblad-Strandberg syndrome.

psilosis (sī-lō′sis): 1. Sprue (*q.v.*). 2. Falling out of the hair.

psittacosis (sit-a-kō′sis): Virus disease of parrots, pigeons and budgerigars which is occasionally responsible for a form of pneumonia in man.

psoas (sō′as): One of two muscles of the loins, the psoas major or the psoas minor.

psoriasis (so-rī′a-sis): A chronic skin condition characterized by bright red, slightly elevated, round or oval areas that are covered with dry adherent scales that leave bleeding points when removed; when scales are scraped they produce a shiny, silvery sheen that is diagnostic. Non-infectious; cause unknown. May occur on any part of the body but characteristic sites are extensor surfaces, especially over the knees and elbows. **GUTTATE P.,** an acute form consisting of teardrop-shaped red, scaly patches 3 to 10 mm in diameter over the entire body; may accompany beta-streptococcal pharyngitis or other upper respiratory infection; unless adequate treatment is instituted, a more severe form of **P.** may develop.—psoriatic, adj.

psoriatic (sō-ri-at′ik): Pertaining to psoriasis. **P. ARTHRITIS** or **ARTHROPATHY,** an arthritic condition associated with psoriasis, often involving the distal interphalangeal joints; may be a variant of rheumatic arthritis, or an unassociated condition.

PSP: Abbreviation for phenolsulfonphthalein (*q.v.*).

PSRO: Abbreviation for Professional Standards Review Organization (*q.v.*).

psych-, psycho-: Combining forms denoting 1) the mind, mental processes; 2) spirit, soul.

psychalgia (sī-kal′ji-a): Mental pain or distress; sometimes caused by mental effort; seen especially in states of melancholia.

psychanopsia (sī-kan-op′si-a): Psychic blindness; the individual is able to see but does not recognize what he sees; usually due to a brain lesion.

psychasthenia (sī-kas-thē′ni-a): A form of psychoneurosis marked by mental fatigue, unreasonable fears, obsessions and compulsion, feelings of inadequacy, lack of self-control, a sensation of unreality of self and surroundings, preoccupation with minor details to the extent that nothing worthwhile is accomplished.

psyche (sī′ke): The mind; the intellect, including both conscious and unconscious mental processes. In psychoanalysis, includes the id, ego, superego, and all their conscious and unconscious processes.

psychedelic (sī-ke-del′ik): 1. Mind-manifesting or mind-expanding. 2. Pertaining to drugs that have the immediate action of producing highly creative and imaginative thought patterns, enlarging the vision, producing freedom from anxiety, and altering sensation or perception, *e.g.*, peyote and LSD. Also psychodelic.

psychiatric (sī-ki-āt′rik): Relating to psychiatry. **PSYCHIATRIC-MENTAL HEALTH NURSE,** see under nurse. **PSYCHIATRIC SOCIAL WORKER;** a specially trained social worker with a masters degree in social work who assists psychiatric patients with problems of employment, housing, family affairs, and other situational adjustments that need to be made following discharge from an institution, and who refers the patient to appropriate helping agencies.

psychiatrist (sī-kī′a-trist): One who specializes in psychiatry (*q.v.*); specifically, a medical school graduate with postgraduate training in the treatment of mental disorders, and licensed to practice psychiatry.

psychiatry (sī-kī′at-ri): That branch of medical science that is devoted to the origin, diagnosis, and treatment of mental, emotional or behavioral disorders; by extension includes problems of personal adjustment and such special fields as mental retardation.—psychiatric, adj.

psychic (sī′kik): 1. Pertaining to the psyche; of the mind; mental. 2. A person who is thought to have unusual sensitivity to non-physical forces; a spiritualistic medium. **P. ENERGIZER,** popular term for a drug that elevates or stimulates the mood of a depressed person. **P. HEALING,** an ancient healing mode often called faith healing because the laying on of hands, which is one aspect of it, often has a religious connotation; the assumption is that a transfer of healing energy passes from the healer to the healee, which is the basis of the modern practice of "therapeutic touch."

psychoactive (sī-kō-ak′tiv): Usually pertains to psychopharmacologic agents that have the ability to alter mood, behavior, and cognitive processes.

psychoanalysis (sī′kō-a-nal′i-sis): A specialized branch of psychiatry founded by Freud. Briefly, the method is based on recall and analysis of a person's past emotional experiences and dreams with the purpose of understanding the origin of the patient's symptoms and furnishing hints as to the kind of psychotherapy that may eventually alleviate the symptoms, which are seen as manifestations of unconscious conflicts.—psychoanalytic, adj.

psychoanalyst (sī-kō-an′al-ist): One who specializes in psychoanalysis (*q.v.*).

psychobiology (sī′kō-bī-ol′o-ji): A school of psychiatric thought that views the biologic, psychologic, and sociologic experiences of an individual as an integrated unit, and that the interactions of body and mind have an important influence on the development of personality. Also called biopsychology.

psychochemotherapy (sī′kō-kē-mō-ther′a-pi): The use of drugs to improve or cure pathological changes in the emotional state.—psychochemotherapeutic, adj.; psychochemotherapeutically, adv.

psychodrama (sī′kō-dra′ma): Therapeutically controlled acting-out. A method of psychotherapy whereby patients act out their personal problems in spontaneous dramatic performances and receive instructive feedback about solving their stressful experiences.

psychodynamic (si-kō-dī-nam′ik): Referring to mental or emotional processes or forces and their effects on behavior and mental states.

psychodynamics (sī-kō-dī-nam′iks): The science of the mental processes, especially of the causative factors in mental activity.

psychoendocrinology (sī′kō-en′dō-kri-nol′o-ji): The study of the interrelationships between endocrine functions and mental states.

psychogenesis (sī-kō-jen′e-sis): The development of mental and emotional traits.

psychogenic (sī-kō-jen′ik): Arising from or originating in the psyche or mind as opposed to having a physical basis. **P. BLADDER**, inability of the bladder to fill to any extent, resulting in incontinence or excessively frequent voiding; due to a number of nervous and/or emotional factors. **P. SYMPTOM**, a neurotic symptom.

psychogeriatric (sī′-ko-jer-i-at′rik): Pertaining to the care and management of geriatric patients with psychological or psychiatric problems. **P. CARE** involves measures to relieve symptoms, treating conditions that are treatable, and providing long-term care when necessary.

psychogeriatrician (sī′-kō-jer-i-a-trish′-un): A psychiatrist who specializes in the treatment of geriatric patients with emotional disturbances or mental illnesses. Also called geropsychiatrist.

psychogeriatrics (sī′-kō-jer-i-at′riks): 1. The branch of medical science dealing with geriatric patients who have psychological or psychiatric disorders. 2. Psychology applied to geriatrics.

psychokinesia (sī′kō-kī-nē′zi-a): Impulsive behavior; a burst of violent behavior, often maniacal, resulting from lack of inhibition.

psychokinesis (sī′kō-ki-nē′sis): The production or alteration of movement by the direct influence of the mind without any somatic influence.—psychokinetic, adj.

psycholepsy (sī′kō-lep-si): A sudden temporary mood change involving mental inertia, feelings of helplessness, confusion, tachycardia; seen in hysterical persons.—psycholeptic adj.

psychologic, psychological (sī-kō-loj′ik, sī-kō-loj′i-kal): Pertaining to psychology. **P. DEPENDENCE**, a craving or psychologic need for an abused substance. **P. TESTING**, the use of diagnostic tools such as cognitive and projective tests by psychologists to aid in assessing and planning treatment for the patient.

psychologist (sī-kol′o-jist): One who specializes in the study of the mind, especially as it affects behavior. **CLINICAL P.**, generally one who holds a doctoral degree in psychology and who has had supervised experience in working with clients who have mental disorders or disturbances

psychology (sī-kol′o-ji): The science that deals with the emotions, mental processes, and behavior of an organism in its environment. Medically, the study of human behavior. **ADLERIAN P.**, individual **P.**; emphasizes man's social nature; emphasizes organic inferiority as a prominent cause of neuroses and the use of compensation and overcompensation to overcome feelings of inferiority and attain superiority. **ANALYTICAL P.**, **BEHAVIORAL P.**, see behaviorism. **DEVELOPMENTAL P.**, deals with changes in human behavior in relation to age. **FREUDIAN P.**, based on the theory that abnormal behavior can be modified or corrected by allowing patients to talk about their early experiences, memories, dreams, and so on, to the therapist who remains ojective and nonjudgmental. **GESTALT P.**, a German school of psychology that teaches that the whole is more than the sum of its parts; that the parts are not put together to make the whole but are derived from it and get their character from it; that humans respond to meaningful entities that cannot be broken down into component parts. From the German word *gestalt,* meaning the whole appearance or shape. **HUMANISTIC P.**, a term invented by Kurt Goldstein to describe an existential approach to psychology, which holds that humans are unique in their subjectivity and their capacity for psychological growth; that humans are innately good and strive for such growth; and that humans control their destiny to a greater extent than was formerly believed possible. **INDUSTRIAL P., P.** that deals with the appplication of psychological principles to the activities and problems that arise in business and industrial situations. **JUNGIAN P., ANALYTIC P.**, utilizing the patient's imagination in the analytic process, often asking patients to paint or draw an image or to act out a fantasy; Jung also considered the libido the will to live rather than an expression of the sex instinct. **PHYSIOLOGIC P.**, deals with the functions of the nervous system as they relate to behavior. **SOCIAL P.**, deals with the cultural, ecologic, and social influences on mental life and mental disorders. **TRANSPERSONAL P.**, an area of psychologic study that investigates experiences that go beyond the ordinary limitations of time and space, including those involving psychic phenomena, biofeedback, meditation, and energy transformation.—psychological, adj.; psychologically, adv.

psychometric (sī-kō-met′rik): Related to or being a measurement of the duration and force of mental processes.

psychometrician (sī-kō-me-trish′-un): A researcher in the field of geriatric health-care services who investigates the methods for assessing and measuring the health status of individuals in long-term care situations; may or may not be a physician.

psychometrics (sī-kō-met′riks): The measurement of mental potential, ability, and functioning by means of psychometric tests (often called intelligence tests).

psychometry (sī-kom′e-tri): The science of testing and measuring psychologic and mental ability and processes.

psychomotor (sī-kō-mō′tor): Pertaining to motor activities initiated by psychic or cerebral activity. **P. EPILEPSY,** recurrent, periodic disturbances of behavior in which the person carries out certain repetitive movements semiautomatically. **P. RETARDATION,** general retardation in both physical and emotional development. **P. TESTS,** usually measure such things as muscular coordination and behavioral activity.

psychoneuroimmunology (sī′-kō-nū′-rō-im′-mū-nol′-o-ji): A relatively new field of science which seeks to find precise connections between the body and mind. It is concerned with such issues as therapeutic touch in which its proponents believe there is a transfer of energy from the healer to the patient.

psychoneurosis (sī-kō-nū-rō′sis): A functional disorder of the mind, usually mild in character, based on psychogenic factors. Neurosis.—psychoneurotic, adj.

psychopath (sī′kō-path): An eccentric, unstable, or mentally ill person with a poorly balanced personality who engages in egocentric, impulsive, immoral, or anti-social behavior, but who knows better and is not insane. See also sociopath and personality, psychopathic.

psychopathology (sī-kō-pa-thol′o-ji): The study of pathology of the mind, or of maladaptive psychological functioning, personality, and/or social adjustment.—psychopathologic, psychopathological, adj.

psychopathy (sī-kop′a-thi): Any disease or disorder of the mind, especially one that is associated with character or personality defect.

psychopharmaceuticals (sī′kō-far-ma-sū′tikals): Drugs used in the treatment of emotional disturbances.

psychopharmacology (sī′kō-far-ma-kol′o-ji): The study of the action of drugs on the emotional state and on behavioral activity. **CLINICAL P.**, includes both the study of drugs and their effects in patients and their use in treatment of psychiatric conditions.—psychopharmacologic, psychopharmacological, adj.

psychophysics (sī-kō-fiz′iks): A branch of experimental psychology dealing with the study of stimuli and the related psychological experiences.—psychophysical, adj.

psychophysiologic (sī′kō-fiz-i-ō-loj′ik): 1. Pertaining to behavior as it relates to physiologic body processes. 2. Denoting an illness that exhibits physical symptoms but has an emotional cause; often called psychosomatic disorder; see psychosomatic.

psychophysiology (sī′kō-fiz-i-ol′ō-ji): The physiology of the mental apparatus or structures.—psychophysiologic, adj.

psychoprophylactic (sī′-kō-prō-fi-lak′tik): That which aims at preventing mental disease; often referring specifically to education programs in preparation for childbirth by the Lamaze method (*q.v.*).—psychoprophylaxis, n.

psychosensory (sī-ko-sen′-sor-i): Pertaining to one's conscious perception of sensation.

psychosexual (sī-kō-seks′ū-al): Pertaining to the emotional aspects of sexuality as contrasted to the physical aspects. **P. DEVELOPMENT,** the characteristic changes that take place in the libido during the years from infancy to adulthood, including the phases described as anal, oedipal, oral, phallic, latent, and genital.

psychosis (sī-kō′sis): A major mental illness of an organic or emotional origin, arising in the mind itself as opposed to a neurosis in which the mind is affected by factors in the environment. Marked by such abnormal mental function or behavior as loss of contact with reality, distortions of perception, diminished control of elementary desires and impulses, delusions, hallucinations. The deterioration of personality may be so great as to be incompatible with self-sustained social adjustment. **AFFECTIVE P.**, **P.** with the predominant disturbance being in the person's emotions and attitude; marked by mood changes ranging from elation to depression, and by disturbances in thinking and behavior; includes 1) cyclothymic disorders which are marked by chronic mood disturbances lasting at least two years, and 2) dysthymic disorders, marked by loss of interest in all activities but not severe enough or sufficiently long lasting to be called depression. **ALCOHOLIC P.**, that caused by excessive use of alcohol; see Wernicke-Korsakoff syndrome. **DEPRESSIVE P.**, that caused by depression; marked by self-doubt, melancholia, guilt feelings, physical symptoms, thoughts of death and/or suicide. **DISINTEGRATIVE P.**, **P.** marked by normal development during the first few years, then loss of speech, social competence and mental acuity; cause sometimes unknown, but may follow measles, encephalitis, or other serious infection. **DRUG P. P.** induced by toxic effects of certain drugs. **FUNCTIONAL P.**, schizophrenic, manic-depressive, and involutional **P.** **GESTATIONAL P.**, **P.** that develops during pregnancy. **HYSTERICAL P.**, **P.** that is characterized by sudden onset, hallucinatory delusions, bizaare behavior; occurs often in self-centered individuals with hysteric personalities. **ICU PSYCOSIS**, intensive care syndrome; a transient state characterized by disorientation, confusion, hallucinations, and sometimes delusions; usually reversible when the patient leaves the ICU. **INVOLUTIONAL P.**, a severe **P.** characterized by depression, insomnia, anxiety, delusions, somatic concerns; occurs in older persons. **MANIC-DEPRESSIVE P.**, a mental disorder characterized by mood swings toward either excitement or depression; not all patients exhibit both phases, and many experience periods of complete recovery between the two phases. Also called bipolar disorder. **ORGANIC P.**, **P.** resulting from brain disorder or injury. **POSTPARTUM P.**, that occurring after delivery; may be organic or toxic in origin. **SCHIZO-AFFECTIVE P.**, that seen in schizophrenic persons who exhibit manic-depressive features. **SENILE P.**, mental deterioration in old age; often accompanied by eccentric behavior and irritability. **TOXIC P.**, that caused by drugs, chemicals, or the presence of toxins in the body.

psychosocial (sī-kō-sō'shul):Pertaining to a person's psychological development in relation to his social environment.

psychosomatic (sī' -kō-sō-mat'ik): Pertaining to the intimate relationship of mental and bodily functions and their effects upon each other. Most commonly used to describe symptoms of illnesses that are at least partly psychic or emotional in origin.

psychosomimetic (sī'kō-sō-mī-met'ik): 1. Pertaining to symptoms that resemble those of psychosis or to drugs that produce psychosis-like symptoms. 2. A hallucinogen. Also psychotomimetic.

psychostimulant (sī-kō-stim'ū-lant): A substance that has psychoactive properties, *e.g.*, amphetamines, coffee, cocaine.

psychosurgery (sī-kō-ser'jer-i): Treatment of severe psychiatric disorders by surgery on the brain, especially by prefrontal lobotomy; once widely used in treatment of schizophrenia (*q.v.*).

psychosynthesis (sī' -kō-sin'the-sis): A lay movement promoting the use of therapy aimed at restoring useful inhibitions; the opposite of psychoanalysis.

psychotherapist (sī' -kō-ther'a-pist): A health care professional who is trained in psychotherapy; may be a psychiatrist, clinical psychologist, nurse, or psychiatric social worker.

psychotherapy (sī' -kō-ther'a-pi): A form of therapy that may be used either in the treatment of organic diseases or of neuroses and psychoses; it is based on psychological methods, *e.g.*, psychoanalysis, hypnosis, suggestion, or persuasion rather than medical, pharmaceutical, or surgical methods. **GROUP P.**, see therapy, group.—psychotherapeutic, adj.

psychotic (sī-kot'ik): 1. Related to or characterized by psychosis (*q.v.*). 2. A person suffering from psychosis, usually out of touch with reality and incapable of reasonable behavior.

psychotogenic (sī-kot' -ō-jen'ik): Producing a condition of psychosis; often refers to certain drugs.—psychotogenesis, n.

psychotomimetic (sī-kot' -ō-mī-met'ik): 1. Pertaining to or capable of producing a state resembling psychosis. 2. An agent that produces symptoms resembling those of psychosis including hallucinations, delusions, and distorted perceptions.

psychotropic (sī-kō-trō'pik): That which exerts its specific influence upon the psyche or mind. Term often used to describe drugs that affect cognitive functioning, such as tranquilizers, antidepressants, and psychotomimetics such as LSD (*q.v.*).

psychro-: Combining form denoting cold, freezing.

psychrometer (sī-krom'e-ter): A device for measuring the relative humidity of the atmosphere.

psychrophile (sī-krō-fīl): An organism that grows best at low temperatures—15–20°C or less.—psychrophilic, adj.

psychrotherapy (sī-krō-ther'a-pi): Treatment of disease by the application of cold.

psyllium (sil'i-um): The seeds of an African plant. They contain mucilage, which swells on contact with water; useful as a bulk-forming laxative.

PT: Abbreviation for: 1. Physical therapy. 2. Physical therapist. 3. Prothrombin time.

pt: Abbreviation for: 1. Patient. 2. Pint.

PTA: Abbreviation for: 1. Post-traumatic amnesia. 2. Prior to admission.

pterion (tē'ri-on): The point on the skull where the frontal, parietal, and temporal bones and the great wing of the sphenoid bone meet; is the thinnest portion of the skull, located about 3 cm behind the outer process of the bony orbit.

pterygium (te-rij'ē-um): 1. Web eye; a triangular patch of mucous membrane and blood vessels, usually seen on the nasal side of the eye with the apex pointing toward the pupil; a benign growth often associated with exposure to wind and sun; encroachment on the cornea results in disturbance of vision. Treatment is surgical. 2. Any fold of skin that extends abnormally from one part of the body to another. **P. COLLI,** a congenital condition in which a tight band of skin extends from the acromion to the mastoid; usually bilateral.

pterygoid (ter'i-goid): Resembling a wing. **P. MUSCLES,** four muscles that originate on the pterygoid process and insert into the mandible; they open and close the jaw and move it forward and from side to side. **P. PROCESS,** one of two processes that extend downward from either side of the sphenoid bone at the junctions of the wings with the body of the sphenoid.

PTH: Abbreviation for parathyroid hormone.

ptilosis (ti-lō'sis): Falling out of the eyelashes.

ptomaine (tō'mān): A chemical substance formed by the putrefactive action of bacteria on protein. **P. POISONING,** term formerly applied to food poisoning.

ptosis (tō'sis): A drooping, falling, or sinking down of an organ or part, particularly the drooping of an upper eyelid. May be an inherited condition or acquired, and may be unilateral, bilateral, or asymmetric. See visceroptosis. **SENILE P.,** usually refers to the ptosis of the upper eyelid; due to weakness of the elevator muscle and the presence of fat in the subcutaneous tissue.—ptotic, ptosed, adj.

-ptosis: Combining form denoting 1) sagging, falling; 2) prolapse of an organ or part.

ptyal-, ptyalo-: Combining forms denoting 1) saliva; 2) salivary gland(s).

ptyalagogue (tī-al'a-gog): An agent that increases the flow of saliva. Also ptyalogogue. Syn., sialagogue.

ptyalin (tī'a-lin): Salivary amylase, an enzyme which in an alkaline medium converts starch into dextrin and maltose.

ptyalism (tī'a-lizm): Excessive flow of saliva; salivation.

ptyalolith (tī'a-lō-lith): A salivary calculus.

ptyalorrhea (tī-a-lō-rē'a): Abnormally heavy flow of saliva.

pubertas (pū'ber-tas): Puberty (*q.v.*). **P. PRAECOX,** premature (precocious) sexual development.

puberty (pū'ber-ti): The age at which the reproductive organs become functionally active and at which the person is potentially able to reproduce. It is accompanied by secondary sex characteristics. Occurs typically between 13 and 16 years of age in boys and 10 and 14 in girls.—pubertal, adj.

pubes (pū'bēz): 1. The hairy region covering the pubic bone. 2. Plural of pubis.

pubescence (pū-bes'ens): Approaching or being at the age of puberty.—pubescent, adj.

pubic (pū-bik): Related to or concerning the os pubis. **P. ANGLE,** that formed at the point where the right and left conjoined rami of the ischium and the pubic bones meet. **P. ARCH,** that formed by the union of the inferior rami of the two pubic bones at the symphysis. **P. BONE,** the os pubis; the lower anterior part of the innominate bone. **P. SYMPHYSIS,** the rather rigid joint at the center of the front of the bony pelvis formed by the union of the two pubic bones by a thick pad of fibrocartilaginous tissue.

pubis (pū'bis): The pubic bone or os pubis; it is the center bone of the front of the pelvis.—pubes, pl.; pubic, adj.

public health: Descriptive of all phases of health promotion and preventive medicine carried on in a community under federal, state, county, or local agencies for the benefit of the public in general. **P. H. NURSE,** see under nurse.

pubococcygeal (pū-bō-cok-sij'ē-al): Pertaining to the pubis and the coccyx or to the pubococcygeus muscle. **P. EXERCISES,** see Kegel exercises. **P. MUSCLE,** the anterior part of the levator ani muscle; helps to support the pelvic viscera.

puddle sign: Observed in patients suffering from ascites. The patient is placed in knee-chest position and remains there for several minutes after which the examiner percusses the umbilical area; a dull sound is indicative of the presence of ascitic fluid.

pudental (pū-den'tal): Of or pertaining to the pudentum. **P. BLOCK,** rendering the pudentum insensitive by the injection of a local anesthetic; used mostly for episiotomy and forceps delivery. See transvaginal. **P. NERVE,** originates in the sacral plexus; branches are distributed to the pudental and anal areas. **P. CANAL,** a passageway through the obturator internus muscle providing for the transmission of the pudental nerve and muscles.

pudentum (pū-den'tum): The external genitalia. In the female, includes the labia majora and minora, mons pubis, clitoris, vestibule of the vagina, perineum, and the vestibular glands. In the male the **P.** includes the penis, testes, and scrotum.

puerilism (pū'er-il-izm): Childishness, particularly that seen in some older individuals; second childhood.

puerpera (pū-er'per-a): A woman who has just delivered a child.

puerperal (pū-er'pe-ral): Pertaining to the puerperium (*q.v.*). **P. ECLAMPSIA,** convulsions that occur during the puerperium. See **eclampsia**. **P. FEVER,** that which occurs after delivery and usually relates to **P.** infection. **P. INFECTION,** a general term for infection of the genital tract after delivery or abortion. Also called childbed fever, lying-in fever, puerperal sepsis. **P. PSYCHOSIS,** a psychotic state that occurs during the puerperium.

puerperium (pū-er-pē'ri-um): The period immediately following childbirth to the time when involution is completed, usually 6 to 8 weeks.—puerperia, pl.

Pulex (pū'leks): A genus of fleas. **P. IRRITANS,** the flea that infests humans, dogs, hogs, and other mammals; may serve as intermediate host for certain types of tapeworm. **PASTEURELLA PESTIS,** the flea that infests rats and may transmit plague to humans.

pulicosis (pū-li-kō'sis): Flea bites causing urticaria, sometimes hemorrhagic.

pulmo-: Combining form denoting lung(s).

pulmonary (pul'mo-ner-i): Pertaining to the lungs. **P. ARTERY,** leaves the right ventricle, divides into right and left branches that carry deoxygenated blood to the right and left lungs, respectively. **P. CIRCULATION,** see **circulation**. **P. DISTRESS SYNDROME,** see **respiratory distress syndrome**. **P. EDEMA,** the extravascular accumulation of fluid in the air sacs and interstitial tissues of the lungs. **P. EMBOLISM,** the blocking or closing of the pulmonary artery by an embolus; a fairly common cause of death. **P. EOSINOPHILIA,** refers to several conditions in which there are shadows on x-ray photographs of the lungs and a very high eosinophil count. **P. FIBROSIS,** see under **fibrosis**. **P. FUNCTION TEST,** any one of several tests to determine the functional ability of normal or diseased lungs, *e.g.*, one series of tests measures the ability of the lungs to move air in and out of the lungs; another series evaluates the ability of the alveoli to diffuse gas across the alveolar capillary membrane, and thus adequately to perfuse the blood with oxygen. **P. HEMOSIDEROSIS,** a rare condition caused by repeated hemorrhage of intra-alveolar capillaries; characterized by anemia and sometimes hemoptysis which may be severe enough to cause death; occurs chiefly in children and young adults. **P. INFARCTION,** a clot occluding a small blood vessel of the lung, causing death of the tissue supplied by the vessel; see **infarction**. **P. PRESSURE,** the pressure in the pulmonary artery. **P. SHUNT,** any condition that allows blood to move from the right side of the heart to the left side without circulating through the lungs. May be anatomical and occur as a congenital anomaly, or physiological, occurring most often in patients with atelectasis, bronchial obstruction, or pulmonary disease, and resulting in anoxia. **P. STENOSIS,** see under **stenosis**. **P. TUBERCULOSIS,** see **tuberculosis**. **P. VALVE,** the tricuspid valve at the junction of the pulmonary artery and the right ventricle. **P. VEINS,** veins that leave each lung and carry oxygenated blood to the left ventricle of the heart. **P. WEDGE PRESSURE,** see under **pressure**. See also **invasive pulmonary disorders** under **invasive**, and **obstructive pulmonary disease** under **obstructive**.

pulmonectomy (pul-mō-nek'to-mi) Pneumonectomy (*q.v.*).

pulmonic (pul-mon'ik): 1. Pertaining to or affecting the lungs. 2. A person suffering from a pulmonary disease. **P. STENOSIS,** see under **stenosis**.

pulmonitis (pul'mo-nī'tis): Inflammation of the lung; pneumonia, pneumonitis.

pulmotor (pul'mō-tor): A portable apparatus for forcing oxygen or air or both, into the lungs and drawing out carbon dioxide; used to induce artificial respiration in emergencies such as drowning, asphyxiation by gas, smoke inhalation, etc. Most local police and fire departments have at least one.

pulp: The soft, interior part of some organs and structures. **DENTAL P.,** found in the **P.** cavity of teeth; carries blood, nerve and lymph vessels. **DIGITAL P.,** the tissue pad at the finger tip.—pulpal, adj.

pulpitis (pul-pī'tis): Inflammation of the pulp of a tooth; usually caused by streptococcal or staphylococcal invasion. Odontitis.

pulsate (pul'sāt): To throb, move, or beat rhythmically; to vibrate.

pulsatile (pul'sa-tīl): Beating, throbbing.

pulsating mattress: Syn., alternating pressure mattress. A mattress made of plastic and consisting of separate cells that are inflated alternately with air about every 3 minutes. Useful for patients who are long confined to bed, debilitated, or subject to decubitus ulcers.

pulsation (pul-sā'-shun): 1. Beating or throbbing, as of the heart or arteries. 2. A single beat of the heart or pulse. 3. Rhythmic contraction, expansion, or vibration.

pulse (puls): The rhythmic impulse transmitted to arteries by contraction of the left ventricle and consequent expansion of an artery; customarily palpated by finger at the radial artery of the wrist. **ABDOMINAL P.**, the **P.** over the abdominal aorta. **ALTERNATING P.**, a regular **P.** with alternating beats of weak and strong amplitude. **ARTERIAL P.**, the **P.** felt in an artery. **BIGEMINAL P.**, coupled **P.**; a **P.** in which the beats occur in pairs, each pair being followed by a prolonged pause. **BOUNDING P.**, one of large volume and force. **CAROTID P.**, one felt in a carotid artery. **CORRIGAN'S P.**, the waterhammer **P.** of aortic incompetence, with high initial upthrust that rapidly falls away; also called collapsing **P.**; triphammer **P.**; waterhammer **P.** **DICROTIC P.**, one with a double beat, the second beat being weaker. **ELASTIC P.**, one felt as full and elastic. **FULL P.**, one that is easily felt and with good expansion of the blood vessel. **HARD P.**, one of high tension. **INTERMITTENT P.**, one characterized by intermittently dropped beats. **PARADOXICAL P.**, one that is markedly lowered in amplitude during inspiration. **QUADRIGEMINAL P.**, a **P.** in which there is a pause after every fourth beat. **QUINCKE'S P.**, pulsations sometimes observable at the arterial end of skin capillaries as, for example, the alternate blanching and flushing of the nail bed, which can be elicited by putting pressure on the nail; also called capillary. **THREADY P.**, a weak, usually rapid and scarcely perceptible **P.** **WATERHAMMER P.**, Corrigan's **P.**

pulse deficit: The difference between the rate of the apical heartbeat, counted by stethoscope, and the **P.** counted at the wrist; occurs when some of the ventricular contractions are too weak to open the aortic valve and hence produce a beat at the heart but not at the wrist.

pulse force or tension: **P.** strength estimated by the force needed to obliterate it by pressure of the finger.

pulse pressure: The difference between the systolic and diastolic pressures. See systolic; disastolic.

pulse rate: The same as the heartbeat; normally about 130 per minute in the newborn infant, 70 to 80 in the adult, and 60 to 80 in the elderly.

pulse rhythm: Refers to **P.** regularity; can be regular or irregular.

pulse volume: Refers to the degree of expansion of the arterial wall during the passage of a pulse wave.

pulse-echo technique: The use of ultrasonic energy directed into the body to obtain a graphic representation of any alterations in the structure of an organ or part.

pulseless disease: A group of disorders characteried by gradual occlusion of one or more arteries above their origin in the aortic arch, resulting in loss of pulse in the neck and arms; other symptoms include headache, fever, dizziness, fainting, claudication, transient hemiplegia, atrophy of the retina, clouding or temporary loss of vision. Also called aortic arch syndrome, Takayasu's disease, progressive obliterative arteritis, and brachiocephalic arteritis.

pulse-wave tracing: Produced by a painless diagnostic procedure which records low-frequency silent vibrations from the jugular vein, carotid artery, or apex of the heart; helps to identify certain heart or circulatory disorders or abnormalities.

pulsimeter (pul-sim'e-ter): An instrument for measuring the rate, rhythm, and force of the pulse beat.

pulsus (pul'sus): Pulse. **P. ALTERNANS,** a pulse beat that alternates between strong and weak. **P. BIGEMINUS,** a pulse in which two beats occur close together, with a longer interval between the pairs. **P. PARADOXUS,** a **P.** that becomes slower on inspiration and faster on expiration; likely to occur in patients with pericarditis. **P. PARVUS,** a **P.** of small amplitude. **P. TARDUS,** a slow pulse. **P. TRIGEMINUS,** a **P.** in which three beats occur followed regularly by a missed beat.

pulv.: Abbreviation for *pulvis* [L.], meaning powder.

pulvis (pul'vis): A powder.

pummeling (pum'mel-ling): A maneuver in massage; consists of mild pounding or thumping with the fist.

pump: An apparatus for forcing or drawing fluid or gas to or from a part. **BREAST P.**, one for withdrawing milk from the breast. **STOMACH P.**, one for withdrawing the contents of the stomach.

pump-oxygenator: An apparatus used during open heart surgery; it substitutes for both the heart and lungs in that it pumps the blood through the body and also oxygenates it.

punch biopsy: See under biopsy.

punch-drunk syndrome: A chronic neuropsychologic disorder, possibly due to repeated head injuries, especially when occurring in individuals who began a boxing career early in life; also occurs in alcoholics. Symptoms include mental, emotional, and motor dysfunction.

punctate (pungk'tāt): Dotted or spotted, *e.g.*, punctate basophilia describes the immature red cells in which there are droplets of blue-staining material in the cytoplasm. **P. ERYTHEMA,** a rash of very fine spots.

punctum (pungk'tum): An extremely small point or spot. **P. LACRIMALE,** the minute opening on either the upper or lower eyelid near the canthus through which excess tears enter the lacrimal duct and are carried to the nasal cavity.—puncta, pl.

puncture (pungk'tūr): 1. A stab wound, hole, or other perforation made with a sharp pointed hollow instrument for the withdrawal or injection of fluid or other substance. 2. To make a stab wound or perforation. **CISTERNAL P.**, insertion of a special hollow needle with stylet through the atlantooccipital ligament between the occiput and atlas, into the cisterna magna. One method of obtaining cerebrospinal fluid. **LUMBAR P.**, insertion of a special hollow needle with stylet either through the space between the third and fourth lumbar vertebrae or lower, or into the subarachnoid space, to obtain cerebrospinal fluid for examination, to remove excess fluid, or to inject a drug, *e.g.*, an anesthetic. **STERNAL P.**, insertion of a special guarded hollow needle with stylet into the body of the sternum for aspiration of a bone marrow sample. **VENTRICULAR P.**, a highly skilled method of puncturing a cerebral ventricle for a sample of cerebrospinal fluid. **P. WOUND**, see wound.

pungent (pun′jent): Sharp, bitter, biting, acrid as to taste or odor.

PUO: Abbreviation for pyrexia of undetermined origin; see under pyrexia.

pupil (pū′pil): The contractile circular opening in the center of the iris that allows the passage of light rays to the retina. **ADIE'S P.**, one characterized by slow accommodation, contracting or dilating only after prolonged stimulation. **ARGYLL ROBERTSON P.**, one that responds to accommodation but not to light. **MARCUS GUNN P.**, see Marcus Gunn phenomenon. **PINHOLE** or **PINPOINT P.**, extremely contracted pupil, sometimes caused by miotics or certain brain disorders.

pupillary (pū′pi-ler-i): Pertaining to or concerning the pupil.

pupillotonia (pū′pil-ō-tō′ni-a): Tonic reaction of the pupil, as seen in Adie's syndrome.

Pure Food and Drug Act: A federal law, originally enacted in 1906 and amended many times since. Sets certain standards for the purity of drugs and manufactured food products, for the purpose of protecting the consuming public.

purgation (pur-gā′shun): Catharsis; vigorous evacuation of the bowels effected by a cathartic drug.

purgative (pur′ga-tive): 1. Causing copious evacuation of the bowels. 2. A drug that causes copious evacuation of the bowels. **DRASTIC P.**, one which causes an unusually copious evacuation of watery feces.

purge (purj): 1. To cause a thorough evacuation of the bowels. 2. A drug that causes such an evacuation.

Purified Protein Derivative: A purified protein derivative of tuberculin, used in intradermal test for tuberculosis. See Mantoux test, tuberculin.

purines (pū′renz): Constituents of nucleoproteins from which uric acid is derived. Gout is thought to be associated with the disturbed metabolism and excretion of uric acid; thus foods of high purine content are excluded in its treatment.

Purkinje (pur-kin′jē): **P. CELLS**, large flask-shaped cells with many branching dendrites, located in the middle layer of the cerebral cortex; they are important efferent neurons. **P. FIBERS**, the terminal fibers of the right and left bundle branches (see bundle of His); they form a dense network in the walls of the chambers of the heart and make up the sinoatrial and atrioventricular nodes; are concerned with the electrical transmission of impulses through the heart. [Johannes E. von Purkinje, Bohemian anatomist. 1787–1869.]

purohepatitis (pū′-rō-hep-a-tī′tis): Inflammation of the liver accompanied by suppuration.

puromucous (pū-rō-mū′kus): Containing both pus and mucus. Syn., mucopurulent.

purple (pur′p'l): A dark color that is a blend of red and blue. **VISUAL P.**, a photosensitive pigment in the rods and cones of the retina; rhodopsin (*q.v.*).

purpura (pur′pū-ra): A physical sign rather than a disease entity, characterized by spontaneous extravasation of blood from the capillaries into the skin and manifest by either small red spots (petechiae) that darken to a purplish color and gradually fade, or large plaques (ecchymoses), or by oozing into the mucous membranes. The condition may be idiopathic, or it can be due to impaired function of the capillary walls or to defective quality or quantity of blood platelets; it may also be associated with any of several infective, toxic, or allergic conditions; see Schönlein's disease. **ALLERGIC P.**, nonthrombocytopenic **P.**, due to ingestion of certain foods or drugs, or to insect bites. **P. HEMORRHAGICA**, thrombocytopenic **P.**, a **P.** characterized by greatly diminished platelet count and prolonged clotting time. **HENOCH'S P.**, a variety of Henoch-Schönlein **P.** Henoch-Schönlein **P.**, a type of idiopathic nonthrombocytopenic **P.** characterized by pain and tenderness in the abdomen, exanthema and purpuric skin lesions, mild fever, joint pains, vomiting of blood, bloody stools, nephritic symptoms; may be due to vasculitis; seen most commonly in male children. Also called Schönlein-Henoch purpura, Henoch-Schönlein syndrome, acute vascular **P. IDIOPATHIC THROMBOCYTOPENIC P.**, an acute or chronic form of **P.**, of unknown cause; characterized by red petechiae that are surrounded by blue-black areas occurring on the mucosa and skin of the face and neck, and upper and lower extremities; destruction of platelets; later symptoms include moon face, bleeding of gums, vomiting of blood, monorrhagia, stiff painful joints, prostration. Also called autoimmune thrombocytopenia. May be fatal. **NONTHROM-**

BOCYTOPENIC P., P. that is characterized by a normal platelet count and clotting time. SENILE P., an ecchymotic eruption seen on the forearms and hands of elderly persons. P. SIMPLEX, a type of non- THROMBOCYTOPENIC P., a common benign recurring disorder not usually accompanied by systemic illness; characterized by bruising following trauma; seen most often on the arms, legs, and trunk. THROMBOCYTOPENIC P., any of the several forms of P. in which the platelet count is decreased; may be primary and idiopathic or secondary. THROMBOTIC THROMBOCYTOPENIC P., a disease of unknown origin characterized by thrombocytopenia, hemolytic anemia, fever, neurological signs, intermittent nasal bleeding, purpura, and thrombosis occurring in terminal arterioles and capillaries; may be secondary to known disease or idiopathic, with prolonged bleeding time in either case; occurs chiefly in children and young adults—Syn., p. hemmorrhagica.

pursed lip breathing: Prolonged slow expiration with the lips pursed as in whistling.

purulence (pū′rū-lens): The state of being purulent, or of containing pus.

purulent (pū′rū-lent): Pertinent to, caused by, resembling, containing, or producing pus; suppurative (*q.v.*). Term is often combined with the part affected, *e.g.*, purulent meningitis.

pus: A thick, opaque fluid or semifluid substance; the product of inflammation; formed in certain infections, and composed of serum, leukocytes, tissue and dead cell debris, living and dead bacteria, fibrin, and various foreign elements; varying in color, odor, and consistency with the particular causative organism.

pustulation (pus-tū-lā′shun): The formation of pustules.

pustule (pus′tūl): A small, circumscribed, superficial inflammatory elevation on the skin containing pus, *e.g.*, the lesions of acne, eczema, smallpox, chickenpox, impetigo.—pustular, adj. MALIGNANT P., cutaneous anthrax (*q.v.*).

putrefaction (pū′trē-fak′shun): The process of rotting; the destruction of organic material by bacteria.—putrefactive, adj.

putrescible (pu-tres′ib-l): Capable of undergoing putrefaction.

putrid (pū′trid): Decayed, rotten.

Putti-Platt operation: An operation to shorten the subscapularis tendon in order to limit lateral rotation; done to correct recurrent anterior dislocation of the shoulder.

PVC: Abbreviation for premature ventricular contraction.

PWP: Abbreviation for pulmonary wedge pressure.

py-, pyo-: Combining forms denoting 1) suppuration; 2) pus; 3) pus-producing infection.

pyarthrosis (pī-ar-thrō′sis): Pus or suppuration in a joint cavity.

pycn-, pycno-: See pykn-, pykno-.

pyel-, pyelo-: Combining forms denoting relationship to the pelvis of the kidney.

pyelitis (pī-e-lī′tis): Inflammation of the pelvis of the kidney. A mild form of pyelonephritis (*q.v.*) with pyuria but minimal involvement of renal tissue. P. on the right side is a common complication of pregnancy.

pyelocystitis (pī-e-lō-sis-tī′tis): Inflammation of the renal pelvis and the urinary bladder.

pyelogram (pī′e-lō-gram): An x-ray photograph of the renal pelvis and ureter. INTRAVENOUS P., a P. in which a radiopaque contrast material is given intravenously and excreted through the kidney, making possible radiographic visualization of the renal pelvis and ureter; abbreviated IVP.

pyelography (pī-e-log′raf-i): Radiographic visualization of the renal pelvis and ureter after injection of a radiopaque liquid. The liquid may be injected into the blood stream whence it is excreted by the kidney (intravenous P.) or it may be injected directly into the renal pelvis or ureter by way of a fine catheter introduced through a cystoscope. Pyelogram, n.; pyelographic, adj.

pyelolithotomy (pī′e-lō-lith-ot′-ō-mi): The operation for removal of a stone from the renal pelvis.

pyelonephritis (pī′e-lō-nē-frī′tis): An acute or chronic infection that spreads outward from the pelvis to the cortex of the kidney. The origin of the infection is usually in or below the ureter, or in the bloodstream. EMPHYSEMATOUS P., a rare, usually fatal disease in which gas produced by bacteria accumulates in the kidney; occurs most often in older people who have diabetes. Nephrectomy is the usual treatment. XANTHOGRANULOMATOUS P., a rare chronic form of P., signs and symptoms include back pain, costovertebral tenderness, fever, weight loss, enlarged kidney with fibrosis of the parenchyma, enlarged histiocytes containing fat and cholesterol, staghorn calculi, diminished or absent kidney function.

pyelonephrosis (pī′e-lō-ne-frō′sis): A pathological condition of the kidney and its pelvis.

pyeloplasty (pī′el-ō-plas-ti): A plastic operation on the kidney pelvis.

pyeloscopy (pī-e-los′ko-pi): Fluoroscopic examination of the pelvis of the kidney after introduction of radiopaque material.

pyelostomy (pī-e-los′to-mi): The operation of making an incision into the pelvis of the kidney and inserting a tube to divert the flow of urine from the ureter. The tube is connected with drainage apparatus in which the urine is collected.

pyelotomy (pī-e-lot′o-mi): An incision into the pelvis of the kidney, usually for the removal of a calculus.

pyemesis (pī-em′e-sis): The vomiting of material containing pus.

pyemia (pī-ē′mi-a): A grave form of general septicemia (*q.v.*) in which blood-borne bacteria from an acute primary focus of infection lodge and grow in distant organs, *e.g.*, brain, kidneys, lungs, or heart, and form multiple abscesses.—pyemic, adj.

pyencephalus (pī-en-sef′a-lus): A purulent effusion or an abscess within the cranium. Also pyocephalus.

pyesis (pī-ē′sis): The formation of pus; suppuration.—Syn., pyosis.

pygmalionism (pig-māl′-yon-izm): A psychopathic disorder in which the individual is in love with something he has created. [Pygmalion, a Greek king and sculptor who fell in love with an ivory figure of a young woman he had carved and which had been endowed with life by Aphrodite, the goddess of love and beauty.]

pygopagus (pi-gop′a-gus): A congenital anomaly in which conjoined twins are united at the sacral region and consequently are back to back.

pykn-, pykno-: Combining forms denoting: 1. Compact, dense, bulk. 2. Frequent.

pyknic (pik′nik): A type of body structure; the **P.** individual has a large head and chest, broad shoulders, large body cavities, generally stocky body with considerable subcutaneous fat. Often associated with a personality that is an extrovert, happy and interested in others. Cf. asthenic body type.

pyknocyte (pik′nō-sīt): A distorted erythrocyte, contracted and sometimes with spicules; small numbers are normally present in the blood of full-term infants; may also be seen in greater numbers in persons with hemolytic disorders.

pyknocytosis (pik′-nō-sī-tō′sis): Noticeable increases in the number of pyknocytes in the circulating blood. **P. INFANTILE,** a transient hemolytic anemia in the newborn; characterized by a high number of pyknocytes among the red cells; cause unknown; symptoms include jaundice, anemia, splenomegaly; usually recovery is spontaneous in a few weeks.

pyknosis (pik-nō′sis): Thickening, inspissation. Refers especially to the degenerative changes in cell nuclei whereby they shrink and condense into a mass of chromatin with no specific structure or form. Also pycnosis.

pyl-, pyle-: Combining forms denoting the portal vein.

pylephlebitis (pī′-lē-flē-bī′tis): Inflammation of the veins of the portal system, usually secondary to intra-abdominal sepsis.

pylethrombosis (pī′-lē-throm-bō′sis): Intravascular blood clot in the portal vein or any of its branches.

pylorectomy (pī′-lō-rek′tō-mi): Surgical removal of the pyloric end of the stomach.

pyloric (pī-lor′ik): Pertaining to the pylorus. **P. ORIFICE,** the lower opening of the stomach into the duodenum. **P. STENOSIS,** see **stenosis, pyloric.**

pyloroduodenal (pī-lor′ō-dū-dē′nal): Pertaining to the pyloric sphincter and the duodenum.

pyloromyotomy (pī-lor′-ō-mī-ot′ō-mi): Incision of the longitudinal and circular muscles of the pylorus to correct congenital stenosis.

pyloroplasty (pī-lor′ō-plas-ti): A plastic operation on the pylorus, designed to widen the passage.

pylorospasm (pī-lor′ō-spazm): Spasm of the pyloric sphincter muscle or of the pyloric portion of the stomach; usually due to the presence of a duodenal ulcer, but is also frequently of emotional origin.

pylorotomy (pī-lō-rot′o-mi): An operation on the pyloric muscle; usually done to relieve pyloric stenosis.

pylorus (pī-lō′rus): The opening of the stomach into the duodenum, encircled by a sphincter muscle.—pyloric, adj.

pyochezia (pī-ō-kē′zi-a): The presence of pus in the feces. Also pyofecia.

pyocolpocele (pī-ō-kol′pō-sēl): An accumulation of pus in the vagina or a vaginal tumor containing pus.

pyocolpos (pī-ō-kōl′pōs): Accumulation of pus in the vagina.

pyocyanin (pī′ō-sī′a-nin): An antibiotic substance that forms blue crystals; produced by a Pseudomonas organism and used in medicine for its action against many bacteria and fungi.—pyocyanic, adj.

pyoderma (pī-ō-der′ma): Any inflammatory disease of the skin that is marked by formation of pus-containing lesions, *e.g.*, impetigo contagiosa, ecthyma. Also called pyodermia. **P. GANGRENOSUM,** a form of **P.** occurring chiefly on the trunk and associated with ulcerative colitis and other wasting disease. **STREPTOCOCCAL P.,** usually occurs in children of school age; spread by person-to-person contact and insect vectors, sometimes by contaminated food.

pyogen (pī′ō-jen): An agent that causes the formation of pus.—pyogenic, pyogenous, adj.; pyogenesis, n.

pyogenic (pī-ō-jen′ik): 1. Pertaining to or characterized by the formation of pus. 2. Pus-forming.

pyometra (pī-ō-mē′tra): Pus retained in the uterus and unable to escape through the cervix; may be due to malignancy or atresia.—pyometric, adj.

pyometritis (pī′ō-mē-trī′tis): Purulent inflammation of the musculature of the uterus.

pyonephritis (pī-ō-nē-frī′tis): Suppurative inflammation of the kidney.

pyonephrolithiasis (pī′ō-nef-rō-lith-ī′a-sis): A condition in which pus and stones are present in the kidney.

pyonephrosis (pī′ō-ne-frō′sis): Distension of the pelvis of the kidney with pus; there is suppurative destruction of the functional structures of the kidney with severe loss of renal function.—pyonephrotic, adj.

pyopericarditis (pī′ō-per-i-kar-dī′tis): Pericarditis with purulent effusion.

pyoperitonitis (pī′ō-per-i-to-nī′tis): Inflammation of the peritoneum, with suppuration.

pyopneumothorax (pī′ō-nū-mō-thō′raks): Pus and gas or air within the pleural sac.

pyopoiesis (pī′ō-poy-ē′sis): Formation of pus.

pyoptysis (pī-op′ti-sis): The spitting of material containing pus.

pyorrhea (pī-or-rē′a): A flow of pus. **P. ALVEOLARIS**, an inflammatory condition involving the gums and the periodontal membrane, often with a discharge of pus from the alveoli; the breath has a foul odor and the teeth often become loose.

pyosalpingitis (pī′ō-sal-pin-jī′tis): Suppurative inflammation of a fallopian tube.

pyosalpinx (pi-ō-sal′pinks): A fallopian tube containing pus.

pyosis (pī-ō′sis): Pus formation. Also pyesis.

pyothorax (pī′ō-thō′raks): Pus in the pleural cavity; empyema (*q.v.*).

pyr-, pyro-: Combining forms denoting 1) fire, heat; 2) fever production.

pyramid (pir′a-mid): Descriptive of anatomical structures that are shaped like a wide-based, pointed cone. **PETROUS P.**, the pyramid-like part of the temporal bone that contains the inner ear structures. **RENAL P.**, one of the cone-shaped structures in the medulla of the kidney; contains the collecting tubules.

pyramidal (pi-ram′id-al): Applied to some conical-shaped eminences in the body. **P. CELLS**, nerve cells in the pre-rolandic area of the cerebral cortex, from which originate impulses to voluntary muscles. **P. TRACTS** in the brain and spinal cord, transmit the fibers arising from the **P.** cells.

pyrectic (pī-rek′tik): 1. An agent that induces fever. 2. Pertaining to fever. 3. Feverish; febrile. Also pyretic.

pyretherapy (pī′re-ther′a-pi): Treatment of disease by artificially inducing fever; may involve the use of diathermy or the injection of malarial organisms. Also called fever therapy, pyrotherapy, pyretotherapy. See **malariotherapy**.

Pyrex (pī′reks): Trade name for a kind of glass that is extremely resistant to heat, chemicals and electricity; much used in laboratories.

pyrexia (pī-rek′si-a): Fever; elevation of the body temperature above normal. **P. OF UNDETERMINED ORIGIN**, a term often used in reference to a fever that occurs before the diagnosis of the condition causing it has been determined; abbreviated PUO. Also often referred to as fever of undetermined origin; see under **fever**.

pyridoxine (pir-i-dok′sin): A water-soluble member of the vitamin B complex; may be connected with the utilization of unsaturated fatty acids and the conversion of tryptophan to niacin. Found in wheat germ, cereal grains, fish liver, meat (especially organ meats), blackstrap molasses; an ordinary diet provides an adequate amount. Deficiency may result in symptoms of nervousness and convulsions (in infants), dermatitis, neuritis, anorexia, nausea, vomiting. Also called vitamin B_6.

pyrimidine (pī-rim′id-in): An organic compound that is the source of several nitrogen compounds found in nucleic acid and in some barbiturates.

pyrogen (pī′rō-jen): A substance capable of producing pyrexia (*q.v.*). **DISTILLED WATER P.**, a substance of unknown nature, found sometimes in distilled water; it causes a rise in the patient's temperature when used in solutions that are injected into the body.—pyrogenic, adj.

pyrolysis (pī-rol′i-sis): Decomposition of an organic substance by the application of heat.

pyromania (pī-rō-mā′ni-a): Excessive preoccupation with fires; compulsive desire to set fires; in psychoanalysis, thought to be due to a desire to obtain erotic gratification.—pyromaniac, n.

pyrosis (pī-ro′sis): Heartburn; water-brash. The eructation of dilute acid content from the stomach into the pharynx or mouth, accompanied by a bitter, burning sensation.

pyruvate (pi-rū′vāt): A salt or ester of pyruvic acid.

pyruvic acid (pī-rū′vik): An important intermediate compound produced during carbohydrate metabolism and dependent upon an adequate supply of thiamin(e) for its proper oxidation.

pyuria (pī-ū′ri-a): Pus in the urine (more than 3 leukocytes per high-power field).—pyuric, adj.

Q

Q: 1. Abbreviation for a) quadrant, b) quality. 2. Symbol for coulomb, the quantity of electricity transferred by one ampere in one second.

q: Abbreviation for *quaque* [L.], meaning every.

Q fever: A mild rickettsial infection somewhat like Rocky Mountain spotted fever, characterized by fever, chills, muscle pain; transmitted by raw milk, contact with infected animals, or by ticks which serve as vectors. The name is derived from the fact that the disease was first desribed in Queensland, Australia.

Q law: The principle that, as temperature decreases chemical activity also decreases, has been utilized in the form of treatment with cold to reduce acid secretion in patients with hemorrhaging gastric ulcer.

Q wave: The first deflection in the QRS complex; if it goes below the baseline it is considered a criterion for the diagnosis of myocardial infarction.

q.d.: Abbreviation for *quaque die* [L.], meaning every day.

q.h.; q.2h.; q.3h., etc.: Abbrevations for *quaque hora* [L.], meaning every hour, every two hours, every three hours, etc.

q.i.d.: Abbreviation for *quater in die* [L.] meaning four times a day.

q.l.: Abbreviation for *quantum libet* [L.], meaning as much as desired.

q.m.: Abbreviation for *quaque matin* [L.], meaning every morning.

q.n.: Abbreviation for *quaque nox* [L.], meaning every night.

q.n.s.: Abbreviation for quantity not sufficient.

q.p.: Abbreviation for *quantum placeat* [L.], meaning as much as you please.

q.q.h.: Abbreviation for *quaque quarta hora* [L.], meaning every four hours.

QRS complex: In the electrocardiogram, represents transmission of a group of waves created by the passage of the cardiac impulse through the ventricles, the R wave being the most prominent. Its width, along with the P-R interval, is important in interpreting cardiac rhythm. It represents depolarization of the ventricles.

q.s.: Abbreviation for 1) *Quantum satis* [L.], meaning as is needed, or 2) *quantum sufficit* [L.], meaning a sufficient quantity. Used in prescription writing.

q-sort: A personality assessment technique in which a person sorts cards carrying representations of certain objects according to his or her interpretation of their meaning.

qt.: Abbreviation for quart.

q.t.h.: Abbreviation for *quaque tertia hora,* [L.], meaning every three hours.

quack (kwak): One who fraudulently represents oneself as having medical skill and knowledge; a medical charlatan; a fraud.

quackery (kwak′er-i): The pretensions and methods employed by a quack (*q.v.*). Charlatanism.

quadr-, quadri-, quadro-: Combining forms denoting four, fourth.

quadrangular (kwah-drang′ū-lar): Having four sides or four angles.

quadrant (kwah′drant): A quarter of a circle. In anatomy, an area that is roughly circular and may be divided into quandrants for descriptive purposes, *e.g.,* the surface of the abdomen.

quadrantanopsia (kwah′drant-an-op′si-a): Loss of vision in approximately one-fourth of the field of vision. Also quadrantanopia.

quadrate (kwah′drat): Square; having four equal sides.

quadratus (kwah-drā′tus): Square. In anatomy, descriptive of skeletal muscles that are more or less four-sided, *e.g.,* the quadratus lumborum, which forms part of the posterior wall of the abdomen.

quadri-: Combining form meaning four.

quadribasic (kwah′dri-bā′sik): Pertaining to an acid that has four replaceable hydrogen atoms.

quadriceps (kwah′dri-seps): Having four heads; denoting the great extensor muscle of the front of the thigh, which has four heads; the quadriceps femoris.

quadricuspid (kwah′dri-kus′pid): Having four cusps; said of 1) a tooth or 2) a semilunar valve (aortic or pulmonary) having four cusps.

quadridigitate (kwah′dri-dij′i-tāt): Having only four fingers or four toes on a hand or foot; tetradactyl.

quadrigeminal (kwah′dri-jem′i-nal): In four parts or forming a group of four. **Q. BODIES,** four small prominences in the midbrain; they are concerned with sight and hearing reflexes; the pineal body lies between the two upper ones. **Q. PULSE,** one in which there is a pause after every four beats. **Q. RHYTHM,** see quadrigeminy.

quadrigeminum (kwah-dri-jem′-i-num): Quadruplet.

quadrigeminy (kwah′dri-jem′i-ni): A cardiac dysrhythmia characterized by heart beats occurring in groups of four, usually a sinus beat followed by three extrasystoles.

quadrilateral (kwah'dri-lat'er-al): 1. Having four sides. 2. A four-sided figure.

quadrilocular (kwah'dri-lok'u-lar): Having four chambers, cavities, or cells.

quadripara (kwah-drip'a-ra): A woman who has had four full term pregnancies.—quadriparous, adj.

quadriparesis (kwah'dri-par'e-sis): Weakness of all four limbs.

quadripartite (kwah'dri-par'tīt): Divided into four parts or having four divisions.

quadriplegia (kwah'dri-plē-ji-a): Paralysis of both arms and both legs.

quadriplegic (kwah'dri-plē'jik): 1. Pertaining to quadriplegia. 2. A person with quadriplegia.

quadrisect (kwah'dri-sekt): To divide into four parts. Also quartisect.—quadrisection, n.

quadritubercular (kwah'dri-tū-ber'kū-lar): Having four tubercles. In dentistry, refers to a molar with four cusps.

quadrivalent (kwah'dri-va'lent): Having a valence of 4.

quadroon (kwah-droon'): The offspring of one white parent and one mulatto parent.

quadruple vaccine: A vaccine to immunize against diphtheria, pertussis, poliomyelitis, and tetanus.

quadruplet (kwah'drū-plet): One of four children born at a single birth.

quale (kwā'lē): The quality of a thing, sensation in particular.

qualitative (kwah'li-tā'tiv): Pertaining to the quality of a thing or substance. **Q. ANALYSIS,** laboratory analysis of a material or compound to determine what kind of substance(s) it is composed of; see also quantitative.

quality (kwah'li-ti): 1. A characteristic, distinguishing property or attribute. 2. A characteristic that denotes excellence, superiority, fineness.

quality assurance: In nursing, involves 1) setting standards for excellent nursing care; 2) taking steps for the achievement of excellent care; 3) utilizing peer review or audit to evaluate the quality of care given both in the past and currently; and 4) taking action to correct deficiencies in care as revealed by the evaluation. The Quality Assurance Program of 1972 (Public Law 92-603), provided for the creation of review organizations to monitor and evaluate health care services to clients receiving care through government-funded programs such as Medicare and Medicaid.

quantitative (kwahn'ti-tā-tiv): Pertaining to amount, degree, or portion. **Q. ANALYSIS,** laboratory analysis of a material or compound to determine how much of a certain kind(s) of substance it contains. See also qualitative.

quantum (kwahn'tum): 1. A definite amount. 2. A unit of radiant energy.

Quant's sign: A T-shaped depression in the occipital bone; often seen in individuals with rickets.

quarantine (kwahr'an-tēn): 1. To detain or isolate a person who has been exposed to a communicable disease for a period of time equal to the longest incubation period. 2. To restrict persons from an area or premises where a case of communicable disease exists. 3. To detain a ship coming from an infected port or carrying passengers who are suspected of having or of having been exposed to a communicable disease, (originally for 40 days). 4. A place where persons under quarantine are kept, *e.g.*, an isolation hospital or ward. 5. To detain or isolate a carrier.

quart: A unit of capacity. Liquid quart is equal to one-fourth of a gallon; 0.9463 of a liter. Dry quart is slightly larger than a liquid quart.

quartan (kwahr'tan): Recurring every fourth day, reckoning inclusively. Malaria in which the paroxysms occur every 72 hours.

quartipara (kwahr-tip'a-ra): Quadripara (*q.v.*).

quasi (kwah'si): Having some resemblance to a given thing; seemingly; in some sense or degree. Often joined by a hyphen to another word element naming the thing or condition that is resembled.

quassation (kwah-sā'shun): In pharmacology, refers to beating or breaking up of crude drug materials, such as leaves or bark of a tree, in the preparation of medicinal substances.

quassia (kwah'shi-a): A substance obtained from the bitterwood tree of Latin America; formerly much used as a bitter tonic and as an enema in the treatment for threadworms.

quaternary (kwah'ter-ner-i): 1. Denoting a chemical compound containing four elements. 2. The fourth in a series. 3. Pertaining to a compound in which four hydrogen atoms have been replaced by organic radicals; many medicinals are quaternary compounds.

Queckenstedt's test: Normally, compression of the veins in the neck, on either or both sides, will result in a rapid rise in the pressure of the cerebrospinal fluid and the quick disappearance of the increase when the pressure is removed. When this maneuver produces little or no change in the pressure, the test is said to be positive for blockage in the spinal canal.

Queen Anne's sign: Loss of the outer portions of the eyebrows; often a sign of myxedema in older persons.

Queensland: **Q. COASTAL FEVER,** tsutsugamushi disease (*q.v.*). **Q. TYPHUS FEVER,** a fever occurring in Queensland Australia where it is transmitted by marsupials and wild rodents; resembles Rocky Mountain spotted fever.

quellung (kwel'lung): Swelling. **Q. REACTION,** swelling of the capsule of a bacterium when it comes into contact with its antigen.

querulent (kwer'ū-lent): Refers to an individual who is always suspicious, complaining, dissatisfied, and in opposition to suggestions of others; characteristic of the paranoid personality.

Quervain's disease: Tenosynovitis due to inflammation of the tendons of the thumb muscles, characterized by swelling, tenderness, and pain.

Queyrat's erythroplasia (ka-rahz' -ē-rith-rō-plā'zi-a): A squamous-cell, precarcinomatous, circumscribed, erythematous lesion, velvety and papular in nature, occurring at the mucocutaneous junctions of the mouth, glans penis, or prepuce, and leading to ulceration and scaling.

Quémi's operation: A thoracoplastic operation for treatment of empyema.

quick: 1. Rapid. 2. Alive. 3. The stage of pregnancy when movements of the fetus can be felt. 4. The eponychium (*q.v.*).

quickening: The first movements of the fetus that are perceptible to the mother; usually occurring at 16 to 18 weeks gestation.

quicklime: Calcium oxide; unslacked lime. Formerly much used as a deordorant and mild disinfectant, particularly for excreta.

quicksilver: Mercury (*q.v.*).

quiescent (kwī-es'ent): Arrested; not active; causing no symptoms. Said especially of a skin disease which is settling under treatment.

quiet: **Q. DELIRIUM**, delirium marked by quiet incoherent mumblings and the absence of uncontrolled psychomotor activity. **Q. NECROSIS**, aseptic necrosis; see under necrosis.

Quincke: **Q.'S DISEASE**, angioneurotic edema (*q.v.*). **Q.'S MENINGITIS**, acute aseptic m., see aseptic m. under meningitis. **Q.'S PULSE**, see under pulse. [Heinrich Quincke, German physician. 1842–1922.]

quinidine (kwin'i-dēn): One of the alkaloids obtained from cinchona bark; an antimalarial; also used in treating arrhythmias.

quinine (kwī'nīn): The chief alkaloid of cinchona, once the standard treatment for malaria. Now largely replaced by more modern drugs.

quininism (kwī'ni-nizm): A condition caused by an idiosyncratic reaction to, or long-continued use of, quinine or cinchona; symptoms include headache, noises in the ears and partial deafness, disturbed vision, and nausea.

quininoderma (kwin-i-nō-der'ma): Dermatitis following ingestion of quinine.

Quinlan's test: A spectroscopic test for the presence of bile.

quinquagenarian (kwin'kwa-jen-ar'i-an): An individual in his fifties.

quinquecuspid (kwin-kwē-kus'pid): A tooth with five cusps.

quinquetubercular (kwin' -kwē-tū-ber'kū-lar): Having five tubercles or cusps.

quinquevalent (kwin' -kwē-vā'lent): Having a valence of 5; pentavalent.

quinsy (kwin'zi): Acute inflammation of the tonsil and surrounding loose tissue, with abscess formation. Peritonsillar abscess.

quint-, quinti-: Combining forms denoting five, fifth.

quintan (kwin'tan): Recurring every fifth day.

quintessence (kwin-tes'ens): The highly concentrated essence of any subtance.

quintipara (kwin-tip'a-ra): A woman who has had five full term pregnancies.—quintiparous, adj.

quintiparity (kwin-ti-par'i-ti): The state of being a quintipara.

quintuplet (kwin'tup-let): One of five children born at a single birth.

quotidian (kwō-tid'i-an): Recurring daily. A form of malaria in which paroxysms recur daily. **DOUBLE Q.**, recurring twice daily.

quotient (kwō'shent): A number obtained by division. **ACHIEVEMENT Q.**, a percentage statement of the amount a child has learned in relation to his inherent intellectual ability. **INTELLIGENCE Q.**, the estimate of intelligence; obtained by dividing the mental age, as determined by standard tests, by the chronological age, and multiplying the result by 100. Expressed as IQ. **RESPIRATORY Q.**, the ratio between the CO_2 expired and the O_2 inspired during a specified time.

q.v.: Abbreviation for *quod vide* [L.], meaning which see, or *quantum vis* [L.], meaning as much as you wish.

R

R: Abbreviation for: 1. Right. 2. Rectal. 3. Respiration. 4. Roentgen.

R wave: In the ECG, an upward deflection following the Q wave.

Ra: Chemical symbol for radium.

rabbeting (rab′et-ing): The fitting together of the jagged ends of a fractured bone.

rabbit fever: Tularemia (*q.v.*).

rabic (rā′bik): Pertaining to rabies.

rabicidal (rā-bi-sī′dal): Destructive to the virus that causes rabies.

rabid (rab′id): 1. Pertaining to rabies. 2. Affected with rabies. 3. Extremely violent, furious.

rabies (rā′bēz): An acute, highly fatal, infectious disease of warmblooded animals, especially the dog, cat, wolf, fox; caused by a filterable virus; attacks chiefly the nervous system; fatal if untreated. May be transmitted to man through the infected saliva of a rabid animal, usually through a bite, primarily dogbite. Characterized by the formation of Negri bodies (*q.v.*) in the brain, central nervous system excitement, wild madness, paralysis, and often, death. Sny., hydrophobia.—rabid, rabic, adj.

rabiform (rā′bi-form): Resembling rabies.

racemose (ras′e-mōs): Resembling a bunch of grapes, as a gland that is divided and subdivided, *e.g.*, a salivary gland.

rachi-, rachio-: Combining forms denoting relationship to the spine.

rachial (rā′ki-al): Pertaining to the vertebral column. Spinal.

rachialgia (rā-ki-al′ji-a): Pain in the spine.

rachianesthesia (rā′ki-an-es-thē′zi-a): Spinal anesthesia; see under anesthesia.

rachicele (rā′ki-sēl): Protrusion of spinal canal contents to the exterior, as in spina bifida (*q.v.*).

rachicentesis (rā′ki-sen-tē′sis): Spinal puncture for the aspiration of fluid. Rachiocentesis.

rachidial (rā-kid′i-al): Spinal.

rachigraph (rā′ki-graf): An instrument for recording the curves of the spine.

rachilysis (rā-kil′i-sis): Forcible mechanical correction of a lateral curvature of the spine by pressure against the convexity of the curve, combined with traction.

rachiocampsis (rā-ki-ō-camp′sis): Curvature of the spine.

rachiochysis (rā-ki-ok′i-sis): The accumulation of fluid in the subarachnoid space of the spinal canal.

rachiodynia (rā′ki-ō-din′i-a): A painful condition of the spinal column.

rachiometer (rā-ki-om′e-ter): An apparatus for measuring curvatures in the spinal column.

rachiomyelitis (rā′ki-ō-mī-e-lī′tis): Inflammation of the spinal cord.

rachiopathy (rā-ki-op′a-thi): Any disease of the spine. Spondylopathy.

rachioplegia (rā-ki-ō-plē′ji-a): Paralysis of the spine.

rachioscoliosis (rā′ki-ō-skō-li-ō′sis): Lateral curvature of the spine.

rachiotomy (rā-ki-ot′o-mi): An incision into the spinal column or into a vertebra. See also laminectomy.

rachis (rā′kis): The spinal column.

rachischisis (ra-kis′ki-sis): A congenital fissure in the spinal column. Spina bifida (*q.v.*).

rachitic (ra-kit′ik): Pertaining to or affected with rickets. **R. ROSARY OR BEADS,** a row of bead-like nodules that form on the ribs at their junctions with the cartilage, sometimes seen in children with rickets.

rachitis (ra-kī′tis): 1. Rickets (*q.v.*). 2. An inflammatory condition of the spine.

rachitogenic (ra-kit-ō-jen′ik): Producing rickets.

raclage (ra-klazh′): 1. Removal of soft tissue or growth by rubbing or scraping. 2. Curettage.

rad: The standard unit of absorbed radiation dose; replaces the term roentgen as the unit of dosage. It is a measure of the x-ray energy absorbed per gram of tissue.

radectomy (rā-dek′to-mi): Surgical removal of all or part of the root of a tooth.

radiad (rā′di-ad): Toward the radius or the radial side.

radial (rā′di-al): In anatomy, pertaining to the radius. **R. ARTERY,** the artery at the thumb side of the wrist. **R. NERVE,** arises in the cervical plexus, runs around the back of the humerus and down the outer side of the forearm; supplies the extensor muscles of the elbow, wrist, and hand. **R. PULSE,** the pulse felt by placing the fingers over the radial artery at the wrist.

radiant (rā′di-ant): Emitting rays or beams of light. **R. ENERGY, ENERGY** that is transmitted in the form of waves, including radiowaves, infrared and ultraviolet rays, visible light, x- and gamma rays.

radiate (rā′di-āte): 1. To spread from a common point or center. 2. To emit radiation.

radiation (rā′di-ā′shun): 1. Divergence in all directions from a common center. 2. In anatomy, a structure made up of divergent elements, particularly a group of nerve fibers which diverge from a common origin. 3. A general term for any form of radiant energy such as that emitted from a luminous body, x-ray tube or radioactive substance such as radium. **R. RECALL,** a condition that occurs several weeks after the simultaneous administration of radiation and chemotherapy; presents as an erythema, with vesicle formation or desquamation and often followed by permanent pigmentation of the skin. **R. SICKNESS,** that which follows the therapeutic use of radioactive substances or x-rays; symptoms include nausea, vomiting, anorexia, headache. The term is now also used in reference to illness resulting from fallout from atomic bombs. **R. THERAPY,** the therapeutic use of roentgen rays, radium, cobalt, or other similar agent.

radical (rad′i-kal): 1. In chemistry, a substance that, when dissolved in water, will dissociate into elements or groups of elements that will each carry a positive or negative charge. 2. A group of atoms that act as a single atom in chemical processes, *e.g.*, the sulfate radical, SO_4. 3. Pertaining to or going to the root of a thing; in medicine, going to the root of a disease process. 4. The smallest branch of a vessel or nerve; a rootlet. **R. OPERATION,** see surgery, radical.

radiculalgia (ra-dik′ū-lal′ji-a): Neuralgia of the sensory root, or roots, of a spinal nerve or nerves; caused by irritation.

radiculectomy (ra-dik′ū-lek′to-mi): Excision of the root of a spinal nerve.

radiculitis (ra-dik-ū-lī′tis): Inflammation of the root of a nerve, particularly a spinal nerve.

radiculography (ra-dik′ū-log′ra-fi): Radiographic examination of the cauda equina and lumbar nerve roots of the spinal cord after injection of a water-soluble radiopaque medium.

radiculomeningomyelitis (ra-dik′ū-lō-me-nin′gō-mī-e-lī′tis): Inflammation of the spinal nerve roots, the meninges, and the spinal cord.

radiculomyelopathy (ra-dik′ū-lō-mī-e-lop′a-thi): Any disease of the nerve roots and spinal cord.

radiculoneuropathy (ra-dik′ū-lō-nū-rop′a-thi): Any disease of the spinal nerve roots and spinal nerves.

radiculopathy (ra-dik′ū-lop′a-thi): Any disease of the spinal nerve roots.

radio-: Combining form denoting: 1. Radiation; radiant energy. 2. The radius. 3. Radium.

radioactive (rā′di-ō-ak′tiv): Pertaining to a substance that gives off penetrating rays due to the spontaneous breaking up of its atoms. **R. DECAY,** the decrease, over time, in the number of radioactive atoms in a radioactive substance. **R. FALLOUT,** a mixture of debris and radioactive particles that fall to earth following a nuclear explosion. **R. GOLD,** see radiogold. **R. IODINE,** see under iodine. **R. ISOTOPES,** substances made up of atoms in which the nuclei have more neutrons than protons; in certain substances the excess of neutrons creates too much energy and the atom proceeds to lose this energy in the form of radiation as alpha, beta, and gamma rays. Artificial isotopes can be made by bombarding stable elements with neutrons in a nuclear reactor. **R. MERCURY,** used in investigation of brain lesions. **R. TECHNETIUM,** used for investigation of visceral lesions. **R. TRACER,** a labeled element that emits radiation and so can be traced throughout a chemical, biological, or physical process.

radioactivity (rā′di-ō-ak-tiv′i-ti): The quality or property of emitting radiant energy; possessed naturally by certain elements such as radium and uranium; certain other elements become radioactive after bombardment with neutrons or other particles. The three major forms of radioactivity are designated as alpha, beta, and gamma.

radioautography (rā′di-ō-aw-tog′ra-fi): A form of photography that reveals the location and distribution of radioactive elements in a test material.

radiobicipital (rā′di-ō-bī-sip′i-tal): Pertaining to the radius and the biceps muscle of the arm.

radiobiology (rā′di-ō-bī-ol′ō-ji): The study of the effects of ionizing radiation on living tissue.—radiobiological, adj.; radiobiologically, adv.

radiocalcium (rā′di-ō-kal′si-um): A radioactive isotope of calcium; used chiefly in studies of calcium metabolism.

radiocarbon (rā′di-ō-kar′bon): A radioactive form of the element carbon used for research into metabolism, for diagnostic procedures, etc.

radiocarcinogenesis (rā′di-ō-kar′si-nō-jen′e-sis): Cancer caused by exposure to radiation.

radiocarpal (rā′di-ō-kar′pal): Pertaining to the radius and the carpus.

radiochemistry (rā′di-ō-kem′is-tri): The branch of chemistry that deals with radioactive substances and their properties.

radiocobalt (rā′di-ō-kō′balt): Any radioactive isotope of cobalt; medical uses include treatment of malignancies.

radiocurable (rā′di-ō-kūr′a-b′l): Refers to a condition that may be curable by radiation therapy.

radiode (rā′di-ōd): A metal container for a radioactive substance used in radiotherapy.

radiodermatitis (rā′di-ō-der-ma-tī′tis): Reddening and irritation of the skin due to overexposure to x-rays or radium.

radiodiagnosis (rā′di-ō-dī-ag-nō′sis): Diagnosis made by use of x ray pictures.

radiodigital (rā′di-ō-dij′i-tal): Pertaining to the radius and the fingers on the radial side of the arm.

radiodontia (rā'di-ō-don'shi-a): Roentgenology of the teeth and associated structures.

radioelectrocardiology (rā'di-ō-ē-lek'trō-kar-di-ol'ō-ji): A technique in electrocardiology whereby the heart impulses of a patient who is engaged in the normal activities of daily living are beamed by radio waves to a receiver placed at a distance from the patient.

radioencephalography (rā'di-ō-en-sef-a-log'ra-fi): Recording of changes in the electrical potential of the brain by radio waves beamed from the patient directly to the recording apparatus.

radioepidermitis (rā'di-ō-ep'i-der-mī'tis): Destructive changes in the skin resulting from overexposure to radiation.

radioepithelitis (rā'di-ō-ep'i-thē-lī'tis): Disintegration and destruction of epithelium caused by exposure to irradiation.

radiogenic (rā'di-ō-jen'ik): Produced by radiation.

radiogold (rā'di-ō-gōld'): A radioactive isotope of gold; has diagnostic and therapeutic uses.

radiogram (rā'di-ō-gram): An image produced on a radiosensitive surface by radiation, particularly by x-rays, or by photographing an image made by a radiopaque substance.

radiography (rā-di-og'ra-fi): The making of a photograph or a record by the action of certain rays on a sensitized surface such as a film; roentgenography. **CONTRAST R.**, a technique involving injection of a radiopaque fluid into a cavity or tissue space before x-ray films are made; utilized in venography, arteriography, arthrography, and myelography. **DIAGNOSTIC R.**, is concerned with obtaining roentgenographic information useful in making diagnoses. **THERAPEUTIC R.**, treatment by radiation from x-rays, radium, or radioisotopes.

radiohumeral (rā'di-ō-hū'mer-al): Pertaining to the radius and the humerus.

radioimmunity (rā'di-ō-im-mū'ni-ti): Reduction of sensitivity to radiation which may be produced by repeated irradiation.

radioimmunoassay (rā'di-ō-im-mu-nō-as'ā): A sensitive investigative procedure utilizing a radioactive material and blood plasma to determine the presence and concentration of the particular hormone or other natural substance under study. Useful in diagnosis and treatment of diabetes, thyroid disease, sterility, growth disorders, certain types of hepatitis, and hormone-producing cancers.

radioiodine (rā'di-ō-ī'ō-dēn): A radioactive isotope of iodine, I^{130} and I^{131} being most frequently used in medicine for diagnosis and treatment of disorders of the thyroid gland. **R. UPTAKE TEST**, a test in which the person is given a small dose of radioactive iodine and the radioactivity of the thyroid gland is subsequently measured. If the gland is overactive, more than 45 percent of the iodine will be taken up by the gland within four hours. If the gland is underactive, less than 20 percent will be taken up after 48 hours.

radioiron (rā' -di-ō-ī'ern): A radioactive isotope of iron; used chiefly in diagnostic studies of iron metabolism.

radioisotope (rā'di-ō-ī'sō-tōp): A radioactive isotope (*q.v.*) of an element; an element that has the same atomic number as another but a different atomic weight, and exhibits the property of spontaneous decomposition. When fed or injected can be traced with a Geiger-Muller counter. **R. SCAN**, pictorial representation of the distribution and amount of radioactive isotope present.

radiolesion (rā'di-ō-lē'zhun): A lesion produced by exposure to radiation.

radiologist (rā-di-ol'ō-jist): One skilled in the use of x-rays and other forms of radiant energy for the diagnosis and treatment of disease.

radiology (rā-di-ol'ō-ji): The science that deals with radioactive substances, particularly that branch of medicine that is concerned with the use of the sources of radiant energy in the diagnosis and treatment of disease.—radiologic, radiological, adj.

radiolucent (rā-di-ō-lū'sent): Being entirely or partially permeable to x-rays or other forms of radiant energy.—radiolucency, n.

radiometer (rā-di-om'e-ter): An instrument used for detecting and measuring radiant energy, particularly small amounts of such energy.

radiomimetic (rā'di-ō-mī-met'ik): Producing effects similar to those of radiotherapy. See cytotoxic.

radiomutation (rā'di-ō-mū-tā'shun): Changes in cells following exposure to radiation.

radion (rā'di-on): One of the radiant particles emitted by a radioactive substance.

radionecrosis (rā'di-ō-nē-krō'sis): Ulceration or destruction of tissue caused by exposure to radiant energy.

radioneuritis (rā'di-ō-nū-rī'tis): Neuritis resulting from exposure to radiant energy.

radionuclide (rā' -di-ō-nū'klīd): 1. An atom of an element that gives off electromagnetic radiation as it disintegrates. 2. A nuclide that exhibits radioactivity.

radiopaque (rā-di-ō-pāk'): Referring to a substance that does not permit the passage of x-rays or other forms of radiation. Areas or organs treated with a **R.** substance prior to taking x-ray pictures appear light or white on the film.—radiopacity, n.

radioparent (rā-di-ō-par'ent): The characteristic of being penetrable by roentgen rays.

radiopasteurization (rā'di-ō-pas'tur-ī-zā'shun): The use of ionizing radiation to preserve foods or to prolong the shelf life of certain fresh food products.

radiopathology (rā′di-ō-pa-thol′o-ji): The pathology of the effects of radioactive substances on cells and tissues.

radiopharmaceutical (rā′di-ō-far-ma-sū′ti-kal): Pertaining to 1) radiopharmacy, or 2) a radioactive chemical or substance used in diagnosis or treatment of disease.

radiopharmacy (rā′di-ō-far′ma-si): The branch of pharmacy that deals with the preparation of radioactive substances used in therapy.

radiophosphorus (rā′di-ō-fos′for-us): One of two radioactive isotopes of phosphorus; ^{32}P has diagnostic and therapeutic uses.

radioreceptor (rā′di-ō-rē-sep′tor): A receptor that is responsive to radiant energy such as heat or light.

radioresistance (rā′di-ō-rē-zis′tans): The resistance of cells or tissues to the effects of radiation, said especially of certain tumors.

radioscopy (rā-di-os′kō-pi): The examination of inner structures of the body by means of x-ray; fluoroscopy.

radiosensitivity (rā′di-ō-sen-si-tiv′i-ti): The condition of being sensitive to the effects of radiant energy; term often used to describe cells that can be destroyed by radiation.—radiosensitive, adj.

radiotelemetry (rā′di-ō-tel-em′e-tri): Transmission of data, including biological data, by means of radio; a technique developed for monitoring vital signs of astronauts while in flight and now adapted for use by hospitals for monitoring patients at a distance.

radiotherapeutics (rā′di-ō-ther-a-pū′tiks): 1. Radiotherapy. 2. The body of knowledge concerning what is known about the therapeutic use of radiation therapy.

radiotherapist (rā′di-ō-ther′a-pist): One who specializes in radiotherapy (*q.v.*).

radiotherapy (rā′di-ō-ther′a-pi): Treatment of disease by x rays, radium, radon seeds, cobalt, sunlight, or other forms of radioactive substances or radiant energy.

radiothermy (rā′di-ō-ther′mi): The use of radiant heat in therapy; short-wave diathermy.

radiotoxemia (rā′di-ō-tok-sē′mi-a): Toxemia produced by exposure to a radioactive substance.

radiotransparent (rā′di-ō-trans-par′ent): Refers to substances through which x rays can pass without hindrance.—radiotransparency, n.

radiotropic (rā′di-ō-trōp′ik): Affected or influenced by radiation.

radioulnar (rā′di-ō-ul′nar): Pertaining to both the radius and ulna, bones of the forearm.

radium (rā′di-um): A rare radioactive element found in pitchblend and other uranium minerals; discovered in 1898 by Marie Curie, a Polish scientist in Paris. Used in radiotherapy, especially in the treatment of malignancies. **R. NEEDLE,** a slender container containing **R.** that is inserted into tissue in treatment of malignant growths. **R. IMPLANTATION,** the implanting of radium in a tumor for therapeutic treatment. **R. THERAPY,** treatment by radium or radon in cancer therapy.

radius (rā′di-us): 1. The bone on the outer side of the forearm. 2. A line radiating from the center to the periphery of a circle or sphere.—radial, adj.

radon (rā′don): A radioactive gas that is an intermediary product of the disintegration of radium. It is used therapeutically for the same purposes as radium. **R. SEEDS,** capsules containing radon gas, designed to be placed where it would not be convenient to place radium or remove it after treatment; the rays lose their effect in a few days and the capsule remains harmlessly in the tissues.

Raeder's syndrome: A rare condition characterized by trigeminal neuralgia followed by sensory loss on the affected side of the face, weakness of facial muscles, miosis, and ptosis of the upper eyelid; usually due to a lesion in the trigeminal ganglion.

ragweed: A common weed the pollen of which is the most frequent cause of asthma and hay fever.

RAI: Abbreviation for radioactive iodine.

rales (ralz): Abnormal, noncontinuous, bubbling, crackling, or gurgling sounds associated with pneumonia, congestive heart failure, and long periods of recumbency; heard at the base of the lungs at inspiration when fluid is present in the small air passages and alveoli. Usually described as moist or dry, or as fine, medium, or coarse. Fine rales are high pitched, crackling, or popping; they are indicative of fluid in the smallest airways. Medium rales are of lower pitch and have a wetter sound; they are indicative of fluid in the bronchioles. Coarse rales are low pitched and loud; they indicate fluid in the bronchi and trachea.

ramify (ram′i-fī): To branch or diverge in different directions.—ramification, n.

ramisection (ram-i-sek′shun): A surgical procedure in which a ramus commmunicans (*q.v.*) of a spinal nerve and a ganglion of the sympathetic trunk are severed.

ramose (rā′mōs): Branching.

Ramsay-Hunt syndrome: See Hunt's syndrome.

Ramstedt's operation: An operation to relieve pyloric stenosis in infants by dividing the pyloric muscle, leaving the mucous lining intact.

ramulus (ram′ū-lus): A small ramus or branch.

ramus (rā'mus): 1. An elongated process of a bone. 2. A branch. Term used to describe the smaller structure formed when a larger one divides or forks; applied to bones, nerves, blood vessels. **MANDIBULAR R.**, the upturned perpendicular part of the mandible on each side.—rami, pl.

Rana: A genus of frogs. **R. PIPIENS,** a species of *Rana* formerly often used in pregnancy tests.

rancid (ran'sid): Having a rank, disagreeable smell or taste; said of fatty substances that are undergoing or have undergone decomposition.—rancidity, n.

range: The difference between the upper and lower limits of a series of values.

range of motion: Refers to the range through which a joint can move or be moved; measured in degrees of a circle. Abbreviated ROM. **ROM EXERCISES,** exercises to restore motion in a joint or to keep joints functioning normally; may be active, *i.e.,* performed by the patient himself, or passive, *i.e.,* performed by a therapist who moves the body part through the possible range.

ranine (rā'nīn): Pertaining to a ranula or to the lower surface of the tongue.

ranula (ran'ū-la): A retention cyst that forms underneath the tongue on either side of the frenum due to obstruction of the duct of a sublingual or mucous gland; contains stringy, mucoid material; surgery is usually needed.—ranular, adj.

Ranvier's nodes (ron-vē-āz'): Regularly spaced constrictions in myelinated nerve fibers; at these points the myelin sheath is absent.

rape (rāp): Unlawful sexual abuse of one person by another, usually a female by a male, and chiefly by force or deception; legally considered an act of violence. **STATUTORY R.**, sexual intercourse with a person who has not reached the age of consent, is mentally retarded, or whose consciousness has been altered by illness, drugs, or sleep.

rape trauma syndrome: A group of symptoms that sometimes develop in women who have been raped. Symptoms that develop immediately include fear, weeping, insomnia, terrifying dreams, nausea, loss of appetite, depression, suicidal behavior; those that develop during the adjustment period include fears and phobias, nightmares, refusal to socialize, complete change in lifestyle.

raphe (rā'fē): A seam, suture, ridge, or crease marking the line of fusion of two similar parts, *e.g.,* the median furrow on the dorsal surface of the tongue.

rapid eye movements (REM): Movements of the eye that occur in certain phases of the sleep cycle. **REM SLEEP,** the period of deep normal sleep when one also has dreams which are thought to be the cause of the rapid eye movements. See also NREM.

rapport (ra-pōr'): A relation characterized by harmony and accord. In psychiatry, a conscious feeling of accord, trust, confidence, and responsiveness to another, particularly the therapist, with willingness to cooperate. Cf., transference.

rapture of the deep: A psychotic experience of deep sea divers, caused by sensory deprivation and disorientation.

raptus (rap'tus): 1. A sudden violent attack; may be physical, as a hemorrhage; or psychological, as an attack of intense nervousness. 2. Rape.

rarefaction (rar-e-fak'shun): Becoming less dense or thinning, but not being reduced in volume, as occurs in some bone diseases.—rarefy, v.

rash: A localized or general temporary skin eruption, often a characteristic of certain infectious diseases. **NETTLE R.**, urticaria (*q.v.*). **SERUM R.**, one following injection of a serum, *e.g.,* antitoxin; due to hypersensitivity.

raspatory (ras'pa-tor-i): A rasp-like instrument used in bone surgery for removing rough margins or the periosteum.

raspberry mark: A congenital hemangioma (*q.v.*).

ratbite fever: A relapsing fever caused by the *Streptobacillus moniliformis* or the *Spirillum minus;* the result of a bite by an infected rat, sometimes an experimental animal. The wound often ulcerates and becomes abscessed.

ratio (rā'shi-ō): The relationship in degree or number between two things. **ALBUMIN-GLOBULIN R.**, the **R.** between the albumin and globulin in the blood serum which is normally 1.5 to 3; when lower than 1, some pathological condition is indicated.

rational (rash'un-al): 1. Of sound mind; not delirious. 2. Reasonable. 3. In medicine, treatment that is based on reason or general principles rather than empiricism. See empirical.

rational emotive therapy (RET): A form of psychotherapy in which the patient is helped and encouraged to change his attitudes, his past ways of solving problems, and his general functioning in society in order to develop a more suitable and satisfying behavior.

rationale (rash-un-al'): The underlying reason or explanation for a practice, opinion, or phenomenon.

rationalization (rash'-un-al-ī-zā'shun): A mental process whereby a person explains an emotionally activated occurrence by substituting one that is more acceptable than the truth, both to himself and to others. The substitution must be plausible enough for self-deception and self-justification. In psychiatry, a defense mechanism used by the individual to justify a threat or event or to make something unreasonable seem reasonable.

rattle: A rale or other sound heard on auscultation of the chest. **DEATH R.**, a gurgling sound heard over the trachea in the dying; may also be heard as a respiratory sound.

Rauwolfia (raw-wol'fi-a): A genus of trees and shrubs found in South America, Africa, and Asia and formerly much used in those areas as the source of a drug used as a tranquilizer, nervous system depressant, and antihypertensive. Now also used in the U.S. for the treatment of such conditions as require the use of drugs with these actions.

rave (rāv): To speak incoherently, as in delirium; irrational speech.

raw: 1. Uncooked. 2. Not pasteurized (*q.v.*), as applied to milk.

ray: 1. A beam of light or other radiant energy. 2. A stream of particles from a radioactive substance. **ALPHA RAYS**, streams of fast-moving positively charged particles emitted from a disintegrating radioactive isotope; they are actually the nuclei of atoms. **BETA RAYS**, particles emitted from radioactive isotopes as streams of electrons; their penetrating power is greater than that of alpha rays. **DIATHERMY RAYS**, produced by an oscillating electric current; used to produce heat in the deeper body tissues. **GAMMA RAYS**, electromagnetic radiation similar to x rays but of greater penetrating power. **INFRARED RAYS**, long invisible rays beyond the red end of the visible spectrum; they emanate from a surface heated to 300–800°C, penetrate the skin and are felt as heat; hence used therapeutically to produce heat in the tissues. **ROENTGEN RAYS**, see under x ray. **ULTRAVIOLET R.**, the invisible rays beyond the violet rays of the spectrum; see ultraviolet.

Raynaud: [Maurice Raynaud, French physician. 1834–1881.] **RAYNAUD'S PHENOMENON**, The occasional spasm of the digital arteries causing paleness and numbness of the fingers and toes. **RAYNAUD'S DISEASE**, idiopathic trophoneurosis, a common vasospastic disorder; characterized by bilateral paroxysmal spasm of the digital arteries producing severe hand-finger pain, numbness, tingling, and pallor of fingers or toes, or both, which become red as circulation returns; repeated attacks may result in osteoporosis of the fingers and toes, atrophy of the nails, and occasionally gangrene. Primarily a disease of young women who are under pressure; is brought on by emotion, any exposure to cold, even eating cold foods, or shock.

RBBB: Abbreviation for right bundle branch block. See bundle branch block.

RBC: Abbreviation for 1) red blood cell (s); 2) red blood cell count. Also written rbc.

RDA: Abbreviation for recommended dietary allowance. Refers to the recommended daily amounts of specific nutrients and/or vitamins and minerals required to maintain health. Lists are published by the Food and Nutrition Board of the National Academy of Science.

RDS: Abbreviation for respiratory distress syndrome (*q.v.*).

re-: Prefix denoting: 1. Again; 2. Back, backward.

Reach to Recovery: A volunteer organization sponsored by the American Cancer Society; founded in 1953. Members are women who have had mastectomies and who provide support and empathy as well as information to help post-mastectomy patients cope with emotional and physical adjustments to breast loss.

react (rē-akt'): 1. To respond to a stimulus in a particular way. 2. To undergo a chemical reaction. 3. To tend to move toward a prior condition. 4. To exert a counteracting or reciprocal influence.

reaction (rē-ak'shun): 1. Response to stimulation. 2. Result of a test to determine acidity or alkalinity of a solution; usually expressed as pH. 3. The interaction of two or more different types of molecules with the production of a new type of molecule. **ADVERSE R.**, an unpleasant or harmful physiological or psychological **R.** to a drug or treatment. **ALLERGIC R.**, (see sensitization) is a hypersensitivity to certain proteins with which the patient is brought into contact through the medium of his skin, or his digestive or respiratory tract, resulting in eczema, urticaria, hay fever, etc. Inheritance and emotion contribute to the allergic tendency. The basis of the condition is probably a local antigen-antibody **R.** **ANAPHYLACTIC R.**, **R.** that occurs following the administration of a substance to which the individual has become sensitized. **DELAYED R.**, a **R.** occurring after more than the usual reaction time. **IDIOSYNCRATIC R.**, an unexpected, unusual **R**; in pharmacotherapy, the opposite **R.** from what was expected. **IMMUNE R.**, a **R.** that indicates the presence of antibodies and probable high resistance to a specific infection. **R. TIME**, the time interval between the application of a stimulus and the response to it. **TRANSFUSION R.**, **R.** that occurs following transfusion of incompatible blood.

reactive (rē-ak' -tiv): 1. Readily responsive to a stimulus. 2. Occurring as a result of stress of emotional upset. **R. DEPRESSION**, an emotional state characterized by a strong feeling of sadness and depression of spirit, usually occurring following an external incident or emotional situation, and is relieved when the incident or situation is removed or understood.

reactivity (rē-ak-tiv'i-ti): The property of reacting or the state of being reactive.

reactor (rē-ak'tor): In medicine, refers to a person who reacts positively to a foreign substance, particularly one who is sensitive to tuberculin (*q.v.*). In physics, an apparatus that houses a device that can initiate and control nuclear fission chain reaction to generate heat or produce radiation.

Read method: A method of preparing for childbirth introduced by Dr. Grantly Dick-Read. The woman learns exercises that foster relaxation and conditioning of the muscles, and slow diaphragmatic breathing; the emphasis is on fearlessness.

reagent (rē-ā'jent): An agent capable of producing a chemical change; when added to a complex solution it may determine the presence or absence of certain substances.

reagin (rē-ā'jin): An antibody associated with allergic reactions; present in the serum of hypersensitive people. It is responsible for the liberation of histamines and other substances that cause symptoms of hay fever and asthma.—reaginic, adj.

reality: The aggregate of all things that have an objective existence; not imaginary, fictitious, or pretended. **R. PRINCIPLE,** in psychoanalytic theory, the awareness that the gratification of instinctual wishes is modified by the inescapable external demands of the physical environment in a way that meets these demands but also allows for gratification at a more appropriate time. **REALITY ORIENTATION,** the performance of measures to increase one's awareness of time, place, and person. **REALITY TESTING,** a function of the ego in which certain actions are explored and their outcomes analyzed so that when the stimulus to act in a given fashion occurs, the individual will know what outcome to expect.

reality shock: In nursing, the phenomenon experienced by newly or recently graduated nurses when they discover that their education and experiential background has not adequately prepared them for coping with the requirements of the work situation or to function at a level that is satisfactory to themselves, to their fellow-workers, or to nursing service directors.

reamer (rē'mer): A surgical instrument designed for gouging out holes or enlarging them; used mostly in bone surgery. One type is designed for use by dentists in root canal treatment.

rebore (rē-bor'): Boring out or recanalizing. See disobliteration.

rebound phenomenon: The reaction that occurs when a limb that is being subjected to resistance moves in the intended direction and then, when the resistance is removed, rebounds in the opposite direction; spastic limbs respond with exaggerated rebound, whereas in patients with cerebellar disturbances, no rebound occurs.

rebreathing bag: A bag attached to a mask and which is used to pump air or an anesthetic gas into the patient's lung when needed; it serves as an accessory source of anesthetic gases during an operation.

recalcitrant (rē-kal'si-trant): Refractory. Describes medical conditions that are resistant to treatment.

recall (rē-kawl'): The process of bringing a past mental image or event into consciousness; to remember. **R.** is one phase of memory, the other two being memorization and retention.

recanalization (rē'kan-a-lī-zā'shun): Reestablishment of patency of 1) a blood vessel, or 2) a bodily tube, *e.g.* the vas deferens.

recapitulation theory: The theory that an embryo goes through the same stages in its development that the species did in developing from lower to higher forms of life.

receptaculum (rē'sep-tak'ū-lum): Receptacle, often acting as a reservoir. **R. CHYLI,** the pear-shaped sac at the lower end of the thoracic duct, in front of the first lumbar vertebra. It receives the digested fat from the intestine.

receptor (rē-sep'tor): Sensory afferent nerve ending capable of receiving and transmitting stimuli. **ALPHA** and **BETA RECEPTORS,** are located on cell surfaces throughout the body; they react to stimulation by acetylcholine, norepinephrine, and epinephrine, **ALPHA-1 RECEPTORS,** when stimulated, cause peripheral vasoconstriction **ALPHA-2 RECEPTORS** respond to stimulation by inhibiting release of norepinephrine at the neuron terminal. **ALPHA-ADRENERGIC RECEPTOR,** any of the adrenergic parts of the receptor of a stimulus that react to certain chemical substances, epinephrine in particular, by causing constriction of peripheral vessels of the skin, mucosa, intestine, and kidney, and contraction of the pupil and pilomotor muscles; the opposite of beta-adrenergic receptor; also called alpha receptor. **BETA-1 RECEPTORS,** when stimulated, cause an increase in heart rate, and heart contractility, and facilitate atrioventricular conduction. **BETA-2 RECEPTORS,** when stimulated, cause relaxation of smooth muscle which results in peripheral and coronary vasodilatation.

recess (rē'ses): A small empty space, depression, or cavity.

recession (rē-sesh'un): The gradual withdrawal of a part or a structure from its normal position.

recessive (rē-ses'iv): Receding; having a tendency to disappear. **R. GENE,** one of a gene pair that determines the character trait in an individual only if the other member of the pair is also recessive. **R. TRAIT,** an inherited characteristic that remains latent when paired with a dominant trait in selective mating. See Mendel's law. Opp. to dominant.

recidivation (rē-sid-i-vā'shun): Relapse of a disease or recurrence of a symptom; or the repetition of a crime or offense; or a tendency to relapse into a previous condition, or; more particularly, the recurrence of an undesirable behavior pattern.

recidivist (rē-sid'i-vist): A person who is inclined toward recidivation.

recipe (res'i-pi): 1. A prescription. 2. A word at the head of a written prescription meaning *take;* usually represented by R_X.

recipient (rē-sip'i-ent): In medicine, one who receives; usually refers to the person who receives blood in a transfusion. **UNIVERSAL R.**, one who can receive any type of blood in a transfusion without harmful effects.

Recklinghausen's disease (rek-ling-howz'enz): Name given to two conditions: 1) osteitis fibrosa cystica—the result of overactivity of the parathyroid glands (hyperparathyroidism), resulting in decalcification of bones and formation of cysts; 2) multiple neurofibromatosis—an hereditary skin disease in which tumors of all sizes appear on the skin along the course of the cutaneous nerves all over the body; the skin is pigmented in various areas; there is mental retardation and skeletal deformity. [Friedrich Daniel von Recklinghausen, German pathologist. 1833–1910.]

Reclus' disease: A painless enlargement of the breast of the cystic disease type.

recombinant (rē-kom'bi-nant): Pertaining to or resulting from a recombination; usually refers to new combinations of genes.

recompression (rē-kom-presh'un): The gradual return to conditions of normal pressure after exposure to diminished atmospheric pressure, a procedure used in treating deep sea divers or caisson workers to prevent decompression sickness after their return to the surface.

reconstructive surgery: Surgery to correct or repair a defect, congenital or acquired.

recovery room: A special room where patients are kept until they recover from anesthesia. It is usually located near the operating suite so that if emergency care is needed it can be given quickly by the anesthesiologist or surgeon. Specially prepared nurses are present at all times to observe the patients and care for them.

recreation therapy: The use of such recreational activities as games, music, or theatre to provide relaxation for physically or mentally handicapped individuals, to improve their quality of life, and to help prepare them to reenter the community following disease or injury.

recrement (rek're-ment): A secretion that performs its function and then is reabsorbed into the blood, *e.g.*, saliva, bile.—recrementitious, adj.

recrudescence (rē-kroo-des'ens): The return of symptoms, or of a pathological state, after a period of apparent improvement.

rectal (rek'tal): Pertaining to the rectum. **R. ANESTHESIA**, introduction of an anesthetic into the rectum to produce local anesthesia, used particularly in labor. **R. FEEDING**, introduction of fluid nutrients into the rectum. **R. REFLEX**, the normal reflex that produces the desire to evacuate the rectum. **R. TUBE**, a rubber tube used to introduce substances into the rectum or to assist in the expulsion of flatus.

rectalgia (rek-tal'ji-a): Proctalgia (*q.v.*).

rectectomy (rek-tek'to-mi): Excision of the rectum.

rectitis (rek-tī'tis): Inflammation of the rectum; proctitis.

recto-: Combining form denoting: 1. Relationship to the rectum. 2. Straight. For words beginning thus see also words beginning procto-.

rectoabdominal (rek'tō-ab-dom'i-nal): Pertaining to the rectum and the abdomen, particularly to a rectal examination in which one hand of the examiner is placed firmly on the abdominal wall while one (or more) finger(s) of the other hand is inserted into the rectum.

rectoanal (rek'tō-ā'nal): Pertaining to the rectum and the anus.

rectocele (rek'tō-sēl): Hernial protrusion of the anterior wall of the rectum through the vagina following injury to the posterior wall; may occur during childbirth or, in later life, by weakening of the muscles of the pelvic floor; usually repaired by posterior colporrhaphy. Proctocele.

rectoclysis (rek-tok'li-sis): Proctoclysis (*q.v.*).

rectocolitis (rek'tō-kō-lī'tis): Inflammation of the rectum and colon. Proctocolitis.

rectoperineal (rek'tō-per-i-nē'al): Pertaining to the rectum and the perineum.

rectoperineorrhaphy (rek'tō-per-i-nē-or'a-fi): Repair of the rectal wall and the perineum.

rectopexy (rek'tō-pek-si): Surgical fixation of a prolapsed rectum.

rectoscope (rek'tō-skōp): An instrument for examining the rectum. Proctoscope. See endoscope.—rectoscopic, adj.

rectosigmoid (rek-tō-sig'moyd): The rectum and sigmoid portion of the colon. Also descriptive of the place where the rectum and the sigmoid join.

rectosigmoidectomy (rek'tō-sig-moy-dek'to-mi): Surgical removal of the rectum and sigmoid colon.

rectostenosis (rek'tō-ste-nō'sis): A narrowing or stricture of the rectum. Proctostenosis.

rectostomy (rek-tos'to-mi): The surgical creation of a permanent opening into the rectum to relieve stricture. Proctostomy.

rectourethral (rek-tō-ū-rē'thral): Pertaining to

the rectum and the urethra. **R. FISTULA,** a fistula between the rectum and the urethra.

rectouterine (rek-tō-ū'ter-in): Pertaining to the rectum and uterus.

rectovaginal (rek-tō-vaj'in-al): Pertaining to rectum and vagina. **R. FISTULA,** one between the rectum and vagina.

rectovesical (rek-tō-ves'i-kal): Pertaining to the rectum and urinary bladder. **R. FISTULA,** one between the rectum and the bladder. **R. POUCH,** the fold of peritoneum that extends between the urinary bladder and the rectum in the male.

rectovulvar (rek-tō-vul'var): Pertaining to the rectum and the vulva. **R. FISTULA,** a fistula between the rectum and the vulva.

rectum (rek'tum): The lower part of the large intestine between the sigmoid colon and anal canal.—rectal, adj.; rectally, adv.

rectus (rek'tus): Straight; in anatomy a straight muscle. **R. ABDOMINIS MUSCLE,** one of a pair of straight muscles that extend from the pubis to the xiphoid process; they compress the abdomen and assist to flex the trunk **R. FEMORIS MUSCLE,** the large muscle on the front of the thigh; it flexes the thigh and extends the leg. The **R. MUSCLES OF THE EYE** include the superior, inferior, lateral and medial; they control the movements of the eyeball.

recumbent (rē-kum'bent): Lying down or reclining.—recumbency, n.

recuperate (rē-kū'per-āt): To regain health or strength.—recuperation, n.

recurrent (rē-kur'ent): Occurring again at intervals after a period of quiescence or abatement, *e.g.,* fever, hemorrhage. **R. BANDAGE,** see bandage.

recurvature (rē-kur'va-chur): A backward curvature or bending.

red: **R. BLOOD CELL,** erythrocyte (*q.v.*). **R. BONE MARROW,** see marrow. **R. NUCLEUS,** a large distinctive oval nucleus in the upper part of the midbrain; it receives fibers from the cerebellum and projects fibers to the brain stem, spinal cord, and thalamus.

Red Cross: 1. Abbreviation for a local, national, or the International Red Cross Society. 2. The insignia adopted by the various Red Cross Societies; consists of a red Geneva cross on a white ground. 3. A sign of neutrality used for protection of the sick and wounded and those caring for them in time of war. See International Red Cross.

reduce (rē-dūs'): 1. To restore something to its normal place or position, as in hernia, fracture or dislocation. 2. In chemistry, to remove oxygen from a chemical substance. 3. To decrease in volume or size.—reduction, n.; reducible, adj.

reductase (rē-duk'tās): Any enzyme that has a reducing action on a chemical compound; a hydrogenase.

reduction (rē-duk'shun): In chemistry, the removal of oxygen or addition of hydrogen to a compound. In medicine, the replacement of a part to its normal position in the body. **CLOSED R.,** refers to reduction of a fracture by manipulation without making an incision. **OPEN R.,** refers to reduction of a fracture after incision of the tissues over the site of the fracture.

Reed-Sternberg cell: An enlarged anaplastic reticuloendothelial cell with multiple hyperlobulated nuclei, characteristic of Hodgkin's disease but also seen in other conditions. Also called Sternberg-Reed cell; Dorothy Reed's cell; Hodgkin's cell; giant cell.

reepithelialization (rē'ep-i-thē'li-al-ī-zā'shun): 1. The regrowth of epithelial tissue over an area that has been denuded of it. 2. The surgical replacement of epithelial tissue over a denuded surface.

referred pain: Pain which is felt as occurring at a place distant from its origin, *e.g.,* the pain felt in the arm during an attack of angina pectoris.

reflection (rē-flek'shun): 1. The turning back of a light ray from a surface that it does not penetrate. 2. A turning or bending back. 3. Deep continued thought on written or oral material, often a devotional act; meditation.

reflex (rē'fleks): In physiology, an unlearned, involuntary response to a stimulus. **R. ACTION,** an involuntary response by the body or any of its parts to a stimulus; the testing of various reflexes provides information on the location and diagnosis of disorders involving the nervous system. **ABDOMINAL R.,** contraction of the underlying muscles when the skin of the abdomen is stroked. **ACCOMMODATION R.,** constriction of the pupils and convergence of the eyes for near vision. **ACHILLES R.,** contraction of the calf muscles causing flexion of the foot when the Achilles tendon is stroked. **BABINSKI'S R.,** movement of the great toe upward (dorsiflexion) instead of downward (plantar flexion) and fanning of the other toes, on stroking the outer border of the sole of the foot. Occurs in young infants and in some cases of disease of the brain or spinal cord. Also called Babinski's sign and Babinski's great toe sign. [Joseph Francois Felix Babinski, French neurologist. 1857–1932.] **BICEPS R.,** contraction of the biceps muscle when the biceps tendon is struck at the elbow. **BLINK R.,** involuntary closing of both eyes when any stimulus is applied to the face; present in parkinsonism and in those with generalized brain disease, and sometimes in normal older persons. **BRACHIORADIALIS R.,** contraction of the brachioradialis muscle when the lower end of the radius is tapped and the arm is held in supination at 45°. **BRUDZINSKI'S R.,** see Brudinzski's sign. **CALORIC R.,** see caloric test. **CAROTID R.,** slowing of the heart rate and decreased blood pressure when pressure is applied to the carotid sinus; see **c. sinus**. **CHADDOCK R.**, extension of the great toe when a stimulus is applied to the area below the external malleolus; an indication of lesion in the pyramidal tract. **CHEMICAL R.**, one initiated by hormones or other chemicals in the blood. **CILIARY R.**, the normal pupillary constriction that occurs in accommodation. **CILIOSPINAL R.**, ipsilateral dilatation of the pupil when a painful stimulus is applied to the skin of the neck; usually present in comatose patients when there is no lesion in the brain stem. **CONDITIONED R.**, one that is not inborn but developed through training and repeated association with a definite stimulus. **CONJUNCTIVAL R.**, involuntary closure of the eyelids when the conjunctiva is touched. **CORNEAL R.**, the reaction of blinking when the cornea is touched lightly. **COUGH R.**, clearing of the air passageways of foreign material; results from impulses carried to the medulla by the vagus nerve. **CREMASTERIC R.**, reaction of the ipsilateral testis when the skin on the inner surface of the thigh is stimulated. **DANCE** or **DANCING R.**, stepping **R.**, **DEEP R.**, a **R.** elicited by irritating a deep structure. **DOLL'S EYE R.**, the involuntary turning of the eyes upward or downward with flexion and extension of the head. **GAG R.**, contraction of the constrictor muscle of the pharynx when the back of the pharynx is touched. **GALANT'S R.**, seen in normal infants during the first months of life; running a finger parallel to the spine from the last rib to the iliac crest will cause the infant to flex its trunk toward the side that is stimulated. **GASTROCOLIC R.**, an increase in intestinal and colic peristalsis following entrance of food into the empty stomach. **GLUTEAL R.**, contraction of the muscles of the buttock when the skin over the area is stroked. **GORDON R.**, extension of the thumb and index finger or all the fingers on pressure on the pisiform bone of the wrist; also called finger phenomenon. **GRASP R.**, contraction of the flexor muscles and resistance to attempts to remove an object placed in the hand of a person with a prefrontal lesion. **HERING-BREUER R.**, a nervous mechanism by which afferent vagal impulses inhibit the inspiratory center in the brain. **HIRSCHBERG'S R.**, adduction of the foot when the sole under the great toe is tickled. **ILEOGASTRIC R.**, the inhibition of gastric motility when the ileum becomes distended. **JAW JERK R.**, a quick closure of the jaws when the chin of a person whose mouth is open is tapped; implies damage to the cerebrum in the area that controls motor activity of the fifth cranial nerve (trigeminal). **KNEE-JERK R.**, see **patellar r.** **MONOSYNAPTIC R.**, any **R.** that involves only one synapse and no internuncial neurons, *e.g.*, the patellar **R.** **MORO R.**, the startle **R.**, tested for in evaluating newborn's status; when a sudden noise is made the infant will throw out its arms and legs and bring them together as if to hold on. Also called the Moro embrace **R.** **NECK-RIGHTING R.**, when an infant's head is forcibly turned to one side the whole body tries to turn to that side; this **R.** disappears at about one year of age. **OCULOCARDIAC R.**, slowing of the rhythm of the heartbeat following pressure on the eyes or on the carotid sinus; a slowing of 5 to 13 beats per minute is considered the normal range. **OCULOCEPHALIC R.**, the doll's eye **R.** **OPPENHEIM'S R.**, dorsiflexion of the great toe on downward stroking of the medial surface of the tibia. **PALMAR R.**, flexion of the fingers when the palm is tickled. **PALMOMENTAL R.**, contraction of the mentalis muscle when a non-painful stimulus is applied to the palm; seen in patients with cerebral arteriosclerosis. **PATELLAR R.**, a forward jerk that occurs when the tendon immediately below the patella is struck; also called the **KNEE-JERK R.** **PLANTAR R.**, the involuntary movement of the toes when the sole of the foot is stroked. **POSTURAL R.**, the ability to maintain body alignment against the effects of gravity. **PUPILLARY R.**, change in size of the pupil in response to a stimulus such as light. **QUADRICEPS R.**, pateller **R.** **RIGHTING R.**, the ability to assume the optimal position when there has been a departure from it, either voluntary or involuntary. **ROOTING R.**, occurs when a newborn's cheek is touched lightly; the infant turns its head toward the direction of the touch and purses its lips in preparation for sucking. **STARTLE R.**, contraction of the leg and neck muscles of an infant when dropped a short distance or in response to a loud noise or jerk. **STEPPING R.**, the stepping or dancing movements made by an infant when held upright with its feet on a flat surface. **SUCKING R.**, sucking movements of the lips, tongue, and jaw in response to contact of the lips with an object; normal in infants. **SUPERFICIAL R.**, one that can be elicited by applying a stimulus such as stroking or scratching to the skin. **SWALLOWING R.**, the act of swallowing when the palate, fauces, or posterior pharyngeal wall are touched. **TENDON R.**, contraction of a stretched muscle when the skin over it is tapped lightly; includes the Achilles, biceps, patellar, and triceps reflexes. **TONIC NECK R.**, a **R.**, in the newborn when the infant, lying on its back with its head forcibly turned, extends the ipsilateral arm and sometimes the leg, in the direction the head is turned, while the contralateral limbs become flexed; this **R.** disappears after about four months. **TRICEPS R.**, extension of the forearm when the triceps tendon is tapped at the elbow while the arm hangs loosely at right angles to the side. **VOMITING R.**, contraction of the abdominal muscles, relaxation of the cardiac sphincter of the stomach and of the throat muscles, elicited by a variety of stimuli, usually applied to the fauces.

reflex arc (rē′fleks ark): A sensory neuron, a connective neuron, and a motor neuron which,

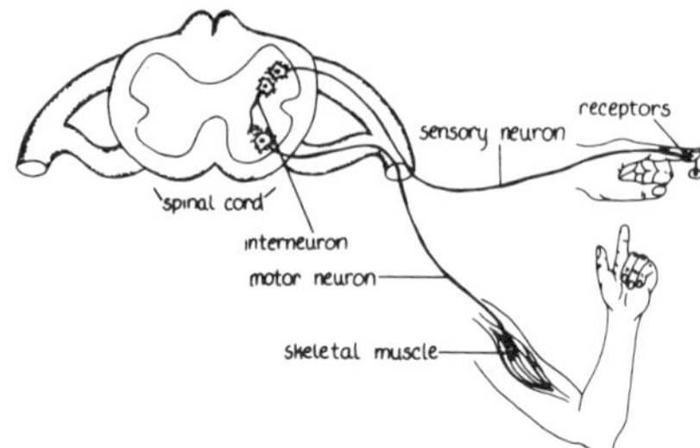

Reflex arc

acting together, constitute the path that an impulse travels from a receptor to an effector organ or gland.

reflexogenic (rē-flek-sō-jen′ik): Producing, increasing, or increasing the tendency to reflex action.

reflexograph (rē-flek′sō-graf): A device for recording a reflex action.

reflexology (rē-flek-sol′o-ji): The study or the science of reflexes.

reflux (rē′fluks): Backward flow or return of a fluid; regurgitation. **GASTROESOPHAGEAL R.,** often due to an incompetent gastroesophageal sphincter and associated with hiatal hernia; characterized by heartburn, regurgitation, anterior chest pain; is aggravated by spicy foods, aspirin, chocolate; complications include esophageal ulcer, hemorrhage, and perforation. **HEPATOJUGULAR R.,** distention of the jugular vein and elevation of blood pressure resulting from pressure on the liver; can be observed in the jugular vein and measured in the arm veins. **VESICOURETERAL R.,** the passage of urine from the bladder back into the ureter. See also **peptic esophagitis.**

refraction (rē-frak′shun): 1. The bending of light rays as they pass through media of different densities. In normal vision, the light rays are so bent that they meet on the retina. 2. The process of measuring errors of refraction in the eyes and correcting them by eyeglass lenses.—refractive, adj.; refract, v.

refractometer (rē′frak-tom′e-ter): An instrument used to measure the degree of refraction in substances that transmit light, particularly those in the eye. Refractionometer.

refractometry (rē-frak-tom′e-tri): In ophthalmology, the use of a refractometer to measure refractive errors in the eye.

refractory (rē-frak′tō-ri): 1. Stubborn, unmanageable, rebellious; resistant to treatment. 2. Unable to accept a stimulus. **ABSOLUTE REFRACTORY PERIOD,** the time immediately after a nerve has been stimulated when the cells are depolarized and the nerve cannot respond to another stimulus, regardless of its strength. **RELATIVE R. PERIOD,** the time period during which a neuron can respond to a stimulus if the stimulus is strong enough.

refracture (rē-frak′chur): The operation of rebreaking a bone that has united improperly after fracture.

refrigerant (rē-frij′er-ant): 1. Allaying heat or fever. 2. An agent that reduces fever and produces a feeling of coolness.

refrigeration (rē-frij-er-ā′shun): Cooling of the body or any part of it, to reduce basal metabolism or to render a part insensitive as is needed for minor surgery. See **hibernation, hypothermia.**

Refsum's disease: A rare autosomal recessive disease characterized by peripheral neuritis with motor and sensory involvement, retinitis pigmentosa, deafness, cerebellar ataxia, ichthyoid skin lesions, and elevation of protein in the cerebrospinal fluid.

refusion (re-fū′zhun): The return of blood to the circulation after it has been temporarily removed from the body or cut off from a part.

regeneration (rē-jen-er-ā′shun): The natural renewal or repair of tissue after injury.—regenerate, v.

Regents College Degree: Originally called the New York State Regents External Degree. This program grants both the associate degree and baccalaureate degree in nursing. Entry into the program is based on the individual's educational and life experience background. The instruction consists of independent study and written examinations followed by a clinical performance examination.

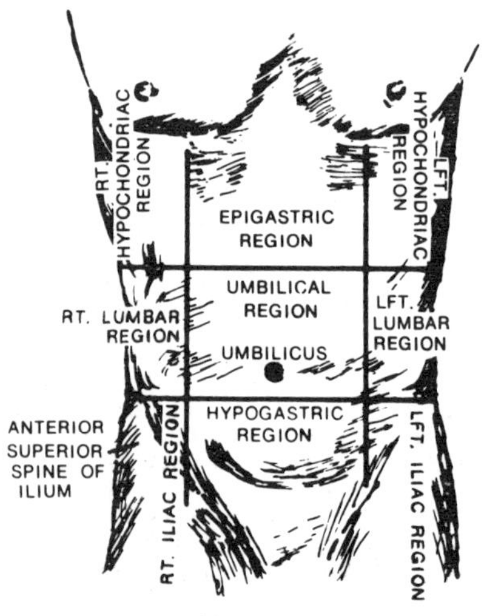

Abdominal regions

regimen (rej′i-men): A systematic plan of diet, medication, and activities designed to restore or maintain a certain state of health or keep a certain condition under control.

region (rē′jun): In anatomy, a limited area of the surface of the body, *e.g.*, the **ABDOMINAL REGIONS** include the epigastric, right and left hypochondriac, umbilical, right and left lumbar, hypogastric, right and left iliac.

Regional Medical Programs: Originally designed to provide for regionalization of medical services for heart disease, cancer, and stroke; fully financed by the federal government; now concerned mostly with improving health services through sponsoring new means of delivering health care services, the training of health paraprofessionals, and continuing education for physicians.

registered nurse: See under nurse.

registration: A process by which qualified individuals are listed on an official roster maintained by a governmental or nongovernmental agency. In nursing, refers to nurses who have passed a qualifying examination to practice as a registered nurse (R.N.).

registry (rej′is-tri): A placement bureau or office where a nurse may list her name as available for nursing duty.

regression (rē-gresh′un): 1. A return to a former state or condition. 2. The subsidence or abatement of symptoms or of a disease condition. 3. In psychiatry, a turning back to an earlier more comfortable stage of development in order to escape a frustrating or unbearable situation; occurs in dementia, especially senile dementia.—regressive, adj; regress, v.

regurgitant (rē-gur′ji-tant): Flowing back or in the opposite direction from normal.

regurgitation (rē-gur-ji-tā′shun): Backward flow, as of stomach contents into or through the mouth, or of blood into the heart or between the chambers of the heart when the valves do not function properly, as in **MITRAL R.** in which blood flows back from the left ventricle into the left atrium, or in **TRICUSPID R.**, in which blood flows back from the right ventricle into the right atrium.—regurgitant, adj.; regurgitate, v.

rehabilitation (rē-ha-bil-i-tā′shun): The restoration of an individual's ability to function as efficiently and normally as his condition will permit following injury, illness, or accident. It involves re-education and retraining of those who have become partially or wholly incapacitated by such conditions as blindness, deafness, heart disease, amputation, paralysis, etc. **R. COUNSELOR**, a health care professional who counsels physically and mentally handicapped persons to help them improve their ability to function optimally in society. **R. ENGINEERING**, the construction and use of a great number of devices used to restore or replace motor and sensory functions. **R. MEDICINE**, all aspects of medicine involved in rehabilitative programs.—rehabilitate, v.

rehabilitee (rē′-ha-bil-i-tē′): One who is undergoing or has undergone rehabilitation (*q.v.*).

Rehfuss' tube (rā′fus): Consists of a graduated syringe attached to a fine-caliber stomach tube that has a bulbous perforated metal tip. Formerly used in obtaining gastric juice for study and for gastric feeding.

rehydration (re-hī-drā′shun): The restoration of water or fluid to a substance that has been dehydrated.—rehydrate, v.

Reichian therapy: A type of psychotherapy chacterized by emphasis on the necessity of full expression of the sexual libido as a cure for neurosis; introduced by Wilhelm Reich, German psychoanalyst [1897–1957].

Reil's island (rīls): See insula.

reimplantation (rē′im-plan-tā′shun): The replacement into its former position of a body part that has been removed.

reinfection (rē′in-fek′shun): A second infection, during convalescence or after recovery from a previous infection by the same or a very similar organism.

reinforcement (rē′in-fors′ment): Increasing the cumulative effect of something by strengthening it through repetition, addition, or similar action. In psychology, the strengthening of a response by offering a reward or by withholding punishment, an important process in operant conditioning.—reinforce, v.

reinfusion (rē′in-fū′zhun): The reinjection of blood serum, or cerebrospinal fluid.

reinnervation (rē′-in-er-vā′shun): The operation of restoring the nerve supply of an organ or muscle by grafting in a living nerve when the motor nerve supply has been lost.

reinoculation (rē′in-ok-ū-lā′shun): A second inoculation with the same virus or infection.

Reiter's syndrome: An arthritis-like syndrome with urethritis, conjunctivitis, and cutaneous lesions; of unknown origin; sometimes mistaken for acute gonorrheal arthritis. Likely to be chronic and to recur. Occurs most often in males. Also called Reiter's disease.

rejection (rē-jek′shun): 1. An immune reaction against a grafted tissue or organ. 2. In psychology, a denial; a refusal to accept, recognize, or grant.

relapse (rē-laps′): The return of a disease or of serious symptoms after the disease has apparently been overcome.

relapsing fever: Louse-borne or tick-borne infection caused by spirochetes of genus Borrelia. Prevalent in many parts of the world. Characterized by a febrile period of a week or so, with apparent recovery, followed by a further bout of high fever.

relaxant (rē-lak'sant): 1. Causing relaxation. 2. An agent that produces relaxation or reduction of tension.

relaxin (rē-lak'sin): A factor secreted by certain pregnant animals and also prepared pharmaceutically for treatment of dysmenorrhea and premature labor and to facilitate labor at term; it produces relaxation of the symphysis pubi and dilatation of the uterine cervix.

REM: Abbreviation for rapid eye movement (*q.v.*).

rem: The amount of ionizing radiation that will have the same effect as 1 rad of x-ray radiation.

remedial (re-mē'di-al): Having curative properties.

remediation (rē-mē-di-ā'shun): The act of remedying.

remedy (rem'e-di): Any agent that prevents, cures, or alleviates a disease or its symptoms.

remission (rē-mish'un): 1. Lessening or abatement of the symptoms of a disease. 2. A period of temporary abatement of the symptoms of a disease, *e.g.*, as in a fever.

remittent (rē-mit'ent): Characterized by periodic intervals of abatement of symptoms of a pathologic condition.

ren (ren): The kidney.—renal, adj.

ren-, reni, reno-: Combining forms denoting the kidney.

renal (rē'nal): Pertaining to the kidney. **R. ASTHMA,** hyperventilation of the lung occurring sometimes during uremia, as a result of acidosis. **R. CALCULUS,** a stone in the kidney. **R. COLIC,** severe pain in the lower back, radiating down the groin and sometimes the leg; caused by a calculus in the kidney or ureter. **R. DIALYSIS,** see hemodialysis. **R. DWARFISM,** dwarfism due to renal failure. **RENAL FAILURE,** failure of the kidney to perform its functions; chronic failure is usually irreversible. **R. GLYCOSURIA,** that which occurs in patients with normal blood sugar and lowered renal threshold for sugar. **R. HEMANGIOPERICYTOMA,** a vascular neoplasm of the kidney in which the capillaries are often obscured by the growing tumor, which may be benign or malignant. **R. HYPERTENSION,** systemic arterial hypertension resulting from kidney disease. **R. INSUFFICIENCY,** inability of the kidney to perform its functions properly. **R. MEDULLA,** the inner darker part of the kidney, composed of the renal pyramids. **R. OSTEODYSTROPHY,** a chronic condition with onset in childhood, due to renal insufficiency, marked by increased resorption of bone with osteomalacia and osteoporosis; also called renal rickets. **R. SHUTDOWN,** R. failure. **R. SYSTEM,** consists of the two kidneys, two ureters, bladder, urethra, renal arteries and veins. **R. THRESHOLD,** the degree of concentration of a substance in the urine at which the kidney begins to excrete it. **R. TUBULAR ACIDOSIS,** a hereditary disorder characterized by inability to produce an acid urine; it occurs chiefly in males in whom it is the result of incomplete reabsorption of bicarbonate in the proximal tubule. **R. UREMIA,** uremia that follows kidney disease in contrast to that caused by a circulatory disorder.

Rendu-Weber-Osler disease: Hereditary hemorrhagic telangiectasia; see under telangiectasia.

renin (rē'nin): A protein substance manufactured in the kidney that acts like an enzyme; when secreted into the bloodstream it acts as a powerful vasoconstrictor and raises the blood pressure; too high a level in the bloodstream will result in blood pressure that is higher than normal.

renin-angiotensin-aldosterone-system: A system by which the kidneys control blood pressure. Renin, released by the kidney when blood pressure falls, combines with a plasma protein to form angiotensin I, then angiotensin II which is a potent vasoconstrictor that stimulates the production of aldosterone by the kidney cortex, which, in turn, promotes the reabsorption of sodium by the kidney tubules and results in the release of potassium and an increase in blood volume. Also called renin-angiotensin system.

renin-sodium profile test: Measures the sodium content in a 24-hour urine specimen during which time salt is restricted, and compares it with the renin content of the blood; useful in planning medical treatment of hypertension.

rennet (ren'et): An extract made of calf's stomach; contains rennin. Used in preparing certain foods and in cheese making.

rennin (ren'nin): A coagulating enzyme occurring in the gastric juice of the calf; the active principle in rennet (*q.v.*). Prepared commercially from the mucous lining of the calf's stomach.

renninogen (ren-in'ō-jen): The inactive precursor of rennin.

renogenic (rē-nō-jen'ik): Originating or arising in the kidney.

renogram (rē'nō-gram): The roentgenographic record showing the rate at which kidneys remove an intravenously injected dose of a radioactive substance from the blood, an aid in evaluating renal function.

renography (rē-nog'ra-fi): Radiography of the kidney.

renomegaly (rē'nō-meg'a-li): Abnormal enlargement of the kidney.

renopathy (rē-nop'a-thi): Any disease of the kidney.

renorenal (rē-nō-rē'nal): Pertaining to or affecting both kidneys. **R. REFLEX,** the mechanism by which pathology in one kidney will affect the functioning of the other kidney.

renotrophic (rē′nō-trōf′ic): Having the ability to cause an increase in the size of the kidney.

renovascular (rē′nō-vas′kū-lar): Pertaining to the blood vessels of the kidney. **R. HYPERTENSION,** see under hypertension.

reorganization (rē-or′ga-nī-zā′shun): Healing by the formation of new tissue similar to that lost through some morbid process.

Reovirus (rē′ō-vī′rus): A genus of RNA viruses closely related to the ECHO viruses (*q.v.*) and the arboviruses (*q.v.*); have been found in the respiratory and intestinal tracts of both healthy and sick people, but not yet associated with any specific disease.

Rep.: See repetatur.

repellent (rē-pel′ent): 1. Capable of reducing a swelling. 2. An agent that is capable of reducing a swelling or edema. 3. Capable of repelling insects or mosquitoes. 4. An agent that repels insects or mosquitoes.

repetatur (re-pe-tā′tūr): Let it be renewed; a Latin term used in prescription writing.

replacement (rē-plās′ment): 1. The infusion of donor blood to replace lost blood. 2. The substitution of a prosthetic device to replace a missing part or one that has been lost by amputation or accident.

replantation (re-plan-tā′shun): Usually refers to the replacement of teeth that have been extracted or otherwise removed.—replant, v.

repletion (rē-plē′shun): The state of having ingested food and drink sufficient to produce satiation. Fullness.

repolarization (rē′pō-lar-ī-zā′shun): The process by which a depolarized cell membrane becomes repolarized by the restoration of a positive charge on the outer surface of the cell and a negative charge on the inner surface.—repolarize, v.

reportable disease: Communicable or other disease of humans or animals that the physician or other responsible person is required by law to report to the appropriate authority. The list of such diseases is made up by each health jurisdiction.

reposition (rē′pō-zish′un): To replace an organ or part to its normal site.

repression (rē-presh′un): In psychiatry, a defense mechanism whereby an individual unconsciously refuses to recognize the existence of urges, thoughts, memories, or feelings that are unacceptable or painful, or in conflict with the person's accepted moral principles; these experiences may not be recalled at will, but may emerge as the source of anxiety neuroses.

reproduction (rē′prō-duk′shun): The process of producing offspring, usually by sexual means, *i.e.*, the union of male and female sex cells; may also occur asexually, *i.e.*, by some means other than the union of male and female sex cells.

reproductive (rē′prō-duk′tiv): Pertinent to or associated with reproduction. **R. SYSTEM,** consists of the organs involved in reproduction. **MALE R. SYSTEM,** includes the testes, efferent ducts, epididymus, ductus deferens, ejaculatory duct, urethra, prostate gland, penis. **FEMALE R. SYSTEM,** includes ovaries, fallopian tubes, uterus, vagina, vulva, and accessory glands.

repulsion (rē-pul′shun): The act of forcing or driving apart or away. Opp. of attraction.

research (re′serch): Scholarly or scientific systematic careful in-depth study and investigation of some field of knowledge in order to establish some principle, to discover facts or test theories, or to find valid answers to questions raised or solutions for problems identified. See nursing research.

resect (rē-sekt′): To cut off or out part of a structure or organ.

resection (rē-sek′shun): Surgical removal of a section or segment of an organ or structure. **SUBMUCOUS R.,** a surgical procedure involving incision of nasal mucosa, removal of deflected nasal septum, and replacement of mucosa. **TRANSURETHRAL R.,** removal of the prostate utilizing an instrument passed through the urethra. **WEDGE R.,** the removal of a small wedgeshaped portion of tissue from an organ or part.

resectoscope (rē-sek′tō-skōp): A tubular instrument for dividing or removing small structures from a body cavity under direct vision, without making an incision other than that used for passing the instrument; used particularly when removing the prostate gland through the urethra.

reserve (rē-serv′): In physiology, something that is held back or stored for future use. **ALKALINE R.,** the amount of alkaline available in the body to act as buffer to maintain the normal pH of the blood. **CARDIAC R.,** the amount of work the heart is able to perform in increasing its output to meet increased physiologic demands.

reservoir (rez′er-vwor): A place where anything is collected or stored. **R. OF INFECTION,** anything that provides a place for infectious agents to live and multiply and from which such agents can transmit an infection to a susceptible host; may be a person, animal, plant, water, soil, or inanimate organic matter.

resident (rez′i-dent): A graduate licensed physician who serves as a house officer in a hospital following his internship in order to gain additional clinical training. So called because formerly he lived in the hospital.

residual (rē-zid′ū-al): Remaining. In physiology, refers to something remaining in a body cavity after normal expulsion has occurred.

Also refers to a disability or deformity that remains after recovery from disease or operation, as a limp or a scar. **R. AIR,** the air remaining in the lung after forced expiration. **R. URINE,** urine remaining in the bladder after micturition. **R. VOLUME,** the volume of air remaining in the lung after a maximal expiration.

residue (rez'i-dū): That which remains after removal of other substances.—residual, adj.

resilient (rē-zil'yent): Elastic. Having a tendency to return to previous shape, position, or condition.—resilience, n.

res ipsa loquitur: A legal term (Latin) that, literally, means "the thing speaks for itself." An important concept in malpractice lawsuits since it means specifically that the person or institution is being sued for an unfavorable or injurious injury or condition which could have been prevented if proper care had been used, *e.g.*, leaving a sponge in the patient's body after surgery.

resistance (rē-zis'tens): 1. Opposition to the passage of an electrical current. 2. Power of opposing an active force. 3. In psychology, the name given to the force that prevents repressed thoughts from reentering the consciousness. **AIRWAY RESISTANCE,** that usually offered to the airflow, mainly by the larynx, trachea, and bronchi. **COGWHEEL R.,** stepwise jerking resistance felt by the examiner on passive stretching of muscle as in passive flexion and extension of the elbow; occurs in patients with parkinsonism. **R. TO INFECTION,** the power of the body to withstand infection; see **immunity. PERIPHERAL R.,** that offered by the capillaries to the blood passing through them.

resolution (rez-ō-loo'shun): The subsidence or spontaneous arrest of an inflammatory process without suppuration; the breaking down and removal or absorption of the products of inflammation, as seen, *e.g.*, in lobar pneumonia when the consolidation begins to liquefy.

resolve (rē-zolv'): To return to a normal state following a pathological condition, particularly when no suppuration has occurred.

resonance (rez'o-nans): The sound elicited when percussing a part that can vibrate freely, as for example, a hollow organ or a cavity containing air. **VOCAL R.,** the reverberating note heard through the stethoscope on auscultation of the chest while the patient is speaking.—resonant, adj.

resorption (rē-sorp'shun): 1. The loss or disappearance of a body process or substance by absorption, lysis, or dissolution, *e.g.*, callus following bone fracture, the root of a tooth, or blood from a hematoma. 2. The act of resorbing or assimilating an excretion, blood clot, pus, or exudative material.

respiration (res-pi-rā'shun): 1. The physical and chemical processs by which the cells and tissues of an organism receive the oxygen needed for carrying on their physiological processes and are relieved of the carbon dioxide resulting from these activities. 2. The movement of gases across the alveolar-capillary membrane in the lungs. 3. The act or function of breathing. **ABDOMINAL R.,** the use of the diaphragm and abdominal muscles in breathing. **APNEUSTIC R.,** characterized by long inspirations and short expirations. **ARTIFICIAL R.,** artificial methods to restore respiration such as mouth-to-mouth breathing, or by the use of a device that intermittently inflates the lungs by forcing either oxygen or air into them. **BIOT'S R.,** jerky, rapid, irregular breathing that is interrupted by apnea after four or five breaths; seen in meninjitis and other conditions resulting from increased intracranial pressure which depresses the respiratory center. **CAVERNOUS R., R.** characterized by prolonged hollow resonance; usually indicates a cavity in the lung. **CHEYNE-STOKES R.,**a type of breathing in which

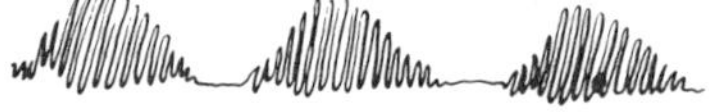

Pattern of Cheyne-Stokes respiration

the respirations gradually increase in depth until they reach a maximum, then gradually decrease in depth, finally ceasing for a period of time after which the cycle is repeated; results from retarded blood flow to the cerebrum and is often seen in congestive heart failure; the prognosis is ominous. **COGWHEEL R.,** jerky, interrupted breathing. **DIAPHRAGMATIC R.,** abdominal **R. EXTERNAL R.,** the exchange between the oxygen in the air in the lungs and the carbon dioxide in the blood in the walls of the capillaries in the alveoli. **INTERNAL R.,** the exchange of oxygen and carbon dioxide in the tissues. **KUSSMAUL R.,** the deep, sighing or gasping respirations characteristic of diabetic acidosis. **PARADOXICAL R.,** inward movement of the chest wall during inspiration and outward movement during expiration; occurs when the lung or part of it is deflated. **STERTEROUS R.,** noisy, rattling **R.** due to breathing with the mouth open which causes vibration of the soft palate; often occurs in comatose patients. **SONOROUS** or **STRIDENT R.,** in which a high-pitched crowing sound is heard; usually indicates a partial airway obstruction. **THORACIC R., R.** accomplished chiefly by the intercostal muscles.

respirator (res'pi-rā-tor): 1. An appliance worn over the nose and mouth and designed to filter out irritating or poisonous substances such as gases, fumes, smoke, or dust, or to warm the air before it enters the respiratory tract. 2. An apparatus that artificially and rhythmically inflates and deflates the lungs as in normal breathing, when for any reason the natural nervous or muscular control of respiration is impaired. The apparatus may work on either positive or negative pressure or on electrical stimulation. **CUIRASS R.,** a **R.** in the shape of a shell; is worn over the front of the trunk; used for patients who have some ability to breathe on their own. **DRINKER R.,** used when it is necessary to supply artificial respiration for a long period of time. Consists of a metal tank that encloses the entire body except the head; commonly called "iron lung."

respiratory (rē-spī'ra-tō-ri): Pertaining to respiration. **R. ACIDOSIS,** see under acidosis. **R. ALKALOSIS,** see under alkalosis. **R. CENTER,** the area in the medulla oblongata that regulates respiratory movements; it is stimulated by carbon dioxide in the blood and cerebrospinal fluid. **R. FAILURE,** functional failure of the lungs and respiratory system to extract enough oxygen from the air to meet the body's needs. **R. FUNCTION TESTS,** numerous available tests for vital capacity, forced vital capacity, forced expiratory volume, and maximal breathing capacity. **R. SYSTEM,** consists of the nose, pharynx, larynx, trachea, bronchi, lungs, and pleura; accessory structures include the diaphragm, pleural sac, and muscles of the chest wall. **R. TRACT,** the group of tubular and cavernous structures that, functioning together, accomplish the exchange of gases between the ambient air and the blood, the principal organs involved being the nose, larynx, trachea, bronchi, bronchioles, and lungs.

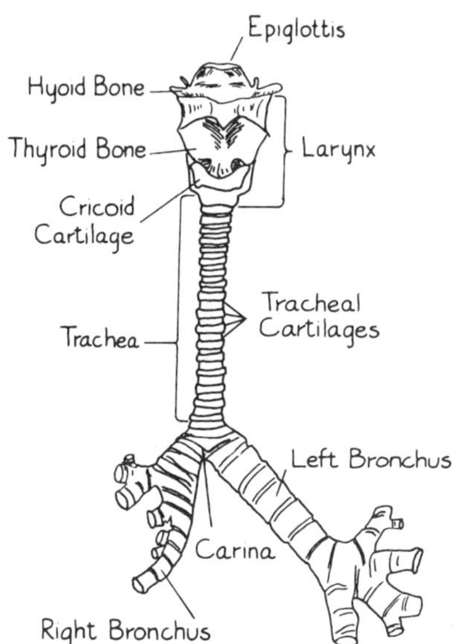

Upper Respiratory Tract—The hyoid bone, larynx, trachea, and bronchi

respiratory distress syndrome: 1. **RESPIRATORY DISTRESS SYNDROME OF THE NEWBORN,** dyspnea in the newly born; formerly called hyaline membrane disease. Occurs most often in those born of diabetic mothers, or by cesarean section. A protein-lipid complex forms in the air spaces of the lungs on the first entry of air causing reduced amounts of lung surfacant (*q.v.*) and atelectasis; the chest wall retreats with every breath, cyanosis develops, the respiration rate increases and a characteristic grunt is heard on expiration. The survival rate is about 40 to 50 percent. 2. **ADULT RESPIRATORY DISTRESS SYNDROME,** the name given to a severe obstructive lung disorder that results from the inflammatory response to such stresses as shock, chest injury, certain drug overdoses, or the effects of a viral, bacterial, chemical, or allergic agent; other causes include inhalation of smoke or corrosive chemicals, aspiration of stomach contents, or drowning. Symptoms are due to formation of a hyaline membrane in the alveoli which prevents formation of surfactant, causing suspension of oxygen-carbon dioxide exchange in the alveoli, which then become filled with exudate and fibrinous material. Symptoms include dyspnea, hypoxia, interstitial edema, and respiratory failure. Also called white lung, wet lung, and shock lung. Abbreviated ARDS.

respiratory sounds: May be 1) normal breath sounds heard on auscultation; often described as low-pitched, non-musical rustlings, or murmurs, or 2) adventitious sounds which are usually indicative of a pathologic condition; may be popping or clicking, squeaking, wheezing, whistling.

respiratory syncytial virus (rē-spī'ra-tō-ri sin-sish'-i-al vī'rus): A virus of the genus *Pneumovirus;* causes bronchitis and bronchopneumonia in children and minor upper respiratory infections in adults.

respiratory therapist: A therapist who administers respiratory therapy to patients as prescribed by a physician; includes the use of various respirators, oxygen dispensers, aerosol dispensers, and nebulizers. Preparation for the work includes a two-year course and passing a qualifying examination.

respiratory tract infection: Any infection affecting the respiratory tract; usually identified as 1) upper respiratory tract infections which includes colds, tonsillitis, pharyngitis, sinusitis, rhinitis, and bronchial infections, and 2) lower respiratory tract infections which include those of the trachea and bronchi, and the various pneumonias.

respire (rē-spīr'): To breathe.

respirometer (res-pi-rom'e-ter): An instrument used for studying and measuring the extent and character of the respiratory movements. Spirometer.

respite care: Regular relief for the families of patients who are being cared for at home; often provided by a community facility and may be on an hourly, daily, or weekly basis.

responaut (res′po-nawt): A person with permanent respiratory paralysis and needing a mechanical breathing device.

respondeat superior: The doctrine that an employer is responsible for wrongful or negligent acts of his employees in certain situations, and that both can be sued.

response (re-spons′): A reaction or movement following the application of a stimulus.

rest cure: Bed rest; usually combined with special diet, massage, physical therapy, etc., to improve muscle tone and circulation and to promote relaxation; usually prescribed for individuals who are convalescing from debilitating illness or nervous system disorder.

rest pain: Pain that occurs mostly at night in patients with peripheral vascular disease; often severe and persistent; due to ischemic neuritis. The peripheral pulses are absent and the toes may be red and tender; gangrene follows easily after injury.

restiform (res′ti-form): In the shape of a rope; ropelike.

restless legs syndrome: A condition characterized by weakness, coldness, and a disagreeable, prickly, creeping sensation in the muscles of the lower legs, and sometimes in the thighs, arms, and hands; begins after the person has gone to bed and can be relieved only by walking; the cause is unknown but thought to be a vascular condition; occurs most often in those suffering from a neurosis and in the elderly.

restoration (res-to-ra′shun): Repair or reconstruction of a part, or a return to a previous state of health.

restorative (rē-stŏr′a-tiv): 1. An agent that serves to restore health, strength, or consciousness. 2. Promoting or tending to restore health, strength, or consciousness.

restraint (rē-strānt′): 1. Forcible restriction of the movements of an excessively restless, irrational or psychotic patient in order to prevent him from injuring himself or others. 2. The means used to restrain a patient who is delirious, irrational, or psychotic; may be a drug or a mechanical appliance. May consist simply of a sheet applied firmly over the thighs and fastened to the bed frame, or cuffs, straps, splints, restraining jacket, etc. Drugs and seclusion rooms are also used.

restrictive pulmonary disease: Any disease or disorder that interferes with lung expansion, *e.g.*, pulmonary fibrosis.

Resusci-Anne: A training manikin that responds to external cardiac massage and mouth-to-mouth resuscitation.

resuscitation (rē-sus-i-tā′shun): The restoration to life of someone who is in cardiac or respiratory failure or shock. **CARDIOPULMONARY R.**, bringing an individual back to consciousness by keeping the airway open, and by mouth-to-mouth breathing or external cardiac massage. **MOUTH-TO-MOUTH R.**, a method of giving artificial respiration in which the rescuer forces air from his own lungs into the mouth of the victim; also called oral resuscitation. **OPEN-CHEST R.**, accomplished by massaging the heart in cases when the patient is in the operating room and the chest is already open, or when the patient is obese or barrel-chested, or in cases of tension pneumothorax or flail chest.—resuscitate, v.; resuscitative, adj.

resuscitator (rē-sus′i-tā-tor): An apparatus used to initiate breathing in persons whose respirations have ceased; consists of a mask that fits over the nose and mouth, a bag or reservoir for air, and a pump that may be electrically or hand-powered.

retardate (rē-tar′dāt): A mentally retarded person.

retardation (rē-tar-dā′shun): Delay; hindrance; slowing down; backwardness. **MENTAL R.**, lack of normal mental development; falling behind the norm mentally for one's age; marked by below-average intellectual functioning that is connected with maladaptive behavior in childhood and early youth; the IQ range is usually considered to be from 20 to 70. **PSYCHOMOTOR R.** abnormal slowness or lack of progress in both mental and physical development.

retch: To make a strong involuntary but ineffective effort to vomit.

retching: Straining at vomiting.

rete (rē′tē): A mesh or network; in anatomy, a network or plexus of nerve fibers or blood vessels.—retia, pl.; retial, adj.

retention: 1. Retaining information and facts in the mind; memory. 2. Accumulation of that which is normally excreted. 3. Keeping within the body that which normally belongs there, particularly food and liquid in the stomach. 4. Keeping in the body that which should normally be discharged. **R. ENEMA,** one given with the intent that it be retained in order to provide nourishment, medication, or anesthesia. **R. OF URINE,** accumulation of urine within the bladder. See catheter, indwelling.

reticular (rē-tik′ū-lar): 1. Resembling a net. 2. Pertaining to the reticuloendothelium (*q.v.*). **R. ACTIVATING SYSTEM,** consists of the reticuloendothelium; maintains the person in the alert conscious state; lesions or chemical dysfunction of the system may produce lethargy, stupor, or coma.

reticulocyte (rē-tik'ū-lō-sīt): A young circulating red blood cell, which still contains traces of the nucleus that was present in the cell when developing in the bone marrow. Increased numbers of reticulocytes in the blood is evidence of active blood regeneration. Reticulocytes normally constitute about 1% of the circulating red blood cells.

reticulocytopenia (rē-tik' -ū-lō-sī-tō-pē'ni-a): A decrease in the normal number of reticulocytes in the circulating blood.

reticulocytosis (rē-tik'ū-lō-sī-tō'sis): A condition in which there is more than the normal number of reticulocytes in the peripheral blood, due either to irritation of the bone marrow or to excessive production; may occur after hemorrhage, in high altitude, and in treatment of some types of anemia.

reticuloendothelioma (rē-tik'ū-lō-en'dō-thē-li-ō'ma): A tumor that is derived from reticuloendothelial tissue.

reticuloendotheliosis (re-tik'ū-lō-en'dō-thē-li-ō'sis): A group of diseases affecting the reticuloendothelial system, including Hand-Schüller-Christian disease and Letterer-Siwe disease. Cause unknown; characterized by the proliferation of histiocytes; symptoms include otitis media, seborrheic rash, lymphoadenopathy, enlarged liver and spleen, anemia.

reticuloendothelium (rē-tik'ū-lō-en'dō-thē'li-um): A system of widely dispersed cells important in immunity because of their ability to remove bacteria, foreign particles, and cellular debris from the blood. Scattered throughout the body, these cells may be fixed or wandering, the fixed cells being found chiefly in connective tissue, thymus gland, lymph glands, bone marrow, liver, spleen, adrenals, hypophysis, and the microglia of the central nervous system, while the wandering cells are found in the blood.—recticuloendothelial, adj.

reticuloma (rē-tik-ū-lō'ma): A tumor consisting chiefly of reticuloendothelial cells.

reticulosarcoma (rē-tik'ū-lō-sar-ko'ma): Sarcoma composed of reticuloendothelial cells.

reticulosis (rē-tik'ū-lō' -sis): Proliferative disease of the reticuloendothelial system. An ill-defined group of fatal conditions of unknown etiology in which glandular and splenic enlargement is commonly found, and of which the three commonest members are Hodgkin's disease (lymphadenoma), lymphosarcoma, and reticulum cell sarcoma. See mycosis.—reticuloses, pl.

reticulum (re-tik'ū-lum): A fine network of cells or of connective tissue fibers; the neuroglia.

retiform (ret'i-form): Resembling a net or network; reticular.

retina (ret'i-na): The delicate, light-sensitive, innermost of the three coats of the eyeball. The optic nerve enters the posterior of the eyeball and then expands to form the retina, which extends forward to the margin of the pupil. Thus it is composed of nerve tissue which receives stimuli from light and transmits them to the visual center in the brain. It is soft in consistency, translucent, of a pinkish color, and made up of layers, the outer one being pigmented and the seven inner ones being nerve tissue, the innermost of which contains the rods and cones, the receptors for light. In the center of the posterior retina is the *macula lutea* or yellow spot, and in the center of it is the *fovea centralis,* the area of most acute vision. DETACHED R., partial or complete separation of the retina from the choroid; may be due to trauma, or to hemorrhage into the choroid.—retinae, pl.; retinal, adj.

retinaculum (ret-i-nak'ū-lum): 1. An instrument for holding tissues out of the way during surgery. 2. A band or structure that holds an organ or tissue in place. 3. A frenum (*q.v.*).

retinal (ret'i-nal): Related to the retina. R. DETACHMENT, see detached r. under retina.

retinene (ret'i-nēn): A pigment extracted from the retina; the chief component of rhodopsin; can be converted into vitamin A by light and resynthesized into rhodopsin in the dark; allows for maximun vision in a dim light.

retinitis (ret-i-nī'tis): Inflammation of the retina. R. CIRCINATA, a condition of inadequate vascularity of the retina; characterized by the deposit of lipids in the pattern of a complete or incomplete ring in the deeper layers of the retina; seen most often in the elderly. R. PIGMENTOSA, a familial degenerative disease that leads to blindness following intraretinal pigmentation, narrowing of vision, and nyctalopia; often associated with other degenerative disorders. R. PROLIFERANS, proliferation of the retinal vessels extending into the vitreous; occurs in retrolental fibroplasia and diabetic retinopathy; usually seen in children and adolescents.

retinoblastoma (ret'i-nō-blas-tō'ma): A malignant tumor of the neuroglial element of the retina, occurring exclusively in children; usually bilateral. Often several in a family are affected.

retinochoroidal (ret'in-ō-kō-roy'dal): Pertaining to both the retina and the choroid.

retinochoroiditis (ret' -in-ō-kō-roy-dī'tis): Inflammation of the retina and choroid. Syn., chorioretinitis.

retinoid (ret'i-noyd): Resembling the retina, or affecting it.

retinomalacia (ret' -i-nō-ma-lā'shi-a): Softening of the retina.

retinopapillitis (ret'i-nō-pap-i-lī'tis): Inflammation of the retina and the optic disk.

retinopathy (ret-i-nop'a-thi): Any noninflammatory disease of the retina. **DIABETIC R.**, that which occurs in diabetic patients; progressive disease of the retinal blood vessels with small punctate hemorrhages and dilation of the veins; severe hemorrhage into the vitreous may lead to visual disturbances or blindness. **HIGH-ALTITUDE R.**, retinal changes associated with symptoms of hypoxia, including retinal hemorrhage. **HYPERTENSIVE R.**, vascular **R.**; associated with arteriosclerosis; characterized by "cotton wool" exudate and linear hemorrhages.

retinopexy (ret'in-ō-pek'si): Fixation of a detached retina by surgery, freezing, laser beam, photocoagulation, or other methods.

retinoschisis (ret'i-nos'ki-sis): Splitting of the retina with the formation of an intra-retinal cyst; a benign and slowly progressive disorder.

retinoscope (ret'i-nō-skōp): Instrument for detection of refractive errors by illumination of the retina using a special mirror.

retinoscopy (ret'i-nos'kō-pi): A method of examining the eye and evaluating refractive errors by projecting a beam of light onto the retina and observing the refraction by the eye of the emergent rays.

retinosis (ret'i-nō'sis): A degenerative condition of the retina; retinomalacia.

retinotoxic (ret'i-nō-tok'-sik): Having an injurious effect on the retina.

Retired Senior Volunteer Program: A program that provides for out-of-pocket expenses for older people who volunteer for any one of many community services; usually covers transportation costs, meals while on the job, etc. Abbreviated RSVP.

retract (rē-trakt'): To draw back, shorten, or contract.

retractile (rē-trak'til): 1. Capable of being drawn back. 2 The state of being drawn back.

retraction (rē-trak'shun): A drawing back or backward. **R. OF NIPPLE**, frequently a sign of breast cancer.

retractor (rē-trak'tor): 1. An instrument for drawing apart the edges of a wound during surgery so as to expose the deeper structures or make them more accessible. 2. A muscle that draws a part backward.

retrad (rē'trad): Toward the back or posterior.

retro-: Combining form denoting: 1. Backward. 2. Located behind. 3. Contrary to a natural or ordinary course.

retroaction (ret'rō-ak'shun): Action in a direction that is the reverse of normal.

retroauricular (ret'rō-aw-rik'ū-lar): Behind the auricle of the external ear.

retrobuccal (ret'rō-buk'al): Pertinent to the back part of the mouth or cheek.

retrobulbar (ret'rō-bul'bar): 1. Behind the medulla oblongata. 2. Pertaining to or located at the back of the eyeball or behind it. **R. NEURITIS**, inflammation of that portion of the optic nerve behind the eyeball.

retrocalcaneobursitis (ret'rō-kal-kā'nē-ō-bur-sī'tis): Achillobursitis (*q.v.*).

retrocecal (ret'rō-sē'kal): Behind the cecum, *e.g.*, a retrocecal appendix.

retrocele (ret' -rō-sēl): Herniation of the rectum through the posterior vaginal wall.

retrocervical (ret'rō-ser'vi-kal): Behind the cervix of the uterus.

retrocession (ret-rō-sesh'un): 1. Going backward; a relapse. 2. A backward displacement, particularly of the uterus as a whole.

retrocolic (ret-rō-kol'ik): Behind the colon.

retrocollic (ret-rō-kol'lik): Relating to the back of the neck. **R. SPASM**, spasm of the muscles of the back of the neck.

retrocollis (ret-rō-kol'is): Retrocollic spasm in which the head is drawn backward.

retrocrural (ret-rō-krū'ral): Pertaining to the back of the leg. See **crus**.

retrodeviation (ret'rō-dē-vi-ā'shun): A bending backward.

retrodisplacement (ret'rō-dis-plās'ment): Backward displacement of an organ or part.

retroflexed (ret'rō-flext): Bent backwards.

retroflexion (ret-rō-flek'shun): The state of being bent backward, specifically the bending backward of the body of the uterus at an acute angle, the cervix remaining in its normal position. Opp. to anteflexion.—retroflexed, adj.

retrognathia (ret-rō-nath'i-a): The condition wherein the jaws are located back of the frontal plane of the forehead.—gnathic, adj.

retrograde (ret'rō-grād): Going backward. **R. AMNESIA**, loss of memory for events that occurred just before trauma, illness, or emotional shock. **R. CONDUCTION**, movement of impulses through the cardiac conduction system in a direction that is the reverse of the usual conduction pattern. **R. PYELOGRAPHY**, see **pyelography**.

retrography (ret-rog'ra-fi): Mirror writing.

retrogression (ret-rō-gresh'un): 1. Reversal in a condition or development. 2. Degeneration; catabolism.

retroinfection (ret'rō-in-fek'shun): Infection of the mother by the fetus.

retrolental (ret'-rō-len'tal): Behind the crystalline lens. **R. FIBROPLASIA**, the presence of fibrous tissue in the vitreous, from the retina to the lens, causing blindness. Noticed shortly after birth, more commonly in premature babies that have had continous oxygen therapy.

retrolingual (ret'rō-ling'gwal): Pertaining to the back of the tongue or the area behind it.

retroorbital (ret'rō-or'bit-al): Behind the orbit of the eye.

retroperitoneal (ret'rō-per-i-tō-nē'al): Behind the peritoneum. **R. SPACE,** the space between the posterior parietal peritoneum and the posterior abdominal wall; contains the kidneys and adrenal glands, the aorta, the vena cava, and the sympathetic nervous system trunk.

retroperitoneum (ret'rō-per-i-tō-ne'um): The space between the peritoneum and the posterior body wall.

retroperitonitis (ret'rō-per-i-tō-nī'tis): Inflammation of tissues in the peritoneal space.

retropharyngeal (ret'rō-fa-rin'jē-al): Behind the pharynx. **R. ABSCESS,** one between the pharynx and the spine.

retropharynx (ret'rō-far'inks): The posterior part of the pharynx.

retroplasia (ret'rō-plā'zi-a): Degeneration of a cell or tissue whereby lack of normal cellular activity results in reversion to an earlier more primitive form, or progresses to necrosis or death.

retroposed (ret'rō-pōzd): Displaced backward but not bent.

retropubic (ret-rō-pū'bik): Behind the pubis. **R. SPACE,** the space immediately above the pubis and between the peritoneum and the posterior side of the rectus abdominis muscle. Also called the space of Retzius.

retropulsion (ret-rō-pul'shun): 1. Forcing back of any part, *e.g.*, the fetal head during labor. 2. The involuntary tendency to walk backward as sometimes occurs in tabes dorsalis or Parkinson's disease.

retrospective (ret'-rō-spek'-tiv): Referring to or pertaining to things in the past. **R. CHART AUDIT,** an examination of patients' charts after care has been given; may take place while they are still in the hospital or after they have been discharged; the purpose is to evaluate the care in comparison to set standards. Nurses may conduct such an audit to evaluate effectiveness of the care that was given and alter their care plans for other patients accordingly. Or, examiners from the American Hospital Associations' Joint Commission on the Accreditation of Hospitals may conduct a retrospective study of patients' care, comparing it with standards set by the Commission for the accreditation of the institution.

retrospondylolisthesis (ret'rō-spon'di-lō-lis-thē'sis): The slipping of the body of a vertebra, making it out of alignment with the other vertebrae; occurs most commonly to a lumbar vertebra; may cause pressure on the spinal cord with resulting paraplegia.

retrosternal (ret-rō-ster'nal): Behind the breastbone.

retrosymphysial (ret-rō-sim-fiz'i-al): Behind the symphysis pubis.

retrotracheal (ret-rō-trā'kē-al): Behind the trachea.

retrouterine (ret-rō-ū'ter-in): Behind the uterus.

retroversioflexion (ret'rō-ver-sĭ-ō-flek'shun): Combined retroversion and retroflexion of the uterus.

retroversion (ret-rō-ver'zhun): Turning or tilting backward. **R. OF THE UTERUS,** tilting of the whole of the uterus and the cervix backward, with the cervix pointing forward; may be developmental, acquired after childbirth, or due to some pelvic pathology such as the presence of a cyst, tumor, or adhesions.

retrovirus (ret-rō-vī'-rus): Any of the *Retroviridae* family of complex viruses some of which induce the development of certain tumors, *e.g.*, lymphoma and sarcoma.

revaccination (rē'vaks-in-ā'shun): Vaccination of an individual who has been successfully vaccinated previously.

revascularization (rē-vas'kū-lar-ī-zā'shun): 1. The regrowth of blood vessels in a tissue or organ after deprivation of the normal blood supply. 2. The reestablishment of the blood supply to a part by the operation of grafting a blood vessel.

reverse isolation: See under isolation.

reversible brain syndrome: Also known as acute brain syndrome or delirium; caused by a variety of biological stressors and characterized by loss of cognition; recovery is possible.

reversion (rē-ver'zhun): 1. The appearance of an inherited characteristic in an individual after several generations in which it has not appeared. 2. A return to a previous state or condition.

Review of Systems: A procedure begun on an individual's admission to a health care facility when the initial interview and the physical examination take place. The examiner makes observations and interviews both the patient and significant others about the patient's various anatomical systems, with particular emphasis on any abnormalities and past or present disorders, starting usually with the skin, then the head, torso, and extremities. This important procedure provides information that all health care personnel who will be giving care to the patient need in making diagnoses and planning care.

Reye's syndrome: A rare, acute, and often fatal illness of children from birth to about age 17. Often follows recovery from a mild virus infection such as chickenpox or flu; is marked by fever, explosive and repetitive vomiting, encephalopathy, and fatty degeneration of the liver; occurs most often in spring and winter; cause unknown; apparently not contagious.

Rh: Symbol of Rhesus, rhesus blood groups in particular.

Rh factor: Rhesus factor. See under rhesus.

Rh hemolytic disease: Erythroblastosis fetalis. See erythroblastosis.

Rh incompatibility: See Rhesus.

Rh sensitivity: The state of being or becoming sensitized to the Rh factor, *e.g.*, as happens when an Rh-negative woman is pregnant with an Rh-positive fetus. See blood groups.

Rhabditis: A genus of small nematode worms, some of which are parasitic to man.

rhabdo-: Combining form denoting rod-shaped, or relationship to a rod.

rhabdocyte (rab′dō-sīt): A band cell; see under cell.

rhabdomyolysis (rab′dō-mī-ol′i-sis): An acute, fulminating disease characterized by destruction of skeletal muscle, accompanied by myoglobulinemia and myoglobulinuria.

rhabdomyoma (rab′dō-mī-ō′ma): A benign tumor of striated muscle cells.

rhabdomyosarcoma (rab′dō-mī-ō-sar-kō′ma): A rare malignant tumor, usually involving the striated muscle cells of the muscles of the extremities and the torso; grows rapidly and metastasizes early.

rhachi-, rhachio-: For words beginning thus see words beginning rachi- and rachio-.

rhacoma (ra-kō′ma): Relaxation of the integument of the scrotum, causing it to become pendulant.

rhagades (rag′a-dēz): Cracks or fissures in the skin, especially around a body orifice, seen in vitamin deficiences and syphilis. When they occur around the nares and mouth in cases of congenital syphilis, they leave superficial elongated scars that are pathognomic for the disease.

-rhage, -rrhage, -rrhagia: Combining forms denoting hemorrhage, a bursting forth, or profuse flow.

-rhaphy, -rrhaphy: Combining forms denoting a joining together in a seam; suturing.

-rhea, -rrhea, -rrhoea: Combining forms denoting flow, discharge.

rhegma (reg′ma): A rupture, fracture, or tear.

rheo-: Combining form denoting flow, or relation to electricity.

rheobase (rē′ō-bās): The minimum voltage required to stimulate a tissue if allowed to flow through it for an adequate time.

rheocardiology (rē′ō-kar-di-ol′o-ji): The technique of measuring and recording the changes in electric conductivity of the body during the cardiac cycle.

rheocythemia (rē′ō-sī-thē′mi-a): The presence of degenerated red blood cells in the peripheral circulation.

rheoencephalography (rē′ō-en-sef-a-log′ra-fi): The measurement of blood flow through the brain.

rheometer (rē-om′e-ter): An instrument for 1) measuring the flow of viscous substances, such as blood, or 2) a galvanometer (*q.v.*).

rheophore (rē′ō-fōr): A cord conducting an electric current, particularly as between a patient and an electrical apparatus; an electrode.

rheoscope (rē′ō-skōp): A device for detecting the existence of an electric current.

rheostat (rē′ō-stat): An apparatus for regulating the resistance in an electric current.

rheotome (rē′ō-tōm): A device for interrupting an electric current at specified intervals.

rheotometry (rē-ō-tom′e-tri): The measurement of blood flow.

Rhesus (rē′sus): A genus of monkey from India much used in medical research and experimentation; *macaca mulatta*. **R. FACTOR,** usually called Rh factor, a substance with antigenic properties that is present in the red blood cells of most people. Blood that has this factor is designated as Rh positive and that which does not is designated Rh negative. If a person with Rh negative blood is given Rh positive blood in transfusion, antibodies develop in the recipient's blood and, in the event of a second transfusion, will cause agglutination of red cells and severe reaction in the patient. If a fetus with Rh positive blood has a mother with Rh negative blood, some of the Rh positive blood enters the mother's bloodstream via the placenta; her blood builds up antibodies against this substance and they enter the fetus's circulation (again via the placenta) where they cause destruction of the red blood cells and the development of erythroblastosis fetalis (*q.v.*) in the infant.

rheum (room): A watery discharge from a mucous membrane, of the nose and eyes in particular.

rheumarthritis (roo-mar-thrī′tis): Rheumatism affecting chiefly the joints.

rheumatalgia (roo-ma-tal′ji-a): Rheumatic pain.

rheumatic (roo-mat′ik): Pertaining to or affected by rheumatism. **R. FACTOR,** an antibody that reacts against human globulin; is diagnostic for rheumatic arthritis when it can be demonstrated in the blood serum. **R. FEVER,** see acute rheumatism. **R. HEART DISEASE,** a serious form of rheumatic fever, consisting of inflammatory changes and damaged heart valves; may occur as an accompaniment to or sequela of that disease; usually involves the endocardium, including the mitral valve, the myocardium, and the pericardium. The heart may be seriously and permanently damaged. A frequent cause of death in children and young adults.

rheumatid (roo′ma-tid): A nodule or other skin eruption that may accompany rheumatism.

rheumatism (roo'ma-tizm): A non-specific term embracing a diverse group of diseases and syndromes that have, in common, disorder or disease of connective tissue and hence usually present with pain, or stiffness, or swelling of muscles and joints. The main groups are rheumatic fever, rheumatoid arthritis, ankylosing spondylitis, nonarticular rheumatism, osteoarthritis and gout. **ACUTE R.** (rheumatic fever), a disorder tending to recur but initially commonest in childhood, classically presenting as fleeting polyarthritis of the larger joints, pyrexia and carditis within 3 weeks following a streptococcal throat infection. Atypically, but not infrequently, the symptoms are trivial and ignored, but carditis may be severe and result in permanent cardiac damage; the most common cause of mitral stenosis in later life because of scar tissue resulting from inflammation of the valve. **GONORRHEAL R.**, that which results from a systemic infection with the gonococcus. **INFLAMMATORY R.**, an acute form (**R.** fever) that tends to affect the heart. **LUMBAR R.**, lumbago. **MUSCULAR R.**, term for a number of muscle conditions characterized by pain, tenderness and local spasm; includes myalgia, myositis, fibromyositis, torticollis. **NONARTICULAR R.**, involves the soft tissues; includes fibrositis. **OSSEOUS R.**, arthritis deformans, see under **arthritis**. **PALINDROMIC R.**, a condition characterized by irregularly occurring attacks of afebrile arthritis and periarthritis of only one joint, which becomes red and swollen; the symptoms disappear within a short time without producing lasting deformity of the joint. **TUBERCULOUS R.**, inflammation of the joints due to the toxins of the tubercle bacillus.

rheumatoid (rōō'ma-toyd): Resembling rheumatism. **R. ARTHRITIS**, a chronic disease of unknown etiology, characterized by polyarthritis affecting mainly the smaller peripheral joints, accompanied by general ill health and resulting eventually in varying degrees of ankylosis, crippling joint deformities, and associated muscle wasting; see **Still's disease**. **R. FACTOR**, a factor found in the serum of patients with rheumatoid arthritis; laboratory tests for its presence are useful in diagnosis.

rheumatologist (roo-ma-tol'ō-jist): A physician who specializes in rheumatic conditions.

rheumatology (roo-ma-tol'ō-ji): The study of rheumatic diseases.

rhexis (rek'sis):Rupture or bursting of an organ, blood vessel, or tissue.

rhigosis (ri-gō'sis): The perception of the sensation of cold.

rhin-, rhino-: Combining forms denoting the nose.

rhinal (rī'nal): Pertaining to the nose.

rhinalgia (rī-nal'-ji-a): Pain in the nose.

rhinallergosis (rīn'al-er-gō'sis): Allergic rhinitis.

rhinedema (rī'nē-dē'ma): Swelling of the nose or of the nasal mucosa.

rhinelcos (rī-nel'kōs): An ulcer in the nose.

rhinencephalon (rī'nen-sef'a-lon): The part of the cerebral cortex concerned with the reception and interpretation of olfactory stimuli.—rhinencephalic, adj.

rhinenchysis (rī-nen'kī-sis): 1. The instillation of a medication into the nose. 2. The washing out of the nasal cavity; nasal douche.

rhiniatry (rī-nī'a-tri): The treatment of nasal defects and disorders of the nose.

rhinism (rī'nizm): A nasal quality of voice; rhinolalia.

rhinitis (rī-nī'tis): Inflammation of the nasal mucous membrane. **ACUTE R.**, coryza; the common cold. **ALLERGENIC R.**, **R.** caused by any effective allergen such as a pollen; usually seasonal but may be perennial. **R. MEDICAMENTOSA**, inflammation of the nasal mucosa resulting from overuse or improper use of topical medications. **VASOMOTOR R.**, congestion of the nasal mucosa that is noninfectious and nonseasonal; catarrh.

rhinoantritis (rī'nō-an-trī'tis): Inflammation of the nose and either or both of the maxillary sinuses.

rhinobyon (rī-nō'bi-on): A nasal tampon or plug.

rhinocanthectomy (rī'nō-kan-thek'tō-mi): Excision of the inner canthus of the eye.

rhinocheiloplasty (rī-nō-kī'lō-plas-ti): Plastic surgery on the nose and upper lip. Also rhinochiloplasty.

rhinocleisis (rī-nō-klī'sis): Any obstruction in the nasal passageways.

rhinodacryolith (rī-nō-dak'ri-ō-lith): A lacrimal concretion formed in the nasal duct.

rhinodynia (rī-nō-din'i-a): Pain in the nose; rhinalgia.

rhinogenous (rī-noj'e-nus): Originating or arising in the nose.

rhinokyphectomy (rī'nō-kī-fek'to-mi): A plastic operation to remove an abnormal hump on the nose.

rhinokyphosis (rī'nō-kī-fō'sis): The presence of an excessively prominent hump on the bridge of the nose.

rhinolalia (rī'nō-lā' -li-a): Having a voice of nasal quality due to some defect of structure or pathology of the nose.

rhinolaryngitis (rī'nō-lar-in-jī'tis): Inflammation of the mucous membrane of the nose and of the larynx, occurring at the same time.

rhinolaryngology (rī'nō-lar-in-gol'ō-ji): The branch of medicine that deals with diseases of the nose and larynx.

rhinolith (rī'nō-lith): A stone that has formed in the nasal passage.

rhinolithiasis (rī'nō-li-thī'a-sis): A condition marked by the formation of nasal stones.

rhinology (rī-nol'o-ji): That branch of medical science that has to do with the nose and pathological conditions of the nose.

rhinomiosis (rī' -nō-mī-ō'sis): A plastic operation for reducing the size of the nose.

rhinomycosis (rī'nō-mī-kō'sis): A fungal infection of the mucous membrane of the nose.

rhinonecrosis (rī'nō-nē-krō'sis): Necrosis of the nasal bones.

rhinopathy (rī-nop'a-thi): Any disease of the nose or nasal structures.

rhinopharyngitis (rī'nō-far'jī'tis): Inflammation of the posterior nares and the upper part of the pharynx.

rhinopharyngocele (rī'nō-far-ing'gō-sēl): A tumor situated in the nasopharynx.

rhinopharyngolith (rī'nō-far-ing'gō-lith): A stone in the nasopharynx.

rhinopharynx (rī'nō-făr'inks): The upper part of the pharynx which lies above the soft palate and communicates with the nasal cavity; the nasopharynx.

rhinophonia (rī'nō-fō'ni-a): Having a voice of nasal quality. Rhinolalia (*q.v.*).

rhinophycomycosis (rī'nō-fī-kō-mī-kō'sis): A fungal infection in which polyps form in the subcutaneous tissues of the nose and sinuses; may extend to paranasal sinuses, the cerebrum, and to the eye, causing blindness.

rhinophyma (rī'nō-fī'ma): A form of rosacea (*q.v.*) characterized by nodular swellings or tumors of the skin of the nose, red coloration, and congestion. May also be called toper's ncse, rum or brandy nose, and rum blossom.

rhinoplasty (rī'nō-plas-ti): Plastic surgery to alter the shape or size of the nose or to repair a defect.

rhinopolypus (rī-nō-pol'i-pus): A polyp on the mucous membrane of the nose.

rhinoreaction (rī'nō-rē-ak'shun): An exudation that appears on the nasal mucous membrane after the application of a tuberculin solution if the individual is affected with tuberculosis.

rhinorrhagia (rī-nō-rā'ji-a): Nosebleed.

rhinorrhea (rī-nō-rē'a): 1. Free discharge of thin watery mucus from the nose. 2. The escape of cerebrospinal fluid through the nose.

rhinosalpingitis (rī'nō-sal-pin-jī'tis): Inflammation of the nasal mucosa and the auditory tube.

rhinoscleroma (rī'nō-sklē-rō'ma): A chronic infectious condition involving the nose, upper lip, and mouth; starts with the development of hard nodules in the nose and extends to the pharynx, larynx, trachea, and bronchi.

rhinoscopy (rī-nos'ko-pi): Examination of the nose by means of an instrument called a rhinoscope.

rhinosporidiosis (rī'nō-spō-rid-i-ō'sis): A fungal infection caused by the *Rhinosporidium,* characterized by the persistent formation of polypi on the mucous membranes of the nose, nasopharynx, soft palate, trachea, larynx, and occasionally the genitalia and conjunctiva. Seen chiefly in India, Pakistan, Ceylon, but also in North and South America.

rhinostenosis (rī'nō-sten-ō'sis): Narrowing or constriction of the nasal passages.

rhinotomy (rī-not'o-mi): Any cutting operation on or in the nose.

rhinotracheitis (rī'nō-trāk-ē-ī'tis): Inflammation of the nasal mucosa and the trachea.

rhinovaccination (rī'nō-vak-si-nā'shun): The application of an immunizing material to the mucous membrane of the nose.

rhinovirus (rī'nō-vī'rus): Any one of a large group of viruses considered to be the cause of common colds. More than 100 varieties have been identified.

rhitid-: For words beginning thus see those beginning **rhytid-**.

rhizo-: Combining form denoting relationship to a root.

rhizoid (rī'zoyd): Resembling a root.

rhizomeningomyelitis (rī'zō-me-nin'gō-mī-e-lī'tis): Radiculomeningomeningitis (*q.v.*).

rhizotomy (rī-zot'o-mi): Surgical division of a root, especially that of a nerve. **ANTERIOR R.,** sectioning of the anterior root of a spinal nerve for the relief of essential hypertension. **POSTERIOR R.,** sectioning of the posterior root of a spinal nerve for the relief of intractable pain. **CHEMICAL R.,** accomplished by injection of a chemical, often phenol.

rhodogenesis (rō-dō-jen'e-sis): The restoration of visual purple to the rhodopsin after it has been bleached by exposure to light.

rhodopsin (rō-dop'sin): The visual purple contained in the retinal rods. Its color is preserved in darkness and bleached by daylight. Formation of rhodopsin is dependent on vitamin A.

rhombencephalon (rom-ben-sef'a-lon): The hind-brain or after-brain; includes the pons, cerebellum, and medulla oblongata.

rhomboid (rom'boyd): A parallelogram in which the angles are oblique and the adjacent sides unequal.

rhomboideus (rom-boy'dē-us): One of the two large muscles of the upper back; they lie under the trapezii and act to draw the scapula upward and toward the median line and to rotate it.

rhonchus (rong'kus): 1. A whistling, turbulent, rattling, rumbling, or sonorous sound heard on auscultation when there is exudate or fluid in the bronchi. 2. A rattling in the throat. See sibilus.—rhonchi, pl.; rhonchial, rhonchal, adj.

Rhus (roos): A large genus of trees and shrubs; includes some that have leaves containing an oil that causes dermatitis on contact with the skin, *e.g.*, poison ivy, poison oak, and poison sumac.

-rhysis: A combining form denoting a flowing out.

rhythm (rith′em): The regular recurrence of a similar feature, action, or situation, *e.g.*, the heartbeat. ALPHA R., rhythm seen as uniform waves on the normal electroencephalogram when the subject's eyes are closed and the brain is at relative rest; average frequency is about 10 per second. BETA R., a rhythm of smaller and faster waves, also seen on the EEG; the average frequency is about 25 per second. BIOLOGIC R., cyclic variations in level of activity, physical and chemical functions of the body, and emotional states. CIRCADIAN R., R. having a cycle of 24 hours. CIRCAMENSUAL R. R. having a cycle of about 30 days. CIRCANNUAL R., R. having a cycle of about one year. CIRCASEPTAL R., R. having a cycle of about seven days. CIRCATRIGINTAN R., R. having a cycle of about 30 days. CIRCAVAGINTAN R., R. having a cycle of about 20 days. DIURNAL R., R. in which fluctuations are confined to the working day. GALLOP R., is of two types: 1) ventricular G., R. that is marked by a three-sound sequence in which two heartbeats occur close together followed by a third louder sound, the sound resembling that of a galloping horse; and 2) atrial R., R. in which a fourth sound is heard when the atrium contracts in resistance to ventricular filling. IDEOVENTRICULAR R., a slow ventricular rhythm controlled by an ectopic center in the ventricle independently of the atrial rhythm. INFRADIAN R., R. having a cycle longer than 28 hours; may be weeks or months. NODAL R., R. initiated in the atrioventricular node and the main bundle of His. R. METHOD, see under method. SINUS R., normal heart rhythm as initiated by electrical impulses in the sinoatrial node. THETA R., the theta wave in the electroencephalogram; see under wave. ULTRADIAN R., R. having a cycle of less than 24 hours.—rhythmic, rhythmical, adj.

rhythmicity (rith-mis′i-ti): The property of rhythmic recurrence of an action or situation. In cardiology, the natural ability of the heart to beat rhythmically.

rhytidectomy (rit-i-dek′to-mi): The surgical removal of wrinkles. Face-lifting. Also called rhytidoplasty.

rhytidosis (rit-i-dō′sis): 1. Wrinkling of the skin of the face. 2. Wrinkling of the cornea. Also spelled rhitidosis.

rib: Any one of the paired bones, 12 on either side, which articulate with the twelve dorsal vertebrae posteriorly and form the walls of the thorax. The upper seven pairs are TRUE R. and are attached to the sternum anteriorly by costal cartilage. The remaining five pairs are the FALSE R. The first three pairs of these do not have an attachment to the sternum but are bound to each other by costal cartilage. The lower two pairs are the FLOATING R. which have no anterior articulation. CERVICAL R. are formed by an extension of the transverse process of the seventh cervical vertebra in the form of bone or a fibrous tissue band; this causes an upward displacement of the subclavian artery; a congenital abnormality. R. CAGE, the bony thorax; consists of the sternum, ribs, and thoracic vertebrae.

riboflavin (rī′bō-flā′vin): Vitamin B_6, a member of the vitamin B complex. Essential for growth and good vision; aids in digestion and carbohydrate metabolism. Found in liver, milk, eggs, kidney, lean meats, malt, yeast, green leafy vegetables, whole grain and enriched flour and cereals; also synthesized. Deficiency may result in lowered resistance and vitality, cracks at corners of mouth and lesions on lips, glossitis, anemia, retarded growth, photophobia, cataracts.

ribonuclease (rī′bō-nū′klē-ās): An enzyme present in various body tissues; is responsible for the breakdown of ribonucleic acid.

ribonucleic acid (RNA) (rī′bō-nū-klē′ik as′id): A nucleic acid substance found in the nucleus and cytoplasm of all living cells and in many viruses; an intermediate of deoxyribonucleic acid (DNA) and the medium by which genetic instructions from the chromosomes in the nucleus are transmitted to the rest of the cell. It is also an important factor in the synthesis of protein within the cells. Differences in the molecular structure of the RNA particles determine the difference between messenger RNA which is believed to transmit the genetic code from the nucleus to the cytoplasm of the cells and transfer RNA which carries amino acid from the nucleus to the ribosomes (*q.v.*) for protein synthesis.

ribonucleoprotein (rī′bō-nū′klē-ō-prō′te-in): Any of a large group of complex molecules which, on hydrolysis, yield ribonucleic acid and protein.

ribose (rī′bōs): A pentose sugar occurring in riboflavin and ribonucleic acids.

ribosome (rī′bō-sōm): One of the small complex particles within the cytoplasm of living cells that contain ribonucleic acid and various proteins, and which synthesize protein within the cell.

ribosuria (rī-bō-sū′ri-a): The presence of ribose in the urine; occurs especially in patients with muscular dystrophy.

rice diet: See under diet.

rice-water stool: The stool of cholera. The "rice grains" are small pieces of desquamated epithelium from the intestine.

Richards, Linda: Credited for being the first "trained nurse" in America; the first graduate of the first training school for nurses at the New England Hospital for Women and Children, established in 1872. [1841–1930.]

ricin (rī′sin): A poisonous substance found in the seeds of the castor bean plant from which castor oil is derived.

ricinism (ris′i-nizm): Poisoning by ricin or castor oil.

Ricinus (ris′i-nus): A genus of plants including the castor plant, the seeds of which are the source of castor oil.

rickets (rik′ets): A disorder of calcium and phosphorus metabolism associated with a deficiency of vitamin D, and beginning most often between the ages of 6 months and 2 years. There is proliferation and deficient ossification of the growing epiphyses of bones, producing bossing, softening and bending of the long weight-bearing bones, muscular hypotonia, head sweating, delayed closure of the fontanelles, degeneration of the liver and spleen and, if the blood calcium falls sufficiently, tetany. **FETAL R.**, see achondroplasia. **RENAL R.**, condition of decalcification of bones (osteoporosis) associated with chronic kidney disease and clinically simulating **R.** It occurs in later age groups than **R.**, and is due to retention of phosphorus in the blood, which prevents absorption of calcium, and is characterized by excessive calcium loss in the urine.

Rickettsia (ri-ket′si-a): A group of small parasitic gram-negative, non-filterable microorganisms that are like bacteria in some ways and like viruses in others. Their natural habitat is the gut of arthropods such as lice, mites, ticks, fleas. They are the vectors of many diseases, transmitting the organisms to man through their bites. One clinical classification, based on groups of *Rickettsiae* according to the diseases they cause, lists four groups: 1. Typhus group, the causative agents in epidemic and endemic typhus. 2. Spotted fever group, the causative agents in Rocky Mountain spotted fever, boutonneuse fever, and rickettsial-pox. 3. Tsutsugamushi group, the causative agents in Tsutsugamuchi disease and in both rural and scrub typhus. 4. Miscellaneous group, the causative agents in trench fever and Q fever.

rickettsialpox (ri-ket′si-al-poks): An acute self-limited febrile disease resembling chickenpox; caused by the bite of a mite that infests house mice. Characterized by chills, fever, myalgia, headache, and a papulovesicular rash; a papule forms at the site of the bite, vesicates, and becomes escharotic. Usually nonfatal.

rickettsiosis (ri-ket-si-ō′sis): Infection with Rickettsia.

rickety (rik′i-ti): Suffering from rickets. **R. ROSARY**, see under rachitic.

RICU: Abbreviation for respiratory intensive care unit.

Riedel: [Bernhard M.C.L. Riedel, German physician. 1846–1916.] **RIEDEL'S LOBE**, a congenital elongation that extends downward from the right lobe of the liver. **RIEDEL'S DISEASE**, thyroiditis associated with enlargement and hardening of the thyroid tissues, which become adherent to surrounding structures, causing pressure on the trachea; a rare condition, often fatal. To be differentiated from cancer of the thyroid.

Rift Valley fever: A highly infectious, virulent, viral disease, primarily of animals but transmissible to humans through many species of mosquitoes or the handling of infected animals; marked by headache, malaise, myalgia, pain in the bones, encephalitis, liver damage, retinitis that can lead to blindness. Seen particularly in certain parts of Africa and the Near East.

Rigg's disease: See periodontitis.

right to die: Refers to a debatable issue concerning the employment by others for "mercy killing" or "involuntary euthanasia" when an individual cannot make that decision because of being in a condition such as irreversible coma, or of having suffered "brain death" and hence cannot be expected to recover.

Right to Life movement: A movement with the primary purpose of prohibiting abortion, by whatever means, including legislation; based on the idea that life begins at conception.

righting reflex: See under reflex.

rigid (rij′id): Firm; hard; unyielding; inflexible.

rigidity (ri-jid′i-ti): Stiffness, inflexibility or rigor, particularly that which is abnormal or pathological. **DECEREBRATE R.**, rigid contraction of the extensor and other muscles involved in maintaining the standing position; due to a lesion in the brain stem. **COGWHEEL R.**, muscle **R.** that progresses from rhythmic jerky movements to passive stretching. **HEMIPLEGIC R.**, **R.** of the paralyzed limbs in paraplegia. **LEAD-PIPE R.**, the muscular rigidity seen in persons with Parkinson's disease. **POSTMORTEM R.**, see rigor mortis under rigor. See also decorticate posture under decorticate.

rigor (rig′or): 1. Stiffness, rigidity. 2. A sudden chill, accompanied by severe shivering. The body temperature rises rapidly and remains high until perspiration ensues and causes a gradual fall in temperature. **R. MORTIS**, the stiffening of the body after death.

Riley-Day syndrome: Familial dysautonomia. A condition characterized by many symptoms of disturbances of the autonomic nervous system. See **dysautonomia.**

rima (rī'ma): A slit, cleft, or fissure between two like parts. **R. GLOTTIDIS,** the slit between the free margins of the vocal cords. **R. PALPEBRARUM,** the slit between the eyelids when the eye is closed.—rimal, adj.

rimose (rīm'os): Fissured; having many cracks going in all directions.

rimula (rim'ū-la): A very small crack or fissure, particularly one in the brain or spinal cord.

ring: In chemistry, a closed chain of atoms in a cyclic compound, *e.g.*, the benzene **R.** In anatomy, a more or less circular structure that surrounds an opening or an area. **EXTERNAL INGUINAL R.,** the opening in the fascia of the transversalis muscle through which the vas deferens or the round ligament passes into the inguinal canal. **INTERNAL INGUINAL R.,** the opening in the aponeurosis of the external oblique muscle through which the spermatic cord or round ligament passes. **WALDEYER'S R.,** the ring of lymphoid tissue in the throat; made up of the lingual, palatine, and pharyngeal tonsils.

Ringer's solution: A sterile isotonic solution containing a mixture of sodium chloride, potassium chloride, and calcium chloride in distilled water; used as a fluid and electrolyte replenisher. **LACTATED RINGER'S SOLUTION,** contains sodium chloride, sodium lactate, potassium chloride, and calcium chloride in distilled water; it has the same uses as Ringer's solution. Also called Hartmann's solution.

ringworm: A broad general term used to describe a group of diseases of the skin and its appendages; caused by a fungus. So called because the common manifestations are circular, scaly patches. See **tinea** and **mycosis.**

Rinne test: Testing of air conduction and bone conduction hearing, by tuning fork. Discriminates between conduction and sensorineural deafness. [Heinrich Rinne, German otologist. 1819–1868.]

RISA: Abbreviation for radio-iodinated serum albumin.

risk: A hazard; the possibility of harm. **R. FACTOR,** an element that increases the possibility or likelihood of harm or of a harmful occurrence.

Risser jacket: A specialized body cast used in correcting structural scoliosis; employs a spica jacket which usually incorporates the head and sometimes the arm; the cast is split on the side of the curve and a turnbuckle is incorporated into the two halves; as the two parts of the cast are opened out by the turnbuckle, correction takes place; when this is accomplished spinal fusion may be performed through a window in the jacket.

risus sardonicus (rī'sus sar-don'i-kus): An expression resembling a grin, caused by spasm of facial muscles; seen in tetanus.

ritual (rich'ū-al): In psychiatry, any psychomotor activity that a person persists in performing when there is no need for it; a means of relieving anxiety. See **obsessional neurosis.**

RLF: Abbreviation for retrolental fibroplasia.

RLQ: Abbreviation for right lower quadrant (of the abdomen).

R.N.: Abbreviation for Registered Nurse. See under **nurse.**

RNA: Abbreviation for ribonucleic acid (*q.v.*).

Robertson's pupil: See **Argyll Robertson pupil.**

Robert's Law of Progression: Describes a condition occurring in the elderly in whom early forgetfulness increases progressively until the individual cannot remember recent events whether or not they are important to his life and safety, but may remember earlier events clearly; the resulting development of hostility and resentment has a marked effect on the person's behavior.

Rochelle salt: Potassium sodium tartrate, formerly much used as a saline cathartic.

Rocky Mountain spotted fever: An infectious rickettsial disease formerly thought to be confined to the Rocky Mountain area, but now known to occur in many parts of the Western hemisphere. It is transmitted by the bite of an infected tick or by contamination of the broken skin with the crushed tissues or feces of an infected tick. It is characterized by fever, headache, conjunctivitis, and a maculopapular rash. Also called Colorado tick fever, tick fever, and spotted fever.

rod: In anatomy, a slender mass of substance, specifically the rodlike bodies found in the retina. See also **cone; Harrington rod.**

rodent (rō'dent): A gnawing animal. **R. ULCER;** see **basal-cell carcinoma.**

rodonalgia (rō-dō-nal'ji-a): A condition characterized by cutaneous vasodilatation of the blood vessels of the feet and sometimes of the hand, causing redness, mottling, neuralgic pain, swelling, and increase in skin temperature of the extremities. Also called erythromelalgia and acromelalgia.

roentgen (rent'gen): The original international unit used in measuring dosage of x or gamma rays. **R. RAYS,** x rays; see **rad.** [Wilhelm Konrad von Roentgen, German physicist. 1845–1923.]

roentgenism (rent'gen-izm): 1. Disease or disorder caused by overexposure to x rays. 2. The use of x rays for therapeutic purposes.

roentgenkymography (rent'gen-kī-mog'ra-fi): Recording the movements of the heart and other organs by means of the x-ray kymograph; see **kymograph.**

roentgenocinematography (rent'gen-ō-sin'-e-ma-tog'ra-fi): Cinematography of x-ray images to show movements of internal organs.

roentgenogram (rent′gen-ō-gram): The shadow picture that is produced on specially sensitized film by roentgen rays or by a radioactive body. Radiograph.

roentgenography (rent′gen-og′ra-fi): Examination of a part of the body by means of a photograph made by exposure of the part to roentgen rays. See **radiography**.

roentgenologist (rent′ge-nol′ō-jist): One skilled in the use of roentgen rays for diagnostic and therapeutic purposes.

roentgenology (rent′ge-nol′ō-ji): The study of the roentgen rays and their diagnostic and therapeutic uses.

rolandic (rō-lan′dik): Pertaining to structures first described by Rolando. **R. AREA,** the area in the cortex of the cerebrum that is concerned with control of motor activities. **R. FISSURE,** the boundary between the frontal and parietal lobes of the cerebrum. [Luigi Rolando, Italian anatomist. 1773–1831.]

role: The kind of behavior expected of a person because of his particular place in his social setting or situation, *e.g.,* the mother's role, nurse's role, etc. Every person assumes or fulfills more than one role on occasion or as demanded by his situation, *e.g.,* the mother role and the nurse role may be enacted simultaneously.

rolfing: A technique, developed by Dr. Ida Rolf, a chemist, based on the theory that the body is not a unit but an aggregate of large structures. It involves manipulating the muscles of the body with the purpose of helping the individual to establish relationships between deep structures that will result in symmetrical balanced functioning of the body when upright.

Rollier's treatment: A method of treating tuberculosis of the joints by exposure to the ultraviolet rays in sunlight; now obsolete.

ROM: Abbreviation for range of motion.

romanopexy (rō-man′ō-pek-si): The surgical procedure of fixing the sigmoid flexure in place to correct prolapse of the rectum.

Romberg: [Mortiz Romberg, German neurologist. 1795–1873.] **ROMBERG'S DISEASE,** facial hemiatrophy, usually progressive and may involve most of the structures of the face. Symptoms may appear early in childhood along with epilepsy, trigeminal neuralgia, and alopecia; reconstructive surgery and orthodontia are often used successfully. **ROMBERG'S SIGN,** a sign of ataxia (*q.v.*); inability to stand erect without swaying when the eyes are closed and the feet together; also called rombergism, Romberg's phenomenon, and Romberg's test.

rongeur (ron-zhur′): A type of forceps designed for cutting bone.

roof: A top covering membrane or structure. **R. OF THE MOUTH,** the bony and muscular structure between the nasal and oral cavities; the palate.

rooming-in: The practice of keeping the neonate in a crib at the mother's bedside for most of the 24 hours; said to have psychological and physical advantages for both mother and infant and to facilitate "on demand" feeding and bonding.

root: In anatomy, 1) the base, foundation, origin, beginning, or lowest part of a structure; 2) the embedded part of a structure; or 3) the proximal end of a nerve. **R. OF THE LUNG,** the bronchus, pulmonary artery and veins, plexuses of pulmonary nerves, lymphatic vessels and lymph nodes, all of which are embedded in mediastinal tissue with the mass entering the lung at the hilus, thus forming the root.

rooting reflex: See under **reflex**.

ROP: Abbreviation for right occipitoparietal (position of the fetus).

Rorschach test (ror′shahk): A psychologic test that also measures the elements of personality; consists of a series of ink blots, which the patient is told to look at and then simply tell what he sees. [Herman Rorschach, Swiss psychiatrist. 1884–1922.]

ROS: Review of systems. A review of the various body systems and the state of their functioning; part of an initial physical examination.

rosacea (rō-zā′shē-a): A chronic skin disease affecting the nose particularly; marked by flushing due to chronic dilatation of the capillaries, often complicated by the appearance of papules and acne-like pustules. Called also acne rosacea, acne erythematosa, brandy face, rum nose, rum blossom. Occurs most often in adult males.

rosaceiform (rō-zā′shē-i-form): Resembling acne rosacea; see under **acne**.

rosary: **RACHITIC R.,** rachitic bead; see under **rachitic**.

rose bengal test: A test for measuring the level of liver activity. A saline solution of rose bengal (a dye) is injected intravenously; under normal conditions it disappears from the blood rapidly; a delay in its disappearance indicates diminished liver activity.

rose cold, rose fever: Seasonal allergy that occurs in the spring or early summer, due to pollens. Symptoms are those of a common cold.

rose spots: The rose-colored papular eruption that appears on the abdomen and loins during the first week of typhoid and paratyphoid fevers; the spots disappear on pressure.

roseola (rō-zē-ō′la): A rose- or scarlet colored rash. **EPIDEMIC R.,** rubella (*q.v.*). **R. INFANTUM,** exanthem subitum, see under **exanthem**. **SYPHILITIC R.,** the rose-colored eruption of early secondary syphilis; usually appears 6–12 weeks after the initial lesion of the disease; spreads over most of the body except for the skin of the hands and face.—roseolous, adj.

Rose-Waaler test: A serological test formerly much used in the diagnosis of rheumatoid arthritis. The presence of rheumatoid factor is detected in the serum by the agglutination of sheep's red blood cells sensitized with rabbit gamma globulin.

rosin (roz'in): The solid resin obtained from several species of pine trees; used in plasters and ointments.

rostellum (ros-tel'um): The anterior part of the head of a tapeworm, a fleshy protrusion with one or more rows of hook-like processes.

rostrate (ros'trāt): Having a beak-like appendage or process.

rostrum (ros'trum): A beak-like or hook-like process.—rostral, adj.

ROT: Abbreviation for right occipitotransverse (position of the fetus).

rot: To decay or decompose.

rotary (rō'-ta-ri): 1. Pertaining to or causing rotation. 2. Resembling a body in rotation. **R. NYSTAGMUS,** rotation of the eyeball around part of the visual axis.

rotate (rō'tāt): To turn about on an axis.

rotating tourniquet: See under tourniquet.

rotation (rō-tā'shun): 1. The act of turning about on an axis that passes through the center of the body, as **R.** of the head. 2. The turning of the fetus' head as it accommodates to the contours of the birth canal. **EXTERNAL R.,** turning the anterior surfaces of a limb outward. **INTERNAL R.,** turning the anterior surface of a limb inward or medially.

rotator (rō'tā-tor): A muscle having the action of turning a part.

rotator cuff: Name given to the tendinous cuff over the shoulder; consists of the upper half of the shoulder joint capsule and the insertion tendons of the supraspinatous, infraspinatous, teres minor, and scapularis muscles; it helps to stabilize the joint. **ROTATOR CUFF INJURIES,** injuries that result from improper overhead or swing motion; occurs in those engaging in such sports as tennis, baseball, volleyball, or softball; also called rotator cuff impingement syndrome.

rotavirus (rō-ta-vī'rus): A recently recognized virus resembling reovirus (*q.v.*); found worldwide; an important cause of infant diarrhea, spread by oral-fecal route.

Rothmund-Thomson syndrome: See poikiloderma congenitale.

Roto-Rest: A bed that automatically turns the patient 60 degrees every 9 minutes; often used to relieve skin pressure, particularly in spinal-cord injured persons.

rotula (rot'ū-la): 1. The patella or any simliar disk-like bony structure. 2. A troche or lozenge.—rotular, adj.

roughage (ruf'ij): Coarse food such as unprocessed bran, fresh fruit, and vegetables, which contain much indigestible fibre composed of cellulose. It provides bulk in the diet and by this means helps to stimulate peristalsis and eliminate waste products. Lack of **R.** may cause atonic constipation. Too much **R.** may cause spastic constipation.

rouleau (roo'lō): A row of red blood cells, resembling a roll of coins.—rouleaux, pl.

round ligament: The ligament that passes from the anterior cornu of the uterus forward and downward through the folds of the broad ligament and the inguinal canal and inserts into the subcutaneous fat of the labia; its function is to help hold the uterus in its proper position of anteversion and anteflexion.

rounds: The practice employed by health care professionals of discussing and evaluating the status and care of patients for whom they are collectively responsible. Rounds may be conducted as "sit-down" conferences or as "teaching" or "walking" rounds during which the patients are visited. Medical rounds are led by the physician in charge of the patients' care and are attended by residents, interns, medical students; nurses and others who have some responsibility for the care of the patients involved may also attend medical rounds. Nursing rounds are attended by members of the nursing staff and are usually conducted at the beginning of a shift; they may or may not include visits to patients' bedside. **GRAND ROUNDS,** formal conferences in which an expert gives a lecture or discussion regarding a clinical issue; slides, films, charts, etc. may be used, and the patient involved may or may not be presented. Or, the conference may be held at the patient's bedside with physicians, nurses, medical students, interns, and other involved caretakers in attendance.

roundworm: One of the more prevalent intestinal worms parasitic to man, especially one of the class *Nematoda;* threadworm. See also Ascharis.

Rous sarcoma: A type of fibrosarcoma that arose spontaneously in fowl and which furnished the basis for study and experimental work on the concept of a viral causation of sarcoma.

Roussy-Levy syndrome: Progressive muscular atrophy associated with cerebellar ataxia and scoliosis.

route: In health care, the path of administration of a medication.

Roux: [Cesar Roux, Swiss surgeon. 1857–1926.] **ROUX-EN-Y DRAINAGE,** a surgically established system for draining the esophagus, pancreas, and biliary tract directly into the jejunum, to prevent peristaltic reflux of intestinal content into these organs. **ROUX-EN-Y JEJUNAL**

LOOP, the segments of the jejunum as rearranged for establishing Roux-en-Y drainage.

Rovsing's sign: Pain in the right iliac fossa when pressure is applied in the left iliac fossa; a sign of acute appendicitis.

rpm: Abbreviation for revolutions per minute.

RPT: Abbreviation for Registered Physical Therapist.

RQ: Respiratory quotient; the relationship between the amount of carbon dioxide produced in the body and the amount of oxygen absorbed.

RR: Abbreviation for recovery room.

RR interval: The period in the electrocardiogram from one R wave to the next.

-rrhacis: Combining form denoting the spine.

-rrhage, -rrhagia: Combining forms denoting excessive flow.

-rrhaphy: Combining form denoting a joining together by sutures.

-rrhea: Combining form denoting discharge or flow.

-rrhexis: Combining form denoting rupture or splitting.

R.T.: Abbreviation for 1. Registered Technician. 2. Reaction time.

rub: 1. Friction occurring when two surfaces are moved against one another. 2. The sound heard when two serous surfaces rub together. **PERICARDIAL FRICTION R.,** a scraping or grating noise heard over the pericardium on auscultation when the pericardium is inflamed. **PLEURAL FRICTION R.,** the creaking or dry scuffing noise heard at the end of inspiration when the pleural membranes are roughened by inflammation, in the presence of a neoplasm, or in the absence or decrease of pleural fluid.

rubedo (rū-bē'dō): Blushing or other temporary reddening of the skin.

rubefacient (rū-bē-fā'shent): 1. Producing redness of the skin. 2. An agent that acts as a counterirritant and produces a reddening when applied to the skin.

rubella (rū-bel'la): An acute, infectious, eruptive fever resembling both measles and scarlet fever, caused by the rubella virus and spread by droplet infection; symptoms include mild fever, coryza, conjunctivitis, a pink rash, possibly enlarged cervical glands, and arthralgia. The course is short and usually uneventful except when contracted in the first three months of pregnancy when it may produce fetal deformities. Also called German measles and three-day measles.

rubella syndrome: A congenital condition due to intrauterine rubella infection; characterized by deafness, cardiac anomalies, cataracts, thrombocytic purpura, hepatitis, retinitis, encephalitis, occasionally glaucoma.

rubeola (ru-bē-ō'la): See measles.

rubeosis (rū-bē-ō'sis): Redness. **R. IRIDIS,** the formation of numerous new blood vessels and connective tissue on the surface of the iris; usually bilateral; may occur in patients with diabetes and those with secondary glaucoma. **R. RETINAE,** the formation of new blood vessels in front of the optic papilla in patients with retinitis; often occurs in diabetics as well as nondiabetics.

ruber (rū'ber): Red.

rubescent (ru-bes'ent): Reddish, or growing red.

rubiginous (rū-bij'i-nus): Having a brownish or rusty color; most often applies to sputum.

Rubin's test: A test for patency of the fallopian tubes; carbon dioxide is insufflated into a tube and, if the tube is patent, the gas will pass out into the abdominal cavity where it can be visualized by x ray. A manometer may be used

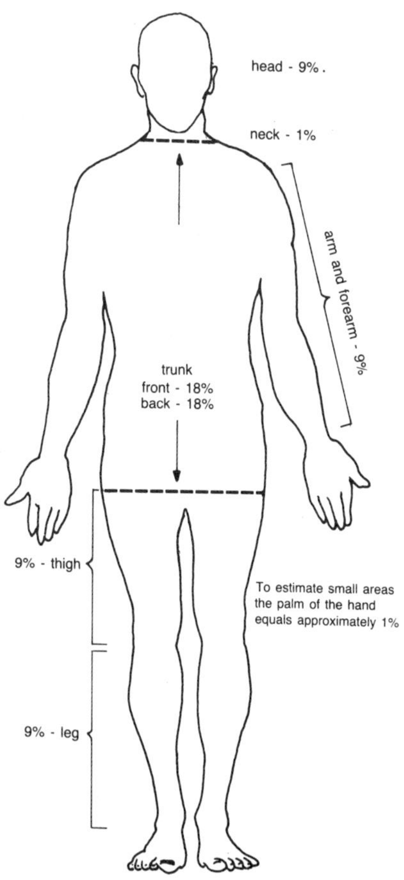

The rule of nines

to determine the pressure of the gas in the tube, which indicates the degree of patency.

rubor (rū'bor): Redness; one of the four classic signs of inflammation, the other three being pain, heat, and swelling.

rubricyte (rū'bri-sīt): An erythroblast (*q.v.*).

rubriuria (rū-bri-ū'ri-a): Red or reddish discoloration of the urine.

ructus (ruk'tus): Belching; eructation. **R. HYSTERICUS,** a condition in which the individual belches air frequently and noisily.—ructation, n.

rudimentary (rū-di-men'ta-ri): Imperfectly or incompletely developed; elementary.

Ruffini's corpuscles (roo-fē'nēz): Specialized encapsulated sensory nerve endings in the subcutaneous connective tissue of the finger; they are sensitive to warmth. [Angelo Ruffini, Italian anatomist. 1864–1929.]

ruga (rū'ga): A wrinkle, corrugation, or fold; often of an impermanent nature and allowing for distention, *e.g.*, the wrinkles and folds seen on the inner surface of the stomach.—rugae, pl.; rugose, rugous, adj.

rugitus (rū'ji-tus): Rumbling sounds in the intestine caused by movement of flatus; borborygmus (*q.v.*).

rule of halves: The rule that states that half of the people in a specific group will take advantage of an available screening program; half of those found to be at high risk will start a prevention program; and half of those who start such a program will reach their set goal.

rule of nines: See Wallace's rule of nines, and Lund and Browder's chart.

rum-blossom: See rhinophyma.

rumination (rū-min-ā'shun): 1. The voluntary regurgitation of food, and the rechewing and reswallowing of it; most often seen in young children with emotional problems; also sometimes seen in the mentally retarded and in psychiatric patients. 2. Chronic vomiting.

ruminative (rū'mi-nā'tiv): 1. Having a tendency to be preoccupied with certain thoughts and ideas. 2. Having a tendency to regurgitate previously swallowed food; see regurgitation.

rump: The gluteal region; the buttocks.

Rumpel-Leede test: A test for capillary fragility. A tourniquet is applied to the upper arm for 5–10 minutes; if petechiae appear on the forearm, the test is said to be positive.

rupia (rū'pi-a): A skin eruption of vesicles and ulcers that appears especially in the tertiary stage of syphilis; the lesions are raised, dark yellow or brown, crusted and adherent, tending to develop into bullae.—rupial; rupoid, adj.

rupture (rup'chur): Tearing, splitting, bursting of a part. A popular name for hernia (*q.v.*).

RUQ: Abbreviation for right upper quadrant (of the abdomen).

rural health centers: Health care centers established in areas distant from metropolitan health care facilities and where there are few physicians in practice; may be financed by the community, by a foundation, or by federal funds; much of the care given is provided by physicians assistants and nurse practitioners.

Rush pin: A pin, rod, or nail used in surgical treatment of major long-bone fractures.

rushes: Vigorous peristaltic movements producing sounds that are longer and higher pitched than normal bowel sounds.

rutilism (rū'ti-lizm): Red-headedness.

RV: Abbreviation for: 1. Right ventricle. 2. Residual volume (of air in the lungs).

Ryle's tube: A small caliber rubber tube, with an olive-shaped end, used for giving a test meal.

R_x: Symbol used at the head of a prescription; stands for the word "recipe." Dates back 5000 years to a picture of the eye of Horus, the Egyptian god of healing. See recipe.

S

S: 1. Abbreviation for *sinister* [L.] meaning left or on the left side. 2. Chemical symbol for sulfur. 3. Abbreviation for *sigma* [L.], let it be written; used in prescription writing.

s wave: The sharp downward deflection in the electrocardiogram that follows the peak of the R wave to the beginning of the upward curve of the T wave.

s: Abbreviation for *semis* [L.], meaning half. Also used as an abbreviation for *sinister* [L.], meaning left or on the left side.

s̄: Abbreviation for *sans* [F.], or *sine* [L.] meaning without.

SA, S-A: Abbreviation for sinoatrial.

Sabin's vaccine (sā'binz vak'sēn): A live, orally administered vaccine prepared from poliovirus and used to produce immunity to poliomyelitis; induces a poliovirus infection in the recipient, stimulating the production of antibodies and thus producing resistance to the disease. Licensed for use in the U.S. in 1961. Also called TOPV (trivalent oral poliovaccine) and often used to immunize children. See also Salk. [Albert Bruce Sabin, Russian born virologist in the U.S. 1906– .]

sabulous (sab'ū-lus): Sandy or gritty.

saburra (sab-bur'a): See sordes.

sac (sak): A small pouch or bag-like cavity. **AIR S.**, an air vesicle of the lung; an alveolus. **AMNIOTIC S.**, the membrane that holds the fetus and amniotic fluid when in utero. **CONJUNCTIVAL S.**, the potential space between the eyeball and the conjunctiva. **HERNIAL S.**, the pouch of peritoneum that contains a hernia. **LACRIMAL S.**, the expanded portion of the upper part of the lacrimal duct. **PERICARDIAL S.**, that formed by the pericardium.—saccular, sacculated, adj.

saccade (sa-kahd'): Rapid jerky movement of the eye as it moves from one fixation point to another, as occurs in reading.—saccadic, adj.

saccate (sak'āt): Shaped like a sac; pouched.

sacchar-, sacchari-, saccharo-: Combining forms denoting relationship to sugar.

saccharase (sak'a-rās): An enzyme that acts as a catalyst in the hydrolysis of sucrose to dextrose and levulose.—Syn., invertase, invertin, sucrase.

saccharic (sak'ar-ik): Pertaining to sugar.

saccharide (sak'a-rīd): 1. A simple sugar such as glucose. 2. A compound made up of sugar and another substance. 3. The carbohydrate grouping contained in each of the various types of carbohydrates which have been classified as monosaccharides, disaccharides, trisaccharides, polysaccharides, and heterosaccharides.

saccharify (sa-kar'i-fī): To make sweet or to convert into sugar.

saccharin (sak'a-rin): 1. A well-known sugar substitute. 2. Excessively sweet; cloying.

saccharine (sak'a-rīn): Sweet.

saccharogalactorrhea (sak'ar-ō-ga-lak'tō-rē'a): The secretion of milk that has a higher than normal amount of lactose.

saccharolytic (sak'ar-ō-lit'ik): Having the capacity to ferment or otherwise disintegrate carbohydrate molecules.

saccharometabolic (sak'a-rō-met-a-bol'ik): Pertaining to the metabolism of sugar.—saccharometabolism, n.

Saccharomyces (sak-a-rō-mī'sēz): A genus of yeasts which includes baker's and brewer's yeast.

saccharomycosis (sak'a-rō-mī-kō'sis): A pathologic condition caused by yeasts, often the of the genus *Saccharomyces*.

saccharose (sak'ar-ōs): Cane sugar; sucrose.

saccharum (sak'ar-um): Sugar.

saccharuria (sak-a-rū'ri-a): The presence of glycose in the urine; syn., glycosuria.

sacciform (sak'si-form): Resembling a sac or bag in shape.

saccular (sak'ū-lar): Sac-shaped.

sacculated (sak'ū-lā-ted): Containing or divided into small sacs. **S. BLADDER**, a condition of the urinary bladder in which small pouches are formed by a pushing out of the mucous membrane lining between the muscular bundles; they contain urine that is not voided with a normal urination; may be caused by overdistention of the bladder or an obstruction in the bladder outlet.

sacculation (sak-ū-lā'shun): The formation of a saccule (*q.v.*).

saccule (sak'ūl): 1. A minute sac. 2. The lower portion of the vestibule of the inner ear.—saccular, sacculated, adj.

sacculus (sak'ū-lus): Saccule (*q.v.*).

sacr-, sacro-: Combining forms denoting sacrum.

sacrad (sā'krad): Toward the sacrum.

sacral (sā'kral): Involving, pertaining to, or in the area of the sacrum. **S. BLOCK**, anesthesia produced by injection of an anesthetic into the sacral canal. **S. NERVES**, the five pairs of nerves attached to the spinal cord at the sacral segment; they innervate the skin and muscles of the lower back and sacral region, pelvic viscera, the perineum, and the genitalia. **S. VERTEBRAE**, the five lowest vertebrae which are fused into a single triangular bone, the sacrum.

sacralgia (sā-kral′ji-a): Pain in the sacral region.

sacrectomy (sā-krek′to-mi): Surgical removal of part of the sacrum.

sacroanterior (sā-krō-an-tē′ri-er): Describing a breech presentation in which the fetal sacrum is directed to one or the other acetabulum of the mother.—sacroanteriorally, adj.

sacrococcygeal (sā′-krō-kok-sij′ē-al): Pertaining to the sacrum and the coccyx.

sacrocoxalgia (sā′-krō-kok-sal′ji-a): Pain in the sacroiliac region or joint.

sacrocoxitis (sā′-krō-kok-sī′tis): Inflammation of the sacroiliac joint.

sacrodynia (sā-krō-din′i-a): Pain in the sacrum.

sacroiliac (sā-krō-il′i-ak): Pertaining to the sacrum and the ilium; or denoting the articulation between the two bones.

sacroiliitis (sā′krō-il-ē-ī′tis): Inflammation of the sacroiliac joint.

sacrolumbar (sā-krō-lum′bar): Pertaining to the sacrum and the loins.

sacroperineal (sā′krō-per-i-nē′al): Pertaining to the sacrum and the perineum.

sacroposterior (sā′krō-pos-tē′ri-or): Describing a breech presentation in which the fetal sacrum is directed to one or the other sacroiliac joint of the mother.—sacroposteriorally, adj.

sacropubic (sā-krō-pū′bik): Pertaining to the sacrum and the pubis.

sacrosciatic (sā′krō-sī-at′ik): Pertaining to both the sacrum and the ischium.

sacrospinalis (sā′krō-spī-nal′is): The long large muscle that passes up on either side of the vertebral column from the sacrum to the head. Extends the trunk, and bends the head and vertebral column to the side.

sacrouterine (sā′krō-ū′ter-in): Pertaining to the sacrum and the uterus. **S. LIGAMENT**, a band of connective tissue that extends backward from the cervix of the uterus, passes on either side of the rectum, and attaches to the posterior wall of the pelvis.

sacrovertebral (sā′krō-ver′te-bral): Pertaining to the sacrum and a vertebra or vertebrae above it.

sacrum (sā′krum): The triangular bone lying between the fifth lumbar vertebra and the coccyx; forms the back of the pelvis. It consists of five vertebrae fused together, and articulates on each side with the innominate bones of the pelvis, forming the sacroiliac joints.—sacral, adj.

saddle: **TURK'S** or **TURKISH SADDLE**, the sella turcica (*q.v.*). **S. BLOCK**, anesthesia produced by introducing an anesthetic low in the dural sac to anesthetize the buttocks, perineum, and inner aspects of the thighs; so called because these areas are in contact with the saddle in horseback riding; sometimes used for anesthesia in childbirth and in surgical procedures on the rectum.

saddlenose: A nose with a flattened bridge; often a sign of congenital syphilis.

sadism (sad′izm, sā′dizm): The obtaining of pleasure from inflicting pain, violence or degradation on another person, or the sexual partner. Opp. to masochism.

sadist (sad′ist, sā′dist): An individual who practices sadism (*q.v.*).

sadistic (sad-is′tik, sā-dis′tik): Pertaining to or marked by sadism.

sadomasochism (sad-ō-mas′ō-kizm, sā-dō-): The coexistence of sadism and masochism in a human relationship; the individual has a strong desire to inflict suffering and, at the same time, invites it.

"safe" period: A misleading term, used to describe the time in the menstrual cycle when conception is least likely to occur; the basis of a method of birth control used when mechanical or chemical means are not acceptable or obtainable; intercourse is avoided from the tenth to the twentieth day of the cycle inclusively.

safflower oil (saf′flow-er): Oil obtained from the safflower plant; used in diets of those in whom it is desirable to keep the blood cholesterol low.

sagittal (saj′it-al): 1. Shaped like an arrow; straight. 2. A lengthwise plane of the body, running from front to back; divides the body into right and left halves. **S. SUTURE**, the immovable joint formed by the union of the two parietal bones.

sailor's skin: Pigmentation and keratosis of exposed areas of the skin due to excessive exposure to sunlight; may lead to squamous-cell carcinoma.

Saint Anthony: **SAINT ANTHONY'S DANCE**, Huntington's chorea; see under chorea. **SAINT ANTHONY'S FIRE**, an old term for certain inflammatory or gangrenous conditions of the skin, including ergotism and erysipelas.

Saint Louis encephalitis: Named for an epidemic in St. Louis, Missouri that was caused by a mosquito-borne arborvirus. See under encephalitis.

Saint Vitus' dance: Chorea (*q.v.*). Named for a third century child martyr who was invoked by sufferers of chorea.

sal: Salt or any substance resembling it.

salicylate (sa-lis′i-lāt): Any of a large group of salts of salicylic acid, commonly used in medicine for their analgesic effects in the treatment of such conditions as rheumatism, dysmenorrhea, arthritis, and a variety of other aches and pains.

salicylic acid (sal-i-sil′ik as′id): A white crystalline substance derived from phenol; the basic component of aspirin.

salicylism (sal′i-sil-izm): A condition of toxicity resulting from large doses of salicylates; symptoms include nausea, vomiting, headache, dizziness, tinnitus, confusion.

saline (sā′lēn, sā′līn): 1. Salty, containing salt, or resembling a salt. 2. A solution containing salt. **NORMAL** or **PHYSIOLOGICAL S.**, a 0.9% solution of sodium chloride in water that is of the same osmotic pressure as the blood. **S. ABORTION**, see under abortion. **S. DEPLETION**, a condition existing when there is a deficiency of both water and sodium in the body; see hypertonic, hypotonic, isotonic.

saline injection technique: A technique sometimes used to induce abortion, especially when the patient has a bronchial disorder and cannot tolerate drugs that produce brochoconstriction.

saliva (sa-lī′va): A secretion produced by the parotid, submaxillary, sublingual, and buccal glands; spittle. It contains water, mucus, and ptyalin. Its function is to keep the inside of the mouth moist, to moisten and dissolve foods, and to start the digestion of carbohydrates.

salivant (sal′i-vant): 1. Stimulating the flow of saliva. 2. An agent that stimulates the secretion of saliva.

salivary (sal′i-ver-i): Pertaining to saliva. **S. AMYLASE**, ptyalin (*q.v.*). **S. CALCULUS**, a stone formed in a salivary duct. **S. DUCT**, one of several ducts that conduct the saliva. **S. GLANDS**, those that secrete saliva, *e.g.*, parotid, submandibular, and sublingual. **SALIVARY GLAND DISEASE**, cytomegalic inclusion disease (*q.v.*).

salivate (sal′i-vāt): To produce an excessive amount of saliva.

salivation (sal-i-vā′shun): An increased secretion of saliva. Ptyalism.

Salk vaccine: An inactivated poliovirus vaccine (IPV) administered subcutaneously to infants, certain children, and unvaccinated adults to produce active artificial immunity to poliomyelitis; booster doses are required periodically. Introduced in 1955. See also Sabin's vaccine. [Jonas E. Salk, American immunologist. 1914– .]

sallow (sal′low): Having a skin that is pale, yellowish, unhealthy looking.

Salmonella (sal′mō-nel′a): A genus of motile rod-shaped, gram-negative bacteria of the family Enterobacteriaseae. Parasitic in many animals and man in whom they are often pathogenic. Some species, such as *S. typhi*, are host-specific, infecting only man. Others may infect a wide range of host species, usually through contaminated foods. Some species cause mild gastroenteritis, others a severe and sometimes fatal food poisoning.

salmonellosis (sal′mō-nel-lō′sis): Infection with a Salmonella organism.

salping-, salpingo-: Combining forms denoting: 1. The fallopian tube(s). 2. Less often, the eustachian tube(s).

salpingectomy (sal-pin-jek′to-mi): Excision of a fallopian tube.

salpingian (sal-pin′ji-an): Of or pertaining to: 1. The uterine tube. 2. The auditory tube.

salpingitis (sal-pin-jī′tis): Acute or chronic inflammation of one or both of the fallopian tubes. The term is also sometimes applied to inflammation of the eustachian tube. **GONOCOCCAL S.**, infection of a fallopian tube(s) with *Neisseria gonorrhoea*.

salpingocyesis (sal-ping′gō-sī-ē′sis): Tubal pregnancy. See ectopic pregnancy under ectopic.

salpingogram (sal-ping′gō-gram): Radiological examination of tubal patency after injecting an opaque substance into the uterus and along the tubes.—salpingography, n.; salpingographic, adj.; salpingographically, adv.

salpingography (sal-ping-gog′ra-fi): Radiographic demonstration of the fallopian tube after it has been filled with a radiopaque medium.

salpingolithiasis (sal′ping-gō-li-thī′a-sis): The collection of calcareous material in the walls of the fallopian tubes.

salpingolysis (sal-ping-gol′i-sis): The breaking up of adhesions involving the fallopian tubes, a surgical procedure.

salpingo-oophorectomy (sal-ping′gō-ō′of-ō-rek′to-mi): Excision of a fallopian tube and ovary.

salpingo-oophoritis (sal-ping′ō-ō′of-ō-rī′tis): Inflammation of both the fallopian tubes and the ovaries.

salpingoperitonitis (sal-ping′gō-per′i-tō-nī′tis): Inflammation of the fallopian tube(s) and the peritoneum.

salpingopexy (sal-ping′gō-pek-si): Surgical fixation of one or both fallopian tubes.

salpingoplasty (sal-ping′gō-plas-ti): Plastic repair of a fallopian tube.

salpingoscope (sal-ping′gō-skōp): An instrument used for examining the nasopharynx and the eustachian tube; nasopharyngoscope.

salpingostomy (sal-ping-gos′to-mi): An operation performed to restore tubal patency.

salpinx (sal′pingks): A tube, especially the fallopian tube or the eustachian tube.

salt: 1. A chemical compound formed by the interaction of an acid and a base. 2. Sodium chloride; common table salt. 3. In the plural, any mineral salt used as a cathartic, *e.g.*, Epsom salts. **IODIZED SALT**, salt that has been treated with sodium iodide, usually 1 part to 10,000 parts of sodium chloride; used as a source of iodine in the diet to prevent the development of goiter.

salt glow: A condition produced by rubbing the body with wet salt following a shower to stimulate the functions of the skin.

salt rheum (room): An old term for any of a variety of skin conditions resembling eczema.

salt-free diet: A diet low in sodium chloride; usually refers to a diet in which no salt is used in cooking, and none is added at the table.

saltpeter (salt-pe′ter): Potassium nitrate, often mistakenly claimed to be useful in decreasing sexual desire; its main effect is diuretic.

salts: Usually refers to a saline cathartic such as magnesium sulfate, Rochelle salt, or sodium sulfate.

salt-wasting disease: Chronic renal malfunctioning characterized by high excretion of sodium.

salubrious (sa-lū′bri-us): Wholesome; healthful. Usually refers to climate or environment.

saluresis (sal′ū-rē′sis): The excretion of sodium and chloride ions in the urine.

saluretic (sal′ū-ret′ik): 1. Pertaining to or causing saluresis. 2. An agent that produces saluresis.

salutary (sal′ū-tā-ri): Healthful; remedial; curative.

salvarsan (sal′var-san): An arsenical preparation, discovered in 1910 to be a specific for syphilis, since it destroys the treponema pallidum; now superseded by penicillin and other antibiotics.

salve (sav): An ointment.

sanative (san′a-tiv): Healing; curative.

sanatorium (san-a-tō′ri-um): An institution, usually private, for the treatment of patients with such chronic disorders as tuberculosis, and who are not extremely ill.

sand bath: See under bath.

sandfly: A fly of the genus *Phlebotomus;* responsible for the "sandfly" fever of the tropics, and for various types of leishmaniasis (*q.v.*).

Sandos Clinical Assessment Guide (SCAG): A rating scale used for differentiating between depression and dementia in older persons.

sane: Of sound mind.

Sanfilippo's syndrome: A congenital condition marked by excessive amounts of heparitin sulfate in the urine, some skeletal abnormalities, neurological deficits, and progressive mental deterioration. See mucopolysaccharidosis.

sangui-: Combining form denoting blood.

sanguifacient (sang′gwi-fā′shent): Forming blood.

sanguinary (sang′-gwin-er-i): Pertaining to, derived from, containing, or consisting of blood.

sanguine (sang′gwin): 1. Full-blooded, bloody, or resembling blood. 2. Hopeful, as of a cheerful temperament; optimistic.

sanguineous (sang-gwin′ē-us): Pertaining to or containing blood.

sanguinopurulent (sang′win-ō-pū′ru-lent): Pertaining to an exudate that contains both blood and pus.

sanguis (sang′gwis): Blood [L.]

sanies (sā′ni-ēz): A thin, greenish, fetid discharge from a wound or ulcer; consists of blood, pus, and serum.

sanitarian (san-i-tā′ri-an): A person who specializes in matters of sanitation, particularly as they relate to public health. Sanitary engineer.

sanitary (san′i-tāri): 1. Healthful; promoting health. 2. Characterized by or readily kept in cleanness.

sanitation (san-i-tā′shun): The science of using measures that prevent diseases and that promote either individual or community health, or both.

sanitize (san′i-tīz): To clean or sterilize something so as to make it sanitary according to public health standards.—sanitization, n.

sanity (san′i-ti): Soundness, particularly of the mind.

San Joaquin Valley fever (san wa-kēn′): Coccidioidomycosis (*q.v.*).

saphenectomy (saf-ē-nek′tō-mi): Excision of a saphenous vein.

saphenofemoral (sa-fē′nō-fem′ō-ral): Pertinent to the saphenous and femoral veins.

saphenous (sa-fē′nus): Apparent; manifest. The name given to the two main superficial veins in the leg, the internal and the external, and to the nerves accompanying them.

sapo (sā′pō): A specially prepared soap with a pure olive oil base.

sapo-: Combining form denoting soap.

saponaceous (sap′ō-nā′shus): Soapy.

saponification (sa-pon′i-fi-kā′shun): Conversion into soap or a soapy substance.

saponin (sap′ō-nin): A glycoside obtained from certain plants growing widespread in the U.S. and Europe; formerly used as a detergent and as an emulsifying agent, now largely replaced by synthetic products.

sapphism (saf′ -izm): Lesbianism (*q.v.*).

sapr-, sapro-: Combining forms denoting 1) rotten, putrid, decayed; 2) dead or decaying organic matter.

sapremia (sa-prē′mi-a): A pathologic condition caused by the absorption into the bloodstream of toxins and breakdown products resulting from the action of saprophytic organisms on dead tissue. Septicemia.

saprogen (sap'rō-jen): Any microorganism that causes putrefaction (*q.v.*).

saprogenic (sap-rō-jen'ik): Causing putrefaction or resulting from it.

saprophagous (sap-rof'a-gus): Denotes an organism that lives on decaying organic matter.

sarapus (sar'a-pus): A flat-footed individual.

sarc-, sarco-, -sarc: Combining forms denoting muscle tissue or resemblance to flesh.

sarcitis (sar-sī'tis): Inflammation of muscle tissue; old term for myositis.

sarcoadenoma (sar'kō-ad-e-nō'ma): See adenosarcoma.

sarcoblast (sar'kō-blast): An embryonic cell that becomes a muscle cell.

sarcocarcinoma (sar'kō-kar-si-nō'ma): Carcinosarcoma (*q.v.*).

sarcocele (sar'kō-sēl: A tumor of the testis.

sarcoid (sar'koyd): 1. Resembling flesh. 2. Sarcoidosis (*q.v.*).

sarcoidosis (sar-koy-dō'sis): A chronic granulomatous disease of unknown etiology, characterized by the presence of tubercles that histologically resemble those of tuberculosis and range in size from that of a pinhead to that of a bean. May affect any organ of the body but most commonly presents as a condition of the skin, lymph nodes, lungs, liver, spleen, or the small bones of the hands and feet. See lupus.

sarcolemma (sar-kō-lem'ma): The delicate outer elastic membranous covering of the striated muscle fibers.

sarcology (sar-kol'o-ji): Study of the soft tissues as distinguished from bone.

sarcoma (sar-kō'ma): A tumor of connective tissue, often highly malignant; tends to grow rapidly and to metastasize early to distant spots; may occur in any part of the body; seen most frequently in children and young adults. The tumor is usually soft, bulky, and highly vascular, and may give rise to ulceration and hemorrhage. The most common type is osteosarcoma, usually of the tibia, femur, or humerus; also called osteogenic **S.** and osteoid **S.** **CHONDROSARCOMA,** a **S.** containing much fibrous tissue. **EPITHELOID S.,** a **S.** composed of a nest of epithelial cells that have sarcomatous properties. **EWING'S SARCOMA,** malignant myeloma of bone, the long bones in particular; characteristic symptoms are pain, fever, swelling, and leukocytosis. **KAPOSI'S S.,** a low-grade benign or malignant idiopathic neoplasm; occurs chiefly in the skin where it presents as purplish papules and nodules, particularly on the toes and feet, but may also affect lymph nodes and viscera where it is often hemorrhagic. **MELANOTIC S.,** a very malignant type of **S.** containing melanin. **NEUROGENIC S.,** neurofibrosarcoma (*q.v.*). **OAT CELL S.,** a **S.** made up of cells that are long and blunted at the ends. **OSTEOGENIC S.,** a malignant primary tumor of bone involving both the bone and cartilage; three subtypes are chondroblastic, fibroblastic, and osteoblastic. **RETICULUM CELL S.,** a malignant tumor of lymphoid tissue in which the predominating cell is an anaplastic, sometimes multinucleated reticulum cell. **ROUND CELL S.** and **GIANT CELL S.,** named for the type of cell that is predominant in the tumor. **SYNOVIAL S.,** see synoviosarcoma.—sarcomatous, adj.; sarcomata, pl.

sarcomatoid (sar-kō'ma-toyd): Resembling a sarcoma.

sarcomatosis (sar-kō'ma-tō'sis): A condition in which many sarcomata develop in the same individual.

sarcomatous (sar-kō'ma-tus): Resembling, or of the nature of, sarcoma.

sarcomphalocele (sar-kom-fal'ō-sēl): A fleshy tumor of the umbilicus.

sarcomyces (sar-kō-mī'sēz): A fleshy, tumorous growth that has a fungoid appearance.

sarcoplasm (sar'kō-plazm): The cytoplasmic substance of muscle in which the muscle fibers are imbedded.

sarcopoietic (sar'kō-poy-et'ik): Forming muscle tissue.

Sarcoptes scabiei (sar-kop'tēz skā'bē-i): The itch mite that causes scabies (*q.v.*).

sarcosine (sar'kō-sēn): An amino acid resulting from the hydrolysis of certain proteins.

sarcosinemia (sar'kō-si-nē'mi-a): An inborn error of metabolism marked by an increased amount of sarcosine (*q.v.*) in the plasma and urine; associated with mental and physical retardation.

sarcosis (sar-kō'sis): 1. The presence of multiple fleshy tumors. 2. Abnormal increase in body mass.

sarcous (sar'kus): Pertaining to muscle tissue or flesh.

sardonic grin (sar-don'ik): See risus sardonicus.

sartorius (sar-tō'ri-us): A long muscle of the thigh; originates on the anterior superior spine of the ilium and inserts on the medial surface of the upper end of the tibia. It adducts the leg and enables one to sit with one leg crossed over the other; so called because tailors formerly sat in this cross-legged position while at their work.

sassafras (sas'a-fras): The dried bark of the root of the *Sassafras albidum* tree; yields a volatile oil formerly much used as a carminative and mild aromatic.

satellitosis (sat'e-lī-tō'sis): A condition marked by the accumulation of neuroglial cells around the neurons of the central nervous system whenever the neurons are damaged by inflammatory or degenerative processes.

satiety (sa-tī′e-ti): The condition of being satisfied or gratified in regard to appetitie or thirst, with no desire to ingest more food or drink; limitation of intake is thought to result from stimulation of a satiety center located in the ventromedial part of the hypothalamus.

saturated (satch′ū-rā-ted): Holding all of a substance that can be absorbed or taken up. **S. FATS,** fats that are thought to encourage formation of plaque in blood vessels when taken in quantity; include animal fats, dairy products, and certain vegetable oils, *e.g.*, coconut oil and palm oils. **S. SOLUTION,** a liquid that contains as much of a solute as it is capable of holding in solution.

Saturday night paralysis: Saturday night palsy. See under palsy.

saturnine (sat′ur-nīn): Pertaining to, resembling, or produced by the absorption of lead.

saturnism (sat′ur-nizm): Lead poisoning; plumbism. See lead.

satyriasis (sat-i-rī′a-sis): Excessive sexual craving in a male. Same as nymphomania in a female.

sauna (saw′na): Steam bath followed by plunge in the snow; originated in Finland and adapted for use in other countries using cold shower as a substitute for snow. Dry heat is also now being used instead of steam.

sauriasis (saw-rī′a-sis): Ichthyosis (*q.v.*).

sausarism (saw′sa-rizm): 1. Dryness of the tongue. 2. Paralysis of the tongue.

Sayre head sling: A type of support for the head of a person in cervical traction.

SBE: Abbreviation for: 1. Subacute bacterial endocarditis; see under endocarditis. 2. Self breast examination.

s.c.: Abbreviation for subcutaneous and subcutaneously.

scab: A dried crust forming over an open wound.

scabicide (skā′bi-sīd): Any agent that is destructive to *Sarcoptes scabiei,* the causative agent of scabies.

scabies (skā′bēz): A parasitic skin disease caused by the itch mite which bores beneath the skin; highly contagious. Characterized by intense itching and eczematous lesions caused by scratching. Sites most affected are the skin between the fingers and toes, axillae, genital region, around the breasts. **NORWEGIAN SCABIES,** a rare infectious form; marked by encrusted skin swarming with mites; may occur in epidemic form in small communities.—Syn., itch; seven-year itch.

SCAG: Sandoz Clinical Assessment-Geriatric: Appears to be a valid and reliable rating form for differentiating between depression and dementia in the elderly.

scag: One of the street names for heroin.

scala (skā′la): Resembling stairs; refers particularly to the various passageways in the cochlea.

scald: 1. A burn caused by moist heat, either steam or a hot liquid. 2. To burn the skin with moist heat.

scale: 1. A small visible flake of skin that is cast off. 2. A system of marks at regular intervals on a strip of metal or glass that serves as a standard of measurement. 3. In dentistry, the removal of tartar from the teeth.

scalene (skā′lēn): 1. Pertains to a structure that has three unequal sides. 2. Part of a name given to any of several muscles with origins at the processes of cervical vertebrae and insertions at the two upper ribs; they act to flex and rotate the neck and assist in respiration by elevating the ribs.—scalenus, adj.

scalenectomy (skā′le-nek′tō-mi): Surgical removal of a scalene muscle.

scalenotomy (skā′lē-not′ō-mi): A surgical procedure in which the scalene muscles are severed close to their insertion into the ribs; the objective is to allow the apical part of the lung to rest; used in the treatment of pulmonary tuberculosis.

scalenus (skā-lē′nus): Descriptive of a structure that has three sides; refers particularly to the three muscles on each side of the neck, the anterior, medial, and posterior scalenus muscles; see scalene. **SCALENUS ANTICUS SYNDROME,** pain over the shoulder radiating up the back or down the arm; caused by pressure on the nerves between the anticus (anterior scalenus) muscle and a cervical rib.

scaling (skā′ling): 1. Desquamation; the production of scales. 2. The removal of calculous material from the exposed part of a tooth.

scalp: Consists of the skin, subcutaneous tissue, muscles, and periosteum that cover the top of the cranium.

scalpel (skal′pel): A small, straight, pointed knife with a sharp edge, used in surgery.

scan: Usually used with another, designating word; *e.g.,* bone scan, brain scan, thyroid scan. See scanning.

scanner (skan′er): An apparatus consisting of a detector that scans a specific body region in a systematic manner to determine the distribution of a radiopaque substance, and a device for recording that distribution. **GAMMA S.,** one in which the camera remains stationary. **RECTILINEAR S.,** one in which the camera moves back and forth over the area being examined.

scanning (skan′ing): 1. Visually examining a small area or several isolated areas in great detail. In **RADIOISOTOPE S.,** a two-dimensional picture is made showing the gamma rays that are emitted by the isotope, which is concentrated in the particular tissue, *e.g.,* brain, thyroid. A useful technique for diagnosis and for detection of infections and lesions such as tumors. 2. The process of making a radioactive scan. **S. SPEECH,** slow, hesitant speech with pronunciation of words a syllable at a time with a pause between each syllable; may be seen in individuals with multiple sclerosis.

scapegoating (skāp'gō-ting): Passing the blame for mistakes, misdemeanors, or problems to a person or persons other than the one(s) responsible.

scaphocephaly (skaf'ō-sef'a-li): A condition in which the skull is unusually long and narrow like the keel of a boat, with a ridge running from front to back; caused by premature closure of the sagittal suture; often associated with mental retardation.

scaphoid (skaf'oyd): Boat-shaped, as the navicular bones of the tarsus and carpus. **S. ABDOMEN,** refers to an abdomen in which the wall is thin, the contents small, and the contour concave rather than flat.

scaphoiditis (skaf-oy-dī'tis): Inflammation of the scaphoid bone.

scapholunate (skaf-ō-lū'nāt): Pertaining to the scaphoid and lunate bones of the wrist.

scapula (skap'u-la): The shoulder blade—a large, flat, triangular bone; it articulates with the clavicle and the humerus.

scapulalgia (skap-ū-lal'ji-a): Pain in the scapular area.

scapular (skap'ū-lar): Pertaining to the scapula. **S. LINE,** in anatomy, a vertical line drawn through the inferior angle of the scapula.

scapuloclavicular (skap'ū-lō-kla-vik'ū-lar): Pertaining to the scapula and the clavicle.

scapulocostal syndrome (skap'ū-lō-kos'tal): Pain in the shoulder girdle radiating to the neck and upper part of the triceps muscles, and numbness and tingling of the hands; caused by trauma, habitually poor posture, or friction between the scapula and the thoracic cage.

scapuloglenohumeral (skap'ū-lō-glen'ō-hū'mer-al): Pertaining to the scapula, glenoid cavity, and the humerus.

scapulohumeral (skap'ū-lō-hū'mer -al): Pertaining to the scapula and the humerus or the shoulder joint, or the muscles of the shoulder girdle.

scapulothoracic (skap'ū-lō-thō-ras'ik): Pertaining to the scapula and the thorax.

scar: The dense, avascular white fibrous tissue, formed as the end result of healing, especially in the skin. Cicatrix. See keloid.

scarf sign: A sign of immaturity if the infant's arm passes the midline of the body when the examiner places the infant's hand as far as possible in the direction of the opposite shoulder.

scarf skin: A popular name for the epidermis.

scarification (skar-i-fi-kā'shun): The making of a series of small superficial incisions or punctures in the skin.—scarify, v.

scarlatina (skar'la-tē'na): Scarlet fever. Acute infection by hemolytic streptococcus, producing a scarlet rash. Occurs mainly in children. Begins commonly with a throat infection, leading to pyrexia and the outbreak of a punctate erythematous eruption of the skin followed by desquamation. Characteristically, the area around the mouth escapes (circumoral pallor).—scarlatinal, adj.

scarlatinella (skar-lat-i-nel'a): Mild scarlet fever, with the rash but not the fever usually associated with scarlet fever. Also called fourth disease because it is the fourth member of a group of specific fevers including scarlet fever, morbilli, and rubella.

scarlet fever: See scarlatina.

scarlet fever test: Dick test (*q.v.*).

scarlet red: A dye with some bacteriostatic action; sometimes used to stimulate epithelial cell growth in treatment of burns, ulcers, and some other wounds, and as a covering for donor sites in skin grafting.

Scarpa's triangle: An anatomical area just below the groin. The base of the triangle is uppermost and is formed by the inguinal ligament. The vessels and nerves passing to and from the thigh are superficial here. [Antonio Scarpa, Italian anatomist and surgeon. 1747–1832.]

SCAT: Abbreviation for sheep cell agglutination test, a test for the presence of rheumatoid factors in the blood.

scat-, scato-: Combining forms denoting feces, dung.

scatacratia (skat-a-krā'shi-a): Incontinence of feces.

scatemia (ska-tē'mi-a): An autotoxic condition of the intestines, due to retained feces.

scatology (ska-tol'o-ji): 1. The study and analysis of feces. 2. Obsession with the obscene, particularly with the function of excretion and excreta.

scatophagy (ska-tof'a-ji): The eating of excrement.

scattering (skat'er-ing): In psychiatry, refers to behavior characterized by lack of relationship between ideas and thoughts expressed; results in meaningless or incomprehensible speech. In nuclear physics, the change in direction of a particle when it collides with another particle.

scavenger cell: See macrophage; phagocyte.

Schaefer's method: A method of performing manual (prone pressure) artificial respiration. [Albert Edward Sharpey-Schaefer, English physiologist. 1850–1935.]

Scheie's syndrome: A rare type of inherited mucopolysaccharidosis resembling Hurler's syndrome (*q.v.*), characterized by progressive clouding of the cornea, bone and joint disorders, and hirsutism, but no mental retardation.

schema (skē'ma): An outline or plan.

schematogram (skē-mat'ō-gram): An outline of the body or of some part of it that can be filled in following surgery or a physical examination.

Scheuermann's disease: Osteochondritis of the vertebral bodies. Occurs chiefly in adolescents. [Holger Werfel Scheuermann, Danish orthopedic surgeon. 1877–1960.]

Schick test: A test for susceptibility to the toxin of the organism that causes diphtheria, *Corynebacterium diphtheriae*. The toxin is injected into the skin of one arm and inactivated toxin is injected into the skin of the other arm. If the individual is susceptible, a red area will develop around the site of the toxin injection and persist for several days.

Schilder's disease: A chronic or subacute form of leukoencephalopathy (*q.v.*), characterized by destruction of white matter of the cerebral hemispheres resulting in progressive mental deterioration, varying degrees of bilateral spasticity, disorders of vision, deafness; occurs chiefly in children. Also called encephalitis periaxialis diffusa. [Paul Schilder, German-American psychiatrist. 1886–1940.]

Schiller's test: A test that involves painting an area, particularly the cervix, with iodine in order to determine from which sites a biopsy should be taken; normal cells stain brown, but abnormal cells do not.

Schilling test: A test for the detection of malabsorption or deficiency of Vitamin B_{12}. Following the oral administration of a small dose of radioactive B_{12}, urine for the test is collected for 24 hours.

Schimmelbusch's disease: Cystic disease of the breast; see under cystic.

Schiötz tonometer: An instrument for measuring intraocular pressure.

Schirmer test: A test used for evaluating the secretion of the lacrimal glands.

schirro-: Combining form denoting hard.

-schisis: A combining form denoting fissure, split, cleft.

schistasis (skis'ta-sis): In anatomy, a split or splitting; usually refers to a congenital anomaly.

schisto-: Combining form denoting split, cleft.

schistocelia (skis-tō-sē'li-a): A congenital anomaly consisting of a fissure of the abdominal wall.

schistocephalus (skis-tō-sef'al-us): A fetus with an unclosed cranium.

schistocyte (skis'tō-sīt): A fragment of a damaged red blood cell containing hemoglobin that appears as an irregularly shaped fragment on a stained glass smear; seen in patients with hemolytic anemia.

schistocytosis (skis-tō-sī-tō'sis): The presence of many schistocytes in the circulating blood.

schistoglossia (skis-tō-glos'i-a): A congenitally cleft tongue.

schistorrhachis (skis-tor'a-kis): A congenital anomaly consisting of a fissure of the spinal column with protrusion of membranes. See spina bifida.

Schistosoma (skis-tō-sō'ma): A genus of trematode worms or flukes that infest man. See schistosomiasis.

schistosome (skis'tō-sōm): Any of the species of the genus *Schistosoma*. **S. DERMATITIS,** "swimmers itch," a dermatitis occurring after exposure to water in some U.S. freshwater lakes, caused by penetration of the skin by a schistosome for which snails are the intermediate hosts.

schistosomiasis (skis-tō-sō-mī'a-sis): Infestation of the human body by certain *Schistosoma*. The worm, often present in contaminated water, penetrates the skin, enters the bloodstream and is carried to other parts of the body, giving rise to dysentery, hematuria, anemia. Bilharziasis. See snail fever.

schistosomicide (skis-tō-sō'mi-sīd): An agent that destroys schistosomes.

schiz-, schizo-: Combining forms denoting split or divided.

schizoaffective (skiz'-ō-af-fek'tiv): Pertains to psychiatric disorders in which the individual exhibits a mixture of schizoid and major affective disorders.

schizogenesis (skiz-ō-jen'e-sis): Reproduction by fission.

schizognathism (skiz-ō-nath'izm): A congenital anomaly in which either the upper or lower jaw is fissured.

schizogony (skiz-og'o-ni): The asexual cycle of sporozoa, particularly the life cycle of the parasite that causes malaria.

schizoid (skit'-zoyd): Resembling schizophrenia. **SCHIZOID DISORDER OF CHILDHOOD OR ADOLESCENCE,** a condition characterized by inability to make or keep friends, belligerence, irritability, seclusiveness, indecision; may be self-limited as the child matures. **SCHIZOID PERSONALITY DISORDER,** a disorder characterized by lack of ability to make and keep friends, coldness, aloofness, withdrawal, seclusiveness, eccentricity, detachment, and indifference to the feelings of others.

Schizomycetes (skiz-ō-mī-sē'tēz): Unicellular vegetable microorganisms that multiply by fission. May be saprophytic, parasitic, or pathogenic to man.

schizont (skiz'ont): A stage in the life cycle of the malarial parasite, *Plasmodium*.

schizonticide (ski-zon′ti-sīd): An antimalarial drug that destroys the parasite in the red blood cell; used to prevent or terminate the clinical attack.

schizonychia (skiz-ō-nik′i-a): Splitting of the nails.

schizophrenia (skiz-ō-frē′ni-a): A large group of mental illnesses characterized by disorganization of the personality, progressive withdrawal from reality, inappropriate responses, and often abnormal behavior; may be a chronic lifelong illness with frequent hospitalizations. The onset, commonly in early life, may be sudden or insidious. Five main types are generally recognized: 1. DISORGANIZED type, in which the person exhibits silly purposeless behavior, mannerisms, and speech; social withdrawal, fragmentary delusions or hallucinations; and incoherence; also referred to as hebephrenic type. 2. CATATONIC type, in which the person goes through stages of excitement alternating with stages of stupor, a peculiar sustained rigidity of the body, and mutism. 3. PARANOID type, a common chronic type characterized by delusions of persecution or of grandeur; anger; intense jealousy, argumentativeness; sometimes violence; and possibly, doubts about one's gender identity. 4. RESIDUAL TYPE, in which the person has had one episode of schizophrenia in which the symptoms were not particularly prominent but signs of the illness still persist in the individual who may exhibit certain eccentric behaviors, social withdrawal, and illogical thinking; this type may be chronic or sub-chronic with remissions and exacerbations. 5. UNDIFFERENTIATED TYPE, in which the person may exhibit symptoms not noted under the other four types or which appear in more than one of them, *e.g.*, disorganized behavior, incoherence, strong delusions, or hallucinations.

schizophrenic (skiz-ō-fren′ik): Pertaining to schizophrenia. S. SYNDROME, in childhood sometimes considered a truer diagnosis than autism or psychosis.

schizophreniform (skiz-ō-fren′i-form): Having some of the characteristics of schizophrenia. S. DISORDER, a condition in which the individual presents with some of the symptoms of schizophrenia, but the onset is acute and the condition responds to treatment within a few weeks or months.

schizophrenogenic (skiz′ō-fren-ō-jen′ik): Having a tendency to result in schizophrenia.

schizotrichia (skiz-ō-trik′i-a): Splitting of the hairs at the end.

schizotrypanosomiasis (skiz′ō-tri-pa-nō-sō-mī′a-sis): Chagas' disease (*q.v.*).

Schlatter's disease: Also Osgood-Schlatter's disease. Osteochondritis of the tibial tuberosity. [Carl Schlatter, Swiss surgeon 1864–1934. Robert Bayley Osgood, American orthopedic surgeon. 1873–1956.]

Schlemm's canal: A lymphaticovenous canal in the inner part of the sclera, close to its junction with the cornea, which it encircles. It receives the aqueous humor from the anterior chamber; obstruction leads to increased intraocular pressure. [Friedrich Schlemm, German anatomist. 1795–1858.]

schmutz pyorrhea (schmootz pī-ō-rē′a): Periodontal pyorrhea, seen in the elderly with very poor oral hygiene; white and yellow necrotic debris accumulates around the necks of the teeth and then peels off leaving a pocket with pus which gives off a foul odor.

Schneider nail: A nail used in surgical treatment of fractures of the femur.

Schneiderian membrane: The mucous membrane that lines the paranasal sinuses and the nasal cavities.

school nurse: See nurse and school nurse practitioner under nurse practitioner.

school phobia: Term used to describe a child's irrational avoidance or fear of school, teachers, and classmates; thought to result from intense separation anxiety caused by dependency on the mother.

Schölz's disease: Genetically determined degenerative disease associated with subnormality; the familial form of juvenile demyelinating encephalopathy.

Schönlein's disease: A form of anaphylactoid purpura occurring in young adults, without apparent cause; associated with damage to the capillary walls and accompanied by swollen, tender joints and mild fever. See Henoch-Schönlein purpura under purpura. [Johann Lukas Schönlein. German physician. 1793–1864.]

Schüffner's spots or dots: Small round yellowish or pink granules that can be seen in stained red blood cells early in malaria.

Schultz-Charlton reaction: A skin test utilized in the diagnosis of scarlet fever; it is positive if the skin around the point of injection blanches when a person with a scarlatinaform rash is given an injection of human scarlet fever immune serum.

Schwabach's test: A tuning fork test in which the bone conduction capability in a pathological ear is compared to the normal.

Schwann: SCHWANN'S CELLS, the cells that make up the neurilemma (*q.v.*). SCHWANN'S SHEATH, the neurilemma. SCHWANN'S TUMOR, a firm encapsulated neoplasm arising in the neurilemma of a nerve fiber; also called schwannoma and neurilemmoma. [Theodor Schwann, German anatomist. 1810–1882.]

schwannoma (shwa-nō′ma): Neurilemmoma (*q.v.*).

SCI: Abbreviation for spinal cord injury.

sciatic (sī-at'ik): Pertaining to the ischium or the region of the hip. **S. NERVE,** the largest nerve in the body; it extends from the hip down the back of the leg after passing under the buttock; at the level of the knee it divides into the tibial and common peroneal nerves. **GREATER SCIATIC NOTCH,** a deep notch below the posterior spine of the ilium through which the sciatic nerve, other nerves, blood vessels, and the piriform muscle pass. **LESSER SCIATIC NOTCH,** a notch between the spine and tuberosity of the ischium through which the tendon of the obturator muscle, nerves, and blood vessels pass.

sciatica (sī-at'i-ka): Pain along the line of distribution of the sciatic nerve (buttock, back of thigh, calf, and foot); may be caused by a herniated vertebral disk or an injury.

science (sī'ens): Any branch of systematized knowledge that is a specific object of study or practice.

scieropia (sī-er-ō'pi-a): A defect in vision in which all objects appear darker than they are.

scillocephaly (sil-ō-sef'a-li): A congenital anomaly in which the head is small and cone-shaped.

scintigram (sin'ti-gram): See **scintiscan.**

scintigraphy (sin-tig'-ra-fi): A non-invasive procedure for obtaining a photographic recording of the distribution of an internally administered radiopaque substance, utilizing a stationary scintillation detector device; may be used instead of renal pyelography to obtain a photographic recording of the renal system following administration of a low dose of radioactive substance.

scintillation (sin'ti-lā'shun): 1. A sensation as of seeing sparks or flashing lights. 2. A flashing or sparkling. 3. A particle emitted when radioactive substances disintegrate. **S. COUNTER,** a device for measuring radiation.

scintiphotography (sin'ti-fō-tog'ra-fi): Radioisotope scanning. **PULMONARY S.,** scanning of the lungs after the patient has inhaled or been injected with radioactive particles.

scintiscan (sin'ti-scan): 1. To use a scintiscanner, *i.e.,* to count by automation the gamma rays emitted by a radioisotope, revealing their concentration and location. 2. The record made on a scintigram.

scintiscanner (sin'ti-skan'er): A device that scans a part of the body, measures the amount and distribution of radioactive tracer substances, and records this information on a grid called a scintigram.

scirrhous (skir'us): Pertaining to or of the nature of a hard tumor; indurated. Usually refers to a type of cancer. **S. CARCINOMA,** chimney-sweep's cancer; see **scrotal epithelioma** under **epithelioma.**

scirrhus (skir'us): A carcinoma which provokes a considerable growth of hard, connective tissue; a hard carcinoma of the breast.—scirrhoid, adj.

scissor gait: An abnormal gait in which the legs are abducted and the thighs cross each other alternately with the knees scraping together; seen in patients with bilateral hip joint disease or spastic diplegia or as a manifestetion of Little's disease (*q.v.*). Also called scissor leg.

scissoring (siz'or-ing): Tendency to cross the legs at the thighs when walking or lying down; due to spastic adductor hip muscles.

scissura (si-sū'ra): A splitting or a fissure; a cleft.

sclera-, sclero-: Combining forms denoting: 1. The sclera. 2. Hard or dry.

sclera (sklē'ra): The "white " of the eye; the opaque bluish-white fibrous outer coat of the eyeball covering the posterior five sixths; it merges into the cornea at the front.—scleral, adj.; sclerae, pl.

scleradenitis (sklē'rad-e-nī'tis): An inflammatory induration or hardening of a gland.

sclerectasia (sklē-rek' -tā'zi-a): A bulging forward of the sclera.

sclerectoiridectomy (sklē-rek'tō-ir-i-dek'tomi): A surgical procedure in which part of the sclera and part of the iris are removed; a treatment for glaucoma.

sclerectomy (sklē-rek'to-mi): 1. Surgical removal of a portion of the sclera of the eye. 2. Operation for the removal of sclerosed parts of the middle ear after otitis media.

scleredema (sklē'rē-dē'ma): A condition of edema and induration of the skin; often follows an acute infection; more common in females than males. Frequently confused with scleroderma.

sclerema (sklē-rē'ma): Hardening of the skin; scleroderma. **S. OF THE NEWBORN,** a usually fatal disease of premature or undernourished children; excessive drying and hardening of the skin with limitation of movement.

scleriritomy (sklē-ri-rit'o-mi): Excision of the sclera and the iris.

scleritis (sklē-rī'tis): Inflammation of the sclera.

sclerochoroiditis (sklē'rō-kō-roy-dī'tis): Inflammation of the sclera and choroid.

scleroconjunctival (sklē'rō-kon-junk-tī'val): Pertaining to both the sclera and the conjunctiva.

scleroconjunctivitis (sklē'rō-kon-junk-ti-vī'tis): Inflammation of both the sclera and the conjunctiva.

sclerocorneal (sklē-rō-kor'nē-al): Pertaining to the sclera and the cornea, as the circular junction of these two structures.

sclerodactylia (sklē'rō-dak-til'i-a): Thickening and hardening of the fingers, often associated with scleroderma.

scleroderma (sklē-rō-der′ma): A progressive disease in which localized edema of the skin is followed by hardening, atrophy, deformity, and ulceration. Occasionally it becomes generalized, producing immobility of the face, contraction of the fingers; diffuse fibrosis of the myocardium, kidneys, digestive tract and lungs. Cause unknown; occurs most often in women between 30 and 50 years of age. **LOCALIZED S., S.** that is characterized by the formation of yellowish or whitish cutaneous patches that have a pinkish or purplish halo; occurs chiefly in women; also called morphea. **LINEAR S.,** linea morphea; a form of **S.** in which the lesions appear in a line or band, singly or as multiple ribbon-like lesions. See also dermatomyositis.

sclerodermatitis (sklē′rō-der-ma -tī′tis): Inflammation and hardening of the skin.

scleroid (sklē′roid): Hard; firm, or of a firm nature.

scleroiritis (sklē′rō-ī-rī′tis): Inflammation of the sclera and iris.

sclerokeratitis (sklē′rō-ker-a-tī′tis): Inflammation of both the sclera and cornea.

scleroma (sklē-rō′ma): A circumscribed area or patch of hardened skin or mucous membrane.

scleromalacia (sklē′rō-ma-lā′shi-a): Softening or thinning of the sclera; sometimes seen in persons with rheumatoid arthritis.

scleronychia (sklē-rō-nik′i-a): Thickening and drying of the nails.

sclerophthalmia (sklē′rof-thal′mi-a): Overgrowth of the cornea over the sclera so that only part of it remains clear.

scleroprotein (sklē′rō-prō′tē-in): A simple protein that is insoluble in water; of fibrous structure; serves a protective and structural function in the body. Also called albuminoid (*q.v.*).

sclerosant (sklē-rō′sant): 1. An agent that hardens tissues. 2. A chemical agent that produces inflammation followed by fibrosis; sometimes used in treatment of varicose veins.

sclerose (sklē-rōs′): To become hardened.—sclerosed, sclerotic, adj.

sclerosis (sklē-rō′sis): Term used in pathology to describe abnormal hardening or fibrosis of tissue. **AMYOTROPHIC LATERAL S.,** hardening of the motor tracts of the lateral columns of the spinal cord; results in progressive atrophy of the muscles; often fatal. Also called Lou Gehrig disease. **DIFFUSE INFANTILE FAMILIAL S.,** a form of **S.** characterized by demyelinization of the cerebrum in infants; tends to affect several family members; also referred to as globoid cell leukodystrophy and Krabbe's disease. **DISSEMINATED S.,** multiple **S.** **LATERAL S., S.** of the pyramidal tracts in the spinal cord; results in slowly progressive weakness and disability of the legs; usually occurs after age 50. **MULTIPLE S.,** a variably progressive chronic disease of the nervous system, most commonly first affecting adults between 20 and 40 years of age; may occur as a sequel to various viral infections including encephalitis, chickenpox, rubella, measles, or herpes; distribution is worldwide with the highest incidence occurring in the colder regions and the lowest in the tropics. The disease begins with patchy degenerative changes occurring in the nerve sheaths in the brain, spinal cord, and optic nerves, followed by the formation of plaques and sclerosis. The disease may remain silent for years, and when the early signs appear they may be quite diverse, but usually include diplopia; nystagmus; numbness, weakness, and unsteadiness of a limb; ataxia; scanning speech; and loss of the sensations of pain and temperature; later signs include partial blindness, emotional lability, disturbances of micturition, and paralysis; remissions and exacerbations are characteristic with the intervals between them becoming progressively shorter. **PROGRESSIVE SYSTEMIC S.,** scleroderma characterized by thickening of tissues and skin of hands and face; fibrosis of tissues of lungs, esophagus, and myocardium; osteoporosis of distal phalanges; dysphagia; dyspnea. **TUBEROUS S.,** see epiloia.

sclerostenosis (sklē-rō-ste-nō′sis): Hardening combined with contraction of tissues.

sclerostomy (sklē-ros′to-mi): A surgical procedure in which an opening is made into the sclera for the relief of glaucoma.

sclerotherapy (sklē-rō-ther′-a-pi): A treatment for varicose veins or hemorrhoids; consists of the injection into the vein of a sclerosing fluid that damages the epithelium and causes an aseptic thrombosis, which progresses to fibrosis and obliteration of the vessel.

sclerothrix (sklē′rō-thriks): Abnormal brittleness or dryness of the hair.

sclerotic (sklē-rot′ik): Relating to 1) the sclera of the eye; 2) sclerosis or the hardening of tissue.

sclerotitis (sklē-rō-tī′tis): Scleritis (*q.v.*).

sclerotomy (sklē-rot′o-mi): Incision of the sclera. **ANTERIOR S.,** incision into the anterior chamber of the eye for the relief of acute glaucoma. **POSTERIOR S.,** incision into the vitreous chamber of the eye for treatment of detached retina or removal of a foreign object.

sclerous (sklē′rus): Indurated or hard.

scolex (skō′leks): The head of the tapeworm which embeds itself in the intestinal wall and from which the segments develop.

scolio-: Combining form denoting twisted, crooked.

scoliokyphosis (skō′li-ō-kī-fō′sis): Combined lateral and posterior curvature of the spine.

scoliolordosis (skō′li-ō-lor-dō′sis): Combined scoliosis and lordosis.

scoliometer (skō′li-ō-mē′ter): An instrument for measuring the degree of curvature in scoliosis.

scoliorachitic (skō′li-ō-ra-kit′ik): Affected with both scoliosis and rickets.

scoliosis (skō-li-ō′sis): An appreciable lateral curve in the spine, causing a compensating deviation of the lumbar spine to the opposite side, and resulting in an S-shaped curve. May be functional and reversible, disappearing on flexion of the trunk, or structural and irreversible. Recognized types are lumbar, thoracolumbar, and thoracic. **COXITIC S., S.** in the lumbar area; caused by hip disease. **HABIT S.,** caused by improper posture. **IDIOPATHIC STRUCTURAL S.,** begins in childhood and increases progressively; cause unknown; often leads to development of marked deformity. **OSTEOPATHIC S.,** caused by disease of the vertebrae. **PARALYTIC S.,** caused by muscular paralysis. **RACHITIC S.,** caused by rickets. **SECONDARY STRUCTURAL S.,** the most common type; causes include congenital hemivertebra, neurofibromatosis, and poliomyelitis.

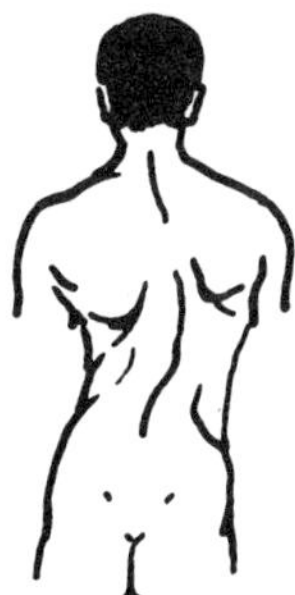

Scoliosis

scoliotic (skol-i-ot′ik): Pertaining to or affected by scoliosis.

-scope: Combining form denoting an instrument for viewing or examining.

scopophilia (skō′pō-fil′i-a): 1. An abnormal desire to be seen. 2. A sexual deviation in which the person derives sexual pleasure from viewing genitalia. 3. Voyeurism.

-scopy: Combining form denoting examination or inspection, usually referring to the use of an instrument for viewing.

scoracratia (skōr-a-krā′shi-a): Incontinence of feces.

scorbutic (skōr-bū′tik): Pertaining to or affected by scurvy (formerly called scorbutus). **S. BEADS.,** a row of nodules at the costochondral junction; seen in patients with scurvy; they differ from rachitic "rosary beads" in that they are sharper.

scorbutigenic (skōr-bū′-ti-jen′ik): Causing scurvy.

scorbutus (skōr-bū′tus): Scurvy (*q.v.*).

scoto-: Combining form denoting darkness.

scotochromogen (skō-tō-krō′mo-jen): Any microorganism whose pigmentation develops as well in the dark as in the light.—scotochromogenic, adj.

scotoma (skō-tō′ma): An area of darkness or blindness within the visual field; may be of varying size and shape; vision is normal in surrounding area. In psychiatry, refers to a "blind spot" in a person's psychological awareness. **ARCUATE S., S.** marked by development of an arc-shaped defect in the field of vision; arises in the area near the blind spot and extends toward it.—scotomata, pl.

scotomization (skō′tō-mī-zā′shun): The development of blind spots or scotomata. In psychiatry, the development of blind spots for things the patient does not want to accept.

scotophilia (skō-tō-fil′i-a): Fondness for the night or for being in the dark. Nyctophilia.

scotopia (skō-tō′pi-a): Night vision.

scotopic vision: The ability to see well in poor light. Dark-adaptation.

scratch test: A test for allergy. The superficial layer of skin is scratched and the suspected allergen rubbed in. If a redness or wheal appears at the site of the scratch the test is said to be negative. A safe test because so little of the allergen is used; as many as 30 may be done at one time.

screening: 1. Fluoroscopy (*q.v.*). 2. Mass examination of the population in a circumscribed area for the detection of such diseases as diabetes or tuberculosis. **HEELSTICK S.,** a test done to screen for hypoglycemia in infants of mothers who are diabetic or toxemic. **MULTIPHASIC S.,** the simultaneous use of several diagnostic tests with medical assessment at the end of the process; used for the detection of various diseases and pathological conditions such as anemia, heart disease, tuberculosis. **S. TEST,** 1) any test that separates those who are not, or who would not be, affected by a disease from those who are at risk for it and who will be given further tests; or 2) a simple test for the purpose of uncovering a disease condition that is treatable.

scrivener's palsy (skriv′nerz pawl′zi): Writer's cramp (*q.v.*).

scrobiculus (skrō-bik′ū-lus): A small pit or cavity.

scrofula (skrof'ū-la): An old term for a constitutional state that predisposes the individual to tuberculosis; also descriptive of primary tuberculosis, particularly of the cervical lymph glands; characterized by enlargement, suppuration, and scarring; seen mostly in the young.—scrofulous, adj.

scrofuloderma (skrof' -ū-lō-der'ma): A skin disease marked by exudative and crusted lesions, often with sinuses, resulting from a tuberculous lesion underneath, as in bone or lymph glands.

scromboid poisoning (skrom'boyd): Poisoning produced by a toxin elaborated by a marine bacterium that infests tuna, mackerel, and several other fishes; symptoms include headache, dizziness, flushing, nausea, vomiting, diarrhea, urticaria.

scrotal (skrō'tal): Pertaining to the scrotum.

scrotectomy (skrō-tek'to-mi): Surgical removal of part of the scrotum.

scrotitis (skrō-tī'tis): Inflammation of the scrotum.

scrotocele (skrō'to-sēl): A hernia into the scrotum.

scrotum (skrō'tum): The pouch in the male which contains the testes and their accessory structures.—scrotal, adj.

scrub: SCRUB NURSE, an operating room nurse who has "scrubbed" (see scrubbing), wears sterile mask, cap, gown, and gloves, and assists during an operation, e.g. by handing the surgeon instruments and other needed items during a surgical procedure. SCRUB TYPHUS, a rickettsial disease occurring mostly in Asia and Australia, characterized by a primary lesion at the site of attachment of an infected mite, fever, headache, conjunctival injection, and maculopapular eruption. Seen mostly in adults who frequent scrub terrain. Mites and various rodents are reservoirs of infection. Syn.—tsutsugamushi disease. See typhus fever.

scrubbing: The thorough cleansing of the hands and nails with soap, water and a brush before carrying out or assisting with a surgical or other procedure requiring aseptic technique (*q.v.*).

scruple (skroo'p'l): A unit of weight in the apothcaries' system; the equivalent of 20 grains or 1.296 grams by weight, or one-third of a dram liquid measure.

SCU: Abbreviation for special care unit.

scultetus binder (skul-tē'tus): A binder (or bandage) with many tails, which are applied overlapping, with each tail overlapping the next in shingle fashion.

scurf (skurf): A flaky desquamation of the epidermis, especially of the scalp; dandruff.

scurvy (skur'vi): A deficiency disease caused by lack of vitamin C (ascorbic acid). Clinical features include fatigue and hemorrhage. Latter may take the form of oozing at the gums or large ecchymoses. Tiny bleeding spots on the skin around hair follicles are characteristic. In children painful subperiosteal hemorrhage (rather than other types of bleeding) is pathognomonic. INFANTILE SCURVY, S. caused by lack of vitamin C in infants whose feeding consists primarily of cow's milk; prevention involves supplementary administration of vitamin C. Also called Barlow's disease.

scutiform (skū'ti-form): Shield-shaped.

scybala (sib'a-la): Rounded hardened masses of fecal matter in the intestine.—scybalum, sing.; scybalous, adj.

scyphoid (sī'foyd): Cup-shaped.

sealant (sē' -lant): A liquid plastic substance brushed on the teeth, covering surface pits and fissures; reduces the number of cavities; used particularly in areas in which the water is not flouridated.

seam: In anatomy, a line of union.

seasickness: See motion sickness.

seatworm: Pinworm; *Enterobius vermicularis* (*q.v.*).

sebaceous (sē-bā'shus): Pertaining to fat or suet. S. CYST, one due to the retention of sebaceous material in a sebaceous follicle; a wen. S. GLANDS, the cutaneous glands which secrete an oily substance called sebum. The ducts of these glands are short and straight and open into the hair follicles.

sebiferous (se-bif'er-us): Producing or secreting a fatty substance.

sebolith (seb'ō-lith): A concretion in a sebaceous gland.

seborrhea (seb-ō-rē'a): A functional disturbance of the sebaceous glands, marked by overactivity and resulting in a greasy condition of the skin of the face, scalp, sternal region, and elsewhere, usually accompanied by itching and burning. The seborrheic type of skin is especially liable to conditions such as alopecia, seborrheic dermatitis, acne, etc.—seborrheal, seborrheic, adj.

seborrheic (seb-ō-rē'ik): Pertaining to or characterized by seborrhea. S. DERMATITIS, see under dermatitis. S. KERATOSIS, see under keratosis.

sebum (sē'bum): The normal secretion of the sebaceous glands; it contains fatty acids, cholesterol and dead cells.

second intention: See healing.

Second Surgical Opinion Program: A program with the objective of inducing patients to get a second opinion to verify the need for elective surgery, for the purpose of preventing unnecessary surgery and reducing the overall cost of medical care; usually voluntary but in some states is mandatory.

secondary: Second or inferior in either time, place, or importance. S. ANEMIA, see under anemia. S. HEALING, see healing, by second intention. S. HEALTH CARE, inpatient care; includes diagnostic, curative, and other services required in long-term care for chronic illnesses and for preventing complications. S. HEALTH CARE SYSTEM, refers to health care given in such facilities as a community hospital where medical, surgical, pediatric, obstetrical, and geriatric services that cannot be provided on an outpatient basis, are given. S. INFECTION, see infection. S. SEX CHARACTERISTICS, those that develop at puberty but are not directly associated with reproduction. S. SEX ORGANS, those that are characteristic of one's sex but are not directly associated with reproduction, *e.g.*, the breasts in the female. S. SHOCK, see under shock. S. SYPHILIS, the second stage of syphilis; usually occurs six weeks to three months after infection.

secreta (sē-krē'ta): The products of glandular secretion; secretions.

secretagogue (sē-krēt'a-gog): An agent that stimulates secretion by a gland.

secrete (sē-krēt'): To produce or elaborate a new product from substances in the blood and either to pass it into the bloodstream or a body cavity, or transport it by a duct to the area where it is required or to the exterior of the body.

secretin (sē-krē'tin): A polypeptide hormone secreted by the mucous lining of the duodenum and the jejunum; in the presence of chyme it stimulates the secretion of pancreatic juice and, to a lesser extent, bile and intestinal juice. S. TEST, a test for pancreatic function; it involves the intravenous administration of secretin, measurement of the pancreatic secretion, and examining it for the level of lipase, trypsin, and chymotrypsin it contains.

secretinase (sē-krē'tin-ās): An enzyme in the blood serum that inactivates secretin (*q.v.*).

secretion (sē-krē'shun): 1. A fluid or substance, formed or concentrated in a gland, and passed into the alimentary tract, the blood or to the exterior. 2. The process of formulating such a substance.

secretory (sē-crē'to-ri): Pertaining to a secretion or a gland that produces a secretion.

section: 1. The act of cutting. 2. A cut surface. 3. A thin slice that has been prepared for microscopic examination. 4. A segment or division of an organ or structure. ABDOMINAL S., laparotomy (*q.v.*). CESAREAN S., incision through the abdominal and uterine walls for the delivery of a fetus. CORONAL S., a section of the skull that is parallel with the coronal suture. FROZEN S., a thin slice that has been cut from tissue that has been frozen; for microscopic study. SAGITTAL S., one that follows the sagittal suture and runs the entire length of the body, dividing it into right and left halves.

secundigravida (sē-kun'-di-grav'i-da): A woman pregnant for the second time.

secundines (sek'un-dins, dēns; sē'kun-dēns): The afterbirth with its membranes which is expelled following delivery of an infant.

secundipara (sek-un-dip'a-ra): A woman who has borne two live children at different labors.

sed.rate: Abbreviation for erythrocyte sedimentation rate; see under sedimentation. Also abbreviated ESR.

sedation (sē-dā'shun): The production of a state of lessened functional activity, especially when it is caused by a sedative drug. Also refers to a state of calmness.

sedative (sed'a-tiv): 1. Quieting; allaying physical activity and excitement. 2. Any agent that quiets, calms, or allays physical activity and excitement, and induces sleep; usually refers to a drug. S. BATH, a prolonged warm bath.

sedentary (sed'en-tar-i): Usually refers to 1) an individual who is inclined to be physically inactive and who sits a great deal of the time, or 2) an occupation that requires the individual to work while seated most of the time.

sedimentation (sed-i-men-tā'shun): The settling of a solid substance in a fluid to the bottom of a container, or causing this to happen by the use of a centrifuge. ERYTHROCYTE S. RATE, the rate at which red blood cells settle to the bottom of a tube of drawn blood; the rate differs in different diseases and in different stages of a disease; determination of the S. rate assists the physician to follow the course of the disease; also called ESR and sed. rate.

seed: 1. The source or origin of anything. 2. Offspring or descendents. 3. Sperm or semen. 4. To plant with seed or to sow seed. In radiotherapy, a small sealed container of radioactive material, often radon, that is inserted into the tissues to be treated. In bacteriology, to inoculate a culture medium with a microorganism one wishes to grow and reproduce for purposes of study.

segment (seg'ment): A small section; a part of an organ or structure.—segmental, adj.; segmentation, n.

segregation (seg-rē-gā'shun): A setting apart, usually for a particular reason, *e.g.*, to put those with the same or similar disease in a particular area.

Seidlitz powders: Consist of potassium sodium tartrate and sodium bicarbonate in one paper and tartaric acid in another paper; when the two are mixed in a solution just prior to taking, effervescence occurs; formerly much used as a cathartic.

seismotherapy (sīz-mō-ther'a-pi): Treatment of disease by mechanical vibration or shaking.

seizure (sē'zhur): 1. A sudden attack or sudden occurrence of symptoms, *e.g.*, convulsions. 2. An epileptic fit. **ABSENCE S.**, occurs chiefly in children; there is no aura, but brief loss of consciousness with staring and twitching of the mouth and hands. **AUDIOGENIC S.**, an epileptic seizure brought on by sound. **CEREBRAL S.**, an epileptic **S. FOCAL S.**, one limited to a particular part of the body or to a single function and without loss of consciousness; often associated with such brain lesions as scars, inflammation, or tumor; may progress to generalized **S. GENERALIZED S.**, affects the entire body and all body functions. **GRAND MAL S.**, see under epilepsy. **JACK-KNIFE S.**, severe muscular contractions causing extreme flexion of the head, neck, and trunk, with extension of the extremities; occurs during the first months of life. **JACKSONIAN S.**, see under epilepsy. **LOCALIZED S.**, focal **S. PETIT MAL S.**, see under epilepsy. **PHOTOGENIC S.**, an epileptic **S.** brought on by light. **PSYCHOMOTOR S.**, psychomotor epileptic **S.**, see under epilepsy.

selective action: 1. The tendency of disease-producing agents to attack certain parts of the body. 2. The ability to kill one group of microbes but not another.

selenium (se-lē'ni-um): A poisonous nonmetallic element resembling sulfur; used in preparations for treating seborrhea of the scalp.

self: The sum total of all that an individual can call his alone, including both mental and physical data. Term used to denote the feeling of self-awareness or personal identity.

self care: The use of one's own knowledge, experience, and preventive practices for maintaining health and for treating health problems that do not necessarily require medical or nursing care or hospitalization. May include procedures such as taking one's own temperature or blood pressure, or taking medications that have been prescribed.

self-abuse: 1) Masturbation. 2) Reproach of oneself.

self-analysis: In psychiatry, the practice of trying to gain insight into one's own psychic state and behavior.

self-breast examination: A procedure in which a woman examines her breasts at regular intervals to determine whether there are any changes that might indicate the presence of any structural change such as a lump or a tumor. Specific instructions for carrying out the procedure are available from the American Cancer Society. Abbreviated SBE.

self-concept: The mental self-image a person has, based on one's ideas and attitudes about oneself and one's personality.

self-demand schedule: A plan of infant feeding based on the infant's behavior rather than following a set time schedule; feeding when the child indicates he is hungry.

self-limited: Descriptive of a pathological condition that runs a definite course regardless of external factors or influences.

sella turcica (sel'a tur'sik-a): Now called pituitary fossa. A depression in the sphenoid bone which contains the pituitary gland; named from its resemblance in shape to a Turkish saddle.

Sellick's maneuver: The procedure of placing pressure on the cricoid cartilage during endotracheal intubation in the anesthetized person in order to prevent regurgitation.

semantic (sē-man'tik): Pertaining to the meaning of words. **S. ALEXIA**, a form of alexia in which the person can read but does not comprehend the meaning of the words he reads. **S. APHASIA**, inability to recognize the broader significance of words and phrases although their individual meanings are understood.

semel (sem'el): Once (Latin).

semelincident (sem'-el-in'si-dent): Happening to or affecting a person only once.

semen (sē'men): The secretion from the testes and acessory male organs, *e.g.*, prostate. It contains the spermatozoa and is discharged during sexual intercourse.

semenuria (sē-me-nū'ri-a): The presence of semen in the urine. Also spelled seminuria.

semi-: Combining form denoting 1) half, in quantity or value; 2) partial, to some extent, incompletely.

semicircular canals (se-mi-sir'kū-lar kanalz'): Three membranous semicircular tubes contained within the bony labyrinth of the internal ear. They are concerned with appreciation of the body's position in space.

semicoma (sem-i-kō'ma): A state of consciousness in which the individual will respond to painful stimuli by drawing away from the stimulus, but not make any spontaneous movements.

semicomatose (sem-i-kō'ma-tōs): Condition bordering on the unconscious. The person appears to be unconscious but can be aroused.

semiconscious (sem-i-kon'shus): Partly conscious.

semilunar (sem-i-lū'nar): Shaped like a crescent or half-moon. **S. CARTILAGES**, the crescentic interarticular cartilages of the knee joint (menisci). **S. VALVES**, those guarding the opening between the right ventricle and the pulmonary artery and between the left ventricle and the aorta.

semimembranous (sem-i-mem'bra-nus): One of the three hamstring muscles of the inner and back part of the thigh.

seminal (sem'i-nal): Pertaining to semen. **S. DUCTS, D.**s that convey the semen and spermatozoa; include the vas deferens and ejaculatory ducts (*q.v.*). **S. FLUID,** the **F.** in which sperm are suspended; includes secretions from the seminal vesicles, prostate, and bulbourethral glands; is ejaculated during sexual excitement. **S. VESICLES,** either of two sacculated glandular secretory structures lying between the male bladder and the rectum.

seminiferous (sem-i-nif′er-us): Carrying or producing semen. **S. TUBULES,** convoluted channels in the testes in which the sperm develop and through which they leave the testes.

seminoma (sem-i-nō′ma): A malignant tumor of the testis; occurs most often in young male adults.—seminomatomata, pl.; seminomatous, adj.

semiography (sē-mi-og′ra-fi): A written description of the signs and symptoms of a disease or pathologic condition.

semiologic (sē-mi-o-loj′ik): Pertaining to the symptoms of a disease.

semiology (sē-mi-ol′o-ji): Symptomatology (*q.v.*).

semipermeable (sem-i-per′me-a-b'l): Pertaining to a membrane that allows the molecules of some substances to pass through, but not others.

semiplegia (sem-i-plē′ji-a): Hemiplegia (*q.v.*).

semis (sē′mis): Half [L.] Used in prescription writing. Abbreviated s̄s̄.

semispinalis (sem-i-spī-nal′is): One of the deeper longitudinal muscles on either side of the spine.

semitendinous (sem-i-ten′di-nus): 1. Partially composed of tendon. 2. Referring to the semitendinosus, one of the three hamstring muscles of the posterior aspect of the thigh.

senescence (se-nes′ens): Normal physcial and behavioral changes that occur with the aging process and lead to decreased power of survival and adjustment; a period when breakdown is not balanced by repair mechanisms.—senescent, adj.

senescide (sen′e-sīd): The practice in some primitive groups of abandoning their elderly or neglecting to care for them as a way of disposing of them.

senescing (sen-es′-ing): The biological processes of aging that accompany the passage of time as shown by the steady decrease of one's capacity for biologic repair; consists of the many changes that occur with aging rather than a single predominant change.

Sengstaken-Blakemore tube: A tube with an attached inflatable balloon that is inserted into the esophagus and retained there to cause pressure on bleeding esophageal varices. [Robert Sengstaken, American neurosurgeon. 1923– . Arthur H. Blakemore, American Surgeon. 1897–1970.]

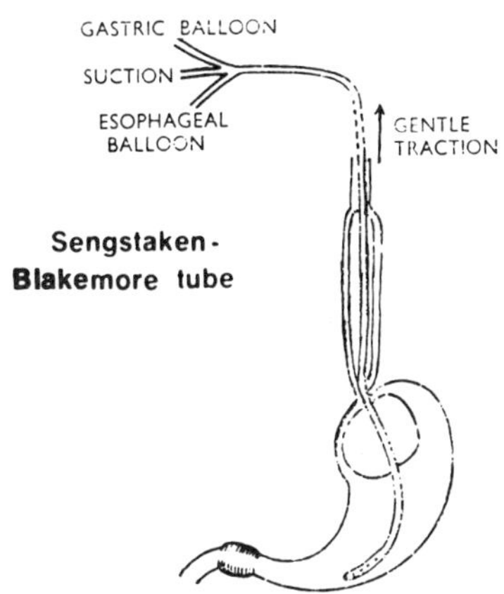

Sengstaken-Blakemore tube

senile (sē′nīl): Pertaining to or characteristic of old age, particularly when associated with mental decline. **S. CATARACT,** a cataract developing in old age due to the aging process. **S. DEMENTIA** or **S. PSYSHOSIS,** loss of intellectual power occurring in the elderly; characterized by loss of memory, irritability, and personality deterioration. **S. LENTIGO,** see under lentigo. **S. VAGINITIS,** see under vaginitis.

senile squalor syndrome: A condition occurring in an older person who withdraws from society, hoards rubbish, lives in filthy conditions; usually occurs in those living alone. Also called Diogenes syndrome.

senilism (sē′nil-izm): Premature aging.

senility (sē-nil′i-ti): 1. Feebleness or deterioration of mind and/or body when it occurs in the aged; progressive and irreversible. 2. Old age.

senna (sen′a): The dried leaves of the plant *Cassia acutifolia;* has long been used as a cathartic.

senopia (sē-nō′pi-a): Improvement of vision in elderly people.

sensate (sen′sāt): Felt or perceived by the senses.

sensation (sen-sā′shun): The perception or mental image produced in the brain by a stimulus which has been carried there by a sensory nerve.

sense: 1. The property of perceiving. 2. Feeling or sensation. **S. ORGAN,** a specialized structure for receiving certain stimuli, *e.g.*, the eye, ear. **SPECIAL S.,** any one of the five senses of feeling, hearing, seeing, tasting, smelling.

sensibility (sen-si-bil′i-ti): Sensitivity; the capacity for feeling or perceiving.

sensible (sen′si-b'l): 1. Endowed with the sense of feeling. 2. Detectable by the senses. **S. PERSPIRATION,** see perspiration.

sensitive (sen′si-tiv): 1. Capable of receiving and responding to a stimulus. 2. Responding to a stimulus. 3. Being unusually aware of factors in interpersonal relations. 4. Being abnormally susceptible to a substance such as a drug or foreign protein.

sensitivity (sen-si-tiv′i-ti): 1. The capacity to feel and react to a stimulus. 2. The quality or state of being sensitive to certain agents such as a drug or antigen. **S. GROUPS,** see encounter groups. **S. TESTS,** tests for sensitization to various allergens; several methods are available: 1) cutaneous, as in the patch test (*q.v.*); 2) percutaneous, as in the scratch test (*q.v.*); 3) intradermal, in which a minute amount of dilute antigen is injected into the skin, usually of the inner arm; a wheal develops at the site to a size that indicates the degree of sensitivity of the person. The percutaneous and intradermal methods may result in such symptoms as nausea, chills, flushing, and dyspnea. **S. TRAINING,** training to identify and deal with one's relationships; employed in group therapy during which groups meet for 8 to 10 hours a day for several days to develop self-assurance, self-awareness, sensitivity, and understanding that will enable the participants to have more satisfactory relationships; see encounter groups.

sensitization (sen-si-tī-zā′shun): Rendering sensitive. Persons may become sensitive to a variety of substances, such as certain foods (*e.g.*, shellfish), bacteria, plants, chemical substances, drugs, sera, etc. The sensitizing agent acts as an antigen leading to the development of antibodies in the blood. See allergy; anaphylaxis.

sensor (sen′sor): 1. A sensory organ or structure. 2. A device that generates a measurable impulse in response to a specific stimulus.

sensorimotor (sen′so-ri-mō′tor): Both sensory and motor; descriptive of a nerve that has both afferent and efferent fibers.

sensorineural (sen′sor-i-nū′ral): Pertaining to a sensory nerve or nerves. **S. HEARING LOSS,** deafness characterized by inability to discriminate sounds; due to damage to the inner ear or to the sensory path from the inner ear to the brain.

sensoristasis (sen′sor-i-stā′sis): A mental state similar to the physical state of homeostasis; the individual receives sufficient sensory stimuli to allow for healthful adaptation to the environment and enjoys an optimum level of well-being.

sensorium (sen-sō′ri-um): A term that implies the presence of memory and orientation to time, place and person; roughly the same as consciousness.—sensorial, adj.

sensory (sen′so-ri): Pertaining to sensation. **S. DEPRIVATION,** being cut off from usual external stimuli by isolation, social withdrawal, loss of hearing or sight. **S. NERVES,** those which convey impulses to the brain and spinal cord. **S. PARALYSIS,** loss of sensation due to pathology of the nerves, their pathways, or centers in the nervous system.

sensory-perceptual alterations—visual, auditory, kinesthetic, gustatory, tactile, olfactory, perception: A nursing diagnosis accepted by the Fourth National Conference on the Classification of Nursing Diagnoses.

sensual (sen′shū-al): Of or pertaining to the senses or to the sensory organs.

sensualism (sen′shū-al-izm): The condition of being unable to control one's emotions or the more primitive bodily appetites, or of being controlled by them.

sentient (sen′shi-ent): Capable of feeling; sensitive.

sentiment: An attitude or thought arising from an emotional experience, *e.g.*, love, hatred, contempt or self-regard, with reference to some particular situation, person or object.

separation anxiety: See under anxiety.

sepsis (sep′sis): The presence of pathogenic bacteria, especially pus-forming bacteria, and their toxins in the bloodstream or tissues.—septic, adj.

sept-, septi-: Combining forms denoting seven; seventh.

sept-, septo-: Combining forms denoting a septum.

septal (sep′tal): Of or pertaining to a septum. **S. DEFECT,** usually refers to a defect in the septum between the right and left sides of the heart, allowing blood to flow from the right side to the left without having circulated through the lungs.

septan (sep′tan): Recurring on the seventh day; often refers to the symptoms of malaria.

septate (sep′tāt): Divided into two or more compartments, usually by a membrane. **S. UTERUS,** a uterus that has a depression in the fundus, giving it the appearance of having two horns. **S. VAGINA,** a vagina that is wholly or partially divided by a longitudinal septum; a congenital anomaly.

septectomy (sep-tek′to-mi): Excision of part or all of a septum; often refers to the nasal septum.

septic (sep′tik): Pertaining to or caused by the presence of pathogenic organisms or their poisonous products; infected. **S. ABORTION,** see under abortion. **S. SHOCK,** see under shock. **S. SORE THROAT,** streptococcic inflammation of the throat, usually accompanied by fever and prostration.

septic-: Combining form denoting poison; sepsis.

septicemia (sep′ti-sē′mi-a): A systemic condition resulting from the invasion of the body by living pathogenic organisms and their persistence and multiplication in the bloodstream.—septicemic, adj.

septigravada (sep'ti-grav'i-da): A woman pregnant for the seventh time.

septipara (sep-tip'a-ra): A woman who has had seven pregnancies resulting in viable infants.

septoplasty (sep'tō-plas-ti): Plastic surgery for reconstruction of the nasal septum.

septostomy (sep-tos'to-mi): The operation of creating an opening in a septum.

septotomy (sep-tot'o-mi): The operation of cutting a septum, the nasal septum in particular.

septum (sep'tum): A thin partition of bone or membrane that separates two cavities. **ATRIOVENTRICULAR S.**, the muscular wall that divides the heart into two sides. **DEVIATED S.**, usually refers to a deviation of the nasal septum from the middle to one side or the other; may be a congenital anomaly, or be due to trauma or fracture. **INTERATRIAL S.**, the partition that separates the two atria. **INTERVENTRICULAR S.**, the partition that separates the two ventricles of the heart. **NASAL S.**, the partition that divides the nasal cavity; is made up of bone, cartilage, and mucous membrane. **RECTOVAGINAL S.**, the membranous partition between the rectum and the vagina. **RECTOVESICAL S.**, the membranous partition separating the rectum from the prostate gland and the urinary bladder.

sequela (sē-kwel'a): Any morbid condition, lesion or affection that occurs following or consequent to a disease.—sequelae, pl.

sequestration (sē-kwes-trā'shun): 1. The separation of tissue and formation of a sequestrum (*q.v.*). 2. Pooling of blood in blood vessels. 3. Isolation of individuals with certain diseases, for treatment and for protection of others.—sequester, v.

sequestrectomy (sē-kwes-trek'to-mi): Excision of a sequestrum (*q.v.*).

sequestrum (sē-kwes'trum): A piece of dead bone that has become entirely or partially detached from the sound bone and remains within a cavity, abscess, or wound. **S. CRISIS**, a situation that occurs in sickle cell anemia, precipitated by decreased oxygen in the red blood cells causing the hemoglobin to crystallize and create obstructions in blood vessels to any of the organs; congestive heart failure or renal failure may ensue.

sequoiosis (sē-kwoy-ō'sis): A type of pneumonitis associated with inhalation of redwood sawdust that contains particles of fungus growth.

serine (ser'ēn): A naturally occurring amino acid, a component of many proteins.

sero-: Combining form denoting: 1. A watery consistency. 2. The blood serum.

serocolitis (sēr-ō-kō-lī'tis): Inflammation of the external serous coat of the colon; pericolitis.

serodiagnosis (sē'rō-dīag-nō'sis): Diagnosis that is based on the results of a test or tests on the serum of the blood or on other serous fluids of the body.

seroenteritis (sē'rō-en-ter-ī'tis): Inflammation of the serous coat of the intestine.

serofibrinous (sē'rō-fī'bri-nus): Both serous and fibrinous in nature; often refers to an exudate.

serologic (sē-rō-loj'ik): Pertaining to serology. **S. TEST**, any test performed on serum.

serologist (sē-rol'o-jist): A person who specializes in serology (*q.v.*).

serology (sē-rol'oj-i): The branch of science dealing with the study of sera.—serologic, serological, adj.; serologically, adv.

serolysin (sē-rol'i-sin): A bactericidal substance normally present in the blood serum.

seroma (sē-rō'ma): An accumulation of serum, usually under the skin, which produces a swelling resembling a tumor.

seromembranous (sē'rō-mem'bra-nus): Pertaining to a serous membrane.

seromucous (sē'rō-mū'kus): Pertaining to a gland which produces a watery mixture that contains both serum and mucus.

seromuscular (sē'rō-mus'kū-lar): Pertaining to both the serous and muscular coats of the intestine.

seronegative (sē'rō-neg'a-tiv): Having a negative reaction to a test for some condition; said especially of serological tests for syphilis.

seroperitoneum (sē'rō-per-i-tō-nē'um): The presence of fluid in the peritoneal cavity; ascites.

seropneumothorax (sē'rō-nū-mō-thō'raks): The presence of a serous effusion, and air or gas in the pleural cavity.

seropositive (sē-rō-pos'i-tiv): Having a positive reaction to a test for some condition; said especially of serological tests for syphilis.

seropurulent (sē'ro-pū'roo-lent): Pertaining to a discharge containing both serum and pus.

seropus (sē-rō'pus): Serum mixed with pus.

serosa (sē-rō'sa): A serous membrane covering a visceral structure, *e.g.*, the peritoneal covering of an abdominal organ.—serosal, adj.

serosanguineous (sē'ro-sang-gwin'ē-us): Descriptive of a discharge or exudate that contains both serum and blood.

serositis (sē-rō-sī'tis): Inflammation of a serous membrane.

serosynovitis (sē'rō-sin-ō-vī'tis): Synovitis accompanied by copious serous effusion.

serotherapy (sē-rō-ther'a-pi): Treatment by injection of serum containing specific antibodies; may be either prophylactic or curative.

serotonin (sēr-ō-tō′nin): A potent vasoconstrictor found particularly in blood platelets, brain, and intestinal tissue; usually acts as a vasoconstrictor to large vessels and dilates arterioles and capillaries. During dissolution of blood platelets serotonin is liberated, along with histamine and, since both are vasoconstrictors, this may aid in the physiological control of blood loss.

serotoxin (sēr-ō-tok′sin): The presence of a toxin in the bloodstream.

serotype (sēr′-ō-tīp): The type of microorganism as identified by the kinds of antigens present in the cell. Used in taxonomy to classify certain sub-types of microorganisms.

serous (sēr′us): Pertaining to, containing, or producing serum. **S. FLUID,** the normal lymph in a serous cavity. **S. MEMBRANE,** one lining a cavity that has no communication with the external air and covering the organs that lie in those cavities.

serpiginous (ser-pij′i-nus): Snake-like; coiled; irregular; term often used to describe the margins of skin lesions, especially ulcers and ringworm which sometimes heal at one side while spreading from the other; also called serpent ulcer.

serpigo (ser-pī′go): Any creeping eruption of the skin.—serpiginous, adj.

serrated (ser′ā-ted): Having a sawtooth-like edge.

Serratia (ser-ā′shi-a): A genus of bacilli often found in water. **S. MARCESCENS,** a gram-negative, motile organism found in milk, water, soil, and human feces; formerly thought to be a harmless saprophyte, now thought to be a cause of pulmonary diseases, septicemia, and hospital infections.

serration (ser-ā′shun): A sawtooth-like notch.—serrated, adj.

serratus anterior (sēr-ā′tus an-tēr-i -or): A muscle that runs around the side of the thorax from the first nine ribs to the vertebral ridge of the scapula; it acts to stabilize, abduct, and rotate the scapula.

serum (sēr′um): 1. Any thin, clear, watery fluid produced by serous membranes and which serves to keep serous surfaces moist. 2. The fluid part of the blood that remains after the blood has clotted and thus removed the corpuscles. 3. The fluid part of the blood of an animal that has been inoculated with a specific microorganism or its toxins and has become immunized against the disease; used to produce passive immunity in exposed or susceptible individuals.—sera, serums, pl. **ANTITOXIC SERUM,** prepared from the blood of an animal that has been immunized by the requisite toxin; it contains a high concentration of antitoxin. **CONVALESCENT S.,** that from a person who has recently recovered from a specific disease; given to exposed or susceptible individuals as a prophylactic measure or to modify the symptoms; used especially in measles, mumps, whooping cough, scarlet fever, chickenpox, poliomyelitis. **S. SICKNESS,** the symptoms arising as a reaction about 10 days after the administration of serum of a different species; symptoms include urticarial rash, pyrexia, joint pains.

serum albumin: The major protein in the blood plasma; present in amounts of 3.5 to 5.5 grams per 100 ml of plasma; important in maintaining the oncotic pressure and viscosity of the blood.

serum alkaline phosphate: Found in almost all body tissues; constantly and rapidly secreted from cells into the interstitial area and then into the blood serum; necessary for hydrolysis of organic phosphates and important in digestion and absorption through the intestinal membrane; eliminated in urine, bile, and feces.

serum glutamic oxaloacetic transaminase (SGOT): See under transaminase.

serum glutamic pyruvic transaminase (SGPT): See under transaminase.

serum gonadotropin (sēr′-um gō-nad-ō-trō′pin): An ovarian-stimulating hormone obtained from the blood serum of pregnant mares. It is used in amenorrhea, often in association with estrogens (*q.v.*).

sesamoid (ses′a-moyd): Resembling a sesame seed. **S. BONES,** small bony masses formed in tendons, *e.g.*, the patella which is the largest sesamoid in the body, and the pisiform bones of the wrist.

sesqui-: Combining form denoting every half hour.

sesquihora (see-kwi-hō′ra): Every one and one-half hours.

sessile (ses′il): Without a peduncle or stalk; having a broad base or attachment.

setaceous (sē-tā′shus): Like a bristle.

setting sun sign: A downward drifting of the eyes when the patient's trunk is raised and then lowered quickly; occurs only if there is cerebral damage.

severe combined immunodeficiency disease (SCID): An inherited disorder consisting of a deficiency of T-cells, B-cells, and macrophages which results in a lack of immunity that is dependent on these cells; the exact cause is unknown. Symptoms, which usually begin in early infancy, include a greatly increased susceptibility to infection, failure to thrive, diarrhea, and respiratory problems. Usually fatal within the first year of life.

Sever's disease: A harmless condition characterized by pain in the back of the heel; tenderness over the calcaneus; occurring usually in children between 8 and 13 years of age;

symptoms subside gradually but spontaneously. Calcaneus apophysitis.

sex: 1. Either of two divisions of organisms that are distinguished as male and female. 2. Coitus. **S. CHROMOSOMES,** the X and Y chromosomes passed down in human reproduction and which determine the sex of offspring. **S. HORMONE,** one having an effect on growth or functions of the reproductive organs or on the development of secondary sex characteristics. **S. LIMITED,** descriptive of conditions that affect one sex only. **S. LINKED,** descriptive of characteristics that are transmitted by genes that are located on the sex chromosomes.

Sex Information and Education Council of the U.S. (SIECUS): A nonprofit organization that provides materials and resources for professionals and others on sexuality and sex education. Address: 84 Fifth Ave., Suite 1011, New York, NY 10011.

sexology (seks-ol′o-ji): That branch of science that deals with sex and relations between the sexes from a biological point of view.

sexopathy (seks-op′a-thi): Abnormality of sexual behavior or expression.

sextan (seks′tan): Recurring every sixth day.

sextipara (seks-tip′a-ra): A woman who has borne six viable infants.

sexual (sek′shū-al): Pertaining to sex. **S. DEVIANCE,** abnormal or unacceptable expression of sexual drives such as sadism, pederasty, exhibitionism, nymphomania, or illegal acts such as rape. **S. INTERCOURSE,** coitus.

sexuality (sek-shū-al′i-ti): The makeup of an individual in relation to sex drives, sexual activity, and other aspects of personality concerned with relationships.

sexually transmitted diseases and disorders: The venereal diseases and disorders, although some of those included in this category are also transmitted by means other than sexual contact. Included are acquired immunodeficiency syndrome (AIDS); condyloma acuminata (genital warts); gonorrhea; herpesvirus hominus (genital infection); nongonococcal urethritis; pediculosis pubis; scabies; syphilis; trichomonas vaginalis. Of these, only gonorrhea and syphilis are reportable.

Sezary syndrome: A condition involving the reticular lymphocytes; characterized by exfoliative erythroderma; associated with alopecia, skin disorders, and nail changes.

SGA: Abbreviation for small for gestational age.

SGOT: Abbreviation for serum glutamic-oxaloacetic transaminase. See under **transaminase**.

SGPT: Abbreviation for serum glutamic-pyruvic transaminase. See under **transaminase**.

shaft: An elongated structure, *e.g.*, the long part of a bone between its wider ends or extremities.

shagreen patches (shā′grēn): The areas of thickened grayish-green to brown skin that appear around the lesions of tuberous sclerosis.

shaking palsy: Paralysis agitans (see **paralysis**).

shamanism (shah′man-izm): A practice among certain ancient peoples of throwing themselves into states of excitement for religious purposes; it developed into a form of ecstatic healing, with the practitioner achieving a heightened state of consciousness; the role of shaman gradually expanded to that of healer and seer and originally was assumed only by women.

shank: The shin or tibia.

sharps: Colloquial term for surgical instruments with a cutting edge.

shear (shēr): An applied force that causes a parallel sliding motion between the planes of an object or of a load, or the result of such application. Bone fractures may be brought about in this way and are referred to as shearing fractures.

sheath (shēth): A tubular or enveloping membrane covering a structure such as a muscle, nerve, or blood vessel. **MYELIN S.,** the covering of many of the axons; composed of lipid and protein molecules; serves to increase the velocity of nerve impulses. **S. OF SCHWANN,** the neurolemma (*q.v.*).

Sheehan's syndrome: Hypopituitarism due to necrosis or dysfunction of the anterior pituitary, occurring as a sequal to postpartum hemorrhage; the thyroid, adrenal, and gonadal glands are all affected. Also called Sheehan's disease.

sheep cell agglutination test (SCAT): A test to determine whether T-lymphocytes are present in sufficient numbers in blood. Human blood cells are mixed with those of sheep and, if the T-lymphocytes are present, the sheep cells will be attracted to them in a characteristic rosette pattern; when this does not occur, or if only a few rosettes form, the reaction is considered diagnostic for certain diseases, *e.g.*, infectious mononucleosis.

sheepskin (shēp′ -skin): May be a real sheep's skin or synthetic; because it absorbs moisture and prevents friction, is used in prevention and treatment of decubitus ulcers.

shell shock: Term first used during World War I to designate a wide variety of psychotic or neurotic disturbances thought to be caused by the noise of bursting shells and other combat experiences. See **shock**.

sheltered workshop: An institution, usually operated by a nonprofit agency, that provides suitable employment for handicapped individuals, some of whom are later able to enter competitive employment. Work may be done on subcontracts from private industry and includes reclaiming and repairing salvage items or manufacturing items that the workshop itself has developed.

shiastic massage (shī-as′tik): Japanese massage, sometimes called acupressure (*q.v.*); pressure is exerted by hand, elbow, or knee along certain pathways, usually for 30 to 60 minutes; may cause discomfort but is not painful.

shield (shēld): A protecting tube or cover. **BULLER'S S.**, a watch glass that is taped over one eye to protect it from infection in the other eye, *e.g.*, in gonorrheal ophthalmia. **LEAD S.**, a lead plate that is placed between the operator and an x-ray machine to protect him from the x rays. **NIPPLE S.**, a device made of a glass dome and rubber teat that is placed over the nipple of a nursing mother to protect it when the infant is suckled.

Shiga's bacillus (*Shigella dysenteriae*): One of the bacteria that produce dysentery. Most common in the Middle and Far East. Infection often serious. [Kiyoshi Shiga, Japanese bacteriologist. 1870–1957.]

Shigella (shi-gel′la): A genus of microorganisms, many of which are the causative agents of various forms of dysentery. The organism is found in the feces of infected persons and carriers; it is also transmitted by infected food and flies; epidemic in underdeveloped areas of the world. **S. FLEXNERI**, the most frequent cause of dysentery epidemics and often of infantile gastroenteritis. **S. SONNEI**, a frequent cause of bacillary dysentery in temperate climates, and of summer diarrhea in children.

shigellosis (shi-gel-ō′sis): Bacillary dysentery caused by one of the Shigella organisms; tends to be endemic in certain lower social and economic areas.

Shiley tube: A tracheostomy tube that has an inner and outer cannula and a pilot balloon to keep the internal cuff inflated.

Shilling test: A test for assessing the ability of the small intestine to absorb vitamin B_{12}; it utilizes cobalt 57.

shin: The front of the leg below the knee. **S. BONE**, the tibia. **S. SPLINT**, pain, discomfort, and swelling along the shin bone caused by strain on the flexor digitoris longus muscle; an athletic injury, but may also be caused by running, jogging, or even walking. See anterior tibial compartment syndrome.

shingles: See herpes.

Shirodkar's suture: A purse-string suture placed around the cervix of a pregnant uterus and left in place until the 38th week of pregnancy after which it is separated, and labor soon begins; done to prevent abortion if the patient has had a previous abortion or has an incompetent cervix.

shock: A grave pathophysiological state in which the vital processes of the body are rapidly and profoundly depressed as a result of inadequate tissue perfusion due to a reduction in blood volume. Its features include a fall in blood pressure; weak, rapid, thready pulse; pallor; restlessness; cold, clammy skin; decreased respiratory depth, and decreased urinary output. **ANAPHYLACTIC S.**, a violent attack of severe symptoms of shock produced when sensitized individuals receive a second injection of serum or foreign protein to which they had been previously exposed; an emergency situation that requires immediate attention. Symptoms include breathlessness; hypotension; pallor; weak, rapid, thready pulse; fever; vascular collapse; sometimes convulsions and unconsciousness. **BACTEREMIC S.**, S. caused by bacterial toxins liberated by bacterial organisms in the circulation. **CARDIOGENIC S.**, S. due to inadequate cardiac output with inadequate peripheral circulation; caused by pump failure; often fatal. **DRUG-INDUCED S.**, may occur following administration of drugs that are incompatible with each other or with some other substance in the blood; occurs chiefly with intravenous administration. **ELECTRIC S.**, the sudden violent convulsive effect of an electric current passing through the body. **ENDOTOXIC S.**, occurs in septicemia as a result of pooling of blood caused by a decrease in effective circulating blood without actual blood loss. **HEMORRHAGIC S.**, S. due to excessive loss of blood. **HYPOVOLEMIC S.**, may be due to hemorrhage, trauma, burns, or diarrhea, any of which may cause a slowly progressive reduction in the volume of circulating blood. **INSULIN S.**, hypoglycemia produced by 1) an overdose of insulin; or 2) a therapeutic measure used in certain psychoses. **IRREVERSIBLE S.**, occurs when prolonged hypoxia causes damage to brain centers. **NEUROGENIC S.**, results from interference with functions of the sympathetic nervous system; may be caused by drugs, anesthesia, spinal injuries. **OLIGEMIC S.**, is associated with severe drop in blood volume. **PRIMARY S.**, occurs immediately following an injury. **SECONDARY S.**, occurs several hours, or even days, after trauma has occurred; often associated with life-threatening injury or illness and may or may not follow primary shock; symptoms include restlessness, weakness, progressive drop in blood pressure and body temperature, profuse sweating, reduced urinary output. **SEPTIC S.**, a syndrome due to vasoconstriction; occurs in severe infections, particularly those caused by gram-negative enteric bacteria; usually develops in persons already debilitated by an underlying disorder; characterized by chills, fever, hypotension, restlessness, irritability, tachypnea, tachycardia, confusion, rapid pulse, gastrointestinal symptoms; may lead to respiratory insufficiency, heart failure, coma, and death. **SHELL S.**, a type of psychoneurosis experienced by soldiers; a form of hysteria in which symptoms often indicate a functional disorder, *e.g.*, blindness, deafness, paralysis. **"SPEED" S.**, **S.** caused by too rapid infusion of intravenous fluids; characterized by shock symptoms and syncope; may lead to cardiac arrest. **SPINAL S.**, follows transection of the spinal cord; results in flaccid paralysis and loss of reflex activity in parts of the body below the lesion; the areflexia may be temporary or permanent. **SURGICAL S.**, a condition in which there is serious impairment of circulation following surgery; may be caused by loss of blood, vasodilatation, prolonged anesthesia, or inadequate cardiac output. **VASOGENIC S.**, **S.** caused by marked vasodilatation. **WARM S.**, occurs particularly in urological patients; characterized by warm, dry skin, fever, normal or excessive urine output; may occur after cystoscopy, urologic surgery, or catheterization.

shock lung syndrome: Occurs after resuscitation following shock or serious insult to the body, when it appears that the patient is recovering. The first sign is rapid pulse followed by hypocapnia, pulmonary insufficiency, and anoxia in spite of the administration of high concentrations of oxygen. Also called adult respiratory distress syndrome, stiff lung, wet lung, respiratory lung, hyaline membrane disease.

shock trousers: See military antishock trousers.

shortsightedness: Myopia (*q.v.*).

shoulder: The part of the body on each side of the base of the neck where the arm joins the trunk and where the clavicle, scapula and humerus meet. **S. BLADE,** the scapula. **S. GIRDLE,** formed by clavicle and scapula on either side. **FROZEN S.**, inability to abduct or rotate the arm due to inflammation of subacromial bursa.

shoulder-hand syndrome: Pain and limitation of motion of the shoulder and hand sometimes seen after injury to the neck or upper extremity, or after myocardial infarction.

show: A popular name for the bloodstained vaginal discharge at the commencement of labor.

shunt: 1. To turn to one side; divert from a normal path or course. 2. A naturally or surgically created passage between two natural channels to divert flow of blood or other body fluid, to allow for healing, or to bypass an obstruction. **ARTERIOVENOUS S.**, passage of blood between an artery and vein, usually between a radial artery and a cephalic vein when repeated access to the arterial blood system is required for hemodialysis. **CARDIOVASCULAR S.**, an abnormal flow of blood between the systemic and pulmonary circulation or between the two sides of the heart. **DENVER S.**, a peritoneo-venous **S.**, similar to the **LAVEEN S.** except that it has a cylindrical pump body instead of the valve that controls the flow rate of acitic fluid. **LAVEEN S.** a peritoneo-venous **S.**, used for treating intractable ascites; the distal end of a tube is placed under the peritoneum and threaded through a channel tunnelled under the subcutaneous tissue to the jugular vein or the vena cava; the ascitic fluid opens a valve when the pressure reaches a certain level allowing the fluid to flow through. **LEFT-TO-RIGHT S.**, diversion of the blood from the left to the right side of the heart through a septal defect or patent ductus arteriosis. **PORTACAVAL S.**, anastomosis of the portal vein with the inferior vena cava. **RIGHT-TO-LEFT S.**, a diversion of the blood from the right to the left side of the heart through a patent ductus arteriosus or in cases of pulmonary stenosis. **SPLENORENAL S.**, an anastomosis of the splenic vein to the left renal vein, accompanied by removal of the spleen; done for the relief of portal hypertension. **VENTRICULOPERITONEAL S.**, a surgically made communication between a lateral ventricle of the brain and the peritoneal cavity by means of a rubber tube, for relief of hydrocephalus. **VENTRICULOATRIAL S.**, the surgical establishment of communication between the ventricles of the brain and a cardiac atrium to shunt cerebrospinal fluid to the heart. **VENTRICULOURETERAL S.**, a surgically created shunt between a lateral ventricle of the brain and a ureter, a measure used in treatment of hydrocephalus.

Shy-Drager syndrome: A form of orthostatic hypotension associated with rigidity, tremor, impotence, atonic bladder, anhidrosis in lower parts of the body, ophthalmoplegia, fasiculations, and degeneration of preanglionic neurons in the sympathetic nervous system.

sial-, sialo-: Combining forms denoting 1) saliva; 2) salivary glands.

sialadenitis (sī'al-ad-e-nī'tis): Inflammation of a salivary gland. Also sialoadenitis.

sialadenoncus (sī'al-ad-e-nong'kus): A tumor of a salivary gland.

sialagogue (sī-al'a-gog): An agent that increases the flow of saliva.

sialic (sīal'ik): Pertaining to saliva.

sialism (sī'a-lizm): Excessive salivation; sialorrhea.

sialoadenectomy (sī'al-ō-ad-e-nek'to-mi): Surgical removal of a salivary gland.

sialoaerophagy (sī'a-lō-ā-er-of'a-ji): The habitual swallowing of saliva and air.

sialoangiectasis (sī'a-lō-an-ji-ek'-ta-sis): The dilatation of a salivary duct.

sialogenous (sī'a-loj'e-nus): Producing or resembling saliva.

sialogram (sī-al′ō-gram): Radiographic picture of the salivary glands and ducts, usually after injection of radiopaque medium.—sialography, n.; sialographic, adj.; sialographically, adv.

sialolith (sī-al′ō-lith): A stone in a salivary gland or duct.

sialolithiasis (sī′ -a-lō-li-thī′a-sis): The formation of calculi within a salivary gland or duct.

sialolithotomy (sī′a-lō-li-thot′o-mi): The surgical removal of a calculus from the salivary duct.

sialoma (sī-a-lō′ma): A tumor of the salivary gland.

sialorrhea (sī′a-lō-rē′a): Excessive salivation.—Syn., sialism, ptyalism.

sialostenosis (sī′a-lō-ste-nō′sis): Stenosis of a salivary duct.

Siamese twins: Twins that are joined together at birth, usually at the head, chest, or hip. When the union is slight it involves skin, muscles and cartilage only; when it is extensive it may involve shared bones and organs. In some cases, surgical separation is possible.

sib: Sibling (*q.v.*).

sibilant (sib′i-lant): Having a dry, high-pitched, shrill, whistling, or hissing sound. **S. RALE,** a whistling sound heard over the bronchi in cases of bronchial narrowing or spasm.

sibilus (sib′il-us): Rhonchus, or dry rale. Whistling sound heard on auscultation of the chest, *e.g.*, in cases of bronchitis, where the bronchi are narrowed by presence of edema or exudate.—sibilant, adj.

sibling (sib′ling): One of a family of children having the same parents. **S. RIVALRY,** jealousy between brothers and sisters, often based on competition for parental affection.

siccant (sik′ant): 1. Drying. 2. A substance that speeds up drying.

siccative (sik′a-tiv): 1. Removing moisture, or drying. 2. An agent that causes drying.

sicchasia (si-kā′zi-a): Nausea; abhorrence of food.

siccus (sik′us): Dry.

sick: 1. Unwell. 2. Nauseated. **SICK HEADACHE,** see migraine.

sick bay: The infirmary or dispensary on a ship.

sickle cell (sik′el): A red blood cell shaped like a crescent. **S.C. ANEMIA,** see under anemia. **S.C. CRISIS,** recurring episodes of acute symptoms developing in patients with S.C. anemia, usually occurring after infection, dehydration, or hypoxia. **S.C. HEMOGLOBINOPATHY,** the red blood cells contain an abnormal amount of hemoglobin and amino acid; results from inheritance of the sickle cell gene; symptoms include hypoesthenia, priapism, pyelonephritis, pallor, weakness, and intermittent crises.

sicklemia (sik-lē′mi-a): The presence of sickle-shaped erythrocytes in the blood; see sickle-cell anemia under anemia.

sickling disease: Sickle cell anemia. See under anemia.

sickness: A disordered, weakened or unsound mental or physical condition; disease. **AIR S.,** see motion S. **ALTITUDE S.,** condition characterized by giddiness, nausea, dyspnea, thirst, prostration; caused by atmosphere that has less oxygen than one is accustomed to breathing. **CAR S.,** see motion S. **DECOMPRESSION S.,** see caisson disease. **FALLING S.,** epilepsy. **RADIATION S.,** see radiation. **SEASICKNESS,** see motion S. **SLEEPING S.,** see African trypanosomiasis.

side effect: A result other than the one for which an agent or drug was administered; sometimes but not always an undesirable effect.

sideboards, siderails: Protective devices attached to the sides of the bed to prevent restless, delirious or aged persons from falling out of bed.

side-chain theory: See Ehrlich's theory of immunity.

sider-, sidero-: Combining forms denoting iron.

sideroblast (sid′er-ō-blast): An immature red blood cell containing granules of iron.

siderocyte (sid′er-ō-sīt): A red blood cell containing granules of free iron.

siderocytosis (sid′er-ō-sī-tō′sis): The presence in the circulating blood of a considerable number of siderocytes.

siderofibrosis (sid′er-ō-fī-brō′sis): Fibrosis combined with multiple small deposits of iron.

sideropenia (sid′er-ō-pē′ni-a): A deficiency of iron in the circulating blood.

sideropenic dysphagia (sid′er-ō-pē′nik dis-fā′ji-a): See Plummer-Vinson syndrome.

siderophil (sid′er-ō-fil): A cell or tissue having an affinity for iron or that contains iron.—siderophilic, siderophilous, adj.

siderophilin (sid′er-ō-fil′in): Transferrin (*q.v.*).

siderosilicosis (sid′er-ō-sil-i-kō′sis): Pneumoconiosis caused by prolonged exposure to silica and iron dust.

siderosis (sid-er-ō′sis): 1. Excess of iron in the blood or tissues. 2. A form of pneumoconiosis caused by the inhalation of iron or other metallic particles.

SIDS: Sudden infant death syndrome (*q.v.*).

Sig: Abbreviation for *signetur* [L.], meaning let it be labeled; used in prescription writing.

sigh (sī): A deep prolonged inspiration followed by a comparatively shorter expiration.

sight (sīt): 1. The act of or the ability of seeing. 2. The special sense involved in seeing.

Sigma Theta Tau: A national honor society with chapters in colleges and universities that have baccalaureate and higher degrees in nursing programs. Organized in 1922, the objectives are to strengthen education for nurses, to promote research in nursing, and to improve health care for all people. Membership is open to RNs with a baccalaureate or higher degree in nursing, and to students in such programs and who are high achievers with potential for leadership in nursing. Publishes the quarterly *Journal of Nurse Scholarship,* and *Image.* Headquarters: 1100 Waterway Blvd., Indianapolis, IN 46202

sigmatism (sig′ma-tizm): 1. A form of stammering in which the individual cannot properly articulate the letter S; lisping. 2. The too frequent enunciation of the letter S.

sigmoid (sig′moyd): Shaped like the letter S, or the Greek sigma. **S. COLON,** the part of the colon between the descending colon and the rectum. **S. FLEXURE,** an S-shaped curve of the intestine joining the descending colon above the rectum below.

sigmoidectomy (sig-moy-dek′to-mi): Surgical removal of part of the sigmoid colon or all of it.

sigmoiditis (sig-moy-dī′tis): Inflammation of the sigmoid colon, especially the sigmoid flexure.

sigmoidopexy (sig-moy′dō-pek-si): An operation to correct prolapse of the rectum.

sigmoidoproctostomy (sig-moy′-dō-prok-tos′to-mi): The surgical creation of an anastomosis between the sigmoid colon and the rectum.

sigmoidorectostomy (sig-moy′dō-rek-tos′to-mi): The surgical creation of an artificial anus at the junction of the sigmoid colon and the rectum; a low colostomy.

sigmoidoscope (sig-moy′dō-skōp): An instrument for visualizing the rectum and sigmoid flexure of the colon. See endoscope.—sigmoidoscopic, adj.; sigmoidoscopy, n.

sigmoidostomy (sig-moy-dos′to-mi): The surgical formation of a colostomy in the sigmoid colon.

sigmoidovesical (sig-moy-dō-ves′i-kal): Pertaining to the sigmoid colon and the urinary bladder. **S. FISTULA,** a fistula between the sigmoid colon and the urinary bladder.

sign (sīn): Any objective evidence of disease. **VITAL SIGNS,** the signs of life, specifically the pulse, respirations, temperature, and blood pressure.

signature (sig′na-tūr): The part of a drug prescription that is placed on the label; it gives the directions for use to be followed by the patient.

silastic (sī-las′tik): A rubbery silicone material with various medical uses including drains, and for replacing certain tissues that have been removed, *e.g.,* breast tissue.

silent: 1. A quiescent state of disease. 2. Not showing the expected symptoms of a disease or disorder. 3. Not responding to stimuli.

silica (sil′i-ka): A substance that occurs naturally and abundantly in the earth in several forms; used in making glass and ceramic products and as an abrasive, adsorbent, and dehydrating agent.

silicon (sil′i-kon): An abundant natural element, found in soil, always found in combination; combines with oxygen to form silica; used in the manufacture of silicone, transistors, solar cells, ceramics.

silicone (sil′i-kōn): A plastic compound of silicon (*q.v.*) with many uses in medicine as a substitute for rubber, as in the manufacture of tubes and implants; also used in the manufacture of sealants, adhesives, and detergents.

silicosiderosis (sil′i-kō-sid-er-ō′sis): A form of pneumonoconiosis caused by inhalation of dust containing particles of silica and iron.

silicosis (sil-i-kō′sis): A form of chronic pulmonary disease characterized by extensive nodular fibrosis of the lung; caused by inhalation of dust containing particles of silica; occurs in miners, metal-grinders, stone workers, and those whose occupations bring them into contact with ceramics, sand, quartz, and other stones.

silicotuberculosis (sil′i-kō-tū-ber′-kū-lō′sis): Tuberculosis occurring in a person who already has silicosis.

silo-filler's disease: An occupational disease; may be due to 1) oxides of nitrogen that are produced by fresh silage; acute form may cause death due to pulmonary edema; chronic form may cause inflammatory reaction in the lung leading to pulmonary disorders; or 2) inhalation of nitrogen oxide; symptoms include headache, nausea, vomiting, respiratory and neurologic symptoms; seldom fatal.

silver (sil′ver): A soft, white, malleable metal; has several uses in medicine. **S. NITRATE,** a compound of **S.** used as 1) a caustic; 2) in a 1 percent solution as a prophylactic to prevent ophthalmia neonatorum (see Credé's method): 3) in treatment of burns, also in 1 percent solution, a disadvantage being that it stains linens an indelible black.

Silvester's method: A manual performance of artificial respiration. An old method, now largely replaced by more efficient techniques. With the patient lying on his back, the rescuer raises the patient's arms up to the sides of his head, holds them there for a few seconds, then brings them down and presses them firmly against the patient's chest. See resuscitation.

simian crease: A single continuous transverse crease in the palm of the hand; often seen in patients with Down's syndrome, but also occurs in some other individuals.

Simmonds' disease: Hypopituitary cachexia. Results from destruction of anterior pituitary lobe with consequent absence of secretions which normally stimulate other endocrine glands, especially the gonads, thyroid, and the adrenal glands. The basal metabolic rate is very low, there is loss of pubic and axillary hair, loss of sexual desire, premature aging, progressive emaciation.

Sims'-Huner test: A test to help determine the cause of infertility; involves examination of postcoital semen from the vaginal pool and endocervix soon after intercourse to ascertain the number and motility of the sperm.

simulation (sim-ū-lā'shun): 1. Malingering (*q.v.*). 2. The imitation of one disease or symptom by another.

Sims' position: See under position.

sinciput (sin'si-put): The front part of the cranium just above and including the forehead, used in reference to the forehead.—sincipital, adj.

sinew (sin'ū): A ligament or tendon.

singer's node: A fibrous nodule that forms on the free margin of the vocal cords; occurs in singers, public speakers, and others who habitually strain their voices.

single blind: Descriptive of an experiment in which the researcher, but not the subject, knows which particular treatment is being used.

singultus (sing-gul'tus): A hiccup.

sinister (sin'is-ter): In anatomy, left, or on the left side.

sinistr-, sinistro-: Combining forms denoting the left; toward the left; on the left side.

sinistrad (sin'is-trad): Toward the left.

sinistral (sin'is-tral): Pertaining to the left side.

sinistrality (sin'is-tral'i-ti): Showing preference for use of the left member of any of the major paired organs or parts, *e.g.*, the eye, ear, hand, foot. Left handedness.

sinistraural (sin'is-traw'ral): Hearing more acutely with the left ear.

sinistrocardia (sin'is-trō-kar'di-a): Displacement of the heart toward the left side of the body.

sinistrocerebral (sin'is-trō-ser'e-bral): Refering to or situated in the left hemisphere of the brain.

sinistrocular (sin'is-trok'ū-lar): Having the tendency to use the left eye when there is a choice as when looking through a microscope.

sinistromanual (sin'is-trō-man'ūal): Left-handed.

sino-, sinu-: Combining forms denoting sinus.

sinoatrial (sī'nō-ā'tri-al): Pertaining to the sinus venosus and the right atrium of the heart. S. NODE, the heart's natural pacemaker; a collection of specialized conductive tissue at the junction of the superior vena cava and the right atrium; it emits regular impulses which control the rate of the heartbeat. S. BLOCK, see under block. Also sinoauricular and sinuatrial.

sinobronchial syndrome (sī'nō-brong'ki-al sin'drom): Bronchitis associated with sinusitis; may be due to aspiration of purulent postnasal discharge; often caused by *Streptococcus pneumoniae* or *Hemophilus influenzae*.

sinobronchitis (sī'nō-brong-kī'tis): Inflammation of the paranasal sinuses and the bronchi.

sinogram (sī'nō-gram): Radiogaphic picture of a sinus after injection of radiopaque medium.

sinography (sī-nog'ra-fi): Roentgenography of any sinus following introduction of a radiopaque medium.

sinopulmonary (sī'nō-pul'mo-ner-i): Pertaining to the paranasal sinuses and the pulmonary airway.

sinus (sī'nus): 1. A hollow or cavity, especially one in a cranial bone. 2. A channel containing blood, *e.g.*, the sinuses of the brain. 3. Any abnormal tract leading from a suppurating area; a fistula. CAROTID S., see under carotid. CAVERNOUS S., a channel for venous blood, on either side of the sphenoid bone; it drains blood from the lips, nose, and orbits. CORONARY S., the dilated portion of the great cardiac vein; it is about one inch in length and opens into the lower part of the right atrium. DERMAL S., a congenital fistula extending from the skin, between the vertebrae, to the spinal canal. ETHMOID S., one of a pair of paranasal sinuses, located in the ethmoid bone. FRONTAL S., one of a pair of paranasal sinuses, located in the frontal bone. INFERIOR SAGITTAL S., a small S. in the dura mater parallel to the superior sagittal S. MAXILLARY S., (the antrum of Highmore) one of a pair of air cavities in the maxillae. PARANASAL S., one of the air spaces in the bones around the nose; they are lined with mucous membrane and communicate with the nasal passages; include the frontal, ethmoid, maxillary, and sphenoid sinuses. PILONIDAL S., a S. containing hairs, usually occurring in the coccygeal region, expecially in the cleft between the buttocks in hirsute people. RECTUS S., a S. of the dura mater; formed by the junction of the great cerebral vein and the inferior sagittal S.; also called straight S. SPHENOID S., one of a pair of paranasal sinuses, located in the anterior part of the sphenoid bone. SUPERIOR SAGITTAL S., located in the sagittal suture of the dura mater. S. OF VALSALVA, three pouches between the wall of the aorta and each of the semilunar cusps of the aortic valve. VENOUS S., a large vein or canal for the circulation of venous blood. S. ARREST, partial or complete obstruction of the heartbeat at its origin. S. BRADYCARDIA, see under bradycardia. **S. HEADACHE**, see under headache. **S. NODE**, see under node. **S. RHYTHM**, see under rhythm. **S. TACHYCARDIA**, see under tachycardia.

sinusitis (si'nū-sī'tis): Inflammation of a sinus, particularly one or more of the paranasal sinuses. **BACTERIAL S.**, may be caused by group A beta-hemolytic streptococci, hemophilus influenzae, hemolytic staphylococcus aureus, pneumococcus. **NONBACTERIAL S.**, may be due to a virus, vasomotor disturbances, obstruction.

sinusoid (sī'nū-soyd): 1. Resembling a sinus. 2. A dilated channel into which arterioles open in some organs and which take the place of capillaries; found in such organs as the heart, spleen, liver, pancreas, and in the suprarenal, parathyroid, and carotid glands.

sinusotomy (sin-ū-sot'ō-mi): An operation in which an opening is made into a sinus to remove pus; a drainage tube may be left in place for several days.

Sipple's syndrome: A condition characterized by pheochromocytoma, cancer of the thyroid, and hyperparathyroidism.

Sippy diet: See under diet.

sirenomelia (si're-nō-mē'li-a): A congenital anomaly in which the lower extremities are fused, and the feet are partially or completely fused; mermaid deformity.

-sis: Combining form denoting 1) a diseased state, or 2) a disease produced by the agent named in the stem, *e.g.*, amebiasis. May appear as aisis, esis, iasis, osis.

sitieirgia (sit-ē-ir'ji-a): Morbid rejection of food; anorexia nervosa (*q.v.*).

sito-: Combining form denoting food; nutrition.

sitology (sī-tol'o-ji): The science of nutrition; dietetics.

sitomania (sī'tō-mā'ni-a): Abnormal craving for food; excessive hunger.

sitotherapy (sī'tō-ther'a-pi): Treatment of disease through diet; dietotherapy.

situs (sī'tus): Site or position.

Sitz bath: A hip bath only; the body from the hips down is immersed in warm water for relief of pain or discomfort from cystitis or pelvic infection, following rectal or vaginal surgery, or after cystoscopy.

Sjögren-Larrson syndrome: Genetically determined congenital ectodermosis. Associated with mental subnormality and spasticity.

Sjögren's syndrome (swā'grens): A condition seen mostly in menopausal or postmenopausal women, characterized by deficient secretion from lacrimal, salivary and other glands; by keratoconjunctivitis, dry tongue, hoarse voice, tenderness of joints, muscular weakness, and anemia. Thought to be due to an autoimmune process, possibly influenced by changes in the functioning of endocrine glands. [Henrik Samuel Conrad Sjögren, Swedish ophthalmologist. 1899–.]

skatole (skā'tol): A strong-smelling nitrogen compound in the human feces; the product of decomposition of proteins in the intestine.

skelalgia (skē-lal'ji-a): Pain in the leg.

skeleton (skel'e-ton): The bony framework of the body supporting and protecting the soft tissues and organs. **APPENDICULAR S.**, the shoulder girdle and upper extremities, and the pelvic girdle and lower extremities. **AXIAL S.**, the skull, spine, ribs, and sternum, forming the bony structure of the trunk.—skeletal, adj.

Skene's ducts: Paraurethral ducts; see under paraurethral.

Skene's glands: Two small mucous glands at the entrance to the female urethra; the paraurethral glands. They empty into the vestibule via Skene's ducts located on either side of the urethra. [Alexander Johnson Chalmers Skene, American gynecologist. 1838–1900.]

skenitis (skē-nī'tis): Inflammation of Skene's glands (*q.v.*).

skia-: Combining form denoting shadow, especially one produced by internal organs on x-ray film.

skiagram (skī'a-gram): An x-ray photograph.

skiagraphy (skī-ag'ra-fi): The making of x-ray pictures.

skiameter (skī-am'e-ter): An instrument for measuring 1) the intensity of x rays, or 2) the refraction of the eye.

skilled nursing facility: A special institution or a department within a health care institution that provides skilled nursing care to patients following hospitalization and during convalescence and rehabilitation, usually on a short-term basis until the patient is ready to assume self-care. Criteria for accreditation are established by the Social Security Act and determine the basis for Medicare and Medicaid reimbursement. Most nursing homes are not considered skilled nursing facilities.

Skillern's fracture: A fracture in the lower one-third of the radius with a greenstick fracture of the ulna in the same region.

skin: The tissue that forms the outer covering of the body; it is an effective barrier against infection and trauma. Consists of the epidermis, or cuticle, the outermost coat which protects the cutis or true skin (cutis vera) which is extremely sensitive and vascular. The cutis contains nerve fibers that respond to pain, pressure, touch, and temperature. Appendages of the skin include hair, nails, sebaceous glands, sweat glands, apocrine and eccrine glands and the mammary glands. **S. GRAFT**, a procedure utilizing healthy skin from another part of the body to replace damaged or defective skin; see graft. **S. TEST**, an injection of a small amount of an antigen to test for immunity to a specific infection.

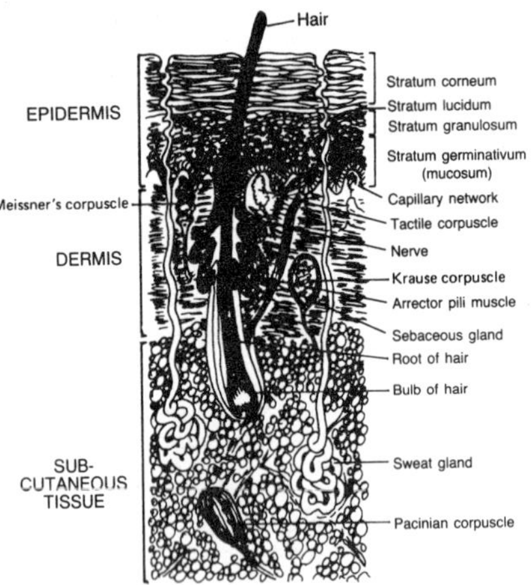

Skin

skin cancer: A fairly common disease among the elderly; may be caused by factors in the cells but is usually due to external factors such as exposure to ultraviolet rays in sunlight; light skinned people are especially affected. Occurs more often in men; farmers and sailors seem to be especially susceptible. Ionizing radiation, including x rays, gamma rays, and ultraviolet rays are common causes. The two most common types of skin cancer are basal cell carcinoma (*q.v.*) and squamous cell carcinoma (*q.v.*).

skin test: A frequently used method of determining induced sensitivity; involves applying an antigen to an abrasion in the skin or injecting it into the skin, and evaluating the inflammatory response this produces.

skinfold (skin′fold): The thickness of a fold of skin pinched between the thumb and forefinger, usually the skin over the ribs; done to help in evaluating the patient's nutritional status. Calibrated calipers are used to measure the thickness of a fold of skin usually of the upper arm or over the lower ribs.

skin-popping: Term used by drug addicts for the subcutaneous injection of drugs; often produces characteristic abscess-like lesions at injection sites.

skull: The bony framework of the head. See cranium.

slant: In microbiology, a test tube containing culture medium set at a slant to provide more area for growth of bacteria.

slapping: 1. A percussion movement in massage, consisting of an alternating series of sharp blows with the palm of the hand. 2. In walking, a gait in which the forefoot slaps the ground forcefully.

SLE: Abbreviation for: 1. Systemic lupus erythematosus. 2. St. Louis encephalitis.

sleep: Recurring periods of rest for the body and mind, usually with the body in a lying-down, immobile position; the person is disengaged from the environment and voluntary acts are suspended. This physiological condition is readily reversible to one of wakefulness and response to external stimuli. Sleep patterns vary with age, state of health, and psychological state, and may be altered by medical regimens; however, scientists have described four stages of sleep as it occurs in the normal healthy adult: Stage 1, the time period immediately after falling asleep, during which the person is responsive to environmental stimuli and cerebral activity continues; lasts about 10 minutes. Stage 2, the time period during which the person is beginning to relax, cerebral activity slows down, with hearing being the last to go, and the individual falls asleep. Stage 3, the time period when the person becomes more relaxed, blood pressure, respirations and pulse decrease, metabolism slows down, and gastrointestinal activity increases. Stage 4, the time period beginning about 30 minutes after the person has fallen asleep; it is marked by deep sleep, very relaxed muscles, an increase in the release of growth hormones, and a very few rapid eye movements (REM). Within 10 to 30 minutes after Stage 4 begins, rapid eye movements become prominent; the person's pulse, respirations, and blood pressure rise, and vivid dreams occur which can often be recalled upon awakening. This REM sleep lasts about 20 minutes and the person then returns to Stage 2 and the cycle is repeated. **TWILIGHT SLEEP**, see twilight state.

sleeping sickness: 1. A disease endemic in Africa, characterized by increasing somnolence; caused by protozoal parasites transmitted by the tsetse fly. 2. Any one of the viral encephalitides that is characterized by somnolence, especially equine encephalitis.

sleepwalking: Somnambulism (*q.v.*).

slide: A glass plate on which the object to be viewed through the microscope is placed.

sliding board: A board of appropriate length that is placed under the buttocks and thighs when transferring a paralyzed individual; also useful for the emergency transfer of a spinal-cord injured person.

sling: A bandage that supports any part of the body, particularly the arm. **PELVIC S.**, see under pelvic.

slipped disc: Herniated disc; see under disc.

slipped femoral epiphysis: See epiphysis, slipped.

slitlamp (slit′lamp): A special instrument for

the microscopic viewing of the eye; it is fitted with a diaphragm with a narrow slit through which an intense beam of light is projected.

slough (sluf): 1. A mass of necrotic tissue that separates from the healthy tissue and is eventually washed away by exudated serum. 2. To separate or cast off necrotic tissue from the healty tissue underneath.

sludge (sluj): To agglutinate or precipitate from a liquid, or the deposit formed by precipitation from a liquid.

slurry (slur'ri): A watery mixture of substances that do not dissolve in water.

SMA: Sequential multiple analyzer. Instrument used for collecting and analyzing data on a large number of chemical determinations and other laboratory tests in screening programs involving large numbers of healthy persons.

small cell carcinoma: See oat cell carcinoma.

small cell lung cancer: Accounts for 20 to 25 percent of annual deaths in U.S. Cigarette smoking is a factor in most cases. Usually starts in the bronchi and disseminates rapidly; symptoms include cough, dyspnea, hoarseness, dysphagia; metastasizes, often to the brain. See oat cell carcinoma.

small for dates: Term used to describe an infant whose birth weight is below the 10th percentile but whose gestation period may be of normal length.

small intestine: The part of the intestine between the stomach and the large intestine; consists of sections named duodenum, jejunum, and ileum; it is concerned chiefly with digestion and absorption of nutriments.

smallpox: Variola. An acute infectious disease caused by a virus indentical with that of vaccinia (cowpox). Endemic in many parts of the world. Headache, vomiting, and high fever precede the eruption of a widespread rash which is papular, vesicular and finally pustular. The eruption follows a set pattern of dissemination, commencing on the head and face. The lesions may be separate and distinct from each other, or they may be confluent and run into each other forming large suppurating masses. When the final stage of dessication is passed, scars (pock marks) are left to disfigure the skin. Prophylaxis against the disease is by vaccination. See vaccine.

smear: A film of material spread on a glass slide and stained for microscopic examination. **BUCCAL S.**, a **S.** containing scrapings from the mucous membrane of the mouth just above the line of the teeth; used in a cytological test for determining the somatic sex of an individual. **VAGINAL S.**, a **S.** from the vagina plated for microscopic examination. **"PAP" S.**, see Papanicolaou.

smegma (smeg'ma): An ill-smelling sebaceous secretion which accumulates under the male prepuce and in the folds of the vagina.

smell: 1. The sense that enables an individual to perceive and discriminate odors. 2. Odor. 3. To emit an odor.

smelling salts: A mixture of compounds usually containing some form of ammonia, which when inhaled acts as a stimulant or restorative, *e.g.*, to prevent or relieve fainting.

Smith-Petersen nail. See under nail.

smoker's cancer: Cancer of the lip, throat, or lung; seen in habitual smokers. **C.** of the lower lip is most often seen in pipe smokers.

S.N.: Abbreviation for student nurse.

SNA: Abbreviation for: 1. Student Nurses' Association. 2. State Nurses' Association.

snail fever: Term used for a type of schistosomiasis (*q.v.*) commonly occurring in the Middle East; a species of snail is the intermediate host. Seen recently in Arabs from the Middle East who have migrated to the U.S.

snare (snār): A surgical instrument with a wire loop at the end; used for removal of polypi, tumors or any soft fleshy projection such as a tonsil.

Snellen's test type: A device employed for testing for acuity of distance vision; consists of block letters of varying sizes arranged on wall charts.

sniffing: Inhaling. In street language, the inhaling of such substances as carbon tetrachloride, gasoline, glue, paint thinner, etc., or cocaine, to produce a state of euphoria; over time, indulgence may result in a pathological condition of liver, kidney, bone marrow or lung.

snore: A rough sound produced during sleep; caused by vibration of the soft palate and the uvula.

snow: Solid carbon dioxide, dry ice. Used for local freezing of the tissues in minor surgery. **S. BLINDNESS**, temporary blindness, with pain in the eyes and photophobia; caused by glare of the sun on snow.

snuffles (snuf'lz): A snorting inspiration due to congestion of nasal mucous membranes when the nasal discharge may be mucopurulent or bloody; seen in newborn infants. May be indicative of congenital syphilis.

SOAP: An acronym used as a guide for recording narrative notes in Problem Oriented Medical Records. It stands for *S*ubjective data, *O*bjective data, *A*ssessment, *P*lan.

soap: A cleansing agent formed by the action of an alkali on fatty acid. **CASTILE S.**, hard soap made with olive oil. **MEDICINAL SOFT S.**, made of vegetable oils; a soft soap used in treating certain skin conditions; also called green soap because of its color.

SOB: Abbreviation for short of breath.

social sciences: The sciences that deal with social institutions, the functioning of human society, and the relationships between individuals in society.

Social Security: The general public retirement pension program established by the Social Security Act of 1935 and administered by the Social Security Administration which functions within the Department of Health and Human Services. Benefits are paid from a fund to which both workers and employers contribute and from which cash benefits are paid to retired or disabled workers who may also receive some help with medical expenses by paying a percentage of supplementary medical insurance premiums.

social service: Organized activities designed to aid the handicapped, sick, and destitute by promoting their social welfare.

socialized medicine: A type of medical care that is controlled, directed, and financed by the state or nation and which provides health care for all the inhabitants.

Society for the Advancement of Nursing (SAIN): An organization for professional nurses with a baccalaureate degree in nursing. Formulated in 1975 with the objective of effecting differentiation between educational preparation for practice for professional and technical careers in nursing, and to support legislation that would lead to different licensure for the two types of nursing practice. Address: Box 307, Cooper Station, New York, NY 10003

sociobiological (sō'si-ō-bī'ō-loj'i-kal): Involving or relating to a combination of social and biological factors.

sociocultural (sō' -si-ō-kul'chur-al): Pertaining to culture in its sociological setting.

sociodemographic (sō'si-ō-dem-ō-graf'ik): Involving or relating to a combination of social and demographic factors.

socioecologic (sō'si-ō-ē'kō-log'ik): Involving or relating to a combination of social and ecologic factors.

socioeconomic (sō'si-ō-ē'kon-om'ik): Concerning or involving both social and economic factors.

sociogram (sō'si-ō-gram): A diagram representing the pattern of relationships between the individuals in a group.

sociology (sō-si-ol'o-ji): The scientific study of interpersonal and intergroup social relationships.—sociological, adj.

sociomedical (sō'si-ō-med'ik-al): Pertaining to the problems of medicine as they are related to society.

sociometry (sō-si-om'e-tri): The branch of sociology that is concerned with the measurement of social relations and behavior of humans.—sociometric, adj.

sociopath (sō'si-ō-path): One who has an aggressively antisocial attitude and behavior.

sociopathic (sō-si-ō-path'ik): Pertaining to or characterized by asocial or antisocial behavior. **S. PERSONALITY**, see under **personality**.

socket (sok'et): **1.** A hollow part or depression into which a part fits, as the eye socket. **2.** The hollow part of a bone at a joint which receives part of another bone. **DRY S.**, term given to a condition that occurs when a clot is lost following a tooth extraction and the bone is exposed to the air, causing considerable pain.

soda: A term often loosely used in reference to the salts of sodium, *e.g*, sodium carbonate (washing soda), sodium bicarbonate (baking soda).

sodium (sō'di-um): A soft white metallic element, many of the salts of which are used in medicine. In the human body it occurs as a cation found chiefly in the extracellular fluid; its main function is to control the water balance in body tissues; its excretion by the kidneys is influenced by antidiuretic hormone and aldosterone. **S. ACETATE**, colorless, odorless crystals with a saline taste, used as a diuretic and laxative. **S. BICARBONATE**, an important constituent of blood; acts as a buffer substance helping to maintain the correct pH of the blood. **S. CHLORIDE**, common salt, also an important constituent of blood and body tissues; an important factor in maintaining the water balance of the body; used for its diuretic effect, as a urinary acidifier, and to restore electrolyte balance. **S. CITRATE**, a white powder, used as an anticoagulant in blood for transfusion. **S. FLUORIDE** a white crystalline powder, used as a dental prophylactic in drinking water. **S. HYDROXIDE,** a compound of sodium that occurs in hard opaque flakes, pellets, or sticks; soluble in water; has a caustic effect; is used in preparation of certain chemicals and pharmaceuticals; not given internally. **S. IODIDE,** a salt resembling potassium iodide, used as a source of iodine. **S. IODOHIPPURATE**, a diagnostic agent used in urinary tract radiology. **S. LACTATE**, a sodium salt of inactive lactic acid; may be administered parenterally to combat acidosis. **S. NITROPRUSSIDE**, a reagent used in analysis to detect the presence of organic compounds. **S. PHOSPHATE**, a form of phosphorus 32, used in treatment of polycythemia vera and certain malignant conditions.

sodomist (sod'o-mist): A person who practices sodomy.

sodomy (sod'o-mi): Sexual relations including 1) anal intercourse between men; 2) copulation with an animal; 3) oral or anal copulation between members of the opposite sex.

soft chancre (shang'ker): Chancroid (*q.v.*).

soft palate: The soft, fleshy structure at the back of the upper part of the mouth; together with the hard palate in the front, it forms the "roof" of the mouth.

soft sore: The primary ulcer of the genitalia occurring in the venereal disease, chancroid (*q.v.*).

sol.: Abbreviation for Solution.

solar (sō'lar): Pertaining to, resembling, or derived from the sun. **S. THERAPY,** treatment by exposure to the sun's rays; heliotherapy.

solar plexus: A large network of sympathetic nerve ganglia, situated behind the stomach and in front of the aorta, that sends nerve fibers to all of the abdominal organs; the pit of the stomach.

solarium (sō-lăr'i-um): 1. A room or porch enclosed by glass; a sun room. 2. A room or place in a hospital where patients may expose their bodies to the sun for therapeutic purposes.

sole: The bottom of the foot.

soleus (sō'lē-us): Muscle at the back of the lower leg; lies over the gastrocnemius with which it unites at the lower end to form the tendon that attaches to the heel.

solipsism (sol'ip-sizm): The belief that the world exists only in one's mind and consists only of the individual and his or her life experiences.

soluble (sol'ū-b'l): Capable of being dissolved.—solubility, adj.

solute (sol'ūt): That which is dissolved in a fluid. **S. LOAD,** refers to the concentration of soluble substances, especially electrolytes, delivered to the kidneys; is higher in artificially fed than breast fed infants.

solution (sō-lū'shun): A fluid that contains one or more dissolved substances that are evenly distributed throughout and chemically unchanged. The dissolving liquid is called the solvent and the dissolved substance is called the solute. **NORMAL SALINE S.,** a solution of distilled water with sodium chloride dissolved in it in the same concentration as occurs in the blood. **SATURATED S.,** one in which as much solid is dissolved as will be held in solution without precipitating or floating. **SUPERSATURATED S.,** one that contains more of an ingredient than can be held in solution permanently, the excess being precipitated when the physical conditions are changed.

solvent (sol'vent): An agent, usually liquid, which is capable of dissolving other substances and holding them in solution.

soma (sō'ma): 1. The body as distinguished from the psyche or the mind. 2. The walls of the body as distinguished from the viscera. 3. The trunk of the body as distinguished from the appendages.

somasthenia (sō-mas-thē'ni-a): General chronic weakness of the body. Also somatasthenia.

somasthetic (sō-mas-thet'ik): Pertaining to the sensations of touch and proprioception (*q.v.*).

somat-, somato-: Combining forms denoting the body.

somatesthesia (sō'ma-tes-thē'zi -a): Being conscious of having a body; being sensitive to bodily sensation. Also somesthesia.

somatic (sō-mat'ik): 1. Pertaining to the body. 2. Pertaining to the trunk. 3. Pertaining to the wall of the body cavity rather than to the viscera. **S. NERVES,** nerves controlling the activity of striated, skeletal muscle. **S. NERVOUS SYSTEM,** see under nervous system. **S. THERAPY,** in psychiatry, the biologic treatment of mental disorders, as in electroconvulsive or psychopharmacologic therapy.

somatization (sō'ma-tī-zā'shun): The conversion of anxiety into physical symptoms, *e.g.*, "butterflies in the stomach, " headache, diarrhea, shortness of breath; an escape mechanism that often releases emotional tensions.

somatogenic (sō'ma-tō-jen'ik): Originating within the body, but resulting from the influence of external forces.

somatology (sō-ma-tol'o-ji): The study of the body, its structure, development, and functions.

somatomedins (sō'ma-tō-mē'dins): A group of hormone-dependent protein compounds synthesized in the liver and found in the circulating blood; they appear to have some insulin-like properties, some effects on growth hormone activity, and to stimulate anabolism in bone.

somatomegaly (sō'ma-tō-meg'a-li): The condition of having an unusually large body; gigantism.

somatometry (sō'ma-tom'e-tri): Measurements of the entire body and the classification of individuals according to their form and size.

somatopathy (sō'ma-top'a-thi): Disorder of the body as distinguished from that of the mind.

somatoplasm (sōmat' -ō-plaz-um): The protoplasm of the cells of the body considered apart from the material constituting the germ cells.

somatopsychic (sō'mat-ō-sī'kik): Relating to states of depression or worry that occur as responses to physical disease states. Opp. of psychosomatic (*q.v.*).

somatoscopy (sō'ma-tos'ko-pi): Physical examination of the body.

somatosensory (sō'ma-tō-sen'sō-ri): Pertaining to the bodily sensations.

somatostatin (so'ma-tō-stat'in): A tetrapeptide hormone produced in the hypothalamus that is capable of inhibiting the release of growth hormone from the anterior lobe of the pituitary gland, and of thyrotropin, as well as the enzymes renin, pepsin, gastrin, and secretin; it also acts on the pancreas to suppress the secretion of both insulin and glucagon.

somatotonia (sō'ma-tō-tō'ni-a): A type of temperament manifested chiefly by enjoyment of activity and vigorous action.

somatotropin (so'ma-tō-trō'pin): The growth-stimulating hormone secreted by the anterior lobe of the pituitary gland; it regulates body growth, stimulates healing of tissues, and lowers the cholesterol level in the body; secretion is increased during sleep. Also called human growth hormone.

somatotype (sō-mat' -ō-tīp): A particular type of body build as identified by certain physical characteristics; see *e.g.*, ectomorph, endomorph, mesomorph.

somite (sō'mīt): Either of the segmented masses of mesoderm that lie alongside the embryonic neural tube, and from which various tissues of the body develop including connective tissue and the skeletal muscles except those of the head and extremities.

somnambulism (som-nam'bū-lizm): Sleep walking; a state of dissociated consciousness in which sleeping and waking states are combined; the individual performs purposeful and often complex acts but has no memory of them upon awakening. Occurs during the third and fourth stages of nonrapid eye movement sleep; see sleep. Considered normal in children but as an illness, having physical or psychological basis, in adults.

somnambulist (som-nam'bū-list): An individual who habitually walks in his sleep.

somni-: A combining form denoting sleep.

somnia-: Combining form denoting a condition resembling sleep.

somnial (som'ni-al): Pertaining to dreams or sleep.

somniculous (som-nik'ū-lus): Sleepy.

somnifacient (som-ni-fā'shent): 1. Causing sleep; hypnotic, soporific. 2. An agent that causes sleep.

somniferous (som-nif'er-us): Producing sleep.

somnific (som-nif'ik): Producing sleep.

somniloquism (som-nil'ō-kwism): Talking in one's sleep.

somnolence (som'nō-lens): Excessive or prolonged sleepiness or drowsiness.—somnolent, adj.

somnus (som'nus): Sleep.

Somogyi: **S. EFFECT** or **PHENOMENON,** hypoglycemia caused by overinsulinization; followed by marked glycosuria and ketonuria resulting from increased production of glucose in the liver; occurs in diabetic patients. **S. METHOD,** either of two methods developed by .Somogyi for detecting amylase in the serum. **S. UNIT,** a measure of diastase or amylase activity in the serum. [M. Somogyi, American biochemist. 1883–1971.]

sonicate (son'i-kāt): To treat with high frequency sound waves.—sonication, n.

sonication (son-i-kā'shun): Exposure to high frequency sound waves.

sonitus (son'i-tus): Tinnitus (*q.v.*).

Sonne dysentery (son'ne dis'en-ter-i): Bacillary dysentery caused by infection with *Shigella sonnei*. [Carl Sonne, Danish bacteriologist. 1882–1948.]

sonochemistry (son'ō-kem-i-stri): The study of the chemical effects of high frequency sound and ultrasonic waves.

sonogram (son'ō-gram): The recording of a diagnostic examination that utilizes ultrasound. See ultrasonography.

sonography (son-og'ra-fi): Ultrasonography (*q.v.*).

sonometer (sō-nom'e-ter): An instrument for testing hearing acuteness.

sonorous (sō-nō' -rus): Being resonant or having a loud sound. **S. RALES,** rales that have a low-pitched or snoring sound; produced by the presence of mucous or viscid secretion in a bronchus.

sophomania (sof'ō-mā'ni-a): The deluded belief in one's own superior wisdom.

sopor (sō'por): Unnaturally deep or profound sleep: stupor.

soporific (sō'pōr-if'ik): 1. An agent that induces profound sleep. 2. Producing sleep.

sorbefacient (sor-be-fā'shent): 1. Causing absorption. 2. An agent that causes or promotes absorption.

sordes (sor'dēz): Dried, fetid brown crusts that form on the teeth, tongue, lips, and around the mouth in illness, especially fevers; consist of saliva, mucus, food particles, epithelial matter, and microorganisms; due to lack of proper oral hygiene.

sore: 1. Painful. 2. A general term for any ulcer or lesion on the skin or mucous membrane. **BEDSORE,** decubitus ulcer (*q.v.*). **CANKER S.,** an ulcer on the mucous membrane of the mouth. **COLD S.,** herpes simplex (*q.v.*). **PRESSURE S.,** decubitus ulcer (*q.v.*). **SOFT S.,** chancroid (*q.v.*). **VENEREAL S.,** any lesion accompanying a venereal infection; usually refers to chancre (*q.v.*). See also Oriental sore.

SOS: Abbreviation for *si opus sit* [L.], meaning, if it is necessary. Term used in written orders, usually for medication. Also written s.o.s.

souffle (soo'f'l): A murmur or soft blowing sound heard on auscultation of the heart. **FUNIC S.,** a high-pitched sound heard on auscultation in pregnancy; it is synchronous with the fetal heart beat and thought to be due to interference in the circulation of blood in the umbilical cord. **UTERINE S.**, soft blowing murmur that can be auscultated over the uterus after the fourth month of pregnancy.

sound: 1. Vibrations that stimulate the receptors and organs of the sense of hearing and result in a mental image. 2. Normal or abnormal noise produced in an organ of the body and audible on auscultation, *e.g.*, heart sound. 3. Sane or healthy. 4. A long, slender, cylindrical instrument to be inserted into a hollow organ for examination or exploration or to detect a foreign body, or into a duct to dilate it.

Southern Regional Education Board (SREB) and Southern Council on Collegiate Education for Nursing (SCCEN): Southern Regional Education Board, established in 1948 consists of 14 state members—Alabama, Arkansas, Florida, Georgia, Kentucky, Louisiana, Maryland, Mississippi, North and South Carolina, Tennessee, Texas, Virginia, and West Virginia. These states are represented on the Board by their governors and other legislators, and, since 1962, by representatives from the Council of Collegiate Education for Nursing. Membership of the Council consists of institutions that have accredited programs in baccalaureate, masters, and/or doctoral programs in nursing. Purposes of the Council: to furnish a means of communication among faculty of member institutions, to conduct seminars and workshops, and to publish material of interest to the members. Address: 1340 Spring St., NW, Atlanta GA 30309

Southey's tube: A small, thin, perforated cannula that is inserted subcutaneously; formerly much used for draining away the fluid from edematous tissues in anasarca or in edema of the legs.

soya bean: A highly nutritous legume that contains high-quality protein and little starch. Is useful in diabetic preparations. Also soybean.

sp gr: Abbreviation for specific gravity. See under specific.

spa (spah): A place in which water, especially that from mineral springs, is used for therapeutic purposes; it is both ingested and used for bathing.

space: 1. A delimited area or region within the body. 2. The world outside or beyond the earth's atmosphere. **S. MEDICINE,** the branch of medicine that deals with the changes and effects on human physiology produced in those who are projected at high velocity through space and then returned to the earth's atmosphere.

space occupying lesions: Lesions such as abscesses, hematomata, or tumors which form in an area where there is little room for expansion and which therefore compress the normal structures in the area; frequently they occur in the skull.

Spallanzani's law: States that the power of cells to regenerate is inversely related to the age of the individual.

spallation (spawl-lā'shun): The process of breaking into small bits or splintering. **S. PARTICLES,** refers to the different chemical elements produced in small amounts in nuclear fission. See fission.

spanemia (spa-nē'mi-a): Thinness of the blood; anemia.

Spanish fly: A species of beetle from which the powerful blistering agent, cantharadin, is derived. Formerly much used as a topical vesicant; not used in modern medicine.

Spansule (span'sūl): Trade name for a delayed-release form of capsule; it is prepared in such a way that some of the granules dissolve almost as soon as the capsule is administered, but the rest are coated with a substance that causes them to dissolve more slowly and farther along in the gut.

spasm (spazm): Convulsive involuntary muscular contraction. **CARPOPEDAL S., S.** of the muscles of the hands, feet, thumbs, or great toe; seen in cases of rickets, tetany due to calcium deficiency, and laryngismus stridulus (*q.v.*). **CLONIC S., S.** in which fairly short periods of contraction alternate with periods of relaxation. **HABIT S.,** an involuntary **S.** which recurs in a muscle that is ordinarily under voluntary control; a tic (*q.v.*). **INFANTILE MASSIVE S.,** jack-knife seizure; see seizure. **NODDING S.,** clonic **S.** of the sternocleidomastoid muscle causing bowing movements of the head. **SALAAM S.,** nodding **S. TETANIC S.,** that which occurs in tentanus. **TONIC S.** that in which rigidity persists for some time. **WINKING S.,** involuntary contraction of the muscles of the eyelid resulting in a wink. **WRITER'S S.,** writer's cramp; see under cramp.

spasmodic (spaz-mod'ik): 1. Recurring at intervals. 2. An agent that produces spasm. 3. Pertinent to or like a spasm.

spasmolygmus (spaz'mō-lig'mus): 1. Spasmodic sobbing. 2. Hiccup.

spasmolytic (spaz'mō-lit'ik): 1. Checking spasm(s). 2. An agent that checks spasm; an antispasmodic.

spasmophemia (spaz'mō-fē'mi-a): Stuttering.

spasmus (spaz'mus): Spasm. **S. NUTANS,** head-nodding spasm.

spastic (spas'tik): 1. Pertaining to spasm(s). 2. In a condition of muscular rigidity or spasm, *e.g.*, spastic diplegia (Little's disease, *q.v.*). **S. BLADDER,** see under bladder. **S. GAIT,** see under gait. **S. PARALYSIS,** see under paralysis.—spasticity, adj.

spasticity (spas-tis′it-i): A condition marked by sudden involuntary muscular spasm or rigidity.

spatula (spat′ū-la): A flat flexible knife with blunt edges for making poultices and spreading ointment. **TONGUE S.** a rigid, blade-shaped instrument for depressing the tongue.

spay: To remove the ovaries by surgery. Term is usually used for animals rather than humans.

special nurse: A private duty nurse; see under nurse.

Special Olympics: A special recreation program for the mentally retarded, for those in wheel chairs, and for blind epileptics. See Paralympics.

specialist: In medicine, a physician who limits his practice to certain diseases or disorders, or a certain type of therapy.

specialty: A branch of nursing (or medicine) for which a health professional has qualified either through advanced study, experience, or having passed a qualifying examination.

species (spē′shēz): A subdivision of genus. A group of individuals having common characteristics and differing only in minor details.

specific (spē-sif′ik): 1. Special; characteristic; peculiar to. 2. Pertaining to a species. 3. A medication that has special curative properties for a particular disease, as quinine for malaria. **S. DISEASE,** one that is always caused by a specified organism.

specific gravity: The weight of a substance, as compared with that of an equal volume of water. The specific gravity of urine is a measure of the relative proportion of the solvents in it.

specimen (spes′i-men): 1. A sample or small part of a substance or a thing taken for the purpose of determining the character of the whole, *e.g.*, urine, sputum, blood, or a small portion of tissue. 2. A preparation of normal or abnormal tissue prepared for study or pathological examination.

spectrocolorimeter (spek′trō-kul-ō-rim′-e-ter): A combined spectroscope and ophthalmoscope used to detect blindness to specific colors.

spectrometry (spek-trom′e-tri): The use of a spectrometer, an optical instrument for measuring the wavelengths of the rays of a spectrum.

spectromicroscope (spek′trō-mi′krō-skōp): A microscope with a spectroscopic attachment. See spectrometry.

spectrophotometer (spek′trō-fō-tom′-e-ter): 1. An apparatus used to measure the amount of coloring matter in a solution by measuring the amount of light that is absorbed as it passes through the solution. 2. An apparatus utilizing a spectrum to measure a person's sense of light.—spectrophotometric, adj.

spectroscope (spek′trō-skōp): A device for producing and observing spectra of light from any source.

spectrum (spek′trum): 1. Range of activity; often refers to antibiotics, *e.g.*, broad-spectrum antibiotics. 2. The components of a wave arranged in a particular order or sequence, such as wavelength or frequency, *e.g.*, x rays, or electric, ultraviolet, or infrared rays.—spectra, pl.; spectral, adj.

speculum (spek′ū-lum): An instrument used to hold the orifice or walls of a cavity apart, so that the interior of the cavity can be examined.—specula, pl.

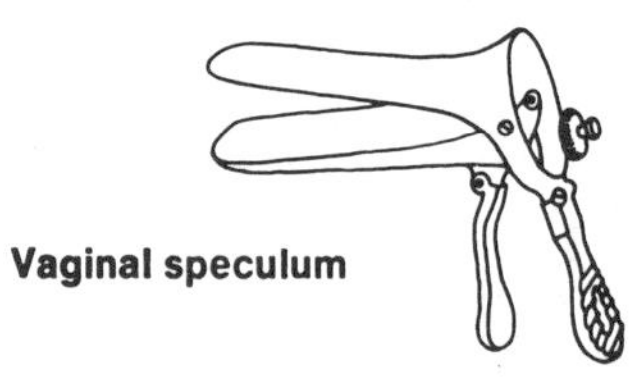
Vaginal speculum

speech: Oral communication of ideas by means of the utterance of vocal sounds. **AUTONOMIC S.**, redundant speaking of words, as repeating the days of the week or months of the year. **S. AUDIOMETRY,** the use of the audiometer to evaluate one's type and degree of hearing loss by testing his ability to discriminate pure tones of differing intensities and frequencies. **S. DYSFUNCTION,** any defect or abnormality in speech including sound production and enunciation, from whatever cause. **ESOPHAGEAL S.**, a technique learned following laryngectomy; the patient swallows air and then regurgitates it, producing vibrations in the column of air against the cricopharyngeal sphincter. **EXPLOSIVE S.**, loud, sudden speech, occurring in patients following nervous system injuries. **INCOHERENT S.**, **S.** in which thoughts expressed are not related. **MIRROR S.** the practice of reversing the order of syllables in words. **S. PATHOLOGY,** the field of study that deals with the evaluation and treatment of communicative disorders such as occur in production of speech, use of language, and voice production. **S. THERAPIST,** a person with special training in helping individuals to overcome their particular speech and language problems. **SCANNING S.**, **S.** in which the speaker pauses between syllables. **STACATTO S.**, **S.** in which each syllable is uttered separately; occurs in persons with multiple sclerosis.

speed: Street term for amphetamine drugs.

sperm: Spermatazoon (*q.v.*).

sperm bank: A facility where a male may deposit a quantity of semen, which is mixed with a protective fluid and stored at a very low temperature. At a later date the material may be thawed and used to induce pregnancy; the procedure is not universally practiced.

sperm-, spermato-, spermo-: Combining forms denoting 1) spermatozoa; 2) semen.

spermatacrasia (sper'-ma-ta-krā'zi-a): A decrease or deficiency of spermatazoa in the semen.

spermatic (sper-mat'ik): Pertaining to or conveying semen. **S. CORD,** suspends the testis in the scrotum and contains the **S.** artery and vein and the vas deferens.

spermatocele (sper-mat'ō-sēl): A localized enlargement of the spermatic cord; contains sperm; usually painless.

spermatocidal (sper-ma-tō-sī'dal): Destructive to spermatazoa.

spermatocide (sper-mat'-ō-sīd): Any agent that kills spermatazoa.

spermatocystitis (sper'ma-tō-sis-tī'sis): Inflammation of the seminal vesicles.

spermatogenesis (sper'mat-ō-jen'e-sis): The formation and development of sperm.—spermatogenetic, adj.

spermatorrhea (sper'ma-tō-rē'a): Frequent involuntary discharge of semen without orgasm.

spermatozoon (sper'ma-tō-zō'on): A mature, male reproductive cell produced in the testes; consisting of a head or nucleus, neck, and tail; about 1/500 of an inch in length.—spermatozoa, pl.

spermaturia (sper'ma-tū'ri-a): The presence of spermatozoa or semen in the urine.

spermicide (sper'mi-sīd): An agent that kills spermatozoa. Also spermatocide.—spermicidal, adj.

spermolith (sper'mō-lith): A concretion in the vas deferens or the seminal vesicle.

sphacelate (sfas'e-lāt): To slough or become gangrenous.—sphacelation, n.; sphacelous, adj.

sphagitis (sfā-ji'tis): 1. Sore throat. 2. Inflammation of a jugular vein.

sphen-, spheno-: Combining forms denoting 1) wedge-shaped; 2) the sphenoid bone.

sphenoethmoid (sfē'-nō-eth'moyd): Pertaining to the sphenoid and ethmoid bones.

sphenofrontal (sfē'nō-fron'tal): Pertaining to the sphenoid and frontal bones or to the line of suture between them.

sphenoid (sfē'noyd): 1. Wedge-shaped. 2. A wedge-shaped bone at the base of the skull, articulating with the occipital bone at the back, the ethmoid in front, and the parietal and temporal bones at the sides. **S. SINUS,** see under sinus.

sphenoiditis (sfē-noy-dī'tis): Inflammation of a sphenoid sinus.

sphenopalatine (sfē-nō-pal'a-tin): Pertaining to the sphenoid bone and the palatine bones.

spherocyte (sfē-rō-sīt): A red blood cell that is round instead of biconcave; characteristic of congenital hemolytic anemia.

spherocytosis (sfē-rō-sī-tō'sis): The presence of spherocytes in the circulating blood. **HEREDITARY S.,** a familial form of hemolytic anemia in which the erythrocytes are abnormally fragile, spherocytes are present in the blood, the patient is jaundiced, and the spleen is enlarged.

sphincter (sfingk'ter): A circular muscle, contraction of which serves to constrict a natural passage or to close a natural orifice. **ANAL S.,** surrounds the anus. **CARDIAC S.,** surrounds the esophagus at its opening into the stomach. **OCULAR S.,** surrounds the eye. **ODDI'S S.,** an intricate muscular structure surrounding the bile and pancreatic ducts, where they join the duodenum. **PUPILLARY S.,** surrounds the pupil. **PYLORIC S.,** surrounds the junction of the stomach and the small intestine. **S. OF BOYDEN,** surrounds the common bile duct just before its junction with the pancreatic duct.

sphincterectomy (sfingk'ter-ek'tō-mi): The excision or resection of a sphincter (*q.v.*).

sphincteroplasty (sfingk'ter-ō-plas-ti): Repair of or plastic surgery on a sphincter muscle.

sphingolipid (sfing'gō-lip'id): Any lipid that, on hydrolysis, yields sphingosine, a fatty acid attached to the nitrogen atom; found in membranes and particularly in brain and nerve tissue.

sphingolipidosis (sfing'gō-lip-i-dō'sis): A collective term for any of several inherited disorders of sphingolipid metabolism including Niemann-Pick disease, Gaucher's disease, and Tay-Sachs disease, which are characterized by the accumulation of certain glycolipids and phospholipids in some of the body tissues. **CEREBRAL S.,** a condition characterized by progressive degeneration of the nervous system, with convulsions, ataxia, spacticity, weakness of extremities, lack of mental development, progressive blindness due to optic atrophy. Formerly called amaurotic familial idiocy.

sphingomyelin (sfing'gō-mī'e-lin): One of a group of phospholipids found in brain, kidney, liver, and egg yolk; is composed of phosphoric acid, choline, a fatty acid, and sphingosine.

sphingosine (sfing'gō-sēn): A basic amino alcohol found as a constituent of sphingomyelin, cerebrosides, and several other phosphatides.

sphygmic (sfig'mik): Pertaining to or relating to the pulse.

sphygmo-: Combining form denoting pulse.

sphygmobolometer (sfig'mō-bō-lom'e-ter): An instrument for measuring and recording the energy of the pulse wave, which is an indirect means of measuring the strength of the systolic beat.

sphygmocardiograph (sfig′mō-kar′di-ō-graf): An apparatus for simultaneous graphic recording of the radial pulse and heartbeat.—sphygmocardiographic, adj.; sphygmocardiographically, adv.

sphygmograph (sfig′mō-graf): An instrument for recording the variations in blood pressure and in the pulse wave.

sphygmography (sfig-mog′ra-fi): The recording of the pulse wave, made with a sphygmograph.

sphygmomanometer (sfig′mō-ma-nom′e-ter): An instrument for measuring the force of the arterial blood pressure indirectly. Consists of an inflatable cuff usually applied to the upper arm and connected by a tube to a bulb used for inflating it; has a gauge that records the arterial pressure in millimeters on a graduated scale of a column of mercury.

sphyrectomy (sfi-rek′to-mi): Excision of the malleus of the ear.

spica (spī′ka): A bandage applied in a figure-of-eight pattern. See under bandage. **S. CAST,** see under cast.

spicule (spik′ūl): A small, spike-like fragment, especially of bone.—spicular, adj. Also spiculum.

spider: S. ANGIOMA, see under angioma. **S. TELANGIECTASIA,** see telangiectasia. See also black widow spider.

spike: The pointed element in a graph or chart that is created by a rising and falling vertical line. The spikes on a fever chart represent the high temperatures that are recorded. The spike in an electroencephalogram represents a brief electrical discharge.

spiloma (spī-lō′ma): A nevus (*q.v.*).

spiloplania (spī-lō-plā′ni-a): Transient redness or erythema of the skin.

spiloplaxia (spī-lō-plak′si-a): A red spot that appears on the skin in leprosy and sometimes in pellagra.

spina bifida (spī′na bif′i-da): A congenital defect in which the vertebral neural arches fail to close properly, so exposing the contents of the vertebral canal posterioraly. The fissure usually occurs in the lumbosacral region. The contents of the canal may or not protrude through the opening; paralysis, loss of sensation in the lower limbs, and bladder and bowel complications may occur; often occurs with other defects such as club feet, scoliosis, or sphincter incontinence. **S.B. CYSTICA,** a protrusion of the meninges and/or the spinal cord through a defect in the spinal column. **S.B. OCCULTA,** occurs when the contents of the spinal cord do not protrude through the fissure in the spinal column.

spinal (spī′nal): Pertaining to a spine or to the vertebral column. **S. ANESTHETIC,** a local anesthetic solution, injected into the subarachnoid space so that it renders the area supplied by the selected **S.** nerves insensitive. **S. BULB,** the medulla oblongata. **S. CANAL,** the central hollow throughout the **S.** column. **S. CARIES,** disease of the vertebral bones. **S. CAVITY,** the **S.** canal. **S. COLUMN,** a bony structure formed by 33 separate bones; the lower ones fuse together; the rest are separated by pads of cartilage; the backbone. **S. CORD,** the continuation of the nervous tissue of the brain down the **S.** canal to the

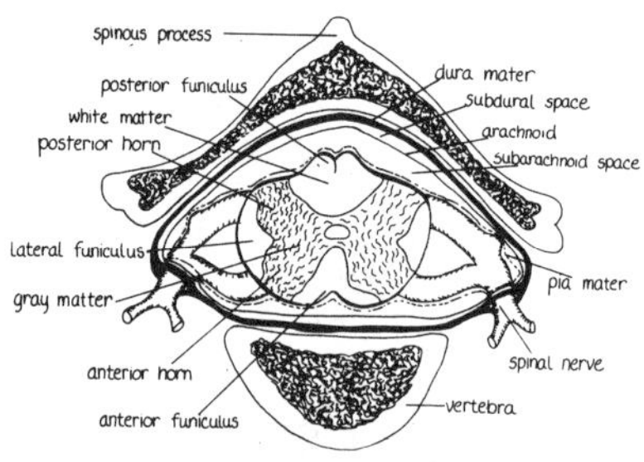

Cross-section of the spinal cord

level of the first or second lumbar vertebra. **S. CURVATURE,** an exaggerated curve in the **S.** column; see kyphosis, lordosis, scoliosis. **S. FLUID,** cerebrospinal fluid (*q.v.*). **S. FUSION,** an operation in which the articulations of vertebrae are destroyed, thus rendering a portion of the spine rigid (ankylosed). **S. GANGLION,** a group of sensory nerve cells on the posterior root of a spinal nerve. **S. NERVES,** 31 pairs leave the **S.** cord and pass out of the **S.** canal to supply the periphery. **S. PUNCTURE,** lumbar puncture (*q.v.*). **S. TAP, S.** puncture.

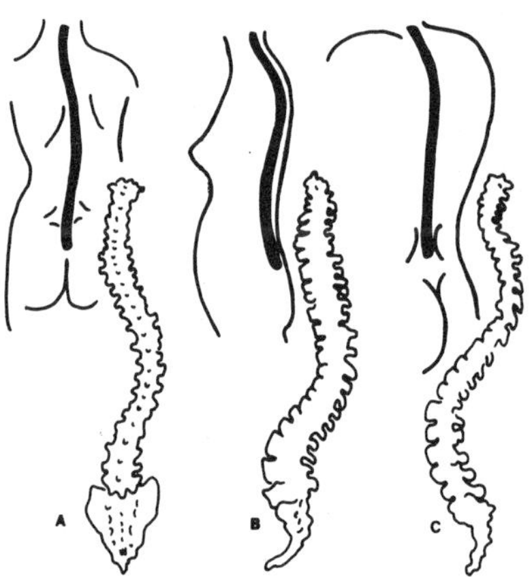

Abnormal spinal curves:
A, scoliosis; B, lordosis; C, kyphosis.

spinalgia (spī-nal′ji-a): Pain in the spinal area.

spine (spīn): 1. A popular term for the bony spinal or vertebral column. 2. A sharp process of bone. **ANTERIOR INFERIOR ILIAC S.**, a blunt projection of the lower part of the anterior edge of the ilium, just superior to the acetabulum. **ANTERIOR SUPERIOR ILIAC S.**, a blunt projection at the anterior end of the crest of the ilium. **S. OF THE SCAPULA**, a triangular plate of bone attached to the back of the scapula; extends from the vertebral edge of the scapula to the shoulder joint.

spinifugal (spī-nif′ū-gal): Conducting or moving in a direction away from the spinal cord, in particular, the efferent fibers of the spinal nerves.

spinipetal (spī-nip′e-tal): Conducting or moving in a direction toward the spinal cord, in particular, the afferent fibers of the spinal nerves.

spinnbarkheit (spin′bark-hīt): The ability of the mucus from the cervical plug to form a thin continuous thread when it is blown onto a glass slide and then drawn out over the slide with a cover glass; a procedure used to determine the time of ovulation and in choosing a day for artificial insemination.

spinobulbar (spī′nō-bul′bar): Pertaining to the spinal cord and the medulla oblongata.

spinocerebellar (spī′nō-ser-e-bel′lar): Pertaining to the spinal cord and cerebellum.

spinocortical (spī′nō-kor′ti-kal): Pertaining to the spinal cord and the cerebral cortex.

spinothalamic (spī′nō-thal′ a-mik): Pertaining to 1) the spinal cord and the thalamus, or 2) the ascending pathways between the spinal cord and the thalamus. **LATERAL S. TRACT**, is made up of nerve fibers that carry impulses for pain and temperature. **VENTRAL S. TRACT**, is made up of fibers that carry impulses for touch and pressure.

spinous (spī′nus): Pertaining to or resembling a spine or a spinelike process. Also spinose.

spintherism (spin′ther-izm): The sensation of sparks appearing before the eyes.

spiradenoma (spī-rad-e-nō′ma): A tumor of the sweat glands.

spirillicide (spī-ril′i-sīd): An agent that destroys spirilla.—spirillicidal, adj.

Spirillum (spī-ril′um): A bacterial genus; the organisms are corkscrew-shaped. Common in water and organic matter. **S. MINUS**, found in rodents and may infect humans, in whom it causes one form of ratbite fever (*q.v.*).—spirilla, pl.; spirillary, adj.

spirit: 1. An alcoholic solution. 2. A distilled solution.

spirochete (spī′rō-kēt): Common term for any motile, slender, spiral-shaped, sometimes flagellated bacterium of the order Spirochaetales; among them are the causative organisms for syphilis, yaws, relapsing fever, and leptospirosis or Weil's disease.

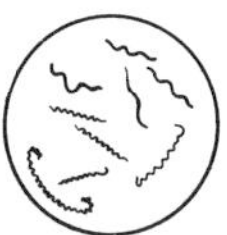

Spirochetes

spirochetemia (spī′rō-kē-tē′mi-a): Spirochetes in the bloodstream. This kind of bacteremia occurs in the secondary stage of syphilis and in the syphilitic fetus.—spirochetemic, adj.

spirocheticide (spī-rō-kē′ti-sīd): An agent that destroys spirochetes.—spirocheticidal, adj.

spirochetosis (spī′ -rō-kē-tō′sis): Infection with spirochetes.

spirogram (spī′rō-gram): A recorded tracing of the chest movements and excursion of the chest during respiration. See **spirograph.**

spirograph (spī′rō-graf): An apparatus which records the depth and rapidity of movement of the lungs.—spirographic, adj.; spirographically, adv.; spirography, n.

spirometer (spī-rom′e-ter): An instrument for measuring the air capacity of the lungs. See **bronchospirometer.**—spirometric, adj.; spirometry, n.

spirometry (spī-rom′e-tri): The measurement, with a spirometer, of the amount of air that can be moved in and out of the lungs.

spironolactone (spī′rō-nō-lak′tōn): A chemical compound in white crystalline form; used in medicine as a steroid diuretic because of its action in blocking the sodium-retaining action of aldosterone.

spissated (spis′āt-ed): Thickened; see inspissated.

spittle (spit'l): Sputum or saliva that is expectorated.

Spitz-Holter valve: A valve used in the tube designed to drain cerebrospinal fluid from the cranium into the internal jugular vein and vena cava, thence into the right atrium, in cases of hydrocephalus.

splanchnic (splangk′nik): Pertaining to or supplying the viscera, especially the abdominal viscera. **S. NERVES**, those of the sympathetic system that supply the abdominal viscera.

splanchnicectomy (splangk-ni-sek′to-mi): Surgical removal of the splanchnic nerves, whereby the viscera are deprived of sympathetic impulses; occasionally performed in the treatment of essential hypertension or for the relief of certain kinds of visceral pain.

splanchnicotomy (splangk-ni-kot′o-mi): The surgical division of a splanchnic nerve; may be done for the relief of hypertension.

splanchno-: Combining form denoting: 1. A viscus. 2. The splanchnic nerve.

splanchnodiastasis (splangk'nō-dī-as'ta-sis): Displacement of a viscus.

splanchnodynia (splangk-nō-din'i-a): Pain in an abdominal organ.

splanchnology (splangk-nol'o-ji): The study of the structure and function of the viscera.

splanchnomegaly (splangk-nō-meg'a-li): Abnormal enlargement of one or more of the viscera.

splanchnopathy (splangk-nop'a-thi): Any disease of the viscera.

splanchnoptosis (splangk'nop-tō'sis): Visceroptosis (*q.v.*).

splayfoot (splā'foot): Flatfoot.

spleen (splēn): An elongated, oval, lymphoid, vascular organ lying in the upper left quadrant of the abdominal cavity, immediately below the diaphragm at the tail of the pancreas and behind the stomach. It is one of the blood-forming organs; stores blood, and acts as a blood filter. Apparently not essential to life as it can be removed without endangering the patient's life.—splenic, adj.

splen-, spleno-: Combining forms denoting the spleen.

splenadenoma (splen-ad-e-nō'ma): Hyperplasia of the spleen.

splenectasia (splē-nek-tā'zi-a): Enlargement of the spleen.

splenectomy (splē-nek'to-mi): Surgical removal of the spleen.

splenic (splen'ik): Pertaining to the spleen. **S. ANEMIA,** Banti's disease (*q.v.*). **S. FLEXURE,** the bend in the colon just beneath the spleen where the transverse colon becomes the descending colon. **S. VEIN,** the vein that transports blood from the spleen to the portal vein.

splenicopancreatic (splē'ni-kō-pan-krē-at'ik): Resembling or pertaining to both the spleen and the pancreas.

splenitis (splē-nī'tis): Inflammation of the spleen.

splenius (splē'nē-us): One of the flat muscles at the back of the neck and upper thoracic region.

splenocaval (splē-nō-kā'val): Pertaining to the spleen and inferior vena cava, usually referring to anastomosis of the splenic vein to the inferior vena cava.

splenocele (splē'nō-sēl): 1. A tumor of the spleen. 2. Hernia of the spleen.

splenocolic (splē'nō-kol'ik): Pertaining to the spleen and the colon; often refers to a fold of peritoneum that lies between the two organs.

splenodynia (splē'nō-din'i-a): Pain in the spleen.

splenogenous (splē-noj'e-nus): Arising in the spleen.

splenogram (splē'nō-gram): Radiographic picture of the spleen after injection of radiopaque medium.—splenograph, splenography, n.; splenographical, adj.; splenographically, adv.

splenohepatomegaly (splē'nō-hep'a-tō-meg'a-li): Englargement of the spleen and the liver.

splenoma (splē-nō'ma): An enlargement of the spleen; may or may not be due to the presence of a tumor.

splenomalacia (splē'nō-ma-lā'-shi-a): Abnormal softness of the spleen.

splenomegaly (splē'nō-meg'a-li): Enlargement of the spleen. **CONGESTIVE S.,** see Banti's disease.

splenomyelogenous (splē'nō-mī-e-loj'e-nus): Formed in both the spleen and the bone marrow. **S. LEUKEMIA,** granulocytic leukemia, see under leukemia.

splenonephroptosis (splē'nō-nef-rop' -tōsis): Downward displacement of the spleen and the kidney.

splenopancreatic (splē'nō-pan-krē- at'ik): Pertaining to the spleen and the pancreas.

splenopathy (splē-nop'a-thi): Any disease or disorder of the spleen.

splenophrenic (sple-nō-fren'ik): Pertaining to the spleen and the diaphragm: often refers to a fold of peritoneum that lies between the two organs.

splenoportal (splē-nō-por'tal): Pertaining to the spleen and portal vein.

splenoportogram (splē'nō-port'ō-gram): Radiographic picture of the spleen and portal vein after injection of radiopaque medium.—splenoportograph, splenoportography, n.; splenoportographical, adj.; splenoportographically, adv.

splenoptosis (splē'nop-tō'sis): Downward displacement of the spleen.

splenorenal (splē'nō-rē'al): Pertaining to the spleen and kidney, as an anastomosis of the splenic vein to the renal vein; a procedure carried out in some cases of portal hypertension. **S. SHUNT,** see under shunt.

splenorrhagia (splē'nō-rā'ji-a): Hemorrhage from a spleen that has ruptured.

splint: An apparatus, usually rigid, used to support, protect, and immobilize an injured part temporarily, or to maintain an injured part in a specific position. **AIRPLANE S.,** a plaster **S.** that holds the arm in elevation and abduction; the **S.** is supported by plaster which extends down the side of the thorax or around it. **BANJO S.,** a device that exerts traction on the fingers; occasionally used to treat certain types of hand injuries; made of a metal rod shaped like a banjo. **BARLOW'S S.,** holds the hips in extension; used for infants with congenital hip dysplasia. **BRAUN S.,** a support that holds the leg in balanced traction eliminating the need for traction equipment attached to the bed. **COCKUP S.**, a **S.** used for treating injury to the wrist or hand or to support the wrist in a position of function in cases of paralysis, *i.e.*, dorsiflexion. **DENIS BROWNE S.**, a metal bar with foot plates at either end to which the feet are attached, usually with shoes riveted to the foot plates. The feet can be rotated internally or externally by using the ratchet mechanism that holds the plates on the bar. Used in a variety of foot and leg problems, *e.g.*, to hold correction obtained by club foot casts, or to correct tibial tortion. **DOLL'S COLLAR S.**, a plaster collar used in treatment of fracture of cervical vertebrae; extends over the occiput, around the ears, over the chin, and down over the shoulders, sternum, and upper part of the back. **DYNAMIC S.**, a **S.** that supplies support for an injured, operated on, or paralyzed part, but allows for controlled motion to prevent stiffness and promote circulation. **GUTTER S.**, a trough-like **S.** of wood or metal in which an injured arm or leg is placed to provide support and immobilization. **HARE S.**, an adaptation of the half-ring Thomas **S.**, has a ratchet mechanism to exert a stable amount of traction on the leg to establish its correct position in the splint. **INFLATABLE S.**, a plastic, first-aid **S.** used to immobilize a fractured leg or arm; is inflated after application to conform to and support the limb. **THOMAS S.**, a ring splint used for fixed traction in emergency care; the ring is placed in contact with the ischium, the leg supported on slings placed on the length of the splint, and the foot and ankle tied to the end of the **S.**, providing traction. May also be used for balanced traction in combination with a Pearson attachment that allows for two lines of traction.

splinting: The application of a splint to provide fixation of a fracture or dislocation. Splinting an incision refers to the practice of pressing a pillow or similar object against the abdomen when the patient coughs, sneezes, or breathes deeply following abdominal surgery.

split: **S. GRAFT**, split-thickness graft, see under graft. **S. PERSONALITY**, see under personality.

spondyl-, spondylo-: Combining forms denoting vertebra(e).

spondylalgia (spon′di-lal′ji-a): Pain in a vertebra.

spondylarthritis (spon-dil-ar-thrī′tis): Arthritis of the vertebrae. **S. ANKYLOPOIETICA**, rheumatoid **S.**; see under spondylitis.

spondyle (e) (spon′dil): A vertebra.

spondylitis (spon-di-lī′tis): Inflammation of one or more vertebrae involving the capsules and intervertebral ligaments; Pott's disease (*q.v.*). **RHEUMATOID** or **ANKYLOSING S.**, a chronic inflammation of unknown etiology, involving primarily the spine and girdle joints, the shoulder, neck, ribs, and jaw; characterized by pain, stiffness, ankylosis progressing upward from the sacroiliac to the intervertebral and costovertebral joints, and rigidity of the spine and thorax. Occurs mostly in men between 20 and 40 years of age; may be hereditary.

spondylizemia (spon′di-lī-zē′mi-a): The downward displacement of a vertebra when the one below it has been destroyed.

spondylodynia (spon′di-lō-dīn′ē-a): Pain in a vertebra.

spondylolisthesis (spon′di-lō-lis-thē′sis): Forward displacement of one of the lower vertebrae on the one below it; more common in men; resulting deformity makes it appear that the trunk has descended into the pelvis.

spondylolysis (spon-di-lol′i-sis): The breaking down of the structure of a vertebra.

spondylopyosis (spon′di-lō-pī-o′sis): Suppuration of a vertebrae.

spondylosis (spon-di-lō′sis): Degeneration of the vertebral bodies or of the intervertebral disks, with an abnormal fusion or growing together of two or more vertebrae. Often called osteoarthritis of the spine. **CERVICAL S.**, degenerative joint disease affecting the cervical vertebrae.

spondylosyndesis (spon′di-lō-sin-dē′-sis): Spinal fusion; surgical immobilization, or ankylosis of the vertebrae.

spondylus (spon′di-lus): A vertebra.

sponge: 1. The elastic, fibrous skeleton of a marine organism. 2. A folded piece of gauze or a piece of cotton used for mopping up fluids, for dressings, etc. **S. BATH**, see under bath.

spongiform (spun′ji-form): Resembling a sponge.

spongioblast (spun′ji-ō-blast): An embryonic cell, the processes of which develop into the neuroglia (*q.v.*).

spongiocytoma (spun′ji-ō-sī-tō′ma): Astrocytoma (*q.v.*).

spontaneous (spon-tān′ē-us): Occurring without apparent cause. **S ABORTION**, unexpected premature delivery of the contents of a pregnant uterus. **S. FRACTURE**, one occurring without apparent injury; sometimes seen in certain diseases of the bone. **S. GENERATION**, an obsolete theory in microbiology that microorganisms arise spontaneously.

spoonerism (spoon′er-izm): A speech or writing defect in which the person tends to transpose letters or syllables of words.

sporadic (spō-rad′ik): Scattered; occurring in isolated cases; not epidemic.—sporadically, adv.

spore (spōr): A phase in the life cycle of a limited number of bacterial genera where the vegetative cell becomes encapsulated and metabolsim almost ceases. These spores are highly resistant to environmental conditions such as heat and desiccation. The spores of important species such as *Clostridium tetani* and *Cl. botulinum* are ubiquitous and can survive for long periods of time without food or water; when water, a suitable food supply, and a suitable temperature become available, the spores grow, mature, and become pathogenic.

sporicidal (spōr-i-sı′dal): Lethal to spores.—sporicide, n.

sporogenesis (spo-rō-jen′e-sis): The formation or reproduction of spores.—sporogenic, adj.

sporogony (spō-rog′o-ni): The sexual cycle of sporozoa; usually refers to the life cycle of the malarial parasite in the stomach and body of the mosquito.

sporonticide (spō-ron′ti-sīd): A drug that inhibits the growth of oocytes in the stomach wall of the mosquito and thus prevents the development of sporozoites (*q.v.*), making transmission of malaria by the mosquito impossible.

sporotrichosis (spōr′ō-tri-kō′sis): A subacute or chronic disease caused by infection of a wound with a fungus (*Sporotrichum schenkii*) that results in a primary sore with lymphangitis and subcutaneous painless granulomata, which tend to break down and become ulcerous. Three forms are recognized: cutaneous lymphatic, disseminated, and pulmonary, with the symptoms varying with the form. Occurs among those working in the soil.

Sporozoa (spō-rō-zō′a): A class of *Protozoa,* some of which are parasitic to man.—sporozoan, adj.

sporozoite (spō-rō-zō′īt): A spore that is formed after fertilization. In malaria, sporozoites are the forms of the causative organism that are liberated in the oocysts in the mosquito host and transferred to man when the mosquito bites.

sport: An organism that varies entirely or partly from others of the same type and which may transmit this variation to its offspring; a mutation.

sporulation (spōr-ū-lā′shun): The formation of spores.—sporulate, v.

spot: In medicine, a circumscribed area that differs from the surrounding area in color, texture, elevation, or other characteristics; a macule. See rose spots, liver spots, Koplik's spots.

spotted fever: 1. A name given to several eruptive fevers that are characterized by the appearance of distinctive spots, including typhus and Rocky Mountain spotted fever. 2. Endemic cerebrospinal fever, caused by meningococcus.

spotting: The loss of a slight amount of blood between menstrual periods.

sprain: Injury to the soft tissues surrounding a joint, caused by forcible wrenching or hyperextension of the joint; sometimes ligaments or tendons are ruptured but the bone is not fractured or dislocated; accompanied by pain, swelling, and discoloration. Classified as first, second, and third degree, according to severity and extent of the injury.

sprue (sproo): A chronic disorder due to malabsorption in the intestinal tract, characterized by glossitis, indigestion, weakness, emaciation, anemia, diarrhea, steatorrhea. **NON-TROPICAL S.,** may be hereditary; characterized by loss of weight, asthenia, depletion of electrolytes, diarrhea with frothy fetid stools; occurs in children and adults; due to ingestion of gluten-containing foods. **TROPICAL S.,** occurs mostly in the tropics and characterized by anemia; due to folic acid deficiency resulting from protein malnutrition.

spur: A calcar (*q.v.*). **CALCANEAN S.,** occurs on the lower surface of the calcaneus; often follows injury and causes pain on walking. **OCCIPITAL S.,** a small bony process on the occipital bone behind the posterior process of the atlas. **OLECRANON S.,** an abnormal process of bone at the insertion of the triceps muscle on the olecranon.

sputum (spū′tum): Excess of secretion from the respiratory passages expectorated through the mouth; consists mainly of mucus and saliva, but may also contain blood, pus, microorganisms. **PRUNE-JUICE S., S.** with a dark reddish brown or bloody color; seen in certain respiratory conditions including lobar pneumonia and cancer of the lung.

sq cm: Abbreviation for square centimeter.

Sq, sq: Abbreviation for subcutaneous or subcutaneously.

squama (skwā′ma): 1. A mass of platelike tissue, especially of bone, as the **S.** of the temporal bone. 2. A flake or scale of the skin.—squamous, adj.

squame (skwām): Squama (*q.v.*).

squamo-columnar (skwā′mō-kol-um′nar): Pertaining to squamous and columnar cells; usually refers to the junction of these two types of cells in the epithelial lining of the uterine cervix.

squamosa (skwā-mō′sa): The squamous part of the frontal, occipital, and, particularly, of the temporal bone.

squamous (skwā′mus): 1. Thin and flat like a fish scale. 2. Consisting of thin flat cells, as in the epithelium. 3. Pertaining to the thin scale-like portion of certain bones, *e.g.*, the temporal bone.

squamous cell carcinoma: See under carcinoma.

squint (skwint): 1. Strabismus. Incoordinated action of the muscles of the eyeball, such that the visual axes of the two eyes fail to meet at the objective point. **CONVERGENT S.,** occurs when the eyes turn toward the medial line. **DIVERGENT S.**, occurs when the eyes turn outward. 2. To partially close the eyes, as in a very bright light.

SR: Abbreviation for sedimentation rate.

s̄s̄: Abbreviation for *semis* [L.], meaning one-half.

s.s.: Abbreviation for soapsuds.

SSI: See Supplementary Security Income.

S-T segment: The interval in the electrocardiogram between the QRS complex and the beginning of the T wave.

stable: Steady, regular, not easily moved or broken down.

staccato speech (sta-ka'tō): A jerky manner of speaking with interruptions between words or syllables; scanning speech (*q.v.*).

stage (stāj): 1. The platform-like part of a microscope upon which a slide is placed for viewing. 2. A phase or period in the course of a disease, in the life of an organism, or in the progress of labor.

staging (stāj'ing): Term used to describe the classification of malignant tumors according to their cellular makeup, their potential for responding to therapy, and the prognosis for the patient.

stain: 1. To discolor. 2. A dye or other pigment or coloring matter used to color microorganisms or tissue for microscopic examination. See acid-fast; counter-stain; differential stain, under differential; Wright's stain.

stalk (stawk): In anatomy, a narrow connecting or supporting structure.

stamina (stam'i-na): Endurance, vigor, strength.

stammer (stam'er): A speech disorder characterized by halting, repeating, mispronouncing, or inability to pronounce certain sounds; most often seen in children; may be caused by excessive nervousness, agitation, being constantly scolded, emotional states such as fear, worry, insecurity.

stammering bladder: Pertains to a condition in which the urinary stream is frequently interrupted; may be a pathologic or psychogenic condition.

standard of care: In the health sciences, a measure against which a professional person's conduct is compared; comprises a list of those acts that a prudent professional person would have performed (or not performed) in like circumstances. In nursing, usually refers to nursing actions that would be performed (or not performed) by other reasonably careful nurses in like circumstances.

Standards of Nursing Practice: A set of eight general standards for carrying out the nursing process; established by the Congress of Nursing Practice of the American Nurses' Association. Consists of guidelines concerning the process and outcomes of nursing practice against which the quality of nursing care can be determined. More specific standards for practice in the various fields of nursing and recommended methods for their implementation are also available.

standardization (stand'dard-ī-zā-shun): The bringing of any drug or other substance into conformity with a set standard of purity, concentration, etc.

standing orders: A written set of general orders prepared for a nursing care unit; to be followed for all patients on the unit. They usually relate to routine care and include instructions for checking vital signs; for monitoring ambulatory patients and those on oxygen therapy; for administration of analgesics, sedatives, and laxatives; may also include restrictions regarding smoking, use of telephone, radio, or television; transfer activities, and so on.

standstill: The stoppage or cessation of a normal activity, as may occur with the heart. **CARDIAC S.**, asystole; may be due to cessation of normal activity of the atrium, the sinoatrial node, or the ventricle; marked by complete absence of waves on the electrocradiogram.

Stanford-Binet test: The Binet-Simon intelligence test as it has been revised and prepared at Stanford University; it is an individually administered test used to measure intelligence.

stapedectomy (stā-pe-dek'to-mi): Surgical removal of stapes in treatment of otosclerosis.

stapediolysis (stā'-pē-dī-ol'i-sis): An operation to mobilize the foot of the stapes in treatment for conduction deafness from otosclerosis.

stapes (stā'pēz): The stirrup-shaped innermost bone of the middle ear. **S. MOBILIZATION,** release of a stapes rendered immobile by otosclerosis.

Staph: Common abbreviation for Staphylococcus.

staphyl, staphylo-: Combining forms denoting: 1. The uvula. 2. A structure or arrangement that resembles a bunch of grapes.

staphyle (staf'i-lē): The uvula.

staphylectomy (staf-i-lek'to-mi): Amputation of the uvula. Uvulotomy.

staphyledema (staf'il-ē-dē'ma): Edema or any enlargement or swelling of the uvula.

staphyline (staf'i-līn): 1. Pertaining to the uvula. 2. Shaped like a bunch of grapes.

staphylitis (staf-i-lī'tis): Inflammation of the uvula.

staphylocide (staf'i-lō-sīd): Destructive to staphylococci.

staphylococcal (staf'i-lō-kok'al): Pertaining to or caused by staphylococci.

staphylococcemia (staf′i-lō-kok-sē′mi-a): The presence of staphylococci in the bloodstream.

staphylococcosis (staf′i-lō-kok-ō′sis): Infection with staphylococci.

Staphylococcus (staf-i-lō-kok′us): A genus of bacteria. Gram-positive cocci occurring in clusters. May be saprophytic or parasitic. Common commensals of man, in whom they are responsible for much minor pyogenic infection and a lesser amount of more serious infection. A common cause of hospital cross-infection. **S. ALBUS,** a white form often found in sputum; occasionally the cause of staphylococcal pneumonia. **S. AUREUS,** produces a golden yellow pigment on culture media; responsible for many diseases and infections in man. **S. EPIDERMIS,** a species of **S.** commonly found on the skin.—staphylococcal, adj.

staphylolysin (staf′i-lol′i-sin): A substance produced by staphylococci that causes hemolysis (*q.v.*).

staphyloma (staf′i-lō′ma): A bulging outward of the cornea or sclera of the eye, caused by an inflammatory reaction.

staphyloncus (staf-i-long′kus): A tumor or other enlargement of the uvula.

staphylopharyngorrhaphy (staf′i-lō-far-in-gor′a-fi): A plastic operation on the palate and pharynx for repair of a cleft palate.

staphyloptosis (staf′i-lop-tō′sis): Elongation of the uvula.

staphylorrhaphy (staf′i-lor′a-fi): The operation for closing or uniting a cleft uvula or cleft palate.

staphylotomy (staf′i-lot′o-mi): Excision of the uvula or of a staphyloma.

starch: A complex carbohydrate, classed as a polysaccharide, found abundantly in nature in rice, corn and other cereals, in vegetables, and in unripe fruits. **S.** bath, a bath using starch for relief of pruritus.

Starling's law of the heart: States that the more the heart muscle is stretched as blood enters the ventricle, the more vigorously it will contract, the result being that a greater amount of blood will be pumped out of the heart.

Starr-Edwards ball valve prosthesis: One of several types of prostheses used in heart surgery; replaces a damaged mitral valve.

"start hesitation": A sudden feeling of one's feet being extremely heavy and of being unable to walk.

startle reflex: See under reflex.

stasibasiphobia (stas′i-bā′si-fō′bi-a): A morbid fear of standing upright or walking. See astasia-abasia.

stasis (stā′sis): Stagnation, cessation, retardation, or stoppage of flow of blood, urine or other body fluid, or of the motion of a part *e.g.*, the intestines. **INTESTINAL S.,** atony or sluggish bowel contractions resulting in constipation, auto-intoxication, neurasthenia and other symptoms. **S. ULCER,** see ulcer.

-stasis: Combining form denoting 1) stoppage; 2) maintenance of a constant level.

Stat: Abbreviation for *statim* [L.], meaning immediately.

State Boards of Nursing: Composed of professional nurses (in some states practical nurses also) who administer the laws regarding nursing; they set the regulations for accrediting schools of nursing; examine candidates for the R.N.; issue licenses to qualified applicants, and discipline those who violate the regulations in their particular jurisdictions.

state medicine: A method of managing medical treatment in which a governmental body supervises medical care and regulates financial aspects of care, the objective being to furnish medical care to all who need it.

State Nurses' Association: A unit or constituent of the American Nurses' Association, organized and conducted at the state level.

static (stat′ik): Not dynamic; not moving; resting.

statim (sta′tim): At once [L.]. Abbreviated Stat. or stat.

station: 1. An individual's attitude or manner when standing, *i.e.,* the position of his body and its parts. 2. A specific location to which the sick or wounded are taken for care.

statistical significance: A measurement or score that is unlikely to have occurred by chance alone and might, therefore, be accounted for by some specific factor, such as an experimental treatment.

statistics (sta-tis′tiks): The science dealing with collecting, tabulating, and interpreting numerical data on any subject.

statoacoustic (stat′ō-a-koos′tik): Pertaining to equilibrium and hearing.

statocyst (stat′ō-sist): One of the sacs of the labyrinth of the ear; thought to be involved in the maintenance of static equilibrium.

statolith (stat′ō-lith): An otolith (*q.v.*).

stature (statch′ūr): The height or tallness of a person when standing; measured from the soles of the feet to the top of the head.

status (stā′tus): A state or condition; in medicine, often used in the sense of implying severe or intractable. **S. ANGIOSUS,** angina that occurs during rest and is resistant to treatment; see angina. **S. ASTHMATICUS,** a prolonged and refractory attack of asthma; an acute emergency condition requiring immediate medical treatment. **S. EPILEPTICUS,** repeated epileptic attacks in rapid succession without recovery between them; an emergency condition. **S. LYMPHATICUS,** a morbid condition found mostly in children, in which there is hypertrophy of lymphoid tissue, particularly of the thymus; sudden death is not unusual in these patients, especially when they are under the influence of an anesthetic.

staunch (stawnsh): To stop the flow of blood; usually refers to bleeding from a wound. Also spelled stanch.

STD: Abbreviation for sexually transmitted diseases (*q.v.*).

steapsin (stē-ap'sin): The lipase of the pancreatic juice, which splits fat into fatty acids and glycerine following emulsification of bile salts.

stearate (stē'a-rāt): Any compound of stearic acid.

stearic acid (ste-ar'ik as'id): A saturated fatty acid derived from animal fat; used in pharmaceutical preparations.

stearo-: Combining form denoting relationship to fat.

steat-, steato: Combining forms denoting fat.

steatitis (stē-a-tī'tis): Inflammation of fatty tissue.

steatolysis (stēa-tol'i-sis): The process by which fats are emulsified in the intestine and prepared for absorption.

steatoma (stē-a-tō'ma): 1. A retention cyst of a sebaceous gland; a wen. 2. A lipoma. Also steatocystoma.

steatomatosis (stē'a-tō-ma-tō'sis): The presence of numerous sebaceous cysts.

steatonecrosis (stē'a-tō-ne-krō'sis): Necrosis of fatty tissue.

steatopathy (stē-a-top'a-thi): Any disease or disorder of the sebaceous glands.

steatopygia (stē-at-ō-pij'i-a): Excessive deposit of fat on the buttocks; most often seen in women. Also sometimes called Hottentot bustle.

steatorrhea (ste-a-tō-rē'a): 1. An increase in sebaceous gland secretion. 2. A syndrome of varied etiology associated with multiple defects in digestion and absorption of fat from the gut; characterized by the passage of pale, bulky, greasy stools.

Steele-Richardson-Olszewski syndrome: Progressive supranuclear palsy; see under palsy.

Stein-Leventhal syndrome: Polycystic ovary syndrome. A group of symptoms, seen most often in women between 15 and 30 years of age; characterized by large polycystic ovaries with small follicles that do not mature enough to ovulate but become cystic. Symptoms include amenorrhea or abnormal bleeding, or both; obesity, infertility, hirsutism.

Steinmann pin: An alternative to the use of a Kirschner wire (*q.v.*) for applying skeletal traction to a limb. [Fritz Steinmann, Swiss surgeon 1872–1932.]

stellate (stel'āt): Star-shaped. **S. GANGLION,** a large collection of nerve cells (ganglion) on the sympathetic chain in the root of the neck.

Stellwag's sign: Occurs in exophthalmic goiter (Graves' disease). Patient does not blink as often as normally, and the eyelids close only imperfectly when he does so; also the upper eyelid is retracted so that the palpebral opening is widened. [Carl Stellwag von Carion, Austrian opthalmologist. 1823–1904.]

stem: 1. A supporting structure; a stalk. 2. To check, as blood flow. 3. To originate in. **BRAIN S.,** all of the brain except the cerebrum and the cerebellum. **S. CELL,** a cell that gives rise to a particular type of cell, as occurs in hematopoiesis.

sten-, steno-: Combining forms denoting narrow, constricted.

stenagmus (ste-nag'mus): Sighing.

Stenger test: A test to expose simulated deafness in one ear only.

stenocardia (sten-ō-kar'di-a): Angina pectoris (*q.v.*).

stenocephaly (sten-ō-sef'a-li): Unusual narrowness of the head or cranium.

stenochoria (sten-ō-kō'ri-a): A narrowing; said especially of the lacrimal duct.

stenopeic (sten-ō-pē'ik): Having a very narrow slit or a tiny hole for admitting light.

stenosed (ste-nozd'): Narrowed, constricted.

stenosis (ste-nō'sis): Abnormal narrowing or stricture of any canal or orifice. **AORTIC S.,** narrowing of the orifice between the heart and the aorta. **AQUEDUCTAL S.,** narrowing or malformation of the aqueduct of Sylvius resulting in an enlarged cranium, and hydrocephalus; may be caused by trauma or meningoencephalitis; characterized by headache, visual disturbances, possibly seizures. **CARDIAC S.,** narrowing of any of the heart cavities or orifices. **MITRAL S.,** narrowing of the biscupid opening between the left atrium and ventricle. **PULMONARY** or **PULMONIC S.,** narrowing of the orifice between the right ventricle and the pulmonary artery. **PYLORIC S.,** narrowing of the orifice between the stomach and the small intestine. **SUBAORTIC S, S.** that obstructs the flow of blood from the left ventricle; due to a lesion subjacent to the aortic valve. **TRICUSPID S.,** narrowing of the orifice between the right atrium and ventricle.—stenotic, stenosed, adj.

stenothermia (sten'ō-ther'mi-a): The condition of being able to develop only within a narrow range of temperature; said of certain bacteria.

stenothorax (sten'ō-thō'raks): An unusually narrow chest.

stenotic (ste-not'ik): Characterized by abnormal narrowing or constriction.

Stensen's duct (sten'sen): The duct leading from the parotid gland and opening into the cheek opposite the upper second molar tooth. [Niels Stensen or Steno, Danish anatomist. 1638–1686.]

stercobilin (ster'kō-bī'lin): The brown pigment of feces; it is derived from the bile pigments.

stercobilinogen (ster'kō-bī-lin'ō-jen) Urobilinogen (*q.v.*).

stercolith (ster'kō-lith): A hard, dry mass of fecal matter in the intestine.

stercoraceous (ster-kō-rā'shus): Consisting of, containing, or resembling feces. Also stercoral. **S. VOMITING,** the vomiting of material that contains feces.

stercoroma (ster-kō-rō'ma): A hard fecal mass in the rectum.

stereo-: Combining form denoting: 1. Special qualities. 2. Three dimensionality. 3. Firm, hard, solid, or a solid medium.

stereoarthrolysis (ster'ē-ō-ar-throl'i-sis): Loosening or manipulation of stiff joints so as to make them movable, especially in ankylosis.

stereognosis (ster' -ē-og-nō' -sis): Perception through the sense of touch; the faculty of being able to appreciate the form and nature of objects by handling them, or the ability to identify writing traced on one's palm by another person's fingers.

stereopsis (ster-ē-op'sis): Stereoptic vision. See **stereoscope.**

stereoroentgenography (ster'ē-ō-rent'gen-og'ra-fi): The making of a stereoscopic roentgenogram.

stereoscope (stē'rē-ō-skōp): An instrument that projects two images of the same object that, when blended, give an impression of depth to a single picture of that object.—stereoscopic, adj.

stereotactic surgery: Electrodes and cannulae are passed to a predetermined point in the brain for physiological observation or destruction of tissue in such diseases as paralysis agitans, epilepsy, multiple sclerosis. Used for the relief of intractable pain also.—stereotaxy, stereotaxis, n.

stereotypy (ster'ē-ō-tī'pi): The persistent repetition of meaningless words or acts, often observed in persons with schizophrenia and in those with some forms of mental retardation.

sterile (ster'il): 1. Free from living microorganisms and their products. 2. Being unable to conceive; barren. **S. TECHNIQUE,** a method of functioning that aims to maintain the sterility of sterilized objects.

sterility (ster-il'i-ti) 1. Freedom from microorganisms. 2. Inability to conceive or bear offspring.

sterilization (ster'i-lī-zā'shun): 1. The process of completely ridding material or tissue of live microorganisms, leaving no viable forms including spores. 2. Rendering an individual incapable of reproduction. **CHEMICAL S.,** destruction of microorganisms by means of a chemical substance. **DRY HEAT S., S.** by subjection to very high temperatures for several hours. **EUGENIC S.,** the process of rendering an individual incapable of producing offspring. **FRACTIONAL S.,** subjection of materials to free-flowing steam for several hours several days in succession to kill spores that might have developed between sterilizations. **GAS S.,** exposure of materials to a gas that kills microorganisms. **MECHANICAL S.,** removing microorganisms by passing a fluid substance containing them through a filter. **RADIATION S.,** utilizes x rays, violet rays, and isotopes to sterilize certain substances. **STEAM S.,** the destruction of microorganisms by exposure to free flowing steam. **STEAM UNDER PRESSURE S.,** utilizes the autoclave (*q.v.*) for sterilizing many materials and articles. **ULTRASONIC S.,** a method of destroying bacteria by exposing articles or materials to be sterilized to a transmitter that emanates ultrasonic waves which shatter the bacteria; used in certain industries and laboratories.

sterilize (ster'i-līz): To render sterile.

sterilizer (ster'i-līz-er): A mechanism, chemical, or method used for making any material or object free of living microorganisms.

stern-, sterno-: Combining forms denoting relationship to the sternum or breast.

sternal (ster'nal): Pertaining to or relating to the sternum. **S. ANGLE,** that formed on the anterior surface of the sternum where the body of the sternum and the manubrium meet. Also called the angle of Louis; an anatomical landmark. **S. PUNCTURE,** aspiration of bone marrow from the sternum for diagnosis of certain diseases of the blood or bone marrow.

sternalgia (ster-nal'ji-a): Pain in the sternum.

sternoclavicular (ster'nō-kla-vik'ū-lar): Pertaining to the sternum and the clavicle. Also sternocleidal.

sternocleidomastoid (ster'nō-klī'dō-mas' -toyd): Pertaining to the sternum, clavicle, and the mastoid process. **S. MUSCLE,** a strap-like muscle arising from the sternum and clavicle, and inserting into the mastoid process of the temporal bone. It draws the head toward the shoulder and assists in flexing the head and neck. See **torticollis.**

sternocostal (ster'nō-kos'tal): Pertaining to the sternum and ribs.

sternodymus (ster-nod'i-mus): Conjoined twins united at the sternum.

sternodynia (ster-nō-din'i-a): Pain in the sternum.

sternohyoid (ster-nō-hī'oyd): Pertaining to the sternum and the hyoid bone.

sternomastoid (ster'nō-mas'toyd): Pertaining to the sternum and the mastoid process of the temporal bone.

sternotomy (ster-not'o-mi): The surgical division of the sternum.

sternum (ster'num): The breastbone; a narrow, flat bone, shaped like a dagger, with a handle (manubrium), blade (body), and tip (xiphoid); the first seven costal cartilages are attached to it on either side, and it articulates with the clavicles above.—sternal, adj.

sternutation (ster'nū-tā'shun): Sneezing, or a sneeze.

steroid (stēr'oyd): A term embracing a naturally occurring group of chemical compounds related to cholesterol, and including sex hormones, adrenal cortical hormones, progesterone, sterols, bile acids; by custom now often implies the natural adrenal glucocorticoids, *i.e.*, hydrocortisone and cortisone, or such synthetic analogs as prednisolone and prednisone.

steroidogenesis (stē-roy'-dō-jen'e-sis): The production of steroids by living tissue.

sterol (stēr'ōl): Any one of a class of solid alcohols widely distributed in nature; they are waxy materials found in plant and animal tissues; cholesterol is the best known of the group.

stertor (ster'tor): A snore. Noisy or laborious breathing as occurs in deep sleep or in coma.—stertorous, adj.

stertorous (ster'tor-us): Pertaining to or characterized by stertor or snoring.

steth-, stetho-: Combining forms denoting relationship to the chest.

stethometer (steth-om'e-ter): An instrument for measuring the expansion of the chest during respiration.

stethoscope (steth'ō-skōp): An instrument used for listening to the various body sounds, especially those of the heart and lungs—stethoscopic, adj.; stethoscopically, adv.

Stevens-Johnson syndrome: A severe type of erythema multiforme of unknown etiology, which affects children and young adults. Sometimes attacks follow administration of sensitizing drugs. It is characterized by the abrupt onset of fever, malaise; and ulcerative lesions of the mouth, pharynx, and anogenital region; conjunctivitis; keratitis; ulceration of the cornea may cause gradual loss of vision. Syn., ectodermosis erosiva pluriorificialis. [Albert Mason Stevens, American pediatrician. 1884–1945. Frank Chambliss Johnson, American pediatrician. 1894–1934.]

sthenia (sthē'ni-a): A condition of normal strength and activity. Opp. asthenia.

sthenic (sthen'ik): Refers to a body type that is well developed, with broad shoulders and athletic appearance.

stheno-: Combining form denoting relationship to strength or power.

"stiff" lung: A lung that has low compliance and resists inflation.

stiff man syndrome: Intermittent, progressive, fluctuating muscular rigidity; cause unknown.

stiff neck: Torticollis; wryneck. Rigidity of neck muscles due to spasm.

stigma (stig'ma): In medicine, 1) a spot or mark on the skin; or 2) any physical or mental mark or characteristic that aids in diagnosis of a particular condition, *e.g.*, the facies of congenital syphilis.—stigmata, stigmas, pl.; stigmatic, adj.

stigmatosis (stig-ma-tō'sis): A skin disease characterized by the appearance of multiple ulcerated spots.

stilette (stī-let'): 1. A thin wire or metal rod for maintaining patency of a hollow instrument or rigidity of a catheter. 2. A small, slender, sharp surgical probe. Also stylet.

stillborn: Born dead.

Still's disease: A form of rheumatoid polyarthritis, of unknown cause, characterized by high fever, skin rashes, abdominal discomfort, progressive pain and tenderness of joints, especially the larger joints; later by lymphadenectomy, splenomegaly, valvular heart disease, ankylosis, especially of the cervical spine, impaired growth and development. Occurs in young children. Also called arthritis deformans juvenilis. [George Frederic Still, English physician. 1868–1941.]

stimulant (stim'ū-lant): 1. Stimulating or promoting mental and physical activities or function. 2. An agent that excites or increases functional activity.

stimulate (stim'ū-lāt): 1. To excite to functional activity or growth. 2. To elicit a response in a special organ or system.—stimulation, n.

stimulus (stim'ū-lus): Anything that is capable of exciting functional activity or producing a response in an organ or part. **ADEQUATE S.**, one that arouses a response in a particular receptor. **INADEQUATE** or **SUBLIMINAL S.**, one that is too weak to arouse a response. **THRESHOLD S.**, one that is just strong enough to arouse an appropriate response.—stimuli, pl.

stippling (stip'ling): A spotted appearance of a membrane or cell; often refers to blood cells. **MALARIAL S.**, characteristic fine dots seen in the red blood cells in quartan malaria; also called Ziemann's stippling.

stirrup bone: The stapes (*q.v.*).

"stir-up" routine: The routine of turning, coughing, and deep breathing; a useful exercise to promote the removal of secretions from the respiratory tract.

stitch: 1. A sudden, sharp, darting pain. 2. A suture. 3. To fix an organ or part in a certain position or to bring the edges of a wound together with a needle and some suture material used as thread. **S. ABSCESS**, one that forms at the site of a stitch in a wound, due to nonsterile suture material or pus-forming bacteria on the skin.

stockinet, stockinette (stok-i-net′): A soft, circular-knit material, usually cotton, having elastic properties and used for bandages, under casts, etc.

stocking: See elastic stocking.

stoic (stō′ik): A person who is indifferent to passion or feeling, or who does not allow pain to interfere with his or her plans and desires.

stoicism (stō′i-sizm): Indifference to pleasure or pain; an attitude of endurance and bravery.

Stokes-Adams syndrome: A fainting (syncopal) attack, commonly transient, which frequently accompanies heart block; characterized by slow and occasionally irregular pulse, vertigo, fainting, sometimes convulsions; Cheyne-Stokes respiration, and unconsciousness. Also Adams-Stokes syndrome. [William Stokes, Irish physician. 1804–1878. Robert Adams, Irish physician. 1791–1875.]

stom-, stoma-, stomo-, stomata-: Combining forms denoting mouth or opening.

stoma (stō′ma): 1. Any minute pore, orifice or opening. 2. The mouth. 3. An artificial opening established surgically between an organ and the exterior or between two organs or parts.—stomal, adj.; stomata, pl.

stomach (stum′ak): The most dilated part of the digestive tube, situated between the esophagus (cardiac orifice) and the beginning of the small intestine (pyloric orifice); it lies just under the diaphragm in the epigastric, umbilical and left hypochondriac regions of the abdomen. The wall is composed of four coats: serous, muscular, submucous, and mucous. **HOURGLASS S.**, one partially divided into two halves by an equatorial constriction following scar formation. **S. PUMP**, a suction pump attached to a flexible tube that is passed into the stomach via the nose or mouth to remove stomach contents. **S. TOOTH**, either of the canine teeth of the lower jaw in the first dentition; informal. **UPSIDE-DOWN S.**, popular name for a **THORACIC S.**, one that is in the thoracic cavity. **S. TUBE**, a tube passed into the stomach through the mouth and used for feeding purposes or for lavage.

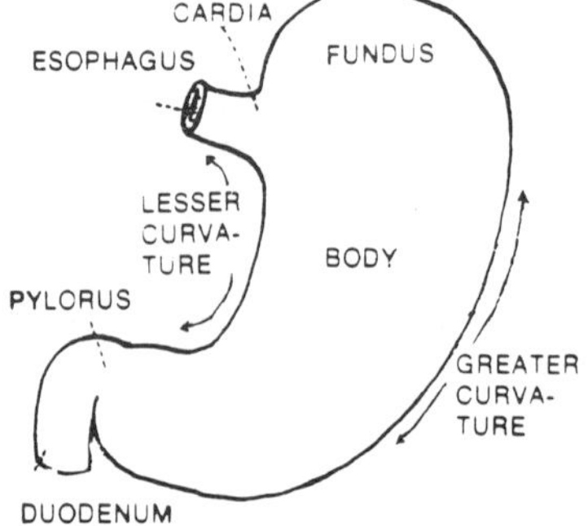

The stomach when full

stomachalgia (stum′a-kal′ji-a): Pain in the stomach.

stomachic (stum-ak′ik): 1. Pertaining to the stomach. 2. An agent that increases the appetite and improves digestion, especially one of the bitters.

stomatic (stōm-at′ik): Relating to the mouth.

stomatitis (stō-ma-tī′tis): Inflammation of the mucous membrane of the mouth. **ANGULAR S.**, fissuring in the corners of the mouth, usually due to riboflavin deficiency, pellagra, or sensitivity to dental materials. **APHTHOUS S.**, recurring crops of small ulcers in the mouth; see apthae. **GANGRENOUS S.**, see cancrum oris. **HERPETIC S.**, an acute infection of the oral mucosa with the formation of vesicles; caused by the herpes simplex virus; also called vesicular **S.** S. NICOTINA, inflammation of the mucous membrane of the palate, due to the irritating properties of tobacco; occurs chiefly in cigarette and cigar smokers. **ULCERATIVE S., S.** characterized by chronically recurring painful, shallow ulcers on cheeks, tongue, and lips. **VINCENT'S S.**, see Vincent's angina under angina. See also thrush.

stomatocyte (stō′mat-ō-sīt): A red blood cell in which a slit or mouth-like area replaces the normal circle of pallor; may be observed in a rare form of hemolytic anemia and in certain liver diseases.

stomatocytosis (stō′ -ma-tō-sī-tō′sis): An uncommon form of congenital hemolytic anemia, characterized by the presence of stomatocytes in the peripheral blood.

stomatodynia (stō′ma-tō-din′i-a): Pain in the mouth.

stomatogastric (stō′ma-tō-gas′trik): Pertaining to the mouth and the stomach.

stomatomalacia (stō′ma-tō-ma-lā′shi-a): Softening of the tissues and structures of the mouth.

stomatomycosis (stō′ma-tō-mī-kō′sis): A fungal infection of the mouth.

stomatonecrosis (stō′ma-tō-nē-krō′sis): Gangrenous stomatitis. Noma.

stomatonoma (stō′ma-tō-nō′ma): Gangrene of the mouth. See noma.

stomatopathy (stō′ma-top′a-thi): Any disease or disorder of the mouth.

stomatoplasty (stō′ma-tō-plas-ti): Plastic surgery of the mouth.

stomatorrhagia (stō′ma-tō-rā′ji-a): Hemorrhage from the gums or other part of the oral cavity.

-stomy: Combining form denoting a surgical opening into a hollow organ or a new opening between two structures.

stone (stōn): Calculus; a hardened mass of mineral matter. **"INFECTION" STONES,** those that form in the urinary tract when the urine is highly alkaline and contains a high concentration of ammonia; commonly occur in patients with long-term indwelling catheters and those with recurrent infections; they damage tissue and encourage bacterial growth.

stool: Feces discharged by the bowels. **ACHOLIC S.,** a **S.** that is whitish in color, due to lack of bile content. **CURRANT-JELLY S.,** a **S.** that contains bloody mucus. **FATTY S.,** one that contains fat; seen in malabsorption syndrome and diseases of the pancreas. **MELANIN S.,** one that is dark colored, often due to medications containing iron. **PEA-SOUP S.,** the liquid **S.** seen in typhoid fever. **RICE-WATER S.** the watery **S.** that is characteristic of cholera. **STEATORRHEAL S.,** fatty **S.** **TARRY S.,** a **S.** that has the color and consistency of tar; may be the result of taking medications containing bismuth, iron, or certain other substances, or of intestinal hemorrhage.

stopcock: A device to prevent fluid from flowing through tubing.

storage disease: A metabolic disorder in which some substances such as fats, proteins, and carbohydrates accumulate in certain body cells in abnormal amounts.

strabismometer (stra-biz-mom'e-ter): An apparatus for measuring the deviation in strabismus.

strabismus (stra-biz'mus): A condition in which the intraocular muscles do not balance, making it impossible for the eyes to function in unison. It is called **CONVERGENT S.** when the eye turns toward the nose (esotropia), and divergent when it turns outward (exotropia). **ACCOMODATIVE S.,** overconvergence caused by excessive accomodation (*q.v.*). **ALTERNATING S.,** a form of **S.** in which either eye may deviate. **VERTICAL S.,** a form of **S.** in which one eye deviates either upward or downward.

strabotomy (stra-bot'o-mi): The cutting of an ocular tendon or muscle in treatment for strabismus.

Strachan's syndrome: A painful neuropathy, thought to be due to a nutritional deficiency; characterized by bilateral loss of sensation and strength in the distal part of the extremities, disturbances of vision and hearing, dizziness, and genital dermatitis.

straight back syndrome: A skeletal deformity marked by loss of the anterior concavity of the upper thoracic part of the spinal column which results in reduction of the anterior-posterior dimension of the upper part of the thorax and compression of the heart between the sternum and the vertebral column.

strain (strān): 1. To exert effort to the limit of one's ability. 2. Weakening or stretching of a muscle at the tendon area, resulting from over-exercise, overuse, or improper use. 3. To over-stretch some muscular part of the body. 4. To filter. 5. A group of microorganisms within a species whose common properties are maintained through successive generations.

strait (strāt): A constricted or narrow space or passage, as of the pelvic canal.

strait jacket: Common name for a device used to restrain irrational or restless patients; consists of a shirt with long sleeves which are fastened so as to restrict movement of the arms.

strangle (strang'g'l): 1. To suffocate, choke, or cause one to be choked by compression or obstruction of the trachea sufficiently to prevent breathing. 2. To deny an organism or a body part of a vital substance such as blood, water, air.

strangulated (strang'gū-lat-ed): The condition of being compressed or constricted so as to cut off the supply of air, blood or other vital substance from a body part. **S. HERNIA,** see **hernia**.

strangulation (strang-gū-lā'shun): 1. Choking caused by compression, constriction or obstruction of air passages with consequent arrest of breathing. 2. Arrest of blood circulation to a part by compression or constriction of the blood vessels.

strangury (strang'gū-ri): Frequent desire to urinate with slow and painful micturition; due to spasm of the urethral muscles.

strapping: The application of strips of adhesive tape that overlap; used to cover, support, exert pressure on, or immobilize a part in such condition as strain, sprain, dislocation or fracture.

stratified (strat'i-fīd): Arranged in layers. **S. EPITHELIUM,** epithelium in which the differently-shaped cells are arranged in distinct strata or layers.

stratum (strā'tum): A lamina or layer, or a sheet-like mass of differentiated tissue, *e.g.*, one of the layers of the skin.—strata, pl., stratified, adj.

strawberry mark: A congenital hemangioma; a bright red, soft, elevated, and often lobulated hemangioma present at birth; see **hemangioma**.

strep throat: Lay term for an infection of the pharynx and tonsils caused by hemolytic *Streptococcus;* characterized by fever, chills, malaise, sore throat; spread by droplet infection; highly communicable.

streph-, strepho-, strepto-: Combining forms denoting twisted or a twisted chain.

strephosymbolia (stref-ō-sim-bō'li-a): The perception of objects as reversed, particularly letters, words, or phrases in reading or writing, *e.g.*, g-o-d for d-o-g; found mainly in children; has been said to result from forcing a left-handed person to use the right hand for eating, writing, etc.

strepticemia (strep-ti-sē′mi-a): Streptococcemia (*q.v.*).

streptococcal (strep′tō-kok′al): Pertaining to or caused by a streptococcus.

streptococcemia (strep′tō-kok-sē′mi-a): The presence of streptococcic organisms in the bloodstream.

streptococci (strep′tō-kok′sī): Plural of streptococcus. **BETA HEMOLYTIC S.**, Lancefield's groups (*q.v.*).

Streptococcus (strep′tō-kok′us): A genus of more or less round, non-sporeforming, nonmotile, gram-positive bacteria that occur in chains of varying length; may be saprophytic or parasitic; some pathogenic species are capable of producing powerful exotoxins. **S. FAECALIS**, an enterococcus normally present in the gastrointestinal tract; may on occasion be the cause of bacterial endocarditis. **S. PNEUMONIAE**, organisms of this group produce lobar pneumonia and other acute pus-forming conditions, including middle ear infections and meningitis. **S. PYOGENES**, organisms from this group produce hemolysis on blood agar medium; includes organisms that cause scarlet fever, septic sore throat, tonsillitis, erysipelas, cellulitis, endocarditis, puerperal fever, rheumatic fever, acute glomerulonephritis, wound infections. **S. SALIVARIUS**, a species normally present in the mouth, nose, and throat; may be associated with tooth abscesses and subacute bacterial endocarditis.

streptodornase (strep-tō-dor′nās): An enzyme used with streptokinase (*q.v.*) in liquefying pus and blood clots, thus promoting healing.

streptokinase (strep-tō-kī′nās): An enzyme derived from cultures of beta-hemolytic streptococci. Because it activates the formation of plasmin, a fibrinolytic enzyme that dissolves fibrin, it is often administered with streptodornase to liquefy and remove clotted blood, or fibrinous or purulent accumulations.

streptolysins (strep-tol′i-sinz): A group of filterable hemolysins (*q.v.*) produced by streptococci, the *Streptocossus pyogenes* in particular. Antibody produced in the tissues against streptolysin may be measured and taken as an indicator of recent streptococcal infection. **STREPTOLYSIN-O**, is antigenic and oxygen-labile. **STREPTOLYSIN-S**, is not antigenic; is insensitive to oxygen but is destroyed by heat and acid.

Streptomyces (strep′tō-mī′sēz): A genus of microorganisms found mostly in the soil but also occasionally on plants and animals; the source of several antibiotics in common use.

streptosepticemia (strep′tō-sep-ti-sē′mi-a): Septicemia (*q.v.*) that is caused by a streptococcal organism.

stress: 1. Intense effort; emphasis; pressure; a constraining force or influence. 2. A condition of strain caused by inability to adjust to factors in the environment, resulting in physiologic tensions; may even contribute to the production of disease. 3. The sum of physiologic and psychologic wear and tear caused by external influences that produce adverse reactions involving the entire body. **S. INCONTINENCE**, see under incontinence. **S. TEST**, Bruce treadmill test; a diagnostic test to determine the body's response to physical exertion; involves taking an ECG, taking blood pressure and pulse, and making observations while the patient is exercising by running in place, jogging, etc. **S. ULCER**, see under ulcer.

stressor (stres′or): An agent or condition that serves as a stress-producing factor; may be biological, psychological, physical, or environmental in character.

stretch marks: See stria.

stretcher (strech′er): A device for carrying and transporting the sick and injured.

stria (strī′a): A streak; stripe; narrow band. **STRIAE GRAVIDARUM**, lines which appear, especially on the abdomen, as a result of stretching of the skin in pregnancy; due to rupture of the lower layers of the dermis. They are red at first and then become silvery white. Striae may also result when the skin of the abdomen is stretched due to weight gained and then lost.—striae, pl.; striated, adj.

striated (strī′āt-ed): Striped. In anatomy, term usually applies to skeletal muscles in which the fibers are marked by cross striations.

stricture (strik′tūr): An abnormal congenital or acquired narrowing of a tube, canal or passage; may be temporary or permanent; usually due to inflammation, infection, injury, scar formation, muscle spasm, or growth of abnormal tissue.

stridor (strī′dor): A harsh, high-pitched sound in breathing, caused by air passing through constricted air passages; often heard in acute constriction of the larynx. In absence of pathology may be due to poorly developed larynx, small glottis, or a large epiglottis.

stridulous (strid′ū-lus): Characterized by stridor (*q.v.*).

strip: 1. To force out the contents of a tube such as a blood vessel or the urethra by pressing a finger along the length of the tube. 2. To remove lengths of large veins or incompetent vessels by use of a stripper (*q.v.*); sometimes the treatment for varicose veins.

stripper: A surgical instrument consisting of a flexible metal tube with a cup or disc at the end; used in excising lengths of veins.

strobila (strō'bil-a): The segmented body of the adult tapeworm.

stroke (strōk): A sudden severe attack, particularly one resulting from the bursting or clogging of a blood vessel in the brain causing damage to nerve centers. **APOPLECTIC S.,** one in which sudden unconsciousness occurs as a result of intracranial hemorrhage, thrombosis or embolism. **HEAT S.,** one resulting from hyperpyrexia due to inhibition of the heat-regulating mechanism in conditions of high temperatures or high humidity or because sweating is interfered with; marked by dry skin, vertigo, headache, nausea, muscular cramps. **PARALYTIC S.,** one in which injury to the brain or spinal cord causes paralysis of some part or parts of the body. **S. VOLUME,** the amount of blood ejected by the left ventricle at each heart beat.

stroke syndrome: Cerebrovascular accident (*q.v.*).

stroking (strōk'ing): A massage maneuver. See effleurage.

stroma (strō'ma): The interstitial substance or supporting framework of a structure as distinguished from its specific functional physiological element.—stromal, stromatic, adj.

stromal (strō'mal): Of or pertaining to the stroma of an organ or structure.

Strongyloides (stron'ji-loy'dez): A genus of widely distributed parasitic intestinal nematodes that infest mammals, including certain animals and rodents as well as humans.

strongyloidiasis (stron'-ji-loy-dī'a-sis): Infestation with *Strongyloides stercoralis,* a roundworm widely distributed in tropical and subtropical areas. The larvae develop in the soil, penetrate the human skin and mucous membrane on contact, pass through the intestinal membrane, get into the bloodstream and are carried to all parts of the body including the lung where they may cause hemorrhage; other symptoms include abdominal pain, nausea, vomiting, and weight loss; severe cases may prove fatal, Occurs in southern U.S., in persons with poor circulation, and those who travel in tropical areas.

strontium (stron'shi-um): A metallic element, similar to calcium in its properties; its various salts are used therapeutically. The isotopes of strontium are used in radioisotope scanning; strontium 90 (^{90}Sr) is the longest-lived of the isotopes having a half-life of 28 years; it is the most dangerous component of atomic fallout. Chemical symbol, Sr.

structuralism (struk'-chur-a-lizm): The branch of psychology that is particularly interested in the basic structure or content of consciousness, including intellect and feeling as well as behavior; the opposite of functionalism (*q.v.*).

struma (stroo'ma): 1. Goiter. 2. Any hardening of tissue. 3. Obsolete term for any enlargement. **STRUMA OVARII,** a rare teratomatous condition in which the ovary consists almost entirely of thyroid tissue. See Hashimoto's disease and Riedel's disease.

strumectomy (stroo-mek'to-mi): Thyroidectomy (*q.v.*).

strumitis (stroo-mī'tis): Thyroiditis.

strumous (stroo'mus): 1. Pertaining to or having the characteristics of a struma. 2. Having goiter.

struvite (strū'vīt): A colorless to yellow or pale brown mineral; the principal constituent of kidney stones.

Strümpell-Marie disease: Rheumatoid spondylitis. See spondylitis.

strychnine (strik'nīn): An alkaloid obtained from the nux vomica plant; formerly much used as a central nervous system stimulant.

Stryker wedge frame (strī'ker): An anterior and posterior frame mounted on a stand with a device by which they can be pivoted and the patient turned from his back to his face. He is placed on the posterior frame, the anterior frame is placed over him and he is securely fastened between the two frames before he is turned. Then the first frame is removed and he remains on his face until it is time to turn him again and the process is repeated. Used in cases where it is necessary to keep the spine immobile, for burn cases and other instances when the patient cannot be turned in the ordinary manner.

Stuart-Prower factor: See factor X.

stump: The remaining distal end of a part that has been amputated.

stun: To render unconscious by a blow or other force; to daze.

stupe (stoop): A piece of cloth, usually woolen, or a sponge, that has been placed in hot water and then wrung almost dry before being applied to a part of the body; a medicament with irritating properties or turpentine may be added to the water. See fomentation.

stupefacient (stū-pē-fā'shent): 1. Inducing stupor. 2. An agent that causes stupor.

stupor (stū'por): A state of marked impairment of mental and physical activity but not complete loss of consciousness; may be due to cerebral vascular insufficiency or damage to brain tissue. The patient shows gross lack of responsiveness, usually reacts only to painful stimuli, and is disoriented as to person, time, and place, but the reflexes remain intact. In psychiatry, three main varieties are recognized—depressive, schizophrenic, and hysterical.—stuporous, adj.

Sturge-Weber syndrome: A genetically determined congenital condition characterized by atrophy and calcification of localized areas of the cerebral cortex, ipsilateral port-wine hemangiomas, and buphthalmos (*q.v.*); often associated with mental retardation.

stutter (stu'ter): To speak with hesitation and spasmodic repetition of the initial consonant of a word or syllable; due to anxiety, nervousness, or an impediment.

sty, stye (stī): Inflammation of one of the sebaceous glands at the edge of the eyelid. Syn., hordeolum.

styl-, styli- stylo-: Combining forms denoting 1) a pillar, or pillar-like; 2) a projecting bony process.

stylet (stī'let): A wire that is inserted into a hollow instrument, tube, or needle to ensure patency or rigidity.

styloglossus (stī'lō-glos'sus): A muscle that arises at the styloid process of the temporal bone and inserts into the tongue.

styloid (stī'loyd): Long and pointed, resembling a pen or stylus. Used especially in reference to a bony process, such as those at the distal end of the radius and of the ulna.

stylomastoid (stī-lō-mas'toyd): Pertaining to the styloid and mastoid processes of the temporal bone.

stylus (stī'lus): In pharmacology, a pencil-shaped stick of some substance containing a medicament such as a caustic.

styptic (stip'tik): 1. Astringent or hemostatic in action. 2. An astringent applied locally to stop bleeding.

sub-: Prefix denoting 1) under, below; 2) near, almost, moderately; 3) less than normal.

subabdominal (sub-ab-dom'i-nal): Below the abdomen.

subacromial (sub-a-krō'mi-al): Situated beneath the acromion.

subacute (sub-a-kūt'): Moderately severe. Often the stage between the acute and chronic phases of a disease. **S. BACTERIAL ENDOCARDITIS**, see endocarditis.

subarachnoid (sub-a-rak'noyd): Beneath the arachnoid membrane. **S. HEMORRHAGE**, Hemorrhage into the subarachnoid space. **S. SPACE**, the space between the arachnoid membrane and the pia mater; it contains cerebrospinal fluid.

subaural (sub-aw'ral): Below the ear.

subception (sub-sep'shun): The reaction to a stimulus that one is not fully aware of having perceived.

subchondral (sub-kon'dral): Below or beneath a cartilage; usually refers to the cartilages of the ribs.

subclavian (sub-klā'vi-an): Beneath the clavicle; usually refers to the subclavian artery or vein.

subclavian steal syndrome: A condition caused by the occlusion of one subclavian artery near the origin of the vertebral artery, causing in turn, a reversal of blood flow through the vertebral artery; manifestations are visual symptoms, lower blood pressure in the involved arm, pain in the occipital and mastoid regions, diminished or absent pulse on the affected side.

subclinical (sub-klin'i-kal): 1. The period in the course of a disease before the symptoms are severe enough to make the disease identifiable. 2. A condition or infection not severe enough to cause the classic identifiable disease.

subconjunctival (sub-con-jungk-tī'val): Under the conjunctiva.—subconjunctivally, adv.

subconscious (sub-kon'shus): 1. That portion of the mind outside the range of clear consciousness, but capable of affecting conscious mental or physical reactions. 2. Partially but not wholly conscious.

subcortical (sub-kor'ti-kal): 1. Beneath the cortex of an organ or structure. 2. Beneath the cerebral cortex.

subcostal (sub-kos'tal): Beneath a rib or ribs.

subcrepitant (sub-krep'i-tant): Only faintly crepitant; said of a rale.

subcutaneous (sub'kū-tā'nē-us): 1. Pertaining to the tissues beneath the skin. 2. Hypodermic.

subcuticular (sub-kū-tik'ū-lar): Beneath the cuticle or epidermis, as a **s.** abscess.

subcutis (sub-kū'tis): The superficial fascia which lies immediately below the skin.

subdermal (sub-der'mal): Subcutaneous (*q.v.*).

subdiaphragmatic (sub'dī-a-frag-mat'ik): Below the diaphragm.—subphrenic, syn.

subdural (sub-dū'ral): Beneath the dura mater; between the dura and arachnoid membranes. **S. HEMATOMA**, see under hematoma. **S. SPACE**, the space between the dura mater and the arachnoid.

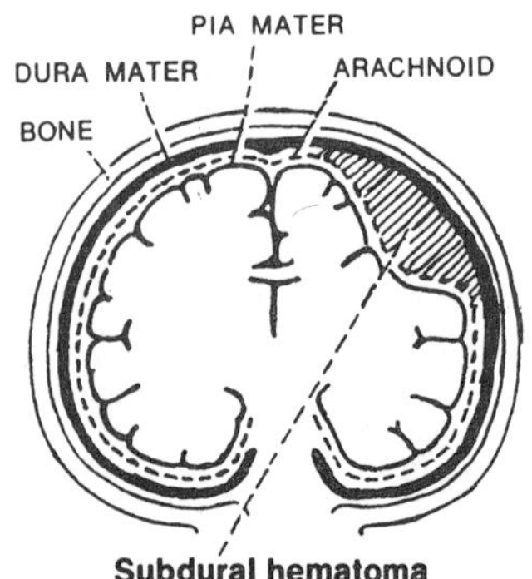

Subdural hematoma

subendocardial (sub-en-do-kar′di-al): Beneath the endocardium, that is, between the endocardium and the myocardium.

suberosis (sū-ber-ō′sis): Pneumoconiosis (*q.v.*), which affects cork workers; characterized by bronchial asthma. Also called cork workers' lung.

subfertility (sub-fer-til′i-ti): A below normal capacity for reproduction.

subgaleal (sub-gal′ē-al): Beneath the galea aponeurotica (*q.v.*).

subglenoid (sub-glē′noyd): Beneath the glenoid cavity.

subglossal (sub-glos′al): Sublingual; under the tongue.

subglossitis (sub-glos-sī′tis): Inflammation of the underside of the tongue and the tissues that lie beneath the tongue.

subglottic (sub-glot′ik): Beneath the glottis. **S. STENOSIS GRANULOMATOUS,** a narrowing below the glottis, usually of cicatricial origin.

subhepatic (sub-hē-pat′ik): Below the liver.

subinvolution (sub-in-vō-lū′shun): The failure of an organ to return to its normal size and condition after enlargement; said especially of the uterus that fails to return to its normal size after childbirth. See involution.

subjacent (sub-jā′sent): Lying below or under something.

subjective (sub-jek′tiv): Internal; personal; arising from the senses and not influenced by the environment or perceptible to others. Opp., objective. **S. EFFECTS,** mental and physical feelings a person reports while undergoing drug or other therapeutic regimen. **S. SYMPTOMS,** those perceived only by the patient and not perceptible to the observer.

sublatio (sub-lā′shi-ō): The removal or detachment of a part; sublation (*q.v.*). **S. RETINAE,** detachment of the retina.

sublation (sub-lā′shun): Detachment, removal, or elevation of an organ or part.

sublethal (sub-lē′thal): Almost fatal. **S. DOSE,** one that contains not quite enough of a toxic substance to cause death.

sublimate (sub′li-māt): 1. A solid deposit resulting from the condensation of a vapor. 2. In psychiatry, to redirect an antisocial drive or primitive desire into some more socially acceptable channel, *e.g.*, a strong tendency to aggressiveness sublimated into athletic activity.—sublimation, n.

sublimation (sub-lim-ā′shun): 1. In psychiatry, an unconscious defense mechanism whereby unacceptable cravings, instinctive wishes, and repressed erotic data are channelled into socially acceptable behavior. 2. In chemistry, the process whereby a solid is converted to a vapor without passing through a liquid state.

subliminal (sub-lim′in-al): Inadequate for perceptible response. Below the threshold of consciousness. See liminal, stimulus.

sublingual (sub-ling′gwal): Beneath the tongue. **S. ADMINISTRATION OF MEDICATION,** a method of administration in which the medication, in tablet form, is placed under the tongue and allowed to dissolve before swallowing; the substance is quickly absorbed by the oral mucosa. **S. DUCT,** a duct leading from the sublingual gland to the oral cavity. **S. GLAND,** a complex of small glands situated on each side of the floor of the mouth; their secretion forms part of the saliva.

sublinguitis (sub-ling-gwī′tis): Inflammation of the sublingual gland.

sublobular (sub-lob′ū-lar): Beneath a lobule. **S. VEINS,** those below the liver that receive the blood from the intralobular veins.

subluxation (sub-luk-sā′shun): Incomplete or partial dislocation of a joint. **S. OF THE ELBOW,** the head of the radius is pulled backward under the edge of a ligament, resulting in obstruction to rotation; often seen in young children. Characterized by sudden acute pain following a traction type force to the forearm, such as lifting a child by the arm; the elbow is held in a fixed position and the hand is pronated.

submandibular (sub-man-dib′ū-lar): Below the mandible.

submaxilla (sub-mak′sil-a): The lower jawbone; the mandible.

submaxillary (sub-mak′sil-a-ri): Beneath the lower jaw. **S. DUCTS,** those that drain the submaxillary gland; they open on the floor of the mouth on either side of the frenum of the tongue; also called Wharton's ducts.

submental (sub-men′tal): Beneath the chin. **S. LIPECTOMY,** the removal of excess fat and tissue from under the chin.

submentobregmatic diameter (sub-men′tō-breg-mat′ik): The measurement from below the chin to the center of the bregma (*q.v.*); it is the presenting diameter in a face presentation of the fetus.

submucosa (sub-mū-kō′za): The layer of areolar connective tissue beneath a mucous membrane that attaches it to the underlying tissues.—submucous, submucosal, adj.

submucous (sub-mū′kus): Beneath a mucous membrane. **S. RESECTION,** an operation for the correction of a deviated septum in the nose.

subnormal (sub-nor′mal): Having less of something than is normal; said especially of intelligence. Being inferior to an accepted standard.

subnormality: A state of arrested or incomplete development of mind, which includes s. of intelligence and is of a nature or degree that requires or is susceptible to medical treatment or other special care or training of the patient. **SEVERE S.**, a state of arrested or incomplete development of mind, which includes s. of intelligence and is of such a nature or degree that the patient is incapable of living an independent life or of guarding himself against exploitation, or be so incapable when of a normal age to do so.

suboccipital (sub-ok-sip′it-al): Beneath the occiput; in the nape of the neck.

suboccipitobregmatic diameter (sub-oks-sip′i-tō-breg-mat′ik): The measurement from the nape of the neck to the center of the bregma (*q.v.*); it is the presenting diameter in a vertex presentation of the fetus.

suborbital (sub-or′bi-tal): Beneath the orbit of the eye.

subpatellar (sub-pa-tel′ar): Beneath the patella.

subpericardial (sub-per-i-kar′di-al): Beneath the pericardium.

subperiosteal (sub-per-i-os′ti-al): Beneath the periosteum of bone.

subperitoneal (sub-per-i-to-nē′al): Beneath the peritoneum.

subpharyngeal (sub-fa-rin′ji-al): Below the pharynx.

subphrenic (sub-fren′ik): Beneath the diaphragm. **S. ABSCESS**, see under abscess.

subpituitarism (sub-pi-tū′i-tar-izm): Hypopituitarism (*q.v.*).

subpleural (sub-ploo′ral): Beneath the pleura.

subpreputial (sub-prē-pū′shi-al): Beneath the prepuce.

subpubic (sub-pū′bik): 1. Situated below the pubic arch. 2. Pertaining to a surgical procedure that is performed below the pubic arch.

subpulmonary (sub-pul′mō-nar-i): Situated, or occurring, below the lungs.—subpulmonic, adj.

subscapular (sub-skap′ū-lar): Beneath the scapula.

subscription (sub-skrip′shun): The part of a prescription that gives directions to the pharmacist as to its preparation.

substance (sub′stans): The material of which something is made; in the body it refers to the materials that make up the organs and tissues to which they owe their characteristic qualities. Matter.

substance abuse: Usually refers to the use of a drug, alcohol, or tobacco to the extent that it interferes with one's health and social functioning.

substandard (sub-stan′dard): Descriptive of something that falls short of the usual or accepted standard of quality.

substantia (sub-stan′shi-a): In anatomy, substance or tissue. **S. COMPACTA**, the compact portion of bone. **S. GELATINOSA**, a network of small nerve cells along the posterior horn of the gray matter of the spinal cord; they have the ability to interfere with incoming nerve impulses. **S. NIGRA**, a broad thick layer of pigmented cells lying between the border of the pons and the hypothalamus. **S. SPONGIOSA**, the cancellous portion of bone.

substernal (sub-ster′nal): Beneath the sternum. **S. GOITER**, one which lies partially beneath the sternum.

substitution (sub′sti-tū′shun): 1. In chemistry, the replacement of one substance in a compound by another substance. 2. Something that is used in place of another substance; may or may not be cheaper or inferior. 3. An artificial product used in place of a natural one; usually to correct a deficiency of the natural product, *e.g.*, a hormone. 4. In psychology and psychotherapy, the person who takes the place of or acts for another person in relation to the patient. 5. The unconscious acceptance of a suitable goal or emotion for one that is unacceptable or unattainable. **S. THERAPY**, see under therapy.

substrate (sub′strāt): A substance upon which an enzyme acts; also called zymolyte.

substratum (sub-strā′tum): A lower stratum or layer; an underlying structure or part.

subsultus (sub-sul′tus): Muscular twitching, jerking or tremor. **S. TENDINUM**, twitching of tendons and muscles, particularly around the wrist in severe fever, such as typhoid.

subtemporal (sub-tem′po-ral): Beneath the temporal area of the skull.

subtendinous (sub-ten′di-nus): Situated beneath a tendon, as a bursa.

subtotal (sub′tō-tal): Somewhat less than total or complete. **S. HYSTERECTOMY**, see hysterectomy.

subungual (sub-ung′gwal): Beneath a finger or toe nail.

Sucaryl: A calorie-free liquid sweetener; a preparation of cyclamate.

succagogue (suk′a-gog): 1. Stimulating a glandular secretion or the flow of a juice. 2. An agent that stimulates glandular secretion or the flow of a juice.

succenturiate (suk-sen-tū′ri-āt): An accessory, or serving as a substitute. **S. LOBE**, a lobe of placental tissue, which is separated from the main placenta but connected to it by blood vessels that cross the placental membranes; may lead to hemorrhage if the vessels lie over the cervical os and are ruptured.

succinic acid (suk-sin′ik): A colorless, crystalline dibasic acid; may be produced synthetically or in the fermentation of alcohol; also found in amber, lignite, and several plants; formerly had several medicinal uses, now used chiefly in treatment of barbiturate poisoning.

succorrhea (suk-ō-rē′a): An abnormal increase in the flow of a secretion or a juice, *e.g.*, saliva, intestinal juice.

succus (suk'us): 1. A fluid secretion; usually refers to a secretion of a digestive fluid. 2. The fluid present in body tissues.

succussion (sū-kush'un): The shaking of a person to determine whether this produces a splashing sound in a body cavity, indicating the pressure of a fluid and gas or air. **HIPPOCRATIC S.**, the splashing sound heard on shaking when fluid accompanies the presence of gas or air in the thorax or the stomach and intestine. **S. SPLASH**, the sound heard when air or fluid moves about in a body cavity or hollow area.

sucking wound: A wound in the chest wall through which air is taken in and expelled.

suckle (suk'l): 1. To suck or draw nourishment from the breast. 2. To feed an infant at the breast.

sucrase (sū'krās): An intestinal enzyme that acts to split sucrose; invertase.

sucrose (sū'krōs): A sugar obtained from sugar cane, sugar beets, or sorghum; a disaccharide; is normally converted into dextrose and levulose in the body.

sucrosemia (sū-krō-sē'mi-a): The presence of sucrose in the blood.

sucrosuria (sū-krō-sū'ri-a): The presence of sucrose in the urine.

suction (suk'shun): The act or process of sucking up or aspirating. **S. ABORTION**, abortion resulting from the use of a suction device inserted into the uterus; a technique utilized during the first trimester of pregnancy. **S. LIPIDECTOMY**, a plastic operation for suctioning fat out of body tissue without leaving scars; a controversial procedure. **WANGENSTEEN S.**, see under Wangensteen.

sudamina (sū-dam'i-na): Minute, transient, whitish vesicles caused by the retention of sweat in the sweat ducts or the corneum of the skin, occurring after profuse perspiration; sweat rash.—sudamen, sing.

sudarium (sū-dā'ri-um): A sweat bath.

sudation (sū-dā'shun): Sweating or excessive sweating.

sudden infant death syndrome: Unexplained crib death; occurs most often during sleep, with no warning cry; occurs chiefly during cold seasons and more often among children from low-income groups; most likely victims are premature or low birth weight infants. Cannot be predicted or prevented; appears to occur more often in boys than girls; thought to be a disorder of sleep. Also called crib death.

Sudek's atrophy: See under atrophy

sudo-, sudor-: Combining forms denoting sweat, perspiration.

sudogram (sū'dō-gram): A graphic representation of the areas of the skin where sweat is produced.

sudomotor (sū-dō-mō'tor): Pertaining to the nerves that stimulate the production of sweat glands. **S. TEST**, sweat test; see under sweat.

sudor (sū'dor): Sweat.—sudoriferous, adj.

sudoresis (sū'do'-rē'sis): Profuse sweating; diaphoresis.

sudoriferous (sū'dō-rif'er-us): 1. Conveying sweat. 2. Producing sweat. **S. DUCT**, the duct leading from a sweat gland to the surface of the skin. **S. GLAND**, a gland in the skin that produces sweat (sudor): see under sweat.

sudorific (sū'dor-if'ik): 1. Promoting the secretion of sweat. 2. An agent that induces sweating; a diaphoretic.

sudorrhea (sū'dō-rē'a): Excessive sweating; hyperhidrosis.

suffocation (suf-ō-kā'shun): Asphyxia (*q.v.*).

suffusion (su-fū'zhun): 1. Extravasation or spreading of blood or other body fluid into surrounding parts. 2. A sudden reddening of the surface as in blushing. 3. The act of pouring a fluid over the body or wetting it.

sugar: A generic name for any of a class of crystalline, sweet-tasting, water soluble carbohydrates, mostly monosaccharides and disaccharides, of animal or vegetable origin; examples are glucose and lactose.

suggestibility (sug-jes'ti-bil'i-ti): Susceptibility to suggestion (*q.v.*); is heightened in hospital patients, due to the dependence on others that illness brings, in children, and individuals with a tendency to hysteria.

suggestion (sug-jest'shun): The implanting in a person's mind of an idea which is accepted by the individual without fully understanding the reason for acceptance. In psychiatric practice, **S.** is used as a therapeutic measure, sometimes under hypnosis or narcoanalysis (*q.v.*). See autosuggestion.

suicide (sū'i-sīd): Any action undertaken by a person with the intention of killing oneself.

suicide post-vention: A term denoting the study of the effects of suicide on survivors, families, and friends.

suicidologist (sū'i-sīd-ol'o-jist): A person who studies and practices suicidology.

suicidology (sū'i-sī-dol'o-ji): The study of all aspects of suicide, its causes and prevention.

sulcus (sul'-kus): A furrow or groove, particularly one separating gyri or convolutions of the brain. **CENTRAL S.**, the rolandic fissure, a groove on the lateral surface of the cerebrum; it separates the frontal from the parietal lobes of the brain. **LATERAL S.**, the fissure of Sylvius, lies between the temporal lobe below and the frontal and parietal lobes above. **PARIETO-OCCIPITAL S.**, marks off the boundaries of the occipital lobe.

sulf-, sulfo-: Combining forms denoting the presence of sulfur in a compound.

sulfa: Denoting tne sulphonamides or sulfa drugs.

sulfanemia (sul-fa-nē'mi-a): Anemia caused by the use of sulfa drugs.

sulfanilamide (sul-fa-nil'a-mīd): The first sulfonamide (*q.v.*), and parent of the other sulfa drugs; derived from coal tar and effective especially against beta-hemolytic streptococci, meningococci, and gonococci; also against *Clostridium welchii* (*q.v.*) and *Escherichia coli* (*q.v.*); Not used as much as formerly because of its toxic reactions; symptoms of toxicity include beta-hemolytic anemia, agranulocytosis.

sulfatase (sul'fa-tās): An enzyme that acts as a catalyst in the hydrolysis of sulfuric acid esters into sulfuric acid and alcohol. A deficiency of sulfatase A is thought to be the cause of metachromatic leukodystrophy; see under leukodystrophy.

sulfate (sul'fāt): Any salt of sulfuric acid.

sulfhemoglobin (sulf-hē'-mō-glō'bin): A greenish substance formed by the action of hydrogen sulfide on hemoglobin; may appear in the blood after the ingestion of sulfanilamide and some other substances. Also called sulfmethemoglobin.

sulfhemoglobinemia (sulf-hē'mō-glō-bi-nē'mi-a): The presence of sulfhemoglobin in the blood.

sulfide (sul'fīd): A compound of sulfur and another element or a base.

sulfite (sul'fīt): Any salt of sulfurous acid.

sulfonamides (sul-fon'a-mīds): A group of synthetic drugs derived from sulfonic acid. Their action is bacteriostatic, thus, they prevent multiplication of bacteria and allow the body to build its defenses against the organisms.

sulfones (sul'fōns): A group of synthetic drugs related to the sulfonamides, useful in treatment of leprosy; also sometimes used in tuberculosis.

sulfonic acid (sul-fon'ik as'id): Any of several acids containing the sulfonic group (—SO_3H).

sulfonylurea (sul'-fō-nil-ū-rē'a): Any one of several chemical agents that are related to the sulfanilamides and that act with the beta cells of the pancreas to stimulate the secretion of insulin; also used as oral antidiabetics.

sulfur (sul'fur): A pale yellow crystalline substance frequently used in various combinations in medicine.

sulfuric acid (sul-fū'rik): Heavy, colorless, odorless, oily liquid; extremely corrosive and caustic.

Sulkowitch's test: A test for determining the presence and amount of calcium in the urine.

sullage (sul'aj): The liquid waste from bathrooms, laundries, kitchens, etc.

sulph-: For words beginning thus, and not found here, see words beginning sulf-

sum: Abbreviation for *sumat,* [L.], meaning let him take. Used in prescription writing.

summer diarrhea: Acute diarrhea; occurs chiefly in children; caused by enteropathogenic bacteria and usually associated with poorly refrigerated food.

sump drain: A double-lumen drain of rubber or plastic with lateral openings and fish-tail end, used to remove accumulated fluids from the stomach, with or without suction; provides for continuous drainage, accurate measurement of drainage material, and prevents irritation to the skin from the gastric secretion.

sun: **S. BATH,** exposure of the body to sunlight for therapeutic purposes. **S. BLINDNESS,** caused by retinal damage from looking at the sun without proper eye protection; may be temporary or permanent.

sunburn: Reddening of the skin or dermatitis, caused by direct exposure to the rays of the sun. The reaction varies with the individual and the degree of exposure.

sundowning (sun-down'ing): A condition seen in some elderly individuals who become disoriented or confused toward the end of the day. These people have some loss of vision and/or hearing and of the sense of touch, and, as daylight fades, the inability to see well increases the handicap imposed by their other sensory losses. Also called sundowner's syndrome.

sunstroke: A condition produced by overexposure to the direct rays of the sun; marked by convulsions, coma, and high temperature of the skin. See stroke.

super-: Combining form denoting 1) situated above, over; 2) extra, in addition; 3) in excess; 4) higher in degree, quantity or quality.

superactivity (sū-per-ak-tiv'i-ti): Hyperactivity.

superacute (sū'per-a-kūt'): Extremely acute.

superalimentation (sū'per-al-i-men-tā'shun): Overfeeding or overeating.

supercilium (sū'per-sil'i-um): The eyebrow.—supercilia, pl.; superciliary, adj.

superego (sū-per-ē'gō): That part of the personality that is concerned with moral standards and ideals, derived mainly from parents, teachers, and others in the environment. The theoretical part of the mind; popularly referred to as the conscience.

superfecundation (sū'per-fē-kun-dā'shun): The fertilization of more than one ovum during one intermenstrual period but at different acts of coitus; results in dizygotic twins.

superfetation (sū'per-fē-tā'shun): The presence of two fetuses of different ages in the uterus; they are not twins but the result of impregnation of two ova released at successive ovulations.

superficial (sū'per-fish'al): 1. At or near the surface. 2. Not serious or dangerous.

superficies (sū-per-fish'i-ez): The outer surface.

supergenual (sū-per-jen'ū-al): Above the knee.

superinfection (sū-per-in-fek'shun): A second infection developing in a person who has not recovered from a different one; caused by a bacterium or fungus that is resistant to the drugs being used to treat the original infection; may occur at the site of the original infection or at a site remote from it.

superior (sū-pēr'i-or): Situated above. In anatomy, the upper of two parts. **S. VENA CAVA**, the venous trunk that drains blood from the head, neck, upper extremities and chest and empties it into the right atrium.

superior vena cava syndrome: A condition characterized by engorgement of the vessels of the upper trunk, flushing of the face, neck, and upper arms; caused by pressure on the superior vena cava and its tributaries; most often seen in lung cancer.

superlactation (sū-per-lak-tā'shun): Excessive secretion of milk or excessive continuance of lactation.

superlethal (sū-per-lē'thal): Extremely lethal; refers to a dose of a drug that is larger than the dose that produces death.

supernatant (sū-per-nā'tant): 1. Above or on the top of something. 2. The upper layer of material, liquid or solid, that remains after the precipitation of a solid part of a mixture.

supernumerary (sū-per-nū'mer-ar-i): In excess of the normal number; additional.

supersaturate (sū-per-sat'ū-rāt): To add more of an ingredient than can be held in solution permanently, the excess being precipitated when the physical conditions are changed.

superscription (sū'per-skrip'shun): The Rx sign at the beginning of a prescription; it stands for recipe.

supersensitive (sū'per-sen'si-tiv): Abnormally sensitive; usually referring to a foreign protein or other antigenic substance.

supervisor (sū'per-vī-sor): In nursing, an administrative or management position between that of the director of nursing and the head nurses of a care unit; now sometimes referred to as clinical director.

supinate (sū'pin-āt): 1. To turn the face upward or to assume the supine position. 2. To turn the palm upward or to turn the sole of the foot inward.

supination (sū'pi-nā'shun): 1. The position of the forearm and hand when the palm is turned up or of the foot when the sole is turned up and inward. 2. The position of lying on the back, face up.

supinator (sū'pin-ā-tor): That which supinates (*q.v.*), usually applied to a muscle of the forearm. Opp., pronator.

supine (sū-pīn'): Lying on the back with the face and palms of the hands turned upward. Having the palm of the hand turned upward or outward. Opp., prone.

supplemental air: That air that remains in the lung after an ordinary expiration but which can be exhaled when one makes a forcible effort to do so.

Supplementary Security Income: A federal assistance program whereby needy Social Security beneficiaries who meet stringent criteria may receive an additional amount arrived at by subtracting any income the individual may have from a federally mandated income floor; this amount is indexed to the cost of living and adjusted annually and may or may not be supplemented by the individual states. Abbreviated SSI.

supportive (sū-por'tiv): Refers to any person, device, or measure that assists, supports, maintains, or in any other way helps a patient. **S. THERAPY**, any form of treatment that reinforces the patient's own defenses or ability to overcome a physical or emotional disability.

suppository (su-poz'i-tō-ri): Medicament in a semi-solid base that remains solid at room temperature but melts at body temperature, for insertion into a body orifice other than the mouth, *e.g.*, rectum, vagina, urethra. Usually shaped like a cone or cylinder made of glycerinated gelatin, certain glycols, or cocoa butter.

suppressant (sū-pres'ant): 1. Having a suppressing effect. 2. An agent that reduces or stops a secretion, excretion, or normal body discharge. In psychoanalysis, the conscious effort to ignore or control feelings, thoughts, or acts that are unacceptable.

suppression (su-presh'un): 1. Holding back; repressing; arresting. 2. Cessation or arrest of a secretion (*e.g.*, urine) or a normal process (*e.g.*, menstruation), as distinguished from retention (*q.v.*). In psychology, the conscious, intentional forcing out of the mind of unacceptable thoughts or feelings; may result in the precipitation of a neurosis (*q.v.*); to be differentiated from repression (*q.v.*).

suppurant (sup'ū-rant): 1. Producing suppuration. 2. Any agent that promotes suppuration.

suppurate (sup'pū-rāt): To form or discharge pus.

suppuration (sup'ū-rā'shun): The formation or discharge of pus.—suppurative, adj.; suppurate, v.

supra-: Combining form denoting 1) a situation above, over, or higher; 2) beyond. Often used interchangeably with super-.

supracondylar (sū-pra-kon′di-lar): Situated above a condyle.

supradiaphragmatic (sū-pra-dī-a-frag-mat′ik): Situated above the diaphragm.

supraglottic (sū-pra-glot′ik): Situated above the glottis.

suprainfection (sū-pra-in-fek′shun): 1. An infection or disease occurring in a patient weakened by another disease. 2. An infection occurring after antibiotic treatment for another infection.

supralethal (sū-pra-lē′thal): More than just enough of a drug or other toxic substance to cause death.

supraliminal (sū-pra-lim′i-nal): Above the threshold of consciousness; referring to a stimulus that is more than just strong enough to be perceived.

supraorbital (sū-pra-or′bit-al): Above the orbits. **S. RIDGE,** the ridge formed by the prominence of the frontal bone; the eyebrows are situated over this ridge.

suprapatellar (sū-pra-pa-tel′ar): Situated above the patella. **S. BURSA,** the bursa that lies between the tendon of the quadriceps muscle and the front of the lower end of the femur. **S. REFLEX,** the sudden upward movement of the patella when the quadriceps muscle contracts in response to a sharp blow on the examiner's finger, which rests on the upper border of the patella with the leg in extension.

suprapubic (sū-pra-pū′bic): Performed or situated above the pubic arch. **S. CYSTOTOMY,** surgical opening of the bladder just above the pubis. **S. PROSTATECTOMY,** see prostatectomy.

suprarenal (sū-pra-rē′nal): 1. Situated above the kidney. 2. Tiny endocrine gland just above each kidney. Syn., adrenal (*q.v.*).

suprarenalectomy (sū′pra-rē-nal-ek′to-mi): Surgical removal of the adrenal gland(s).

suprascapular (sū-pra-scap′ū-lar): Situated above or in the upper part of the scapula.

supraspinal (sū-pra-spī′nal): Situated above a spine or the spinal column.

suprasternal (sū-pra-ster′nal): Situated above the sternum. **S. NOTCH,** the U-shaped curve at the top of the manubrium of the sternum.

supraumbilical (sū-pra-um-bil′i-kal): Situated above the navel.

supraventricular (sū-pra-ven-trik′ū-lar): Located, occurring, or originating above a ventricle of the heart or above the branching of the bundle of His. **S. RHYTHM,** any rhythm originating above the bifurcation of the bundle of His. **S. TACHYCARDIA,** an arrhythmia characterized by atrial contractions at a very fast rate.

supravergence (sū-pra-ver′jens): The upward movement of one eye while the other eye remains stationary.

sura (sū′rah): The calf of the leg.—sural, adj.

surdimutitas (sur-di-mū′tī-tas): Deafmutism.

surditas, surdity (sur′di-tas, sur′di-ti): Deafness.

surface: The exterior of any solid body. **S. TENSION,** see under tension.

surfactant (sur-fak′tant): A lipoprotein substance that is manufactured in the alveoli of the lungs and lines them; it serves to decrease the surface tension of pulmonary fluids and permits the lungs to expand during inspiration and prevents them from collapsing during exhalation. In the newborn it reduces the adhesion between the unexpanded walls of the alveoli. See respiratory distress syndrome.

surfer's nodules: Traumatic nodules that form on the front of the legs and feet, due to repeated bumping from a surf board or other activity in which the leg is repeatedly hit.

surgeon (sur′jun): A medical practitioner who treats disease, disorders, or deformities by operative procedures.

surgery (sur′jer-i): The branch of medicine that treats diseases, deformities, and injuries, wholly or in part, by manual or operative procedures; usually involves making an opening in the body to remove, replace, or repair a part in order to cure or correct a pathologic condition or damage caused by trauma, or to give the patient a period of remission from a disease. **ASEPTIC S.,** that performed in a field kept free of pathogenic bacteria. **CLOSED S.,** that done without making an incision, as in reducing a fracture. **CLOSED HEART SURGERY,** that in which the myocardium is not invaded and normal cardiac circulation is maintained; can be utilized in performing valvulotomy. **CONSERVATIVE S.,** that in which injured or diseased parts are repaired but removal is avoided if possible. **ELECTIVE S.,** that which can be done at the patient's or physician's convenience when the delay would not endanger the health status or life of the patient. **MAJOR S.,** important and serious operations that may involve risk to life. **MINOR S.,** simpler, less serious operations that do not usually involve risk to life. **OPEN-HEART S.,** involves opening the heart and establishing extra-corporeal circulation; utilized in heart transplant operations, insertion of prosthetic heart valves, correction of congenital anomalies, or repair of ruptured aortic aneurysm. **ORAL S.,** that done to treat disorders of the mouth and teeth; a branch of dentistry. **ORTHOPEDIC S.,** that which treats diseases or deformities of the skeletal system. **PLASTIC S.,** that which repairs or reconstructs a tissue or part by such methods as skin grafting or transplanting of other tissue. **RADICAL S.,** that which is extensive and thorough enough to be curative rather than palliative; often said of mastectomy that includes removal of the entire breast along with the pectoral muscles, axillary lymph nodes, and contiguous lymph tissue. **TRANSSEXUAL S.,** that which alters the external appearance and characteristics of a person so as to make them resemble those of the opposite sex.

surgical (sur'ji-kal): Pertaining to or involving surgery.

surgi-center (sur' -ji-sen-ter): An independent operating facility that provides care for patients having surgery that does not require overnight hospitalization.

Surgi-lift: A special lifting device designed for use when transferring spinal-cord injured persons.

surrogate (sur'ō-gāt): A substitute or replacement for something or someone.

sursumduction (sur-sum-duk'shun): The turning upward of a part, especially the upward turning of one eye but not the other.

susceptibility (sus-sep-ti-bil'i-ti): The opposite of resistance. Usually refers to a disposition to infection.

suspension (sus-pen'shun): 1. Temporary cessation, as of a vital process. 2. A mixture in which finely divided particles are dispersed throughout a liquid and remain undissolved even after stirring or shaking vigorously. 3. A method of treatment whereby a part or the whole of a person's body is suspended in a desired position. 4. The fixation of an organ or part in correct position by suturing it to other tissues, *e.g.*, suspension of the uterus.

suspensory (sus-pen'so-ri): 1. Descriptive of a structure, often a ligament, that functions to hold an organ or part in correct position, *e.g.*, the suspensory ligament of the eye, which passes from the lens to the ciliary body and holds the lens in place. 2. A bandage or other material used to support a dependent part or organ, *e.g.*, the scrotum.

sustenance (sus'ten-ans): That which sustains life; nourishment; food.

sustentacular (sus'ten-tak'ūlar): Supporting or sustaining; said of cells, fibers, tissues.

susurrus (su-sūr'us): A soft murmur.

sutura (sū-tū'ra): An immovable joint in which the bones are united by fibrous tissue that is continuous with the periosteum covering the bones, *e.g.*, the joints in the skull bones. Also called suture.

suture (sū'chur): 1. The jagged line of union of cranial bones. 2. A stitch or series of stitches used to close a wound. 3. The act of stitching to close a wound. 4. The material used to close a wound by stitching; see ligature. **ABSORBABLE S.**, one made with a material that is liquefied in the body and absorbed. **CONTINUOUS S.**, one of a series of sutures made with one length of material. **INTERRUPTED S.**, one of a series of sutures each one being made with a separate piece of material. **MATTRESS S.**, strong nonabsorbable suture that goes through the deeper tissues either vertically or parallel to the skin sutures; used to maintain strong repair in obese patients and those with weak musculature. **NONABSORBABLE S.**, one that is not liquefied and absorbed by the body; made of cotton, silk, or nylon thread, or stainless steel; remains in the tissues when great strength is needed. Screws and plates used in bone repair are the equivalent of nonabsorbable sutures in other tissues. **PURSE-STRING S.**, a stitching around the edge of a circular opening that is then drawn up tightly to close the opening.

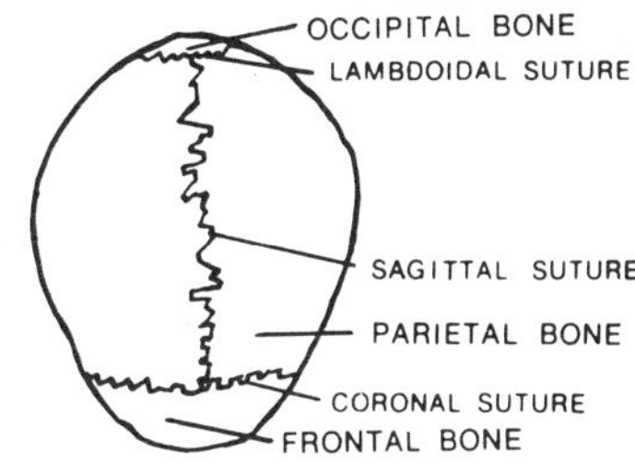

Sutures of the skull

swab (swob): 1. To use a small tuft of cotton or similar material to cleanse an area or a cavity, absorb an exudate, or apply a medication. 2. A small piece of cotton or similar material wound firmly around one or both ends of a shaft of wire or wood; used to cleanse a cavity, apply a medication, or collect a specimen for laboratory examination; in the latter case it is sterilized and within a protective tube.

swage (swāj): A tool used for bending or shaping cold metal. In medicine, to fuse suture material to a needle, or a type of suture made by fusing the suture material to the needle.

swallow: To pass food or any other material through the mouth, pharynx, and esophagus into the stomach. **BARIUM S.**, see under barium.

swan neck deformity: 1. A finger deformity in which the distal interphalangeal joint is flexed while the proximal joint is extended, giving the finger the appearance of a swan's neck. 2. An abnormality of the convoluted part of the kidney tubules which is distorted into the shape of a swan's neck; associated with rickets.

Swan-Ganz catheter: See under catheter.

swathe (swath): To envelop, cover, wrap or bind tightly as with a bandage.

swayback: Increased lumbar lordosis accompanied by compensatory kyphosis.

sweat: 1. Sudor; a clear fluid secreted by the sweat glands in the skin; consists of water, salt, and waste products from the blood; is eliminated through channels that end in pores in the skin. 2. To perspire or sweat. **S. TEST**, a diagnostic procedure used in cystic fibrosis of the pancreas; it is a measurement of the sodium and chloride in the sweat; see cystic fibrosis.

MINOR'S S. TEST, a sweat test used to demonstrate lesions in the nervous system. **NIGHT S.,** profuse sweating while asleep; often a symptom of pulmonary tuberculosis and of AIDS and AIDS Related Complex. See perspiration and bromhidrosis.

sweetbread: The pancreas of an animal, usually the calf, used as a food.

swelling (swel'ling): A transient, abnormal elevation or enlargement of a body part or area, usually on the surface, that is not caused by new growth or proliferation of cells; may be due to injury, inflammation, or edema.

swimmer's ear: Otitis media caused by an infection contracted in water, often that in swimming pools.

"swimmer's" shoulder: A syndrome sometimes seen in long-distance swimmers; the rotator cuff impinges over the shoulder and catches on the under surface of the coracoacromial ligament.

"swimming-pool conjunctivitis": See under conjunctivitis.

swineherd's disease: A disease caused by the *Leptospira pomona,* an organism that is harbored in swine; may be transmitted to man, causing a form of leptospirosis characterized by aseptic meningitis.

swoon: A faint. See syncope.

sycoma (sī-kō'ma): A large soft wart-like growth.

sycosis (sī-kō'sis): A skin disease in which inflammation of the hair follicles, usually by a staphylococcal organism, results in papules, pustules, and scab formation. **S. BARBAE,** see barbers' itch. **S. NUCHAE,** folliculitis at the nape of the neck which leads to keloid thickening (acne keloid).

Sydenham's chorea: See under chorea.

syllepsiology (si-lep-si-ol'o-ji): The branch of medical study that deals with conception and pregnancy.

syllepsis (si-lep'sis): Pregnancy.

sylvatic (sil-vat'ik): Pertaining to or found in the woods. **SYLVATIC PLAGUE,** a disease that is prevalent in wild rodents worldwide, especially in the wild squirrels of western U.S.; it may be transmitted to man by the bite of an infected flea.

Sylvius (sil'vi-us): **FISSURE OF S.,** a deep fissure at the side of each cerebral hemisphere; the temporal lobe lies below it.—sylvian, adj. [Franciscus de le Boë Sylvius, Dutch physician. 1614–1672.]

sym-: Combining forms denoting: 1. Together; union of; association; similar. 2. At the same time.

symbiosis (sim-bi-ō'sis): In biology, close relationship between two similar organisms, or between organisms of different species, when this is necessary for the survival of both. In the family, **S.** usually refers to the relationship between mother and child. In psychiatry, **S.** refers to a close relationship between two disturbed individuals who are emotionally dependent on each other.

symblepharon (sim-blef'a-ron): Adhesion of one or both of the lids to the eyeball.

symbol (sim'bol): A letter, mark, or sign that represents an idea or word(s) or, in chemistry, an atom or group of atoms of an element.

symbolia (sim-bō'li-a): The ability to recognize objects through the sense of touch.

symbolization (sim'bōlī-zā'shun): In psychiatry, the unconscious substitution of a symbol to express thoughts or ideas that the individual had previously been unable or unwilling to accept or express.

symmetrical (sim-et'rik-al): Even; balanced; the same on both sides; in anatomy, refers to parts of the body.

symmetry (sim'e-tri): Correspondence or equality of size, shape, location, and general characteristics of things, or, in anatomy, of two parts of the body.—symmetric, symmetrical, adj.

sympathectomy (sim-pa-thek'to-mi): Surgical excision of a sympathetic nerve or surgical interruption of sympathetic nerve pathways which results in dilatation of blood vessels and increased blood flow to a part.—sympathectomize, v.

sympathetic (sim-pa-thet'ik): 1. Exhibiting sympathy. 2. Influenced by or produced by disease in another part of the body. **S. NERVOUS SYSTEM,** see under nervous system.

sympathin (sim'pa-thin): An old name for chemical substances liberated by sympathetic nerve endings; now known to be epinephrine and norepinephrine.

sympatholytic (sim'path-ō-lit'ik): 1. An adrenergic blocking agent (*q.v.*). 2. Having an antagonistic effect on activity produced by a stimulant to the sympathetic nervous system.

sympathomimetic (sim-path-ō-mī-met'ik): Capable of producing changes similar to those produced by stimulation of the sympathetic nerves. **S. AMINES,** a group of specific drugs that act as vasoconstrictors, bronchodilators, and sympathetic nervous system stimulants.

symphysiotomy (sim-fiz'i-ot'o-mi): The surgical separation of the mother's pubic bone, at its symphysis, to facilitate the birth of a living child.

symphysis (sim'fi-sis): A very slightly movable joint in which there is a fibrocartilaginous union of bones, as occurs between the two parts of the pubic bone, the vertebrae, and the sacrum and ilium.—symphysiac, symphyseal, symphysial, adj.; symphyses, pl.

symptom (simp'tom): Any morbid phenomenon, condition, or other perceptible evidence of disease. **CARDINAL S.**, a major **S.**, especially one that pertains to temperature, pulse, or respiration. **DEFICIENCY S.**, one that indicates reduction in or lack of secretion of an endocrine gland, or lack of a vital element in the patient's diet. **OBJECTIVE S.**, one apparent to the observer. **PRESENTING S.**, the **S.** or group of **S'S.** the patient complains of most. **PRODROMAL S.**, one that precedes the diagnostic **S'S.** of a disease. **SUBJECTIVE S.**, one that is apparent only to the patient. **SYMPTOM COMPLEX**, a group of symptoms which, occurring together, typify a particular disease or syndrome. **WITHDRAWAL S.**, any of the physiologic or psychologic symptoms that occur when a drug or chemical to which an individual has become habituated, is withdrawn; also called abstinence syndrome.

symptomatic (simp′tō-mat′ik): Pertaining to, constituting, or of the nature of a symptom or symptoms.

symptomatology (simp′tom-a-tol′o-ji): 1. The branch of medicine concerned with symptoms. 2. The combined symptoms typical of a particular disease.

symptothermal method: Term used to describe a rhythm method of natural family planning based on the woman's ability to recognize and keep a record of changes in basal body temperature, and changes in the cervical mucus during the menstrual cycle.

syn-: Combining form denoting with, together, union of, or association with.

synapse (sin′aps): The point of communication between two neurons; it is where the axon of one neuron comes into close proximity to the dendrites or cell body of another neuron and an impulse is chemically transmitted; impulses travel only in one direction at the synapse.—synapses, pl.; synaptic, adj.

synapsis (si-nap′sis): The pairing of homologus chromosomes during the early stage of meiosis (*q.v.*).

synarthrosis (sin′ar-thrō′sis): An immovable articulation of bones that are held tightly together by fibrous connective tissue; two types of **S.** are sutures, as occur between the flat bones of the skull, and syndesmoses, as occur between the distal ends of the tibia and fibula.

synchondrosis (sin′kon-drō′sis): A type of joint in which the bones are held together by cartilage which, in certain joints, is eventually replaced by bone, as occurs in the epiphyses of long bones; the cartilage that joins the ribs to the sternum is not replaced by bone and is a permanent synchondrosis.—synchondroses, pl.

synchronous (sin′kro-nus): Occurring at the same time or together; simultaneous.

synchysis (sin′ki-sis): A degenerative condition of the vitreous body of the eye which renders it fluid. **S. SCINTILLANS**, the appearance of flashes of reflected light caused by the presence of fine crystals in the vitreous; they are usually cholesterol or fatty acid crystals.

synclitism (sin′kli-tizm): The condition existing when the sagittal suture of the presenting fetal skull lies in line with the transverse diameter of the mother's pelvis, midway between the symphysis pubis and the sacral prominence. Also called parallelism.

syncope (sin′kō-pi): A faint, or temporary loss of consciousness, caused by cerebral ischemia. May be a symptom of disease or may result from a sudden change to the upright position, or may be associated with an emotional experience such as fright when the peripheral blood vessels dilate and drain the blood from the brain. The loss of consciousness is usually temporary.—syncopal, adj.

syncretio (sin-krē′shi-ō): The growing together, or development of adhesions between two opposing inflamed serous surfaces.

syncytiotrophoblast (sin-sish′ī-ō-trō′fō-blast): The outer layer of the trophoblast (*q.v.*), consisting of a syncytium (*q.v.*).

syncytium (sin-sish′i-um): A mass of protoplasm with multiple nuclei, produced by the merging of cells.—syncytial, adj.

syndactyly (sin-dak′ti-li): A congenital anomaly in which the fingers and/or toes are webbed. Also syndactylism, syndactylia.—syndactylous, adj.

syndesis (sin-dē′sis): The condition of being bound or fused together; see arthrodesis.

syndesmitis (sin-des-mī′tis): 1. Conjunctivitis. 2. Inflammation of a ligament.

syndesmorrhaphy (sin-des-mor′a-fi): Suturing of a ligament.

syndesmosis (sin′des-mō′sis): A fixed joint (synarthrosis) in which the surfaces of the bones are joined to each other by fibrous connective tissue, with the opposing surfaces being relatively far apart as occurs, *e.g.*, in the joints at the distal ends of the tibia and fibula.

syndrome (sin′drōm): A group of symptoms and/or signs that, occurring together, produce a pattern or symptom complex that is typical of a particular disease, disturbance, disorder, or lesion.—syndromic, adj.

synechia (si-nek′i-a): Abnormal union of parts, especially adhesion of the iris to the cornea in front, or to the lens capsule behind.—synechiae, pl.

syneresis (si-ner′e-sis): The action of drawing together the dispersed particles of a substance, as occurs in clotting of blood. **S. OF THE VITREOUS**, liquefaction of the vitreous of the eye.

synergism (sin′er-jizm): Synergy (*q.v.*).

synergist (sin′er-jist): One of the partners in a synergistic action, *i.e.*, a drug, substance, or organ that stimulates or augments the action of another drug, substance, or organ. See synergy.—synergistic, adj.

synergy (sin′er-ji): 1. In pharmacology, the combined action of two agents which is usually greater or more effective than the sum of their individual actions. 2. In anatomy, the coordination of actions of muscles and organs by the central nervous system, to produce specific motions or functions.—synergic, adj.

synesthesia (sin-es-thē′zi-a): A secondary or concomitant sensation accompanying a sensory response, or one perceived by a sense organ other than the one stimulated as happens, *e.g.*, when a certain sound produces a sensation of color.

synkinesis (sin-ki-nē′sis): Involuntary movements of paralyzed synergic muscle or groups of muscles accompanying voluntary movements of an unparalyzed muscle or group of muscles.—synkinetic, adj.

synophthalmus (sin′of-thal′mus): Cyclops (*q.v.*).

synorchism (sin′-or̄-kizm): Congenital fusion of the testes into one mass, usually within the abdomen.

synostosis (sin′os-tō′sis): The fusion of adjacent bones that are normally separate; also synosteosis.

synovectomy (sin′-ō-vek′tō-mi): Excision of synovial membrane. Current early treatment for rheumatoid arthritis, especially of the hands and of the knees.

synovia (si-nō′vi-a): The transparent, alkaline, viscous fluid secreted by the membrane lining a joint cavity; its function is to lubricate and thus minimize friction during joint movement. Syn., synovial fluid.

synovial (sin-ō′vi-al): Pertaining to or containing synovia (*q.v.*). **S. BURSA,** in anatomy, a small synovia-filled sac that lies between two parts that move upon each other. **S. CAPSULE,** the fibrous sheet that encloses a synovial joint. **S. CHONDROMATOSIS,** an uncommon condition in which folds of the **S.** membrane change to cartilaginous bodies that often become calcified and then separate, becoming freely movable. **S. FLUID,** synovia. **S. JOINT,** a freely movable joint, as the elbow or hip. **S. MEMBRANE,** the fluid-secreting membrane that lines a joint capsule.

synovioma (sin-nō-vi-ō′ma): A tumor of synovial membrane origin. **BENIGN S.,** a giant-cell tumor of a tendon sheath. **MALIGNANT S.,** synoviosarcoma; arises in the synovial membrane of joints, and sometimes in the synovial cells of tendons and bursae.

synoviosarcoma (si-nō′vi-ō-sar-kō′ma): Malignant synovioma (*q.v.*).

synovitis (sin-ō-vī′tis): Inflammation of a synovial membrane.

synovium (si-nō′vi-um): A synovial membrane lining a joint cavity.

synthesis (sin′the-sis): The forming of a complex substance by combining chemical elements or simpler compounds.—synthetic, adj.; synthesize, v.

synthesize (sin′the-sīz): To make or form chemically by means of synthesis.

synthetic (sin-thet′ik): Produced by artificial means.

syntonic (sin-ton′ik): Refers to a stable personality that responds to the various elements in the environment in a normal manner, as contrasted with the schizoid type of personality.

syphilid (e) (sif′i-lid): General term for any syphilitic skin lesion.

syphilis (sif′il-is): [Syphilis, syphilitic shepherd in poem by Fracastorius (1530), in which the term first appears.] A severe contagious venereal disease, caused by the *Treponema pallidum*. Infection is acquired, commonly by sexual intercourse, or the fetus may acquire it from the mother while in utero. **CONGENITAL S.,** present at birth; marked by coryza, skin eruptions, malformed teeth, wasting of the tissues, and craniotabes (*q.v.*). **ACQUIRED S.,** manifests in: 1) The primary stage; appears 4 to 5 weeks (or later) after infection when a primary chancre associated with swelling or local lymph glands appears; 2) The secondary stage in which the skin eruption appears; 3) The third (tertiary) stage occurs 15 to 30 years after initial infection; gummata appear, or neurosyphilis and cardiovascular **S.** intervene. The commonest types of nervous system involvement are general paralysis of the insane and tabes dorsalis (locomotor ataxia). Cardiovascular involvement produces cerebrovascular disasters, aortic aneurism, or destruction of the aortic valve. **LATENT S., S.** for which there is serological or historical evidence but no other symptoms. **MENINGOVASCULAR S., S.** affecting the meninges, with narrowing of the cerebral arteries in the leptomeninges, which may lead to occulsion and infarcts in the brain and spinal cord.—syphilitic, syphilous, adj.

syphilitic (sif-i-lit′ik): Of, pertaining to, affected with, or caused by, syphilis.

syphiloid (sif′i-loyd): 1. Resembling syphilis. 2. A condition resembling syphilis.

syphiloma (sif-i-lō′ma): A tumor of syphilitic origin; a gumma.

syrigmus (si-rig′mus): Ringing in the ears.

syringadenoma (sir′ing-ad-e-nō′ma): An adenoma of a sweat gland.

syringe (si-rinj′): An instrument for injecting or withdrawing liquids; of differing sizes and designs depending upon the specific purpose for which it is used.

syringitis (sir′in-jī′tis): Inflammation of the eustachian tube(s).

syringobulbia (si-ring′gō-bul′bi-a): The presence of a fluid-filled cavity or cavities in the medulla oblongata.

syringomyelia (si-ring′gō-mī-ē′li-a): An uncommon progressive disease of the nervous system of unknown cause that may be due to trauma or defective embryonic development, beginning mainly in early adult life. Cavitation and surrounding fibrous tissue reaction, in the upper spinal cord and brain stem, interfere with sensations of pain and temperature, and sometimes with the motor pathways. The characteristic symptom is painless injury, particularly of the exposed hands. Touch sensation is intact.

syringomyelocele (si-ring′gō-mī′e-lō-sēl): Most severe form of meningeal hernia (spina bifida). The central canal is dilated and the thinned-out posterior part of the spinal cord is in the hernia which protrudes through a defect in the dorsal aspect of the vertebral column.

syrinx (sir′ingks): 1. A pathologic tube or pipe. 2. A fistula. 3. The cavity that forms in spinal cord or brainstem in syringomyelia.

syrup: A concentrated solution of sugar and water usually containing a drug.

system (sis′-tem): 1. A network of things so connected as to form a whole. 2. An established way of doing something; a method. 3. In anatomy, a) a group of organs that work together to perform a particular function, or b) the entire (physical) body organism.—systemic, systematic, adj.

systemic (sis-tem′ik): 1. Related to a particular system of the body. 2. Related to the body as a whole. **S. CIRCULATION,** circulation of the blood through all parts of the body except the lungs.

SYSTEMIC LUPUS ERYTHEMATOSUS, see under lupus.

systems theory: A method of scientific inquiry whereby a particular entity involving human relationships is considered on the basis of resources, input, and outcomes, with feedback at each level leading to progress to the next level and allowing for ongoing evaluation. In nursing, the use of systems theory can be helpful in providing direction for assessment of patients, as well as planning and implementing care.

systole (sis′to-le): The contraction phase of the cardiac cycle; the total ventricular process. **EXTRA-SYSTOLE,** a premature contraction of an atrium or ventricle, or both, which does not alter the fundamental rhythm of contractions.—systolic, adj.

systremma (sis-trem′a): A cramp in the muscles of the leg, the calf muscles in particular.

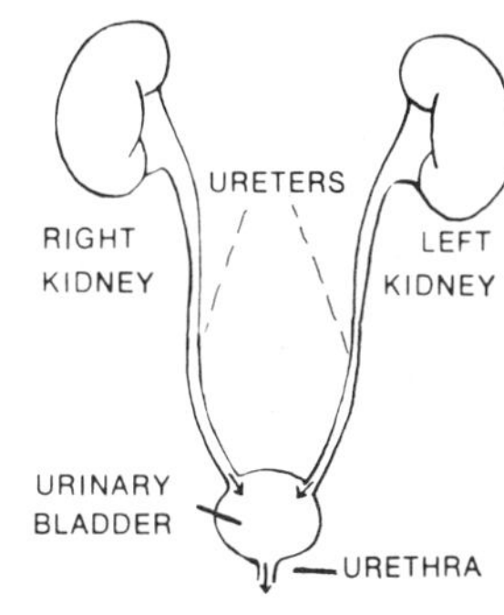

Urinary system

T

T: Abbreviation for: 1. Temperature. 2. Tension.

T and A: Abbreviation for tonsillectomy and adenectomy.

T piece: A T-shaped tube that may be used in conjunction with a tracheostomy tube to provide for delivery of humidity along with oxygen or air.

T tube: A self-retaining drainage tube made in the shape of the letter T. **T-TUBE CHOLANGIOGRAPHY,** see cholangiography.

T wave: In electrocardiology, the deflection that represents ventricular depolarization during which time the ventricles are in a relatively refractory period; it follows the QRS complex.

T's and blues: Street term for a combination of the analgesic pentazocine hydrochloride and the antihistamine tripelennamine hydrochloride; used by addicts as a substitute for heroin; may cause severe cutaneous damage, hepatitis, septicemia, and endocarditis; withdrawal symptoms are severe.

TA: Abbreviation for toxin-antitoxin. Also written T.A.

TAB: A mixed vaccine containing killed *Salmonella typhi, Paratyphi A* and *B;* used to produce immunity to typhoid and paratyphoid fever; usually given in 3 ascending doses a week apart; confers immunity for varying lengths of time, usually one to three years.

Tab: Abbreviation for tablet.

tabacosis (tab-a-kō'sis): A chronic form of tobacco poisoning; usually caused by inhalation of tobacco dust.

tabella (ta-bel'a): A medicated troche or tablet.

tabes (tā'bēz): Progressive emaciation; wasting away. Term usually used in connection with tabes dorsalis. **T. DORSALIS** (locomotor ataxia), a variety of neurosyphilis in which there is progressive sclerosis of the posterior (sensory) columns of the spinal cord, the sensory nerve roots and the peripheral nerves. It is marked by muscular incoordination, ataxia (*q.v.*), anesthesia, joint disorders, neuralgia, sometimes paralysis; usually occurs after middle life. **T. MESENTERICA,** tuberculous enlargement of the peritoneal lymph nodes; seen in children.

tabescense (ta-bes'ens): The state of wasting away, or progressive emaciation; atrophy.—tabescent, adj.

tabetic (ta-bet'ik): 1. Pertaining to tabes. 2. Affected with tabes. **T. ARTHROPATHY,** Charcot's joint (*q.v.*). **T. GAIT,** the ataxic gait of tabes dorsalis.

tabetiform (ta-bet'i-form): Resembling tabes dorsalis.

tablature (tab'la-tūr): The division or separation of the main cranial bones into two tables or plates which are separated by a layer of cancellous bone.

table: 1. In anatomy, the external or internal layer of compact bone, separated by a layer of cancellous bony tissue (diploe), that make up the main bones of the cranium. 2. An orderly presentation of numerical data or steps in an experiment, arranged in rows or columns showing the essential facts, for quick reference and comparison.

tablespoon: A large spoon used in household measurements; holds approximately 4 fluid drams or 15 milliliters.

tablet: In pharmacology, a small disk of varying size and thickness, containing a dose of a medication, in either pure or diluted form. **BUCCAL T.,** a **T.** that is inserted into the buccal pouch where it dissolves quickly and the essential ingredients are absorbed directly by the buccal mucosa. **ENTERIC-COATED T.,** a **T.** coated with a material that delays release of the essential ingredients until after the tablet has left the stomach. **SUBLINGUAL T.,** a **T.** that is placed under the tongue and held there until it is dissolved.

taboo, tabu (ta-boo'): 1. Any behavior regarded as unacceptable or harmful to the social welfare. 2. A prohibition imposed by social usage or for the protection of the group. **INCEST T.,** pertaining to sexual activity between persons so closely related that marriage is prohibited.

taboparesis (tā'bō-par-ē'sis): A condition in which the spinal cord shows the same lesions as in tabes dorsalis (*q.v.*) and general paresis. Also called taboparalysis.

TABS: A useful acronym in checking the newborn's adjustment to the environment; refers to *t*emperature, *a*irway, *b*reathing, *s*ugar (blood glucose level).

tabular (tab'ū-lar): 1. Laminated or table-like, or having a flat surface. 2. Arranged in the form of a table, or resembling a table.

tache (tahsh): A macule, blemish, spot, or any circumscribed area of discoloration on the skin or mucous membrane.—tachetic, adj.

tachistoscope (ta-kis'tō-skōp): An apparatus used in psychologic testing; it presents visual images for a short period of time to test the subject's time rate for appreception.

tachogram (tak'ō-gram): The graphic record made by tachography.

tachography (ta-kog'-ra-fi): The recording of movement and velocity of arterial blood flow. Also tachygraphy.

tachometer (ta-kom′e-ter): An instrument for measuring the speed of a moving object or substance. Also tachymeter.

tachy-: Combining form denoting rapid, swift, accelerated.

tachyarrhythmia (tak′i-a-rith′mi-a): A heartbeat of 100 or more per minute; may or may not be regular.

tachycardia (tak′i-kar′di-a): Very rapid heart action (over 100 beats per minute in adults) with resulting increase in the pulse rate; some of the causes are heart disease, hyperthyroidism, high fever, toxemia. **PAROXYSMAL ATRIAL T.**, regular heart rhythm with an atrial rate of 150–250 per minute; often associated with acute respiratory disorders and with most forms of heart disease. **PAROXYSMAL T.**, sudden marked increase in the pulse rate, lasting for various lengths of time and then disappearing; sometimes accompanies failing heart muscle action, but in some people it is of nervous origin. **SINUS T.**, **T.** that originates in the sinoatrial node. **SUPRAVENTRICULAR T.**, rapid heartbeat caused by an ectopic pacemaker located above the ventricles; see ectopic, beat. **VENTRICULAR T.**, rapid regular heartbeat due to an ectopic stimulus in the conduction system of the ventricle.—tachycardiac, adj.

tachycrotic (tak′i-krot′ik): Relating to, causing, or characterized by an increased pulse rate.

tachylalia (tak-i-lā′li-a): Rapidity of speech.

tachylogia (tak-i-lō′ji-a): Extremely rapid or voluble speech.

tachyphagia (tak-i-fā′ji-a): Abnormally rapid eating, bolting of food.

tachyphrasia (tak-i-frā′zi-a): Volubility; extremely rapid flow of speech; may be seen in certain nervous disorders. Also tachyphasia.

tachyphrenia (tak-i-frē′ni-a): Hyperactivity of the mental processes.

tachyphylaxis (tak-i-fi-lak′sis): The progressive decrease in response to a drug or other substance that produces a physiologic action, following repeated administration of small doses.

tachypnea (tak-ip-nē′a): Abnormal frequency of respiration, *i.e.*, over 20 per minute, in response to low oxygen or high carbon dioxide content of the blood; often seen in hysteria, neurasthenia, high fevers, respiratory infection; sometimes but not always accompanied by dyspnea (*q.v.*). Also spelled tachypnoea.—tachypneic, adj.

tachypsychia (tak-i-sī′ki-a): Rapidity of psychic or mental responses or processes.

tachyrhythmia (tak-i-rith′mi-a): See tachycardia.

tachysystole (tak-i-sis′tō-lē): Tachycardia.

tachytrophism (tak-i-trō′fizm): Unusually rapid metabolism.

tactile (tak′til): 1. Pertaining to the sense of touch. 2. Perceptible through the sense of touch. 3. Real, tangible. **T. AGNOSIA,** loss of the ability to recognize objects by touch due to a cerebral lesion. **T. ANESTHESIA,** loss of the ability to perceive touch. **T.** corpuscles, see Meissner's corpuscles. **T. SENSATION,** a sensation produced through the sense of touch.

taction (tak′shun): 1. The sense of touch. 2. The act of touching.

tactometer (tak-tom′e-ter): An instrument for measuring an individual's acuity for the sense of touch.

tactual (tak′tū-al): Pertaining to or caused by touch.

tactus (tak′tus): Touch; the sense of touch.

Taenia (tē′ni-a): A genus of flat, parasitic worms; cestodes or tapeworms. In **T. ECHINOCOCCUS,** the adult worm lives in the intestines of dogs (the definitive host) and humans (the intermediate host) are infested by swallowing food contaminated by eggs from the dog's excrement. These become embryos in the human small intestine, pass via the bloodstream to organs, particularly the liver, and develop into hydatid cysts. **T. SAGINATA** larvae are present in infested, undercooked beef. In the human intestinal lumen they develop into the adult tapeworm, which, by its four suckers attaches itself to the gut wall. It grows to 12–25 feet in length and is the most common tapeworm in humans in the U.S. Consists of a head and numerous segments, each one being capable of independent existence, consequently, in any treatment, it is necessary for the head to be expelled. **T. SOLIUM** resembles **T. SAGINATA,** but has hooklets as well as suckers. The larvae are ingested in infested, undercooked pork; humans can also be the intermediate host for this worm by ingesting eggs which, developing into larvae in the human stomach, pass via the bowel wall to reach organs, and there develop into cysts. In the brain these may give rise to epilepsy.

tag: 1. A label; tracer. 2. To incorporate into a compound a substance that is more readily visible. 3. A small appendage, polyp, or outgrowth of skin.

tail: 1. The caudal extremity of an animal. 2. Anything resembling a tail, such as an elongated part of an organ. **T. OF SPENCE,** the tissue of the mammary gland that extends into the axillary region; may become enlarged premenstrually or during lactation.

tailor's ankle: An abnormal condition of the bursa over the lateral malleolus of the tibia; due to sitting on the floor in a crossed-leg position.

tailor's bottom: Weaver's bottom (*q.v.*).

taint (tānt): 1. Putrefaction or infestation. 2. A local discoloration or blemish. 3. A hereditary disposition to some pathological condition or unattractive attribute.

Takayasu's disease: Pulseless disease (*q.v.*).

take: In medicine, a successful vaccination or inoculation. In plastic surgery, a successful transplantation of tissue, as a skin graft.

talalgia (ta-lal'ji-a): Pain in the heel.

talar (tā'lar): Of or pertaining to the talus.

talc, talcum: A naturally occurring soft white powder consisting of magnesium silicate.

talcosis (tal-ko'sis): A pulmonary disorder resembling silicosis (*q.v.*); occurs as an occupational disease of people who work in the talc industry.

taliped (tal'i-ped), **talipedic** (tal-i-pēd'ik): Clubfooted.

talipes (tal'i-pēz): Descriptive of several types of congenital foot deformities, especially clubfootedness, of which there are four main types: 1) **T. CALCANEUS,** dorsal flexion of the foot that results in walking with only the heel touching the ground; 2) **T. EQUINUS,** hyperflexion of the foot, which results in walking with only the toes touching the ground; 3) **T. VALGUS,** eversion of the foot, which results in walking on the inner edge of the foot; and 4) **T. VARUS,** inversion of the foot, which results in walking on the outer edge of the foot only (opp. of valgus). Other types include: 1) **T. CALCANEOVALGUS,** a deformity in which the heel is turned outward and the anterior part of the foot is held elevated; 2) **T. CALCANEOVARUS,** a deformity in which the heel is held toward the midline of the body and the anterior part of the foot is held in elevation; 3) **T. EQUINOVALGUS,** the heel is held elevated and turned outward from the midline; 4) **T. EQUINOVARUS,** the foot is plantar flexed, with the sole turned inward toward the midline; the heel does not touch the ground when the person is walking; this is the most common type of clubfoot. See also **pes.**

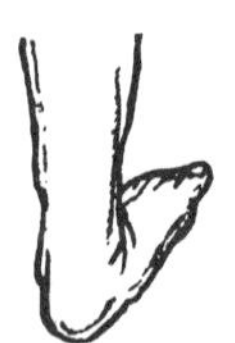

talipes calcaneus

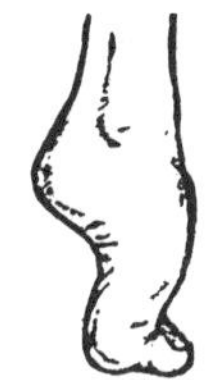

talipes equinus

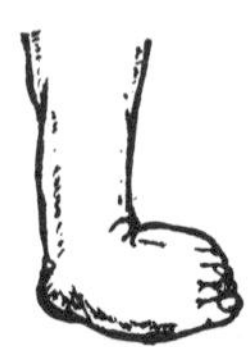

talipes valgus

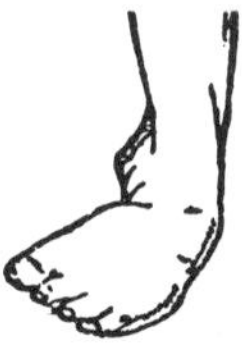

talipes varus

talipomanus (tal-i-pom'a-nus): A congenital or acquired fixed deformity of the hand that is analagous to clubfoot, *i.e.*, the hand is fixed in a position of strong flexion and adduction; also called clubhand.

talo-: A combining form denoting the talus.

talocalcaneal (tā' -lō-kal-kā'nē-al): Pertaining to the talus and the calcaneus. Also talocalcanean.

talocalcaneonavicular (tā'lō-kal-kā'nē-ō-na-vik'ū-lar): Pertaining to the talus, calcaneus, and navicular bones.

talocrural (tā'lō-kroo'ral): Pertaining to the talus and the leg bones. **T. ARTICULATION,** the ankle joint.

talofibular (tā'lō-fib'ū-lar): Pertaining to the talus and the fibula.

talomalleolar (tā'lō-ma-lē'o-lar): Pertaining to the talus and the malleolus.

talonavicular (tā'lō-na-vik'ū-lar): Pertaining to the talus and the navicular bone.

talotibial (tā'lō-tib'i-al): Pertaining to the talus and the tibia.

talus (tā'lus): The astragalus; situated between the tibia proximally and the calcaneus distally, thus directly bearing the weight of the body. It is the second largest bone of the ankle.

tama (tā'ma): Swelling of the feet and legs.

tampon (tam'pon): 1. A ball of absorbent cotton, gauze, sponge or similar substance used to pack or plug a cavity or canal to restrain hemorrhage, absorb secretions, or apply medication. 2. A type of sanitary napkin to be worn internally to absorb menstrual fluid.

tamponade (tam-po-nod'): 1. The surgical insertion of a tampon as a device for checking internal hemorrhage by compression of a viscus. 2. Pathological compression of an organ as in cardiac **T. BALLOON T.,** esophagogastric **T.,** utilizing a device consisting of a three-lumen tube and two inflatable balloons. **CARDIAC T.,** the accumulation of fluid in the pericardial sac, impairing heart function and resulting in decreased heart output, hypertension, tachycardia; may result in heart failure. **ESOPHAGOGASTRIC T.,** exertion of pressure against a bleeding esophageal varix using a tube-shaped balloon; see also **varix. PERICARDIAL T.,** compression of the cardiac muscle by fluid accumulated in the pericardial sac; cardiac **T.**

tamponment (tam-pōn'ment): The insertion of a tampon.

tandem gait: See under **gait.**

tangentiality (tan-jen'shi-al'i-ti): In conversational speech, a pattern characterized by divergence from the original topic, often leading to an entirely different chain of thought. Also called loose association.

Tangier disease: A familial condition in which the lipoprotein in the blood serum is greatly reduced and cholesterol esters are deposited in the reticuloendothelial system; marked by enlarged, yellowish gray tonsils, lymphadenopathy, and splenomegaly. In adults, the vascular and neurologic systems are also involved.

tank: A large receptacle for fluid substances. **HUBBARD T.**, a **T.** used for underwater exercises, for treatment of certain skin conditions, and for burn therapy.

tanner's disease: Anthrax (*q.v.*).

tannic acid (tan'ik as'id): A substance derived from tannin, which is obtained from nutgalls that form on twigs of certain trees, including the oak; used in medicine as a styptic and astringent, and sometimes in the treatment of burns.

tantalum (tan'ta-lum): A rare, noncorrosive, malleable metallic element; used sometimes as wire sutures or as flat plates to repair skull injuries, or for making prosthetic devices.

tantrum: An unreasoning fit of anger accompanied usually by violent physical gestures, seen in children and sometimes in mentally disturbed patients. **TEMPER T.**, loud, annoying behavior, usually seen in children; thought by behavioral psychologists to result from failure of less violent ways of obtaining attention of parents or other significant persons.

tanyphonia (tan-i-fo'ni-a): Weakness or thinness of the voice.

tap: 1. A quick blow used in massage or by the physician during examination. 2. Paracentesis (*q.v.*).

tapetum (ta-pē'tum): A covering or roof-like structure or a layer of cells. In neuroanatomy, a thin sheet of fibers in the roof and lateral walls of the posterior horn and in the lateral walls of the inferior horn of the lateral ventricle of the cerebrum.

tapeworm: See taenia.

taphophilia (taf'ō-fil'i-a): A morbid attraction to graves and burial places.

taphophobia (taf'ō-fō-bi-a): A morbid fear of being buried alive.

tapinocephaly (ta-pi-no-sef'a-li): The condition of having a flattened or depressed skull.—tapinocephalic, adj.

tapotement (ta-pōt-mon'): A percussive or tapping movement in massage, usually performed with the side of the hand.

tar: A dark-colored viscous substance obtained from bituminous coal or the wood of certain trees. **COAL T.**, used as a base for some ointments and solutions used in treating skin disorders. **PINE T.**, has several uses in medicine because of its antibacterial and irritant properties.

tarantism (tar'an-tizm): A mania occurring during the Middle Ages, most often in southern Europe; was believed to be caused by the bite of a tarantula, and that it could be cured by dancing.

tarantula (ta-ran'tū-la): A large hairy spider not significantly poisonous to man.

tarassis (ta-ras'is): The name given to hysteria occurring in a male person.

tardive (tar'div): Late; tardy. **T. DYSKINESIA**, see under dyskinesia.

tarry (tah'ri): Having the consistency and appearance of tar. **T. STOOLS**, usually due to intestinal hemorrhage, but also occur when the patient is receiving certain medications that contain iron or bismuth.

tars-, tarso-: Combining forms referring to: 1. The eyelid. 2 The tarsus of the foot.

tarsadenitis (tar'sad-e-nī'tis): Inflammation of the tarsal edges of the eyelid and of the meibomian glands.

tarsal (tar'sal): 1. Relating to the eyelid or the plates of cartilage in the eyelid. 2. Relating to the seven bones of the tarsus (*q.v.*). **T. PLATE**, the firm framework of connective tissue of the upper and lower eyelids which gives them their shape.

tarsal tunnel syndrome: Pain and sensory loss in the medial anterior part of the foot and great toe; may be due to pressure on the medial plantar nerve or pressure on, or damage to, the posterior tibial nerve.

tarsalgia (tar-sal'ji-a): Pain in the tarsus or ankle.

tarsectomy (tar-sek'to-mi): 1. Excision of a segment of the cartilaginous plate of the eyelid. 2. Excision of one or more of the tarsal bones.

tarsitis (tar-sī'tis): 1. Inflammation of the tarsal edge of the eyelid; blepharitis. 2. Inflammation of the tarsus or ankle.

tarsochiloplasty (tar-sō-kī'lō-plas-ti): Plastic surgery of the eyelid, the borders in particular.

tarsoclasis (tar-sok'la-sis): Surgical fracture of the tarsus of the foot in an operation for correction of clubfoot.

tarsomalacia (tar'sō-ma-lā'shi-a): Softening of the cartilaginous part of the eyelid.

tarsometatarsal (tar-sō-met'a-tar-sal): Pertaining to the tarsal and metatarsal regions.

tarso-orbital (tar'sō-ōr'bit-al): Pertaining to the eyelid and the orbit of the eye.

tarsophalangeal (tar-sō-fa-lan'jē-al): Pertaining to the tarsus and the toes.

tarsophyma (tar-sō-fī'ma): Any tarsal neoplasm.

tarsoplasty (tar'sō-plas-ti): Any plastic operation on the eyelid.

tarsoptosia (tar-sop-tō'si-a): Flatfootedness; falling of the tarsus.

tarsorrhaphy (tar-sor′ra-fi): Suturing together of the eyelids, partially, or entirely to shorten the palpebral fissure or to protect the cornea temporarily when there is paralysis of the obicularis muscle or to allow healing in case of chronic ulcer. Also blepharorrhaphy.

tarsotibial (tar-sō-tib′i-al): Pertaining to the tarsus and the tibia.

tarsus (tar′sus): 1. The part of the foot that is behind the metatarsals; made up of seven bones; the calcaneus or heel bone, the talus or ankle bone, and the cuboid, navicular, and first, second and third cuneiform bones. 2. The thin elongated plates of dense connective tissue found in each eyelid, contributing to its form and support.—tarsal, adj.

tartar: A hard yellowish deposit that forms on the teeth.

tartaric acid (tar-tar′ik): A clear, colorless, crystalline acid found in vegetables and certain fruits; also produced commercially as a soluble white powder from potassium bitartrate, found in grape juice; has several pharmacological uses.

tartrate (tar′trāt): Any salt of tartaric acid.

tasikinesia (tas-i-kī-nē′zi-a): An uncontrollable desire to get up and walk about; inability to remain seated quietly.

taste: 1. The power to perceive and distinguish flavors. 2. The sensation produced when the specialized nerve endings in the taste buds are stimulated. **T. BUDS**, small clusters of specialized cells located in the epithelium of the tongue and the inside of the mouth, epiglottis, and parts of the pharynx; they connect with the surface by small pores through which substances in solution enter and stimulate the nerve endings contained in the buds thus giving rise to the sensation of taste. They are classified according to the composition of the substance to which they are sensitive: sweet, acid, salty, bitter.

TAT: Abbreviation for: 1. Thematic apperception test. 2. Toxin-antitoxin. 3. Tetanus antitoxin.

tatoo (ta-tōō′): The insertion of permanent coloring matter into the skin by puncture. **ACCIDENTAL T.**, the accidental imbedding of small particles of foreign material into the skin.

taurine (taw′rin): An acid found in human bile; small amounts are also found in tissues of the lungs and muscles.

taurocholemia (taw-rō-kō-lē′mi-a): The presence of taurocholic acid in the blood.

taurocholic acid (taw-rō-kō′lik): A bile acid that, on hydrolysis, splits into taurine and cholic acid.

taut (tawt): Tightly drawn or tensely stretched; not loose or flabby.

tauto-: A combining form meaning the same.

tautology (taw-tol′o-ji): The needless repetition of a word, phrase, or idea.

tautomenial (taw-tō-mē′ni-al): Pertaining to the same menstrual period.

-taxia, -taxis, taxy: Combining forms denoting order, arrangement.

taxis (tak′sis): 1. The restoration of a displaced part to its normal position by manual manipulation; term often used in relation to the reduction of a hernia by manipulation. 2. The reflex movement that occurs in response to a stimulus; term is usually attached to a word that designates the kind of stimulus, *e.g.*, chemotaxis, thermotaxis.

taxonomy (taks-on′-o-mi): The scientific and orderly classification of plants and animals, or the principles and laws upon which such classification is made.—taxonomic, adj.

Tay-Sachs disease: Amaurotic familial idiocy (*q.v.*). Thought to be an error of fat metabolism resulting in cerebral lipoidosis. Symptoms usually appear at about 6 months of age. Characterized by bright red spots on the retina and often blindness, neurological deterioration, and death within three to five years. [Warren Tay, English physician. 1843–1927. Bernard Sachs, American neurologist. 1858–1944.]

TB: Abbreviation for: 1. Tubercle bacillus. 2. Tuberculosis. Also T.b. and t.b.

T-bandage: See bandage. Also called T-binder.

TBSA: Abbreviation for total body surface area.

tbsp: Abbreviation for tablespoon, tablespoonful.

Tc: Chemical symbol for technetium.

TCDB: Abbreviation for turn, cough, deep breathe.

T-cell: See under cell.

teaching hospital: A hospital that is usually large, located in a medical center, and near a medical school; it is where medical students, interns, and residents receive clinical instruction and experience during their attendance at medical school.

tear: 1. Laceration; a break in the continuity of a substance. 2. To pull apart by force.

tearing (tēr′ing): Excessive production of more tears than are carried off by the lacrimal duct, resulting in "watering" of the eyes.

tears (tērz): The clear, slightly alkaline secretion constantly being formed by the lacrimal gland, and spread by blinking; function is to keep the conjunctiva moist. Contains the enzyme lysosome, which acts as an antiseptic. See lacrimal.

tease: To draw or pull out or separate into fine threads or minute shreds; refers especially to preparation of tissue for microscopic examination.

teaspoon: A spoon of small size used in household measurements; contains approximately 1 fluidram or 4 milliters.

teat (tēt): A nipple.

technetium (tek-nē'shi-um): A radioactive metallic element. Its most stable isotope is technetium 99m (^{99m}Tc) used in diagnostic tests and in scanning; has a half-life of only 6 hours.

technic, technique (tek-nēk'): The detailed systematic manner in which a specific procedure, such as a mechanical or surgical operation or a test, is performed. **ISOLATION T.**, the methods used to prevent the spread of pathogenic organisms or infection from a patient to other individuals.

technical (tek'ni-kal): Pertaining to technique, or requiring a special skill.

technician (tek-nish'un): One who has had training in and uses the techniques required for carrying out the specific procedures of a particular profession. In the health sciences the title often indicates the particular area in which the individual works, *e.g.*, histology technician.

technologist (tek-nol'o-jist): An individual who works in a particular technology (*q.v.*); often used with the name of the technology involved, *e.g.*, radio-therapy technologist.

technology (tek-nol'o-ji): The practical application of the knowledge and techniques of a profession or science.

tectocephaly (tek-tō-sef'a-li): A condition in which the skull is abnormally long and narrow as a result of premature closing of the sagittal suture; usually associated with mental retardation.—tectocephalic, adj.

tectonic (tek-ton'ik): Pertaining to the reconstruction of a part by plastic surgery or the restoration of a lost part by grafting.

tectorial (tek-tor'i-al): 1. Forming a roof or covering. 2. Of the nature of a roof or cover.

tectospinal (tek-tō-spī'nal): **T. TRACT**, a tract of white nerve fibers that pass from the tectum of the midbrain through the medulla oblongata to the spinal cord.

tectum (tek'tum): A roof-like structure. **T. MESOENCEPHALI**, the membranous roof of the midbrain.

teenage (tēn'āj): The years between childhood and adulthood; usually considered to begin at about age 13 and to last until about age 19.

teeth: See tooth.

teething (tēth'ing): Dentition, the eruption of teeth; usually applied to eruption of the first or deciduous set.

Teflon (tef'lon): A synthetic material used in the manufacture of many medical and surgical supplies and prostheses, ranging from *Band-aids* to grafting material for blood vessels.

tegmen (teg'men): A structure that covers or roofs over a part.

tegmentum (teg-men'tum): 1. A covering. 2. That part of the brain stem that lies behind the peduncles that connect the cerebrum with the pons.—tegmental, adj.

tegument (teg'ū-ment): The skin or covering of the animal body; the integument.—tegumental, tegumentary, adj.

teichopsia (tī-kop'si-a): The sensation of seeing flashing or shimmering lights appearing suddenly before the eyes in a zigzag pattern; may be associated with migraine headache and stress.

tel-, tele-, telo-: Combining forms denoting far off; at a distance; over a distance.

tela (tē'la): In anatomy, any web-like structure; a thin, delicate tissue.—telae, pl.

telalgia (tel-al'ji-a): Referred pain.

telangiectasia (tel-an'ji-ek-tā'zi-a): Abnormal dilatation of the terminal skin capillaries; seen in certain disorders of the circulation, polycythemia, alcoholism, overexposure to sunlight; often in the shape of a spider or a Medusa's head; see caput medusae. **HEREDITARY HEMORRHAGIC T.**, hereditary **T.** characterized by the presence of multiple areas of **T.** and a tendency to hemorrhage, especially from the nose; develops chiefly after puberty. Also called Osler's disease, Osler-Welser-Rendu disease, and spider angioma..

telangiectasis (tel-an'ji-ek'ta-sis): Discoloration of the skin where the capillaries have dilated in telangiectasia (*q.v.*).

telangiectoma (tel-an'ji-ek-tō'ma): An angioma formed from dilated capillaries or arterioles.

telangiitis (tel-an'ji-ī'tis): Inflammation of capillaries.

telangioma (tel-an'ji-ō'ma): An angioma made up of dilated terminal capillaries.

telangiosis (tel-an'ji-ō'sis): Any disease of capillaries.

tele-: Combining form denoting: 1. At the end. 2. At a distance; far away.

telecanthus (tel-e-kan'thus): Increased breadth between the medial canthi of the eyelids, making the eyes appear wide-set.

telecardiography (tel'e-kar-di-og'ra-fi): The recording of an electrocardiogram utilizing an apparatus for transmitting the impulses to a point some distance from the patient.

telecardiophone (tel-e-kar'di-ō-fōn): A specially constructed stethoscope for making heart sounds audible to a listener at some distance from the patient.

Telecare: A program in which volunteers telephone participating elderly clients daily; in cases of no answer, they alert a relative or someone previously designated by the patient to go to the patient's home and investigate the reason for no answer.

teleceptor (tel′e-sep-tor): Sensory nerve terminals or receptors that have the ability to respond to stimuli that originate at a distance, as those in the eyes and ears.—teleceptive, adj.

teleconsultation (tel′ē-kon-sul-tā′shun): Consultation conducted by two-way television.

telecurietherapy (tel′e-kū-rē-ther′a-pi): Treatment with radium placed at a distance from the patient.

telediagnosis (tel′e-dī-ag-nō′sis): Diagnosis made at a distance from the patient by means of data transmitted from the patient's monitoring equipment to a central monitoring station or an intensive care unit.

telefluoroscopy (tel′e-floo-ō-ros′kō-pi): Transmission by television of images on a fluoroscopy screen for observation at a distant point.

telemetry (te-lem′e-tri): Making measurements of a property such as blood pressure or temperature and transmitting the findings by radio signal to a receiver at a distance for interpretation and recording.

telencephalon (tel-en-sef′a-lon): The anterior part of the embryonic forebrain which develops into the cerebral cortex, corpus striatum, and olfactory lobes.

teleneuron (tel-e-nū′ron): A nerve ending.

teleology (tē-lē-ol′o-ji): The belief that all physical phenomena can be explained in terms of their purpose.—teleological, adj.

teleopsia (tē-lē-op′si-a): A visual disorder in which close objects appear to be far away, or objects perceived in space appear much denser than they are.

teleorganic (tel-e-or-gan′ik): Necessary to organic life.

telepathy (te-lep′a-thi): Mental communication, without any obvious means, between people who are at a distance from each other. Thought transference. Also called extrasensory perception.

teleradium (tel-e-rā′di-um): Radium whose radiation is directed into the body from an external source; radium beam.

telesthesia (tel-es-thē′zi-a): Extrasensory perception (*q.v.*).

teletherapeutics (tel′e-ther-a-pū′tiks): The use of hypnotic suggestion as a mode of treatment.

teletherapy (tel-e-ther′a-pi): 1. The external administration of radiotherapy; the radiation is delivered by an isotope placed in a mold or other container and applied to the skin, or by an external beam machine. 2. By custom, often refers to treatment by teleradium.

telethermometer (tel′e-ther-mom′e-ter): A device for registering temperature at a distance from the patient under observation.

telo-: Combining form denoting end.

telodendron (tel-ō-den′dron): One of the fine terminal branches in the arborization at the end of an axon.—telodendria, pl.

telogen (tel′ō-jen): The final, quiescent stage in the cycle of hair in the follicle, lasting from the time the hair ceases to grow until it is shed. See anagen. **T. EFFLUVIUM,** transient loss of hair following a febrile illness, general anesthesia, childbirth, or chemotherapy.

telognosis (tel′og-nō′sis): Diagnosis by examination of radiographs transmitted by special telephonic means.

telolemma (tel-ō-lem′ma): The membranous covering of a motor end plate in a striated muscle fiber.

telophase (tel′ō-fāz): The final stage in cell mitosis when the chromosomes have been grouped at the ends of the cell and the cell divides, forming two new cells.

temp: Abbreviation for temperature.

temperament (tem′per-a-ment): The habitual mental and emotional attitude of an individual as distinct from mood, which is temporary. Historically, four types were identified: sanguine, phlegmatic, bilious or choleric, and melancholic.

temperature (tem′per-a-chur): The degree of heat or coldness of an object or substance as measured by a thermometer. **AXILLARY T.,** that registered on a thermometer placed in the axilla. **BODY T.,** refers to the internal or core temperature of vital organs *i.e.*, the heart, brain, lungs, abdominal viscera; remains constant regardless of environmental temperature. **INVERSE BODY T., T.** that is lower in the evening than in the morning. **MEAN T.,** the average **T.** of the atmosphere in an area over a period of time. **NORMAL T.,** usually refers to that considered normal for the human body, 36.9°C or 98.4°F. **ORAL T.,** that registered on a thermometer placed in the mouth. **RECTAL T.,** that registered on a thermometer placed in the rectum. **ROOM T.,** the ordinary **T.** of the atmosphere in a room. **SHELL T.,** the **T.** at or near the surface of the body; more variable than the core **T.,** and more responsive to environmental influences. **SUBNORMAL T.,** refers to body **T** that is below the normal **T.** See also fever; pyrexia.

temple: 1. The flattened area on either side of the head lying between the outer angle of the eye and the top of the ear flap. 2. One of the side supports for a pair of spectacles.

tempolabile (tem-pō-lā′bil): Having a tendency to change with the passage of time.

temporal (tem′por-al): 1. Limited in time or pertinent to time. 2. Relating to the temple (*q.v.*). **T. ARTERITIS,** giant-cell arteritis, see under arteritis. **T. BONES,** one on either side of the head below the pareital bones; contain the middle ear. **T. LOBE**, one of the five lobes of each hemisphere of the cerebrum; lies under the temporal bone and contains the auditory center. **T. LOBE EPILEPSY**, see under **epilepsy**.

temporofrontal (tem'pō-rō-fron'tal): Pertaining to the temporal and frontal regions or bones.

temporomandibular (tem'po-rō-man-dib'ū-lar): Pertaining to the temporal region or bone and the lower jaw. **T. JOINT SYNDROME**, often seen in the elderly who have ill fitting dentures or degeneration of the soft tissue of the gums following tooth extraction; the pain may radiate to the ear, the mastoid area, or the mandible; sometimes causes trismus, tinnitus, and decreased hearing; also called temporomandibular-pain dysfunction syndrome.

temporomaxillary (tem'po-rō-mak'si-lar-i): Pertaining to the temporal and maxillary regions or bones.

temporo-occipital (tem'pō-rō-ok-sip'i-tal): Pertaining to the temporal and occipital regions or bones.

temporoparietal (tem'pō-rō-pa-rī'e-tal): Pertaining to the temporal and parietal regions or bones.

temporospatial (tem'pō-rō-spā'shul): Pertaining to time and space.

temporosphenoidal (tem'pō-rō-sfē-noy'dal): Pertaining to the temporal and sphenoid regions or bones.

tempostabile (tem'pō-stā'bil): Not subject to change over time.

tenacious (te-nā'shus): 1. Sticky, adhesive, holding fast. 2. Thick and viscid, usually said of sputum or other body fluid.

tenacity (te-nas'i-ti): The characteristic of being tough or resistant.

tenaculum (te-nak'ū-lum): 1. A hook-like instrument with a sharp point. 2. In anatomy, a fibrous band that helps to hold a part in its proper position and place.—tenacula, pl.

tenalgia (te-nal'ji-a): Pain in a tendon.

tenderness: Unusual sensitivity to touch or pressure. **REBOUND T.**, a condition in which pain is felt when pressure over a part is released.

tendinitis (ten-din-ī'tis): Inflammation of tendons and of the tendon-muscle attachments. **BICIPITAL T.**, swelling and enlargement of the biceps muscle sheath, causing discomfort in the upper anterior area of the tendon of the biceps muscle; caused by repetitive movements that put stress on the tendon. Also tendonitis; tenontitis.

tendinoplasty (ten'di-nō-plas-ti): Plastic surgery on a tendon. Also tendoplasty.

tendinous (ten'din-us): Pertaining to, resembling, or composed of tendon.

tendon (ten'don): A band or cord of firm, white, inelastic, fibrous connective tissue that forms the termination of a muscle and attaches it to a bone or other structure. **T. OF ACHILLES**, the **T.** that attaches the gastrocnemius and the soleus muscles to the heel bone; see also **Achilles**. **KANGAROO T.**, **T.** from the tail of a kangaroo; used for sutures when delay of absorption of sutures is desired, as in orthopedic surgery. **T. REFLEX**, see under **reflex**. Syn., sinew.—tendinous, adj.

tendovaginitis (ten-dō-vaj-i-nī'tis): See **tenosynovitis**.

tenectomy (te-nek'to-mi): Excision of part of a tendon. Also tenonectomy.

tenesmus (te-nez'mus): Painful, ineffectual straining to empty the bowel or bladder.—tenesmic, adj.

tenia (tē'ni-a): 1. An organism of the genus Taenia (*q.v.*). 2. A flat band or strip of soft tissue. **T. COLI**, three flat bands running the length of the large intestine and consisting of longitudinal muscle fibers; they pucker the walls of the colon to form pouches (haustra).

teniacide (tē'ni-a-sīd): An agent that destroys tapeworms.—teniacidal, adj.

teniaform (tē'ni-a-form): 1. Shaped like a band or ribbon. 2. Shaped like a tapeworm.

teniafuge (tē'ni-a-fūj): An agent that causes expulsion of tapeworms from the intestine.

teniasis (tē-nī'a-sis): Infestation with Taenia (*q.v.*). Also Taeniasis.

tennis elbow: Pain and tenderness at the outer side of the elbow due to injury of the lateral epicondyle of the humerus and resulting from violent twisting of the hand as often occurs in playing tennis. Epicondylitis.

tennis leg: Severe burning pain in the popliteal area or calf; due to rupture or partial rupture of any of the muscles of the leg or popliteus; usually an athletic injury.

teno-: Combining form denoting tendon.

tenodesis (te-nod'e-sis): The fixation of a tendon, as to a bone, or the transferring of a tendon to a new point of attachment.

tenodynia (ten'ō-din'i-a): Pain in a tendon. Tenalgia.

tenomyoplasty (ten-ō-mī'ō-plas-ti): Plastic surgery on a tendon and a muscle.

tenonitis (ten-o-nī'tis): 1. Inflammation of Tenon's capsule (*q.v.*). 2. Inflammation of a tendon.

tenonometer (ten-o-nom'e-ter): An instrument for measuring the amount of pressure exerted by the substances within the eyeball. Also tonometer.

Tenon's capsule: The thin membrane that envelopes the eyeball from the optic nerve to the ciliary region and which forms a capsule or socket within which the eyeball moves. [Jacques R. Tenon, French anatomist and oculist. 1724–1816.]

tenoplasty (ten′ō-plas-ti): A plastic operation on a tendon.—tenoplastic, adj.

tenorrhaphy (te-nor′a-fi): Suturing together the cut or torn ends of a tendon.

tenositis (ten-ō-sī′tis): Inflammation of a tendon.

tenostosis (ten-os-tō′sis): Ossification of a tendon.

tenosuspension (ten′ō-sus-pen′shun): The surgical procedure of suturing, with tendon, the head of the humerus to the acromian for treatment of recurrent dislocation of the shoulder.

tenosynovectomy (ten′ō-sin-ō-vek′tō-mi): The surgical removal of a tendon sheath.

tenosynovitis (ten′-ō-sin-ō-vī′tis): Inflammation of a tendon sheath; may be caused by irritation or by bacterial infection. **DEQUERVAIN'S T.**, see DeQuervain's disease.

tenotomy (ten-ot′-ō-mi): Division or cutting of a tendon; usually done to correct a deformity caused by a too short muscle, *e.g.*, as occurs in strabismus.

tenovaginitis (ten′ō-vaj-i-nī′tis): Mild chronic inflammation or thickening of a tendon sheath; most often affects tendons of the finger, thumb, or wrist; cause unknown.

tense: Tight; strained.

tension: 1. The act of stretching. 2. The state of being stretched. 3. In psychology, a condition of inner unrest, striving or turmoil with a feeling of psychological stress, often manifested in increased muscular tone and other physiological signs of emotional imbalance. **ARTERIAL T.**, that exerted by the blood on the arterial walls. **INTRAOCULAR T.**, that exerted by the contents of the eyeball on the tunics of the eye. **PREMENSTRUAL T.**, see premenstrual syndrome. **SURFACE T.**, the force that exists between two substances that do not mix; due to differences in molecular attraction. **T. PNEUMOTHORAX**, see under pneumothorax.

tensor: Any muscle that stretches or causes tension in a part.

tent: 1. A conical cylinder of sponge, cotton, or similar material to be introduced into a canal or sinus to dilate it or keep it open. 2. A canopy of material arranged like a tent over a bed or part of a bed. **CROUP T.**, a canopy arranged over the head of the bed in such a way as to maintain a high degree of moisture within it; used in treatment of croup. **FACE** or **HOOD T.**, fits over the head, ties under the chin; used chiefly for providing high humidity for children on oxygen therapy. **ISOLATION T.**, a **T.** placed over a patient's bed as a means of achieving reverse isolation; see under isolation. **HUMIDITY T.**, a covering that may enclose the entire body or just the head; serves to prevent dispersal of mist created to assist in the delivery of oxygen to the terminal alveoli. **OXYGEN T.**, a covering arranged over the bed or the head of it so as to maintain a high degree of oxygen when this is used in therapy.

tentacle (ten′ta-c'l): A slender process on an invertebrate, for prehension or locomotion; may also function as a sense organ.

tentiginous (ten-tij′i-nus): Lascivious; insanely lustful.

tentigo (ten-tī′gō): Lust.

tentorial (ten-tō′ri-al): Pertaining to the tentorium of the cerebrum. **T. HERNIATION**, the herniation of the uncus and other surrounding structures into the tentorium; caused by excess pressure from above as occurs in severe cerebral edema.

tentorium (ten-tō′ri-um): An anatomical part that resembles a tent in shape. **T. CEREBELLI**, that part of the dura mater that forms a partition between the cerebellum and the cerebrum; it covers the cerebellum and supports the occipital lobes.—tentorial, adj.

tephromalacia (tef′rō-ma-lā′shi-a): Softening of the gray matter of either or both the brain and spinal cord.

tepid (tep′id): Lukewarm.

ter-: Combining form denoting three, threefold, three times.

teras (ter′as): A monster; a fetus with grossly malformed parts.—terata, pl.

terat-, terato-: Combining forms denoting a teras (monster).

teratic (ter-at′ik): Pertaining to a teras (*q.v.*).

teratism (ter′a-tizm): The congenital anomaly of being a teras (monster).

teratoblastoma (ter′a-tō-blas-tō′ma): See teratoma.

teratocarcinoma (ter′a-tō-kar-si-nō′ma): 1. A malignant tumor most often occurring in the testis. 2. A malignant epithelioma (*q.v.*) arising in a teratoma (*q.v.*).

teratogen (ter′a-tō-jen): Anything capable of disrupting normal fetal growth and producing malformation, *e.g.*, drugs, poisons, radiation, physical agents such as electroconvulsive shock, infections.—teratogenic, adj.; teratogenicity, teratogenesis, n.

teratogenesis (ter′a-tō-jen′e-sis): Embryonic development leading to gross physical abnormalities; may be the result of the mother's ingestion of chemicals or biologicals, of radiation or of infection during pregnancy.

teratology (ter-a-tol′o-ji): The scientific study of monstrosities, malformations, and other deviations from normal development.—teratologist, n.; teratological, adj.; teratologically, adv.

teratoma (ter-a-tō′ma): A tumor of embryonic origin, composed of various kinds of tissues, including epithelial and connective, none of which are native to the part where the tumor occurs; most commonly found in the ovaries where it is usually benign, and in the testes where it is usually malignant.—teratomata, pl., teratomatous, adj.

teratophobia (ter'a-tō-fō'bi-a): Abnormal fear of 1) deformed people, or 2) of giving birth to a deformed infant.

terebrachesis (ter' -e-brā-kē'sis): The surgical procedure of shortening the round ligament of the uterus.

teres (tē'rēz): Round, smooth and long; usually denotes certain muscles and ligaments.

tergal (ter'gal): Relating to the back.

tergum (ter'gum): The back.

term: In obstetrics, refers to an infant born any time between the thirty-eighth week and the end of the forty-first week of gestation. Also spoken of as full term. See preterm; postterm.

terminad (ter'mi-nad): Toward a terminus.

terminal (ter'min-al): 1. Situated at or forming an end or extremity. 2. Related to the end, as the **T.** stage of a disease. **T. CARE,** care given to the dying patient. **T. DISINFECTION,** that which is done following a patient's illness, discharge from the hospital, or death; involves disinfecting any substance or object that has been used by the patient or been in contact with him. **T. ILLNESS,** one from which the patient is not expected to recover. **T. INFECTION,** infection with a pathogenic organism that occurs during the course of a chronic disease and causes death.

terminology (ter-mi-nol'o-ji): The particular words or expressions used in a special field of endeavor or science.

ternary (ter'na-ri): Denoting a compound containing three elements or three radicals.

terror (ter'er): Excessive fear; fright. **NIGHT T.,** that which occurs in sleep, especially in children; nightmare.

tertian (ter'shun): Occurring every third day, inclusive. See malaria.

tertiary (ter'shi-ar-i): 1. Third in order. 2. Recurring every third day. 3. Pertinent to a third stage or order; often refers to the third stage of syphilis. **T. HEALTH CARE,** includes services of specialists for serious long-term conditions and for treating complications of illnesses; often provided at regional medical centers. **T. HEALTH CARE SYSTEM,** refers to the context in which care is given, usually large hospitals where critical, coronary, intensive, neonatal, and oncological care are given; the hospitals are often associated with universities and also engage in research and experimental work.

tertigravida (ter-ti-grav'ida): A woman who is pregnant for the third time.

tertipara (ter-tip'a-ra): A woman who has had three pregnancies resulting in viable offspring.—tertiparous, adj.

test: 1. A means of examination. 2. A procedure done to determine the presence or absence of a substance. 3. To analyze a substance by the use of chemical reagents. 4. A trial. **T. MEAL,** one given for later removal from the stomach for gastric analysis.

test tube: A slender tube of thin glass, closed at one end; has many uses in scientific laboratories. **TEST TUBE BABY,** one that results from impregnation of the mother by artifical insemination. See insemination.

test type: Letters of various sizes on cards used in testing visual acuity. **SNELLEN'S T.T.,** square black letters on cards, commonly used for testing distance vision.

testalgia (tes-tal'ji-a): Pain in the testes.

testectomy (tes-tek'to-mi): Removal of a testis. Also orchidectomy.

testicle (tes'ti-k'l): Testis.—testicular, adj.

testis (tes'tis): One of two glandular bodies contained in the scrotum of the male; they produce spermatozoa and also the male sex hormones. **UNDESCENDED T.,** refers to the condition existing when a testis remains in the pelvis or inguinal canal; cryptorchism (*q.v.*).—testes, pl.; testicular, adj.

testitis (tes-tī'tis): Inflammation of the testes; orchitis.

testopathy (tes-top'a-thi): Any disease of the testes.

testosterone (tes-tos'te-rōn): 1. The hormone derived from the testes and responsible for the development of the secondary male characteristics. 2. A synthetic product prepared from cholesterol and used in treating carcinoma of the breast, to control uterine bleeding, and in male underdevelopment.

tetanic (te-tan'ik): 1. Characterized by or relating to tetanus. 2. Producing tonic muscle spasm. 3. An agent that produces tonic muscle spasm.

tetaniform (te-tan'i-form): Resembling tetany or tetanus.

tetanigenous (tet'a-nij'e-nus): Tending to produce tetanus or tetanic spasms.

tetanize (tet'a-nīz): To produce tetany or tetanic muscle spasms.

tetanode (tet'a-nōd): The period of quiet between the tonic spasms of tetany.

tetanoid (tet'a-noyd): Resembling the muscle spasms of tetanus.

tetanometer (tet-a-nom'e-ter): An instrument for measuring the force of tonic muscle spasms.

tetanospasmin (tet'a-nō-spaz'min): The potent exotoxin produced by the form of *Clostridium tetani* that causes tetanus and is responsible for the principle symptoms of that disease.

tetanus (tet'an-us): 1. Lockjaw. An acute infectious disease induced by the toxin of *Clostri-*

dium tetani, an anaerobic organism growing at the site of injury to body tissues; because the organism is present sometimes in road dust, manure, and cultivated soil, accidental wounds, particularly penetrating wounds, may become infected by it. **T.** is characterized by painful muscular contractions, chiefly of the face and neck, hence the appellation "lockjaw." Muscles of the back may become involved and result in opisthotonos (*q.v.*). 2. Sustained tonic spasm of a muscle or muscles, produced by repetition of stimuli so often that the muscle does not have a chance to relax between their application. **CEPHALIC T.**, occurs following a head injury involving the facial, trigeninal, oculomoter, or hypoglossal nerve or all of them; spreads rapidly and seizures develop. **DRUG T.**, **T.** that is produced by a drug such as strychnine. **PUERPERAL** or **POSTPARTAL T.**, **T.** that develops from infection of the obstetrical wound.

tetanus antitoxin: Antibody to tetanus toxin, prepared from the serum of horses that have been hyperimmunized against the exotoxin of *Clostridium tetani;* produces passive immunity; used in prevention and treatment of wounds that may have become contaminated with the organism. Abbreviated TAT.

tetanus immune globulin: Used for short term immunization when one may have been exposed to the causative organism of tetanus; prepared from the globulin of an immune person.

tetanus toxoid: Detoxified tetanus toxin; used to produce active immunity against tetanus in well individuals and those who may be at risk of developing tetanus following a dirty wound. Given by repeated subcutaneous doses. Is one of three components of triple vaccine, along with diphtheria toxoid and pertussis vaccine, given routinely to infants.

tetany (tet'a-ni): 1. A condition of muscular hyperexcitability, due to abnormal calcium metabolism, in which mild stimuli produce cramps and spasms (carpopedal spasm). Seen in parathyroid deficiency, potassium deficiency, vitamin D deficiency, alkalosis, sprue. In infants it is associated with gastrointestinal upset and rickets. 2. Tetanus; see definition 2 under **tetanus**.

tetartanopia (tet'ar-ta-nō'pi-a): 1. Loss of vision in the corresponding quandrant in each field of vision. Also tetartanopsia. 2. A rare type of blue-yellow color blindness.

tetr-, tetra-: Combining forms denoting four or having four parts.

tetra-amelia (tet'ra-a-mē'li-a): Absence of both upper and lower extremities.

tetrabrachius (tet'ra-brā'ki-us): A malformed fetus or individual with four arms.

tetrachirus (tet-ra-kī'rus): A malformed fetus or individual having four hands.

tetrachloroethylene (tet'ra-klor-ō-eth'-i-lēn): A clear colorless liquid chemical used as an anthelmintic for hookworm.

tetrachromic (tet-ra-krō'mik): Pertaining to vision that is normal for four colors.

tetrad (tet'rad): A group of four.

tetradactyly (tet-ra-dak'ti-li): The condition of having only four digits on a hand or foot.—tetradactylous, adj.

tetrahydrocannabinol (tet'ra-hī'drō-ka-nab'i-nol): The active ingredient in marijuana; has sedative and hallucinogenic effects. Abbreviated THC.

tetralogy of Fallot: A form of congenital heart defect which includes four abnormalities—narrowing of the pulmonary artery, a septal defect between the ventricles, hypertrophy of the right ventricle, and displacement of the aorta to the right. The condition results in deficient oxygenation of the blood with cyanosis, dyspnea, polycythemia, clubbing of the fingers. [Etienne Louis Arthur Fallot, French physician. 1850–1911.]

tetramastia (tet-ra-mas'ti-a): The condition of having four breasts.—tetramastous, adj.

tetramelia (tet-ra-mē'li-a): Congenital absence of all four extremities. See **amelia**.

tetrapeptide (tet-ra-pep'tid): A polypeptide composed of four amino acid groups.

tetraphocomelia (tet'ra-fō-kō-mē'li-a): Phocomelia affecting all four extremities; see **phocomelia**.

tetraplegia (tet-ra-plē'ji-a): Paralysis of all four limbs. Quadriplegia.

tetrapus (tet'ra-pus): A fetal monster having four feet.

tetrascelus (tet-ras'e-lus): A fetal monster having four legs.

tetravaccine (tet-ra-vak'sēn): A vaccine containing dead cultures of the organisms causing typhoid, paratyphoid A, paratyphoid B and cholera.

tetravalent (tet-ra-vā'lent): Having a valence of four.

tetter (tet'er): A lay term often used for such skin diseases as eczema, herpes, ringworm, or other eruptions, or for a blister or pimple.

texiform (teks'i-form): Web-like; forming a mesh.

texis (tek'sis): Childbirth or childbearing.

textus (teks'tus): A tissue.

thalamectomy (thal-a-mek'tō-mi): Destruction of part of the thalamus by a chemical agent or by surgery.

thalamic (thal'a-mik): Pertaining to the thalamus. **T. SYNDROME**, a condition characterized by mild hemiplegia and hemitaxia, pain with choreoathetoid movements of the affected side, and astereognosis; due to a lesion in the lateral part of the thalamus; is aggravated by fatigue, stress, and emotional disturbances.

thalamo-: Combining form denoting thalamus.

thalamotomy (thal-a-mot'o-mi): Usually operative (stereotaxic) destruction of a portion of the thalamus, sometimes done in treatment of psychotic disorders that have an emotional basis, or for relief of intractable pain.

thalamus (thal'a-mus): A collection of gray matter at the base of the cerebrum. Sensory impulses from the whole body (except olfactory) pass through on their way to the cerebral cortex.—thalami, pl.; thalamic, adj.

thalassemia (thal-a-sē'mi-a): An ethnic, hereditary, genetically transmitted hemolytic anemia in which there is interference with synthesis of hemoglobin; several types are recognized, according to the symptoms. There is no known cure; treatment consists of regular blood transfusions. Most victims are children of Greek or Italian descent; death usually occurs before the age of 25. The disease is marked by severe anemia, headache, anorexia, darkened skin, enlargement of the liver, spleen, and bones. Also called Cooley's anemia, Mediterranean anemia, familial erythroblastic anemia. **BETA ZERO T.**, a type of **T.** characterized by defective structure of hemoglobin causing it to be fragile and break down easily; results in bone and heart problems and usually death in midlife. [Name derived from the Greek word *thalassa,* meaning *sea;* the disease was first described in people in the Mediterranean Sea area.]

thalassophobia (thal'a-sō-fō'bi-a): Morbid fear of the sea.

thalassotherapy (thal'a-sō-ther'a-pi): The treatment of diseases by sea bathing or sea air.

thalidomide (tha-lid'o-mīd): A drug formerly used as a sleeping tablet and sedative; was the cause of several types of birth defects, primarily limb malformations, in infants born to mothers who took the drug during early pregnancy; it is no longer sold.

thallitoxicosis (thal'i-toks-i-kō'sis): Poisoning by thallium (*q.v.*).

thallium (thal'i-um): A bluish-white lustrous metallic element, the salts of which are poisonous, *e.g.,* **T. SULFATE**, is an ingredient of rat poisons. Chemical symbol, Tl.

thamuria (tha-mū'ri-a): Too frequent urination.

thanat-, thanato-: Combining forms denoting death.

thanatognomonic (than'a-tō-nō-mon'ik): Indicating the approach of death; having a fatal prognosis.

thanatologist (than'a-tol'ō-jist): One who specializes in the study of the various aspects of death and dying.

thanatology (than'a-tol'o-ji): The study of the phenomenon of physical death.

thanatophoric (than'a-tō-for'ik): Lethal; causing death.

thanatopsia (than'a-top'si-a): Examination of the body after death; autopsy. Also thanatopsy.

thanatos (than'a-tōs): In psychoanalysis, the death instinct.

Thayer-Martin medium: A culture medium consisting of several antibiotics which will isolate and promote the growth of meningitides and *Neiserria gonorrhoea;* used in screening tests for asymptomatic gonorrhea.

theaism (thē'a-izm): A toxic state caused by excessive tea drinking.

The Basic Four: A nutrition guide that classifies the foods needed to provide an adequate diet into four basic groups: the milk group, the meat group, the vegetable-fruit group, and the bread-cereal group.

thebesian (thē-bē'zi-an): **T. VEINS**, the smallest of the coronary veins; they open into the cavities of the heart.

theca (thē'-ka): An enclosing or covering sac, capsule, or membrane, or the sheath of a tendon. **T. FOLLICULI**, the external connective tissue wall of an ovarian follicle; consisting of an external fibrous layer, the theca externa, and an internal vascular layer, the theca interna; it produces estrogen and contributes to the formation of corpus luteum. **T. VERTEBRALIS**, the dura mater of the spinal cord.—thecal, adj.

thecal (thē'kal): Pertaining to a capsule or sheath, often to a tendon sheath.

thecitis (thē-sī'tis): Inflammation of the sheath of a tendon.

thecoma (thē-kō'ma): A benign ovarian tumor. Also called thelioma.

theine (thē'in): Caffeine.

thelalgia (thē-lal'ji-a): Pain in the nipple.

thelarche (thē-lar'ke): The beginning of breast development at puberty; may occur precociously in girls as young as eight years.

thele (thē'lē): The nipple.

theleplasty (thē'lē-plas-ti): Plastic surgery on the nipple.

thelerethism (thē-ler'e-thizm): Erection of the nipple.

thelitis (thē-lī'tis): Inflammation of a nipple.

thelium (thē'li-um): 1. Nipple. 2. A papilla.

theloncus (thē-longk'us): Tumor of a nipple.

thelorrhagia (thē-lō-rā'ji-a): Hemorrhage from a nipple.

thematic apperception test: A test used in psychiatry. The patient is asked to interpret a series of drawings that depict life scenes and situations and the interpretations given are thought to be indicative of the patient's moods and personality.

thenad (thē′nad): Toward the thenar eminence or toward the palm of the hand.

thenal (thē′nal): Pertaining to the palm of the hand or to the thenar eminence.

thenar (thē′nar): 1. Pertinent to the palm of the hand or the thumb. 2. The fleshy mound at the base of the thumb, called the thenar eminence.

theobroma oil: A yellowish-white solid obtained from the roasted seeds of the *Theobroma cacao* tree; contains the glycerides of oleic, palmitic, stearic, and lauric acids; used in preparation of emollients, ointments, and suppositories. Syn., cocoa butter.

theobromin (thē-ō-brō′-min): An alkaloid derived from the seeds of the *Theobroma cacao* tree; has effects similar to those of caffeine; has been used in medicine as a vasodilator, heart stimulant, diuretic, and smooth muscle relaxant.

theomania (thē′ō-mā′ni-a): A type of religious insanity, especially one in which one imagines oneself to be God or to have divine attributes.

theory (thē′ō-ri): A reasoned proposed explanation of an occurrence or something that will occur or will be produced and for which absolute proof is lacking; a theory is conjectural in nature but less speculative than a hypothesis.

theotherapy (thē-ō-ther′a-pi): Treatment of disease by prayer or other religious expression.

therapeutic (ther-a-pū′tik): 1. Pertaining to the treatment of disease. 2. Curative. 3. Descriptive of an agent that has healing or curing properties. **T. ABORTION,** one induced because of poor health of the mother. **T. COMMUNITY,** a specially structured treatment and rehabilitative hospital milieu in which patients with severe behavior problems are encouraged to assume responsibility for their own behavior and to behave in a way that is socially acceptable. **T. DOSE,** the amount of a drug or other therapeutic agent prescribed; usually considered safe. **T. INDEX,** the margin between the maximum tolerated dose of a drug and the minimal curative dose; based on kilograms of body weight. **T. MILIEU, T.** community. **T. RATIO,** the ratio of the minimal dose of a drug to its therapeutic dose; often used to estimate the safety of a drug. **T. TOUCH,** a mode of treatment or a procedure based on an ancient practice, "the laying-on of hands." Modern health care practitioners have added the concept that the body is an energy field that is constantly being influenced by forces outside itself and that body energies can be transferred from the hands of a person who has been trained to assume the role of healer to the body of the person who has some physical or mental disorder or condition that requires change. The procedure is not based on any religious tenet, nor is it performed in a religious context, but the psychological status of both healer and healee are considered fundamental to the outcome of the procedure.

therapeutics (ther-a-pū′tiks): The branch of medical science dealing with the treatment of disease.—therapeutic, adj.; therapeutically, adv.

therapist (ther′a-pist): A person who is trained and skilled in the treatment of a disease or the effects of disease. The word is often used in combination with another that names the disorder being treated or the type of treatment employed, *e.g.,* speech **T.**, physical **T.**

therapy (ther′a-pi): The treatment of disease, or the means used in treating disease. **AEROSOL T.**, see **aerosol. ART T.**, the therapeutic use of any art form to assist individuals who cannot express their feelings verbally. **AVERSION T.**, sometimes used in treatment of alcoholism; a powerful emetic is administered, followed by alcohol; the effect often conditions the person against alcohol. **COGNITIVE T.**, **T.** involving the correction of erroneous beliefs. **COLLATERAL T.**, **T.** carried on with any two persons involved in a crisis, *e.g.,* mother and daughter. **CORRECTIVE T.**, exercises and other medically prescribed activites to help correct physical impairments; administered by a therapist. **CONJOINT T.**, **T.** carried out with couples to help correct maladaptive relationships. **CONVULSIVE T.**, electric shock **T. CRISIS GROUP T.**, **T.** with a group of unrelated and unacquainted people who meet together, usually for about six sessions, and try to solve their individual problems; most of these groups are open-ended and people can enter or leave when they wish. **DANCE T.**, the use of rhythmic body movement to disclose and express feelings and emotional conflicts, usually conducted in groups. **ELECTROLYTE T.**, **T.** to correct electrolyte imbalance in the body; usually connected with intravenous **T. EMPIRIC T.**, that based on practical experience rather than scientific reasoning. **ENDOCRINE T.**, treatment with hormones or glandular secretions. **FAMILY T.**, group psychotherapy with a family or individual therapy applied to all family members simultaneously. **FEVER T.**, treatment of disease by inducing high body temperatures. **GOLD T.**, treatment of rheumatoid arthritis utilizing a solution containing gold given intramuscularly, in increasing doses, until symptoms abate. **GROUP T.**, **T.** given to small groups of people who discuss their feelings and problems openly. **HEAT T.**, **T.** utilizing some form of heat. **IMPLOSIVE T.**, a counter-conditioning **T.** in which a great deal of anxiety is aroused and overcome; see **flooding. INHALATION T.**, the administration of water vapor, gases, anesthetics, and drugs by inhalation. **INSULIN T.**, shock **T**; consists of the injection of insulin in amounts sufficient to produce coma, followed by administration of glucose to restore consciousness; utilized in some psychoses. **INTRAVENOUS T.**, the administration of medications and other substances by infusion into a vein. **MILIEU T.**, psychiatric **T.** in a carefully constructed environment in which all elements enhance the medical **T.** and help the patient toward rehabilitation by developing needed social skills. **MUSIC T.**, consists of participating in brass bands, opera groups, and choirs, as well as passive listening; used primarily in psychiatric patients. **OCCUPATIONAL T.**, the use of some occupation, usually hand crafts, for remedial effects. **OXYGEN T.**, treatment that makes an increased amount of oxygen available to the patient. **PARENTERAL T.**, refers to administration of therapeutic agents by injection or intravenously to maintain nutrition, or to replace water or other essential substances. **PHYSICAL T.**, the use of such physical agents as massage, exercise, etc. in treatment. **PLAY T.**, a method of psychiatric treatment in which the child expresses himself through play and thus enables the psychiatrist to establish communication with him. **REPLACEMENT T.**, used to replace loss of or deficient formation of body products; natural or synthetic substances are administered. **ROENTGEN T.**, treatment by x-ray or other radioactive substances. **SHOCK T.**, use of electric shock or a convulsant drug as a palliative or therapeutic measure in some psychoneurotic and psychotic disorders. **SPEECH T.**, the treatment of speech disorders. **SPECIFIC T.**, that which is directed toward the eradication of the specific cause of a disease. **STEROID T.**, therapy utilizing various steroid hormones especially those secreted by the adrenal cortex; patients on steroids must be closely monitored because of the many possible side effects. **SUBSTITUTION T.**, **T.** that supplies a substance that is deficient or lacking in the body. **SUPPORTIVE T.**, **T.** in which the therapist gives direct help and encouragement. **SYMPTOMATIC T.**, **T.** directed toward relief of symptoms rather than their cause. **WORK T.**, therapeutic use of work, either for or without compensation. **ZONE T.**, treatment by stimulating a body area in the same longitudinal zone as the particular disorder.

therm: An indefinite term for a unit of heat. It may represent a small calorie, a large calorie, 1000 large calories, or 100,000 British thermal units.

therm-, thermo-: Combining forms denoting relationship to heat.

thermacogenesis (ther′ma-kō-jen′e-sis): The elevation of body temperature resulting from drug action.

thermacotherapy (ther′ma-kō-ther′a-pi): Treatment of disease by the application of heat, especially hot air.

thermal (ther′mal): Pertaining to heat. **T. BURNS,** burns caused by hot liquid or flame. **T. DISTURBANCES,** local or systemic reactions to the application or exposure to heat or cold in excessive amounts, as occurs in burns or frostbite.

thermalgesia (therm-al-jē′zi-a): Excessive sensitivity to heat, even heat of a fairly low degree. Also thermoalgesia.

thermalgia (ther-mal′ji-a): Burning pain.

thermelometer (ther′mel-om′e-ter): An electric thermometer.

thermistor (ther′mis-tor): A device for measuring small changes in temperature.

thermoanesthesia (ther′mō-an-es-thē′zi -a): Loss or lack of the ability to recognize the sensations of heat and cold, or to distinguish between them; often due to spinal cord injury. Also thermanesthesia.

thermocauterectomy (ther′mō-kaw-ter-ek′tō-mi): The destruction of tissue by thermocautery.

thermocautery (ther′mō-kaw′ter-i): Cauterization by use of an instrument with a heated wire or point, or the instrument itself.

thermocoagulation (ther′mō-kō-ag′ū-lā-shun): Coagulation of tissue by electrocautery or by the passage of a high-frequency current.

thermodialysis (ther′mō-dī-al′i-sis): A technique utilized in producing hyperthermia therapeutically whereby the patient's blood is shunted through a controlled heat exchange and then returned to the body.

thermoesthesia (ther′mō-es-thē′zi-a): The ability to recognize sensations of heat and cold and to distinguish between them. Also thermesthesia.

thermogenesis (ther′mo-jen′e-sis): The production of heat, specifically in the body.—thermogenetic, adj.

thermogenic (ther-mō-jen′ik): Pertaining to the production of heat. **T. ACTION,** the action of certain foods and drugs that cause an increase in body temperature.

thermogram (ther′mō-gram): A regional surface area map of the body or part of it obtained by an infrared sensing device; it measures the radiant heat from the part and hence blood flow.

thermograph (ther′mō-graf): 1. The device or apparatus used in thermography (*q.v.*). 2. An instrument for recording variations in temperature.

thermography (ther-mog′ra-fi): A photographic technique that utilizes an infrared detector to measure variations in the surface temperature of the body; sometimes used in diagnosing underlying pathology such as tumors. Has also been used to differentiate pain of psychogenic origin from that of organic origin since a painful disorder or injury may cause the temperature of the surrounding tissues to be lower than that in other parts of the body.—thermogram, n.

thermohyperesthesia (ther′mo-hī-per-es-thē′zi-a): The condition of being extremely sensitive to variations in temperature.

thermolabile (ther-mō-lā′ -bil): Subject to being easily altered or destroyed by heat.

thermolysis (ther-mol′i-sis): 1. The loss of body heat through evaporation, radiation, exhaled air, etc. 2. Chemical decomposition of a substance by use of heat.—thermolytic, adj.

thermomammography (ther′mō-mam-og′ra-fi): The use of thermography to examine for lesions of the breast.

thermomassage (ther′mō-mas-sazh′): A physical therapy technique utilizing a combination of heat and massage.

thermometer (ther-mom′e-ter): A device for determining termperature; consists of a substance such as mercury which expands and contracts with changes in temperature and which is enclosed in a sealed tube, usually glass, that is marked with a graduated scale. **BATH T.**, one used for determining temperature of bath water; usually protected by a wooden case. **CELSIUS T.**, centigrade **T. CENTIGRADE T.**, one marked with a 100-unit scale in which 0° is the freezing point and 100° the boiling point; the scale on the clinical Centigrade **T.** is from 34° or 36° to 42°, with increments of 0.02. **CLINICAL T.**, one used for measuring the temperature of the body. **FAHRENHEIT T.**, one marked with a 180-unit scale in which the freezing point is 32° and the boiling point is 212°; the scale on the clinical Fahrenheit **T.** is from 94° or 95° to 108° or 110°, with increments of 0.2. **FEVER T.**, a clinical **T. ORAL T.**, one used for taking temperature of the body by mouth. **RECTAL T.**, one used for taking temperature of the body by rectum. **ROOM T.**, one used for determining the temperature of the air in a room.

thermoneurosis (ther′ -mō-nū-rō′sis): Elevation of body temperature caused by vasomotor reactions to emotional influences.

thermonuclear (ther′mō-nū′klē-ar): Pertinent to or involving the nuclear fusion reaction that takes place between the molecules of a gas, hydrogen in particular, with the accompanying liberation of energy, when heated to temperatures of several million degrees.

thermophile (ther′mō-fīl): A microorganism that thrives best at a relatively high temperature.—thermophilic, adj.

thermoplegia (ther′mō-plē′ji-a): Sunstroke; heat stroke.

thermopolypnea (ther′mō-pol-ip-nē′a): Rapid respirations caused by exposure to excessive heat or fever.

thermoreceptor (ther′mō-rē-sep′tor): A nerve ending that is sensitive to heat.

thermoregulation (ther′mō-reg-ū-lā′shun): In physiology, the regulation of body temperature by an interrelated system consisting of the hypothalamus, the autonomic nervous system, and the cardiovascular system, which regulate the amount of heat produced or the amount lost, or both.—thermoregulatory, adj.

thermoresistant (ther′mō-rē-zis′tant): The quality of not being greatly affected by heat.

thermostable (ther′mō-stā′b′l): Remaining unaltered at a high temperature, which is usually specified.—thermostability, n.

thermostat (ther′mō-stat): A device that automatically regulates the temperature of a substance or area.

thermosterilization (ther′mō-ster-i-lī-zā′shun): Sterilization by the use of heat.

thermotaxis (ther-mō-tak′sis): 1. The normal regulation of the body temperature. 2. The reaction that occurs in an organism when stimulated by heat.

thermotherapy (ther′mō-ther′a-pi): Treatment of disease by the application of any form of heat including hot water, hot water bottle, hot wet pack, electric heating pad, infrared radiation, and diathermy. Body temperature may also be raised by artifical means such as induced fever, and decreased by induced hypothermia.

theta wave: See under **wave**.

thiamin(e) (thi′a-mēn): Vitamin B_1 (aneurine hydrochloride), a member of the vitamin B complex; essential for metabolism of carbohydrates and fats, and for normal growth and healthy appetite; found in whole grain cereals and flour, wheat germ, nuts, yeast, liver, lean pork, heart, kidney, milk, egg yolk, legumes, leafy vegetables, fruit; also produced synthetically; is slowly destroyed by heating. Deficiency may result in retardation of growth, loss of appetite, fatigue, mental apathy, impaired functioning of the nervous, digestive, muscular, circulatory, and endocrine systems, and, if severe and long-lasting, beriberi.

thiazides (thī′a-zīds): A group of chemical compounds that promote the formation and excretion of urine; often used in treatment of hypertension and edema; they tend to disturb the electrolyte balance in the body by increasing the excretion of sodium and potassium.

thigh (thī): The part of the leg between the hip and the knee. **T. BONE,** the femur.

thigh-lacer (thī′lā-ser): A device used to permit early ambulation following fixation of fracture of the femur. **THIGH-LACER CUFF,** a device attached to a prosthesis that fits over the stump of a below-the-knee amputation.

thigmesthesia (thig′mes-thē′zi-a): Having sensitivity to touch.

thio-: Combining form denoting the presence of sulfur. Usually refers to the replacement of the oxygen in a compound by sulfur.

thionine (thī′ō-nin): A dark green powder that gives a purple color in solution; used as a stain in microscopic studies.

third: THIRD DEGREE BURN, see under burn. THIRD DEGREE HEART BLOCK, see under block. THIRD HEART SOUND, a sound heard at the end of rapid filling of the ventricles; also called ventricular filling sound. THIRD INTENTION, see under healing. THIRD NERVE PALSY, palsy of the oculomotor nerve which affects certain extrinsic and intrinsic muscles of the eye.

third-party payment: Full or partial payment for health care services by private insurance companies or organizations such as Blue Cross/ Blue Shield or Medicare and Medicaid, on behalf of the individual consumer, with reimbursement usually based on costs rather than negotiated rates. Most third-party payees pay only for services that are illness-related; prevention and health promotion services are not covered.

Third space syndrome: A condition marked by dehydration; due to a deficit of extracellular fluid, although the total body fluid remains normal; caused by the pooling of fluid in the abdomen in patients with ascites, in the tissues in cases of cellulitis, in blood vessels that are occluded, or in the intestine when there is an obstruction.

thirst: A sensation of dryness in the mouth and throat, accompanied by a desire for drink.

thobbing (thob'ing): Emotional thinking. Term coined from *th*inking, *o*pining, *b*elieving.

Thomas: THOMAS COLLAR, a stiff high collar, usually made of metal and covered with leather, used as a support for the head in injuries of the neck and upper spine. THOMAS SPLINT, a metal splint used for emergency treatment or transporting a patient with a fractured leg or arm; it is shaped like a hairpin, the open end being equipped with a padded ring that is placed in the groin or axilla when the splint is applied; it is so constructed that traction can be applied to the limb. [H.O. Thomas, Scottish orthopedic surgeon. 1834–1891.]

Thomsen's disease: Myotonia congenita (*q.v.*).

Thomson's sign: In scarlet fever, the appearance of pinkish or red lines across the inner side of the bend of the elbow before the rash has erupted; they persist throughout the course of the disease and, after desquamation, appear as pigmented lines. Also called Pastia's lines.

thorac-, thoraci-, thoraco-: Combining forms denoting chest or chest wall.

thoracectomy (thō-ra-sek'to-mi): Resection of all or part of a rib through an incision in the chest wall.

thoracentesis (thō'ra-sen-tē'sis): Surgical puncture of the chest wall, usually with a large-bore needle, for the drainage of accumulated fluid; paracentesis. Also thoracocentesis.

thoracic (thō-ras'ik): Pertaining to the thorax. T. BREATHING, breathing in which the chest movements predominate; occurs in patients with certain gastric or abdominal conditions and those with paralysis. T. CAGE, the bony framework that encloses the chest. T. CAVITY, the space above the diaphragm; occupied by the thoracic artery and duct, the pulmonary veins and artery, vena cava, lungs, bronchi, mediastinum, heart, thymus gland, trachea, esophagus. T. DUCT, the duct that begins on the posterior abdominal wall in the cisterna chyli at the level of the second lumbar vertebra, and continues upward along the bodies of the vertebrae to its termination at the junction of the left subclavian and left internal jugular veins; it drains lymph from the entire part of the body below the diaphragm and the upper left side of the structures above the diaphragm.

thoracic outlet syndrome: A group of painful symptoms including weakness, coldness, and paresthesia in the hand and arm, pain in the chest wall, and discomfort in the shoulder and neck muscles; may be caused by compression of a cervical disk or compression of a brachial plexus and subclavian artery by muscles of the clavicle and first rib.

thoracicoabdominal (thō-ras'-i-kō-ab-dom'in-al): Pertaining to the thorax and abdomen. Also thoracoabdominal.

thoracocyllosis (thō'rak-ō-si-lō'sis): Deformity of the thorax.

thoracodorsal (tho'ra-kō-dor'sal): Pertaining to the thorax and the back.

thoracodynia (thō'-ra-kō-din'i-a): Pain in the chest.

thoracolaparotomy (thō'ra-kō-lap-a-rot'o-mi): A surgical procedure involving the opening of both the thorax and the abdomen.

thoracolumbar (thō-ra-kō-lum'bar): Pertaining to, arising in, or involving the thoracic and lumbar regions. Term often used in reference to the thoracic and lumbar spinal ganglia and their fibers that go to make up the sympathetic part of the autonomic nervous system.

thoracomyodynia (thō'ra-kō-mi-ō-din'-i-a): Pain in the muscles of the chest.

thoracopagus (thō-ra-kop'a-gus): Conjoined twins united at the thoracic or epigastric region.

thoracopathy (thō-rā-kop'a-thi): Any disease of the organs of the thorax.

thoracoplasty (thō'ra-kō-plas-ti): 1. Plastic surgery on the chest. 2. An operation on the thorax in which the ribs are resected to allow the chest wall to collapse and the lung to rest; used in the treatment of pulmonary tuberculosis. Also thoracopneumoplasty.

thoracoschisis (thō-ra-kos'ki-sis): A congenital fissure of the thorax.

thoracoscope (thō-rak'ō-skōp): A lighted instrument that can be inserted into the pleural cavity through a small incision in the chest wall to permit inspection of the pleural surface and treatment under visual control.

thoracostomy (tho-ra-kos′to-mi): The establishment of a surgical opening into the chest cavity to drain off accumulated fluid. **T. TUBE,** one inserted through an opening in the chest wall; may be used in applying suction to the pleural cavity.

thoracotomy (thō-ra-kot′o-mi): Any surgical incision into the chest wall.

thorax (thō′raks): The chest cavity; that part of the trunk situated below the neck and above the diaphragm, and within a bony framework formed by the sternum, ribs and thoracic vertebrae. Contains the trachea, bronchi, lungs, heart and esophagus.—thoracic, adj.; thoraces, pl.

thorium (thō′ri-um): A radioactive metallic element. Various compounds of **T.** are used in medicine. Chemical symbol, Th.

Thorkildsen's procedure or shunt: See ventriculocisternostomy.

thought transference: Mental telepathy.

threadworm: Enterobius (Oxyuris) vermicularis, a nematode parasite in the colon of children. Pinworm.

thready: Describes a pulse that can barely be felt.

three-day measles: See rubella.

threonine (thrē′ō-nin): A naturally occurring amino acid essential to human nutrition; found in most proteins.

threpsology (threp-sol′o-ji): The science of nutrition.

threshold (thresh′old): The lowest point at which a stimulus will evoke a response. **PAIN T.,** the strength or amount of stimulus required to produce a sensation of pain or discomfort. **RENAL T.,** the plasma level of a substance at which it begins to be excreted in the urine. **T. DOSE,** the minimum dose that will produce a detectable response. **T. STIMULUS,** see stimulus.

thrill: A fine vibration felt by the examiner on palpation over incompetent heart valves or an aneurysm.

thrix: Hair.

-thrix: Combining form denoting hair(s).

throat: The pharynx and fauces; the anterior part of the neck. **SEPTIC SORE T.,** severe inflammation of the fauces and tonsils, usually caused by a streptococcal organism.

throb: 1. To beat or pulsate. 2. A beating or pulsation.

throe (thrō): A severe pain or pang, by custom referring to the pains of childbirth.

thromb-, thrombo-: Combining forms denoting 1) a blood clot; 2) the clotting of blood.

thrombasthenia (throm′bas-thē′ni-a): A rare hereditary platelet abnormality characterized by large platelets, prolonged bleeding time, defective clot formation, epistaxis, easy bruising, and excessive bleeding during or following surgery or other trauma. Also called thromboasthenia and Glanzmann's disease.

thrombaxane (throm-bak-sān′): Any of a number of chemical substances synthesized from arachidonic acid that appear to be related to prostaglandins (*q.v.*), and have the effect of causing platelets to clump and arteries to constrict.

thrombectomy (throm-bek′to-mi): Surgical removal of a thrombus from within a blood vessel.

thrombin (throm′bin): An enzyme in shed blood that converts fibrinogen to fibrin; formed when prothrombin combines with calcium salts. Also called thrombase.

thrombinogen (throm-bin′ō-jen): Prothrombin (*q.v.*).

thromboangiitis (throm′bō-an-ji-ī′tis): Inflammation of the inner coat of a blood vessel with formation of a clot. **T. OBLITERANS** (syn., Beurger's disease), an uncommon disorder of unknown cause, occurring mainly in young adult males, characterized by patchy, inflammatory, obliterative, vascular disease, principally in the limbs (sometimes in the cardiac or cerebral vessels), and presenting usually as calf pains, or more severely as early gangrene of the toes and following a chronic progressive course.

thromboarteritis (throm′bō-ar-ter-ī′tis): Inflammation of an artery with clot formation.

thromboblast (throm′bō-blast): A precursor of the thrombocyte; a giant megalocyte.

thromboclasis (throm-bok′la-sis): Thrombolysis (*q.v.*).

thrombocyte (throm′bō-sīt): Blood platelet; small non-nucleated disk-like body normally present in the blood in concentrations of approximately 300,000 per cu mm; its chief function is to assist in coagulation of the blood.

thrombocythemia (throm′bō-sī-thē′mi-a): An increase in the normal number of circulating blood platelets; thrombocytosis.

thrombocytolysis (throm′bō-sī-tol′i-sis): Destruction of blood platelets.

thrombocytopathy (throm′bō-sī-top′a-thi): Refers to any disorder of the clotting mechanism that is caused by dysfunction of the blood platelets.

thrombocytopenia (throm′bō-sī-tō-pē′ni-a): A reduction in the number of platelets in the circulating blood. **ACUTE IMMUNE T.,** may be caused by certain drugs, viruses, or bacteria. **CHRONIC IMMUNE T.,** may be associated with such immune disorders as Hodgkins disease or lupus erythematosus. **ESSENTIAL T.,** idiopathic thrombocytopenic purpura; see under purpura.

thrombocytosis (throm′bō-sī-tō′sis): An increase in the number of blood platelets.

thromboembolectomy (throm'bō-em-bō-lek'tō-mi): The surgical removal of an embolus of thrombic origin or of part of a thrombus.

thromboembolia (throm'bō-em-bō'li-a): Thromboembolism.

thromboembolism (throm'bō-em'bō-lizm): Obstruction of a blood vessel by a thrombus that has become detached from the site where it was formed and carried to another vessel which it blocks.—thromboembolic, adj.; thromboemboli, pl.

thromboendarterectomy (throm'bō-end-ar-ter -ek'to-mi): Operation for removal of a thrombus that is obstructing an artery.

thromboendarteritis (throm'bō-end-ar-ter-ī'tis): Inflammation of the inner lining of an artery with clot formation.

thrombogen (throm'bo-jen): Prothrombin (*q.v.*).

thrombogenesis (throm'bō-jen'e-sis): The formation of a blood clot.

thrombogenic (throm'bō-jen'ik): 1. Producing or capable of producing thrombi. 2. Capable of clotting blood. 3. Pertaining to thrombogen.—thrombogenicity, n.; thrombogenetic, adj.; thrombogenetically, adv.

thromboid (throm'boyd): Pertaining to or resembling a thrombus.

thrombokinase (throm'bō-kī'nas): Thromboplastin (*q.v.*).

thrombolymphangitis (throm' -bō-lim-fan-jī'tis): Inflammation of a lymph vessel associated with the formation of a lymph clot.

thrombolysis (throm-bol'i-sis): The dissolving of a thrombus.—thrombolytic, adj.

thrombopathy (throm-bop'a-thi): Any disorder of the blood platelets that results in defective thromboplastin formation. Most often seen in kidney disease but also occurs in liver disease, and may be idiopathic.

thrombopenia (throm-bō-pē'ni-a): Thrombocytopenia (*q.v.*).

thrombophilia (throm-bō-fil'i-a): A tendency for thrombi to occur.

thrombophlebitis (throm'bō-flē-bī'tis): Inflammation of the wall of a vein with formation of a clot in the involved segment; sometimes caused by trauma to the vein as by an intravenous needle; may result in embolism. **T. MIGRANS,** a form of recurring **T.** affecting principally the superficial veins; may occur at several sites at the same time or at intervals.

thromboplastin (throm'bō-plas'tin): A group of lipid and protein substances found in tissues, blood platelets and leukocytes, and which have an enzyme-like action in the conversion of prothrombin to thrombin in the clotting of blood.

thromboplastinogen (throm'bō-plas-tin'ō-jen): Factor VIII. See under factor.

thromboplastinogenase (throm'bō-plas-tin'o -je-nās): An enzyme in the blood that acts as a catalyst in the conversion of inactive thromboplastinogen to thromboplastin.

thromboplastinogenemia (throm'bō-plas-tin'ō-je-nē'mi-a): The presence of thromboplastinogen in the blood.

thrombopoiesis (throm-bō-poy-ē'sis): The formation of thrombocytes.

thrombosed (throm'bōs'd): 1. Clotted. 2. Describing a blood vessel that contains a clot.

thrombosis (throm-bō'sis): The intravascular formation or presence of a clot, or other deposit that blocks an artery. **CEREBRAL T., T.** occurring in a cerebral vessel; may result in cerebral infarction. **CORONARY T., T.** occurring in a coronary artery and occluding it, thereby depriving the coronary muscle it serves of blood and usually leading to ischemia and infarction of the myocardium. **MARASMIC T., T.** that occurs usually in the longitudinal sinus of infants suffering a wasting disease; may also occur in the elderly. **MESENTERIC T., T.** occurring in a blood vessel of the mesentery. **PUERPERAL T., T.** occurring in a uterine vessel following childbirth. **TRAUMATIC T., T.,** that occurs following injury to a part. **VENOUS T., T.** occurring in a vein.—thrombotic, adj.

thrombostasis (throm-bos'ta-sis): Stasis of blood in a vessel leading to, or resulting from, the formation of a thrombus.

thrombotic (throm-bot'ik): Pertaining to or affected by thrombosis. **THROMBOTIC PHLEGMASIA,** see phlegmasia alba dolens under phlegmasia. **THROMBOTIC THROMBOCYTOPENIC PURPURA,** see under purpura.

thrombotonin (throm-bō-tō'nin): Serotonin (*q.v.*).

thrombus (throm'bus): An intravascular clot composed of fibrin and solid blood elements that is formed by the coagulation of blood and that remains in the location in which it was formed; may more or less occlude a blood vessel or a heart cavity.—thrombi, pl.; thrombic, thrombotic, adj.

thrush: A disease associated with white spots on the mucous membranes of the mouth, which later become ulcerous; caused by *Candida albicans*. Occurs in malnourished children who feed from unclean nipples and bottles and may involve the esophagus and diaper area. Also sometimes seen in older patients with debilitating diseases when they lack good oral hygiene.

thrypsis (thrip'sis): A comminuted fracture; see under fracture.

thumb: The first digit on the radial side of the hand; differs from the other digits in having only two phalanges and in having a freely movable metacarpal bone.

thym-, thymo-: Combining forms denoting: 1.The thymus gland. 2. The mind; emotions.

thymectomy (thī-mek'to-mi): Surgical excision of the thymus; usually done for removal of a tumor or in treatment of certain disease conditions such as myasthenia gravis.

thymelcosis (thī-mel-kō'sis): Ulceration or suppuration of the thymus gland.

-thymia: Combining form denoting mind or spirit.

thymic (thī'mik): Pertaining to the thymus gland. **T. APLASIA,** a congenital disorder characterized by absence of the thymus and parathyroid glands, by cardiovascular deformities, susceptibility to fungal and viral infection, and tetany; often fatal. **T. DYSPLASIA,** congenital lymphocytopenia characterized by early onset and susceptibility to viral and fungal infections; may be fatal.

thymitis (thī-mī'tis): Inflammation of the thymus.

thymocyte (thī'mō-sīt): A lymphocyte developed in the thymus; participates in the body's immune defenses. Also called T-lymphocyte and T-cell; see under cell.

thymol (thī'mōl): A substance found in thyme oil and other volatile oils; also produced synthetically; used locally as a bactericide and fungicide.

thymoleptic (thī-mō-lep'tik): 1. Pertaining to agents that influence mood or spirit, particularly those that counteract depression. 2. A drug with mood-elevating action that counteracts depression.

thymoma (thī-mō'ma): A tumor arising in the thymus; usually benign; may be associated with myasthenia gravis.

thymopathy (thī-mop'a-thi): Any disease or disorder of the thymus gland.

thymosin (thī' -mō-sin): A hormone with immunologic properties, secreted by the thymus gland during childhood and decreasing as the person ages.

thymus (thī'mus): A gland-like structure lying behind the manubrium of the sternum and extending upward as far as the thyroid gland. It is well developed in infancy and attains its greatest size toward the onset of puberty; then the lymphatic tissue slowly regresses and is replaced by fatty tissue. It has an immunological role in that it controls the production of T-cells (*q.v.*), one of the body's defenses against viruses, fungal infections, some bacterial infections, and cancer. See also lymphokines.

thyr-, thyro-: Combining forms denoting the thyroid gland.

thyroadenitis (thī-rō-ad-e-nī'tis): Inflammation of the thyroid gland.

thyroaplasia (thī'rō-a-plā'zi-a): Imperfect development and functioning of the thyroid gland.

thyrocalcitonin (thī'rō-kal-si-tō'nin): A polypeptide hormone containing 32 amino acids, secreted by the thyroid gland; acts to prevent resorption of bone; used therapeutically in treatment of Paget's disease. Formerly called calcitonin.

thyrocardiac (thī' -rō-kar'di-ac): 1. Pertaining to the thyroid gland and the heart. 2. Pertaining to disease of the thyroid gland in which cardiac symptoms predominate.

thyrocele (thī'rō-sēl): Enlargement of the thyroid gland; goiter.

thyrocervical (thi'rō-ser'vi-kal): Pertaining to the thyroid gland and the neck.

thyroepiglottic (thī'rō-ep-i-glot'ik): Pertaining to the thyroid gland and the epiglottis.

thyrogenic (thī-rō-jen'ik): Originating in the thyroid gland.

thyroglobulin (thī-rō-glob'ū-lin): An iodine-containing glycoprotein secreted in the follicular cells of the thyroid and stored in the colloid substance of the gland; is concerned with the synthesis of thyroid hormones.

thyroglossal (thī-rō-glos'al): Pertaining to the thyroid gland and the tongue.

thyrohyoid (thī-rō-hī'oid): Pertaining to the thyroid cartilage and the hyoid (*q.v.*) bone.

thyroid (thī'roid): 1. Shaped like a shield. 2. The dried, powdered thyroid gland of the ox, sheep, or pig, used in the treatment of cretinism, myxedema, and other conditions caused by thyroid dysfunction. 3. The ductless gland situated in front of and on either side of the upper end of the trachea, in the front part of the neck. It secretes thyroxin(e) which controls body growth and metabolism. **T. CARTILAGE,** the large cartilage of the larynx, commonly called Adam's apple. **T. CRISIS,** a serious condition resulting from the sudden increase in the basal metabolism rate due to hyperthyroidism. **T.HORMONE,** see thyroxine, lipothyronine, triiodothyronine, and thyrocalcitonin. **LINGUAL T.,** a mass of thyroid tissue at or just beneath the base of the tongue; may or may not be associated with a normally situated thyroid gland. **RETROSTERNAL T.,** a mass of thyroid tissue situated behind the sternum. **T.-STIMULATING HORMONE,** see thyrotropin. **T. STORM,** a sudden increase in symptoms of thyrotoxicosis, particularly when it occurs following thyroidectomy; thyroid crisis.

thyroid stimulating hormone (TSH): A substance secreted by the thyroid gland that stimulates the synthesis and release of thyroid hormone.

thyroidectomy (thī-roid-ek'to-mi): Surgical removal of the thyroid gland. **SUBTOTAL T.,** removal of less than the entire thyroid gland.

thyroidism (thi'roy-dizm): Old term for a pathological condition caused either by overdoses of thyroid extract or by overactivity of the thyroid gland.

thyroiditis (thī-roy-dī′tis): Inflammation of the thyroid gland. **HASHIMOTO'S T.**, see Hashimoto's disease. **RIEDEL'S T.**, a chronic fibrosis of the thyroid gland; ligneous goiter. **SUBACUTE T.**, usually occurs in association with viral diseases or upper respiratory infections; characterized by tenderness of the gland, malaise, fever, sore throat, pain that radiates to the ear and jaw; usually self-limited.

thyroidomania (thī′roy-dō-mā′ni -a): Mental disturbance due to hyperthyroidism.

thyrolytic (thī′rō-lit′ik): Destructive to thyroid tissue.

thyromegaly (thī′rō-meg′a-li): Enlargement of the thyroid gland.

thyroncus (thī-rong′kus): Goiter; thyrocele.

thyroparathyroidectomy (thī′rō-par-a-thī′roy-dek′tō-mi): Surgical removal of the thyroid and parathyroid glands.

thyropathy (thī-rop′a-thi): Any disease of the thyroid gland.

thyropenia (thī′ -rō-pē′ni-a): Diminished activity of the thyroid gland.

thyroprival (thī′rō-prī′val): Pertaining to the effects of removal of the thyroid gland, or of loss of thyroid functioning.

thyroptosis (thī-rop-tō′sis): Downward displacement of the thyroid gland.

thyrosis (thī-rō′sis): Any disorder resulting from a malfunctioning thyroid gland.

thyrotherapy (thī-rō-ther′a-pi): Treatment of thyroid disorders with preparations of the thyroid gland obtained from domesticated animals.

thyrotoxic (thī-rō-tok′sik): Pertaining to or affected by markedly increased thyroid gland activity. **T. CRISIS**, sudden increase in the symptoms of thyrotoxicosis with extreme tachycardia, fever, sweating, weight loss; usually fatal. **T. HEART DISEASE**, a condition characterized by precardial pain, weakness, sweating, weight loss; caused by hyperthyroidism which increases the work load of the heart and the amount of oxygen needed by the body.

thyrotoxicosis (thī′ -rō-tok-si-kō′sis): A condition due to excessive production of the thyroid gland hormone, thyroxine; signs and symptoms include increased metabolic rate, anxiety, nervousness, tachycardia, sweating, heat intolerance, emotional lability, increased appetite and loss of weight, a fine tremor of the hands when outstretched, and prominence of the eyes. In older patients, cardiac irregularities may be a prominent feature. Removal of the thyroid gland is usually necessary. **APATHETIC T.**, occurs in a small percentage of cases in the elderly; characterized by severe apathy and inactivity; the classic symptoms of **T.** are often absent; cardiac and other organ pathology may be present. **MASKED T.**, features of classic **T.** are absent but signs and symptoms of pathology affecting other organ systems may be evident.

thyrotropic (thī′rō-trō′pik): 1. Directly affecting the secretory function of the thyroid gland. 2. A substance that stimulates the gland to activity, *e.g.*, the **T.** hormone secreted by the anterior pituitary gland.

thyrotropin (thī-rot′rō-pin): A hormone originating in the anterior lobe of the pituitary gland; has the specific function of stimulating the thyroid gland. **T. RELEASING FACTOR**, a hormone that originates in the hypothalamus of the brain; controls release of thyrotropin by the pituitary gland which, in turn, acts upon the thyroid gland causing it to release thyroid hormone; important in the diagnosis and treatment of disorders of the thyroid gland.

thyroxin (e) (thī-rok′sin, -sēn): An iodine containing amino acid that is the chief active principle of the hormone secreted by the thyroid gland; essential for normal growth and metabolism. It is also prepared synthetically for use in disorders due to inadequate functioning of the thyroid gland.

TIA: Abbreviation for transient ischemic attack (*q.v.*).

tibia (tib′i-a): The shinbone; the inner, thicker of the two bones of the leg below the knee; it articulates with the femur, fibula, and talus.

tibial (tib′i-al): Pertaining to the tibia. **T. NERVE**, a branch of the sciatic nerve; supplies the muscles of the back of the leg.

tibialgia (tib-i-al′ji-a): Pain in the tibia or shin.

tibiocalcaneal (tib′i-ō-kal-kā′nē-al): Pertaining to the tibia and the calcaneus.

tibiofemoral (tib-i-ō-fem′o-ral): Pertaining to the tibia and the femur.

tibiofibular (tib-i-ō-fib′ū-lar): Pertaining to the tibia and the fibula.

tibionavicular (tib-i-ō-na-vik′ū-lar): Pertaining to the tibial and navicular bones.

tibiotalar (tib-i-ō-tā′lar): Pertaining to the tibia and the talus of the ankle, or to the articulation of these bones.

tibiotarsal (tib-i-ō-tar′sal): Pertaining to the tibia and the tarsal bones.

tic (tik): Minor, purposeless, repetitious, quick, involuntary gestures or muscular movements and twitchings, most often of the face, head, neck or shoulder, due to habit usually but also may be associated with a psychological factor. **T. DOULOUREUX**, trigeminal neuralgia; severe, brief but intense spasms of excruciating pain in an area supplied by one of the branches of the trigeminal nerve, especially the face or mouth.

tick (tik): A mite larger than others of the same class of bloodsucking arthropods. Some of them are transmitters of disease. See relapsing fever, Q fever, Rocky Mountain spotted fever, typhus, tularemia.

t.i.d.: Abbreviation for *ter in die,* [L.] meaning three times a day.

tidal (tī'dal): **T. AIR,** see under air. **T. DRAINAGE,** a method for continuous irrigation, most commonly used in treatment of a paralyzed bladder; sometimes used for irrigating the chest after empyema. **T. VOLUME,** the amount of air that flows in and out of the lungs with one breath at any level of activity.

TIDES: An acronym useful in diagnosing zygomatic arch fracture; refers to *t*rismus, *i*nfraorbital hypesthesia, *d*iplopia, *e*pistaxis, *s*ymmetry (of the cheeks).

Tietze's syndrome (tet'zēs): Low-grade costochondritis, characterized by pain in the costal cartilages that may radiate to the shoulder, neck, and arm, and resemble that of coronary heart disease; usually benign and self-limited. [Alexander Tietze, German surgeon. 1864–1927.]

tilt table: A table on which the patient lies prone and which can be rotated to a vertical position or various degrees between horizontal and vertical; used in several examining and therapeutic procedures.

tilt test: A test to determine degrees of shock; the patient is rapidly raised from the lying to the sitting position and the change in blood pressure and pulse rate are noted immediately; the degree of decrease in blood pressure and increase in pulse rate allow the observer to classify the shock state as mild, moderate, or severe.

timbre (tim'b'r): The characteristic musical quality of a sound.

tincture (tink'-chur): An alcoholic pharmaceutical preparation made by extracting the useful principle from a vegetable material or a chemical substance; the amount of drug in the solution varies according to set standards for each drug.

tine test: A skin test for tuberculosis. See Heaf multiple puncture test.

tinea (tin'ē-a): A general term for several fungus infections of the skin; ringworm. **T. BARBAE,** ringworm of the beard; barber's itch. **T. CAPITIS,** ringworm of the scalp. **T. CRICINATA** or **CORPORIS,** ringworm of the non-hairy surfaces of the body. **T. CRURIS,** ringworm of the inner sides of thigh, perineal area or groin; more common in males; see Dhobi itch. **T. PEDIS,** chronic fungal infection of the feet, principally the areas between the toes; marked by intense itching, scaling, maceration and cracking of the skin; commonly called athlete's foot. **T. UNGUIUM,** ringworm of the nails; see onchomycosis. **T. VERSICOLOR,** a common chronic disorder seen most often in tropical regions; usually symptomless and noninflammatory; marked by the occurrence, usually on the trunk, of many macular patches of varying sizes and shapes which vary from white on darkly pigmented skin to faun-colored or brown on pale skin.

Tinel's sign: Used to detect a partial lesion or early regeneration of a nerve; percussing over the nerve trunk will produce a tingling sensation that extends up to the site of the lesion or regeneration but not beyond it. [Jules Tinel, French neurosurgeon. 1879–1952.]

tingle: A slight, prickling, stinging, or throbbing sensation.

tinkles: Very high pitched bowel sounds that have a musical quality.

tinnitus (ti-nī'tus): Subjective noises such as buzzing, thumping, ringing, roaring, clucking, or humming that accompany certain types of hearing disorders. May also be a sign of impacted cerumen or of Ménière's disease (*q.v.*).

tissue (tish'ū): A collection of similar cells and the intercellular material surrounding them that form a structure, which, in turn, performs a particular function in the body. The five main classes of tissue are connective, epithelial, glandular, muscular, and nervous. **ADIPOSE T.,** connective tissue containing masses of fat cells. **AREOLAR T.,** loosely arranged, widely dispersed connective tissue. **CANCELLOUS T.,** bony tissue that is spongy in appearance. **COMPACT T.,** bony tissue that is dense and hard. **CONNECTIVE T.,** made up of an interlacing mass of fibers; pervades, supports and binds together tissues and organs; includes areolar, adipose, fibrous, elastic, and lymphoid tissues, cartilage and bone, blood and lymph. **ENDOTHELIAL T.,** a single layer of flattened cells that lines serous cavities, blood vessels and lymphatics. **EPITHELIAL T.,** one or more layers of flattened cells with little intercellular substance; lines tubes or cavities that connect with the exterior and covers the surface of the body. **MUSCULAR T.,** made up of fibers that are capable of contracting and expanding; classified as skeletal, smooth or visceral, and cardiac. See muscle. **NERVOUS T.,** made up of highly differentiated cells that compose nerves and their fibers and the tissues that support them. **PARENCHYMATOUS T.,** the specialized tissue of an organ that makes up its functioning part as differentiated from supporting tissues. **SUBCUTANEOUS T.,** that found directly underneath the skin; it is a type of loosely organized connective **T.**

tissue culture: The culture of tissue cells in the laboratory.

tissue perfusion, alteration in: A nursing diagnosis accepted by the Fourth National Conference on the Classification of Nursing Diagnoses.

tissular (tish'ū-lar): Pertaining to the tissues of the body.

titanium (tī-tā'ni-um): A dark grey hard metallic element. **T. DIOXIDE,** an opaque white powder, used in creams and powders to protect the skin against irritation and solar rays. An alloy of the metal is used in making various orthopedic prostheses.

titer, titre (tī′tur): The strength of a solution or the quantity of a particular constituent of a solution as determined by titration (*q.v.*). A standard of strength or purity.

titillation (tit-il-lā′shun): Tickling, or the sensation of tickling.

titrate (tī′trat): To determine the strength of a solution, or the concentration of a substance in a solution, in terms of the amount of known concentration required to bring about a given effect in a reaction with a known volume of the test solution.

titration (tī-trā′shun): Determination of the quantity of a given constituent in a substance by observing the volume of a standard solution needed to change the constituent to a completely different form.—titrate, v.

titubation (tit′ū-bā′shun): Incoordination, unsteadiness, and stumbling manifested when walking.

TLC: Abbreviation for: 1. Tender loving care (informal). 2. Total lung capacity; the amount of air in the lungs at maximum inspiration.

t.o.: Abbreviation for telephone order.

toco-: Combining form relating to obstetrics or childbirth.

tocodynamometer (tō′kō-dī-na-mom′-e-ter): An instrument for measuring the frequency, strength, and duration of contractions of the uterus; used particularly during labor.

tocography (tō-kog′ra-fi): A process of recording uterine contractions graphically using a device called a tocograph or parturiometer.

tocologist (tō-kol′o-jist): An obstetrician.

tocology (tō-kol′o-ji): Obstetrics.

tocomania (tō-kō-mā′ni-a): Puerperal psychosis; see under puerperal.

tocopherol (tok-of′er-ol): Any of a group of fat-soluble compounds containing vitamin E, of which alpha-tocopherol is the most physiologically active; is necessary for normal reproduction and believed to be necessary also for certain other physiological processes. Widely distributed in foods including wheat germ, some seeds, peanuts, cereal grains, rice, egg yolk, margarine, vegetable oils, milk, beef liver, fat and lean meats, all leafy green vegetables. Deficiency results in muscle degeneration, anemia, infertility, liver and kidney damage.

tocophobia (tō-kō-fō′bi-a): Undue fear of childbirth.

Todd's paralysis: A transient paralysis that sometimes occurs in epileptics following a focal seizure; usually clears within 24 hours.

toe: Any of the digits of the feet. **HAMMER-T.**, a claw-like deformity caused by the permanent flexion of the joint between the second and third phalanges; most often involves the second toe; may be congenital or caused by ill-fitting shoes. **PIGEON T.**, deformity causing toeing in or walking with the toes turned toward the center line of the body.

toeing in: Walking with the toes or the feet pointed toward the midline of the body; pigeon-toed.

togovirus (tō′ga-vī-rus′): Any of a subgroup of arboviruses (*q.v.*) including some that are transmitted by arthropods, especially ticks and mosquitoes; they cause hemorrhagic fever, yellow fever, dengue, and encephalitis; so called because they are encapsulated in an envelope or toga.

toilet: 1. The cleansing of a wound area after surgery or delivery of an obstetric patient. 2. A device for collecting and disposing of urine and feces, or the room in which such a device is housed. 3. The various activities involved in dressing and grooming. **TOILET TRAINING**, teaching a child to control bowel and bladder function. Training methods used, parents' attitude about these, and the child's responses, are thought to influence the development of personality.

tolerance (tol′e-rans): 1. The ability to endure the administration of unusually large amounts of a substance, usually a drug, without ill effects. 2. Resistance to the effects of a medication administered over a period of time so that increasingly larger doses are required to get the effect of the original dose. **CROSS T.**, the carrying over of tolerance for one drug to tolerance for another drug. **PAIN T.**, the maximum amount of stimulation required to produce the sensation of pain or discomfort. **REVERSE T.**, a condition in which response to a specific dose of a drug increases with repeated use so that smaller doses may be taken and still produce the effects that resulted from larger doses. **SUGAR T.**, the amount of sugar a person can metabolize before it begins to appear in the urine.

tolerant (tol′er-ant): 1. Possessing tolerance for the beliefs, opinions, and practices of others. 2. The state of being resistant to the effects of continued or increasing use of a drug. 3. The ability to survive and grow in a specific environment; said of bacteria particularly.

-tome: Combining form denoting cutting or sectioning, or a cutting instrument.

tomo-: Combining form denoting section or sectional.

tomogram (tōm′ō-gram): A radiographic study that provides segmental visualization of structures at selected levels by blurring structures in all other planes.

tomograph (tō′mō-graf): A device for obtaining an x-ray image of an organ or tissue at a selected plane or layer in a specified region of the body while blurring images of structures in other planes. Can be a series of films taken at different depths.—tomography, n.; tomographic, adj.

tomography (tō-mog′ra-fi): The x-ray photographic process that produces a tomograph (*q.v.*); sectional radiography. **AXIAL T., T.** in which a series of cross-sectional images are combined to produce a three-dimensional scan. **COMPUTED** or **COMPUTERIZED AXIAL T.**, a method of producing an image by using a computer to reconstruct the anatomic features revealed by axial **T.**; abbreviated CAT. **POSITRON EMISSION T.**, a diagnostic procedure utilizing a computerized radiographic technique that depicts function rather than structure. The patient is placed in a supine position and given an intravenous injection of radioactive glucose that emits positively charged particles; these particles combine with negatively charged electrons in certain body cells and emit gamma rays that are converted into color-coded video images that depict the metabolic activity of the organ under study. Useful in diagnosing cancer, in locating brain tumors precisely, and in studies of functional disorders of the brain. Abbreviated PET.

tomomania (tō′mō-mān′i-a): An abnormal desire to 1) perform surgery, or 2) to have surgery performed on one's self.

tomotocia (tō′mō-tō′si-a): Cesarean section.

-tomy: Combining form denoting incision; a cutting operation.

tone (tōn): 1. A particular quality or sound of voice. 2. The normal firmness and strength of tissues. 3. The normal healthy degree of tension in resting muscles.

tongs: In orthopedics, a device with points that engages the skull and is attached to a traction apparatus; used for treatment of cervical fractures. Several types are available, the most common being Burton, Crutchfield, and Vincke.

tongue (tung): The mobile, muscular organ contained in the mouth; it is concerned with speech, mastication, swallowing, and taste. **BIFID T.**, a **T.** in which the anterior part is divided by a longitudinal cleft. **BLACK T.**, a **T.** with a black to brown fur-like patch at the back part where the papillae have become elongated, seen especially after the individual has been treated with antibiotics. **COATED T.**, a **T.** covered with a layer of yellowish or whitish material consisting of bacteria, food debris, etc.; associated with high fever, and digestive disorders. **ENCRUSTED T.**, a **T.** heavily coated with yellowish material. **FURRED T.**, a **T.** coated with a surface that resembles white fur; due to extensive change in the papillae. **GEOGRAPHIC T.**, a **T.** covered with migratory denuded patches that are surrounded by elevated thickened epithelium. **HAIRY T.**, a **T.** in which the papillae have blackened and become elongated; may occur in individuals who have sucked on antibiotic lozenges. **MAGENTA T.**, a purplish-red **T.**, due to deficiency of riboflavin. **RASPBERRY T.**, the **T.** is bright red, not coated, has elevated papillae; seen in scarlet fever after the rash has been present for several days. **SMOKER'S T.**, leukoplakia (*q.v.*) of the **T. STRAWBERRY T.**, a **T.** that has a whitish coat with reddened papillae; characteristic of scarlet fever during the first 24 hours after the rash has appeared.

tongue-tie: Shortness of the frenum resulting in limited mobility of the tongue and interference with sucking and articulation.—tongue-tied, adj.

-tonia: Combining form denoting degree or condition of tonus.

tonic: 1. A state of continuous or sustained contraction, said of muscles. 2. Increasing or restoring physical or mental tone or strength. 3. A drug that invigorates or restores strength. **T. SPASM**, refers to a prolonged muscle spasm as differentiated from a clonic spasm; see **clonus**.

-tonic: A combining form denoting: 1. The degree or quality of muscular contraction, *e.g.*, isotonic. 2. The concentration of a substance in solution, *e.g.*, hypertonic.

tonic-clonic: Pertains to muscle spasms, especially those seen in generalized seizures in which there is both a tonic and clonic stage. See **tonic**, **clonic**. Also tonicoclonic, tonoclonic.

tonicity (tō-nis′i-ti): 1. The condition of possessing tone. 2. The state of normal tension or tone of a muscle or muscles. 3. The osmotic pressure or tension of a solution.

tono-: Combining form denoting: 1. Tone. 2. Tension. 3. Pressure.

tonography (tō-nog′ra-fi): Continuous recording of pressure using an electric tonometer (*q.v.*); used particularly for measuring intraocular pressure.

tonometer (tō-nom′e-ter): An instrument for measuring pressure, specifically intraocular pressure. **SCHIÖTZ T.**, a hand-held instrument for measuring intraocular pressure. **GOLDMAN APPLANATION TONOMETER**, an exceptionally sensitive instrument for measuring intraocular pressure but requires the use of an expensive biomicroscope.

tonometry (tō-nom′e-tri): The measurement of pressure or tension, particularly the use of a tonometer to measure intraocular pressure.

tonsil (ton′sil): By custom referring to one of two small almond-shaped lymphoid bodies lying between the pillars of the fauces on either side of the oropharynx and covered with mucous membrane; called palatine tonsils.

CEREBELLAR T., one of a pair of rounded masses on the inferior surface of the cerebellum. LINGUAL T., an aggregation of lymph follicles at the root of the tongue. PHARYNGEAL T., an aggregation of lymphoid tissue situated in the roof and posterior wall of the nasopharynx. See Waldeyer's ring.—tonsillar, tonsillary, adj.

tonsillectomy (ton'si-lek'to-mi): Usually refers to the surgical removal of one or both of the palatine tonsils.

tonsillitis (ton'si-lī'tis): Inflammation of the tonsils. FOLLICULAR T., inflammation of the tonsils involving the crypts, with development of projecting yellow or white spots.

tonsilloadenoidectomy (ton'sil-ō-ad'-e-noyd -ek'to-mi): Surgical removal of the palatine tonsils and the adenoids.

tonsillolith (ton-sil'ō-lith): Concretion arising in the body of a tonsil.

tonsillopharyngitis (ton'sil-ō-făr-in-jī'tis): Inflammation of the palatine tonsils and the pharynx.

tonsillotome (ton-sil'ō-tōm): An instrument used for excision of tonsils.

tonsure (ton'shur): Shaving of the hair from the crown of the head.

tonus (tō'nus): The normal condition of slight continuous contraction in body tissues, muscles in particular, when in a state of rest.

tooth: Any of the small bone-like structures that are set in the jaws and used for chewing; they also assist in articulation. Each tooth is made up of a pulp cavity which contains a soft pulpy substance that supports blood vessels and nerves, and a solid outer part consisting of dentin or ivory which is covered above the gum with enamel—the hardest substance in the body—and below the gum with cementum. The part outside the gum is called the crown and the part inside is the root. In man, the deciduous, baby or milk teeth erupt between the 6th and 24th months of life and are shed by the age of approximately 7 years. The permanent set, 32 in number, is usually complete in the late teens and consists of 4 incisors, 2 canines (cuspids), 4 premolars (bicuspids), and 6 molars (tricuspids). CANINE or EYE T., a T. with a sharp fang-like edge for tearing food. IMPACTED T., a T. so placed that it cannot erupt into its normal position. INCISOR T., a T. with a knife-like edge for biting food. HUTCHINSON'S T., see Hutchinson's teeth. PREMOLAR and MOLAR T., a T. that has a squarish termination for chewing and grinding food. STOMACH T., the lower canine T., one on each side. WISDOM T., the third and last molars, one at either side of each jaw.

tooth grinding: See bruxism.

toothache: An aching pain in a tooth or near a tooth; may be caused by trauma, infection, or caries. Odontalgia.

top-, topo-: Combining form denoting place; locality.

topagnosis (top'ag-nō'sis): 1. Inability to locate the exact point at which some part of the body is touched. 2. Inability to find one's way about in a familiar location.

topalgia (tō-pal'ji-a): Localized pain.

topectomy (tō-pek'to-mi): Modified frontal lobotomy to treat a psychosis.

toper's nose: Rhinophyma (*q.v.*).

topesthesia (tōp'es-thē'zi-a): The ability to localize a tactile sensation precisely.

tophaceous (tō-fā'shus): Gritty; sandy. T. GOUT, see under gout.

tophus (tō'fus): A small, hard concretion forming in the earlobe, or in the tissues about the joints of the phalanges, etc., as in gout.—tophi, pl.

topical (top'ik-al): 1. Pertaining to a definite spot; local. 2. Term often used to describe a substance that is to be applied to the surface of the body for its local effect as distinguished from one that is given internally for its systemic effect.

topognosis (top'og-nō'sis): The ability to localize a tactile sensation. Topesthesia.

topography (tō-pog'ra-fi): In anatomy, a description of the regions of the body.—topographical, adj.; topographically, adv.

topology (top-ol'o-ji): 1. Regional anatomy. 2. The description of the relation of the presenting part of a fetus to the pelvic canal.

toponarcosis (top'ō-nar-kō'sis): Loss of sensation or the development of anesthesia in a localized area.

TOPS: Take Off Pounds Sensibly, an organization similar to Weight Watchers (*q.v.*).

TOPV: Abbreviation for *t*rivavlent *o*ral *p*oliovirus *v*accine, a live attenuated vaccine that includes all three strains of poliovirus; most recipients are protected after a single dose.

TORCH syndrome: The clinical manifestation of any of a certain group of disease-producing agents, including *T*oxoplasma gondii, *o*ther, *r*ubella virus, *c*ytomegalovirus, and *h*erpes simplex virus in the fetus or newborn infant.

tormina (tor'mi-na): Gripping intestinal pains.—torminal, torminous, adj.

torpid (tor'pid): Sluggish; not reacting with normal vigor or ease.

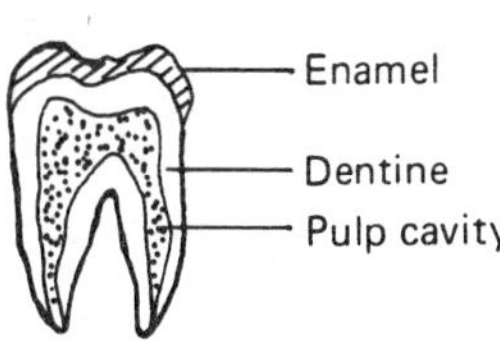

Tooth

torpor (tōr′por): Sluggishness, inactivity, stupor, apathy, numbness; absence or slowness of reaction to ordinary stimuli.

torque (tork): The measurement of the force capable of producing rotation or tortion about an axis; a twisting force.

torr: A unit of measurement of gas pressure; sometimes substituted for mm Hg. [Evangelista Torricelli, Italian physicist and mathematician. 1608–1647.]

torsion (tor′shun): A twisting. **T. OF THE OVARY,** a twisting of the ovary caused by the presence of an ovarian cyst or teratoma, resulting in severe pain, constipation, vomiting, and the presence of an adnexal mass. **T. OF THE TESTICLE,** a twisting of the testicle on its mesentery, causing pain and interference with the blood supply. **T. OF THE UMBILICAL CORD,** more than the normal eight or ten twists of the cord; may follow death of the fetus.—torsive, adj.

torso (tor′sō): The trunk of the body without the head and extremities.

torticollis (tor′ti-kol′is): Wryneck; persistent involuntary contraction of the muscles on one side of the neck; the head is slightly flexed and drawn toward the contracted side, with the face rotated over the shoulder. **CONGENITAL T.,** due to birth injury of the sternocleidomastoid muscle on one side only. **INFANTILE T.,** arises during the first six months of life; due to a tight sternocleidomastoid muscle; the chin points to the opposite foot. **MUSCULAR T.,** associated with fibrosis of the sternocleidomastoid muscle. **MYOGENIC T.,** due to muscular contraction, particularly in rheumatism. **NEUROGENIC T.,** due to irritation of the accessory nerve. **STRUCTURAL T.,** due to congenital hemivertebra.—torticollar, adj.

tortuous (tor′chū-us): Twisted, full of curves, turns and twists.

tortuosity (tor-chū-os′i-ti): 1. The quality of being bent, twisted, or winding. 2. Something twisted, winding, or curved.

torulus (tor′ū-lus): A minute projection or elevation; a papilla.—toruli, pl.

torus (tō′rus): An elevation or prominence. **T. PALATINUS,** the bony elevation along the midline of the hard palate.—tori, pl.; toric, adj.

total hip replacement: Reconstruction of both the head of the femur and the acetabulum and replacement of the head with a metal ball cemented onto the shaft of the femur with methyl methacrylate.

total parenteral nutrition: Parenteral hyperalimentation. A way of supplying essential nutrients via intravenous infusion of a solution containing glucose, amino acids, vitamins, electrolytes, and water, to meet the nutritional needs of the particular patient; used for patients with anorexia nervosa, burns, severe infections, colitis, severe vomiting or diarrhea, or for infants with congenital anomalies that interfere with normal feeding. Abbreviated TPN.

touch: 1. The special sense by which contact with objects makes one aware of their qualities. 2. To examine by touching with the finger or hand. **THERAPEUTIC T.,** see under therapeutic.

Tourette syndrome: See Gilles de la Tourette syndrome.

tourniquet (toor′ni-ket): An apparatus for the temporary compression of the blood vessels of a limb. Designed for compression of a main artery to control bleeding. A **T.** is also often used to obstruct the venous return from a limb and so facilitate the withdrawal of blood from a vein. Tourniquets vary from a simple rubber band to a pneumatic cuff. **ROTATING T.,** a system of treatment in which tourniquets are applied to all four extremities in turn, as near the trunk as possible; every 10–15 minutes, the tourniquets are rotated so that a different arm or leg is free and three tourniquets are always in place.

tourniquet test: A test for capillary resistance. A blood pressure cuff on the patient's arm is inflated to a point midway between diastolic and systolic pressure and the pressure maintained for ten minutes; if petechiae appear on the forearm, the test is positive. Used in diagnosing diseases marked by capillary fragility, *e.g.,* scurvy, thrombocytopenic purpura, and purpura accompanying severe infections.

tox-, toxi-, toxo-: Combining forms denoting toxic, toxin, poison, poisonous.

toxanemia (toks′a-nē′mi-a): Anemia resulting from poisoning by a hemolytic agent.

toxemia (tok-sē′mi-a): Generalized poisoning due to the accumulation of toxins in the bloodstream, usually as a result of bacterial action but may also be due to other causes. **ALIMENTARY T., T.** due to absorption of toxins generated in the gastrointestinal tract. **ECLAMPTIC T., T.** of pregnancy. **HYDATID T., T.** caused by the escape of fluid from a hydatid mole into the peritoneal cavity; see mole, hydatidiform. **T. OF PREGNANCY,** a condition due to a disturbance of metabolism and characterized by hypertension, edema, albuminuria, and sometimes eclampsia (*q.v.*).—toxemic, adj.

toxic (toks′ik): 1. Poisonous. 2. Resulting from or caused by a poison. 3. Pertaining to a toxin. Syn., poisonous.

toxic shock syndrome: A rare, serious, potentially fatal condition characterized by high fever, headache, nausea, vomiting, diarrhea, myalgia, erythematous rash, hypovolemia, rapid drop in blood pressure, thrombocytopenia; resembles disorders caused by bacterial toxins. About 70 percent of cases have occurred in women using a certain brand of tampon, but also occurs in persons with infections of other origin. *Staphylococcus aureus* has been the usual causative organism.

toxic storm: A severe condition characterized by acute hypermetabolism. See **thyroid crisis** under **thyroid**, and **thyrotoxicosis**.

toxic-, toxico-: Combining forms denoting poison.

toxicant (toks'i-kant): A toxic or poisonous substance.

toxicity (tok-sis'i-ti): The quality or degree of the poisonousness of a substance.

Toxicodendron (toks'i-kō-den'dron): Any of a group of plants or shrubs that cause dermatitis on contact with the skin; includes poison ivy, poison oak, and poison sumac. Also classified as *Rhus*.

toxicoderma (toks'i-kō-der'ma): Any skin disease caused by a toxin or poison.

toxicodermatitis (toks'i-kō-der-ma-tī'tis): Inflammation of the skin due to a poison.

toxicogenic (toks'ik-ō-jen'ik): 1. Caused by a poison. 2. Producing or capable of producing a poison.

toxicoid (toks'i-koyd): Resembling a poison, or having an action like that of a poison.

toxicologist (toks-i-kol'o-jist): A person who specializes in the study of poisons.

toxicology (toks-i-kol'o-ji): The science dealing with poisons and poisonings.—toxicological, adj.; toxicologically, adv.

toxicomania (toks'i-kō-mā'ni-a): A periodic or chronic state of intoxication, produced by repeated consumption of a drug harmful to the individual or society. Characteristics are: uncontrollable desire or necessity to continue using the drug and to try to get it by any means; tendency to increase the dose; and psychic and physical dependency as a result.

toxicopathy (toks-i-kop'a-thi): Any disease condition caused by a poison.—toxicopathic, adj.

toxicopexis (toks'i-kō-pek'sis): The neutralization of a poison in the body.

toxicosis (toks-i-kō'sis): The condition of systemic poisoning by a toxin or poison.

toxiferous (tok-sif'er-us): Poisonous.

toxigenicity (toks'i-je-nis'i-ti): The degree of ability of an organism to produce toxic substances that may be injurious to human cells.

toxin (toks'in): Any poisonous substance produced by a plant or animal organism, usually referring to one produced by pathogenic organism.

toxin-antitoxin: A mixture of diptheria toxin and its antitoxin that was formerly used to produce immunity to diphtheria, now largely replaced by diphtheria toxoid (*q.v.*).

toxinemia (toks-in-ē'mi-a): Toxemia (*q.v.*).

toxinfection (toks-in-fek'shun): Infection caused by a toxin rather than a microorganism. Also called toxoinfection.

toxinic (tok-sin'ik): Pertaining to a toxin.

toxinosis (toks'in-ō'sis): Any pathologic condition caused by the action of a toxin.

Toxocara (tok'sō-kar'a): A genus of nematode worms that are parasitic in humans, dogs (*T. canis*), and cats (*T. cati*).

toxocariasis (tok'sō-kar-ī'a-sis): A disease due to infection with the nematode worm of the genus *Toxocara,* which enters the circulation through the intestinal wall; characterized by inflammation, hemorrhage, and necrosis of the tissues of the organs to which the larvae of the worm migrate; may affect the brain, liver, heart, great vessels, or retina.

toxoid (tok'soyd): A bacterial toxin altered in such a way that it has lost its poisonous properties but retained its antigenic properties and thus is capable of producing active immunity. **DIPHTHERIA T.**, that used to produce active immunity against diphtheria; it is prepared from products of the growth of *Corynebacterium diphtheriae*. **TETANUS T.**, used to produce active immunity against tetanus; prepared from the products of the growth of *Clostridium tetani*.

toxophore (tok'sō-fōr): The particular chemical group in the molecules of a poison that give it its toxic characteristics.

Toxoplasma (tok-sō-plaz'ma): A genus of protozoal parasites. *Toxoplasma gondii* causes toxoplasmosis (*q.v.*).

toxoplasmosis (tok'sō-plas-mō'sis): Infection by *Toxoplasma gondii,* a protozoan parasite, which commonly infects birds and mammals, including humans. Intrauterine fetal as well as infant infections are often severe, producing encephalitis, convulsions, hydrocephalus, and eye disease, resulting in death or, in those who recover, mental retardation and impaired sight. Infection in older children and adults may result in pneumonia, nephritis, or skin rashes. **OCULAR T.**, posterior granulomatous uveitis, characterized by chorioretinitis, pain, photophobia.

TPI test: *Treponema pallidum* immobilization test. A highly specific test for syphilis in which syphilitic serum immobilizes and kills spirochetes grown in pure culture.

TPN: Abbreviation for total parenteral nutrition (*q.v.*).

TPR: Abbreviation for temperature, pulse, and respirations.

trabecula (tra-bek'ū-la): In anatomy, one of the fibrous bands or septa of connective tissue that extend into the interior of an organ from its wall or the capsule that covers it, and that serve to hold the functioning cells of the organ in position.—trabeculae, pl.; trabecular, adj.; trabeculum, sing.

trabeculation (tra-bek-ū-lā'shun): The formation or presence of trabeculae in a part of the body.

trabeculectomy (tra-bek'ū-lek'to-mi): A microsurgical procedure for the relief of glaucoma; involves the excision of a small rectangle of the sclera.

trace elements: Metals and other elements that are regularly present in very small amounts in the tissues and thought to be essential for normal metabolism (*e.g.*, copper, cobalt, manganese, fluorine, iodine, zinc).

tracer (trā'ser): 1. An instrument used for dissecting blood vessels and nerves. 2. A substance or instrument used to gain information. 3. A radioactive substance added in minute amounts to a given substance that is introduced into the body in certain x-ray examinations; useful in tracing the outline of organs or structures and determining the presence of tumors.

trach-, trachea-, tracheo-: Combining forms denoting the trachea.

trachea (trā'kē-a): The windpipe; the fibrocartilaginous tube lined with ciliated mucous membrane passing from the larynx to the bronchi. It is about 4.5 in. long and about 1 in. wide.—tracheal, adj.

tracheal (trā'kē-al): Pertaining to the trachea. **T. BREATH SOUNDS,** bronchial breath sounds; see under breath sounds. **T. INTUBATION,** the insertion of a tube through the larynx into the trachea to maintain an airway; used especially in cardiopulmonary resuscitation and in patients having general anesthesia.

trachealgia (trā-kē-al'ji-a): Pain in the trachea.

tracheitis (trā-kē-ī'tis): Inflammation of the mucous membrane lining the trachea. Also spelled trachitis.

trachel-, trachelo-: Combining forms denoting 1) the neck, or 2) a neck-like structure.

trachelagra (trā'ke-lag'ra): A gouty or rheumatic condition of the neck characterized by torticollis.

trachelectomy (trā'ke-lek'to-mi): Surgical removal of the neck of the uterus.

trachelismus (trā'ke-liz'mus): 1. Spasm of the neck muscles. 2. Bending backward of the neck, a sign that sometimes signals the imminence of an epileptic attack.

trachelitis (trā'ke-lī'tis): Inflammation of the cervix of the uterus.

trachelocystitis (trā'ke-lō-sis-tī'tis): Inflammation of the neck of the urinary bladder.

trachelokyphosis (trā'ke-lō-kī-fō'sis): An abnormal anterior curvature of the cervical vertebrae; humpback.

trachelopexy (trā'ke-lō-pek'si): An operation for fixation of the neck of the uterus.

trachelophyma (trā'ke-lō-fī'ma): A swelling or tumor of the neck.

tracheloplasty (trā'ke-lō-plas-ti): Surgical repair of lacerations or other injuries to the neck of the uterus.

trachelorrhaphy (trā'ke-lor'a-fi): Operative repair of a lacerated uterine cervix.

trachelos (trā'ke-lōs): The neck.

tracheo-: Combining form denoting trachea.

tracheobronchial (trā'kē-ō-brong'ki-al): Pertaining to the trachea and the bronchi. **T. TREE,** consists of the trachea, the bronchi, and their branching structures; a system of bifurcating tubes made up of muscular, cartilaginous, and elastic tissues.

tracheobronchitis (trā'kē-ō-brong-kī'tis): Inflammation of the trachea and bronchi.

tracheobronchomegaly (trā'kē-ō-brong'kō-meg'a-li): A rare condition or syndrome of greatly enlarged lumen of the trachea and main bronchi, characterized by recurrent and chronic respiratory tract infections; thought to be congenital.

tracheobronchoscopy (trā'kē-ō-brong-kos'-ko-pi): Inspection of the interior of the trachea and one or both of the bronchi by means of a bronchoscope.

tracheoesophageal (trāk'ē-ō-ē-sof-a-jē'al): Pertaining to the trachea and esophagus. **T. FISTULA,** see under fistula.

tracheography (trā'kē-og'ra-fi): The process of making an x-ray picture of the trachea after instillation of a contrast medium.

tracheolaryngeal (trā'kē-ō-lar-in'jē-al): Pertaining to the trachea and the larynx.

tracheomalacia (trā'kē-ō-ma-lā'shi-a): Softening and destruction of the walls of the trachea, especially of the cartilaginous rings.

tracheopharyngeal (trā'kē-ō-far-in'jē-al): Pertaining to the trachea and the pharynx.

tracheophony (trā'kē-of'o-ni): The sound heard when auscultating over the trachea.

tracheoplasty (trā'kē-ō-plas-ti): Plastic surgery on the trachea.

tracheopyosis (trā'kē-ō-pī-ō'sis): Tracheitis with purulent effusion.

tracheorrhagia (trā'kē-ō-rāj'i-a): Hemorrhage from the trachea.

tracheorrhaphy (trā-kē-or'ra-fi): Suturing of the trachea.

tracheoscopy (trā'kē-os'ko-pi): Inspection of the interior of the trachea with a special instrument called a tracheoscope.—tracheoscopic, adj.

tracheostenosis (trā' -kē-ō-ste-nō'sis): Narrowing or constriction of the trachea.

tracheostoma (trā'kē-ō-stō'ma): An opening made into the trachea through the neck.

tracheostomy (trā-kē-os'to-mi): The surgical creation of a stoma or an opening into the trachea through the neck for the purpose of facilitating passage of air into the lungs or to remove secretions from the trachea; usually a tube is inserted to keep the opening patent and to facilitate passage of air or evacuation of secretions. **T. TUBE,** a curved tube inserted into the trachea following a tracheostomy.

tracheotome (trā'kē-ō-tōm): A tracheotomy knife, used for incising the trachea.

tracheotomize (trā'ke-ot'o-mīz): To perform a tracheotomy upon.

tracheotomy (trā-kē-ot'o-mi): The operation of making an incision into the trachea; may be done to remove a foreign body, secure a specimen for biopsy, or for exploratory purposes.—tracheotomize, v.

trachoma (tra-kō'ma): A chronic communicable disease of the cornea and conjunctiva, caused by the *Chlamydia trachomatis;* of worldwide distribution but occurs chiefly in the Middle East, Asia, and the Mediterranean area where it is the principal cause of blindness; of insidious or sudden onset and of long duration when untreated. Most often occurs in association with poverty, poor hygiene, crowded living conditions and exposure of the eyes to sun and sand in hot dry dusty regions; is transmitted by flies, fingers, and fomites. Symptoms include pain, tearing, photophobia, inflammation of the eyelids and conjunctiva with the formation of lesions that terminate in granulation and scar tissue, deformities of the eyelids, progressive visual disability, and, frequently, blindness.

trachyphonia (trak'i-fō'ni-a): Roughness or hoarseness of the voice.

tracing (trās'ing): A recording or pattern of lines made by a pointed instrument on paper or other surface to show movement or activity.

tract: In anatomy, 1) an area or region that is longer than it is wide, or 2) a path or track. May consist of a number of separate organs arranged serially and engaged in performing a common function; or may consist of a bundle of nerve fibers that have the same origin, termination, and function. **ASCENDING TRACTS,** tracts that transmit afferent nerve impulses up the spinal cord to the brain; they include 1) the funiculus gracilis and funiculus cuneatus, which carry impulses of position movement, and touch-pressure, and terminate in the medulla oblongata; 2) the ventral spinothalamic **T.** which carries proprioceptive impulses and terminates in the thalamus; 3) the dorsal spinocerebellar **T.,** which carries impulses of crude touch and pressure to the cerebellum; 4) the lateral spinothalamic **T.,** which carries impulses of pain and temperature to the thalamus. **DESCENDING TRACTS,** tracts that carry efferent impulses from the brain down the spinal cord; they include 1) the corticospinal **T.,** which transmits impulses from the cerebral cortex to the muscles of the extremities, with some fibers going to the neck and trunk; 2) the vestibulospinal **T.,** which transmits efferent impulses from the medulla oblongata that are concerned with the maintenance of muscle tone and equilibrium (also called extrapyramidal tracts); 3) the reticulospinal **T.** which extends from the brainstem to the sympathetic ganglia and provides innervation for unconscious muscle coordination.

tractability (trak-ta-bil'i-ti): Refers to the condition of being easily handled, managed, or controlled.

traction (trak'shun): A steady drawing or pulling exerted manually or with a mechanical device to overcome muscle spasm, so that a fracture may be reduced, to keep the ends of fractured bones in position until healing can take place, to prevent deformities or contractures from fractures or other conditions, or to correct or lessen deformities such as scoliosis. Many of the types of apparatus used to produce a steady pulling on a part involve the use of pulleys and weights. **BUCK'S T.** or **EXTENSION;** an apparatus for obtaining extension of a fractured hip or femur; consists of a system of weights, ropes, and pulleys, and adhesive straps; also used in treatment of contractures and to realign the vertebrae in cases of scoliosis. **CERVICAL T.,** continuous **T.** to immobilize the cervical spine in treatment of whiplash injuries or conditions due to arthritis; may consist of a head halter, sling, or tongs inserted into the skull. **COTREL'S T.,** continuous opposing **T.** with a pelvic sling and a special head halter with a pulley system that allows the patient to increase the amount of **T.** by extending the legs which are placed in stirrups attached to the **T.** This **T.** plus exercises is used to stretch the muscles on the concave side of a scoliotic curve in preparation for casting or surgical treatment for scoliosis. **FIXED T., T.** exerted between two fixed points as, *e.g.*, on a Hare splint or **T.** between Steinmann pins that are incorporated in a cast. **HALO T.,** consists of a halo (circular band attached to the skull with surgical pins) which may be attached to direct **T.** or to a frame that is supported by the body; used to support the spine after injury or surgery; also used in postoperative treatment of scoliosis. **HALO-PELVIC T.,** applied to the spine by means of two metal hoops; one attached to the skull and one to the pelvis, joined by extension rods; used to correct deformity from scoliosis prior to fusion. **HALTER T.,** a leather halter attached to a bar above the head and to a string that goes over a pulley to weights; the patient may be either sitting or lying down; used for treatment of cervical lesions. **INTERMITTENT T., T.** applied for certain periods each day; may be removed for performance of activites of daily living; used to relieve muscle spasm or to correct certain deformities. **MANUAL T.,** a pull exerted by the hands. **MECHANICAL T.,** skin or skeletal **T.** with weights to exert the necessary pull. **SKELETAL T., T.** exerted directly upon the skeleton with devices attached to pins or tongs inserted into the bone; used when long-term **T.** is necessary and when the amount of weight required is greater than the skin can tolerate, or when skin **T.** is counterindicated. **SKIN T., T.** attached to the skin and held in place with elastic bandage which compresses the soft tissue enough to exert indirect **T.** on the skeleton. **SKULL T.,** used in dislocation or fracture-dislocation of the cervical spine; calipers are inserted into the temporal bones under anesthesia, and a cord with a weight attached runs from the calipers over a pulley and then over the head of the bed, which is elevated. See also Balkan frame.

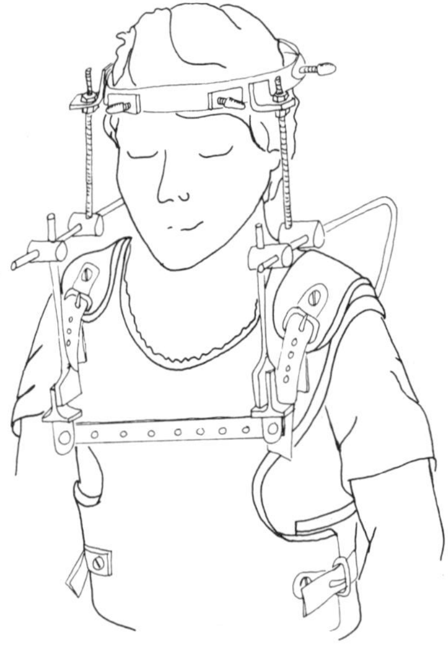

Halo vest and traction

tractotomy (trak-tot'o-mi): The operation of severing or making an incision into a nerve tract. Sometimes done for the relief of intractable pain.

trade name: Also called proprietary name. Usually refers to one registered by the U.S. Patent Office and is applied to a drug instead of the official name. Sometimes there are several trade names for the same drug since each pharmaceutical manufacturer may choose a different name for the same preparation.

tragacanth (trag'a-kanth): The dried gummy exudation of a shrub of the genus *Astralagus;* used in medicine as a demulcent and as an emulsifying, suspending, and thickening agent for medications. Gum tragacanth.

tragus (trā'gus): The small cartilaginous projection just anterior to the external auditory meatus, or one of the hairs at the entrance of the meatus.—tragi, pl.; tragal, adj.

trait (trāt): A distinctive, enduring aspect of an individual's personality, reflecting his or her pattern of interpersonal relationships and adaptation to the environment, *e.g.,* friendliness, orderliness, punctuality. **X-LINKED T.,** a genetically determined trait caused or controlled by a gene located on the X chromosome.

trance (trans): A state of profound unnatural stupor or sleep from which the patient cannot be aroused easily, or of partially suspended animation; may be induced by hysteria, catalepsy, hypnotism, or alcoholic indulgence; not due to organic disease. **MYSTIC T., T.** experienced by those practicing intense meditation.

tranquilizer (trang'kwi-lī-zer): Any of a large group of drugs that act by alleviating agitation and anxiety without inducing hypnosis or narcosis, while calming the patient; they induce drowsiness, greatly exaggerate the effects of alcohol, and may result in drug dependency. **MAJOR TRANQUILIZERS,** drugs used in treatment of psychoses. **MINOR TRANQUILIZERS,** drugs used primarily in treatment of tension, mild anxiety, convulsive disorders, psychic distress, and, sometimes, in cases of alcohol withdrawal.

trans-: Prefix denoting 1) through, across; 2) to the other side.

transaminase (trans-am'i-nās): An enzyme important in the catabolism of amino acids; found in large quantities in the cells of heart, liver, kidney, pancreas, and muscles; becomes elevated when any disease of these organs exists. **SERUM GLUTAMIC OXALOACETIC T.,** an enzyme normally present in the blood serum and some body tissues, the heart and liver in particular; increases in certain liver diseases and when the heart muscle is damaged, as in infarction, severe arrhythmias, or angina, and following cardiac catheterization; may increase from 4 to 10 times the normal during the first 24 hours after infarction. Abbreviated SGOT. **SERUM GLUTAMIC PYRUVIC T.,** an enzyme normally present in the body, especially in the liver; the blood level increases markedly in hepatitis or following tissue injury of the liver. Abbreviated SGPT.

transamination (trans-am'-in-ā'shun): A reaction in which one or more amino groups transfer from one amino acid compound to another, or from one molecule to another in a substance.

transamniotic (trans-am-ni-ot'ik): Through the amniotic fluid, as a **T.** transfusion of the fetus for hemolytic disease.

transanimation (trans-an'i-mā'shun): 1. Resuscitation. 2. Resuscitation by mouth-to-mouth breathing.

transcortical (trans-kor'ti-kal): Through or across the cortex of an organ; often refers to association tracts in the cortex of the brain.

transcutaneous (trans-kū-tā'nē-us): Pertaining to the passage of a substance through the unbroken skin, as occurs in inunction. Percutaneous.

transdermal (trans-der'mal): Through the skin; usually refers to a medication applied to the skin either by inunction or by application of a gauze dressing that is impregnated with the medication which is released over time.

transdiaphragmatic (trans-dī'a-fra-mat'ik): Through or across the diaphragm.

transducer (trans-dū'ser): A device that converts one form of energy into another. In electronics, an electrode (attached to an individual) that converts the energy created by certain body functions into electrical impulses that can be transmitted to an oscilloscope and displayed as waves that can be measured by a monitoring device. **DOPPLER ULTRASONIC T.**, a device that detects changes in the frequency of sounds along a blood vessel.

transect (tran-sekt'): To cut across or divide by cutting across.

transection (tran-sek'shun): A cutting made across the long axis of a structure. A cross section.

transfer: The moving of a patient from one surface to another, *e.g.*, from bed to chair. **ACTIVE T.**, **T.** in which the patient assists with the moving. **PASSIVE T.**, **T.** in which the patient is unable to assist and the moving is done entirely by another person(s) or by a lifting device. **T. FACTOR**, see under factor.

transfer RNA: Certain RNA molecules found in many varieties of cells and which enter into the formation of certain protein molecules in which the amino acid arrangement is determined by the DNA in the chromosomes.

transferase (trans'fer-ās): Any of several kinds of enzymes that act as catalysts in the transfer of atoms or groups of atoms from one molecule to another.

transference (trans-fer'ens): 1. The conveying or shifting of something from one place to another. 2. The shifting of symptoms from one side of the body to the other; sometimes occurs in certain hysterical states. 3. The displacement by the patient of mental attitudes or emotions formerly directed to one object or person, often to the psychotherapist. **THOUGHT T.**, the transfer of thoughts from one person to another; telepathy.

transferrin (trans-fer'in): A globulin of the blood serum concerned chiefly with the binding and the transportation of iron from the intestine to the bloodstream.

transfix (trans-fiks'): To pierce through completely, as with a sharp instrument.

transformation (trans'for-mā'shun): A decided change in structure, form, function, or behavior. In cell biology, the conversion of a normal cell into one that is susceptible to carcinogenic influences.

transformer (trans-for'mer): An electrical apparatus that transfers electric energy from one or more alternating current circuits to one or more other circuits, with a change in voltage, current, phase, or other characteristic.

transfusion (trans-fū'zhun): The introduction of a fluid such as plasma, blood, saline or other solution directly into the bloodstream of the patient. **BLOOD T.**, the transfer of blood, directly or indirectly, from one person into the vein of another person. **DIRECT T.**, **T.** of blood from donor to donee via a tube connecting two of their arteries; also called arterial **T.** and immediate **T.** **EXCHANGE T.**, alternate withdrawal of part of the recipient's blood and replacement with donor blood until the greater part has been exchanged; used for Rhesus babies affected with erythroblastosis fetalis. **INDIRECT T.**, **T.** of blood that has been previously collected and stored under suitable conditions. **INTRAUTERINE T.**, **T.** of Rh-negative blood directly into the peritoneal cavity of the fetus in treatment of erythroblastosis fetalis. **PERITONEAL T.**, the infusion of saline solution into the peritoneal cavity. **PLATELET T.**, **T.** of platelets; used in treatment of individuals with severe thrombocytopenia (*q.v.*). **TOTAL T.**, see exchange **T.**—transfuse v.

transfusion reaction: The response of a recipient to the transfusion of blood that is in some way incompatible with his or her own; may be due to erythrocyte incompatibility, an allergic condition, or some preservative substance in blood that has been stored. Symptoms begin early in the procedure and include headache, rapid thready pulse, dyspnea, fever, cold clammy skin, and, possibly, shock.

transient (tran'shent): Passing quickly into and out of existence.

transient ischemic attack: A sudden episode of ischemia resulting in neurological signs that usually last from 5 minutes to several hours; incidence increases with age; recurrence is common. Symptoms include disturbance of vision, numbness of an extremity or of one side of the body, slurred speech, dizziness. May be associated with atherosclerosis or vertebrobasilar circulation. Incidence increases with age; recurrence is common.

transiliac (trans-il'i-ak): Passing from one ilium to the other, or extending from one iliac spine to the other.

transillumination (trans-i-lū-mi-nā'shun): The transmission of light through a cavity or sinus for diagnostic purposes.

transit time: Usually refers to the time it takes for ingested material to appear in the feces.

transitional (tran-sish'un-al): Pertaining to or characterized by change. **T. CELL CARCINOMA,** a malignant tumor containing anaplastic transitional cells.

translucent (trans-lū'sent): Intermediate between opaque and transparent; describing a substance that allows the passage of light, but which diffuses the light so that objects are not clearly distinguishable through it.

transmigration (trans-mī-grā'shun): A wandering across or through; usually refers to the passage of blood cells through a vessel wall; see diapedesis. **OVULAR T.,** the passage of an ovum from an ovary to the fallopian tube on the opposite side.

transmissible (trans-mis'si-b'l): Capable of being transferred from one person to another; said of certain diseases.

transmission (trans-mish'un): 1. The transfer of a disease from one person to another. 2. The passing on of an inheritable quality from parent to offspring. 3. The passage of a nerve impulse along a neural pathway or across a synapse.

transmural (trans-mū'ral): Through the wall, *e.g.*, of a cyst, organ or vessel.—transmurally, adv.

transmutation (trans-mū-tā'shun): A transformation or change in form, appearance, or nature. In physics, the conversion of one element into another by one or a series of nuclear reactions, or the changes of one nuclide into another.

transorbital (trans-or'bit-al): Passing through the eye socket.

transpeptidase (trans-pep'ti-dās): An enzyme that acts as a catalyst in the transfer of an amino or a peptide group from one molecule to another.

transperitoneal (trans'per-i-tō-nē'al): Through the abdominal wall or the abdomen.

transpiration (tran-spī-rā'shun): The giving off of vapor or moisture through the skin or a membrane, or of air through the lungs.—transpire, v.

transplacental (trans-pla-sen'tal): Through or across the placenta.

transplant (trans-plant', trans'plant): 1. To transfer living tissue from one part to another, or an organ from one person to another. 2. The tissue or organ that is transplanted from one part, or person, to another.

transplantar (trans-plan'tar): Denotes extension across the sole of the foot, particularly with reference to muscles and ligaments.

transplantation (trans-plan-tā'shun): Grafting, on to one part, tissue or an organ taken from another part or another body, *e.g.*, heart, kidney, tendon.—transplant, v.

transpleural (trans-ploo'ral): Through the pleura or across the pleural cavity.

transpose (trans-pōz'): To change from one location to another; may refer to a tissue or an organ.

transposition (trans-pō-zish'un): 1. The location or displacement of an internal organ to the side of the body that is opposite its usual site. 2. An exchange of atoms within a molecule. 3. The attachment of a tissue flap to a new site without separating it from the old one until it has united with the tissues at the new location. **T. OF THE GREAT VESSELS,** a congenital heart defect in which the aorta arises from the right rather than the left ventricle and the pulmonary artery arises from the left rather than the right ventricle. In embryology, the shifting of gentic material from one chromosome to another, resulting in a congenital anomaly.

transseptal (trans-sep'tal): Through or across a septum. **T. CARDIAC CATHETERIZATION,** performed by puncturing the atrial septum in order to perform left heart studies.

transsexual (trans-seks'u-al): Term applied to persons who have the body and generative organs of one sex, but are convinced that they were meant to be a member of the other sex. Such persons distinguish themselves from homosexuals and transvestites and are often obsessed with wanting to be physically changed to the opposite sex; this is sometimes attempted through surgery and hormonal treatment.

transsynaptic (trans-si-nap'tik): Refers to the passage of a nerve impulse over a synapse.

transtelephone surveillance: Term applied to a home-based program that provides for telephone monitoring of persons who have a pacemaker and who are suspected or known to have cardiac arrhythmia; a useful diagnostic tool that can also identify pacemaker problems and initiate emergency care as well as routine treatment for patients with a pacemaker.

transthoracic (trans-thō-ras'ik): Across or through the chest wall or chest cavity.

transtracheal (trans-trā'kē-al): Refers to a surgical procedure performed by passage through the wall of the trachea.

transudate (trans'ū-dāt): A liquid substance that has passed over a membrane or through some other permeable substance. See **transude.**

transude (trans-ūd'): To ooze or pass through a membrane or permeable substance, *e.g.*, the oozing of blood serum through intact vessel walls.—transudation, n.

transureteroureterostomy (trans-ū-rē′ter-ō-ū-rē-ter-os′to-mi): The surgical procedure of transposing a ureter across the midline and suturing it to the opposite ureter in order to bypass an obstruction.

transurethral (trans-ū-rē′thral): By way of the urethra. **T. RESECTION,** prostatectomy or removal of part of the lower urinary tract by means of an instrument passed through the urethra; see prostatectomy.

transvaginal (trans-vaj′in-al): Through or across the vagina; surgery performed through the vagina.—transvaginally, adv.

transventricular (trans-ven-trik′ū-lar): Through a ventricle. Term used mainly in connection with surgery on cardiac valves.—transventricularly, adv.

transverse (trans-vers′): Crosswise or situated at right angles to the long axis of the body or of a part. **T. FRACTURE,** a fracture in which the line of fracture is at right angles to the long axis of the bone. **T. COLON,** the section of the large intestine that crosses the abdomen from the right to the left. **T. LIE** or **PRESENTATION,** a crosswise position of the fetus in the uterus that must be altered before the child can be born normally.

transversectomy (trans-ver-sek′tō-mi): The surgical removal of a transverse process of a vertebra to relieve pressure on a nerve root.

transversus abdominis (trans-ver′sus ab-dom′i-nis): A muscle that forms part of the muscular wall of the side of the abdomen.

transvesical (trans-ves′i-kal): Through the bladder, by custom referring to the urinary bladder.—transvesically, adv.

transvestite (trans-ves′tīt): One who practices tranvestitism (*q.v.*).

transvestitism (trans-ves-ti-tism): A sexual deviation in which one has the desire to wear the clothes of and in other ways masquerade as a member of the opposite sex.

trapeze (tra-pēz′): A triangular device hung from the ceiling or from a bar over the bed which can be adjusted to the patient's reach; assists the person to change his position in bed or to sit up.

trapezium (tra-pē′zi-um): An irregular four-sided figure; specifically the first bone on the thumb side of the second row of carpal bones. Also called the greater multangular bone.—trapezial, trapeziform, adj.

trapezius (tra-pē′zi-us): The large flat, triangular superficial muscle on either side of the posterior part of the neck and upper thorax; it draws the head backward, raises, depresses and rotates the scapula and draws it backward toward the spine.

trapezoid (trap′e-zoyd): Resembling a trapezium (*q.v.*); specifically the second bone in the second row of carpal bones. Also called the lesser multangular bone.

Traube's semilunar space: An area on the lower left front side of the chest where percussion will produce tympanic sounds when there is air in the stomach.

trauma (traw′ma): A wound or injury caused by external force or violence. **BIRTH T.,** injury to an infant during its delivery or, in psychology, the injury to the infant's psyche from the process of being born. **PSYCHOLOGICAL T.,** an emotional shock or an experience that has a more or less permanent effect upon the mind, especially the subconscious mind.—traumatic, adj.; traumatize, n.

traumasthenia (traw-mas-thē′ni-a): Nervous exhaustion or neurosis following injury or violence.

traumatic (traw-mat′ik): Related to or caused by an injury or wound.

traumatize (traw′ma-tīz): To produce injury or trauma through accident or by carelessness.

traumatogenic (traw′ma-tō-jen′ik): Capable of causing a wound or injury.

traumatology (traw-ma-tol′o-ji): The branch of surgery that deals with wounds or accident surgery.

traumatopathy (traw-ma-top′a-thi): Any pathologic condition resulting from injury or violence.

traumatophilia (traw′ma-tō-fil′i-a): The unconscious tendency to become injured, or the craving for injury.

traumatophobia (traw′-ma-tō-fō′bi-a): Morbid fear of being injured.

traumatosepsis (traw′ma-tō-sep′sis): Infection of or following a wound.

travail (tra-vāl′): The labor of childbirth.

travel sickness: See motion sickness.

Treacher-Collins syndrome: Mandibulofacial dysostosis; see under dysostosis.

treadmill (tred′mil): A walkway that moves while the subject "walks" on it while remaining in place. **T. TEST,** Bruce treadmill test (*q.v.*).

treat: To give aid to a person suffering from a pathological, traumatic, or psychiatric condition by means of medical, surgical, nutritional, corrective, curative, or rehabilitative measures.

treatment: Medical or surgical care of an ill person, aimed at relieving symptoms of a disease or curing the disease. **CONSERVATIVE T.,** that in which surgery or other drastic measures are withheld if, and as long as, possible. **CURATIVE T.,** that aimed at curing a disease. **EMPIRIC T.,** that based on measures that experience has shown to be effective in the particular condition. **KENNY'S T.,** see Kenny. **MEDICAL T., T.** by drugs, hygienic and other methods, that are distinguished from surgical methods. **PALLIATIVE T.**, that which aims to relieve pain and distress but does not attempt to cure the causative disease. **PROPHYLACTIC T.**, that which aims to prevent a person from being attacked by a specific disease; also called **PREVENTIVE T.** **SHOCK T.**, consists of induction of coma or convulsions by injection of insulin or other drug or by passing an electric current through the brain. **SIPPY T.**, see Sippy diet, under diet. **SPECIFIC T.**, that which is aimed at removing the specific cause of a disease; frequently refers to diseases caused by bacteriological invasion. **SURGICAL T.**, includes **T.** by cutting operations and manual procedures such as reducing fractures without making an incision. **SYMPTOMATIC T.**, **T.** of symptoms as they arise in the course of a disease rather than treating the cause.—treat, v.

Trematoda (trem'a-tō'da): A class of parasitic fluke-worms that includes many pathogens of humans, such as the Schistosoma of bilharziasis.

trematodiasis (trem'a-tō-dī'a-sis): Infestation with a trematode.

tremens (trē'mens): Trembling; shaking. **DELIRIUM T.**, a form of acute mental disturbance caused by excessive use of alcohol and marked by hallucinations, memory disturbances, sweating, restlessness, mental confusion, severe tremor.

tremograph (trem'ō-graf): A device for recording tremor.

tremolabile (trē'mō-lā'bil): Easily destroyed or inactivated by agitation or shaking.

tremor (trem'or): Involuntary, purposeless, rhythmic contraction of agonist and antagonist muscles causing trembling or quivering of a body part; may be due to disorders of the brain, *e.g.*, Parkinson's disease, emotional disorders, effect of alcohol and other drugs on the nervous system, fear, or aging. **ANXIETY STATE T.**, a fine tremor, usually of the hands, which may be cold and clammy. **COARSE T.**, violent **T.** in which the vibrations are not over six or seven per second. **CONTINUOUS T.**, that which occurs constantly as seen in paralysis agitans. **ESSENTIAL T.**, fine, isolated tremor, possibly familial; exaggerated by ingestion of alcohol, activity, and sedatives; disappears during rest. **FINE T.**, slight trembling in which the vibrations may be 10 or 12 per second; seen in the outstretched hand of persons with thyrotoxicosis; the hands are usually warm. **INTENTION T.**, occurs when voluntary movement is attempted; characteristic of disseminated sclerosis. **PASSIVE T.**, occurs only when the person is at rest; disappears when active movement is undertaken; also called resting tremor. **SENILE T.**, a benign **T.** that occurs in older persons often without other symptoms; involves the head, jaw, and hands; at first seen only when the person uses the affected part; is increased by cold, fatigue, emotional states. **TOXIC T.**, may be fine or coarse with no rigidity; seen in alcoholism and other drug intoxications.—tremulous, adj.

tremostable (trē'mō-stā'b'l): Not easily destroyed or inactivated by agitation or shaking.

tremulous (trem'ū-lus): Trembling; quivering; exhibiting tremor.—tremulousness, n.

trench: **T. FEVER**, a rickettsial infection caused by the bite of an infected body louse; a major medical problem of World War I when the soldiers were in trenches for long periods of time with no opportunity to practice personal hygiene. **T. FOOT**, a condition resembling frostbite; also a medical problem during World War I when men stood in trenches for long periods of time with wet, cold feet. **T. MOUTH**, see angina, Vincent's.

Trendelenburg: **T. GAIT**, a gait that develops following paralysis of the gluteus medius muscle; the person leans the trunk toward the affected side with each step. Also called gluteal gait. **T'S. OPERATION**, ligation of the long saphenous vein in the groin at its junction with the femoral vein. Used in treatment of varicose veins. **T. POSITION**, the **P.** in which the patient is supine on an inclined plane with the head lowered and the knees elevated at a 45° angle, thus causing the pelvic and abdominal organs to drop toward the thoracic cavity. **T.'S SIGN**, seen in congenital dislocation of the hip, when the patient stands on the dislocated leg and flexes the hip and knee on the unaffected side, that side will sag, whereas in normal conditions it would rise. **T.'S TEST**, test for competency of the veins of the leg; with the patient lying down, the leg is held upright until the veins are empty; then the leg is lowered and the patient quickly stands up; if the veins are normal they will fill from below, if not, they will fill from above. [Friederich Trendelenberg, German surgeon. 1844–1924.]

trepanation (trep'a-nā'shun): The surgical procedure of trephining. Trephination.

trephination (tref'i-nā'shun): The operation of trephining; usually refers to opening the skull with a trephine. In dentistry, the surgical creation of an opening through the gum tissues to the root of a tooth.

trephine (trē-fīn'): 1. An instrument with saw-tooth-like edges used to remove a circular piece from a structure, *e.g.*, cornea or skull. 2. To perform an operation with a trephine. Also trepan.

trepidant (trep'i-dant): Exhibiting tremor; trembling.

Treponema (trep'ō-nē'ma): A genus of motile, slender, spiral-shaped bacteria, some of which are pathogenic to man. **T. PALLIDUM**, the causative organism of syphilis (*q.v.*) in man. **T. PERTENUE**, the causative organism of yaws (*q.v.*).

treponematosis (trep'ō-nē-ma-tō'sis): Infection caused by a variety of treponema. See yaws.

treponemicidal (trep'ō-nē-mi-sī'dal): Destructive to any organism of the genus *Treponema*.

trepopnea (trē-pop'nē-a): An uncommon term that describes a situation in which breathing is comfortable in one position but not another; usually occurs when the patient is turned to the left side.

-tresia: A combining form denoting perforation.

tresis (trē'sis): Perforation.

TRF: Abbreviation for thyrotropin-releasing factor. See under thyrotropin.

tri-: Combining form denoting three, three times.

triad (trī'ad): A group of three related objects or elements.

triage (trē'ahzh): The prompt sorting out and classification of injured or seriously ill persons in war, disaster, or emergency situation, whether in hospital or in the field, to determine who should be cared for, in what order, and where. In war, this, along with giving first aid, is done at the front before evacuating casualties to the rear. Casualties are classified as 1) those who need immediate treatment in order to survive, 2) those who will survive without immediate treatment, and 3) those who cannot be expected to survive under any circumstances.

triageur (trē-a-juhr'): A health professional who has been trained in triage assessment and procedures, who may work in a hospital emergency room, a mobile emergency care unit, or in the field; may be a nurse, paramedic, emergency medical technician, or a physician.

trial-and-error learning: The apparently random, haphazard activity that may precede acquisition of knowledge; may be overt and observable or covert and mental in character.

triamelia (trī'a-mē'li-a): The congenital anomaly characterized by the absence of three limbs.

triangle (trī'ang-g'l): A geometric figure having three sides and three angles. In anatomy, a three-sided area the sides of which may be determined by natural structures or represented by arbitrarily drawn lines.

triangular (trī-ang'ū-lar): Resembling or having the shape of a triangle. **T. BANDAGE,** see under bandage.

tribasic (trī-bā'sik): Refers to a substance that has a valence of 3.

TRIC: Acronym for agents that cause *t*rachoma and *i*nclusion *c*onjunctivitis which is widespread in tropical areas where trachoma is a common cause of blindness associated with poor living conditions and lack of hygiene. In temperate climates these agents cause conjunctivitis as well as urethritis and cervicitis.

tricephalus (trī-sef'a-lus): A fetal monster having three heads.

triceps (trī'seps): Three-headed; specifically the three-headed muscle on the back of the upper arm that extends the forearm, and the triceps surae on the back of the lower leg (the gastrocnemius and soleus muscles considered as one), that flexes the leg and extends the foot. **T. TENDON REFLEX,** see under reflex. **T. SKINFOLD,** the skinfold measurement at midarm, used to determine the amount of stored fat.

trich-, thricho-: Combining forms denoting: 1. Hair. 2. Filament.

trichatrophia (trik-a-trō'fi-a): A brittle dry state of the hair due to atrophy of the hair bulbs.

trichauxis (trik-awk'sis): Excessive growth of the hair.

-trichia: A combining form denoting hairiness, or the condition of the hair.

trichiasis (tri-kī'a-sis): Inversion or ingrowing of an eyelash causing irritation from friction on the eyeball.

Trichinella (trik'i-nel'la): A genus of nematode worms that infest both humans and animals. **T. SPIRALIS,** the nematode that causes trichinosis in man.

trichinosis (trik'i-nō'sis): A disease that results from eating raw or undercooked meat, pork in particular, that is infested with a parasitic worm, the *Trichinella spiralis*. The female worms live in the small intestine and produce larvae which invade the body and, in particular, form cysts in skeletal muscles; the usual symptoms are abdominal pain, diarrhea, nausea, fever, facial edema, fatigue, muscular pains, and stiffness. Also called trichiniasis and trichenelliasis.

trichitis (tri-kī'tis): Inflammation of the hair bulbs.

trichloride (trī-klō'rīd): A chloride having a valence of 3.

trichloroacetic acid (trī'klor-ō-a-sē'tik): An astringent and caustic escharotic used chiefly to remove warts.

trichloromethane (trī'klor-ō-meth'ān): Chloroform.

trichobezoar (trik'ō-bē'zōr): A hairball; a concretion found in the stomach or intestine and containing hairs.

Trichocephalus (trik'o-sef'ah-lus): Old name for a genus of nematodes, now called *Trichuris*. See Trichuris trichuria.

trichoclasia (trik'ō-klā'zi-a): Brittleness and breaking off of the hair.

trichocryptomania (trik'ō-krip-tō-mā'ni-a): An abnormal desire to pull out one's hair, usually that of the scalp.

trichocryptosis (trik'ō-krip-tō'sis): Any disease of the hair follicles.

trichoepithelioma (trik′ō-ep-i-thē-li-ō′ma): A small benign nodule, usually multiple, occurring on the skin, particularly that of the face, that has its origin in a hair follicle.

trichoesthesia (trik′ō-es-thē′zi-a): 1. The sensation one feels when a hair is touched. 2. A form of paresthesia in which one has a sensation as of hair being on the conjunctiva, the skin, or the mucous membrane of the mouth.

trichogen (trik′ō-jen): An agent that promotes growth of hair.—trichogenous, adj.

trichoglossia (trik′ō-glos′i-a): "Hairy" tongue; see under **tongue**.

tricholith (trik′ō-lith): A concretion forming on the hair.

trichologia (trik-ō-lō′ji-a): Constant pulling at the hair.

trichoma (tri-kō′ma): 1. Trichiasis (*q.v.*). 2. Trichomatosis (*q.v.*).

trichomatosis (tri-kō′ma-tō′sis): A matted, filthy condition of the hair, due to neglect, lack of hygiene, and infestation by parasites.

Trichomonas (tri-kom′ō-nas): A genus of flagellated protozoa, certain of which are parasitic in the intestinal tract, mouth, vagina, or urethra of humans. **T. VAGINALIS,** the causative agent of a common chronic disease of the genitourinary tract, trichomoniasis (*q.v.*).

trichomoniasis (trik′ō-mō-nī′a -sis): Infection of the genitourinary tract with the protozoal parasite Trichomonas (*q.v.*). Characterized in women by vaginitis and profuse, foamy, yellowish discharge with a foul odor; in men the agent lives in the urethra, prostate, and seminal vesicles, and seldom causes objective symptoms. Transmitted through sexual intercourse.

trichomycosis (trik′ō-mī-kō-sis): Formerly thought to be any disease of the hair that is caused by a fungus; now known to be caused by a Nocardia (*q.v.*).

trichonosis (trik′ō-nō′sis): Any disease of the hair.

trichophagy (tri-kof′a-ji): The nervous habit of biting or eating hair.

Trichophyton (tri-kof′i-ton): A genus of fungi found on the skin, hair, and nails; often a cause of allergy; a causative agent in ringworm or tinea. **T. RUBRUM,** causes chronic superficial infections of the skin and nails. **T. TONSURANS,** a species of ringworm fungus that causes tinea capitis; see **tinea**.

trichophytosis (trik′ō-fī-tō′sis): Infection with a Trichophyton fungus, *e.g.*, ringworm of the hair or skin.

trichorrhea (trik′ō-rē′a): Rapid or excessive falling out of the hair.

trichorrhexis (trik′ōr-rek′sis): Brittleness of the hair with a tendency to break. **T. NODOSA,** the appearance of small white areas on the hairs that look like nodes but are actually places where the hair has partially fractured and split, leaving brush-like ends.

trichosiderin (trik-ō-sid′er-in): An iron containing pigment found in red human hair.

trichosis (trī-kō′sis): Any disease or abnormal condition of the hair.

Trichosporon (tri-kos′pō-ron): A genus of fungi that grow on the hair shaft.

trichosporosis (trik′ō-spō-rō′sis): A fungal infection of the hair shaft.

trichotillomania (trik′ō-til-lō-mā′ni-a): An uncontrollable compulsion to pull out one's own hair.

trichotomy (trī-kot′-o-mi): Being divided into three parts.

trichotrophy (trī-kot′rō-fi): Nutrition of the hair.

trichromatopsia (tri-krō′ -ma-top′si-a): Normal color vision.

trichromic (trī-krō′mik): 1. Having three colors. 2. Being able to perceive three colors; red, green, and blue.

trichuriasis (trik-ū-rī′a-sis): Infestation with *Trichuris trichiura,* a whipworm; a syndrome occurring most frequently in the tropics and often causing no symptoms although in some cases there is diarrhea, vomiting, nervous disorders, and loss of weight.

Trichuris (trik-ū′ris): A genus of roundworms of the class Nematoda that infest humans. **T. TRICHURA,** a whipworm with a coiled head that is parasitic in the large intestine of mammals including humans.

tricipital (trī-sip′i-tal): 1. Pertaining to a triceps muscle. 2. Having three heads.

tricrotic (trī-krot′ik): Pertinent to a pulse in which three waves are palpated during each heartbeat.

tricuspid (trī-kus′pid): Having three cusps or points. **T. VALVE,** that between the right atrium and ventricle of the heart; it allows blood to flow freely from the right atrium into the right ventricle and prevents backflow of blood from the ventricle into the atrium during ventricular contraction. **T. TOOTH,** a tooth having three cusps on the crown, as may occur on the second or third upper molar.

trifacial (trī-fā′shal): Denoting the 5th pair of cranial nerves. See **trigeminal**.

trifid (trī′fid): Split into three or having three corresponding parts.

trifocal (trī′fō-kal): Refers to eyeglasses that have three refractive powers in the same lens; to correct vision for distant, intermediate, and close objects.

trifurcation (trī′fur-kā′shun): A division into three prongs or branches.—trifurcate, adj.

trigastric (trī-gas′trik): Having three bellies; usually said of a certain muscle.

trigeminal (trī-jem′in-al): Triple; separating into three sections, *e.g.*, the **T. NERVES**, the 5th pair of cranial nerves, which have three branches and supply the skin of the face, tongue and teeth. **T. NEURALGIA**, see tic douloureux. **T. PULSE**, pulsus trigeminus, see under pulsus.

trigeminy (trī-jem′i-ni): 1. Occuring in threes. 2. A type of heartbeat in which the beats occur in groups of three.

trigger (trig′er): 1. An act or impulse that initiates an action. 2. To initiate an action. **T. FINGER**, a condition in which the finger can be bent but cannot be straightened without help; usually due to a thickening on the tendon which prevents free gliding. **T. THUMB**, tenderness at the base of the thumb and sometimes snapping or triggering movements; due to tenosynovitis of the pollicis longus muscle, often an occupational injury. **T. POINT**, an area of hyperexcitability where the application of a stimulus will provoke pain or other phenomenon to a greater degree than in the surrounding area. **T. ZONE**, an area of hypersensitivity where a stimulus will elicit a specific response.

triglyceride (trī-glis′er-īd): Any of a group of naturally occurring esters, composed of glycerol and three fatty acids (stearic, oleic, palmitic); found in most animal and vegetable fats; the chief constituent of adipose tissue and the major form in which fat is stored in the body.

trigone (trī′gōn): A triangular area, especially applied to the bladder base bounded by the ureteral openings at the back, and the urethral opening at the front.—trigonal, adj.

trigonitis (trī′gō-nī′tis): Inflammation of the trigone of the urinary bladder; characterized by frequency, urgency, and dysuria.

triiodothyronine (trī′ī-ō-dō-thī′rō-nēn): Either of two hormones present in the thyroid. See liothyronine and thyroxine.

trilateral (trī-lat′er-al): Having three sides.

trilobate (trī-lō′bāt): Having three lobes.

trilocular (trī-lok′ū-lar): Having three cells or chambers.

trilogy of Fallot: A congenital anomaly consisting of an atrial defect, pulmonic stenosis, and right ventricular hypertrophy. See tetralogy of Fallot.

trimensual (trī-men′sū-al): Occurring at intervals of three months.

trimester (trī-mes′ter): A period of 3 months. Usually refers to one-third of the length of a pregnancy.

triolism (trī′ō-lizm): Sexual practices involving three people, one of whom is usually a homosexual who engages in voyeurism by watching his usual partner in a sexual act with the third person.

triorchid (trī-or′kid): 1. Having three testes. 2. An individual who has three testes.

trip: In drug culture, an hallucinogenic drug experience. **BAD T.**, temporary or chronic psychosis or a panic reaction following use of a hallucinogen (*q.v.*).

tripanopia (trip-a-nō′pi-a): Color blindness for the color blue, the third of the primary colors.

tripara (trip′a-ra): A woman who has had three pregnancies resulting in three live offspring. Also written Para III.

tripeptide (trī-pep′tīd): A peptide that yields three peptides on hydrolysis.

triplegia (trī-plē′ji-a): 1. Hemiplegia with one limb on the opposite side also affected. 2. Paralysis of the face and an upper and a lower extremity.

triplet: One of three children born at the same birth.

triploidy (trip′loy-di): In humans, the presence of 69 chromosomes instead of the normal 46; a condition commonly seen in abortuses.

triplopia (trip-lō′pi-a): A defect of vision in which one sees three images of a single object.

tripsis (trip′sis): 1. Trituration (*q.v.*). 2. Massage.

-tripsy: A combining form denoting a crushing.

trisaccharide (trī-sak′a-rīd): A carbohydrate that yields three monosaccharide molecules on hydrolysis.

trismus (triz′mus): Spasm in the muscles of the mastication caused by motor disturbance of the trigeminal nerve; an early sign of lockjaw.—trismic, adj.

trisomy (trī′sō-mi): A chromosomal anomaly; a state in which one of the chromosomes is present in triplicate rather than in a pair, *i.e.*, in human trisomy, the total number of chromosomes is 47 instead of the normal 46. Three main types are recognized: 1) **TRISOMY 13**, or **TRISOMY D**, is relatively rare; the extra chromosome is from the 13–15 group, usually 13; in this condition there is cleft lip and palate, microcephaly, abnormalities of forehead, nose and eyes; polydactyly, mental deficiency, failure to thrive; and a poor prognosis for life, with death occurring usually during the first year; also called Patau's syndrome. 2) *Trisomy 18*, or *trisomy E*, usually occurs in children of parents over 30; characterized by low birth weight, abnormal facies with low-set malformed ears, micrognathia, heart defects, hypertonicity, severe mental deficiency, and poor prognosis for life. Occurs most often in female children; also called Edwards' syndrome. 3) Trisomy 21, Down's syndrome (*q.v.*).

tristimania (tris-ti-mā′ni-a): Melancholia.

tritium (trit′i-um): A radioactive isotope of hydrogen; used as a tracer in metabolic studies.

triturate (trit′ū-rāt): To make into a fine powder.

trituration (trit′ū-rā′shun): The process of reducing a substance to a fine powder.

trivalent (tri-vā′lent): Having a valence of 3. **TRIVALENT ORAL POLIOVACCINE (TOPV),** see Sabin's vaccine.

trocar (trō′kar): A sharply pointed tube that fits inside a cannula that is used for withdrawing fluid from a cavity; after the instrument is inserted, the rod is withdrawn. The term is sometimes used to designate both the cannula and the trocar. Also trochar.

trochanter (trō-kan′ter): One of two bony prominences on the upper end of the femur. The **MAJOR** or **GREATER T.** is on the outer side of the femur; the **MINOR** or **LESSER T.** is on the inner side of the femur between the shaft and the neck; they serve for the attachment of muscles. **T. ROLL,** a large towel or other material rolled and placed under the greater trochanter of the patient in supine position; used to prevent external rotation of the lower limb.—trochanteric, adj.

troche (trō′ke): A medicated disk, tablet, or lozenge in a flavored sweetened mucilaginous substance that is held under the tongue or in the cheek until it is dissolved.

trochlea (trok′lē-a): An anatomical term used to describe a part or structure that is like a pulley in function or appearance; usually a tendon or projection on a bone.—trochlear, adj.

trochlear (trok′lē-ar): 1. Pertaining to a trochlea. 2. Name given to the 4th pair of cranial nerves; important in coordination and control of movements of the eyeball.

trochoides (trō-koy′-dēz): A joint in which the only movement allowed is pivotal, *i.e.*, rotation around the longitudinal axis of the bone; an example is the rotation of the first cervical vertebra around the odontoid process of the second cervical vertebra.

troph-, tropho-: Combining forms denoting nutrition or food.

trophic (trō′fik): Pertaining to nutrition.

-trophic: A combining form denoting 1) nutrition, or 2) a specific type of nutrition.

trophoblast (trof′ō-blast): A layer of ectodermal tissue that serves to attach the ovum to the wall of the uterus and supply nourishment to the embryo.—trophoblastic, adj.

trophoblastoma (trof-ō-blas-tō′ma): Choriocarcinoma (*q.v.*).

trophoneurosis (trof′ō-nū-rō′sis): Any trophic disorder such as atrophy or hypertrophy, caused by failure of nutrition resulting from disease or injury to the nerves of a part. See Raynaud's disease.—trophoneurotic, adj.

trophopathy (trō-fop′a-thi): Any disease or disorder of nutrition.

trophotherapy (trof-ō-ther′a-pi): Diet therapy.

trophotropism (trō-fot′rō-pizm): Repulsion or attraction to various nutritive substances, a characteristic of certain cells.

trophozoite (trof-ō-zō′īt): The active feeding stage of a protozoan as contrasted with the nonmotile encapsulated stage.

tropia (trō′pi-a): An abnormal turning or deviation of the eye; strabismus (*q.v.*).

-tropia: Combining form denoting deviation in the visual axis.

-tropic: Combining form denoting: 1. Turning; changing. 2. Attraction to a specific tissue, organ, or system.

tropical: Pertaining to or common to tropic areas. **T. DISEASE,** one which occurs with greater frequency and/or severity in tropical parts of the world. **T. MEDICINE,** the branch of medicine that deals with diseases that most commonly occur in tropical or subtropical areas of the world.

tropism (trō′pizm): An innate tendency to react in a definite manner to specific stimuli.

tropomyosin (trō-pō-mī′ō-sin): A muscle protein that acts to inhibit muscle contraction.

troponin (trō′pō-nin): A protein found in skeletal muscle; it assists in controlling heart muscle contraction.

Trousseau's sign: Carpopedal spasm; see under carpopedal. [Armand Trousseau, French physician. 1801–1867.]

truncal (trung′kal): Pertaining to the trunk of the body or of a nerve, artery, etc.

truncate (trung′kāt): To cut off; amputate. To cut off at right angles to the long axis of the part.—truncated, adj.

truncus arteriosus (trung′kus ar-ter-i-o′-sis): An arterial trunk arising from the fetal heart; it develops into the pulmonary artery and the aorta and normally does not persist after birth.

trunk: 1. The torso or main part of the body to which the head and extremities are attached. 2. The main, undivided part of a nerve, blood vessel or duct. **NERVE T.,** a collection of nerve fibers closely bound together and enclosed within a sheath of epineurium.

truss: An appliance consisting usually of a belt and a pressure pad, worn over a hernia to keep it in place after it has been reduced.

truth serum: Common name for a drug that acts to inhibit the nervous system and which is given to a person from whom it is desirable to obtain information not otherwise revealed.

trypanocide (tri-pan′ō-sīd): An agent that destroys trypanosomes; see Trypanosoma.

Trypanosoma (tri-pan′ō-sō′ma): A genus of parasitic protozoa; a limited number of species are pathogenic to humans. The species that is the vector of trypanosomiasis (*q.v.*) in Africa lives part of its life cycle in the tsetse fly (*q.v.*)

and is transferred to new hosts, including humans, in the salivary juices when the fly bites.

trypanosome (trī-pan′ō-sōm): One of any of the species of *Trypanosoma;* the protozoa are flagellated and live in the tissues and blood of the host.

trypanosomiasis (trī-pan′ō-sō-mī′a-sis): Disease produced by infection with Trypanosoma. In humans this may be *T. rhodesiense* in East Africa or *T. gambiense* in West Africa; both are transmitted by the tsetse fly and produce the illness known as African sleeping sickness, a severe, often fatal, disease marked by fever, intense headache, lymph node enlargement, anemia, wasting, and somnolence. Not found in the U.S., but Chagas' disease, caused by *T. cruzi* that is transmitted by bites of bloodsucking insects, is found in certain parts of South America.

trypsin (trip′sin): A proteolytic enzyme formed in the intestine when the trypsinogen from the pancreatic juice is acted upon by the enterokinase of the intestinal juice; it is the chief protein-digesting enzyme in the human.

trypsinogen (trip-sin′o-jen): The precursor of trypsin (*q.v.*), secreted by the pancreas; it is converted into trypsin when it comes into contact with enterokinase in the small intestine.

tryptophan (trip′tō-fān): One of the essential amino acids; necessary for optimal growth and for tissue repair; found in varying amounts in many proteins.

tryptophanuria (trip′tō-fan-ū′ri-a): The presence of tryptophan in the urine.

tsetse fly (tset′sē): A blood-sucking fly found in Africa; the vector of Trypanosoma (*q.v.*). Also tzetze.

TSH: Abbreviation for thyroid-stimulating hormone; see thyrotropin.

tsp: Abbreviation for teaspoon; teaspoonful.

tsutsugamushi disease (tsoo-tsū-ga-moosh′ē): Scrub typhus that occurs in Japan; transmitted by mites.

tubal (tu′bal): Pertaining to a tube. **T. ABORTION,** one in which an extrauterine pregnancy is terminated by rupture of the fallopian tube. **T. FEEDING,** see under feeding. **T. INSUFFLATION,** insufflation of the uterine tubes to test for patency; see Rubin's test. **T. LIGATION,** sterilization of a woman by closing off the uterine tubes with a ligature; may also involve crushing or severing the tubes. **T. PREGNANCY,** see ectopic.

tube: An elongated, cylindrical structure or apparatus. For particular tubes, see Abbott-Miller, auditory, bronchial, Cantor, digestive, drainage, endotracheal, esophageal, eustachian, Ewald, fallopian, feeding, gastric, intubation, Lanz, Levin, nasogastric, nephrostomy, neural, rectal, Rehfuss', Ryle's, Sengstaken-Blakemore, Shiley, Southey's, stomach, T, test, thoracostomy, tracheostomy, Wangensteen.

tube feeding: Usually refers to feeding an unconscious patient or one who has a throat problem by introducing pureed or blenderized food directly into the stomach via a tube that is inserted through either the nose or the esophagus. May also refer to hyperalimentation (*q.v.*).

tubectomy (tū-bek′to-mi): Plastic repair or excision of a tube, a fallopian tube in particular; salpingectomy.

tuber: A localized swelling, knob, protuberance.

tubercle (tū′ber-k′l): 1. A small solid elevation or nodule on the skin, mucous membrane, or surface of an organ. 2. A small rounded eminence on a bone. 3. The specific lesion produced by the *Mycobacterium tuberculosis.*—tubercular, adj. See Ghon's focus.

tuberculation (tū-ber′ -kū-lā′shun): The development of tubercles.

tuberculides (tū-ber′kū-līds): A group of erythematous, papular, or other skin manifestations thought to be due to the presence of tuberculosis elsewhere in the body.

tuberculin (tūber′kū-lin): A sterile extract of either crude (old **T.**) or refined (Purified Protein Derivative; P.P.D.) complex protein constituents of the tubercle bacillus. Its most common use is in determining whether a person has or has not previously been infected with the tubercule bacillus, by injecting a small amount into the skin and reading the reaction, if any, in 48 to 72 hours: may be done by the Mantoux method, jet injection, or multiple injections (see Mantoux and tine test): negative reactors are those who have escaped previous infection. **OLD T.,** a concentrated filtrate made from a 6-week-old culture of the tubercle bacillus; it does not contain the microorganisms, only the soluble products of bacterial growth.

tuberculitis (tū-ber′kū-lī′tis): Inflammation of a tubercle.

tuberculization (tū-ber′kū-lī-zā′shun): The formation of tubercles.

tuberculocele (tū-ber′kū-lō-sēl): Tuberculosis of a testis.

tuberculocidal (tū-ber′kū-lō-sī′dal): Having the ability to kill *Mycobacterium tuberculosis* (*q.v.*).

tuberculoid (tū-ber′kū-loid): Resembling tuberculosis or a tubercle.

tuberculoma (tū-ber′kū-lō′ma): 1. A large caseous tubercle, its size suggesting a tumor. 2. A tuberculous abscess. 3. Any new growth or nodule of tuberculous origin.

tuberculosis (tū-ber′kū-lō′sis): A specific, chronic, infectious disease caused by the *Mycobacterium tuberculosis,* characterized by the formation of tubercles in the tissues. Often asymptomatic at first; later the local symptoms depend upon the part affected, and general symptoms are those of sepsis, *i.e.*, fever, sweats, emaciation. In humans the disease most commonly affects the lungs but may also affect the meninges, joints, bones, lymph nodes, kidney, intestine, larynx, or skin. **AVIAN T.**, endemic in birds and rarely seen in humans. **BOVINE T.**, endemic in cattle and transmitted to humans via cow's milk, causing **T.** of glands but rarely of the lungs; less common than formerly. **MILIARY T.**, a generalized acute form of **T.** in which, as a result of bloodstream dissemination, minute, multiple tuberculous foci are scattered throughout many organs of the body; it is often rapidly fatal. **PRIMARY T.**, infection with *Mycobacterium tuberculosis* for the first time; characterized by the formation, usually in the lung, of a local lesion that is most often benign, self-limited, and heals spontaneously; also called childhood **T.** **PULMONARY T.**, **T.** of the lung; the most common site of the disease in man; also called consumption, phthisis. **SECONDARY T.**, the adult type as distinguished from the primary or childhood type.—tuberculous, adj.

tuberculostatic (tū-ber′kū-lō-stat′ik): Inhibiting the growth of *Mycobacterium tuberculosis* which is the causative agent of tuberculosis, or an agent that inhibits such growth.—tuberculostat, n.

tuberculous (tū-ber′kū-lus): Pertaining to or affected by tuberculosis, or caused by the *Mycobacterium tuberculosis*. **T. MENINGITIS**, see under meningitis.

tuberculum (tū-ber′kū-lum): The anatomical term for a small eminence, nodule, knot or tubercle.—tubercula, pl.; tubercular, adj.

tuberosity (tū-be-ros′i-ti): A small rounded elevation or protuberance, particularly one from the surface of a bone.

tuberous (tū′ber-us): Knotty, knobby, covered with tubers.

tubo-: Combining form denoting a tube, or relationship to a tubal structure.

tuboabdominal (tū′bō-ab-dom′i-nal): Pertaining to the fallopian tube and the abdomen. **T. PREGNANCY**, the development of a fertilized ovum in the ampulla of a fallopian tube and extending into the peritoneal cavity.

tubo-ovarian (tū′bō-ō-vā′ri-an): Pertaining to or involving both a fallopian tube and an ovary, *e.g.*, a tubo-ovarian abscess.

tubo-ovariectomy (tū′bō-ō-vā-ri-ek′to-mi): Excision of the uterine tubes and ovaries. Salpingo-oophorectomy.

tubo-ovariotomy (tū′bō-ō-vā-ri-ot′to-mi): Surgical removal of a fallopian tube and an ovary; usually refers to both right and left tube and ovary.

tubo-ovaritis (tū′bō-ōvā-rī′tis): Inflammation of the uterine tubes and the ovaries.

tuboperitoneal (tū′bō-per-i-tō-nē′al): Pertaining to the uterine tubes and the peritoneum.

tuboplasty (tū′bō-plas-ti): Plastic surgery for repair of a uterine tube.

tuborrhea (tū-bō-rē′a): A discharge from the auditory tube.

tubotympanic (tū′bō-tim-pan′ik): Pertaining to the auditory tube and the tympanic cavity.

tubouterine (tū′bō-ū′ter-in): Pertaining to the uterine tubes and the uterus.

tubovaginal (tū′bō-vag′in-al): Pertaining to the uterine tubes and the vagina.

tubular (tū-bū-lar): In the form of or resembling a tube.

tubule (tū′būl): A small tube. **COLLECTING T.**, straight tube in the kidney medulla conveying urine to the kidney pelvis. **CONVOLUTED T.**, coiled tube in the kidney cortex. **SEMINIFEROUS T.**, coiled tube in the testis. **URINIFEROUS T.**, syn., nephron (*q.v.*).

tubulocyst (tū′bū-lō-sist): A cyst-like dilatation in an occluded duct or tube.

tubulointerstitial nephritis (tū′bū-lō-in-ter-stish′al nef-rī′tis): An inflammatory disease of the kidney characterized by destruction of the tubules.

tubulus (tū′bū-lus): A small tube.

tuftsin (tuft′sin): A tetrapeptide that coats white blood cells; it promotes phagocytosis of particulate matter, bacteria, and aged cells.

tularemia (tū′la-rē′mi-a): An endemic disease of rodents, caused by *Pasteurella tularensis;* transmitted by biting insects and acquired by humans either in handling infected animal carcasses, by the bite of an infected insect, or the bite of an infected animal such as the coyote. Suppuration at the inoculation site is followed by inflammation and suppuration of draining lymph glands and severe constitutional upset which may involve the spleen, liver, gastrointestinal organs, or lungs; symptoms include prolonged remittent fever, nausea, vomiting, lassitude, headache, myalgia; complications include pericarditis, bronchopneumonia, meningitis. Also called rabbit fever, deer fly fever, tick fever, and O'Hara's disease.

tulle gras (tūl′grah): A kind of dressing; used chiefly in France. Consists of mesh material impregnated with olive oil, paraffin, and balsam of Peru. Does not stick to the skin; useful in treatment of burns.

tumefacient (tū′me-fā′shent): 1. Swollen or swelling. 2. Causing swelling.

tumefaction (tu′me-fak′shun): 1. A swelling. 2. The condition of being or becoming swollen, puffy, or edematous.

tumefy (tū′me-fī): To swell or cause to swell.

tumentia (tū-men′shi-a): A swelling.

tumescence (tū-mes′ens): A state of swelling; turgidity.—tumescent, adj.

tumid (tū′mid): Swollen.

tumor (tū′mor): 1. A swelling. 2. A mass of abnormal tissue which resembles the normal tissue in structure, but which fulfills no useful function and grows at the expense of the body. Many types are described, often being named for the tissues from which they originate. **BENIGN T.**, a simple, innocent, encapsulated T., that does not infiltrate adjacent tissue or cause metastases and is unlikely to recur if removed. **MALIGNANT T.**, one that is not encapsulated, is likely to infiltrate adjoining tissue and to cause metastases, to progress, and ultimately to destroy life. See cancer.—tumorous, adj.

tumoricidal (tū′mor-i-sī′dal): 1. Destructive to tumors. 2. An agent that is destructive to tumors.

tumorigenic (tū′mor-i-jen′ik): Initiating or promoting the growth of tumors.—tumorigenesis, n.

tumorous (tū′mor-us): Resembling a tumor.

tumultus (tū-mul′tus): Overaction; agitation; commotion.

Tunga penetrans: A sand flea found in Africa and in America; a chigger; it attacks between the toes causing a lesion that develops into a painful ulcer.

tungiasis (tung-gī′a-sis): A pustular skin disorder caused by the bite of the sand flea, *Tunga penetrans*.

tunic: A covering, coat, or lining, particularly of a hollow or tubelike structure. See tunica.

tunica (tū′ni-ka): Anatomical term for a lining membrane or a coat, especially of a tubular structure; usually named for the structure of which it is a part or for its location in that structure; also called tunic. The three tunica of the blood vessels are the **T. ADVENTITIA** or **EXTERNA**, the outer supportive coat of blood vessels, which is thicker in arteries than veins; the **T. INTIMA**, the smooth inner lining of elastic endothelial tissue which also forms the valves in veins; and the **T. MEDIA**, the middle coat, made up of muscular and elastic tissue which contains nerve fibers concerned with the regulation of the caliber of the vessels. **T. DARTOS**, a layer of cutaneous tissue in the scrotum; helps form the septum of the scrotum **T. VAGINALIS TESTIS**, the serous membrane covering the testis and epididymus, and lining the cavity of the scrotum.

tuning fork: A small two-pronged forklike instrument, usually of steel, that gives off a musical note when struck. Used in some hearing tests.

tunnel (tun′el): A closed passageway through a solid structure; of varying length; open at the ends for entrance and exit. See carpal tunnel syndrome.

TUR: Abbreviation for transurethral resection. Usually refers to prostatectomy performed through the urethra.

turbid (tur′bid): Cloudy, unclear.

turbidity (tur-bid′i-ti): Cloudiness; usually refers to a solution in which the solid solutes have been disturbed.

turbinado sugar (tur-bin-ā′dō): Cane sugar that has been washed and dried but not bleached; said to retain the natural enzymes and to be more wholesome than bleached sugar.

turbinate (tur′bin-āt): Shaped like a top or inverted cone. **T. BONES**, situated on either side of the nose, forming the lateral nasal walls. Syn., concha nasalis.

turbinated: Scroll-shaped, as the three bony prominences that project from the lateral nasal walls.

turbinectomy (tur′bi-nek′to-mi): Removal of a turbinate bone.

turgescence (tur-jes′ens): Swelling; distention; inflation.—turgescent, adj.

turgid (tur′jid): Swollen; firmly distended, as with blood by congestion.—turgescence, n.; turgidity, n.

turgor (tur′gor): Fullness, tension, resiliency. Usually refers to the skin and is exhibited when the skin springs back after being pinched.

Turk's saddle: Sella turcica (*q.v.*).

turnbuckle cast: See under cast.

Turner's syndrome: Gonadal dysgenesis; there are 45 chromosomes in a cell instead of the normal 46, the missing one being a sex chromosome. The individual is usually brought up as a girl though a genetic male. Such a person is short of stature, has small female genitalia, scanty pubic hair, atrophic ovaries, webbed neck, and valgus of the elbows. [Henry H. Turner, American endocrinologist. 1892–1970.]

turning frame: See Stryker frame.

TURP: Abbreviation for transurethral resection of the prostate gland.

turpentine (tur′pen-tīn): A thin volatile oil obtained from the distillation of wood from certain pine trees; has several uses in medicine, *e.g.*, in stimulating liniments and ointments, and as a vermifuge, counterirritant, diuretic, and expectorant.

tussiculation (tus-sik′ -ū-lā′shun): A hacking cough.

tussis (tus′sis): A cough.

tussive (tus′iv): Pertaining to or due to a cough. **T. SYNCOPE**, occurs when prolonged coughing causes increased intrathoracic pressure resulting in inadequate return of blood to the heart; cardiac output falls and cerebral blood flow is diminished, causing syncope.

TV: Abbreviation for tidal volume (*q.v.*).

twang: A nasal quality of the voice.

twilight state: A condition of indistinct or distorted consciousness and amnesia induced by the injection of morphine and scopolamine, in which awareness to pain is dulled and memory of it is dimmed or effaced, without total loss of consciousness; used chiefly in childbirth.

twin: One of two children produced in the same pregnancy resulting from the fertilization of either one ovum or two ova at the same time.

twinge (twinj): A sudden sharp fleeting pain.

twinning (twin′ing): The simultaneous production of 1) two identical structures, by division, or 2) two embryos.

twitch: A brief spasmodic contraction of a muscle or muscle fiber. Resembles a tic but usually involves a larger muscle and is more noticeable.

two-point discrimination: The ability to recognize two punctate stimuli applied to the skin simultaneously when the eyes are closed.

two-step test: An exercise test of cardiac function, consisting of repeatedly stepping up and down two steps.

tylectomy (tī-lek′tō-mi): Surgical removal of a local lesion only, usually referring to a partial mastectomy in which only a carcinomatous lesion is removed.

tyloma (tı′lō′ma): Localized keratosis, as a callus.

tylosis (tī-lō′sis): See **keratosis.**

tympanectomy (tim′pa-nek′to-mi): Surgical removal of the tympanic membrane.

tympania (tim-pan′i-a): Tympanitis (*q.v.*).

tympanic (tim-pan′ik): Pertaining to the tympanum. **T. MEMBRANE** (membrana tympani), the eardrum.

tympanites (tim′pa-ni′tēz): Abdominal distension due to accumulation of gas in the intestine. Also called tympanism.

tympanitis (tim-pa-nī′tis): Inflammation of the tympanum and/or the tympanic membrane. Otitis media. Myringitis.

tympanocentesis (tim′pa-nō-sen-tē′sis): Surgical puncture of the tympanic membrane.

tympanoeustachian (tim′pa-nō-ū-stā′shi-an): Pertaining to both the tympanic cavity and the eustachian tube.

tympanomandibular (tim′pa-nō-man-dib′ū-lar): Pertaining to the tympanum and the mandible.

tympanomastoiditis (tim′pa-nō-mas-toy-dī′tis): Infection of the middle ear and the mastoid cells.

tympanoplasty (tim′pa-nō-plas-ti): A plastic operation involving the hearing mechanism of the middle ear.

tympanosclerosis (tim′pa-nō-sklē-rō′sis): The collection of masses of calcified connective tissue around the ossicles of the middle ear; may lead to deafness.

tympanotomy (tim-pa-not′o-mi): Incision of the tympanic membrane. Myringotomy.

tympanous (tim′pa-nus): Distended with gas, usually referring to the abdomen.

tympanum (tim′pa-num): The cavity of the middle ear.

tympany (tim′pa-ni): The drum-like resonant sound heard when a cavity containing air is percussed, *e.g.*, an abdomen distended with gas; may be diagnostic.—tympanitic, adj.

typhemia (tī-fē-mi-a): The presence of typhoid bacilli in the blood.

typhinia (tī-fin′i-a): Relapsing fever (*q.v.*).

typhl-, typhlo-: Combining forms denoting: 1. The cecum. 2. Blindness.

typhlectasis (tif-lek′ta-sis): Dilatation of the cecum.

typhlectomy (tif-lek′tō-mi): Excision of the cecum.

typhlitis (tif-lī′tis): Inflammation of the cecum; cecitis. Term formerly used for appendicitis.

typhlodicliditis (tif′lō-dik-li-dī′tis): Inflammation of the ileocecal valve.

typhloempyema (tif′lō-em-pī-ē′ma): The presence of an abscess in the cecum; may be associated with appendicitis or a sequela of cecitis.

typhloenteritis (tif-lō-en-ter-ī′tis): Inflammation of the cecum.

typhlolexia (tif-lō-lek′si-a): Word blindness; inability to recognize or comprehend words in written material.

typhlolithiasis (tif′lō-li-thī′a-sis): The presence of fecal concretions in the cecum.

typhlology (tif-lol′ō-ji): The study of blindness.

typhlomegaly (tif′lō-meg′a-li): Enlargement of the cecum.

typhlon (tif′lon): The cecum.

typhlopexy (tif′lō-pek′si): The surgical fixation of the cecum to the abdominal wall.

typhloptosis (tif′lō-tō′sis): Downward displacement of the cecum.

typhlosis (tif-lō′sis): Blindness.

typhlostenosis (tif′lō-ste-nō′sis): Stricture or narrowing of the cecum.

typhlostomy (tif-los′tō-mi): A colostomy into the cecum; a cecostomy.

typhloureterostomy (tif′lō-ū-rē′ter-os′tō-mi): An anastomosis between the ureter and the cecum.

typhoid fever (tī′foid): A worldwide, often epidemic, systemic infectious disease caused by the *Salmonella typhi,* which is transmitted by direct or indirect contact with a patient or carrier. Usual vehicles for spread of the disease are contaminated water or food, milk, milk products, or shellfish; flies are sometimes vectors. Average incubation period is 10–14 days.

A progressive febrile illness marks the onset of the disease; there is anorexia, malaise, slow pulse, and rose spots (*q.v.*) on the abdomen and back. As the organism invades the lymphoid tissue, ulceration of Peyer's patches (*q.v.*) and enlargement of the spleen occur. Constipation is more often a symptom than diarrhea, but when the latter occurs it is profuse with "pea soup" stools which may become frankly hemorrhagic. Recovery usually begins at about the end of the third week. Protection is secured through scrupulous personal hygiene when in contact with patients or carriers and by inoculation with the appropriate vaccine. Community control is secured through public health measures concerning the disposal of sewage, purification of water supply, inspection and control of food handlers, and discovery of carriers. See TAB.—typhoidal, adj.

typhous (tī′fus): Pertaining to typhus fever.

typhus (tī′fus): A group of acute, infectious, endemic diseases, many of which are named for the area in which they occur; caused by a rickettsial organism transmitted by arthropods; characterized by high fever, a skin eruption that may be macular or papular, severe headache, mental depression; lasts about two weeks. Spread by lice, fleas, and ticks; is a disease of war, famine, and castrophe when large groups of people are concentrated in a small area and facilities for personal hygiene are lacking. Protection is secured by immunization with the appropriate vaccine. Community control during epidemics is secured through vigilant public health measures. **MURINE T., T.** transmitted to man through the bite of the rat flea or rat louse. **SCRUB T.**, seen mostly in Japan and the Orient; transmitted by a larval mite; marked by sudden onset and a rash that occurs several days after the first symptoms; tsutsugamushi disease (*q.v.*).

typing (tīp′ing): Classifying an individual microorganism, object, or substance in the category in which it belongs. **BLOOD T.**, see blood groups.

tyremesis (tī-rem′e-sis): The vomiting of curd-like or cheese-like material by infants.

tyriasis (ti-rī′a-sis): 1. Elephantiasis (*q.v.*). 2. Alopecia (*q.v.*).

tyroma (tī-rō′ma): A tumor composed of caseous material.

tyromatosis (tī-rō-ma-tō′sis): Cheesy degeneration of tissue.

tyrosine (tī-rō′sēn): An amino acid found in many proteins that is concerned with growth and is an essential element in any diet; may be present in the urine in some diseases, especially diseases of the liver. **T. IODINASE**, an enzyme in the thyroid; important in the production of thyroxine.

tyrosinemia (tī-rō-si-nē′mi-a): A disorder of tyrosine metabolism in which there is an abnormally high level of tyrosine in the blood and urine; occurs in two forms 1) transient **T.**, seen in the newborn and 2) hereditary **T.**, which is associated with cirrhosis of the liver, glycosuria, and rickets.

tyrosinosis (ti′rō-si-nō′sis): A condition due to abnormal metabolism of tyrosine; *p*-hydroxyphenylpyruvic acid, an intermediate product of this metabolism is excreted in the urine. See phenylketonuria.

tyrosinuria (tī′rō-si-nū′ri-a): The presence of tyrosine in the urine.

tyrosis (tī-rō′sis): 1. The curdling of milk. 2. Tyremesis (*q.v.*).

U

U: 1. Chemical symbol for uranium. 2. Abbreviation for unit, units.

u: Symbol for micron, one millionth of a meter. Usually written μ.

U wave: A deflection in the electrocardiogram that sometimes follows the T wave.

uberus (ū'ber-us): Fruitful; plentiful; fertile.

UGI: Abbreviation for upper gastrointestinal.

ul-, ule-, ulo-: Combining forms meaning: 1. Gingivae, or gums. 2. Scar.

ula (ū'la): The gums.

-ula, -ulum, -ulus: Suffixes denoting: 1. Abounding in. 2. Small one, *e.g.*, formula, capitulum, tubulus.

ulalgia (ū-lal'ji-a): Pain in the gums.

-ular: Suffix in adjectives denoting relationship to the thing named in the stem *e.g.*, cellular.

ulatrophia (ū-la-trō-fi-a): Shrinkage of the gums.

ulcer (ul'ser): An open circumscribed lesion on the surface of the skin, or on serous or mucous membrane, due to destruction of tissue; characterized by necrosis, sometimes suppuration, and slow healing. **BURROWING U.**, usually caused by microaerophilic streptococci and coexisting staphylococci; characterized by necrosis of large skin areas; may produce sinus tracts in underlying tissues. **CORNEAL U.**, one occurring on the cornea of the eye. **CURLING'S U.**, a peptic **U.** associated with extensive burns and scalds or severe bodily injury. **CUSHING'S U.**, an acute **U.** of the stomach or duodenum; associated with central nervous disease. **DECUBITUS U.**, bedsore (*q.v.*). **DUODENAL U.**, one on the mucous membrane lining of the duodenum; peptic **U. GASTRIC U.**, one on the mucous membrane lining of the stomach; peptic **U. GRAVITATIONAL U.**, an **U.** of the leg that develops as a result of incompetency of the valves in varicosed veins. **HARD U.**, chancre (*q.v.*). **INDOLENT U.**, one with hard elevated edges and little or no granulation; occurs most frequently on the leg; very slow healing. **MOOREN'S U.**, chronic, progressive, usually bilateral ulceration of the marginal cornea; seen in the elderly; cause unknown. **PENETRATING U.**, a locally invasive **U.**, may involve the wall of an organ, or may erode a blood vessel and result in hematemesis if the **U.** is in the stomach or duodenum. **PEPTIC U.**, a **U.** that occurs in the mucous lining of the stomach or duodenum; caused by the action of the acidic gastric juice. **PERFORATING U.**, one which erodes through the wall of an organ. **RODENT U.**, one which grows slowly and is locally invasive of the skin, usually of the face; see **basal cell carcinoma. SERPENT U.**, serpiginous **U.**, **SERPIGINOUS U.**, an **U.** that erodes at one margin while extending at another thus creating an undulating margin. **STASIS U.**, a chronic ulcerative lesion, usually on the lower leg; due to venous stasis; a varicose **U.**, **STRESS U.**, an **U.** that occurs in people who experience long periods of physiological or environmental stress; usually occurs in the stomach or duodenum and is usually multiple. **SYPHILITIC U.**, chancre (*q.v.*). **VARICOSE U.**, an indolent **U.** in which there is loss of skin surface in the area of a varicose vein; usually occurs on the lower third of the leg; also called stasis **U.** or gravitational **U. VENEREAL U.**, chancroid (*q.v.*).

ulcerate (ul'ser-āt): 1. To undergo ulceration. 2. To form an ulcer.

ulceration (ul-ser-ā'shun): 1. The process of forming and developing an ulcer. 2. An ulcer or ulcers.

ulcerative (ul'ser-a-tiv): Pertaining to, or of the nature of an ulcer. **U. BLEPHARITIS.** see under **blepharitis. U. COLITIS**, see under **colitis.**

ulcerogenic (ul'ser-ō-jen'ik): Ulcer-producing or capable of producing an ulcer.

ulcerous (ul'ser-us): Affected with, resembling, or pertaining to an ulcer.

-ule: Suffix denoting little or diminutive, *e.g.*, capsule.

ulectomy (ū-lek'to-mi): 1. The surgical removal of diseased gingival (gum) tissue. 2. The surgical removal of scar tissue, as in iridectomy.

ulemorrhagia (ū'lem-ō-rā'ji-a): Bleeding from the gums.

-ulent: Suffix denoting abounding in, or full of, *e.g.*, corpulent.

uletic (ū-let'ik): Pertaining to the gums.

ulitis (ū-lī'tis): Inflammation of the gums; gingivitis.

ulna (ul'na): The bone on the inner side of the forearm extending from the elbow to the wrist parallel to the radius.

ulnar (ul'nar): Pertaining to the ulna. **U. ARTERY,** originates in the brachial artery; is distributed to the forearm, wrist, and hand. **U. NERVE,** runs down the inner side and middle of the forearm; supplies the flexor muscles of the wrist and hand.

ulnocarpal (ul'nō-kar'p'l): Pertaining to the ulna and the ulnar side of the wrist.

ulnoradial (ul'nō-rā'di-al): Pertaining to the ulna and the radial side of the wrist.

ulo-: Combining form denoting the gums.

uloncus (ū-long'kus): A tumor or swelling on the gums.

ulorrhea (ū-lō-rē'a): Bleeding from the gums.

ulotrichous (ū-lot′ri-kus): Having wooly hair or curly hair.

ulotripsis (ū-lō-trip′sis): Stimulation of the gums by massage.

ultra-: A prefix denoting 1) excess, excessive; 2) beyond in space, range, or limits; 3) beyond what is normal, ordinary, or natural.

ultrafiltration (ul′tra-fil-trā′shun): 1. The separation, by an ultrafilter, of all except the very smallest particles of a mixture. 2. The separation, by ultrafilters, of colloids or crystalloids from the medium in which they are dispersed or dissolved. See colloid; crystalloid.

ultramicroscope (ul-tra-mī′krō-skōp): A microscope for viewing objects too small to be seen with an ordinary microscope; it utilizes refracted instead of direct light.—ultramicroscopic, adj.; ultramicroscopy, n.

ultramicrotome (ul-tra-mī′krō-tōm): A cutting instrument for cutting sections of tissue extremely thin for examination under the electron microscope.

ultrasonic (ul′tra-son′ik): Relating to energy waves that are similar to sound waves but which have such a high frequency that they are inaudible to the human ear (above 20,000 cycles per second). **U. STERILIZATION,** see under sterilization.

ultrasonogram (ul-tra-son′ō-gram): The image obtained by ultrasonography. See also echogram.

ultrasonography (ul′tra-so-nog′ra-fi): A diagnostic technique utilizing ultrasound; when ultrasound waves are passed over a body area the reflection or echo of the sound waves as they pass over the junction of tissues of differing intensities is converted into a visual pattern. Also called sonography. See also echoencephalography.

ultrasound (ul′tra-sownd): Sound waves that are of such high frequency that they are inaudible to the human ear (over 20,000 vibrations per second); when they strike living tissue their energy is changed to heat which is reflected in differing degrees by various tissues. These reflections or echoes, which may be recorded pictorially, are used in making diagnoses since they detect heart abnormalities, delineate the deep body structures and determine the size and location of abnormal tissues or foreign bodies, *e.g.*, tumors, gallstones, foreign objects in the eye. Therapeutically, **U.** is utilized to destroy tissue, as in cancer treatment; in brain surgery; in physiotherapy for joint diseases; and in treatment of such conditions as Ménière's disease. **U.** is also useful in detecting multiple pregnancies and for determining fetal size, maturity, position, and abnormalities. See also echoencephalography

ultrastructure (ul-tra-struk′chur): 1. Very fine structure or particles seen with ultramicroscope. 2. The invisible ultimate structure of protoplasm.

ultraviolet (ul-tra-vī′ō-let): Denoting radiant energy waves that are beyond the violet end of the spectrum. **U. RAYS,** invisible natural component of the sun's radiation; may also be produced artificially by a special lamp; important in the synthesis of vitamin D in the body, and for normal growth and development; also used in treatment of certain skin diseases and for their indirect effect in treatment of rickets and anemia; their bacteriostatic effect has been utilized for degerming inanimate objects and air in enclosed areas but is no longer widely used for this purpose.

ultravirus (ul-tra-vī′rus): A very small virus (*q.v.*).

ululation (ūl-ū-lā′shun): The loud, inarticulate wailing or crying of hysterical or emotionally disturbed persons.

umbilectomy (um-bil-ek′tō-mi): Excision of the umbilicus. Also called omphalectomy.

umbilical (um-bil′i-kal): Pertaining to the umbilicus. **U. CORD,** the structure that connects the umbilicus of the fetus to the placenta in the gravid uterus; contains the umbilical arteries and vein; approximately two feet long and about one-half inch in diameter. **U. HERNIA,** see under hernia.

umbilicated (um-bil′i-kāt-ed): Having a central depression, *e.g.*, a smallpox vesicle.

umbilicus (um-bil′i-kus): The scar or pit in the center of the abdominal wall left by the separation of the umbilical cord after birth; the navel. See cord.—Also called navel and belly-button.

umbo (um′bō): 1. A boss (*q.v.*). 2. Any central eminence on the surface of a structure. **U. OF THE TYMPANIC MEMBRANE,** the elevated point in the tympanic membrane to which the manubrium of the malleus is attached.

un-: A prefix denoting 1) not, in-, non-; 2) contrary to, opposite of; 3) to remove, release, or free from.

unciform (un′si-form): Shaped like a hook. **U. BONE,** the hamate bone, one of the eight bones of the carpus.

Uncinaria (un′si-nā′ri-a): A genus of the nematodes, including one of the causative agents of hookworm disease.

uncinariasis (un′-sin-a-rī′as-is): Hookworm disease (*q.v.*).

uncinate (un′sin-āt): 1. Being hooked or barbed; unsiform. 2. Pertaining to the uncinate gyrus in the cortex of the brain; see gyrus. **U. SEIZURE,** a psychomotor or temporal lobe seizure that is preceded by an aura involving an olfactory and gustatory hallucination of something unpleasant, often of something burning; occurs in epileptics and others suffering from a lesion in the region of the uncus or hippocampus. Also called uncinate fit.

unconditioned reflex: A reflex that is inborn, *e.g.*, salivation at the sight of food.

unconscious (un-kon'shus): 1. Insensible; not aware of, or perceiving, factors in the environment. 2. State of being unable to receive stimuli or to have subjective experiences. 3. A psychoanalytic term for that part of the mind that consists of personality factors and physiological drives of which one is unaware and that are not accessible to memory, although they may be studied by psychoanalytic techniques. COLLECTIVE U., according to Jung, the accumulated memories and urges of the entire human race.

unconsciousness (un-kon'shus-nes): A physiological and psychological state of being unconscious (*q.v.*); lack of awareness and ability to perceive; insensibility. May result from shock, severe trauma, serious illness, alcoholism, overdose of certain drugs, sunstroke, toxemia.

unction (ungk-shun): 1. The application of a soothing ointment, salve or oil. 2. An ointment.

unctuous (ungk'shu-us): Fatty; oily; greasy.

uncus (ung'kus): A hook-shaped structure or process, specifically the hooked process of the anterior end of the hippocampal gyrus.

underwater: U. SEAL DRAINAGE, see under drainage. U. EXERCISE, exercise performed under water in a pool or large tub; the buoyancy afforded by the water increases the effectiveness of the exercise.

undescended: Not descended; refers specifically to a testis that does not descend into the scrotum but remains within the abdomen.

undine (un'dīn): A small, thin glass flask used for irrigating the eyes.

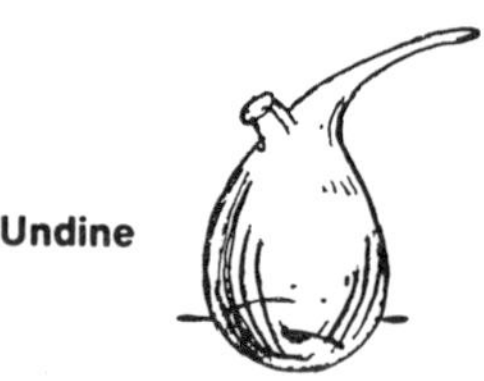

Undine

undulant (un'dū-lant): Characterized by rising and falling, or wave-like motion. U. FEVER, brucellosis (*q.v.*).

ung: Abbreviation for *unguent* (ointment).

ungual (ung'gwal): Pertaining to the fingernails or toenails.

unguent (ung'gwent): Ointment. Also unguentum.

unguis (ung'gwis): A fingernail or toenail.—ungues, pl.; ungual, adj.

uni-: Combining form denoting one; single.

uniarticular (ū'ni-ar-tik'ū-lar): Involving only one joint.

unicellular (ū-ni-sel'ū-lar): Consisting of only one cell.

unicornous (ū-ni-kor'nus): Having only one horn or cornu.

unigravida (ūn-i-grav'i-da): A woman who is pregnant for the first time.

unilateral (ū-ni-lat'er-al): Related to, or involving, only one side of a structure or of the body.—unilaterally, adv.

uniocular (ū-ni-ok'ū-lar): 1. Pertaining to, affecting, or involving only one eye. 2. Having only one eye.

union (ūn'yun): The process of healing or growing together, as occurs between the edges of a wound or the ends of fractured bones. DELAYED U., that in which the speed of callus formation following fracture is slower than usual. See intention.

uniovular (ū-ni-ov'ū-lar): Pertaining to, or arising from, one ovum; descriptive of certain twin pregnancies that result in identical twins. Cf. binovular.

unipara (ū-nip'a-ra): A woman who has borne only one child.—uniparous, adj.

unit: 1. A single person or thing. 2. A measurement of quantity, weight, or other quality that has been adopted as standard for that particular substance. U. DOSE, a pharmacologic preparation of a medication that contains the prescribed amount for a single dose.

United Nations International Children's Fund (UNICEF): A fund established by the United Nations in 1946 to provide help for children in areas of the world that have suffered the devastation of war or other catastrophic event; provides food and clothing and acts to prevent such diseases as tuberculosis and diphtheria; children of over 50 nations have benefitted from the Fund.

United States Pharmacopeia (USP): The legally recognized pharmacopeia for the United States; a compendium of information about pharmaceutical agents, their strengths and standards of purity, their uses and dosages; first compiled in 1820 and now revised every five years by a committee of pharmacists, physicians, and scientists and kept up to date by interim supplements.

United States Public Health Service (USPHS): A group of federal agencies in the Department of Health and Human Services that, under the direction of the Surgeon General, sponsors the development of public health problems and is concerned with health and health care problems that are not handled by state and local governments. In addition to the office of the Assistant Secretary for Health, the USPHS includes the National Institutes of Health; the Food and Drug Administration; the Centers for Disease Control; the Health Resources Administration; the Health Services

Administration; the Alcohol, Drug Abuse, and Mental Health Administration; and the Health Care Financing Administration.

univalent (ū-ni-vā'lent): Having a valence (chemical combining power) of one.

universal: Without limit; including or covering every member of the class, genus, or group being considered. **U. ANTIDOTE,** consists of a solution in warm water of 50 percent charcoal, 25 percent magnesium oxide, and 25 percent tannic acid; considered useful in many types of poisoning including that from acids, alkaloids, certain heavy metals, and glycosides. **U. DONOR,** an individual whose blood group is O and therefore compatible with most other blood types. **U. RECIPIENT,** in transfusions, an individual whose blood group is AB and therefore compatible with A, B, and O types. See blood groups.

unmedullated (un-med'ū-lāt-ed): Descriptive of a nerve fiber that has no myelin sheath.

Unna's boot (o͞o'naz): A semirigid cast-like casing, using a paste made of glycerin, zinc oxide, and gelatin; applied to the entire leg or the lower leg and foot and covered with a spiral bandage, then more paste; this process is repeated until rigidity is obtained. Used in treating varicose veins and ulcers, edema, and, sometimes, fractures of the ankle. [Paul Unna, German dermatologist. 1850–1929.]

unsaturated (un-sat'ū-rāt-ed): Descriptive of a solution that is capable of dissolving more of a solvent; not saturated.

unsex: To deprive an individual of the gonads, thus making reproduction impossible. To castrate.

unstriated (un-strī'ā-ted): Unstriped, referring usually to smooth muscle fibers.

untoward (un-tward'): Undesirable, adverse, unexpected, unfortunate; descriptive of effects of a drug or treatment.

upper GI series: The examination of the stomach and duodenum by x-ray, following the administration of a barium "swallow."

upper motor neuron: A neuron that has its cell in the brain cortex and which conducts impulses to the nuclei of the cerebral nerves or to the ventral gray columns of the spinal cord. See lower motor neuron.

upper respiratory tract: Composed of the nose and nasal cavity; the ethmoid, sphenoid, frontal, and maxillary sinuses; and the larynx and trachea; abbreviated URT. **URT INFECTION,** infection confined to the structures of the upper respiratory tract.

ups or uppers: Slang for drugs that produce elated feelings, or "highs."

uptake: In medicine, a term used to describe the absorption of some substance by a tissue, *e.g.*, iodine by the thyroid gland.

ur-, uro-: Combining forms denoting; 1. Urine; urination; urinary tract. 2. Urea.

urachus (ū'rak-us): The stem-like structure connecting the bladder with the umbilicus in the fetus; in postnatal life it is represented by a fibrous cord situated between the apex of the bladder and the umbilicus, known as the median umbilical ligament.—urachal, adj.

uracratia (ū-ra-krā'shi-a): The inability to retain urine in the bladder.

uragogue (ū'-ra-gog): A diuretic (*q.v.*).

uran-, urano-: Combining forms denoting the palate or roof of the mouth.

uraniscoplasty (ū'ran-is'kō-plas-ti): Plastic surgery of a cleft palate. Also uranoplasty.

uraniscus (ū'ra-nis'kus): The palate.

uranium (ū-rā'ni-um): A hard, heavy, silvery-white, radioactive metallic element of the radium group; found chiefly in pitchblende; important in the work on atomic energy. Some of its isotopes have uses in medicine.

uranorrhaphy (ū-ran-or'-a-fi): An operation involving suturing of a cleft palate. Palatorrhaphy.

uranoschisis (ū-ran-os'ki-sis): Cleft palate; uraniscochasm.

urarthritis (ū'rar-thrī'tis): Inflammation of the joints, as occurs in gout.

urate (ū'rāt): Any of several salts of uric acid. Urates are present in blood and urine and are constituents of stones or concretions formed in the body, *e.g.*, tophi (*q.v.*).

uraturia (ū'ra-tū-ri'a): Excess of urates in the urine.—uraturic, adj.

urea (ū-rē'a): A white, crystalline substance, the major nitrogenous end waste product of protein metabolism; it is synthesized in the liver and carried to the kidneys by the blood, thus is a normal constituent of blood, lymph and urine. The chief nitrogenous constituent of urine. Used in medicine as a diuretic. **U.** clearance, **U.** concentration, and **U.** range tests are all procedures for measuring the efficiency of kidney function. **U. CYCLE,** a cyclic series of reactions involving several substances including arginine and ornithine, the end product being urea; this is the major route of removal from the body of the ammonia formed in the liver and kidney during metabolism of amino acids.

Ureaplasma urealyticum (ū-rē'a-plaz'ma ū-rē'a-lit'i-kum): A small gram-negative sexually transmitted microorganism found in both male and female genitourinary tracts and sometimes in the rectum and the pharynx; infections with the organism may be symptomless but may also be associated with non-gonorrheal urethritis in the male and with genitourinary tract infections, puerperal infections, and reproductive failure in the female, and with prematurity and neonatal death.

urease (ū'rē-ās): An enzyme elaborated by various microorganisms, it catalyzes the change of urea into ammonia and carbon dioxide and is found in the mucus in urine of patients with inflammation of the bladder.

urecchysis (ū-rek'i-sis): Extravasation of urine into tissue, as may occur in rupture of the bladder caused by fracture of the pelvis.

uremia (ū-rē'mi-a): A clinical syndrome due to renal failure resulting from either disease of the kidneys themselves, or from disorder or disease elsewhere in the body, which induces kidney dysfunction, and which results in gross biochemical disturbance in the body, including retention of urea and other nitrogenous substances in the blood. Depending on the cause it may or may not be reversible. The fully developed syndrome is characterized by nausea, vomiting, headache, hiccough, weakness, dimness of vision, convulsions, and coma. Also called azotemia.—uremic, adj.

uremic (ū-rē'mik): Pertaining to or affected with uremia. **U. FROST,** whitish flakes that appear on the skin of some patients with advanced renal failure; due to inability of the kidneys to excrete urea compounds which are then excreted by the small capillaries in the skin where they collect on the surface.

uresis (ū-rē'sis): Urination.

ureter (ur're-ter, u-rē'ter): The tube that passes from each kidney to the bladder for the conveyance of urine; its average length is approximately 30 cm (10–12 inches).—ureteric, ureteral, adj.

ureterectasia (ū-rē'ter-ek-tā'si-a): Dilation of a ureter.

ureterectomy (ū-rē-ter-ek'to-mi): Excision of a segment or all of a ureter.

ureteric (ū-rē-ter'ik): Pertaining to a ureter. **U. CATHETER,** a fine caliber catheter that can be passed up the ureter to the pelvis of the kidney in order to collect a specimen of urine. **U. TRANSPLANTATION,** an operation in which the ureters are separated from the bladder and implanted in the ileus or colon; done to correct a congenital defect or because of a malignant growth.

ureteritis (ū-rē-ter-ī'tis): Inflammation of a ureter.

uretero-: Combining form denoting ureter.

ureterocele (ū-rē'ter-ō-sēl): Prolapse and sacculation of the ureter at its junction with the bladder, resulting from stenosis of the meatus; may lead to hydronephrosis and kidney damage.

ureterocolic (ū-rē'ter-ō-kol'ik): Pertaining to the ureter and colon, especially to an anastomosis between the two structures when there is a pathological condition of the lower urinary system.

ureterocolostomy (ū-rē'ter-ō-kō-los'to-mi): Surgical transplantation of the ureters from the bladder to the colon so that urine is passed by the bowel.

ureteroenterostomy (ū-rē'te-ō-en-ter-os'to-mi): The formation of an anastomosis between a ureter and the intestine.

ureteroileostomy (ū-rē'ter-ō-il-ē-os'to-mi): The formation of an anastomosis between a ureter and the ileum. Also called ileoureterostomy.

ureterolith (ū-rē'ter-ōlith): A stone in a ureter.

ureterolithotomy (ū-rē'ter-ō-li-thot'o-mi): Surgical removal of a stone from a ureter.

ureteroneocystostomy (ū-rē'ter-ō-nē'ō-sis-tos'to-mi): A surgical procedure in which the upper end of a divided ureter is implanted into the urinary bladder; most often performed during kidney transplant operation.

ureteronephrectomy (ū-rē'ter-ō-nef-rek'to-mi): Removal of a kidney and its ureter.

ureteropathy (ū-rē'ter-op'a-thi): Any disease or disorder of a ureter.

ureteropelvic (ū-rē'ter-ō-pel'vik): Pertaining to a ureter and the pelvis of the kidney to which it is attached.

ureteroplasty (ū-rē'ter-ō-plas-ti): Plastic surgery for repair of a ureter.

ureteroproctostomy (ū-rē'ter-ō-prok-tos'to-mi): The establishment of an anastomosis between a ureter and the rectum.

ureteropyelonephritis (ū-rē'ō-pī'e-lō-ne-frī'tis): Inflammation of a ureter, the pelvis of the kidney, and the kidney substance.

ureterosigmoidostomy (ū-rē'ter-ō-sig-moyd-os'to-mi): The surgical implantation of a ureter into the sigmoid colon.

ureterostenosis (ū-rē'ter-ō-ste-nō'sis): Stricture or narrowing of a ureter.

ureterostomy (ū-rē-ter-os'tō-mi): The formation of a permanent fistula through which the ureter discharges urine. **CUTANEOUS U.,** transplantation of the ureter to the skin in the iliac region.

ureterouterostomy (ū-rē'ter-ō-ūrē'ter-os'to-mi): The establishment of an anastomosis between the two ureters.

ureterovaginal (ū-rē'ter-ō-vaj'i-nal): Pertaining to a ureter and the vagina. **U. FISTULA,** one between the ureter and the vagina; may be congenital or the result of a pathological condition such as cancer of the cervix.

ureterovesical (ū-rē'ter-ō-ves'ik-al): Pertaining to a ureter and the urinary bladder.

urethr-,urethro-: Combining forms denoting urethra.

urethra (ū-rē'thra): The channel leading from the bladder through which urine is excreted; in the female it measures about 1½ inches; in the male 8 to 9 inches.—urethral, adj.

urethralgia (ū-rē-thral′ji-a): Pain in the urethra.

urethrectomy (ū-rē-threk′to-mi): The surgical removal of all or part of the urethra.

urethremphraxis (ū′rē-threm-frak′sis): An obstruction preventing the free flow of urine through the urethra.

urethritis (ū-rē-thrī′tis): Inflammation of the urethra, characterized by pain on urination; often associated with an infection in the kidney or bladder. **GONORRHEAL U.**, that caused by gonococcal infection. **GOUTY U.**, that due to gout. **NONSPECIFIC U.**, that not due to a gonococcal or other specific organism.

urethrocele (ū-rē′thrō-sēl): In the female, 1) a prolapse of the urethra through the meatus urinarius, or 2) a pouch-like protrusion of the urethral walls into the vaginal canal.

urethrocystitis (ū-rē′thrō-sis-tī′tis): Inflammation of the urethra and urinary bladder.

urethrocystography (ū-rē′thrō-sist-og′ra-fi): X ray of the urethra and bladder after the injection of a contrast medium. **MICTURATING U., U.** in which the bladder is filled with radiopaque fluid and several x rays are taken with the bladder at rest, and during and after voiding; done to determine the efficiency of the internal sphincter of the bladder and the angle of the posterior junction of the urethra and the bladder.—urethrocystogram, n.

urethrogram (ū-rē′thrō-gram): An x-ray view of the urethra, usually following the introduction of a contrast medium. **VOIDING U.**, a **U.** taken while the patient is voiding.

urethrography (ū-rē-throg′ra-fi): X-ray examination of the urethra. See **urography**.

urethroplasty (ū-rē′thrō-plas-ti): Any plastic operation on the urethra.—urethroplastic, adj.

urethrorectal (ū-rē′thrō-rek′tal): Pertaining to the urethra and the rectum.

urethrorrhea (ū-rē′thrō-rē′a): Any abnormal discharge from the urethra.

urethroscope (ū-rē′thrō-skōp): An instrument designed to allow visualization of the interior of the urethra.—urethroscopic, adj.; urethroscopically, adv.; urethroscopy, n.

urethrostenosis (ū-rē′thrō-ste-nō′sis): Urethral stricture.

urethrostomy (ū-rē-thros′to-mi): The surgical creation of an artificial opening into the urethra in cases of severe stricture.

urethrotomy (ū-rē-throt′o-mi): Incision into the urethra; usually part of an operation for stricture.

urethrotrigonitis (ū-rē′thrō-trī-gō-nī′tis): Inflammation of the urethra and the trigone of the urinary bladder; often due to damage to the urethra during sexual intercourse; marked by lower abdominal discomfort, frequent urination with pain and burning on voiding. See **trigone**.

urethrovaginal (ū-rē′thrō-vaj′i-nal): Pertaining to the urethra and the vagina.

urethrovesical (ū-rē′thrō-ves′ik-al): Pertaining to the urethra and the urinary bladder.

-uretic: Combining form denoting urine.

urgency (ur′jen-si): Sudden strong desire to urinate.

urhidrosis (ūr-hī-drō′sis): The presence of urinous substances such as urea or uric acid in the sweat. The crystals of uric acid may be deposited on the skin as fine white particles.

URI: Abbreviation for upper respiratory infection.

-uria: Combining form denoting 1) urine; 2) some characteristic of urine.

uric acid (ū′rik as′id): An acid formed in the breakdown of nucleoproteins in the tissues, and excreted in the urine. It is relatively insoluble and liable to give rise to stones. Present in excess in the blood in gout.

uricaciduria (ū′rik-as-i-dū′ri-a): The presence of more than the normal amount of uric acid in the urine. Uricemia.

uricase (ū′ri-kās): An enzyme that acts as a catalyst in the decomposition of uric acid.

uricosuria (ū′rik-ō-sū′ri-a): Excessive excretion of uric acid in the urine.

uricosuric (ū′ -rik-ō-sū′rik): An agent that enhances the excretion of uric acid in the urine; such substances are often used in treatment of chronic gout.

uridrosis (ū-ri-drō′sis): Urhidrosis (*q.v.*).

urin-, urino-: Combining forms denoting urine.

urinal (ū′rin-al): A vessel or container for receiving urine.

urinalysis (ū′ri-nal′i-sis): A systematic examination and study of the physical, chemical, and microscopic properties of urine to obtain data that will be helpful in making diagnoses, serving as a guide for further tests, or checking on the progress of patients under treatment.

urinary (ū′ri-ner-i): Pertaining to urine. **U. BLADDER**, the sac-like pelvic organ that serves as a reservoir for the collection of urine to be voided through the urethra. **U. CALCULUS**, a concretion formed in the urinary tract. **U. DIVERSION**, see **ileal conduit**. **U. FREQUENCY**, the urge to void more often than usual although the overall amount of urine voided is not increased; often associated with infection in the urinary tract and accompanied by pain or a burning sensation. **U. INCONTINENCE**, the involuntary voiding of urine; may be neurogenic or psychogenic in origin. **U. OUTPUT**, the amount of urine secreted by the kidneys. **U. RETENTION**, accumulation of urine in the bladder due to inability to void. **U. STASIS**, the remaining still or pooling of urine as may occur in the kidney or bladder. **U. SYSTEM**, consists of the kidneys, ureters, urinary bladder, and the urethra. **U.**

TRACT, the urinary system. U. TRACT INFECTION, infection of any of the structures in the urinary system. U. UNIDIVERSION, an operation to reestablish continuity of the urinary tract following the creation of an ileal conduit.

urinate (ū'rin-āt): To discharge urine from the body.

urination (ū-ri-nā'shun): The discharge or passing of urine from the body; micturition.

urine (ū'rin): The amber-colored fluid that is secreted by the kidneys, conveyed to the bladder by the two ureters, and stored there until it is discharged from the body. It has a normal pH of 4.5 to 8.0, and a specific gravity of 1.005 to 1.030, and consists of 96 percent water and 4 percent solids, the most important of which are urea and uric acid. Other solids normally found in urine include sodium chloride, potassium chloride, ammonia, hippuric acid, sulfuric acid, phosphoric acid, creatine. Solids that may be found in the urine of patients with various pathological conditions include bacteria, bile, blood, fat, glucose, ketone bodies, pus. The daily output varies, depending on various environmental factors, but the average is about 3 pints.

uriniferous (ū'ri-nif'er-us): Conveying urine; denoting particularly the tubules of the kidney.

urinogenital (ū'rin-ō-jen'it-al): See urogenital.

urinoma (ū'ri-nō'ma): A cyst that contains urine.

urinometer (ū'rin-om'e-ter): An instrument for estimating the specific gravity of urine.

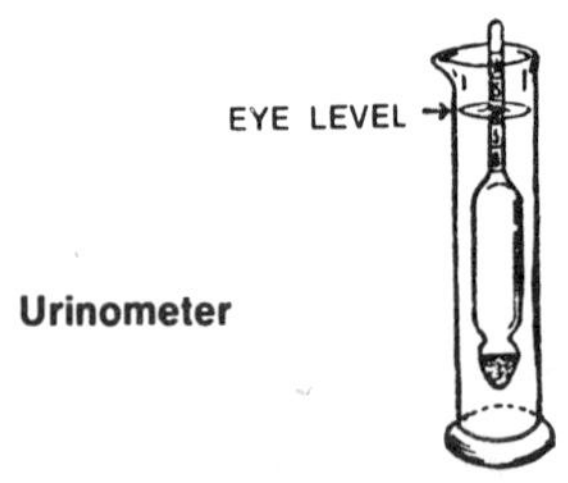

Urinometer

urinous (ū'rin-us): Having the characteristics of urine.

uro-, urono-: Combining forms denoting 1) urine; 2) urination; 3) urinary tract.

urobilin (ū'rō-bī'lin): A brownish pigment formed by the oxidation of urobilinogen and excreted in the urine and feces.

urobilinogen (ū'ro-bī-lin'ō-jen): A pigment formed from bilirubin in the intestine by the action of bacteria. It may be reabsorbed into the circulation and converted back to bilirubin in the liver. Small amounts are excreted in the urine and large amounts in the feces.

urobilinuria (ū'rō-bī-lin-ū'ri-a): The presence of increased amounts of urobilin in the urine.

urocele (ū'rō-sēl): The escape of urine into the scrotal sac.

urochesia (ū-rō-kē'zi-a): The excretion of urine from the anus.

urochrome (ū'rō-chrōm): The brownish or yellowish pigment that gives the urine its normal color.

urodynamics (ū-rō-dī-nam'iks): The study of the forces involved in moving the urine along the urinary tract.

urodynia (ū-rō-din'i-a): Pain on urination; dysuria.

urogenital (ū-rō-jen'it-al): Pertaining to the urinary and the genital organs.

urogenous (ū-roj'e-nus): Producing or excreting urine.

urogram (ū'rō-gram): The graphic recording of a radiograph of the urinary tract or any part of it, after injection of contrast medium.

urography (ū-rog'ra-fi): Radiologic examination of any part of the urinary tract; usually involves use of a contrast medium. CYSTOSCOPIC U., U. with the contrast fluid being injected into the bladder. EXCRETORY U., U. with the contrast medium being taken by mouth. INTRAVENOUS U., U. with the contrast fluid being injected into a vein. RETROGRADE U., cystoscopic U.

urokinase (ū'rō-kī'nās): An enzyme normally found in the urine; important in the conversion of plasminogen to plasmin which acts as a fibrolytic enzyme.

urolagnia (ū-rō-lag'ni-a): Sexual stimulation produced by association with urine, *e.g.*, watching people urinate, or wishing to urinate on another person.

urolith (ū'rō-lith): A stone in the urinary tract, or one passed in the urine.

urolithiasis (ū-rō-li-thī'a-sis): A state in which there is marked tendency toward the formation of urinary stones.

urologist (ū-rol'ō-jist): A physician who specializes in urology (*q.v.*).

urology (ū-rol'o-ji): That branch of medical science that deals with disorders of the female urinary tract and the male genitourinary tract.—urologic, urological, adj.; urologically, adv.

uromelus (ū-rom'e-lus): Sirenomelus (*q.v.*).

uropathogen (ū'rō-path'o-jen): Any microorganism that causes disease of the urinary tract.

uropathy (ū-rop'ath-i): Any disease or disorder of the urinary tract or of any part of it.

uropoiesis (ū'rō-poy-ē'sis): The formation or secretion of urine.

uroporphyria (ū'rō-por-fir'i-a): See porphyria.

uroporphyrin (ū′rō-por′fir-in): Any of the several porphyrins found in small amounts in normal urine and feces; all contain four acetic acid groups and four proprionic acid groups.

uropsammus (ū-rō-sam′us): Calcareous sediment in the urine.

urorubin (ū-rō-ru′bin): A red pigment in urine.

uroschesis (u-ros′ke-sis): 1. The retention of urine in the bladder. 2. The suppression of urine.

urosepsis (ū-rō-sep′sis): Septicemia resulting from the retention and absorption by the tissues of substances normally excreted in the urine.

urtica (ur′ti-ka): An herbaceous weed; nettle. The leaves produce an intense stinging sensation on contact with the skin; has some uses in medicine.

urticaria (ur-ti-kā′ri-a): A skin eruption characterized by circumscribed, smooth, itchy, raised wheals that are either redder or paler than the surrounding skin, developing very suddenly, usually lasting a few days, and leaving no visible trace. Common provocative agents in susceptible subjects are ingested foods such as shellfish, injected sera, and contact with, or injection of, antibiotics such as penicillin and streptomycin. Also called nettle rash or hives. **ACUTE U., U.** accompanied by mild constitutional symptoms. **ALLERGIC U.,** wheals due to sensitization and reexposure to allergenic substances, usually from ingestion. **CHOLINERGIC U.,** small wheals produced by heat created by exercise or emotion. **CHRONIC U.,** a form in which wheals appear frequently or are persistent. **COLD U., U.** due to exposure to cold. **GIANT U.,** angioneurotic edema (*q.v.*). **U. MEDICAMENTOSA, U.** due to ingestion of certain drugs. **NEONATAL U.,** ill defined white or yellow wheals surrounded by blotches of bright erythema. **U. PIGMENTOSA,** a form of **U.** seen in mastocytosis (*q.v.*) in which the lesions have a brown or reddish color when stroked. **SOLAR U., U.** occurring in certain individuals on exposure to sunlight.

urtication (ur-ti-kā′shun): 1. The development or production of urticaria (*q.v.*). 2. The sensation of having been stung with nettles.

urushiol (ū-roo′shē-ol): The irritating substance in certain plants, poison ivy, poison oak, and poison sumac in particular, that causes contact dermatitis and/or allergic reaction in susceptible individuals.

uter-, utero-: Combining forms denoting uterus.

uteralgia (ū-ter-al′ji-a): Pain in the uterus.

uterectomy (ū-ter-ek′to-mi): Excision of the uterus; hysterectomy.

uterine (ū′ter-in): Pertaining to the uterus. **U. DYSFUNCTION,** inertia uteri (*q.v.*). **U. PROLAPSE,** see prolapse. **U. TUBE,** see fallopian. See also anteflexion, anteversion, retroflexion, retroversion.

uteritis (ū-ter-ī′tis): Inflammation of the uterus. Also called metritis.

uterocervical (ū′ter-ō-ser′vi-kal): Pertaining to the uterine cervix, or to the uterus and the cervix.

uterofixation (ū′ter-ō-fik-sā′shun): Hysteropexy (*q.v.*).

uterography (ū-ter-og′ra-fi): X-ray examination of the uterus.

uterolith (ū′ter-ō-lith): A calculus in the uterus.

uteropexy (ū′ter-ō-pek-si): Hysteropexy (*q.v.*).

uteroplacental (ū′ter-ō-pla-sen′tal): Pertaining to the uterus and placenta. **U. APOPLEXY,** see Couvelaire uterus and uterus.

uteroplasty (ū′ter-ō-plas-ti): Any plastic operation on the uterus.

uterorectal (ū′ter-ō-rek′tal): Pertaining to the uterus and the rectum. See Douglas' pouch.

uterosacral (ū′ter-ō-sā′kral): Pertaining to the uterus and sacrum. **U. LIGAMENT,** the thickened pelvic fascia that curves along beside the lateral wall of the pelvis from the cervix to the front of the sacrum.

uterosalpingography (ū′ter-ō-sal-ping-gog′raf-i): X-ray examination of the uterus and fallopian tubes after injection of a contrast medium.

uterotonic (ū′ter-ō-ton′ik): Giving tone to the muscles of the uterus, or an agent that gives tone to uterine muscles.

uterotubal (ū′ter-ō-tū′bal): Pertaining to the uterus and the fallopian tubes. **U. INSUFFLATION,** the blowing of air into the fallopian tubes via the uterus; a test for tubal patency.

uterotubography (ū′ter-ō-tū-bog′ra-fi): Roentgenography of the uterus and fallopian tubes after the injection of a radiopaque material.

uterovaginal (ū′ter-ō-vaj′i-nal): Pertaining to the uterus and the vagina.

uterovesical (ū′ter-ō-ves′ik-al): Pertaining to the uterus and the bladder.

uterus (ū′ter-us): The womb; a hollow, pear-shaped muscular organ into which the ovum is received through the uterine tubes, and where it is retained during development, and from which the fetus is expelled through the vagina. Situated in the pelvic cavity, between the bladder and the rectum, it is about 3 in. long and 2 in. wide at the widest part; is divided into 3 parts, the *fundus* or upper broad part, the cavity or *body,* and the neck or *cervix;* it opens into the vagina below and the fallopian tubes above; it is maintained in position by ligaments, and lined with mucous membrane called endometrium. **BICORNUATE U.,** a uterus with two horns. **COUVELAIRE U.,** a serious condition involving separation of the placenta and infiltration of blood into the uterine musculature; may occur in association with abruptio placentae (q.v.); also called utero-placental apoplexy. [Alexandre Couvelaire, French obstetrician. 1873–1948.] **GRAVID U.**, a pregnant uterus.—uteri, pl.; uterine, adj.

UTI: Abbreviation for urinary tract infection.

utricle (ū'trik-l): 1. A little sac or pouch. 2. The small, delicate sac in the bony vestibule of the ear; the semicircular canals open into it.

uvea (ū'vē-a): The pigmented middle coat of the eye, including the iris, ciliary body and choroid.—uveal, adj.

uveitis (ū-vē-ī'tis): Inflammation of the uvea or any part of it.

uveomeningitis (ū'vē-ō-men-in-jī'tis): A condition marked by lesions of the uvea, accompanied by meningeal signs.

uveoparotid fever (ū'vē-ō-pa-rot'id): A form of sarcoidosis with symptoms of fever, uveitis, enlargement of the parotid gland, and sometimes temporary facial palsy. Also uveoparotitis.

uvula (ū'vū-la): Any dependent fleshy mass; term usually refers to the central tag-like structure hanging down from the posterior of the soft palate.—uvular, adj.

uvulectomy (ū'vū-lek'to-mi): Excision of the uvula.

uvulitis (ū'vū-lī'tis): Acute swelling and inflammation of the uvula; also called staphylitis.

uvuloptosis (ū'vū-lop'tō-sis): A falling or relaxed condition of the palate.

uvulotomy (ū'vū-lot'o-mi): The operation of cutting off all or part of the uvula. Staphylotomy.

V

V: Abbreviation for: 1. Volt. 2. Volume. 3. Vision or visual acuity.

v: Abbreviation for volt.

vaccinate (vak′sin-āt): 1. To inoculate with a vaccine to produce immunity to smallpox. 2. To inoculate with a vaccine to produce immunity to the corresponding infectious disease.

vaccination (vak′sin-ā′shun): Originally, the process of inoculating persons with discharge from cowpox to protect them from smallpox. Now applied to the inoculation of any antigenic material for the purpose of producing active artificial immunity.

vaccine (vak-sēn′): A suspension or extract of the organisms that cause a disease, either killed or modified so as to reduce their power to cause the disease while retaining their power to cause the body to form antibodies against the disease. Used chiefly in prophylactic treatment of certain infections by producing active immunity; sometimes used for amelioration or treatment of certain infectious diseases. **AUTOGENOUS V.**, one prepared from a culture of bacteria taken from the patient who is to receive the vaccine. **MIXED V.**, one prepared from two species of bacteria. **POLYVALENT V.**, one prepared from more than two species of bacteria. **QUADRUPLE V.**, one that protects against diphtheria, tetanus, whooping cough, and poliomyelitis. **SMALLPOX V.**, one prepared from the skin lesions of vaccinia in healthy calves that have been inoculated with smallpox virus. **TRIPLE V.**, one that protects against diphtheria, tetanus, and whooping cough. Vaccines are available for protection against many other diseases including cholera, influenza, measles, mumps, plague, rabies, typhoid and typhus fever, and yellow fever. See also Sabin's v.; Salk's v.; BCG.

vaccinia (vak-sin′i-a): 1. Cowpox; a contagious disease of cattle, transmissible to humans. 2. A disease of humans that is usually limited to the site of inoculation with the virus of cowpox, either accidentially or for the purpose of conferring immunity to smallpox.

vacciniola (vak-sin-i-ō′la): A secondary vesicular eruption that sometimes occurs after vaccination; it resembles the eruption of smallpox.

vacuole (vak′ū-ōl): A very small space in the protoplasm of a cell, containing air or fluid.—vacuolar, vacuolated, adj.; vacuolation, n.

vacuolization (vak′-ū-ō-lī-zā′shun): The formation of vacuoles. Also called vacuolation.

vacuum (vak′ū-um): An empty enclosed space from which all air has been extracted. **V. ASPIRATION**, the use of a vacuum extractor to assist in aborting the products of conception; done before the 14th week of pregnancy. **V. EXTRACTION**, the employment of suction instead of obstetrical forceps in the second stage of labor.

vagal (vā′gal): Pertaining to the vagus nerve (*q.v.*).

vagectomy (vā-jek′to-mi): Excision of a portion of the vagus nerve.

vagin-, vagini-, vagino-: Combining forms denoting the vagina.

vagina (va-jī′na): 1. A sheath or sheath-like structure. 2. The musculomembranous genital canal in the female lying between the urinary bladder and the rectum and extending from the cervix uteri to the vulva; it measures about 3 in. along the anterior wall and 3½ in. along the posterior wall.—vaginal, adj.

vaginal (vaj′i-nal): 1. Like a sheath. 2. Pertaining to the vagina. **V. HYSTERECTOMY**, surgical removal of the uterus by way of the vagina. **V. SPECULUM**, an instrument used to open the vagina so as to facilitate inspection of it. **V. SPERMICIDES**, contraceptives that are inserted into the vagina before coitus; they act by interfering with the viability of the sperm; available without prescription in the form of foams, jellies, and suppositories.

vaginate (vaj′in-āt): To ensheath, or to be enclosed in a sheath. See invagination.

vaginectomy (vaj-i-nek′tō-mi): Colpectomy; excision of the vagina or part of it.

vaginismus (vaj-in-iz′mus): Painful spasm of the muscular wall of the vagina preventing satisfactory sexual intercourse.

vaginitis (vaj-i-nī′tis): A nonspecific inflammation of the vagina. **ATROPHIC V.**, characterized by a watery discharge, burning and itching of the vulva; usually occurs during and after menopause; may progress to kraurosis vulvae; often associated with leukoplakia. **CANDIDAL V.**, caused by *Candida albicans,* a fungus; fairly common in pregnant women, diabetics, debilitated persons, and those taking oral contraceptives; characterized by a thick, curd-like discharge and severe pruritus. **GONOCOCCAL V.**, caused by infection with *Neisseria gonorrhoea;* characterized by a thick yellow purulent discharge. **HEMOPHILUS V.**, caused by a gram-negative organism, *Hemophilus vaginalis;* characterized by a scanty, malodorous, thin, creamy, gray discharge of frothy material; consistency and color may vary. **MONILIAL V.**, Candidal **V.** **SENILE V.**, relatively common in older women; may be accompanied by profuse purulent or bloody discharge causing soreness;

sometimes seen in cancer of the uterus. **TRICHOMONAL V.**, caused by *Trichomonas vaginalis;* characterized by frothy, greenish or yellowish copious discharge, intense itching and burning of vulva.

vaginocele (vaj′in-ō-sēl): Colpocele (*q.v.*).

vaginodynia (vaj′i-nō-din′i-a): Pain in the vagina; colpodynia.

vaginofixation (vaj′in-ō-fik-sā′shun): Surgical fixation of the vagina to the abdominal wall to correct vaginal relaxation or prolapse.

vaginohysterectomy (vaj′i-nō-his-ter-ek′to-mi): The surgical removal of the uterus through the vagina without any abdominal incision.

vaginolabial (vaj′i-nō-lā′bi-al): Pertaining to the vagina and the labia.

vaginomycosis (vaj′in-ō-mī′kō′sis): Infection of the vagina caused by a fungus.

vaginopathy (vaj-i-nop′a-thi): Any pathological condition of the vagina; colpopathy.

vaginoperineal (vaj′in-ō-per-in-ē′al): Pertaining to both the vagina and perineum.

vaginoperineorrhaphy (vaj′in-ō-per-i-nē-or′a-fi): Surgical repair of a lacerated or ruptured vagina and perineum.

vaginoperineotomy (vaj′i-nō-per-i-ne-ot′o-mi): An incision at the outlet of the vagina and the adjoining perinuem; done to facilitate childbirth.

vaginopexy (vaj-ī′nō-pek-si): Vaginofixation (*q.v.*).

vaginoplasty (vaj-īnō-plas-ti): Reparative plastic surgery on the vagina.

vaginovesical (vaj′i-nō-ves′i-kal): Pertaining to the vagina and the urinary bladder.

vagitis (va-jī′tis): Inflammation of the vagus nerve.

vagitus (va-jī′tus): The cry of an infant while being born or while still in the uterus.

vagolysis (vā-gol′i-sis): Surgical destruction of the vagus nerve.

vagolytic (vā-gō-lit′ik): 1. Pertaining to or causing vagolysis. 2. An agent that neutralizes the effect of a stimulated vagus nerve.

vagomimetic (vā′gō-mī-met′ik): Having an effect resembling that produced by vagal stimulation.

vagotomy (vā-got′o-mi): 1. Surgical division of the vagus nerve. 2. Interruption of the impulses carried by the vagus nerve.

vagotonia (vā-gō-tō′ni-a): A condition of hyperexcitability of the vagus nerve; may result in vasomotor instability, sweating, bradycardia, constipation.—vagotonic, adj.

vagus (vā′gus): The parasympathetic pneumogastric nerve; the tenth pair of cranial nerves, composed of both motor and sensory fibers, with a wide distribution in the neck, thorax, and abdomen, sending important branches to the heart, lungs, stomach, etc.—vagal, adj.; vagi, pl.

valence (vā′lens): The degree of combining power of one atom of an element or a radical, using the combining power of one atom of hydrogen as the unit of comparison.

valetudinarian (val′e-tū-di-ner′i-an): An individual who is in chronically poor health; an invalid.

valgus (val′gus): Twisted or bent outward, denoting a displacement or angulation away from the midline of the body; term is used in connection with the noun it describes, *e.g.*, hallux valgus. Opp. of varus.—valgoid, adj.

valine (val′ēn, vā′lēn): One of the essential amino acids; found in most protein foods; is synthesized in the body and considered essential for growth and development in infants and for maintaining nitrogen balance in adults.

vallate (val′āt): Cupped; describing a depression that is surrounded by an elevated rim. **V. PAPILLAE**, the papillae that occur in a V-shaped arrangement on the surface of the posterior part of the tongue.

vallecula (va-lek′ū-la): In anatomy, a shallow depression or furrow. **V. CEREBELLI**, the depression on the under surface of the cerebellar hemispheres in which the medulla oblongata lies. **V. EPIGLOTTICA**, a depression between the lateral and median folds on each side of the epiglottis. **V. UNGUIS**, the fold of skin at the sides and base of the nails—vallecular, adj.

valley fever: Coccidiomycosis (*q.v.*).

Valsalva: V. MANEUVER, forceful expiration of air against a closed glottis, which increases thoracic pressure, impedes venous return to the heart, and slows the heart rate; occurs normally in individuals when lifting heavy objects, straining at stool, or changing position when lying down; sometimes employed in treating paroxysmal tachycardia. **V. TEST**, a test for patency of the auditory tube; when the patient exhales forcefully while holding the nose and mouth tightly closed, air should pass into the middle air cavity and the person should hear a popping sound if the tube is patent. **V. SINUSES**, three small dilatations of the aorta behind the flaps of the valves at the opening of the aorta in the left ventricle. [Antonio Mario Valsalva, Italian anatomist. 1666–1723.]

valve (valv): In anatomy, a fold of membrane in a passage or tube, permitting the flow of contents in one direction only. **AORTIC V.**, the **V.** between the left ventricle and the ascending aorta. **ATRIOVENTRICULAR V.'S**, either of the two **V.**'s between the atria and ventricles of the heart. **BICUSPID V.**, one that has two cusps, *e.g.*, the **V.** between the left atrium and left ventricle; also called the mitral **V. HOUSTON'S V.**'s, three or four folds of crescent-shaped membranous folds in the rectum; also called Houston's folds and rectal valves. **ILEOCECAL V.**, a **V.** consisting of membranous folds between the ileum and the large intestine; it prevents fecal matter from moving back into the ileum. **MITRAL V.**, the bicuspid **V.** between the left atrium and left ventricle. **PULMONARY V.**, the **V.** between the right ventricle and the pulmonary trunk. **PROSTHETIC V.**, usually refers to a prosthetic heart valve used to replace a defective natural **V.** **PYLORIC V.**, a membranous fold at the junction of the stomach and the duodenum. **SEMILUNAR V.**, a **V.** having three cusps, as the aortic and pulmonary **V'S.** **TRICUSPID V.**, a valve having three cusps, as the right atrioventricular **V.** **VENOUS V.**, **V'S** found in most veins except the vena cavae and the intestinal veins; they are semilunar pockets on the inner surface of the veins, with their free edges lying centrally in the direction of blood flow and preventing reversal of the direction of flow; most numerous in the lower extremities.

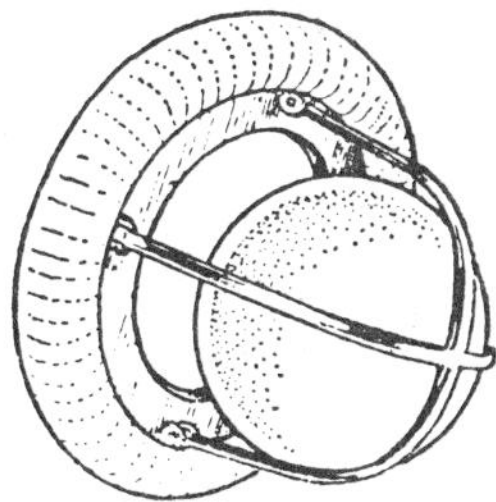

Prosthetic heart valve

valvoplasty (val'vō-plas-ti): A plastic operation on a valve, usually reserved for the heart; includes valve replacement and valvulotomy (*q.v.*).

valvotomy (val-vot'om-i): See **valvulotomy**.

valvulae conniventes (val'vū-lē kon-i-ven'tēz): Circular membranous folds that project into the lumen of the small intestine, retarding the passage of food along the intestine and providing a larger area for absorption; they persist even during distention of the bowel.

valvular (val'vū-lar): Pertaining to or resembling a valve. **V. DISEASE OF THE HEART**, a condition resulting from deformity or constriction of one or more of the heart valves, making it impossible for them to reclose completely and allowing blood to regurgitate; may be congenital but more often a sequel of endocarditis resulting from rheumatic fever. **V. PNEUMOTHORAX**, tension pneumothorax, a condition in which an open chest wound acts as a valve allowing inspired air to enter the pleural cavity but preventing its escape during exhalation.

valvulitis (val-vū-lī'tis): Inflammation of a valve, particularly one in the heart.

valvulotomy (val-vū-lot'o-mi): Surgical incision of a valve, by custom referring to a valve of the heart; specifically the operation of correcting a deformed or narrowed heart valve.

van den Bergh's test: A laboratory test for the presence of bilirubin in the blood serum.

vanillylmandelic acid (van'i-lil-man-del'ik): A metabolite of epinephrine and norepinephrine; its measurement in the urine is used as a test for pheochromocytoma. Abbreviated VMA.

vapor (vā-por): The gaseous state of a liquid or solid, *e.g.*, steam, mist, gas, or an exhalation.

vaporizer (vā'por-ī-zer): An apparatus for converting a liquid, particularly a medicated liquid, into a vapor that can be inhaled; frequently used in treatment of bronchial conditions.

vapors (vā-pors): An obsolete term applied to hysterical nervousness, thought to be caused by bodily exhalations.

Vaquez's disease (va-kāz): Polycythemia vera (*q.v.*). [Louis Henri Vaquez, French physician. 1860–1936.]

variable (va're-ah-b'l): In research, any factor, characteristic, quality, or attribute under study. **DEPENDENT V.**, the variable under investigation which the researcher wishes to observe so as to note the effect of an independent variable on it. **INDEPENDENT V.**, the **V.** that the researcher manipulates or introduces into the situation.

varic-, varico-: Combining forms denoting varix (a twisted, tortuous vein, sometimes dilated).

varicella (var'i-sel'la): Chickenpox (*q.v.*).—varicelliform, adj.

varices (var'i-sēz): Pl. of varix (*q.v.*).

varicoblepharon (var'i-kō-blef'a-ron): A varicose swelling or tumor of the eyelid.

varicocele (var'i-kō-sēl): Varicosity of the veins of the spermatic cord.

varicogaphy (var'i-kog'ra-fi): Roentgenology of a varicose vein.

varicophlebitis (var'i-kō-flē-bī'tis): Inflammation of a varicose vein.

varicose (var'i-kōs): 1. Unnaturally swollen or distended. 2. Related to or exhibiting varices (see **varix**). **V. VEINS**, dilated veins that have lost their elasticity and in which the valves have become incompetent so that blood flow may be reversed or become static; may be due to trauma, thrombosis, inflammation, or heredity; usually seen in the lower legs, rectum (hemorrhoids) or lower esophagus (esophageal varices).

varicosity (var-i-kos'i-ti): 1. The state or condition of being varicose. 2. A varix (*q.v.*).

varicotomy (var-i-kot'o-mi): Excision of a varicose vein.

variola (va-rī'ō-la): Smallpox (*q.v.*).—variolar, variolic, variolous, adj.

varioloid (var′i-ō-loyd): 1. An attack of smallpox modified by previous vaccination or attack of the disease. 2. Resembling smallpox.

varix (var′iks): A dilated, tortuous (or varicose) vein; less often an artery or lymphatic vessel.—varices, pl.

varus (vā′rus): Bent inward; denoting a displacement or angulation toward the midline of the body; term is used in connection with the noun it modifies, *e.g.*, talipes varus (*q.v.*).

vas: A vessel or canal for carrying a fluid.—vasa, pl. **V. DEFERENS,** the excretory duct of the testes; it unites with the excretory duct of the seminal vesicle to form the ejaculatory duct. Also called ductus deferens.

vas-, vasi-, vaso-: Combining forms denoting a channel or vessel, especially a blood vessel.

vasa (vas′a, vā′za): **V. PRAEVIA,** 1) blood vessels that lie below the presenting part in labor; if they rupture there is danger of blood loss; 2) prolapsed umbilical cord; the cord precedes the infant in delivery. **V. VASORUM,** the minute nutrient vessels in the outer and inner coats of the larger veins and arteries.

vascular (vas′kū-lar): Related to, supplied with, or containing vessels, referring especially to blood vessels. **V. BED,** the total blood supply to an organ or body part, including arteries, veins, and capillaries. **V. HEADACHE,** headache caused by painful dilatation of branches of the external carotid artery; see **migraine**. **V. INSUFFICIENCY,** lack of adequate peripheral blood flow; may be due to damaged, blocked, or diseased vessels, causing cyanosis and swelling of an extremity, and intermittent claudication. **V. SYSTEM,** the cardiovascular and lymphatic systems considered together.

vascularity (vas-kū-lar′i-ti): The condition of being supplied with blood vessels.

vascularization (vas′kū-lar-ī-zā′shun): The acquisition of a blood supply through the formation of new blood vessels in a part. The process of becoming vascular.

vasculature (vas′kū-la-chūr): The arrangement of the blood vessels in a structure or a part of the body.

vasculitis (vas′kū-lī′tis): Inflammation of a blood or lymph vessel.—vasculitides, pl.

vasectomy (vas-ek′to-mi): Surgical excision of the vas deferens or a part of it.

vasitis (vas-ī′tis): Inflammation of the vas deferens.

vasoactive (vas-ō-ak′tiv, vā′zō-): 1. Having an influence on the tone and caliber of the blood vessels. 2. A condition of blood vessels when they respond to various stimuli by changing their caliber.

vasoconstriction (vas-ō-kon-strik′shun, vā′zō): Narrowing or diminution of the caliber of the blood vessels, particularly the smaller ones, resulting in reduced blood flow to a part.

vasoconstrictor (vas-ō-kon-strik′tor, vā′zō-): Any agent that causes a narrowing of the lumen of blood vessels.

vasodepressor (vas-ō-dē-pres′or, vā′zō-): Any agent that depresses circulation by lowering the blood pressure.

vasodilation (vas-ō-dī-lā′shun, vā′zō-): Dilation of the blood vessels.

vasodilator (vas-ō-dī′lā-tor, vā′zō-): Any agent that causes a widening of the lumen of blood vessels.

vasoepididymostomy (vas′ō-ep-i-did-i-mos′-to-mi, vā′zō-): An anastomosis between the vas deferens and the epididymus.

vasogenic (vas-ō-jen′ik, vā′zō-): Vascular in origin. **V. SHOCK,** see under **shock**.

vasography (vas-og′ra-fi, vā-sog′): Radiography of blood vessels.

vasoinhibitor (vas-ō-inhib′i-tor, vā-zō-): Any agent that interferes with or depresses the action of vasomotor nerves, thus causing dilation of the blood vessels.—vasoinhibitory, adj.

vasoligation (vas-ō-lī-gā′shun, vā-zō-): Ligation of a vessel, the vas deferens in particular.

vasomotor (vas-ō-mō′tor, vā-zō-): Pertaining to or affecting the nerves and muscles that control the contraction and expansion of blood vessels.

vasopressin (vas-ō-pres′in, vā′zō-): The antidiuretic hormone formed in the hypothalamus and stored in the posterior lobe of the pituitary; also prepared synthetically. **V.** stimulates the muscular coat of the smaller blood vessels, thus raising the blood pressure, stimulates contraction of intestinal muscles, thus increasing peristalsis, has some effect on the muscles of the uterus, and has an antidiuretic effect. May be used in treatment of diabetes insipidus.

vasopressor (vas-ō-pres′sor, vā′zō): Stimulating contraction of the musculature of the blood vessels, especially the smaller vessels, or an agent that has this effect.

vasoresection (vas-ō-rē-sek′shun, vā′zō-): Surgical division of the vas deferens.

vasospasm (vas′ō-spazm, vā′zō-): Constricting spasm of vessel walls, the smaller blood vessels in particular. Syn., vasoconstriction.—vasospastic, adj.

vasostomy (va-sos′to-mi, vā-zos′): The operation of making an opening into the vas deferens. Also vasotomy.

vasotonia (vas-ō-tō′ni-a, vā′zō): The tone of blood vessels, the smaller ones in particular.—vasotonic, adj.

vasotripsy (vas′ō-trip-si, vā′zo-): The arrest of hemorrhage by crushing an artery with a strong forceps. Angiotripsy.

vasovagal (vas-ō-vā′gal, vā-zō-): Referring to the vagus nerve and its action on the blood vessels. **V. SYNDROME,** an autonomic nervous system response which may be caused by extreme fear; marked by faintness, pallor, sweating, anxiety, epigastric distress, feeling of impending death, respiratory difficulty, syncope. When part of the post-gastrectomy syndrome, it occurs a few minutes after a meal.

vasovasostomy (vas'-ō-va-sos'to-mi, vā'zō): The surgical anastomosis of two cut ends of the vas deferens; usually done to restore fertility after a previous vasectomy.

vasovesiculectomy (vas'ō-ve-sik-ū-lek'to-mi, vā'zō-): Surgical removal of the vas deferens and the seminal vesicles.

vasovesiculitis (vas'ō-ve-sik-ū-lī'tis, vā'zō-): Inflammation of the vas deferens and the seminal vesicles.

vastus (vas'tus): Large or great. **V. MUSCLES,** the large muscles of the thigh, named for their location: **V.** externus, **V.** intermedius, **V.** internus, **V.** lateralis, and **V.** medialis.

Vater: Ampulla of **V.**, see under ampulla.

vault (vawlt): An anatomical part resembling an arched roof. **PALATINE V.**, the roof of the mouth. **VAGINAL V.**, the upper end of the vaginal canal into which the cervix inserts.

VC: Abbreviation for vital capacity.

VD: Abbreviation for venereal disease.

VDRL: Abbreviation for Venereal Disease Research Laboratories (*q.v.*).

VE: Abbreviation for volume (of air) exhaled per minute at rest.

vection (vek'shun): The carrying of the organisms of a disease from an infected to an uninfected person; the transmission may be direct or through an intermediate host.

vector (vek'tor): 1. A living carrier of disease that transmits the organisms causing a disease from one host to another; often an arthropod, *e.g.*, mosquito, fly, flea, louse. 2. A quantity that expresses direction, magnitude, and polarity; may be represented by a straight line, and used to express velocity, force, or momentum.

vectorcardiogram (vek'tor-kar'di-ō-gram): A graphic record of the magnitude and direction of the heart's electric currents.

vectorcardiography (vek'tor-kar-di-og'ra-fi): Three-dimensional electrocardiography utilized for determining the direction and magnitude of the electrical forces of the heart.

vegan (vej'an): An individual whose diet excludes all animal products.

vegetarian (vej-e-tā'ri-an): A person whose diet consists entirely of foods of vegetable or plant origin, *i.e.*, vegetables, fruits, nuts, grains, and sometimes animal products such as milk or cheese.

vegetation (vej-e-tā'shun): A growth or accretion of any kind, especially a clot made up of fibrin and platelets occurring on the edge of the cardiac valves in endocarditis.

vegetative (vej'e-tā-tiv): 1. Pertaining to growth or nutrition. 2. Pertaining to the nonsporing stage of a bacterium. 3. Functioning involuntarily or unconsciously. 4. In psychiatry, describing a state of inactivity or sluggishness.

vehicle (vē'i-k'l): An inert or inactive substance, *e.g.*, water or syrup, used as a carrier for a drug that has a therapeutic action.

veil (vāl): 1. In anatomy, any veil-like structure. 2. A caul (*q.v.*).

vein (vān): A vessel carrying deoxygenated blood back to the heart (with the exception of the pulmonary veins). It has the same three coats as an artery, *i.e.*, inner, middle, and outer, but they are not as thick and they collapse when cut. Many veins have valves that prevent backflow of blood. All except the pulmonary veins carry dark, venous, deoxygenated blood.

velamentous (vel'a-men'tus): 1. Being covered with a veil-like membrane. 2. Veil-like or membranous. **V. PLACENTA,** a **P.** with the umbilical cord arising from the outer border.

Velcro: A textile used for closing a garment, appliance, or dressing; consists of two layers of material that adhere to each other.

vellication (vel-i-kā'shun): Spasmodic involuntary twitching of muscle fibrils.

vellus (vel'us): The fine downy hair that appears on all parts of the body except palms of the hands and soles of the feet. See also lanugo.

velocity (ve-los'i-ti): Rapidity of motion; the rate of motion in a particular direction in relation to time.

Velpeau's bandage (vel-pōz'): A shoulder bandage; see under bandage.

velum (vē'lum): In anatomy, 1) any structure that resembles a veil or curtain; 2) the muscular portion of the roof of the mouth; it is elevated when one is speaking or swallowing, thus closing off the nasal passages.

ven-, veni-, veno-: Combining forms denoting 1) veins; 2) the vena cava.

vena (vē-na): Vein [L.] **V. CAVA,** one of the two large veins which empty their contents into the right atrium of the heart. **INFERIOR V. C.**, the vein which receives blood from the trunk of the body and lower extremities; it is formed by the union of the two common iliac veins. **SUPERIOR V. C.**, the large vein which collects blood from the head, chest, and upper extremities; it is formed by the junction of the two innominate veins.—venae and venae cavae, pl.

venacavography (vē'na-kā-vog'ra-fi): Radiography of the vena cava; usually refers to the inferior vena cava.

venectasia (ven-ek-tā'si-a): Dilatation of a vein or veins.

venectomy (ven-ek'to-mi): The excision of part of a vein, a procedure sometimes used in treatment of varicose veins. Phlebectomy.

venenation (ven-e-nā'shun): Poisoning, or the condition of being poisoned.

veneniferous (ven-e-nif'er-us): Carrying or conveying poison.

venenific (ven-i-nif'ik): Poison producing.

venenous (ven'e-nus): Poisonous.

venepuncture (vē'ne-pungk-tūr): Venipuncture (*q.v.*).

venereal (ve-nēr'-ē-al): Pertaining to or transmitted by sexual contact. **V. DISEASE,** a contagious disease most often acquired by sexual contact, intercourse in particular; includes gonorrhea, syphilis, chancroid, lymphogranuloma venereum, granuloma inguinale, balanitis gangrenosa, herpes simplex, Type 2. **V. SORE,** see chancre. **V. WART,** see condyloma lata and wart.

Venereal Disease Research Laboratories (VDRL): A federal agency within the Centers for Disease Control in Atlanta, GA. **VDRL TEST,** a serological test for syphilis; is not considered definitive unless supported by positive results in other tests for syphilis. Yaws and several other diseases caused by the *Treponema* organism also give positive results in the VDRL test.

venereologist (ve-nēr'ē-ol'o-jist): A specialist in the study and treatment of venereal diseases.

venereology (ve-ner-ē-ol'-o-ji): The study of venereal diseases.

venereophobia (ve-nēr'ē-ō-fō'bi-a): Morbid fear of contracting a venereal disease.

venesection (vēn-e-sek'shun): Phlebotomy; opening the cubital vein with a scalpel for the purpose of letting blood; formerly a common clinical procedure. Also spelled venisection.

venin (ven'in): Any one of the various toxic substances in snake venom (*q.v.*).

venin-antivenin (ven-in-an'ti-ven-in): A mixture of venin and antivenin, used as a vaccine in the treatment of bites by venomous snakes.

venipuncture (vē'ni-pungk-tūr): The puncturing of a vein, through the skin, usually with the needle of a syringe or a cannula to introduce a catheter for any purpose, most often to administer a medication or other fluid or to withdraw a blood sample. Also venepuncture.

venoclysis (vē-nok'li-sis): The slow, continuous introduction of nutrient or medicinal fluids into a vein. See clysis.

venogram (vē'nō-gram): A radiogram of veins after injection of a radiopaque substance.

venography (vē-nog'ra-fi): X-ray visualization of a vein or veins after injection with an opaque medium.—venographic, adj.; venographically, adv.

venom (ven'um): A poison, particularly the substance secreted by certain snakes, insects, and other arthropods, or animals, and that is transmitted to humans by a bite or sting.

venomous (ven'ō-mus): Poisonous. Secreting or containing venom.

venoperitoneostomy (vē'nō-per-i-tō-nē-os'to-mi): The surgical procedure of inserting a cut end of the saphenous vein into the peritoneum to drain ascitic fluid from the cavity into the vein.

venosclerosis (vē'nō-scler-ō'sis): Fibrous hardening of venous walls. Phlebosclerosis.

venostasis (vē-nō-stā'sis): 1. Slowing of the blood flow in the venous system. 2. A procedure for temporarily checking the return flow of blood by applying compression to the veins of the four extremities. See rotating tourniquet under tourniquet.

venotomy (vē-not'o-mi): Surgical incision into a vein. Phlebotomy.

venous (vē'nus): Pertaining to the veins or the circulation within them. **V. HUM,** a continuous humming sound normally heard on auscultation in children and some healthy adults with high cardiac output. **V. LAKES,** single or multiple bluish-black vascular lesions seen on exposed areas of the ears, face, and neck. **V. PRESSURE,** the pressure of blood in the veins, often measured in the superior vena cava or right atrium and reported as central venous pressure; See central venous pressure under pressure. **V. RETURN,** the blood that is returning to the heart through the great veins. **V. STAR,** a small reddish blue starlike spot often seen on the legs of elderly persons. **V. STASIS,** the impairment or stoppage of blood flow in a vein or veins. **V. THROMBOSIS,** the formation of a thrombus in a vein.

venovenostomy (vē-nō-vē-nos'to-mi): The surgical creation of an anastomosis between two veins.

venter (ven'ter): Any of the great cavities of the body, *e.g.*, the abdomen.

ventilate (ven'ti-lāt): 1. To remove stale air and supply fresh air to take its place; may be done artificially by mechanically propelling and extracting the air or naturally by opening windows, doors, etc. 2. To oxygenate the blood and remove the carbon dioxide from it; a function carried out by the capillaries and the alveoli in the lungs. 3. In psychiatry, to discuss problems and grievances.—ventilation, n; ventilatory, adj.

ventilation (ven'ti-lā'shun): 1. The process of bringing fresh air into the environment, *i.e.*, air with a higher oxygen content and lower carbon dioxide content than the air being replaced. 2. In physiology, the movement of air or a gas mixture in or out of the lungs. 3. In psychiatry, the opportunity to express one's emotional problems verbally. **ALVEOLAR V.,** see under alveolar. —ventilatory, adj.

ventilator (ven'til-a-tor): Any of several available devices used in respiratory therapy to augment the respiratory exchange of gases in the lungs; a respirator (*q.v.*). Three main types are 1) **VOLUME-CYCLED V.**, a **V.** that ends inspiration when a pre-set volume has been reached; 2) **PRESSURE-CYCLED V.**, a **V.** that ends inspiration when a pre-set pressure has been reached, and 3) **TIME-CYCLED V.**, a **V.** that ends respiration when a pre-set time interval has been reached.

ventilometer (ven-ti-lom'e-ter): A device for measuring the volume of air breathed in and out at various times during the respiratory cycle, and the capacity of the lungs under different environmental conditions.

ventr-, ventri-, ventro-: Combining forms denoting 1) the belly; 2) the anterior aspect of the body.

ventrad (ven'trad): Toward the ventral aspect of the body.

ventral (ven'tral): Pertaining to the abdomen or the anterior surface of the body. Opp., dorsal.—ventrally, adv.

ventricle (ven'trik-l): A small belly-like cavity. **V.'S OF THE BRAIN,** four cavities filled with cerebrospinal fluid within the brain. **V.'S OF THE HEART,** the two lower muscular chambers of the heart.—ventricular, adj.

ventricular (ven-trik'ū-lar): Pertaining to a ventricle. **V. ANEURYSM,** see cardiac aneurysm under aneurysm. **V. FIBRILLATION,** rapid, irregular, uncoordinated twitchings of muscle fibers that replace the normal contractions of the muscular walls of the ventricles. **V. GALLOP,** a sound heard over the right ventricle early in diastole; caused by early rapid filling of the ventricle with limited extensibility; the sound is likened to the word Ken-tuk'key. **V. SEPTAL DEFECT,** a defect of the septum between the two ventricles, usually congenital. **V. TACHYCARDIA,** see under tachycardia.

ventriculitis (ven-trik'ū-lī'tis): Inflammation of a ventricle, particularly one in the brain.

ventriculo-: Combining form denoting ventricle.

ventriculoatrial shunt (ven-trik'ū-lō-ā'tri-al): The surgical establishment of communication between a cerebral ventricle and the right atrium of the heart, to drain cerebrospinal fluid from the brain in cases of hydrocephalus. See shunt.

ventriculocisternostomy (ven-trik'ū-lō-sis-ter-nos'to-mi): The surgical establishment of communication between the lateral ventricle of the brain and the subarachnoid cisterns, usually the cisterna magna; used in the treatment of hydrocephalus. See shunt.

ventriculogram (ven-trik'ū-lō-gram): A radiograph of the brain after the injection of a gas or an opaque medium into the cerebral ventricles.

ventriculography (ven-trik-ū-log'ra-fi): Radiography of the ventricles of the brain after injection of gas or an opaque medium into the ventricles to displace the cerebrospinal fluid normally present.

ventriculoperitoneal (ven-trik'ū-lō-per-i-tō-nē'al): Pertaining to a ventricle of the brain and the peritoneal cavity. **V. SHUNT,** a shunt between the lateral ventricle of the brain and the peritoneal cavity; used in treatment of hydrocephalus. See shunt.

ventriculoscope (ven-trik'ū-lō-skōp): An instrument for viewing the inside of the ventricles of the brain.

ventriculostomy (ven-trik-ū-los'to-mi): An artificial opening into a ventricle. Usually refers to a drainage operation for hydrocephalus.

ventriculotomy (ven-trik-ū-lot'o-mi): Surgical incision into a ventricle, *e.g.*, into a ventricle of the heart for repair of a cardiac defect or into the third ventricle of the brain for the relief of hydrocephalus.

ventriculoureteral (ven-trik'ū-lō-ū-rē'ter-al): Pertaining to a ventricle of the brain and the ureter, particularly to a shunt between these two structures, used in treatment of hydrocephalus. See shunt. Also called ventriculoureterostomy.

ventrofixation (ven'trō-fik-sā'shun): Surgical fixation of a displaced organ to the abdominal wall.

ventrohysteropexy (ven'trō-his'ter-ō-peks-i): Surgical fixation of a displaced uterus to the abdominal wall.

ventrolateral (ven-trō-lat'er-al): Situated or occurring both ventrally and somewhat laterally.

ventrosuspension (ven'trō-sus-pen'shun): A surgical procedure in which the round ligaments are shortened to hold a retroplaced uterus forward. Also ventrofixation.

Venturi effect: A principle stating that as the velocity of a fluid going through a constricted section of a tube increases, the pressure decreases; applies when measuring the flow of a fluid.

Venturi mask: A mask designed to mix room air with oxygen so that varying percentages of oxygen can be administered.

venule (vēn'ūl): A minute vein; the smallest division or branch of a vein, continuous at one end with the vein and at the other end with a capillary.—venulae, pl.; venular, adj.

verbigeration (ver-bij-er-ā'shun): The constant uncontrollable repetition of meaningless words, phrases or sentences as seen in states of mental disorientation.

verbomania (ver-bō-mā'ni-a): A mania for words or for talking.

vergence (ver′jens): A turning; usually said of one eye which turns vertically or horizontally as compared with the other eye.

vermicide (ver′mi-sī′d): An agent that kills intestinal worms.—vermicidal, adj.

vermiform (ver′mi-form): Worm-like in form. **V. APPENDIX,** the vestigial, hollow, worm-like structure that is attached to the cecum, commonly called the appendix.

vermifuge (ver′mi-fūj): An agent that causes intestinal worms or parasites to be expelled. An anthelmintic.

vermin (ver′min): External parasites; usually refers to insects such as lice or bedbugs. Broadly speaking, noxious, disgusting small animals or insects that are hard to control, *e.g.*, mice, rats, fleas, flies.

vermis (ver′mis): 1. A worm. 2. The narrow middle part of the cerebellum; it lies between and connects the two hemispheres of the cerebellum.

vernix (ver′niks): A covering. **V. CASEOSA,** the fatty substance which covers the skin of the fetus at birth and keeps it from becoming sodden by the liquor amnii.

verruca (ve-ru′ka): Wart. **V. ACUMINATA,** a nonvenereal wart that appears on the external genitalia. **V. NECROGENICA,** develops as a result of accidental inoculation with tuberculosis. **V. PLANA JUVENILIS,** the common, multiple, flat, tiny warts often seen on childrens' hands and knees. **V. PLANTARIS,** a flat wart on the sole of the foot; plantar wart. **V. SEBORRHEICA,** the brown, greasy wart commonly seen on the chest or back of seborrheic subjects. **V. SENILIS,** superficial warty lesions that appear on the hands or face of older people, due to exposure to sunlight; may become malignant. **V. VULGARIS,** the common wart of the hands, of brown color and rough pitted surface.—verrucous, adj.; verrucae, pl.

version (ver′zhun): A change of direction; a tilting, or turning. In gynecology, refers to a displacement or tilting of the uterus; varieties include anteversion, lateroversion, and retroversion. In ophthalmology, refers to the simultaneous rotation of both eyes in the same direction; may be upward, downward, or to the right or the left. In obstetrics, applies to the maneuver of altering the position of the fetus in utero from an abnormal to a normal or more favorable position; may occur spontaneously or by manual manipulation. Varieties of **V.** in obstetrics include: **CEPHALIC V.,** turning the fetus so that the head presents; **EXTERNAL V.,** turning the fetus by manipulation through the abdominal wall; **INTERNAL V.,** turning the fetus with one of the obstetrician's hands in the uterus and the other on the mother's abdomen; **PODALIC V.,** turning the fetus to a breech presentation.

vertebr-, vertebro-: Combining forms denoting 1) a vertebra, or 2) the vertebral column.

vertebra (ver′te-bra): One of the 33 small bones forming the vertebral (spinal) column. There are seven cervical, twelve thoracic, five lumbar, five sacral, and four coccygeal vertebrae. The sacral and coccygeal groups are fused in the adult.—vertebrae, pl.; vertebral, adj.

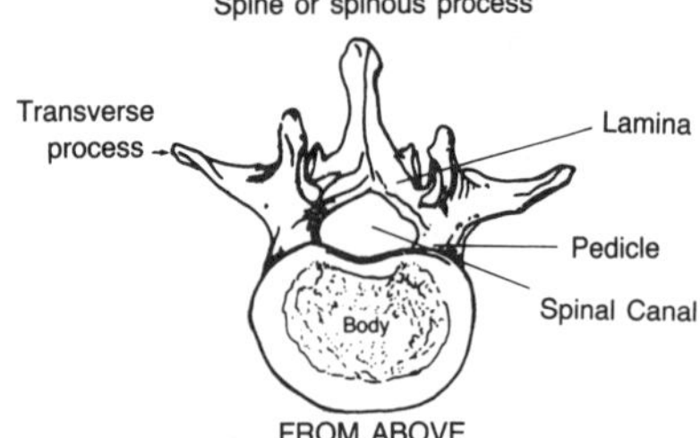

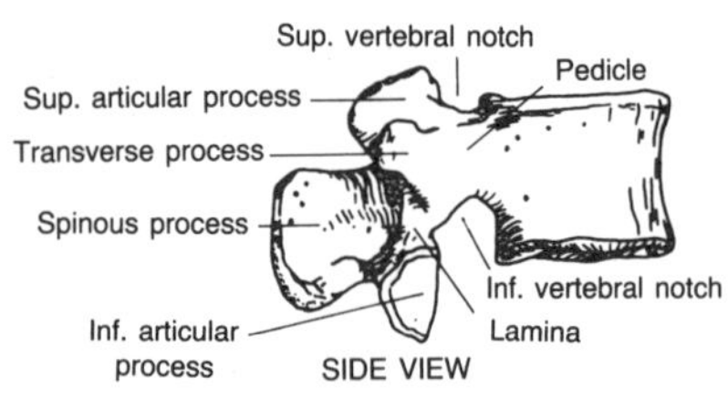

Vertebra

vertebral (ver′te-bral): Pertaining to the vertebrae. **V. ARTERY,** either of two arteries, right and left, that arise in the subclavian artery and which supply the deep muscles of the neck, the spinal cord and its membranes, and the cerebellum. **V. BODY,** the short column of bone in the vertebrae that forms the weight-bearing part of the spine. **V. CANAL,** that formed by the foramina of the vertebrae; contains the spinal cord and its meninges. **V. COLUMN,** the vertebrae from the cranium through the coccyx; the spine. **V. CURVES,** seen when viewed from the side, the **V.** column curves slightly inward in the area of the cervical vertebrae, outward in the area of the thoracic vertebrae, and inward at the area of the lumbar vertebrae; exaggeration of the thoracic (posterior) curve causes kyphosis (hunchback); of the lumbar curve (anterior) causes lordosis (swayback); normally there are no lateral curvatures, but when this does exist it is called scoliosis.

vertebrate (ver′te-brāt): Having a vertebral column or referring to an animal that has a vertebral column.

vertebrobasilar (ver′te-brō-bas′i-lar): Pertaining to the vertebral and basilar arteries. **V. INSUFFICIENCY,** a syndrome caused by lack of sufficient blood to the hindbrain; may be progressive and episodic; symptoms include vertigo, nausea, ataxia, blindness, diplopia, hemiplegia due to transient cerebral ischemia, drop attacks and signs of cerebellar dysfunction.

vertebrocostal (ver'te-brō-kos'tal): Pertaining to a vertebra and a rib.

vertex: A summit or top. In anatomy, refers usually to the top of the head. In obstetrics, the part of the fetus' head that is bounded in front by the anterior fontanel, behind by the posterior fontanel, and laterally by the two parietal eminences.

vertiginous (ver-tij'i-nus): Pertaining to or affected with vertigo.

vertigo (ver'ti-gō): A sensation as of whirling, either of oneself in space or of the world around one; may be a symptom of disease of the inner ear, eyes, stomach, heart, or brain, or of toxemia. Also often a precursor to an epileptic seizure. Not the same as dizziness or faintness. **BENIGN POSTIONAL V.**, occurs chiefly in the elderly, usually when walking, turning suddenly, or changing position of the head; may be due to peripheral neuropathy, cervical spine disease, or vestibular dysfunction; often associated with hearing loss and diminished vision.

vesic-; vesico-: Combining forms denoting: 1. A bladder. 2. A blister.

vesica (ves'i-ka): 1. A hollow organ or sac. 2. A bladder; a hollow organ with a musculomembranous structure that serves as a reservoir for a fluid, *e.g.*, the gallbladder or the urinary bladder.

vesical (ves'i-kal): Pertaining to a bladder, the urinary bladder in particular.

vesicant (ves'i-kant): 1. Causing blisters. 2. An agent that produces blisters.

vesication (ves-i-kā'shun): A blister or blisters, or the production of a blister or blisters.

vesicle (ves'ik-l): 1. A small bladder, cell, or hollow structure. 2. A small circumscribed superficial elevation on the skin containing clear or nonpurulent serous fluid. **SEMINAL V.**, one of two small sacs that store the seminal fluid until it is ejaculated.—vesicular, adj.

vesicocele (ves'i-kō-sēl): Hernia of the bladder.

vesicocervical (ves-i-kō-ser'vi-kal): Pertaining to the urinary bladder and the cervix. **V. FISTULA**, one between the bladder and the uterine cervix.

vesicocolonic (ves'i-kō-kō-lon'ik): Pertaining to the urinary bladder and the colon. **V. FISTULA**, one between the urinary bladder and the colon.

vesicoenteric (ves'i-kō-en-ter'ik): Vesicointestinal (*q.v.*).

vesicofixation (ves'i-kō-fiks-ā'shun): Surgical fixation of 1) the urinary bladder to the abdominal wall; 2) the uterus to the urinary bladder.

vesicointestinal (ves'i-kō-in-tes'tin-al): Pertaining to the urinary bladder and the intestine. **V. FISTULA**, see under fistula.

vesicopapular (ves'i-kō-pap'ū-lar): Pertaining to an eruption that consists of both vesicles and papules.

vesicoprostatic (ves'i-kō-pros-tat'ik): Pertaining to both the urinary bladder and the prostate gland.

vesicopustular (ves'i-kō-pus'tū-lar): Pertaining to an eruption that consists of both vesicles and pustules.

vesicorectal (ves-i-kō-rek'tal): Pertaining to the urinary bladder and the rectum. **V. FISTULA**, one between the urinary bladder and the rectum.

vesicostomy (ves-i-kos'to-mi): Cystostomy (*q.v.*). **CUTANEOUS V.**, a surgical procedure to divert drainage from the urinary bladder onto the anterior abdominal wall to which a collection bag is attached.

vesicotomy (ves-i-kot'o-mi): An incision into the urinary bladder.

vesicoureteral (ves'i-kō-ū-rē'ter-al): Pertaining to the urinary bladder and the ureters. **V. REFLUX**, the backflow of urine from the bladder into the ureter.

vesicourethral (ves'i-kō-ū-rē'thral): Pertaining to the urinary bladder and the urethra.

vesicouterine (ves'i-kō-ū'ter-in): Pertinent to the urinary bladder and the uterus. **V. POUCH**, the fold of peritoneum that extends downward between the urinary bladder and the uterus.

vesicovaginal (ves-i-kō-vag'i-nal): Pertaining to the urinary bladder and the vagina.

vesicular (ve-sik'ū-lar): Pertaining to or composed of vesicles. **V. BREATH SOUNDS**, see breath sounds.

vesiculation (ve-sik' -ū-lā'shun): 1. The presence of vesicles. 2. The formation of vesicles.

vesiculectomy (ve-sik'ū-lek'to-mi): Resection of all or part of both seminal vesicles; produces sterility.

vesiculitis (ve-sik'ū-lī-tis): Inflammation of a vesicle, particularly a seminal vesicle.

vesiculography (ve-sik'ū-log'ra-fi): X ray of the seminal vesicles.

vesiculopapular (ve-sik'ū-lō-pap'ū-lar): Pertaining to or exhibiting both vesicles and papules.

vesiculoprostatitis (ve-sik'ū-lō-pros-ta-tī'tis): Inflammation of the urinary bladder and the prostate gland.

vesiculopustular (ve-sik'ū-lō-pus'tū-lar): Pertaining to or exhibiting both vesicles and pustules.

vessel (ves'el): A tube, duct or canal, holding or conveying fluid, especially blood and lymph.

vestibular (ves-tib'ū-lar): 1. Pertaining to a vestibule. 2. Pertaining in particular to the vestibular part of the eighth cranial nerve that is concerned with equilibrium. **V. GLANDS,** four small glands located in the vestibule of the vagina; two, called major or Bartholin's glands, are located on either side of the vaginal orifice; two, called minor **V.** glands, are located in the mucous membrane around the urethral opening. **V. NEURONITIS,** a disorder of the vestibular nerve that causes extreme vertigo but the hearing is not affected. **V. SENSE,** the sense of balance, needed for maintaining posture, walking, and running. **V. SYSTEM,** the structures in the vestibule of the inner ear that have to do with the maintenance of equilibrium.

vestibule (ves'ti-būl): 1. The middle part of the internal ear, lying between the semicircular canals and the cochlea. 2. The triangular area between the clitoris and the inner surfaces of the labia minora; it forms the entrance to the vagina. **V. OF THE MOUTH,** the part between the teeth and alveolar ridges and the lips.

vestibulo-: Combining form denoting vestibule.

vestibulocochlear (ves-tib'ū-lō-kok'lē-ar): Pertaining to the vestibule and the cochlea of the inner ear. **V. NERVE,** the acoustic **N.**, see under acoustic.

vestibulotomy (ves-tib'ū-lot'o-mi): Operation of making an opening into the vestibule of the inner ear.

vestibulourethral (ves-tib'ū-lō-ū-rē'thral): Pertaining to the vestibule of the vagina and the urethra.

vestigial (ves-tij'i-al): Rudimentary; indicating a remnant of something formerly present.

Veterans Administration: An independent agency of the federal government; functions directly under the President; operates the largest centrally directed hospital and clinic system in the U.S.; about 14 percent of the population is eligible to receive care in these facilities. Provides hospital and outpatient care for veterans who 1) have service-connected disabilities; 2) cannot pay for hospital services; 3) are over 65 years of age; or 4) receive VA pensions. Abbreviated VA.

VF: Abbreviation for ventricular fibrillation; see fibrillation.

viability (vī-a-bil'i-ti): Ability to live, grow, and develop. **LEGAL V.,** term applies to a fetus of at least 20 weeks gestation. **MEDICAL V.,** term applies to a fetus of 24 to 28 weeks gestation or of at least 400 grams in weight, or to an infant who weighs at least 1000 grams at birth.

viable (vī'a-b'l): Capable of living a separate existence, said particularly of the ability of a fetus to live after birth.

vial (vī'al): A small bottle for medicines or drugs; also spelled phial. **VIAL OF LIFE,** a small vial which contains a listing of the person's nearest relative and physician, and vital medical information; at home, it is usually placed in the refrigerator because there it is least likely to be misplaced; a small sign is pasted on the refrigerator door indicating its presence. Paramedics are instructed to look for this, particularly if the person is aged, infirm, or unconscious, and living alone.

vibex (vī'beks): A linear mark or streak; a linear hemorrhage under the skin.—vibices, pl.

vibration (vī-brā'shun): 1. A rapid to-and-fro motion. 2. A maneuver in massage. 3. A therapeutic procedure in which the body is shaken rapidly.

vibrator (vī'brā-tor): A hand-held device that is set into vibration by an electric current; held over the thorax to assist in postural drainage or over a paralyzed muscle to stimulate contraction.

Vibrio (vib'ri-ō): A genus of curved, motile microorganisms. **V. CHOLERAE** or **COMMA** causes cholera. **V. PARAHAEMOLYTICUS,** an organism found worldwide that causes food poisoning from eating contaminated seafood, raw vegetables, or meat; characteristic symptoms are stomach pain, vomiting, diarrhea, fever, chills.

vibrissae (vī-bris'ē): The hairs growing in the vestibule of the nose.—vibrissa, sing.

vicarious (vī-kar'i-us): 1. Acting as a substitute for something. 2. Occurring in an unexpected or abnormal situation. **V. MENSTRUATION,** bleeding from the nose or other part of the body when menstruation is abnormally suppressed.

videognosis (vid'-ē-ō-og-nō'sis): Diagnosis made at a clinical center to which x-ray photographs have been transmitted by television.

villous (vil'us): Pertaining to, resembling, or furnished with villi. **V. ADENOMA,** a slow growing neoplasm of the intestinal mucosa, usually occurring in the colon; potentially malignant. **V. CARCINOMA,** carcinoma of the intestinal mucosa involving the villi.

villus (vil'us): A microscopic finger-like projection, such as is found in the mucous membrane of the small intestine, or on the outside of the chorion of the embryonic sac.—villi, pl.; villous, adj.

Vincent's angina: See angina.

Vincke tongs: See tongs.

vinculum (ving'kū-lum): A bandlike structure, ligament; or frenum (*q.v.*).

violaceous (vī'ō-lā'shē-us): Refers to a violet discoloration, usually of the skin.

violence (vī'ō-lens): Unwarranted, extremely rough physical force or action exerted with the intent to injure or destroy oneself or another person. Rape is considered a form of violence. "Violence, potential for: self-directed or directed at others" was accepted as a nursing diagnosis at the Fourth National Conference on the Classification of Nursing Diagnoses in 1980.

viral (vī'ral): Pertaining to, caused by, or resembling a virus (*q.v.*). **V. HEPATITIS,** see under hepatitis. **V. INFECTION,** see under infection. **V. PNEUMONIA,** see under pneumonia.

viremia (vī-rē'mi-a): The presence of virus in the bloodstream.—viremic, adj.

virgin (ver'jin): 1. A female who has never experienced sexual intercourse. 2. A person of either sex who has never experienced sexual intercourse.—virginity, n., virginal, adj.

viricidal (vi-ri-sī'dal): Virucidal (*q.v.*).

virile (vir'il): 1. Energetic; vigorous; possessed of characteristics usually considered as belonging to men. 2. Specifically capable of functioning as a male in copulation.

virilism (vir'i-lizm): 1. Masculinity. 2. The appearance of secondary male characteristics in a woman.

virility (vi-ril'i-ti): The state of being a male; having the nature and characteristics of an adult male.

virilization (vir-il-ī-zā'shun): The acquisition of masculine characteristics by a female, *e.g.*, lowering of the voice pitch, loss of hair in the temporal area, amenorrhea, hypertrophy of the clitoris. See adrenogenital syndrome.—virilizing, adj.

virion (vī'ri-on): A minute virus particle that consists of either deoxyribonucleic acid (DNA) or ribonucleic acid (RNA) contained within a protein coat called a capsid which, collectively, forms subunits called capsomeres. DNA is found in plant viruses, RNA in bacterial viruses, and both DNA and RNA in animal viruses.

virologist (vī-rol'o-jist): One who studies viruses and viral diseases.

virology (vī-rol'o-ji): The study of viruses and the diseases caused by them.—virological, adj.

virucidal (vī' -rū-sī'dal): Destructive or lethal to a virus. 2. Capable of destroying a virus.

virulence (vir'ū-lens): Infectiousness; the disease-producing power of a microorganism; the relative degree of the power of a microorganism to overcome host resistance and produce disease.—virulent, adj.

virulent (vir'ū-lent): 1. Extremely harmful or poisonous. 2. Having the power to overcome the host's defenses and produce disease.

virus (vī'rus): Any of a large group of disease-producing agents so small that they can be seen only under the electron microscope; are capable of passing through a filter that would hold back ordinary bacteria; can live and propagate only in the presence of living cells; and which produce a variety of pathologic conditions. The virus particle, or virion, consists of a core of either DNA (*q.v.*) or RNA (*q.v.*) that is enclosed in a protein sheath called a capsid; it varies greatly in size and shape. Viruses may gain entrance to the body through droplet infection from the respiratory tract; ingestion by the gastrointestinal system; blood transfusion; or a break in the skin including bites by insect or animal carriers. Viruses that have been classified according to several characteristics; the list according to anatomic area affected include: 1) dermatropic (smallpox, chickenpox, measles); 2) pneumotropic (common cold, influenza, atypical pneumonia); 3) neurotropic (rabies, poliomyelitis, herpes zoster, encephalitis); 4) viscerotropic: (yellow fever and mumps).

viscera (vis'er-a): Plural of viscus (*q.v.*).

visceral (vis'er-al): Pertaining to a viscus or the viscera.

visceralgia (vis-er-al'ji-a): Pain in a viscus or viscera.

viscero-: Combining form denoting viscera.

visceromegaly (vis'er-ō-meg'a-li): Abnormal enlargement of the viscera.

visceroperitoneal (vis'er-ō-per-i-tō-ne'al): Pertaining to the viscera and the peritoneum.

visceroptosis (vis'er-op-tō'sis): Downward displacement or falling of the abdominal organs.

viscerotonia (vis' -e-rō-tō'ni-a): A temperamental trait manifested chiefly by enjoyment of physical pleasures such as eating, relaxation, sociability, and comfortable situations.

viscerotonic (vis'er-ō-ton'ik): Pertaining to the behavior of a somatotype individual; characterized by love of food, sociability, friendliness, general relaxation.—viscerotonia, n.

viscid (vis'id): Glutinous or sticky.

viscidity (vi-sid'i-ti): Adhesiveness; stickiness.

viscosity (vis-kos'i-ti): The quality of being glutinous, sticky, viscous. In physics, the tendency of a fluid to resist flow, due to the friction created by cohesion of its molecules.

viscous (vis'kus): Having a glutinous or ropy consistency and the quality of sticking or adhering.

viscus (vis'kus): Any one of the internal organs, especially those in the trunk of the body.—viscera, pl.

vision: Sight; the special sense concerned with the perception of the particular qualities of an object, *e.g.*, color, size, shape. **ACHROMATIC V.,** colorblindness. **BINOCULAR V.,** the normal perception of a single image when viewed with both eyes. **DOUBLE V.,** diplopia (*q.v.*). **NIGHT V.,** ability to see in dim light.

visiting nurse: See under nurse.

visual: Pertaining to vision. **V. ACUITY,** acuteness of sight. **V. CELLS,** usually refers to the rods and cones of the retina. **V. FIELD,** the area within which objects can be seen. **V. MEMORY,** see under **memory**. **V. PURPLE**, the light-sensitive purple substance contained in the rods of the retina; syn., rhodopsin (*q.v.*).

visuoauditory (vizh′ū-ō-aw′di-to-ri): Pertaining to both vision and hearing.

visuognosis (vizh′ū-og-nō′sis): The recognition and understanding of what is seen.

vital (vī′tal): Pertaining to or necessary to the maintenance of life. **V. CAPACITY**, the maximal amount of air expelled from the lungs after a maximal inspiration. **V. FUNCTIONS**, those necessary for the maintenance of life. **V. SIGNS**, temperature, pulse, respiration, and blood pressure. **V. STATISTICS**, records of births, deaths, marriages, and incidence of diseases in a specific area.

vitality (vī-tal′i-ti): 1. Vigor, liveliness, energy. 2. The power of surviving, living, and growing.

Vitallium (vī-tal′i-um): An alloy that, in the form of nails, plates, tubes, prostheses, etc., can be left in the tissues. Often used to make knee and hip joint replacement.

Vitalograph (vī-tal′ō-graf): An instrument used for spirometry; portable, can be used at the bedside. See **spirometer**.

vitals (vī′tals): Name sometimes given to the viscera.

vitamin (vī′ta-min): Any one of several complex chemical substances found in minute quantities in certain foodstuffs. As a group, vitamins are essential to life, growth, reproduction, good health, and resistance to infection. Sometimes classified as fat soluble and water soluble. Some can now be synthesized. Their absence or deficiency in the diet causes a variety of deficiency diseases. (See individual vitamin listings.)

vitamin A: A fat-soluble anti-infective vitamin that is necessary for growth, reproduction, the maintenance of healthy skin and mucous membranes, and for the formation of rhodopsin and prevention of night blindness. A carotene derivative, it is found in all animal fats, fish liver oils, egg yolk, liver, milk, butter, some leafy green vegetables, some yellow vegetables, carrots in particular, some fruits; also produced synthetically. Deficiency results in night blindness, xerophthalmia, keratinization of the skin and mucous membranes, predisposition to infections of the skin, bladder, and bronchi due to altered epithelial membranes in these organs, and retarded growth. Overdosage is possible, resulting in headache, anorexia, sparsity of hair, and certain bone changes as seen on x ray. Also known as the anti-infective vitamin. See also **provitamin** and **carotene**.

vitamin B complex: An important group of water-soluble vitamins all of which are found in liver and yeast; various members of the group are also found in kidney, heart, pork, fish, egg yolk, nuts, soybeans, whole grain cereals, leafy green vegetables, dairy products, blackstrap molasses. All are destroyed by heat or long cooking. Substances belonging to the complex, or that may be found associated with it include biotin, choline, folic acid, para-aminobenzoic acid, riboflavin, thiamine.

vitamin B_1: See **thiamin**.

vitamin B_2: Old term for riboflavin (*q.v.*).

vitamin B_3: See **pantothenic acid**.

vitamin B_6: See **pyridoxine**.

vitamin B_{12}: See **cyanocobalamin**.

vitamin C: A water-soluble vitamin found in citrus and other fruits and fruit juices, the leafy green vegetables, tomatoes, sweet potatoes; also prepared artificially. Necessary for building strong teeth and bones; for strengthening small blood vessels, muscles, and connective tissue; for formation of intercellular cement; important in combating infections and preventing scurvy; facilitates absorption of iron. Deficiency results in sore bleeding gums, pyorrhea, dental caries, sore joints, anemia, tendency to bruise easily, scurvy. Also known as ascorbic acid, antiascorbic vitamin, and cevitamic acid. See **ascorbic acid**.

vitamin D: A fat-soluble vitamin necessary for the absorption of calcium and phosphorus from the gut and for the proper development of bones and teeth. Found in fish liver oils, especially that of salmon, tuna, cod, and herring; milk and milk products, especially those which have been irradiated; oysters; and yeast. Deficiency results in rickets, osteoporosis, osteomalacia, and osteodystrophy. Overdosage is possible, producing anorexia, vomiting, diarrhea, headache, drowsiness, high blood calcium, calcareous deposits in walls of blood vessels, heart and kidney tissues. Sometimes called the "sunshine" vitamin because it can be produced synthetically by irradiation of ergosterol as occurs when the skin is exposed to sunlight. **VITAMIN D_2**, calciferol (*q.v.*).

vitamin E: See **tocopherol**.

vitamin H: Name formerly designating biotin.

vitamin K: Any of a group of fat-soluble vitamins that are essential for the formation of prothrombin and the clotting of blood and which are absorbed only in the presence of bile; found in fish liver and meal, animal liver, alfalfa, cabbage, spinach, tomatoes, all leafy vegetables, green vegetables, soybean oil, fats, pork, cheese, egg yolk; also produced synthetically. Also called prothrombin factor and antihemorrhagic factor.

vitamin P: Bioflavinoid; a group of pigments and related compounds occurring in the rind of citrus fruits and in other fruits and plants; considered necessary for maintaining stability of capillary walls by decreasing their permeability and fragility; also considered essential for the absorption and metabolism of ascorbic acid.

vitaminology (vī'ta-min-ol'o-ji): The scientific study of vitamins.

vitelliform macular dystrophy (vī-tel'i-form mak'ū-lar dis'trō-fi): A familial disease marked by degeneration of the macula lutea; bilateral; affects individuals between 10 and 25 years of age. Vision may be minimally or markedly affected. Also called Best's disease.

vitellin (vi-tel'in): The chief protein in egg yolk.

vitiate (vish'ē-āt): To contaminate or corrupt.

vitiation (vish-i-a'shun): 1. Contamination or injury. 2. Lessening of efficiency or impairment of usefulness.

vitiligo (vit-i-lī'gō): A skin disease characterized by formation of smooth, white, circumscribed irregular patches, with normal or increased pigmentation of the surrounding skin which darkens on exposure to sunlight. Occurs chiefly on the hands, most often in the elderly. Cause unknown. Most commonly seen in tropical zones.

vitrectomy (vī-trek'tō-mi): A microsurgical procedure for removing an opacity (usually consisting of old blood and protein) from the vitreous cavity of the eye.

vitreoretinal (vit'rē-ō-ret'i-nal): Pertaining to both the vitreous humor and the retina.

vitreous (vit'rē-us): 1. Resembling glass. 2. Resembling jelly. **V. BODY,** the semifluid, transparent jelly-like substance filling the posterior cavity of the eye. Also called vitreous humor.

vivax malaria: Tertian malaria; see malaria.

vivi-: Combining form denoting alive; living.

viviparous (viv-ip'ar-us): Bringing forth or bearing the young alive.

vivisection (viv-i-sek'shun): The act of cutting or performing surgery on a living animal for purposes of research or experimentation; often extended to mean any form of animal experimentation.

v.o.: Abbreviation for verbal order.

vocal (vō'kal): Pertaining to the voice or the organ that produces voice. **V. CORDS,** membranous folds enclosing ligaments that stretch anterioposteriorly across the larynx; usually referred to as **TRUE** and **FALSE VOCAL CORDS** depending on their place of attachment to the thyroid and arytenoid cartilages. Sound is produced by their vibration as air from the lungs passes between them. **V. CORD NODULE,** see singers' node. **V. FREMITUS,** see fremitus.—vocalization, n.

vocalis (vō-kal'is): A muscle situated just beneath the true vocal cord; the musculus vocalis.

vocalization (vō'ka-lī-zā'shun): Use of the voice as in speaking or singing.

Vogt-Koyanagi-Haranda syndrome: Uveomeningitis (*q.v.*) involving the iris and the choroid, associated with loss of pigment in the eyebrows and lashes and in patches of skin;

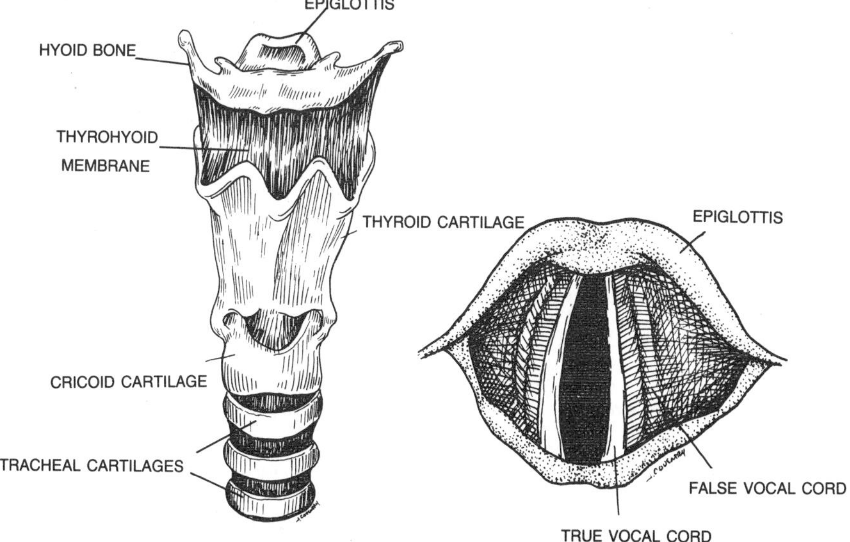

The larynx and upper trachea **Vocal cords**

detached retina, and sometimes tinnitus and hearing loss.

voice box: See larynx.

void: 1. To cast off or out, as waste matter from the body. 2. To urinate.

vola (vō'la): The palm of the hand or the sole of the foot.

volar (vō'lar): Pertaining to the palm of the hand or the sole of the foot.

volatile (vol'a-til): 1. Having a tendency to evaporate quickly. 2. Having an explosive or violent nature or tending to change suddenly.

volition (vō-lish'un): The conscious act or power of adopting or refraining from a certain line of action.—volitional, adj.

volitional (vō-lish'un-al): Voluntary; describing an act of will.

Volkmann's contracture: See under contracture.

volt: The standard measure of intensity of an electric current.

voltage (vol'tej): Potential electromotive force measured in volts.

volubility (vol-ū-bil'i-ti): Garrulousness; loquaciousness; talkativeness.

volume (vol'yum): Amount. 1. The measure of a quantity of a substance. 2. The space occupied by a substance, mass, bulk. BLOOD V., the total amount of blood circulating in the body. MINUTE V., the amount of air exhaled per minute; or the amount of cardiac output per minute. RESIDUAL V., the amount of air that remains in the lungs after a maxiumum exhalation. STROKE V., the amount of blood the left ventricle ejects with each heartbeat; usual amount is about 75 cc per minute. TIDAL V., the amount of air that is breathed in and out in normal respiration.

voluntary (vol'un-ter-i): Under the control of the will; free and unrestricted; as opposed to reflex or involuntary. V. HEALTH CARE AGENCY, one that is organized and controlled by individuals who are not salaried and who may or may not be professional health care givers; may be supported by governmental or voluntary financing. V. MUSCLES, striated muscles that perform activities that are initiated and controlled by the individual.

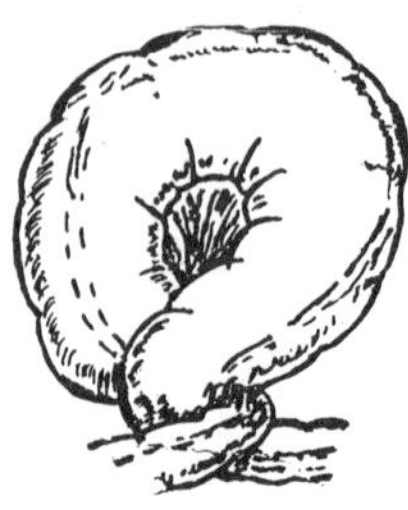

Volvulus

volvulus (vol'vū-lus): A twisting of a section of bowel, so as to occlude the lumen. It causes obstruction of the bowel.

vomer (vō'mer): The thin plowshare-shaped bone that forms the inferior and posterior part of the nasal septum.

vomit (vom'it): 1. To forcibly eject the stomach contents through the mouth. 2. Stomach contents ejected forcibly through the mouth.

vomiting (vom'i-ting): Forcible ejection of stomach contents through the mouth. CYCLIC V., recurrent spasms of vomiting. DRY V., retching and attempting to vomit without being able to do so. FECAL V., vomiting of matter that contains feces. PERNICIOUS V., uncontrollable V.; severe V. of pregnancy. PROJECTILE V., ejection of stomach contents with great force. PSYCHOGENIC V., V. without apparent physical cause; presumed to be of psychologic origin. STERCORACEOUS V., FECAL V. V. OF PREGNANCY, see hyperemesis.

vomitus (vom'i-tus): Vomited matter. COFFEE-GROUND V., that which contains broken-down blood mixed with matter from the stomach; occurs in malignancy and some other diseases of the stomach.

von Gierke's disease: Glycogen storage disease, Type I; a hereditary condition characterized by hypoglycemia, hepatomegaly, acidosis, and hyperuricemia.

von Hippel-Lindau disease: A hereditary condition involving the retina and cerebellum and sometimes the spinal cord; usually seen in association with lesions of the kidney, adrenal gland, pancreas, or other organ; characterized by seizures and lack of mental development. See also angiophacomatosis.

von Pirquet test: A skin test for tuberculosis. [Clemens Freiherr von Pirquet, Austrian pediatrician. 1874–1929.]

von Recklinghausen's disease: *See* Recklinghausen's disease.

von Willebrand's disease: A hereditary disorder in which the bleeding time is increased. There is a deficiency of Factor VIII and blood platelet abnormality. Symptoms include epistaxis, bleeding from the gastrointestinal tract, gums, uterus, and surgical incisions. Other names include von Willebrand's syndrome, Willebrand-Jurgens syndrome, angiohemophilia, and vascular hemophilia.

Voorhees' bag: A hydrostatic bag formerly often used in obstetrics; it was inserted into the cervix to induce labor.

voyeur (vwah'yer): One who derives sexual satisfaction from seeing the sexual organs of another or from watching sexual acts. A Peeping Tom.

voyeurism (vwah′yer-izm): The characteristics, tendencies or acts of a voyeur (*q.v.*).

vulgaris (vul-gar′is): Ordinary.

vulnus (vul′nus): A wound or injury.

vulsellum (vul-sel′um): A forceps with claw-like hooks at the end of each blade.

vulva (vul′va): 1. The labia minora and majora. 2. The pudendum (*q.v.*).—vulval, vulvar, adj.

vulvectomy (vul-vek′to-mi): Excision of the vulva. **RADICAL V.**, excision of the vulva and of tissues from the anus to a few centimeters above the symphysis pubis, including the labia majora and minora, and the clitoris.

vulvismus (vul-viz′mus): Vaginismus (*q.v.*).

vulvitis (vul-vī′tis): Inflammation of the vulva. **DIABETIC V.**, **V.** occurring in women with diabetes. **LEUKOPLAKIC V.**, kraurosis **V.**, see under kraurosis.

vulvo-: Combining form denoting 1) a covering, or 2) the vulva.

vulvopathy (vul-vop′a-thi): Any disorder of the vulva.

vulvorectal (vul-vō-rek′tal): Pertaining to the vulva and the rectum, as a **V.** fistula.

vulvovaginal (vul-vō-vag′in-nal): Pertaining to the vulva and the vagina. **V. GLANDS**, see Bartholin's glands.

vulvovaginitis (vul′vō-vaj-in-ī′tis): Inflammation of the vulva and vagina or of the vulvovaginal glands.

W

w: Abbreviation for: 1. Watt. 2. Week.

Waardenburg's syndrome: A congenital hereditary syndrome, marked by lateral displacement of the inner canthi, widened bridge of the nose, white forelock and eyelashes, nonpigmented patches on the skin, premature graying of the hair, cochlear deafness.

waddle: To walk with short steps and a swinging side-to-side movement of the upper part of the body, seen in certain neurological disorders.

wafer: A two-layered disk made of flour paste, with a dose of medicine between the layers; a cachet.

Wagner-Meissner corpuscles: Meissner's corpuscles (*q.v.*).

WAIS: Abbreviation for Wechsler Adult Intelligence Scale (*q.v.*).

waist (wāst): The small part of the trunk of the body below the thorax and above the hips.

Waldenström's disease: 1. Osteochondritis deformans juvenilis. See under osteochondritis. 2. Macroglobulinemia (*q.v.*).

Waldeyer's ring: A circle of lymphoid tissue that encircles the pharynx, the part above being called the pharyngeal tonsil, that on the sides the palatine tonsils, and that on the lower part the lingual tonsil. [Wilhelm von Waldeyer-Hartz, German anatomist. 1836–1921.]

wale (wāl): A linear wheal, especially one produced by a stick or whip.

walker: A light, cage-like metal frame that rests steadily on the floor and partially encircles the body at waist height, has four legs and supports for the hands; often made so that it can be folded for storage and sometimes fitted with casters; used as an aid in standing and walking. The patient lifts and advances the walker, then steps forward either with the feet together or one after the other.

walking: W. CAST, a cast so constructed as to allow the patient to be ambulatory. SLEEP W., somnambulism (*q.v.*). W. TYPHOID, a mild case of typhoid fever in which the patient is not confined to bed.

wall: The structures that cover or surround an anatomical unit such as a cell or an organ, or that enclose a cavity, *e.g.*, the chest cavity or the abdominal cavity.

wall climbing: An exercise prescribed for postmastectomy patients to prevent contraction of shoulder muscles and to restore full range of motion of the arm; the patient stands facing the wall, places her hands on the wall and moves them upward until she reaches the point of pain, marks that place on the wall, and the next time she exercises tries to overreach it.

Wallace's rule of nines: A rule for expressing the size of burns as a percentage of the body surface area involved; the head is estimated at 9% (4½% each for the anterior and posterior surface); the upper extremities at 9% (4½% each for anterior and posterior surfaces); the anterior and posterior trunk, 18% each; the lower extremities at 18% each (9% for each anterior and posterior surface). The perineum is estimated at 1%. See also Lund and Browder's chart.

Wallenberg's syndrome: A condition characterized by occlusion of the posterior inferior cerebellar artery, which results in contralateral loss of temperature and pain sensation; occurs in fifth, ninth, and eleventh nerve palsies and in nystagmus, dysarthria, and dysphagia.

wallerian degeneration: See under degeneration.

walleye: 1. Opacity of the cornea. 2. A condition in which the iris is white or pale colored. 3. A strabismus in which the eye turns outward.

wandering: Moving about; not fixed in place. W. KIDNEY, floating kidney; see under kidney.

Wangensteen: W. SUCTION, a widely used method of continuous siphonage by suction, for the purpose of draining fluid from a body cavity, *e.g.*, the stomach, employing a device that consists of a nasogastric catheter and a suction apparatus that operates on the principle of negative pressure. It is most commonly used for evacuating gas and fluids from the stomach and upper intestine. W. TUBE, the catheter part of the Wangensteen suction device. [Owen Wangensteen, American surgeon. 1898–1981.]

ward: A room in a hospital with beds for several patients. PSYCHOPATHIC W., a W. in a general hospital that is occupied by patients with mental disorders.

ward clerk or **secretary:** An assistant to the ward or unit manager; assists with paper work, mans the telephones, takes messages, orders supplies, etc.; is usually trained on the job.

ward or **unit manager:** A person on the administrative staff of a hospital who is responsible for the general management of a ward or unit; may or may not be assisted by a ward clerk or secretary.

warfarin (war'fa-rin): A chemical substance that acts as an anticoagulant; in medicine, useful in prevention and treatment of such conditions as coronary thrombosis and pulmonary embolism. W. POISONING, may occur as a result of overdosage of warfarin, or accidental ingestion of certain rodenticides that contain the chemical; marked by internal bleeding, epistaxis, hematuria; treatment is aimed at reestablishing normal coagulability of the blood.

wart: A benign horny projection on the skin caused by hypertrophy of the papillae of the corium. May also occur on mucous membrane. Believed to be caused by a virus; usually painless. Many varieties are described. See verruca. GENITAL W., appears on the vulva especially during pregnancy; can be spread sexually; also called venereal W. and condyloma acuminatum. PERIUNGUAL W., a W. occurring commonly around or under a fingernail; may become fissured and painful. PLANTAR W., see under plantar. SEBORRHEIC W., seborrheic keratosis; see under keratosis.

wash: A lotion for application to the skin or mucous membrane.

Wassermann test: The first serological test for syphilis; utilizes a complement-fixation technique; no longer in general use.

waste: In physiology, material that is of no use to the body and is cast off as refuse. W. THEORY, the theory that aging occurs as a result of the collection of chemical wastes in the body, which interferes with normal cell functioning.

wasting: Emaciation; pronounced loss of body weight, accompanied by decreased physical and mental activity.

water: A colorless, odorless, and almost tasteless liquid; makes up a large part of the body substance; boils at 212°F (100°C) and freezes at 32°F (0°C). W. BALANCE, the condition that exits when the intake of water equals the output. W. BED, a sealed rubber sack filled with water and used as a mattress for such purposes as preventing decubiti. W. BRASH, see pyrosis. W. DEPLETION, refers to loss of water alone as differentiated from dehydration, which may refer to loss of water and salt; is prevented by the sensation of thirst and drinking to relieve it; occurs chiefly in the person whose sensation of thirst is blunted or who is mentally or physically unable to respond to it. DISTILLED W., W. that has been heated to boiling, vaporized, and condensed into liquid form; the condensate has a pH of 7.0 and contains no minerals. HARD W., W. that contains calcium and magnesium ions which combine with fatty acids and prevent soap from making a lather in it. HEAVY W., W. in which most of the hydrogen atoms are heavy hydrogen (^{2}H), giving it properties that differ from those of ordinary W. W. OF HYDRATION, W. in combination in a substance, but that may be expelled from it without any change in composition. W. INTOXICATION, a condition produced by the intake and retention of abnormal amounts of water and marked by subnormal temperatures, vomiting, depression, and possibly irreversible coma and death. LIME W., CALCIUM HYDROXIDE. MINERAL W., contains certain mineral salts in sufficient quantity to be tasted and is considered to have some therapeutic properties. POLLUTED W., W. that is unfit for human consumption. POTABLE W., W. that is suitable for drinking. W. MATTRESS, see water bed under bed. SODA W., W. that has been charged with carbon dioxide gas. SOFT W., W. that does not contain calcium and magnesium ions and in which soap will lather readily. VICHY W., W. from springs in Vichy, France; has a diuretic action.

water cure: Hydrotherapy.

water on the knee: Lay term for synovitis of the knee joint; a sign of some underlying problem; not a diagnosis.

water-borne: Said of diseases that are spread largely by drinking-water, *e.g.*, cholera, typhoid fever.

water-hammer pulse: The full, bounding pulse felt in patients with aortic insufficiency. Also called Corrigan's pulse.

Waterhouse-Friderichsen syndrome: A fulminating meningococcal infection marked by headache, chills, fever, vomiting, diarrhea, purpura, joint pain, shock, adrenal insufficiency, respiratory distress, convulsions; occurs mainly in children, especially those under ten years of age; an emergency condition.

waters: Usually refers to the amniotic fluid (liquor amnii, *q.v.*). BAG OF W., the closed sac that encloses the amniotic fluid.

water-seal drainage: A method of drainage in which the end of the tube is in water, thus allowing fluid and air to escape but preventing air from entering; used especially for draining and collecting fluid from the pleural space.

Waterson procedure: A surgical procedure performed on patients with tetralogy of Fallot; involves creating an anastomosis between the ascending aorta and the right pulmonary artery.

Watson-Crick helix: See helix.

watt: The standard unit of electrical power.

wave: 1. A continuous, uniformly advancing, undulating rhythmic motion or series of movements that pass along a surface or through the air. 2. BRAIN WAVES, the fluctuations in the electrical current set up in the cortex of the brain by brain action; they may be recorded during electroencephalography. ALPHA WAVES, in the EEG, occur chiefly in the occiput of the normal person, awake and at rest at a rate of about 8 to 13 per second. BETA WAVES, in the EEG, occur chiefly in the frontal and parietal areas during periods of intense nervous system activity, at a rate of about 18 to 30 per second. DELTA WAVES, in the EEG, occur during deep sleep and in serious brain disorders, at a rate of about 3 to 3.5 per second. F or FF WAVES, regular rapid atrial waves seen in the ECG; occur in cases of atrial flutter. J. WAVE, a positive deflection at the junction of the QRS and ST segments of the electrocardiogram of some patients with hypoglycemia. P. WAVE, in the electrocardiogram, represents the depolarization of the atria. **PULSE WAVE,** the beat felt with the finger over an artery or shown on a sphygmograph. **Q WAVE,** in the ECG, the first downward deflection in the QRS complex; represents the beginning of depolarization of the ventricles. **R. WAVE,** in the ECG, an upward deflection, following the Q wave. **S. WAVE,** in the ECG, the negative deflection in the QRS complex, following the R wave. **T. WAVE,** in the ECG, is due to repolarization of the ventricles. **THETA WAVES,** in the EEG, occur chiefly in adults under stress and in children at a rate of about 4 to 7 per second. **U WAVE,** in the ECG, a low amplitude upward deflection following the T wave; not always present.

wavelength (wāv′length): In physics, the distance from a given point in the progression of a wave cycle to the corresponding point in the next wave cycle in a wavelength having the same phase in two consecutive cycles.

wax: A solid fatty substance secreted by insects and obtained from plants; also made synthetically. **EAR WAX,** cerumen (*q.v.*). **PARAFFIN W.,** a wax prepared from petrolatum. **BEESWAX,** a yellow wax secreted by bees; used as a base for ointments.

waxy flexibility: The condition of muscles that exists when a patient's limbs are held indefinitely in any position in which they are placed. See catatonia and cerea flexibilitas.

WBC: Abbreviation for 1) white blood cell; 2) white blood cell count.

wean: 1. To discontinue feeding a child at the breast and substitute other methods of providing nutrition. 2. To discontinue use of a respirator by gradually lessening the time the patient uses it; an important nursing responsibility to prevent the patient from becoming emotionally and physically dependent on artificial ventilation. 3. To assist a person in withdrawing from something on which the person has become dependent.

wear and tear theory: A theory of aging that poses the idea that the body is like a machine, and that various parts wear out, and that physiological functions deteriorate until, finally, they are unable to sustain life.

weaver's bottom: Inflammation of the bursa over the ischial tuberosity; occurs in sedentary people, especially those who sit cross-legged much of the time.

webbed: A congenital condition in which adjacent structures are connected by an abnormal band of tissue.

Weber-Christian syndrome: A disorder characterized by the formation of nodules and plaques in the subcutaneous fatty layer of the skin affecting chiefly the trunk and extremities, the thighs and legs in particular, and resulting in atrophy; malaise, fever, hepatomegaly and aplenomegaly may be present.

Weber's test: Tuning fork test for the diagnosis of conduction deafness. [Friedrich Eugen Weber, German otologist 1832–1891.]

Wechsler-Bellevue Intelligence Scale: Widely used in verbal and performance tests, for persons between 16 and 64 years of age, in converting test results into a conventional intelligence quotient. Comprises 11 subtests in various areas. Other scales developed by Wechsler are the **WECHSLER INTELLIGENCE SCALE** (WAIS), **WECHSLER INTELLIGENCE SCALE FOR CHILDREN,** and **WECHSLER PRESCHOOL AND PRIMARY SCALE OF INTELLIGENCE.** [David Wechsler, American psychologist. 1896–1981.]

wedge pressure: See pulmonary wedge pressure under pressure.

weep: To exude, drop by drop, tears or other fluid such as serum.

weeping eczema (wē′ping ek′ze-ma): A type of eczema in which there is a vesicular eruption with the vesicles exuding serum.

Wegener's granulomatosis: Thought to be a variant of polyarteritis nodosa; a progressive disorder characterized by necrotizing lesions in the upper respiratory tract, the lungs, and arterioles; inflammation of all the organs of the body; and glomerulonephritis, which frequently results in renal failure and death.

Weigert's law: States that when a part of an organic structure is lost or destroyed, the repair and regeneration process is likely to result in overproduction of tissue.

Weight Watchers: A behavioral self-management support group; the objective of members is to gain and retain control of their weight.

Weil-Felix reaction: Agglutination reaction useful in diagnosis of rickettsial diseases such as epidemic, marine, and scrub typhus; Rocky Mountain spotted fever; various other tick fevers. [Edmund Weil, German physician in Prague. 1880–1922. Arthur Felix, Prague bacteriologist. 1887–1956.]

Weil's disease (wīlz): A type of jaundice with fever and splenic enlargement caused by a small spirochete voided in the urine of rats. A disease of miners, sewer workers, etc., who work in dirty water. Syn., Spirochetosis ictohemorrhagica, leptospiral jaundice. [Adolph Weil, German physician. 1848–1916.]

Welch's bacillus: *Clostridium perfringens,* the most common causative agent of gas gangrene.

well baby clinic: A clinic devoted to the health care of well infants and children, usually through the first three years of life; provides guidance for parents regarding the child's nutrition, growth and development, immunizations, and general health care. May be free standing or connected with a doctor's office or a neighborhood health care facility.

wellness: For the adult, a state of emotional, social, and spiritual health that permits clients, within the limits of their abilities and disabilities, to function effectively in their particular social group and to enjoy life. "Wellness is a process of moving toward greater awareness of onself and the environment, leading to ever increasing planned interactions with the dimensions of nutrition, fitness, stress, interpersonal relationships, and self-care. A Wellness Center is a facility that assists clients to self-assess and self-evaluate their progress in the interacting dimensions of wellness and where a wellness practitioner facilitates the clients' movement toward wellness." [C. C. Clark.]

welt: A raised ridge left on the skin by a slash or a blow, as of a whip. A wheal.

Welterntergang dreams: May occur in schizophrenic patients; the sense of the real world is lost and the patient becomes fearful and panicky and creates a substitute world made up of things and people that have meaning only for the individual.

wen: A retention cyst of a sebaceous gland of the skin. See cyst.

Wenckebach phenomenon: A second degree atrioventricular heart block in which the P-R interval in the electrocardiogram becomes progressively longer until the P wave finally disappears and the sequence begins again; often a forerunner of complete heart block.

Werdnig-Hoffman syndrome or **disease:** A hereditary form of infantile muscular atrophy resulting from degeneration of the anterior horn cells of the spinal cord; characterized by wasting of the muscles, flaccid paralysis, and early death; usually occurs in siblings, rather than successive generations. Also called infantile spinal muscular dystrophy and Werdnig-Hoffman paralysis.

Werlhof's disease: Idiopathic thrombocytopenic purpura; see under purpura.

Wermer's syndrome: A rare hereditary condition characterized by hyperplasia of more than one endocrine tissue, involving most often the pituitary and parathyroid glands and the islands of Langerhans. Polyendocrine adenomatosis. Also called multiple endocrine adenomatosis.

Werner's syndrome: A condition involving many body systems, characterized by early senescence; cataracts; osteoporosis; scleroderma; and glandular dysfunction, particularly hypogonadism.

Wernicke-Korsakoff syndrome: Wernicke's encephalopathy and Korsakoff's syndrome, which often occur together, particularly in alcoholics; due to nutritional deficiency, specifically of vitamin B_1.

Wernicke's syndrome: Wernicke's encephalopathy. See under encephalopathy.

Wertheim's hysterectomy (his-ter-ek'to-mi): An extensive operation for removal of carcinoma of the cervix, where the uterus, cervix, upper vagina, tubes, ovaries, and regional lymph glands are removed. [Ernst Wertheim, Austrian gynecologist. 1864–1920.]

Westergren method: A laboratory test for determining the erythrocyte sedimentation rate; see sedimentation.

western equine encephalomyelitis: See under encephalomyelitis.

wet dreams: The discharge of semen during sleep, a natural occurence during adolescence; may or may not be accompanied by a pleasurable dream.

wet lung syndrome: A condition of the lungs characterized by persistent cough and rales heard at the base of the lung; seen in those whose work exposes them to irritating dust, fumes, or vapor.

wet nurse: A woman who breast-feeds a child who is not her own offspring.

Wharton: WHARTON'S DUCT, that of the submaxillary salivary gland. WHARTON'S JELLY, a jelly-like substance contained in the umbilical cord. [Thomas Wharton, English physician. 1616–1673.]

wheal (hwēl): The characteristic lesion of urticaria, but may follow insect bites or stings, or exposure to substances to which the person is allergic. Consists of an edematous, circumscribed raised area of the skin, irregular in shape, redder or paler than the surrounding skin; usually accompanied by intense itching and usually transitory.

wheelchair: A chair mounted on wheels for individuals who cannot walk; may be propelled by hand or be motor driven; some are collapsible for transportation by a vehicle.

wheeze: 1. To breathe noisily and with difficulty. 2. The hoarse whistling sound heard in conditions in which breathing is difficult; caused by partial obstruction of one or more of the air passages, may result from inflammation, trauma, presence of a foreign body, tumor.

whiplash injury (whip'lash in'jer-i): A popular term for injury of one or more of the cervical vertebrae, resulting from sudden jerking of the head. Symptoms are pain, swelling and limitation of motion.

Whipple's disease: A generalized disease involving the lymphatics and intestinal wall; marked by arthritis, steatorrhea, emaciation, and lymphadenectomy. Syn., intestinal lipodystrophy.

Whipple's operation: A radical surgical procedure done in cases of carcinoma of the head of the pancreas and the area of the papilla of Vater; involves removal of the distal part of the stomach, duodenum, head of the pancreas, and the common bile duct.

whipworm: See Trichuris trichiura.

whirlpool bath: A bath in which the water is agitated and injected with air by a power device.

white blood cell: A blood cell that does not contain hemoglobin. A leukocyte (*q.v.*). The main types of white blood cells are polymorphonuclear, lymphocyte, and monocyte.

white matter: Nerve tissue that is whitish in color as opposed to the gray matter. Consists of myelinated nerve fibers of the neurons and makes up the conducting matter of the brain and spinal cord.

whitehead (whīt′hed): A small white papule, seen particularly on the face; probably caused by a blockage of a pilosebaceous follicle. See also milia.

whiteleg (hwīt′leg): Phlegmasia alba dolens; see under phelgmasia.

whitlow (hwit′low): A felon (*q.v.*). MELANOTIC W., a malignant tumor that is characterized by changes about the border of the nail and in the nail bed. See paronychia.

whoop: The characteristic crowing intake of breath following a paroxysm of coughing in whooping cough. See pertussis.

whooping cough: Pertussis (*q.v.*).

whorl (hworl): A twist or spiral turn such as in the cochlea of the ear, in the muscle fibers at the apex of the heart, in the arrangement of the ridges in a fingerprint, or in an area in which the hairs grow in a radial manner.

Widal test or reaction: An agglutination test useful in diagnosing typhoid fever. Also called Gruber-Widal reaction.

will: The faculty of conscious and deliberate action; the power of choosing one's own actions.

Willis: See circle of Willis.

willow fracture: Greenstick fracture; see under fracture.

Wilms' tumor: A congenital, highly malignant tumor of the kidney, occurring chiefly in children; develops from abnormal epithelial tissue in the embryo; may start to grow before birth and may affect any part of the kidney; symptoms include hypertension, fever, anorexia, lethargy; metastasizes early to the lungs, liver, and long bones. [Max Wilms, German surgeon. 1867–1918.]

Wilson-Mikity syndrome: A condition of progressive pulmonary insufficiency seen in infants of low birth weight; characterized by dyspnea, tachypnea, cyanosis; often fatal.

Wilson's disease: Hepatolenticular degeneration (*q.v.*).

winding sheet: A sheet used to wrap a dead body. A shroud.

window: An opening in a structure or a wall, especially a window in the inner ear (oval window, round window).

windpipe: The trachea.

wink: The involuntary opening and closing of the eyelids, a protective action by which the tears are spread over the front of the eyeball keeping the conjunctiva moist; can also be a voluntary act.

winter itch: Pruritus occurring in cold weather; affects chiefly the elderly and those with dry skin.

Winterbottom's sign: Enlargement of the posterior cervical lymph nodes, as seen in trypanosomiasis (*q.v.*).

wiring: Fastening the ends of a fractured bone together with wire sutures. See Kirschner's wire.

Wirsung: [Johann Georg Wirsung, German physician. 1600–1643.] W.'S DUCT, the main excretory duct of the pancreas; runs the length of the pancreas and collects pancreatic secretions from many small ductules; usually joins the common bile duct before emptying into the duodenum. Also called the canal of W. and hepatopancreatic duct.

wisdom tooth: The third molar on each side of the lower and upper jaws; wisdom teeth are the last to erupt, usually between the 17th and 21st years of age.

Wiskott-Aldrich syndrome: Hereditary immunodeficiency; a familial condition transmitted by a sex-linked recessive trait; characterized by anemia, thrombocytopenic purpura, leukopenia, chronic eczema, chronic otitis media and other recurrent infections, bloody diarrhea, and incomplete development of the thymus.

witch hazel: A shrub or small tree found in damp places in Asia and eastern and central North America. The dried leaves as well as an alcoholic solution have been used for treating minor wounds such as a bruise or contusion, inflammation, and headache, and for treatment of hemorrhoids. Also used as a skin toner.

withdrawal (with-draw′al): In medicine, the discontinuance of a medication or therapy. In psychiatry, the process by which a person retreats physically and/or psychologically to escape an emotionally disturbing situation. W. METHOD, coitus interuptus; see under coitus. W. SYNDROME, the group of physical and psychological signs and symptoms exhibited by a drug addict upon withdrawal from an addictive drug; severity depends on the particular drug, the length of time of the addiction, and the size of the doses the person has been taking.

WNL: Abbreviation for within normal limits.

wogging: Term meaning walking and jogging; walking at different rates from brisk to rapid.

Wohlfart-Kugelberg-Welander disease: A familial condition that may appear in childhood or later; a form of spinal muscular atrophy which is first noticed in the proximal muscles of the arms and legs and becomes a slowly progressive lifelong disorder.

wolffian (woolf'i-an): 1. W. BODIES, two small organs in the embryo that represent the primitive kidney. 2. W. DUCTS, embryonic structures that in the male develop into the epididymis, ductus deferens, ejaculatory duct, seminal vesicle, and the efferent ducts of the testes.

Wolff-Parkinson-White syndrome: An electrocardiographic pattern in which the PR interval is shortened and the QRS complex is lengthened; sometimes seen in paroxysmal tachycardia.

Wolman's disease: A rare inborn error of lipid metabolism characterized by large deposits of cholesterol, esters, and glycosides in the viscera, particularly the liver.

womb (woom): The uterus.

Women's Health Movement: Began in 1970 with the objectives of changing the attitude of physicians and others toward women's health problems and care, obtaining more participation by women in governing boards of hospitals and other community health care facilities, and providing literature and courses to inform women about their bodies and about health care services they may require.

Wood: WOOD'S RAYS, ultraviolet rays. WOOD'S GLASS, a light filter that transmits only ultraviolet rays; useful in identifying fungi that are the causative agent in certain skin and scalp diseases.

wood alchohol: Methyl alcohol.

wood tick: Any one of several varieties of ticks that cling to bushes and fasten themselves to the body of an animal or person; the place of attachment often becomes an infected lesion. One variety is the vector for Rocky Mountain spotted fever.

wool test: A test for detecting color blindness. The person is asked to select skeins of wool of matching colors.

woolsorter's disease: Pulmonary anthrax; an occupational disease that occurs in persons who handle the wool of animals that have had anthrax.

word blindness: A type of speech disturbance in which one is unable to perceive or understand certain sounds, syllables, or phrases.

word salad: Term used to describe speech in which words and phrases are so combined that they have no logical coherence or comprehensive meaning; frequently seen in schizophrenic individuals.

workaholism (work'a-hol-izm): A state of exhaustion and a group of symptoms resulting from chronic compulsive overworking.—workaholic, n.

work-up: Usually refers to the process of evaluating the patient's medical history; doing a complete physical examination, including any tests required; and gathering all possible data on the patient's present condition for the purpose of diagnosis and planning for his care.

World Health Organization (WHO): A 150-member agency of the United Nations, founded in 1948, the objective being the attainment, by all people of the world, of the highest possible level of health. Collects, analyzes, and distributes data and statistics on health and environmental problems. It is a directing and coordinating authority on international health; supports and coordinates research in health problems and the control of communicable diseases; sets standards for the production of vaccines and bacteriological products; sets international sanitary regulations; supports the fight against pollution of air, water, and soil; provides technical assistance to member nations in the improvement of their health services. Headquarters are in Geneva, Switzerland.

wormian bones (wer'mi-an): Small, isolated, irregular bones found along the sutures of the skull.

worms: See Ascarides, Taenia, Trichuris trichuria.

wound (woond): An injury to the body that involves a break in the continuity of tissues or of body structures; results from trauma or from a surgical procedure. CONTUSED W., one made with a blunt object and in which the skin is not broken. GUNSHOT W., one made by a bullet from a gun or small firearm. INCISED W. one made by a sharp cutting instrument. INFECTED W., one contaminated by microorganisms, or from debris, bits of clothing, etc. LACERATED W., one in which the tissues are torn. OPEN W., one that opens to the surface. PENETRATING W., one that causes damage to subcutaneous tissues; has a W. of entrance but no W. of exit. PUNCTURE W., deep, narrow W. caused by penetration with a pointed object. SEPTIC W., one infected with pus-producing organisms. SUCKING W., a penetrating chest wound through which air is drawn in and out. WOUND HEALING, see healing.

WPW: Abbreviation for Wolff-Parkinson-White syndrome (*q.v.*).

wrench (rench): 1. To twist something suddenly and forcibly. 2. A painful sudden violent twist, as of an ankle or wrist.

Wright's stain: A stain containing eosin and methylene blue; used for staining formed elements in the blood such as blood corpuscles and the parasites that cause malaria, for microscopic examination.

wrist (rist): The joint between the forearm and the hand; the carpus. Made up of eight carpal bones, the navicular, lunate, triangular, pisiform, greater multangular, lesser multangular, capitate, and hamate bones. **W. DROP** or **WRIST-DROP,** paralysis of the extensor muscles of the hand and fingers causing the hand to hang down at the wrist. Syn., carpus.—carpal, adj.

writer's cramp: An occupational neurosis characterized by painful spasmodic cramps of the muscles of the fingers, hand or forearm whenever an attempt is made to write.

wryneck (wrī'nek): Torticollis (*q.v.*).

Wuchereria (voo-ker-ē'ri-a): A genus of filarial worms that are parasitic in humans, inhabitating chiefly the lymphatic vessels; includes the causative parasite of tropical elephantiasis (*q.v.*).

wuchereriasis (voo-ker' -e-rī' -a-sis): Infestation with worms of the Wuchereria genus. Filariasis.

X

X chromosome: A sex chromosome that appears paired (XX) in each female human zygote and singly in each male zygote; carries the factors for femaleness. It is the differentiating chromosome for the female sex.

x ray: 1. Roentgen ray; electromagnetic rays of short length and high frequency. X rays produce a photographic effect and thus are useful in diagnosis; they also penetrate deeply, making them useful in therapy. So called because their nature was not known at the time of their discovery (1895). 2. **X-RAY PHOTOGRAPH,** a radiographic image of organs or structures projected into a photographic plate.

xanth-, xantho-: Combining forms denoting yellow or yellowish color.

xanthelasma (zan-the-laz′ma): Old term for a variety of zanthoma (*q.v.*). **X. PALPEBRARUM,** old term for a condition in which small yellowish plaques appear on the eyelids, occurring most frequently in elderly people.

xanthine (zan′thin): A yellow-white compound found in the liver, spleen, pancreas, muscle tissue, and in blood and the urine where it sometimes forms into calculi; it is formed during metabolism of nucleoproteins and is a precursor of uric acid.

xanthinuria (zan-thin-ū′ri-a): The presence of abnormally large amounts of xanthine in the urine.

xanthism (zan′ thizm): A congenital anomaly in Negroes characterized by reddish colored skin and hair.

xanthochromatic (zan-thō-krō-mat′ik): Having a yellow or yellowish color.

xanthochromia (zan-thō-krō′mi-a): 1. Yellow discoloration of the skin. 2. Yellow discoloration of the spinal fluid; due to hemolysis of blood in the subarachnoid space following subarachnoid hemorrhage.

xanthocyanopia (zan′thō-sī-an-ō′pi-a): A type of color blindness in which the person cannot distinguish red and green but is able to discern yellow and blue. Also xanthocyanopsia.

xanthoderma (zan-thō-der′ma): Yellow colored skin.

xanthodontous (zan-thō-don′tus): Having yellowish colored teeth.

xanthogranuloma (zan′thō-gran-ū-lō′ma): A tumor that has characteristics of both granuloma and xanthoma (*q.v.*).

xanthogranulomatosis (zan′thō-gran′ ū-lō-ma-tō′sis): A form of xanthomatosis (*q.v.*), in which the lipid deposits are granulomatous and are found chiefly in the skull bones. Also called Hand-Schuller-Christian disease (*q.v.*).

xanthoma (zan-thō′ma): A condition characterized by a collection of histiocytes appearing as papules, nodules, or plaques under the skin around the orbital area, or around tendons and joints, and producing a yellow discoloration; several varieties are recognized; occurs chiefly in middle or later life and more often in women than men.

xanthomatosis (zan-thō-ma-tō′sis): A condition of faulty metabolism of cholesterol, characterized by yellowish or brownish discoloration of skin and other tissues and sometimes by formation of fatty tumors; may affect general health. See Gaucher's disease, Niemann-Pick disease.

xanthomatous (zan-thō′ma-tus): Pertaining to xanthoma.

xanthopia (zan-thō′pi-a): A condition in which all objects appear yellow or yellowish. Also xanthopsia.

xanthoproteic (zan-thō-prō′tē-ik): **X. TEST,** a laboratory test for 1) dextrose; 2) protein. Mulder's test.

xanthoprotein (zan-thō-prō′tē-in): An orange pigment produced by treating protein with hot nitric acid.

xanthopsia (zan-thop′si-a): A condition in which all things are seen as yellow or yellowish; may occur in jaundice, digitalis poisoning, or picric acid poisoning.

xanthopsis (zan-thop′sis):Yellow pigmentation of the skin; seen especially in certain malignancies.

xanthosis (zan-thō′sis): Yellowish discoloration of the skin. Sometimes seen in degenerating tissues of malignant neoplasms. May also occur temporarily due to eating large quantities of foods containing carotene or from taking quinine over a long period of time.

xanthous (zan′thus): Of a yellow or yellowish color.

xanthuria (zan-thū′ri-a): Xanthinuria (*q.v.*).

xeno-: Combining form denoting 1) strange; 2) foreign material.

xenogenesis (zen-ō-jen′e-sis): 1. The production of offspring unlike either parent. 2. Heterogenesis (*q.v.*).—xenogenic, adj.

xenogenous (ze-noj′e-nus): Caused by a foreign body or substance, or originating outside of the organism.

xenograft (zen′ō-graft): Transplantation of an organ or tissue from one species to another. Heterograft.

xenology (ze-nol′o-ji): The study of parasites that affect humans.

xenomenia (zen-ō-mē′ni-a): A condition in

which 1) the physical changes that accompany menstruation occur, but there is no blood flow, or 2) menstrual blood is discharged from a part of the body other than the uterus.

xenon (zē'non): An inert gaseous element. Radioactive xenon is used in blood-flow clearance tests. Chemical symbol, Xe.

xenophobia (zen-ō-fō'bi-a): Morbid fear of strangers or foreigners.

xenophonia (zen-ō-fō'ni-a): An alteration in the voice, due to a speech defect.

xenophthalmia (zen-of-thal'mi-a): Conjunctivitis caused by a foreign body or trauma.

Xenopsylla cheopis (zen-op-sil'a che-op'is): The rat flea that transmits bubonic plague.

xer-, xero-: Combining forms denoting dry; dryness.

xeransis (zē-ran'sis): Gradual loss of moisture from the body tissues.—xerantic, adj.

xerasia (zē-rā'zi-a): Dryness and brittleness of the hair.

xerocheilia (zē-rō-kī'li-a): Dryness of the lips. Also xerochilia.

xeroderma (ze'rō-der-ma): Also xerodermia. Dryness of the skin. See Ichthyosis. **X. PIGMENTOSUM,** Kaposi's disease, a familial dermatosis thought to be caused by photosensitization. Pathological freckle formation (ephelides) may give rise to keratosis, neoplastic growth and a fatal termination. [Moritz Kaposi, Hungarian dermatologist. 1837–1902.]

xerodermatosis (zē'rō-der-ma-tō'sis): Sjögren's syndrome (*q.v.*).

xerography (zē-rog'ra-fi): A technique for obtaining an x-ray image utilizing a plate coated with selenium.

xeroma (zē-rō'ma): Abnormal dryness of the conjunctiva; xerophthalmia.

xeromammography (zē'rō-mam-og'ra-fi): Xeroradiography of the breast, a method that subjects the patient to less radiation than ordinary x ray.

xeromenia (zē-rō-mē'ni-a): The presence of the usual physical disturbances that occur during menstruation but without the usual flow of blood.

xeronosus (zē-ron'o-sus): Dryness of the skin, mucous membranes, or conjunctiva.

xerophagia (zē-rō-fā'ji-a): Subsisting on dry foods only.

xerophthalmia (zē-rof-thal'mi-a): A serious disease of the eyeball, associated with vitamin A deficiency. The eyelids become inflamed, the conjunctiva dry and marked by appearance of yellow spots; the cornea becomes dry and ulcerated; night blindness develops and total blindness may develop in untreated cases.

xerosis (zē-rō'sis): Dryness. **X. CONJUNCTIVAE,** see Bitot's spots.

xerostomia (zē'rō-stō'mi-a): Dryness of the mouth from lack of saliva.

xerotocia (zē'rō-tō'si-a): Dry labor.

xiph-, xipho: Combining forms denoting the xiphoid process.

xiphisternum (zif-i-ster'num): The ensiform cartilage or process; the end section of the sternum. It is subject to much variety as to direction, shape and degree of ossification.—xiphosternal, adj.

xiphocostal (zif-ō-kos'tal): Pertaining to the xiphoid process and the ribs.

xiphodynia (zif-ō-din'i-a): Pain in the xiphoid process.

xiphoid (zif'oyd): Shaped like a sword. **X. PROCESS,** the pointed process of cartilage at the lower end of the sternum; also called the xiphisternum and the ensiform process.

xiphoidalgia (zif-oy-dal'ji-a): A syndrome characterized by pain of a neuralgic character and tenderness over the xiphoid process.

xiphoiditis (zif-oy-dī'tis): Inflammation of the ensiform cartilage.

xylene (zī'lēn): A clear inflammable liquid resembling benzene. Has been used as an ointment in pediculosis.

xylol (zī'lol): A hydrocarbon, derived from coal tar; used as a clarifier in microscopy. Also xylene.

xylophobia (zī'lō-fō'bi-a): An abnormal fear of woods and trees.

xylose (zī'lōs): A pentose sugar found in woody materials; has a sweet taste; soluble in water and alcohol; used as a nonnutritive sweetener.

xylosuria (zī'lō-sū'ri-a): The presence of xylose in the urine.

Y

Y: Chemical symbol for yttrium.

y chromosome (krō′mō-sōm): One of a pair of chromosomes (X and Y) carried in one-half of the male gametes and none of the female gametes; important in the determination of the sex of the offspring, since it is the differentiating chromosome for the male sex.

yawning: The often involuntary act of opening the mouth widely, breathing in deeply, and then breathing out as the involved muscles relax; often due to suggestion or to sleepiness, but may also be a sign of vital depression following hemorrhage.—yawn, n.; v.

yaws: An infectious, non-venereal disease of the tropics, caused by the spirochete *Treponema pertenue* and marked by fever, rheumatic pains and a characteristic lesion called a yaw. Lesions appear on hands, face, feet, and external genitalia and are described as raspberry-like tubercles with a caseous crust; they may run together in fungus-like masses, form pustules and ulcerate. The organism enters through a break in the skin. Penicillin is the treatment of choice. Syn., frambesia tropica, pian, bouba, parangi. This and other diseases caused by the same organism closely resemble syphilis. The general name for this group of diseases is treponematosis.

yeast (yēst): Saccharomyces. A unicellular fungus which reproduces by budding only. Used to produce alcoholic fermentation, leaven bread, and in some cases as a remedy. Some yeasts are pathogenic to man, *e.g.*, the species causing thrush. **BREWER'S YEAST,** a by-product from the brewing of beer; a crude but adequate and complete source of vitamin B complex.

yellow bone marrow: See under bone marrow.

yellow fever: An acute, specific, infectious, febrile illness of the tropics, of short duration and varying intensity, caused by a virus. The urban type is transmitted from person to person by the bite of the *Aedes aegypti* mosquito; the sylvan type is transmitted from monkey to human by the bite of the forest mosquito. Characteristic features of a mild attack include headache, malaise, fever, bradycardia, jaundice, and proteinuria. More severe cases are characterized by icterus, hemorrhagic tendencies, liver necrosis, black vomit, anuria. Mortality rate is about 5 percent in victims who are native to areas of the world where the disease is endemic, but much higher for those from other areas. Vaccination with 17D strain of the virus produces immunity for several years. An attack of the disease results in lifetime immunity.

yellow spot: Macula lutea (*q.v.*).

yerba (yer′ba): An herb. **Y. MATE,** the dried leaves of certain species of Ilex; grows in Paraguay and Brazil; contains caffeine and tannin and used as a diaphoretic and diuretic, also as a beverage.

Yersinia: A genus of small bacilli, aerobic or anaerobic, that are pathologic to animals and humans. **Y. ENTEROCOLITICA,** a coccobacillary organism that causes enterocolitis and mesenteric lymphadenitis in humans. **Y. PESTIS,** a bacillary organism that causes plague in humans. **Y. PSEUDOTUBERCULOSIS,** the cause of lymphadenosis in humans.

yoga: A philosophy that emphasizes, among other concepts, the practice of a system of isometric exercises, breathing education, relaxation, and the assumption of certain positions, with the aim of achieving bodily, mental, and emotional well-being. The term is from the Sanskrit, meaning union, and refers to the union of the human spirit with the infinite.

yogurt, yoghurt (yōg′hert): A form of curdled milk produced by the action of Lactobacillus bulgaricus.

yolk sac: The embryonic membrane that connects to the midgut (*q.v.*).

Young's rule: A formula for determining the fraction of an adult dose of a drug that is the correct dose for a child;

$$\frac{\text{age of child}}{\text{age of child} + 12} = \text{Fraction of adult dose}$$

the fraction of the adult dose that should be given. [Thomas Young, English physician, physicist, mathematician and philologist. 1773–1829.]

youth: The period of life between childhood and maturity.

yttrium 90 (Y^{90}) (it′ri-um): A rare metallic substance emitting beta particles with a half-life of 64 hours; some of its radioactive isotopes are used in treatment of certain cancers.

Z

Zakrzewsky, Marie: Polish-German midwife; earned an M.D. in the U.S.; in 1872 organized the first school of nursing in America at the New England Hospital for Women and Children in Roxbury, Massachusetts; it was a one-year program; Linda Richards is credited with being the first graduate.

Zeis's glands: The sebaceous glands associated with the cilia at the edges of the eyelids.

Zellweger's syndrome: A hereditary disorder characterized by low birth weight, lack of muscle tone, and anomalies of the skeleton including abnormal craniofacial development, osteoporosis, and spontaneous fractures; and disorders of the heart, liver and kidneys. Also called cerebrohepatorenal syndrome and Fanconi-Albertini-Zellweger syndrome.

Zenker's diverticulum: A diverticulum of the pharynx occurring at its junction with the esophagus; also called hypopharyngeal diverticulum and pharyngoesophageal diverticulum.

Zephiran: Benzalkonium chloride. A soluble powder used in solutions of 1:1000 to 1:20,000 as a surface detergent and antiseptic. Its effectiveness is neutralized by soap but since it is an effective cleansing agent it can be used as both a detergent and antiseptic. Effective against many bacteria.

zero (zir'ō, zē'rō): **1.** Nothing; naught. **2.** The numeral or symbol 0. **3.** The point from which negative and positive quantities are measured on a graduated scale, as in a thermometer.

Ziehl-Neelsen procedure: A widely-used laboratory method for detecting acid-fast bacteria, particularly the tubercle bacillus, *Mycobacterium tuberculosis*. [Franz Ziehl, German bacteriologist. 1857–1926. Friedrich Karl Adolf Neelsen. 1854–1894.]

Zieve's syndrome: A condition associated with excessive intake of alcohol; characterized by enlargement of the liver and spleen, jaundice, cirrhosis, hyperlipemia and hypercholesterolemia, anemia, lesions of the sclera, epigastric pain, and telangiectasia; the symptoms tend to disappear once the drinking stops.

zinc (zink): A bluish-white metallic element; many of its salts are used for their antiseptic and astringent action on skin and mucous membranes; made up in powder, solution and ointment forms. Chemical symbol Zn.

Zn: Symbol for zinc.

zo-, zoo-: Combining forms denoting 1) animal; 2) animal kingdom.

zoanthropy (zō-an'thro-pi): The delusion that one has become a dog or horse, or any other of the lower animals.

zoetic (zō-et'ik): Pertaining to life; vital.

Zollinger-Ellison syndrome: A familial condition characterized by tumor of the pancreatic islets of Langerhans, hypersecretion of gastric acid, fulminating ulceration of esophagus, stomach, duodenum, and jejunum. Frequently accompanied by diarrhea. [Robert M. Zollinger, American surgeon. b.1903. E.H. Ellison, American physician. 1918–1970.]

zona (zō'na): **1.** In anatomy, a delineated area in the body having characteristic structure or properties; a zone or girdle. **2.** Herpes zoster (*q.v.*). **Z. FACIALIS,** herpes zoster of the face. **Z. OPHTHALMICA,** herpes zoster occurring along the distribution of the ophthalmic nerve. **Z. ORBICULARIS COXAE,** a thickening of the fibers of the capsule of the hip joint that form a ring around the neck of the femur. **Z. PELLUCIDA,** the thick transparent membrane surrounding the ovum.

zone (zōn): A small belt or area. **EROGENOUS,** or **EROTOGENIC Z.,** an area of the body that produces a sexual response when stimulated. **GERMINATIVE Z.,** the deepest layer of the epidermis, lying just above the dermis; made up of the stratum spinosum and the stratum basale. **Z. THERAPY,** see under **therapy**.

zonesthesia (zō-nes-thē'zē-a): A sensation of constriction about the body resembling that produced by a tight girdle or cord.

zonifugal (zō-nif'ū-gal): Passing outward from within a zone.

zonipetal (zō-nip'i-tal): Passing into a zone from without.

zonula (zon'ū-la): A small zone, belt, or girdle. **ZONULA CILIARIS,** suspensory ligament attaching periphery of lens to ciliary body (*q.v.*). Also zonule.—zonular, adj.

zonule (zon'ūl): A small zone or area. **Z. OF ZINN,** the suspensory ligament that holds the crystalline lens in place.

zonulitis (zon-ū-lī'tis): Inflammation of the zonule of Zinn.

zonulolysis (zon-ū-lol'i-sis): Breaking down the zonula ciliaris—sometimes necessary before intracapsular extraction of the lens; often accomplished by injecting alpha chymotrypsin into the zonula.

zonulysin (zon-ū-lī'sin): A proteolytic enzyme used in surgery to dissolve the suspensory ligament of the crystalline lens.

zooblast (zō'ō-blast): An animal cell.

zoogenous (zō-oj'e-nus): Obtained or derived from animals.

zoograft (zō'ō-graft): A graft of tissue from a lower animal to man.

zoolagnia (zō-ō-lag'ni-a): Sexual attraction of an individual to animals.

zoologist (zo-ol'ō-jist): A person who specializes in the science of zoology.

zoology (zō-ol'o-ji): The science that deals with the study of animals.

zoomania (zō'ō-mā'ni-a): Excessive love of animals.

zoonoses (zō-ō-nō'sēz): Diseases or infections of animals that may be transmitted to humans.—zoonosis, sing.; zoonotic, adj.

zooparasite (zō-ō-par'a-sīt): An animal that exists as a parasite.

zoophagus (zō-of'a-gus): Carniverous; living on animal foods only.

zoophilic (zō-ō-fil'ik): Preferring animals to humans.

zoophilism (zō-of'i-lizm): Abnormal fondness for animals. Antivivisectionism. **EROTIC Z.**, deriving sexual pleasure from handling animals.

zoophobia (zō-ō-fō'bi-a): Abnormal fear of animals.

zooplasty (zō'ō-plas-ti): Transplantation of skin or other tissue from one of the lower animals to man.

zoopsia (zō-op'si-a): A hallucination or delusion in which the individual thinks he sees animals.

zootoxin (zō'ō-tok'sin): A toxic substance produced by an animal, *e.g.*, snake or spider venom.

zoster (zos'ter): Herpes zoster; see under **herpes**.

zosteriform (zos-ter'i-form): 1. Resembling herpes zoster; see **herpes**. 2. Referring to lesions that appear in bands following the course of a nerve.

Z-plasty (zē'plas-ti): A plastic operation for relieving the contraction of scar tissue in which a Z-shaped incision is made over the contracted scar.

Z-track: A method of intramuscular injection that prevents seeping of a medication into subcutaneous tissues or leakage from an injection site. The skin is pulled down and towards the median and held there while the injection is given; after 10 seconds the needle is removed and the skin returns to its normal position leaving a zigzag track from the point of insertion. Also called zigzag method.

zyg-; zygo-: Combining forms denoting joined or yoked.

zygodactyly (zī-gō-dak'ti-li): Syndactyly. The webbing or fusion of one or more fingers or toes.

zygoma (zī-gō'ma): The cheek bone.—zygomatic, adj.

zygomatic (zī'gō-mat'ik): Pertaining to the zygoma. **Z. ARCH**, the bony arch formed by the zygomatic process of the temporal bone and the temporal process of the zygomatic bone that forms the prominence of the cheek. **Z. PROCESSES**, projections on the frontal bone, maxilla, and temporal bone, all of which articulate with the zygoma.

zygote (zī'gōt): 1. The fertilized ovum before cleavage. 2. The organism produced by the union of two gametes (*q.v.*). See **dizygote, monozygote**.

zylose (zī'los): A pentose sugar that is not metabolized in the body.

zymase (zī'mās): 1. An enzyme. 2. The enzyme in yeast that causes alcoholic fermentation.

zymogen (zī'mō-jen): The inactive granular precursor, with the secretory cell, of enzymes.

zymogenic (zī-mō-jen'ik): Causing fermentation.

zymologist (zī-mol'o-jist): One who specializes in the study of ferments.

zymology (zī-mol'o-ji): The study of fermentation.

zymolysis (zī-mōl'ī-sis): Digestion or fermentation brought about by an enzyme.

zymosis (zī-mō'sis): 1. Fermentation. 2. The process by which infectious diseases are thought to develop. 3. Any infectious disease.

zymotic (zī-mot'ik): 1. Relating to zymosis. 2. A general term sometimes used to designate endemic or epidemic infectious diseases that are caused by microorganisms.

zymurgy (zī'mer-ji): The science involved with the industrial uses of enzymes.

Appendix I
Weights and Measurements

METRIC SYSTEM

LINEAR MEASURE

1 millimeter (mm)		0.001 M
10 millimeters	= 1 centimeter (cm)	0.01 M
10 centimeters	= 1 decimeter (dm)	0.1 M
10 decimeters	= 1 meter (m)	1 M
10 meters	= 1 decameter (dcm)	10 M
10 decameters	= 1 hectometer (hm)	100 M
10 hectometers	= 1 kilometer (km)	1000 M

WEIGHT

1 milligram (mg)		0.001 gram (gm)
10 milligrams	= 1 centigram (cg)	0.01 gm
10 centigrams	= 1 decigram (dg)	0.1 gm
10 decigrams	= 1 gram (g)	1 gm
10 grams	= 1 decagram (dcg)	10 gm
10 decagrams	= 1 hectogram (hg)	100 gm
10 hectograms	= 1 kilogram (kg)	1000 gm

VOLUME

1 milliliter		0.001 L
10 milliliters	= 1 centiliter (cl)	0.01 L
10 centiliters	= 1 deciliter (dl)	0.1 L
10 deciliters	= 1 liter (L)	1 L
10 liters	= 1 decaliter (dcl)	10 L
10 decaliters	= 1 hectoliter (hl)	100 L
10 hectoliters	= 1 kiloliter (kl)	1000 L

U.S. APOTHECARIES' SYSTEM

WEIGHT

1 grain (gr)
20 grains = 1 scruple (scr, ʒ)
3 scruples = 1 dram (dr, ʒ) (60 gr)
8 drams = 1 ounce (oz, ʒ) (480 gr)
12 ounces = 1 pound (lb) (5760 gr)

VOLUME

1 minim (m)
60 minims = 1 fluid dram (fl dr, fʒ)
8 fluid drams = 1 fluid ounce (fl oz, fʒ)
16 fluid ounces = 1 pint (0, pt)
2 pints = 1 quart (qt)
4 quarts = 1 gal (C, gal)

AVOIRDUPOIS SYSTEM OF WEIGHTS

1 grain (gr)
27.34 grains = 1 dram (dr)
16 drams = 1 ounce (oz)
16 ounces = 1 pound (lb)

DOMESTIC SYSTEM OF WEIGHTS AND MEASUREMENTS

LINEAR MEASURE

1 inch (in)
12 inches = 1 foot (ft)
3 feet = 1 yard (yd)
5½ yards = 1 rod (rd)
5280 feet = 1 mile (mi)

DRY MEASURE

1 pint (pt)
2 pints = 1 quart (qt)
8 quarts = 1 peck (pk)
4 pecks = 1 bushel (bu)

LIQUID MEASURE

1 gill (gl)	
4 gills	= 1 pint (pt)
2 pints	= 1 quart (qt)
4 quarts	= 1 gallon (gal)

GENERAL RULES FOR CONVERSION FROM ONE SYSTEM TO ANOTHER

Metric to Apothecary or Avoirdupois

Millimeters to inches: Multiply number of millimeters by 10 and divide by 254.

Kilograms to pounds (avoir.): Multiply number of kilograms by 1000 and divide by 454.

Grams to ounces (avoir.): Multiply number of grams by 20 and divide by 567.

Grams to grains: Multiply number of grams by 15.

Milligrams to grains: Divide number of milligrams by 60.

Liters to U.S. gallons: Multiply number of liters by 265 and divide by 1000.

Liters to pints: Multiply number of liters by 21 and divide by 10.

Cubic centimeters to fluid drams: Divide number of cubic centimeters by 4.

Cubic millimeters to minims: Multiply number of cubic millimeters by 100 and divide by 6.

Millileters to minims: Multiply number of milliliters by 16.7

Milliliters to fluid ounces: Divide number of milliliters by 30.

Apothecary or Avoirdupois to Metric

Inches to millimeters: Multiply number of inches by 254 and divide by 10.

Pounds (avoir.) to kilograms: Multiply number of pounds by 454 and divide by 1000.

Ounces (avoir.) to grams: Multiply number of ounces by 567 and divide by 20.

Grains to grams: Divide number of grains by 15.

Grains to milligrams: Multiply number of grains by 60.

U.S. gallons to liters: Divide number of gallons by 265 and multiply by 1000.

Fluid drams to cubic centimeters: Multiply number of fluid drams by 4.
Minims to cubic centimeters: Multiply number of minims by 6 and divide by 100.
Minims to milliliters: Multiply number of minims by .06.

CONVERSION FACTORS*

METRIC		APOTHECARY
1 milligram (mg)	=	1/64 grain (gr)
64.79 (65) milligrams	=	1 grain
1 gram (G, g)	=	15.43 (15) grains
1 cubic centimeter (cc or ml)	=	16.2 (16) minims (m)
3.88 (4) cubic centimeters	=	1 dram (dr)
31.103 (32) cubic centimeters or grams	=	1 ounce (oz)
473 (500) cubic centimeters	=	1 pint (pt)

*1 cubic centimeter is the equivalent of 1 milliliter.
1 minim is the approximate equivalent of 1 drop.

LINEAR MEASURE: METRIC TO DOMESTIC

METERS	CENTIMETERS	MILLIMETERS	FEET	INCHES
1.0	100.0	1000.0	3.2808	39.37
.01	1.0	10.0	0.03281	0.3937
.9144	91.44	914.40	3.0	36.0
0.3048	30.48	304.8	1.0	12.0
.0254	2.54	25.4	0.0833	1.0

WEIGHT: METRIC TO AVOIRDUPOIS

GRAMS	KILOGRAMS	OUNCES	POUNDS
1	.001	.0353	.0022
1000	1	35.3	2.2
28.35	.02835	1	1/16
454.5	.4545	16	1

WEIGHT: METRIC TO APOTHECARY

GRAMS	MILLIGRAMS	GRAINS	DRAMS	OUNCES	POUNDS
1	1000	15.4	.2577	.0322	.00268
.001	1	.0154	.00026	.0000322	.00000268
.0648	64.8	1	1/60	1/480	1/5760
3.888	3888	60	1	1/8	1/96
31.1	31104	480	8	1	1/12
373.5	373248	5760	96	12	1

VOLUME: METRIC TO APOTHECARY

MILLILITERS	MINIMS	FLUID DRAMS	FLUID OUNCES	PINTS
1	16.2	.27	0.333	.0021
.0616	1	1/60	1/480	1/7680
3.697	60	1	1/8	1/128
29.58	480	8	1	1/16
473.2	7680	128	16	1

FAHRENHEIT AND CELSIUS EQUIVALENTS: BODY TEMPERATURE RANGE

The freezing point on the Fahrenheit scale is 32°; the boiling point is 212°.

The freezing point on the Celsius scale is 0°; the boiling point is 100°.

To convert from Fahrenheit to Celsius, subtract 32 from the F temperature and multiply by 5/9.

To convert from Celsius to Fahrenheit, multiply the C temperature by 9/5 and add 32.

Centigrade degrees are the same as Celsius degrees.

F	C	C	F
92	33.33	33.0	91.4
93	33.89	33.5	92.3
94	34.44	34.0	93.2
95	35.0	34.5	94.1
96	35.56	35.0	95.0
97	36.11	35.5	95.9
98	36.67	36.0	96.8
99	37.22	36.5	97.7
100	37.78	37.0	98.6
101	38.33	37.5	99.5
102	38.89	38.0	100.4
103	39.44	38.5	101.3
104	40.0	39.0	102.2
105	40.56	39.5	103.1
106	41.11	40.0	104.0
107	41.67	40.5	104.9
108	42.22	41.0	105.8
109	42.78	41.5	106.7
110	43.33	42.0	107.6
		42.5	108.5
		43.0	109.4
		43.5	110.3

APPROXIMATE HOUSEHOLD MEASUREMENTS: EQUIVALENTS (LIQUID)

1 teaspoon	1 fluidram ⅛ fluidounce 60 drops	5 ml
1 tablespoon	3 teaspoons	15 ml
1 fluidounce	2 tablespoons 6 teaspoons	30 ml

1 cup	8 fluidounces	240 ml
	16 tablespoons	
1 pint	2 cups	480 ml
	16 fluidounces	
1 quart	2 pints	960 ml
	4 cups	
	32 fluidounces	
1 gallon	4 quarts	3840 ml
	8 pints	
	16 cups	
	128 fluidounces	

Appendix II
Height and Weight Tables

1983 METROPOLITAN HEIGHT AND WEIGHT TABLES*

Men

Height Feet	Height Inches	Small frame	Medium frame	Large frame
5	2	128–134	131–141	138–150
5	3	130–136	133–143	140–153
5	4	132–138	135–145	142–156
5	5	134–140	137–148	144–160
5	6	136–142	139–151	146–164
5	7	138–145	142–154	149–168
5	8	140–148	145–157	152–172
5	9	142–151	148–160	155–176
5	10	144–154	151–163	158–180
5	11	146–157	154–166	161–184
6	0	149–160	157–170	164–188
6	1	152–164	160–174	168–192
6	2	155–168	164–178	172–197
6	3	158–172	167–182	176–202
6	4	162–176	171–187	181–207

Women

Height		Small frame	Medium frame	Large frame
Feet	Inches			
4	10	102–111	109–121	118–131
4	11	103–113	111–123	120–134
5	0	104–115	113–126	122–137
5	1	106–118	115–129	125–140
5	2	108–121	118–132	128–143
5	3	111–124	121–135	131–147
5	4	114–127	124–138	134–151
5	5	117–130	127–141	137–155
5	6	120–133	130–144	140–159
5	7	123–136	133–147	143–163
5	8	126–139	136–150	146–167
5	9	129–142	139–153	149–170
5	10	132–145	142–156	152–173
5	11	135–148	145–159	155–176
6	0	138–151	148–162	158–179

*Courtesy of the Metropolitan Life Insurance Company.

Appendix III
Common Laboratory Values

ABBREVIATIONS USED IN THE TABLES OF LABORATORY VALUES*

↑	increased
↓	decreased
<	less than
>	greater than
cm^3	cubic centimeter
cu mm	cubic milliliter
cu μ	cubic micron
dL, dl	deciliter
EU	expected utility (or EV, expected value)
g, gm	gram
hr, h	hour(s)
Ig A, B, E, G, M	immunoglobulins A, B, E, G, M
IU	International Unit
kg	kilogram
kPa	kilopascal (IU)
L, l	liter
mol	mole
m^2	square meter
μg	microgram
mCi	millicuries
mEq	milliequivalent
mg	milligram
mg/dl	milligrams per deciliter
min	minute(s)
mIU	milliInternational Unit

*Laboratory values may differ from one laboratory to another depending on the laboratory and the particular tests used.

ml	milliliter
mm	millimeter
mm^3	cubic millimeter
mmHg	millimeters of mercury
mmol	millimole
mOsm	milliosmole
mμ	millimicron
ng	nanogram
nmol	nanomole
Pco_2	carbon dioxide pressure
pg	picogram
pH	hydrogen ion concentration
Po_2	partial pressure of oxygen
s	second(s)
SIU	Standard International Unit(s)
U	Units
μ	micron
μg	microgram
Uh	Units per hour
μl	microliter
μmol	micromole

BLOOD

FORMED ELEMENTS IN THE BLOOD

Erythrocytes, adult	
Male	4.6–6.0 million/mm^3
Female	4.0–5.0 million/mm^3
Leukocytes, adult	4,300–10,000/mm^3
Basophils	40–100 mm^3 (0.4–1.0%)
Eosinophils	100–300 mm^3 (1.0–3.0%)
Monocytes	200–600/mm^3 (4.0–6.0%)
Neutrophils	2500–7000/mm^3 (50–70%)
Band	0–500/mm^3 (0–5%)
Segmented	2500–6500/mm^3 (50–65%)
Lymphocytes, adult	1700–3400/mm^3 (25–35%)
Platelets, adult	150,000–400,000/mm^3 (mean 250,000/mm^3)
Reticulocytes, adult	25,000–75,000/mm^3 (0.5–1.5 of RBC count)

HEMATOLOGIC VALUES

Test	Biological Fluid	Reference Value
Bleeding time (Duke)	Blood	1–3 min
(Ivy)		1–6 min
Coagulation time (Lee-White)	Blood	5–15 min
Erythrocyte sedimentation rate (Westergren)	Blood	
Males, <50 yrs		0–15 mm/h
Females, <50 yrs		0–20 mm/h
Hematocrit	Blood	
Males		40–54 ml/100 ml
Females		36–46 ml/100 ml
Hemoglobin	Blood	
Males		13.5–17.5 g/dL
Females		12.0–16.0 g/dL
Fetal		Less than 1% of total
Hemoglobin	Plasma	0–5 mg/100 ml
Partial thromboplastin time	Blood	60–70 sec depending on method
pH	Blood, arterial	7.35–7.45
Prothrombin time, one-stage method (Quick)	Blood, arterial	11–15 sec

CHEMICAL CONSTITUENTS: WHOLE BLOOD, SERUM, OR PLASMA

Component	Reference Value
Acetone	0.3–2.0 mg/dL
Aldolase	3–8 Sibley-Lehninger units; child, 12–24 IU/dL
Aldosterone	1–9 ng/dL (supine position)
Ammonia	40–80 μg/dL
Amylase	60–160 Somogyi U/dL
Ascorbic acid	0.6–1.6 mg/dL
Bicarbonate (art.)	21–28 mmol/L
Bilirubin (total)	0.2–1.0 mg/dL

Component	Reference Value
Blood Gases	
P_{CO_2}	35–45 mmHg
P_{O_2}	75–100 mmHg
Calcium	8.5–10.0 mg/dL (adult)
Carbon dioxide	24–30 mEq/L
Ceruloplasmin	23–50 mg/dL
Chloride	95–105 mEq/L
Cholesterol	150–250 ug/dL
Copper (total)	70–155 ug/dL
Creatine kinase	Male: 17–148 U/L Female: 10–79 U/L
Creatinine	0.6–1.5 mg/dL
Estrogen	Male: 12–34 pg/ml Female: Varies with menstrual cycle
Fatty acids	190–420 mg/dL
Glucose (fasting)	70–110 mg/dL
Iodine, protein-bound	4.0–8.0 ug/dL
Iron (total)	50–100 μg/dL
Lactic dehydrogenase	45–90 U/L
Lead	50 μg/dL or less
Lipase	14–280 mIU/ml
Magnesium	1.3–2.1 mEq/L
Nonprotein nitrogen	15–35 mg/dL
Oxygen content	95–99% arterial blood
Phospholipids	150–380 mg/dL
Potassium	3.5–5.1 mEq/L
Proteins (total)	6.0–8.0 g/dL
Protoporphyrin (RBC)	15–50 pg/dL
Pyruvic acid	0–0.11 mEq/L
Sodium	135–145 mEq/L
Testosterone	Male: 300–1000 ng/dL Female: 30–100 ng/dL
Thyroid-stimulating hormone	2–5.4 uIU/ml
Urea nitrogen	8–25 mg/dL
Uric acid	7.6–7.8 mg/dL
Vitamin A	20–80 ug/dL
Vitamin B_{12}	205–876 pg/ml

BONE MARROW ASPIRATE DIFFERENTIAL NUCLEATED CELL COUNT: NORMAL ADULTS

	% Normal Mean
Myeloblasts	0.1–5.0
Promyelocytes	0.5–8.0
Myelocytes	
Neutrophilic	4.2–8.9
Eosinophilic	0.1–3.0
Basophilic	Up to 0.5
Metamyelocytes	
Neutrophilic	10.0–32
Eosinophilic	0.2–7.0
Basophilic	Up to 0.3
Lymphocytes	12.7–24
Plasmacytes	0.1–0.5
Monocytes	Up to 2.7
Reticulum cells	0.1–2.0
Megakaryocytes	0.1–0.5
Pronormoblasts	0.2–4.0
Normoblasts	
Basophilic	1.5–5.8
Polychromatophilic	5.0–26.4
Orthochromic	1.6–21

CEREBROSPINAL FLUID

Volume: 100–160 ml
Appearance: Clear or colorless
Pressure: 75–175 mmH_2O
Specific gravity: 1.006–1.008
pH: 7.35–7.70
Cells: 0.5 cells/mm^3, leukocytes

Component	Range
Albumin	10–30 mg/dL
Chloride	118–132 mmol/mEq/L
Creatinine	0.4–1.5 mg/dL
Glucose	40–80 mg/dL
Protein (lumbar)	15–45 mg/dL

FECES

Bulk: Solid or semisolid
Wet weight: 197.5 g/24 hr
Dry weight: 66.4 g/24 hr
Fat: 6g/24 hr
Lipids, as fatty acids: 2–5 g/24 hr
Nitrogen: 1–2 g/24 hr
Urobilinogen: 40–280 mg/24 hr
Bile, occult blood, leukocytes, and mucus normally negative

GASTRIC FLUID

Residual volume, fasting	<30–70 ml/h
Reaction	pH, <2.0
Basic acid output (fasting)	
Males	3.0 ± 2.0 mEq/h
Females	2.0 ± 1.8 mEq/h
Acid output after histamine stimulation	
Males	23 ± 5 mEq/h
Females	16 ± 5 mEq/h

URINE - 24 HR

Volume: 600–3500 ml/24 hr
Appearance: Clear to pale yellow; darkens on standing
Specific Gravity: 1.00–1.030
pH: 4.5–8 (average 6)
Total solids: 55–70 g/24 h

Component	Reference value
Albumin	50–150 mg/24 h
Aldosterone	6–25 μg/24 h
Amylase	35–260 Somogyi U/h
Calcium (average Ca diet)	100–250 mg/24 h
Catecholamines	100 μg/24 h

Component	Reference value
Epinephrine (adult)	10 ng/24 h
Norepinephrine (adult)	100 ng/24 h
Chloride	110–150 mEq/24 h
Copper	0–100 ug/24 h
Creatine	Under 100 mg/24 h
Creatinine	
Male	20–26 mg/kg/24 h
Female	14–22 mg/kg/24 h
Estriol, range during 38–40 weeks pregnancy	18–60 mg/24 h
Estrogens	
Male	4–25 μg/24 h
Female	Varies with the ovulation cycle
Follicle-stimulating hormone	
Male, adult	4–25 μIU/ml
Female, menopausal phase	50–250 μIU/ml
17–hydroxycorticosteroids	
Male	5–25 mg/24 h
Female	3–13 mg/24 h
Child	Differs with age
5-Hydroxyindoleacetic acid	2–10 mg/24 h
17-Ketosteroids	
Male	2–25 mg/24 h
Female	5–15 mg/24 h
Child	Differs with age
Lead	120 μg/24 h, or less
Phosphorus (inorganic)	Average, 1 g/24 h
Porphyrins	
Coproporphyrin	50–250 μg/24 h
Uroporphyrin	0–30 μg/24 h
Porphyrobilinogen (quantitative)	0–1 mg/24 h
Potassium (average range)	40–80 mEq/24 h
Pregnanediol	
Male	0.1–1.5 mg/24 h
Female (varies with menstrual cycle and pregnancy)	0.1–7 mg/24 h
Protein	15–150 mg/24 h
Sodium	40–220 mEq/L/h
Urea nitrogen	6–17 g/24 h

Component	Reference value
Uric acid	250–270 mg/24 h
Urobilinogen	0.05–2.5 mg/24 h
Vanillymandelic acid	
Adult	1.5–7.5 mg/24 h
Child	Similar to adult

Appendix IV Abbreviations Used in Prescription Writing

ABBREVIATION	DERIVATION*	MEANING
a; $\overline{aa}$; aa	ana	of each
ac	ante cibum	before meals
ad	ad	to; up to
ad hib	adhibendus	to be administered
ad lib	ad libitum	freely; as desired
agit a us	agita ante usum	shake before using
ante	ante	before
aq	aqua	water
aq dest	aqua destillata	distilled water
aq pur	aqua pura	pure water
bib	bibe	drink
bid	bis in die	twice a day
bin	bis in nocte	twice a night
BT; bt		bedtime
c; c̄	cum	with
cap	(1) capiat	let him take
cap	(2) capsula	a capsule
coch mag	cochleare magnum	a tablespoonful
coch parv	cochleare parvum	a teaspoonful
comp	(1) componere	compound
comp	(2) compositus	compounded of
D	dosis	dose
d	dies	a day
d; det	da; detur	give
DC		discontinue

*Latin unless otherwise indicated.

ABBREVIATION	DERIVATION*	MEANING
dent tal dos; dtd	dentur tales doses	give of such doses
det	detur	let it be given; give
dieb alt	diebus alternis	every other day
dieb tert	diebus tertiis	every third day
dil	dilue, dilutus	dilute, diluted
dim	dimidius	one half
dos	dosis	dose
dur dolor	durante dolore	while the pain lasts
elix	elixir	elixir
et	et	and
ext	extractum	extract
feb	febris	fever
fl	fluidus	fluid
fldext	fluidextractum	fluid extract
ft or f	fiat	make; let it be made
G, g, gm	gramma	gram
gr	granum, grana	grain, grains
gt, gtt	gutta, guttae	drop, drops
H		hypodermic
h; hor; hr	hora	hour
hs; h som	hora somni	hour of sleep; bed-time
IM		intramuscular
inf	infusum	infusion
inj	injectio	injection
IV		intravenous
liq	liquidium; liquor	liquid; a solution
M	misce	mix (thou)
m	minimum	minim
man	mane	in the morning
man prim	mane primo	first thing in the morning
mcg		microgram
m dict; mor dict	more dicto	as directed
m et n	mane et nocte	morning and night
mist	mistura	mixture

ABBREVIATION	DERIVATION*	MEANING
ml		milliliter
mg		milligram
n or noct	nocte	night, at night
noct maneq	nocte maneque	night and morning
non	non	not
n rep or repet	non repetatur	not to be repeated
O	octarius	pint
OD	oculo dextra	in the right eye
od	omni die	every day
oh	omni hora	every hour
ol	oleum	oil
omn hor	omni hora	every hour
omn man	omni mane	every morning
omn noct	omni nocte	every night
OS	oculo sinister	in the left eye
os	os	mouth
ou	oculo uterque	on each eye
oz	uncia	oz
pc	post cibum	after meals
pil	pilula	a pill
po	per os	by mouth
prn	pro re nata	when required; as occasion arises
q or qq	quaque	every
qd	quaque die	every day
qh	quaque hora	every hour
q (2,3,4) h		every (2,3,4) hours
qid	quater in die	four times a day
ql	quantum libit	as much as you please
qs	quantum sufficit	a sufficient quantity
qt		quart
quotid	quotidium	daily
R_x	recipere	take
S, s, $\bar{s}$	sine	without
S; Sig	signa; signetur	let it be labeled
sc		subcutaneous

ABBREVIATION	DERIVATION*	MEANING
sos	si opus sit	one dose if need exists
ss, $\overline{ss}$	semis	a half
stat	statim	immediately
sum	sumat; sume	to be taken; let him take
syr	syrupus	syrup
tab	tabillae	tablets
ter	ter	three times
tid	ter in die	three times a day
tin	ter in nocte	three times a night
tr or tinct	tinctura	tincture
troch	trochiscus	lozenge
ung	unguentum	ointment
ut dict	ut dictum	as directed
vin	vinum	wine
ʒ	drachma	dram
℥	uncia	ounce

Appendix V
Nursing Diagnoses Approved by the North American Nursing Diagnosis Association, 1988

This list represents the NANDA approved nursing diagnostic categories for clinical use and testing (1988), along with the taxonomic code for each diagnosis.

PATTERN 1: EXCHANGING

1.1.2.1	Altered Nutrition: More than body requirements
1.1.2.2	Altered Nutrition: Less than body requirements
1.1.2.3	Altered Nutrition: Potential for more than body requirements
1.2.1.1	Potential for Infection
1.2.2.1	Potential Altered Body Temperature
** 1.2.2.2	Hypothermia
1.2.2.3	Hyperthermia
1.2.2.4	Ineffective Thermoregulation
* 1.2.3.1	Dysreflexia
† 1.3.1.1	Constipation
* 1.3.1.1.1	Perceived Constipation
* 1.3.1.1.2	Colonic Constipation

*New diagnostic categories approved 1988.

**Revised diagnostic categories approved 1988.

†Categories with modified label terminology.

†1.3.1.2	Diarrhea
†1.3.1.3	Bowel Incontinence
1.3.2	Altered Patterns of Urinary Elimination
1.3.2.1.1	Stress Incontinence
1.3.2.1.2	Reflex Incontinence
1.3.2.1.3	Urge Incontinence
1.3.2.1.4	Functional Incontinence
1.3.2.1.5	Total Incontinence
1.3.2.2	Urinary Retention
†1.4.1.1	Altered (Specify Type) Tissue Perfusion (Renal, cerebral, cardiopulmonary, gastrointestinal, peripheral)
1.4.1.2.1	Fluid Volume Excess
1.4.1.2.2.1	Fluid Volume Deficit (1)
1.4.1.2.2.1	Fluid Volume Deficit (2)
1.4.1.2.2.2	Potential Fluid Volume Deficit
†1.4.2.1	Decreased Cardiac Output
1.5.1.1	Impaired Gas Exchange
1.5.1.2	Ineffective Airway Clearance
1.5.1.3	Ineffective Breathing Pattern
1.6.1	Potential for Injury
1.6.1.1	Potential for Suffocation
1.6.1.2	Potential for Poisoning
1.6.1.3	Potential for Trauma
*1.6.1.4	Potential for Aspiration
*1.6.1.5	Potential for Disuse Syndrome
1.6.2.1	Impaired Tissue Integrity
†1.6.2.1.1	Altered Oral Mucous Membrane
1.6.2.1.2.1	Impaired Skin Integrity
1.6.2.1.2.2	Potential Impaired Skin Integrity

PATTERN 2: COMMUNICATING

2.1.1.1	Impaired Verbal Communication

PATTERN 3: RELATING

3.1.1	Impaired Social Interaction
3.1.2	Social Isolation

†3.2.1	Altered Role Performance
3.2.1.1.1	Altered Parenting
3.2.1.1.2	Potential Altered Parenting
3.2.1.2.1	Sexual Dysfunction
3.2.2	Altered Family Processes
*3.2.3.1	Parental Role Conflict
3.3	Altered Sexuality Patterns

PATTERN 4: VALUING

4.1.1	Spiritual Distress (distress of the human spirit)

PATTERN 5: CHOOSING

5.1.1.1	Ineffective Individual Coping
5.1.1.1.1	Impaired Adjustment
*5.1.1.1.2	Defensive Coping
*5.1.1.1.3	Ineffective Denial
5.1.2.1.1	Ineffective Family Coping: Disabling
5.1.2.1.2	Ineffective Family Coping: Compromised
5.1.2.2	Family Coping: Potential for Growth
5.2.1.1	Noncompliance (Specify)
*5.3.1.1	Decisional Conflict (Specify)
*5.4	Health Seeking Behaviors (Specify)

PATTERN 6: MOVING

6.1.1.1	Impaired Physical Mobility
6.1.1.2	Activity Intolerance
*6.1.1.2.1	Fatigue
6.1.1.3	Potential Activity Intolerance
6.2.1	Sleep Pattern Disturbance
6.3.1.1	Diversional Activity Deficit
6.4.1.1	Impaired Home Maintenance Management
6.4.2	Altered Health Maintenance
†6.5.1	Feeding Self Care Deficit

6.5.1.1	Impaired Swallowing
*6.5.1.2	Ineffective Breastfeeding
†6.5.2	Bathing/Hygiene Self Care Deficit
†6.5.3	Dressing/Grooming Self Care Deficit
†6.5.4	Toileting Self Care Deficit
6.6	Altered Growth and Development

PATTERN 7: PERCEIVING

†7.1.1	Body Image Disturbance
†**7.1.2	Self Esteem Disturbance
*7.1.2.1	Chronic Low Self Esteem
*7.1.2.2	Situational Low Self Esteem
†7.1.3	Personal Identity Disturbance
7.2	Sensory/Perceptual Alterations (Specify) (Visual, auditory, kinesthetic, gustatory, tactile, olfactory)
7.2.1.1	Unilateral Neglect
7.3.1	Hopelessness
7.3.2	Powerlessness

PATTERN 8: KNOWING

8.1.1	Knowledge Deficit (Specify)
8.3	Altered Thought Processes

PATTERN 9: FEELING

†9.1.1	Pain
9.1.1.1	Chronic Pain
9.2.1.1	Dysfunctional Grieving
9.2.1.2	Anticipatory Grieving
9.2.2	Potential for Violence: Self-directed or directed at others
9.2.3	Post-Trauma Response
9.2.3.1	Rape-Trauma Syndrome

9.2.3.1.1	Rape-Trauma Syndrome: Compound Reaction
9.2.3.1.2	Rape-Trauma Syndrome: Silent Reaction
9.3.1	Anxiety
9.3.2	Fear

Appendix VI Nomenclature for Diagnosis of Mental Disorders as Identified in the *Diagnostic and Statistical Manual of Mental Disorders (DSM III-R)*, *Axes I and II**

The revised third edition of the *Diagnostic and Statistical Manual of Mental Disorders (DSM III-R)*, published by the American Psychiatric Association in 1987, presents an official nomenclature for diagnosis of mental disorders. It provides a more specific guide for clinicians and others who give psychiatric care in identifying psychiatric disorders than is provided by the *International Classification of Diseases (ICD-9-CM)*. Health care workers, including clinicians and research investigators use this nomenclature when reporting mental disorders, and those filing insurance claims for patients are now also expected to use these terms.

DSM III-R consists of a multiaxial evaluation of psychiatric disorders on the basis of their clinical manifestations, introduces new names for many disorders, redefines them, assigns code numbers to them, and establishes criteria for the diagnosis of many of them. Each complete diagnosis has five parts or Axes which refer to a different class of information, the first three of which constitute the official diagnostic assessment:

*Reprinted with permission from the *Diagnostic and Statistical Manual of Mental Disorders, Third edition, Revised*. Washington, DC. American Psychiatric Association, 1987.

Axis I: Clinical Syndromes and V Codes
Axis II: Developmental Disorders and Personality Disorders
Axis III: Physical Disorders and Conditions
Axis IV: Severity of Psychosocial Stressors
Axis V: Global Assessment of Functioning

Thus, the diagnoses in Axes I and II reflect the current clinical symptoms of the disorders rather than their causes. When the information for Axis III is added, the official diagnosis is complete. When both Axis I and Axis II describe a specific problem for which the individual seeks treatment, Axis I is usually considered the principal disorder, although in some instances the individual will have more than one principal disorder.

The following list consists of the Classification of Mental Disorders as based on Axes I and II. Specific information regarding coding and diagnostic criteria, as well as associated features, will be found in *DSM III-R*.

DSM-III-R CLASSIFICATION OF MENTAL DISORDERS AXES I AND II, CATEGORIES AND CODES†

DISORDERS USUALLY FIRST EVIDENT IN INFANCY, CHILDHOOD OR ADOLESCENCE DEVELOPMENTAL DISORDERS (Note: These are coded on Axis II)

Mental Retardation

317.00 Mild Mental Retardation
318.00 Moderate Mental Retardation
318.10 Severe Mental Retardation
318.20 Profound Mental Retardation
319.00 Unspecified Mental Retardation

Pervasive Mental Disorders

299.00 Autistic Disorder. *Specify* if childhood onset
299.80 Prevailing developmental disorder, NOS

†NOS: Not Otherwise Specified.
Codes followed by a * are used for more than one DSM-III-R diagnosis or subtype in order to maintain compatibility with ICD-9-CM.
A long dash following a diagnostic term indicates the need for a fifth digit subtype or other qualifying term.
All official DSM-III-R codes are included in ICD-9-CM.

Specific Developmental Disorders

Academic skills disorders

315.10 Developmental arithmetic disorder
315.80 Developmental expressive writing disorder
315.00 Developmental reading disorder

Language and speech disorders

315.39 Developmental articulation disorder
315.31* Developmental expressive language disorder
315.31* Developmental receptive language disorder

Motor skills disorder

315.40 Developmental coordination disorder
315.90* Specific developmental disorder, NOS

Other Developmental Disorders

315.90* Developmental disorder, NOS

Disruptive Behavior Disorders

314.01 Attention-deficit hyperactivity disorder

Conduct disorder

312.20 group type
312.00 solitary aggressive type
312.90 undifferentiated type
313.81 Oppositional defiant disorder

Anxiety Disorders of Childhood or Adolescence

309.21 Separation anxiety disorder
313.21 Avoidant disorder of childhood or adolescence
313.00 Overanxious disorder

Eating Disorders

307.10 Anorexia nervosa
307.51 Bulimia nervosa
307.52 Pica
307.53 Rumination disorder of childhood
307.50 Eating disorder. NOS

Gender Identity Disorders

302.60 Gender identity disorder of childhood
302.50 Transsexualism
Specify sexual history; asexual, homosexual, heterosexual, unspecified
302.85* Gender disorder of adolescence or adulthood, nontranssexual type
Specify sexual history: asexual, homosexual, heterosexual, unspecified
302.85* Gender identity disorder NOS

Tic Disorders

307.23 Tourette's disorder
307.22 Chronic motor or vocal tic disorder
307.21 Transient tic disorder
Specify: single episode or recurrent
307.20 Tic disorder NOS

Elimination Disorders

307.70 Functional encopresis
Specify: primary or secondary type
307.60 Functional enuresis
Specify: primary or secondary type
Specify: nocturnal only, diurnal only, nocturnal and diurnal

Speech Disorders Not Elsewhere Classified

307.00* Cluttering
307.00* Stuttering

Other Disorders of Infancy, Childhood, or Adolescence

313.23 Elective mutism
313.82 Identity disorder
313.89 Reactive attachment disorder of infancy or early childhood
307.30 Stereotypy/habit disorder
314.00 Undifferentiated attention-deficit disorder

ORGANIC MENTAL DISORDERS

Dementia Arising in the Senium and Presenium

Primary degenerative dementia of the Alzheimer type, senile onset

209.30 with delirium
200.20 with delusions
200.31 with depression
200.00* uncomplicated
(Note): Code 331.00 Alzheimer's disease on Axis III

Code in fifth digit:
1 = with delirium
2 = with delusions
3 = with depression
0* = uncomplicated

290.1x Primary degenerative dementia of the Alzheimer type, presenile onset ______
(Note): Code 331.00 Alzheimer's disease on Axis III
290.4x Multi-infarct dementia______
290.00* Senile dementia NOS
Specify etiology on Axis III if known
200.10 Presenile dementia NOS
Specify etiology on Axis III if known (e.g., Pick's disease, Jakob Kreutzfeldt disease)

Psychoactive Substance-Induced Organic Mental Disorders

Alcohol

303.00 intoxication
291.40 idiosyncratic intoxication
291.80 Uncomplicated alcohol withdrawal
291.00 hallucinosis
291.30 amnestic disorder
291.10 Dementia associated with alcoholism
305.70* intoxication
292.00* withdrawal
292.81* delirium
292.11* delusional disorder

Caffeine

305.90* intoxication

Cannabis

305.20* intoxication
292.11* delusional disorder

Cocaine

305.60* intoxication
292.00* withdrawal
292.81* delirium
292.11* delusional disorder

Hallucinogen

305.30* hallucinosis
292.11* delusional disorder
292.84* mood disorder
292.89* posthallucinogen perception disorder

Inhalant

305.90* intoxication

Nicotine

292.00* withdrawal

Opioid

305.50* intoxication
292.00 withdrawal

Phenylcyclidine (PCP) or similarly acting arylcyclohexylamine

305.90* intoxication
292.81* delirium
292.11* delusional disorder
292.84* mood disorder
292.90* organic mental disorder NOS

Sedative, hypnotic, or anxiolytic

305.40* intoxication

292.00* Uncomplicated sedative, hypnotic, or anxiolytic withdrawal
292.00* withdrawal delirium
292.83* Amnestic disorder

Other or unspecified psychoactive substance

305.90* intoxication
292.00* withdrawal
292.81* delirium
292.82* dementia
292.83* amnestic disorder
292.11* delusional disorder
292.12 hallucinosis
292.84* mood disorder
292.89* anxiety disorder
292.89* personality disorder
292.90* organic mental disorder NOS

Organic Mental Disorders associated with Axis III physical disorders or conditions, whose etiology is unknown

293.00 Delirium
294.10 Dementia
294.00 Amnestic disorder
293.81 Organic delusional disorder
293.82 Organic hallucinations
293.83 Organic mood disorder
Specify: manic, depressed, mixed
294.80* Organic anxiety disorder
310.10 Organic personality disorder
Specify if explosive type
294.80* Organic mental disorder NOS

PSYCHOACTIVE SUBSTANCE USE DISORDERS

Alcohol

303.90 dependence
305.00 abuse

Amphetamine or similarly acting sympathomimetic

304.40 dependence
305.70* abuse

Cannabis

304.30 dependence
305.20* abuse

Cocaine

304.20 dependence
305.60* abuse

Hallucinogen

304.50* dependence
305.30* abuse

Inhalant

304.60 dependence
305.90* abuse

Nicotine

305.10 dependence

Opioid

304.00 dependence
305.50* abuse

Phenylcyclidine (PSP) or similarly acting arylcyclohexylamine

304.50* dependence
305.90* abuse

Sedative, hypnotic, or anxiolytic

304.10 dependence
305.40* abuse
304.90* Polysubstance dependence
304.90* Psychoactive substance dependence NOS
305.90* Psychoactive substance abuse NOS

SCHIZOPHRENIA

Code in fifth digit:, 1 = subchronic, 2 = chronic, 3 = subchronic with acute exacerbation, 4 = chronic with acute exacerbation, 5 = in remission

Schizophrenia

295.2x catatonic,______
295.1x disorganized,______
295.3x paranoid,______. *Specify* if stable type
295.9x undifferentiated
295.6x residual,______. *Specify* if late onset

DELUSIONAL (PARANOID) DISORDER

297.10 Delusional (Paranoid) disorder
Specify type: erotomanic
grandiose
jealous
persecutory
somatic
unspecified

PSYCHOTIC DISORDERS NOT ELSEWHERE CLASSIFIED

298.80 Brief reactive psychosis
295.40 Schizophreniform disorder
Specify: without good prognostic features or with good prognostic features
295.70 Schizoaffective disorder
Specify: bipolar type or depressive type
297.30 Induced psychotic disorder
298.90 Psychotic disorder NOS

MOOD DISORDERS

Code current state of Major Depression and Bipolar Disorder in fifth digit:

1 = mild
2 = moderate
3 = severe, without psychotic features
4 = with psychotic features (*specify* mood congruent or mood incongruent)
5 = in partial remission
6 = in full remission
0 = unspecified

For major depressive episodes, *specify* if chronic and *specify* if melancholic type.

For Bipolar Disorder, Bipolar Disorder NOS, Recurrent Major Depression, and Depressive Disorder NOS, *specify* if seasonal pattern.

Bipolar Disorders

Bipolar disorder

296.6x mixed,______
296.4x manic,______
296.5x depressed,______
301.13 Cyclothymia
296.70 Bipolar disorder NOS

Depressive disorders

Major Depression

296.2x single episode,______
296.3x recurrent,______
300.40 Dysthymia (or Depressive neurosis)
Specify: Primary or secondary type
Specify: early or late onset
311.00 Depressive disorder NOS

ANXIETY DISORDERS (or Anxiety and Phobic Neuroses)

Panic Disorder

300.21 with agoraphobia
Specify current severity of agoraphobia avoidance
Specify current severity of panic attacks
300.01 without agoraphobia
Specify current severity of panic attacks
300.22 Agorophobia without history of panic disorder
Specify with or without limited symptom attacks
300.23 Social phobia
Specify if generalized type
300.29 Simple phobia
300.30 Obsessive compulsive disorder (or Obsessive compulsive neurosis)
309.89 Post-traumatic stress disorder
Specify if delayed onset
300.02 Generalized anxiety disorder
300.00 Anxiety disorder NOS

SOMATOFORM DISORDERS

300.70* Body dysmorphic disorder
300.11 Conversion disorder (or Hysterical neurosis, conversion type)
Specify: single episode or recurrent
300.70* Hypochondriasis (or Hypochrondriacal neurosis)
300.81 Somatization disorder
307.80 Somatization pain disorder
300.70* Undifferentiated somatoform disorder
300.70* Somatoform disorder NOS

DISSOCIATIVE DISORDERS (or Hysterical Neuroses, Dissociative Type)

300.14 Multiple personality disorder
300.13 Psychogenic fugue
300.12 Psychogenic amnesia
300.60 Depersonalization disorder (or Depersonalization neurosis)
300.15 Dissociative disorder

SEXUAL DISORDERS

Paraphilias

302.40 Exhibitionism
302.81 Fetishism
302.89 Frotteurism
302.20 Pedophilia
Specify: same sex, opposite sex, same and opposite sex
Specify if limited to incest
Specify: exclusive type or nonexclusive type
302.83 Sexual masochism
302.84 Sexual sadism
302.30 Transvestic fetishism
302.82 Voyeurism
302.90* Paraphilia NOS

Sexual Dysfunctions

Specify psychogenic only, or psychogenic and biogenic (Note: if biogenic only, code on Axis III)
Specify: lifelong or acquired
Specify: generalized or situational

Sexual desire disorders

302.71 Hypoactive sexual desire disorder
302.79 Sexual aversion disorder

Sexual arousal disorders

302.72* Female sexual arousal disorder
302.72* Male erectile disorder

Orgasm disorders

302.73 Inhibited female orgasm
302.74 Inhibited male orgasm
302.75 Premature ejaculation

Sexual pain disorders

302.76 Dyspareunia
306.51 Vaginismus
302.70 Sexual dysfunction NOS

Other Sexual Disorders

302.90* Sexual disorder NOS

SLEEP DISORDERS

Dyssomnias

Insomnia disorder

307.42* related to another mental disorder (nonorganic)
780.50* related to known organic factor
307.42* Primary insomnia

Hypersomnia disorder

307.44 related to another mental disorder (nonorganic)
780.50* related to a known organic factor
780.54 Primary hypersomnia

Hypersomnia disorder

307.42* related to another mental disorder (nonorganic)
780.50* related to known organic factor
307.42* Primary insomnia

Hypersomnia disorder

307.44 related to another mental disorder (nonorganic)
780.50* related to known organic factor
780.54 Primary hypersomnia
307.45 Sleep-wake schedule disorder
Specify: advanced or delayed phase type, disorganized type, frequently changing type
Other dyssomnias
307.40* Dyssomnia NOS

Parasomnias

307.47 Dream anxiety disorder (Nightmare disorder)
307.46* Sleep terror disorder
307.46* Sleepwalking disorder
307.40* Parasomnia NOS

FACTITIOUS DISORDERS

Factitious disorder with physical symptoms

301.51 with physical symptoms
300.16 with psychological symptoms
300.19 Factitious disorder NOS

IMPULSE CONTROL DISORDERS NOT ELSEWHERE CLASSIFIED

312.34 Intermittent explosive disorder
312.32 Kleptomania
312.31 Pathological gambling
312.33 Pyromania
312.39* Trichotillomania
312.39* Impulse control disorder

ADJUSTMENT DISORDER

Adjustment disorder

309.24 with anxious mood
309.00 with depressed mood
309.30 with disturbance of conduct
309.40 with mixed disturbance of emotions and conduct

309.28 with mixed emotional features
309.82 with physical complaints
309.83 with withdrawal
309.23 with work (or academic) inhibition
309.90 Adjustment disorder

PSYCHOLOGICAL FACTORS AFFECTING PHYSICAL CONDITION

316.00 Psychological factors affecting physical condition
Specify physical condition on Axis III

PERSONALITY DISORDERS

Note: These are coded on Axis II.

Cluster A

301.00 Paranoid
301.20 Schizoid
301.22 Schizotypal

Cluster B

301.70 Antisocial
301.83 Borderline
301.50 Histrionic
301.81 Narcissistic

Cluster C

301.82 Avoidant
301.60 Dependent
301.40 Obsessive compulsive
301.84 Passive aggressive
301.90 Personality disorder NOS

V CODES FOR CONDITIONS NOT ATTRIBUTABLE TO A MENTAL DISORDER THAT ARE A FOCUS OF ATTENTION OR TREATMENT

V62.30 Academic problem
V71.01 Adult antisocial behavior
V40.00 Borderline intellectual functioning (Note): This is coded on Axis II

V71.02	Childhood or adolescent antisocial behavior
V65.20	Malingering
V61.10	Marital problem
V15.81	Noncompliance with medical treatment
V62.20	Occupational problem
V61.20	Parent–child problem
V62.81	Other interpersonal problem
V61.80	Other specified family circumstances
V62.89	Phase of life problem or other life circumstance problem
V62.82	Uncomplicated bereavement

Appendix VII
State Nurses' Associations and State Boards of Nursing*

Alabama State Nurses Association—360 N. Hull St., Montgomery 36197. Tel. 205-262-8321. Ex. dir., Elizabeth Barker. **Board of Nursing**—Suite 203, 500 Eastern Blvd., Montgomery 36117. Tel. 205-261-4060. Ex. off., Shirley J. Dykes.

Alaska Nurses Association—237 East 3rd Ave., Suite 3, Anchorage 99501. Tel. 907-274-0827. Pres., Constance Trollan. **Board of Nursing Licensing**—Dept. of Commerce & Economic Development, Division of Occupational Licensing, PO Box D-LIC, Juneau 99811-0800. Tel. 907-465-2544. Lic. exam., Nancy Ferguson; ex. sec., Gail M. McGuill. Tel. 907-561-2878.

Arizona Nurses Association—1850 E. Southern Ave., Suite 1, Tempe 85282-5832. Tel. 602-831-0404. Ex. dir., Denise Hallfors. **Board of Nursing**—Suite 103, 5050 N. 19th Ave., Phoenix 85015. Tel. 602-255-5092. Ex. dir., Fran Roberts.

Arkansas State Nurses Association—117 S. Cedar St., Little Rock 72205. Tel. 501-664-5853. Pres., Mary Goza; ex. dir., Carolyn Shannon. **Board of Nursing**—University Tower Bldg., Suite 800, 1123 S. University Ave., Little Rock 72204. Tel. 501-371-2751. Ex. dir., June Garner.

California Nurses Association—1855 Folsom St., Suite 670, San Francisco 94103. Tel. 415-864-4141. Ex. dir., Myra C. Snyder. **Board of Registered Nursing**—PO Box 944210, 1030 13th St., Suite 200, Sac-

*From *American Journal of Nursing, 88,* 562–570, April 1988.

ramento 94244-2100. Tel. 916-322-3350. Ex. officer, Catherine Puri. **Board of Vocational Nurse & Psychiatric Technician Examiners**—1020 N. St., Rm. 406, Sacramento 95814. Tel. 916-445-0793. Ex. off., Billie Haynes.

California, United Nurses Associations of, (UNAC)—170 W. San Jose Ave., Suite 102, Claremont 91711. Tel. 714-625-7931.

Colorado Nurses Association—5453 E. Evans Pl., Denver 80222. Tel. 303-757-7483. Ex. dir., Lola M. Fehr. **Board of Nursing**—1525 Sherman St., Rm. 132, State Services Bldg., Denver 80203. Tel. 303-866-2871. Prog. admin., Karen Brumley.

Connecticut Nurses Association—1 Prestige Dr., Meriden 06450. Tel. 203-238-1207. Ex. dir., Karen S. Ponton. **Board of Examiners for Nursing**—150 Washington St., Hartford 06106. Tel. 203-566-1041. Chp., Bette Jane M. Murphy.

Delaware Nurses Association—2634 Capitol Trail, Suite C, Newark 19711. Tel. 302-368-2333. Ex. dir., Patrina Smith. **Board of Nursing**—Margaret O'Neill Bldg., Federal & Court Sts., Dover 19901. Tel. 302-736-4522. Ex. dir., Rosalee Seymour.

District of Columbia Nurses Association—5100 Wisconsin Ave. NW, Suite 306, Washington 20016. Tel. 202-244-2705. Pres., Dorothy Hararas, ex. dir., Evelyn Sommers. **DC Board of Nursing**—614 H St. NW, Washington 20001. Tel. 202-727-7468. Chp., Barbara J. Hatcher, vice chp., John H. Word.

Florida Nurses Association—Box 536985, Orlando 32853. Tel. 305-896-3261. Ex. dir., Paula Massey. **Board of Nursing**—111 E. Coastline Dr., Suite 504, Jacksonville 32202. Tel. 904-359-6331. Ex. Dir., Judie K. Ritter.

Georgia Nurses Association—1362 W. Peachtree St. NW, Atlanta 30309. Tel. 404-876-4624. Ex. dir., Susan Williamson. Pres., Lynda McSwain. **Board of Nursing**—166 Pryor St. SW, Suite 400, Atlanta 30303. Tel. 404-656-3943. Ex. dir., Carolyn Hutcherson. **Board of Licensed Practical Nurses**—166 Pryor St. SW, Atlanta 30303. Tel. 404-656-3921. Ex. dir., Patricia N. Swann.

Guam Nurses Association—Box 3134, Agana 96910. Pres., Lourdes Leon Guerrero. **Board of Nurse Examiners**—Box 2816, Agana 96910. Nurse examiner admin., Teofila P. Cruz.

Hawaii Nurses Association—677 Ala Moana Blvd. #601, Honolulu 96813. Tel. 808-531-1628. Ex. dir., Geri Marullo. **Board of Nursing**—Box 3469, Honolulu 96801. Tel. 808-548-3086. Ex. sec., Jerold Sakoda.

Idaho Nurses Association—1134 N. Orchard #8, Boise 83706. Tel. 208-323-0103. Ex. dir., Nancy Leslie. **Board of Nursing**—500 S. 10th St., Suite 102, Boise 83720. Tel. 208-334-3110. Ex. dir., Phyllis T. Sheridan.

Illinois Nurses Association—20 N. Wacker, Suite 2520, Chicago 60606. Tel. 312-236-9708. Pres., Mary Beth Badura; acting ex. dir., Joan Bundley. **Department of Registration and Education**—320 W. Washington St., Springfield 62786. Tel. 217-785-0800. Dir., Gary Clayton, 100 W. Randolph St., 9th Fl., Chicago 60601. Tel. 312-917-4500.

Indiana State Nurses Association—2915 North High School Rd., Indianapolis 46224. Tel. 317-299-4575. Ex. dir., Naomi R. Patchin. **Indiana State Board of Nursing,** Health Professions Bureau—One American Sq., Suite 1020, PO Box 82067, Indianapolis 46282-0004. Tel. 317-232-2960. Liaison from Health Professions Service Bureau, Bd. admin., Linda D. McClain.

Iowa Nurses Association—100 Court Ave., Suite 9LL, Des Moines 50309. Tel. 515-282-9169. Ex. dir., Judith Banta. **Board of Nursing**—1223 E. Court, Des Moines 50319. Tel. 515-281-3255. Ex. dir., Ann E. Mowery.

Kansas State Nurses Association—Rm. 520, 820 Quincy St., Topeka 66612. Tel. 913-233-8638. Ex. dir., Terri Rosselot. **Board of Nursing**—Landon State Office Bldg., 900 SW Jackson, Rm. 551, Topeka 66612-1256. Tel. 913-296-4929. Ex. admin., Dr. Lois R. Scibetta.

Kentucky Nurses Association—PO Box 2616, Louisville 40201. Tel. 502-637-2546. Ex. dir., Jean P. Duncan. **Board of Nursing**—4010 Dupont Circle, Suite 430, Louisville 40207. Tel. 502-897-5143. Ex. dir., Sharon M. Weisenbeck.

Louisiana State Nurses Association—712 Transcontinental Dr., Metairie 70001. Tel. 504-889-1030. Ex. dir., Barbara L. Morvant. **Board of Nursing**—Rm. 907, 150 Baronne St., New Orleans 70112. Tel. 504-568-5464. Ex. dir., Merlyn M. Maillian. **Board of Practical Nurse Examiners**—1440 Canal St., Suite 2010, New Orleans 70112. Tel. 504-568-6480. Ex. dir., Terry L. DeMarcay.

Maine State Nurses Association—283 Water St., PO Box 2240, Augusta 04330. Tel. 207-622-1057. Acting ex. dir., Anna Gilmore. **Board of Nursing**—295 Water St., Augusta 04330. Tel. 207-289-5324. Ex. dir., Jean C. Caron.

Maryland Nurses Association—5820 Southwestern Blvd., Baltimore 21227. Tel. 301-242-7300. Pres., Kathleen M. White; ex. dir., Robin Platts. **Board of Nursing**—201 W. Preston St., Baltimore 21201. Tel. 301-225-5880. Ex. dir., Donna Dorsey.

Massachusetts Nurses Association—340 Turnpike St., Canton 02021. Tel. 617-821-4625. Ex. dir., Anne G. Hargreaves. **Board of Registration in Nursing**—Rm. 1519, 100 Cambridge St., Boston 02202. Tel. 617-727-7393. Ex. sec., Mary H. Snodgrass.

Michigan Nurses Association—120 Spartan Ave., E. Lansing 48823. Tel. 517-337-1653. Ex. dir., Carol Franck. **Board of Nursing**—PO Box 30018, Lansing 48909. Tel. 517-373-1600.

Minnesota Nurses Association—Rm. N-377, 1821 University Ave., St. Paul 55104. Tel. 612-646-4807. Ex. dir., Ruth L. Hass. **Board of Nursing**—2700 University Ave. W, #108, St. Paul 55114. Tel. 612-642-0567. Ex. dir., Joyce M. Schowalter.

Mississippi Nurses Association—135 Bounds St., Suite 100, Jackson 39206. Tel. 601-982-9182. Pres., Faye Anderson. **Board of Nursing**—Suite 101, 135 Bounds St., Jackson 39206. Tel. 601-354-7349. Ex. dir., Marcella McKay.

Missouri Nurses Association—206 E. Dunklin St., PO Box 325, Jefferson City 65102-0325. Tel. 314-636-4623. Ex. dir., Caroline Davis. **Board of Nursing**—3523 N. Ten Mile Dr., PO Box 656, Jefferson City 65102. Tel. 314-751-2334. Ex. dir., Florence B. McGuire.

Montana Nurses Association—PO Box 5718, 715 Getchell, Helena 59604. Tel. 406-442-6710. Ex. dir., Barbara Booher. **Board of Nursing**—Dept. of Commerce, 1424 9th Ave., Helena 59620. Tel. 406-444-4279. Ex. sec., Phyllis McDonald.

Nebraska Nurses Association—Suite 711, 941 "O" St., Lincoln 68508. Tel. 402-475-3859. Ex. dir., Mary Ann Sak. **Board of Nursing**—Box 95007, Lincoln 68509. Tel. 402-471-2115. Nursing practice consultant, Vicky Burbach.

Nevada Nurses Association—3660 Baker Lane, Suite 104, Reno 89509. Tel. 702-825-3555. Office mgr., Lori Crocker. **Board of Nursing**—Suite 116, 1281 Terminal Way, Reno 89502. Tel. 702-786-2778. Ex. dir., Lonna Burress.

New Hampshire Nurses Association—48 West St., Concord 03301. Tel. 603-225-3783. Interim ex. dir., V. Lee Pope. **Board of Nursing**—Div. of Public Health Services, Health & Welfare Bldg., 6 Hazen Dr., Concord 03301-6527. Tel. 603-271-2323. Ex. dir., Doris E. Nay.

New Jersey State Nurses Association—320 W. State St., Trenton 08618. Tel. 609-392-4884. Ex. Dir., Barbara W. Wright. **Board of Nursing**—1100 Raymond Blvd., Rm. 319, Newark 07102. Tel. 201-648-2490. Ex. dir., Sr. Teresa L. Harris.

New Mexico Nurses Association—525 San Pedro NE, Suite 100, Albuquerque 87108. Tel. 505-268-7744. Ex. dir., Judith Brown. **Regulation and Licensing Department/Nursing**—4125 Carlisle NE, Albuquerque 87107. Tel. 505-841-6524. Ex. dir., Nancy L. Twigg.

New York State Nurses Association—2113 Western Ave., Guilderland 12084. Tel. 518-456-5371. Ex. dir., Martha L. Orr. **Board for Nursing**—State Education Dept., Cultural Education Center, Albany 12230. Tel. 518-474-3843. Ex. sec., Milene A. Megel.

North Carolina Nurses Association—Box 12025, Raleigh 27605-2025. Tel. 919-821-4250. Ex. dir., Clare LaBar. **Board of Nursing**—Box 2129, Raleigh 27602. Tel. 919-828-0740. Ex. dir., Carol A. Osman.

North Dakota Nurses Association—212 N. 4th St., Bismarck 58501. Tel. 701-223-1385. Ex. dir., Betty Maher. **Board of Nursing**—919 S. 9th St., Suite 504, Bismarck 58501. Tel. 701-224-2974. Ex. Dir., Karen MacDonald.

Ohio Nurses Association—4000 E. Main St., PO Box 13169, Columbus 43213-2950. Tel. 614-237-5414. Ex. dir., Joanne F. Easterling. **Board of Nursing Education and Nurse Registration**—65 S. Front St., Rm. 509, Columbus 43266-0316. Tel. 614-466-3947. Ex. sec., Rosa Lee Weinert.

Oklahoma Nurses Association—6414 N. Santa Fe, Suite A, Oklahoma City 73116. Tel. 405-840-3476. Ex. dir., Frances Waddle. **Board of Nurse Registration and Nursing Education**—2915 N. Classen Blvd., Suite 524, Oklahoma City 73106. Tel. 405-525-2076. Ex. dir., Sulinda Moffett.

Oregon Nurses Association—Suite 200, 9700 SW Capitol Hwy., Portland 97219. Tel. 503-293-0011. Ex. dir., Paula A. McNeil. **Board of Nursing**—1400 SW 5th Ave., Rm. 904, Portland 97201. Tel. 503-229-5653. Ex. dir., Dorothy J. Davy.

Pennsylvania Nurses Association—2578 Interstate Dr., PO Box 8525, Harrisburg 17105-8525. Tel. 717-657-1222. Ex. admin., David R. Ranck. **Board of Nursing**—PO Box 2649, Harrisburg 17105-2649. Tel. 717-783-7146. Ex. sec., Miriam H. Limo.

Colegio de Professsionales de la Enfermeria de Puerto Rico—PO Box 3647, San Juan 00936. Pres., Carmen Bigas; sec., Andrea Velázquez.

Puerto Rico Board of Nurse Examiners—800 Roberto H. Todd Ave., Stop 18, Santurce 00908. Tel. 809-725-8161. Pres., Melba Febus Bernardini; ex. dir., Irza Torres Aguiar.

Rhode Island State Nurses Association—345 Blackstone Blvd., Providence 02906. Tel. 401-421-9703. Ex. dir., Judy L. Sheehan. **Board of Nurse Registration and Nursing Education**—Rm. 104, Cannon Health Bldg., 75 Davis St., Providence 02908. Tel. 401-277-2827. Ex. sec., Bertha Mugurdichian.

South Carolina Nurses Association—1821 Gadsden St., Columbia 29201. Tel. 803-252-4781. Ex. dir., Judith Curfman Thompson. **Board of Nursing**—1777 St. Julian Pl., Suite 102, Columbia 29204. Tel. 803-737-6594. Ex. dir., Renatta Loquist.

South Dakota Nurses Association—1505 S. Minnesota, Suite 6, Sioux Falls 57105. Tel. 605-338-1401. Ex. dir., Kate Heligas. **Board of Nursing**—304 S. Phillips Ave., Suite 205, Sioux Falls 57102. Tel. 605-334-1243. Ex. sec., Carol Stuart.

Tennessee Nurses Association—Suite 400, 1720 West End Ave., Nashville 37203. Tel. 615-329-2511. Ex. dir., Louise Browning. **Board of Nursing**—Bureau of Manpower and Facilities, 283 Plus Park Blvd., Nashville 37219-5401. Tel. 615-367-6232. Ex. dir., Elizabeth Lund.

Texas Nurses Association—Community Bank Bldg., 300 Highland Mall Blvd., Suite 300, Austin 78752-3718. Tel. 512-452-0645. Ex. dir., Clair B. Jordan. **Board of Nurse Examiners**—1300 E. Anderson Lane, Bldg. C, Suite 225, Austin 78752. Tel. 512-835-4880. Ex. sec., Louise Sanders. **Board of Vocational Nurse Examiners**—1300 E. Anderson Lane, Bldg. C, Suite 285, Austin 78752. Tel. 512-835-2071. Ex. dir., Joyce A. Hammer.

Utah Nurses Association—1058 E. 9th S., Salt Lake City 84105. Tel. 801-322-3439. Ex. dir., Colleen Price. **Division of Occupational & Professional Licensing—Board of Nursing**—Heber M. Wells Bldg., 4th Fl., 160 E. 300 S., PO Box 45802, Salt Lake City 84145. Tel. 801-530-6733.

Vermont State Nurses Association—500 Dorset St., S. Burlington 05403. Tel. 802-864-9390. Pres., Kathleen A. Mariak. **Board of Nursing**—Redstone Bldg., 26 Terrace St., Montpelier 05602. Tel. 802-828-2396. Chrm., Dennis Ross.

Virgin Islands Nurses Association—PO Box 2866, Charlotte Amalie, St. Thomas 00801. Pres., Lucia Mitchell; ex. sec., Verna C. Garcia. **Board of Nurse Licensure**—Knud-Hansen Complex, Charlotte Amalie, St. Thomas 00801. Tel. 809-774-9000. Ex. sec., Juanita Molloy.

Virginia Nurses Association—1311 High Point Ave., Richmond 23230. Tel. 804-353-7311. Ex. dir., Jan M. Johnson. **Board of Nursing**—1601 Rolling Hills Dr., Richmond 23229. Tel. 804-662-9909.

Washington State Nurses Association—83 S. King St., Suite 500, Seattle 98104. Tel. 206-622-3613. Ex. dir., Joyce Pashley. **Board of Nursing Licensing Information**—Division of Professional Licensing, Box 9649, Olympia 98504. Tel. 206-753-2206. Ex. sec., Constance E. Roth. **Board of Practical Nursing Licensing Information**—Division of Professional Licensing, PO Box 9649, Olympia 98504. Tel. 206-753-3728.

West Virginia Nurses Association—PO Box 1946, Charleston 25327. Tel. 304-342-1169. Ex. dir., Linda Plemons. **Board of Examiners for Registered Nurses**—Rm. 309, Embleton Bldg., 922 Quarrier St., Charleston 25301. Tel. 304-348-3596. Ex. sec., Garnette Thorne. **Board of Examiners for Licensed Practical Nurses**—Rm. 506, Embleton Bldg., 922 Quarrier St., Charleston 25301. Tel. 304-348-3572.

Wisconsin Nurses Association—6117 Monona Dr., Madison 53716. Tel. 608-221-0383. Ex. admin., JoAnn Hanaway. **Board of Nursing**—Rm. 174, PO Box 8935, Madison 53708. Tel. 608-266-3735. Dir., Ramona Weakland Warden.

Wyoming Nurses Association—Majestic Bldg., Suite 305, 1603 Capitol Ave., Cheyenne 82001. Tel. 307-635-3955. Pres., Marcia Dale; ex. dir., Lola Fehr. **Board of Nursing**—Barrett Bldg., Suite One, 2301 Central Ave., Cheyenne 82002. Tel. 307-777-7601. Ex. dir., Joan C. Bouchard.

Appendix VIII
Nursing and Nursing-Related Organizations, Councils, Committees and Agencies

INTERNATIONAL

International Association for Enterostomal Therapy
International Childbirth Education Association
International Committee of Catholic Nurses and Social Assistants
International Committee of the Red Cross
International Council of Nurses and the Florence Nightingale International Foundation
International Council on Women's Health Issues
International Hospital Association
Pan American Health Organization
People to People Health Foundation (Project Hope)
Sigma Theta Tau, International Honor Society of Nursing
World Federation of Mental Health
World Health Organization

NATIONAL

Alpha Tau Delta, National fraternity for professional nurses
American Academy of Ambulatory Nursing Administrators
American Academy of Nurse Practitioners
American Academy of Nursing
American Assembly for Men in Nursing
American Assembly of Hospital Schools of Nursing
American Association of Colleges of Nursing

American Association of Critical Care Nurses
American Association for the History of Nursing
American Association of Nephrology Nurses and Technicians
American Association of Neuroscience Nurses
American Association of Nurse Anesthetists
American Association of Nursing Assistants
American Association of Nurse Attorneys
American Association of Occupational Health Nurses
American Association of Rehabilitation Therapy
American Association of Spinal Cord Injury Nurses
American Cancer Society
American College Health Association
American College of Nurse-Midwives
American Heart Association
American Holistic Nurses' Association
American Hospital Association, Division of Nursing
American Nephrology Nurses' Association
American Nurses' Association. Comprises the 50 State Nursing Organizations and those of the District of Columbia, Guam, and the Virgin Islands.
American Nurses' Foundation
American Nursing Federation
American Occupational Therapy Association
American Organization of Nurse Executives
American Physical Therapy Association
American Psychiatric Nurses' Association
American Public Health Association
American Radiological Nurses' Association
American Red Cross
American School Health Association
American Society of Allied Health Professionals
American Society of Childbirth Educators
American Society of Hospital Service Administrators
American Society of Ophthalmic Registered Nurses
American Society of Plastic and Reconstructive Surgical Nurses
American Society of Post-Anesthesia Nurses
American Thoracic Society
American Urological Association, Allied
Assembly of Hospital Schools of Nursing

Association for the Care of Children's Health
Association for the Care of Children in Hospitals
Association of Diploma Schools of Professional Nursing
Association of Operating Room Nurses
Association of Pediatric Oncology Nurses
Association for Practitioners in Infection Control
Association of Rehabilitation Nurses
Cassandra: Radical Feminist Nurses Network
Catholic Health Association of the United States
Chi Eta Phi Sorority
Commission on Graduates of Foreign Nursing Schools
Committee on Nursing of the Catholic Hospital Association
Council of Associate Degree Programs in Nursing
Council of Nurse Healers
Department of School Nurses, National Education Association
Dermatology Nurses Association
Drug and Alcohol Nursing Association
Emergency Department Nurses' Association
Federation of Nurses and Health Professionals
Frontier Nursing Service
Hospice Link
Intravenous Nurses' Society, Inc.
Joint Commission on Accreditation of Health Care Organizations
Lesbian and Gay Nurses' Alliance
Mid-Atlantic Regional Nursing Association
Midwest Alliance in Nursing
National Alliance of Nurse Practitioners
National Association of Colored Graduate Nurses
National Association for Health Care Recruitment
National Association of Hispanic Nurses
National Association for Home Care
National Association for Mental Health
National Association of Neonatal Nurses
National Association of Nurse Recruiters
National Association of Orthopaedic Nurses
National Association of Pediatric Nurse Associates and Practitioners
National Association of Physicians' Nurses
National Association for Practical Nurse Education and Service
National Association of School Nurses

National Black Nurses' Association
National Center for Nursing Ethics
National Council of Licensure Examination
National Council of State Boards of Nursing
National Council of Homemaker Services
National Federation of Licensed Practical Nurses
National Federation of Specialty Nursing Organizations
National Flight Nurses' Association
National Intravenous Therapy Association
National Joint Practice Commission
National League for Nursing
National Maternal and Child Health Clearinghouse
National Nurses for Life
National Nurses' Society on Addictions
National Nurses' Society on Alcoholism
National Organization for Advancement of A.D. Education
National Organization of World War Nurses
National Student Nurses' Association
New England Organization for Nursing
North American Nursing Diagnosis Association
Nurses Against Misrepresentation
Nurses' Alliance for the Prevention of Nuclear War
Nurses' Association of the American College of Obstetricians and Gynecologists
Nurses' Christian Fellowship
Nurses' Coalition for Action in Politics
Nurse Consultants' Association
Nurses' Educational Funds, Inc.
Nurses' Environmental Health Watch
Nurses in Transition
Nurses' House, Inc.
Oncology Nursing Society
Public Health Nursing/American Public Health Association
Retired Army Nurse Corps Association
Sex Information and Education Council of the United States
Society for the Advancement of Nursing
Society for Gastrointestinal Assistants, Inc.
Society for Nursing History
Society for Otorhinolaryngology and Head/Neck Nurses

Society of Retired Air Force Nurses
Southern Council on Collegiate Education for Nursing
Southern Regional Education Board
Transcultural Nursing Society
United Nurses' Associations of California
Visiting Nurse Associaton of America
Western Council on Higher Education for Nursing
Western Institute of Nursing

U.S. Government Services
Peace Corps
Air Force Nurse Corps
Army Nurse Corps
Navy Nurse Corps
Veterans Administration Nursing Service
Department of Health and Human Services
  Public Health Service
    Alcohol, Drug Abuse and Mental Health Administration
    Centers for Disease Control
    Food and Drug Administration
    Health Resources and Services Administration
    Indian Health Service
    National Institutes of Health
  Health Care Financing Administration

Appendix IX
Health-Care-Related Organizations

Addicts Anonymous
Al-Anon
Alcoholics Anonymous
Allergy Foundation of America
Alexander Graham Bell Association for the Deaf
American Academy of Hearing
American Academy of Pediatrics
American Academy of Physical Medicine and Rehabilitation
American Academy of Physicians' Assistants
American Anorexia Nervosa Association
American Association for the Care of Childrens' Health
American Association for the Deaf
American Association of Diabetes Educators
American Association of Pathologists and Bacteriologists
American Association of Respiratory Therapy
American Association of Retired Persons
American Association of Sex Educators, Counselors, and Therapists
American Association of Suicidology
American Burn Association
American College of Obstetricians and Gynecologists
American College of Physicians
American College of Radiologists
American College of Sports Medicine
American Council for the Blind
American Dental Association
American Dermatology Association
American Diabetes Association
American Dietetic Association

American Foundation for the Blind
American Geriatrics Society
American Health Care Association
American Lung Association
American Medical Association
American Medical Writers Association
American Nursing Home Association
American Parkinson's Disease Association
American Rehabilitation Committee
American Rheumatism Association
American Social Hygiene Association
American Speech, Language, and Hearing Association
Amyotrophic Lateral Sclerosis Society of America
Arthritis Foundation
Asthma and Allergy Foundation of America
Better Hearing Institute
Catholic Hospital Association
Committee to Combat Huntington's Disease
Cystic Fibrosis Foundation
Deafness Research Foundation
Emergency Care Research Institue
Epilepsy Foundation of America
Eye Bank Association of America
Family Service Association of America
Gerontological Society of America
Institute for Cancer Research
International Association of Laryngectomees
International Federation on Aging
Juvenile Diabetics Foundation
La Leche League, International
Leukemic Society of America
Muscular Dystrophy Association of America
Narcotics Education
National Association for Health Care Recruitment
National Association for Home Care
National Association for Mental Health
National Cerebral Palsy Association
National Council on Aging
National Council on Alcoholism

National Cystic Fibrosis Foundation
National Easter Seal Society of Crippled Children and Adults
National Epilepsy League
National Foundation for the March of Dimes
National Health Council
National Hemophilia Foundation
National Hospice Organization
National Interagency Council on Smoking and Health
National Institute on Alcohol Abuse and Alcoholism
National Institute of Arthritis and Metabolic Diseases
National Institute of Burn Medicine
National Kidney Foundation
National Mental Health Association
National Multiple Sclerosis Foundation
National Paraplegic Foundation
National Parkinson's Disease Foundation
National Psoriasis Foundation
National Rehabilitation Foundation
National Reye's Syndrome Foundation
National Safety Council
National Society for the Prevention of Blindness
National Tuberculosis and Respiratory Disease Association
Society of Gastrointestinal Assistants
Society of Otolaryngology
United Cerebral Palsy Association
United Nations Internationl Childrens' Emergency Fund
Western Division of Council of University Hospitals
Women Organized Against Rape

Governmental Departments, Administrations, Centers, Institutes, Services

Department of Health and Human Services
***

Administration on Aging
Alcohol, Drug Abuse, and Mental Health Administration
Food and Drug Administration
Health Care Financing Administration
Health Resources and Services Administration
Veterans Administration

***

Centers for Disease Control
Center for Health Statistics
National Institute on Aging
National Institute on Aging, Work, Retirement
National Institute of Child Health and Human Development
National Institute of Environmental Health Sciences
National Institutes of Health
National Institute of Neurological Disorders and Stroke
National Institute of Occupational Safety and Health

***

Appendix X
Nursing and Nursing-Related Periodicals

AANA Journal; bimonthly. Official journal of the American Association of Nurse Anesthetists. Charles B. Slack, Inc.

AAOHN Journal; bimonthly. Official journal of the American Association of Occupational Health Nurses. Charles B. Slack, Inc.

AD Nurse; bimonthly. Data Design, Inc.

Advances in Nursing Science; quarterly. Aspen Publishers, Inc.

Alumni Magazine. Journal of the Johns Hopkins Alumni Association, Inc.

Alumni Magazine; 3 × yr. Journal of the Columbia-Presbyterian Hospital School of Nursing Alumni Association, New York, N.Y.

American Journal of Hospice Care; bimontly. Journal of the American Health Care Association. Prime National Publishing Co.

American Journal of Infection Control; bimonthly. Journal of the Association for Practitioners in Infection Control. C.V. Mosby Co.

American Journal of Mental Deficiency; 6 × yr. Journal of the American Association on Mental Deficiency

American Journal of Nursing; monthly. Professional journal of the American Nurses' Association. The American Journal of Nursing Company

American Journal of Occupational Therapy; monthly. Journal of the American Occupational Therapy Association, Inc.

American Journal of Primary Health Care; bimonthly. Health Sciences Media and Research Services, Inc.

American Journal of Public Health; monthly. Journal of the American Public Health Association

American Nurse Newspaper; 10 × yr. Official newspaper of the American Nurses' Association

ANNA Journal; 7 × yr. Journal of the American Nephrology Nurses' Association. Anthony J. Jannetti, Inc.

Annual Review of Nursing Research. Springer Publishing Company

AORN Journal; monthly. Journal of the Association of Operating Room Nurses, Inc. Charles B. Slack, Inc.

Applied Nursing Research; quarterly. W. B. Saunders and Co.

Archives of Psychiatric Nursing; bimonthly. Grune & Stratton, Inc.

Aspen's Advisor for Nursing Executives; monthly. Aspen Publishers, Inc.

Birth: Issues in Perinatal Care and Education; 4 × yr. Blackwell Scientific Publications

Briefs; 10 × yr. From the Maternity Center of New York. Charles B. Slack, Inc.

Canadian Nurse; 11 × yr. Professional journal of the Canadian Nurses' Association

Cancer Nursing; bimonthly. The Raven Press

Cardiovascular Nursing; bimonthly. A journal of the American Heart Association

Caring; monthly. The journal of the National Association for Home Care

Childbirth Educator; quarterly. American Baby, Inc.

Childrens' Health Care; quarterly. Journal of the Association for Care of Childrens' Health

Clinic-Alert; 24 × yr. Science Editors, Inc.

Communicating Nursing Research; quarterly. Western Interstate Commission for Higher Education

Community Mental Health Journal; quarterly. The journal of the National Council of Community Mental Health Centers, Inc. Human Sciences Press

Computers in Nursing; bimonthly. J.B. Lippincott Co.

Critical Care Nurse; bimonthly. Hospital Publications, Inc.

Critical Care Nursing Quarterly. Aspen Publishers, Inc.

Critical Care Update; monthly. Journal of the National Critical Care Institute of Education

The Dean's Note. Newsletter for Deans and Directors of Schools of Nursing

Death Education Quarterly. Hemisphere Publishing Corp.

Death Studies; quarterly. Hemisphere Publishing Corp.

Diabetes Care; bimonthly. Journal of the American Diabetes Association, Inc.

Diabetes Educator. The journal of the American Association of Diabetes Educators

Diet and Nutrition Health Letter; monthly. Tufts University Press

Dimensions in Critical Care Nursing; bimonthly. J.B. Lippincott Co.

Dimensions in Oncology Nursing. A publication of the Nursing Staff Services, Anderson Hospital and Tumor Institute, Houston, Texas

Emergency Nurse Legal Bulletin; quarterly. Med/Law Publishers, Inc.

Emergency Nursing Reports; monthly. Med/Law Publishers, Inc.

Emphasis: Nursing. A publication of the Department of Nursing, UCLA Medical Center

EMT Journal; bimonthly. Journal of the National Association of Emergency Medical Technicians. C.V. Mosby Co.

Family and Community Health; quarterly. Aspen Publications, Inc.

Focus on Critical Care; bimonthly. Journal of the American Association of Critical Care Nurses. C.V. Mosby Co.

Frontier Nursing Service Quarterly Bulletin. Journal of the Frontier Nursing Service, Inc.

Geriatric Nursing; American Journal of Care for the Aging; bimonthly. The American Journal of Nursing Company

Harvard Medical School Health Letter; monthly.

Health; monthly. Family Media

Health Care Education; bimonthly. Woodbury Communications, Inc.

Health Care Forum. Journal of the Association of Western Hospitals

Health Care Recruiter: monthly. Prime National Publishing Co.

Health Care Supervisor. Aspen Publications, Inc.

Health Care for Women, International; bimonthly. Hemisphere Publishing Corp.

Health Education Quarterly. John Wiley & Sons, Inc.

Health Education; bimonthly. Journal of the Association for the Advancement of Health Education, the American Alliance for Health, Physical Education and the Dance.

Heart and Lung: Journal of Critical Care; bimonthly. Official publication of the American Association of Critical Care Nurses. C.V. Mosby Co.

Holistic Health Review; quarterly. Journal of the Holistic Health Organizing Committee

Holistic Nursing Practice; quarterly. Aspen Publishers, Inc.

Home Healthcare Nurse; bimonthly. Hospital Publications, Inc.

Home Health Care Services; quarterly. The Haworth Press, Inc.

Home Health Review; quarterly. Journal of the National Home Health Care Agencies

Homecare; monthly. Miramar Publishing Co.

Hospice Journal; quarterly. The journal of the National Hospice Organization. The Haworth Press, Inc.

Hospital Formulary; monthly. Harcourt, Brace, Jovanovich Publications

Hospital Topics; bimonthly. Official journal of the National Hospital Nursing Supervisor Management Conference and the National Central Service Conference

Hospitals; semi-monthly. The journal of the American Hospital Association

Image: The Journal of Nursing Scholarship; 4 × yr. The journal of Sigma Theta Tau, International Honor Society of Nursing

Imprint: 5 × yr. Newsletter of the National Student Nurses' Association

Infection Control; monthly. Charles B. Slack, Inc.

International Journal of Nursing Studies; quarterly. (Text in English, Spanish, French, Russian). The Pergamon Press

International Nursing Index; quarterly. The American Journal of Nursing Company in cooperation with the National Library of Medicine

International Nursing Review; bimonthly. The journal of the International Council of Nurses. Published in Geneva, Switzerland

Issues in Comprehensive Pediatric Nursing; bimonthly. Hemisphere Publishing Corp.

Issues in Emergency Nursing; bimonthly. The journal of the Emergency Department Nurse's Association

Issues in Health Care of Women; 6 × yr. Hemisphere Publishing Corp.

Issues in Mental Health Nursing; quarterly. Hemisphere Publishing Corp.

Johns Hopkins School of Nursing Alumni Magazine; quarterly

Journal of Allied Health; quarterly. The journal of the American Society of Allied Health Professionals. RAM Associates, Ltd.

Journal of Ambulatory Care Management; quarterly. Aspen Publishers, Inc.

Journal of the American Association of Nephrology Nurses and Technicians; bimonthly. Published by Pitman

Journal of American College Health; bimonthly. The journal of the American College Health Association. Hildreth Publications

Journal of the American Physical Therapy Association; monthly

Journal of the Association for the Care of Children in Hospitals; quarterly. Charles B. Slack, Inc.

Journal of Burn Care and Rehabilitation; semi-monthly. JAC Publishing Co.

Journal of Christian Nursing; quarterly. Journal of the Nurses' Christian Fellowship

Journal of Community Health; quarterly. Human Sciences Press

Journal of Community Health Nursing; bimonthly. Charles B. Slack, Inc.

Journal of Continuing Education in Nursing; bimonthly. Charles B. Slack, Inc.

Journal of Emergency Nursing; bimonthly. Journal of the Emergency Departmrnt Nurses' Association. C.V. Mosby Co.

Journal of Enterostomal Therapy; quarterly. Journal of the International Association for Enterostomal Therapy. C.V. Mosby Co.

Journal of Gerontological Nursing; bimonthly. Charles B. Slack, Inc.

Journal of Intravenous Therapy; bimonthly. Medical Education Consultants

Journal of Long-Term Care Administration; quarterly. The journal of the American Nursing Home Administration

Journal of the National Intravenous Therapy Association. Lippincott, Harper & Row

Journal of Nephrology Nursing; bimonthly. Phoenix Educational Systems, Inc.

Journal of Neuroscience Nursing; quarterly. The journal of the American Association of Neuroscience Nurses.

Journal of Nurse-Midwifery; bimonthly. The journal of the American College of Nurse Midwives. Elsevier North Holland, Inc.

Journal of Nursing Administration; 11 × yr. Charles B. Slack, Inc.

Journal of Nursing Care; monthly. The journal of the National Federation of Licensed Practical Nurses. Technomic Publishing Co.

Journal of Nursing Education; 9 × yr. Charles B. Slack, Inc.

Journal of Nursing Quality Assurance; quarterly. Aspen Publishers, Inc.

Journal of Nursing Staff Development; quarterly. J. B. Lippincott Co.

Journal of Obstetric, Gynecologic and Neonatal Nursing; bimonthly. The journal of the Organization for Obstetric, Gynecologic and Neonatal Nursing. J.B. Lippincott Co.

Journal of Ophthalmic Nursing and Technology; bimonthly. Charles B. Slack, Inc.

Journal of Pediatric and Neonatal Nursing; quarterly. Aspen Publishers, Inc.

Journal of Pediatric Nursing: Nursing Care of Children and Families; bimonthly. Grune & Stratton, Inc.

Journal of Pediatric Psychology; quarterly. Plenum Publishing Co.

Journal of Perinatal and Neonatal Nursing; quarterly. Aspen Publishers, Inc.

Journal of Post-Anesthesia Nursing; quarterly. The journal of the American Society of Post-Anesthesia Nurses. Grune & Stratton, Inc.

Journal of Practical Nursing; quarterly. The journal of the National Association for Practical Nurse Education and Practice, Inc.

Journal of Prevention; quarterly. Human Sciences Press

Journal of Professional Nursing; bimonthly. The journal of the American Association of Colleges of Nursing. W.B. Saunders Co.

Journal of Psychosocial Nursing and Mental Health Services; monthly. Charles B. Slack, Inc.

Journal of Rehabilitation; quarterly. Journal of the National Rehabilitation Association

Journal of School Health; 10 × yr. The journal of the American School Health Association

Journal of School Psychology; quarterly. Human Sciences Press

Law, Medicine and Health Care; quarterly. The journal of the American Society of Law and Medicine

Licensed Practical Nurse; quarterly. Journal of the National Federation of Licensed Practical Nurses. McClain Publishing Co.

Life Support Nursing; bimonthly. Barlin Publishing Co.

Long-Term Care Management; 36 × yr. McGraw Hill Publishing Co.

Maternal-Child Nursing Journal; quarterly. Published by the Departments of Maternity Nursing and Nursing Care of the University of Pittsburgh

Mayo Clinic Health Letter; published by the Mayo Clinic, Rochester, Minnesota, 55905.

MCN: American Journal of Maternal-Child Nursing; bimonthly. The American Journal of Nursing Co.

NAACOG Newsletter; monthly. Newsletter of the Nurses' Association of the American College of Obstetricians and Gynecologists

The Nation's Health; monthly. Official Newspaper of the American Public Health Association. 12 × yr.

NITA; bimonthly. Official journal of the National Intravenous Therapy Association. J.B. Lippincott Co.

NLN News: monthly. News magazine of the National League for Nursing

Nurse Practitioner: The American Journal of Primary Health Care; monthly. Vernon Publications, Inc.

Nurses' Drug Alert; monthly. Michael J. Powers & Co.

Nursing: Title appears with the current year; monthly. Springhouse Corp.

Nursing Administration and Law Manual; semi-annually. Aspen Publishers, Inc.

Nursing Administration Quarterly. Aspen Publishers, Inc.

Nursing and Health Care; 10 × yr. Official journal of the National League for Nursing.

Nursing Clinics of North America; quarterly. W. B. Saunders Co.

Nursing Digest; quarterly. Concept Development Co.

Nursing Economics; monthly. Anthony J. Jannetti, Inc.

Nursing Forms Manual; semi-annually. Aspen Publishers, Inc.

Nursing Forum; quarterly. Nursing Publications, Inc.

Nursing Job News; monthly. Prime National Publishing Corp.

Nursing Law and Ethics; monthly. Journal of the American Society of Law and Medicine. Charles B. Slack, Inc.

Nursing Life; bimonthly. Springhouse Corp.

Nursing Management; monthly. S-N Publications, Inc.

Nursing Outlook; bimonthly. Official journal of the American Academy of Nursing. Pub. by The American Journal of Nursing Co.

Nursing Report: monthly. Recom Publishing Co.

Nursing Research; bimonthly. Sponsored by the American Nurses' Association and the National League for Nursing. Pub. by the American Journal of Nursing Co.

Nursing Success Today; monthly. Charles B. Slack, Inc.

Occupational Health Nursing; monthly. Charles B. Slack, Inc.

Oncology Nursing Forum; bimonthly. The journal of the Oncology Nursing Society.

Orthopaedic Nursing; monthly. Journal of the National Association of Orthopaedic Nursing. Anthony J. Jannetti, Inc.

Pediatric Clinics of North America; quarterly. W. B. Saunders Co.

Pediatric Nurse Practitioner Newsletter; monthly. A publication of the National Association of Pediatric Nurse Associates and Practitioners

Pediatric Nursing; bimonthly. The journal of the National Association of Pediatric Nurse Associates and Practitioners. Anthony J. Jannetti, Inc.

Perioperative Nursing; quarterly. Aspen Publishers, Inc.

Perspectives in Psychiatric Care; quarterly. Nursing Publications, Inc.

Physical Therapy; monthly. Journal of the American Physical Therapy Association

Physical and Occupational Therapy in Geriatrics; quarterly. Haworth Press, Inc.

Physical and Occupational Therapy in Pediatrics; quarterly. Haworth Press, Inc.

Plastic Surgical Nursing. Journal of the American Society of Plastic and Reconstructive Surgical Nurses

Primary Care Quarterly. W. B. Saunders Co.

PROVIDER: For Long-Term Care Professionals; monthly. The journal of the American Health Care Association

Public Health Nursing; monthly. Blackwell Scientific Publications, Inc.

Public Health Reports; bimonthly. Journal of the Department of Health Education, U.S. Public Health Service. Superintendent of Documents, Washington D.C.

Regan Report on Nursing Law; monthly. Media Press

Rehabilitation Nursing; bimonthly. The journal of the Association of Rehabilitation Nurses. AMC Publishers

Research in Nursing and Health; quarterly. John Wiley & Sons, Inc.

Respiratory Care; monthly. The journal of the American Association of Respiratory Therapy

RN: National Magazine for Nurses; monthly. Medical Economics Co.

Scholarly Inquiry for Nursing Practice; An International Journal; 3 × yr. Springer Publishing Co.

School Health; bimonthly. The journal of the American School Health Association

School Nurse: quarterly. The journal of the Department of School Nurses of the National Education Association

Seminars in Oncology Nursing; quarterly. Grune & Stratton, Inc.

Senior Nurse; monthly; John Wiley & Sons, Inc.

Sexually Transmitted Disease Bulletin; quarterly. J. B. Lippincott Co.

State Nursing Legislation; quarterly. The American Nurses' Association Center for Research.

Today's Nursing Home; monthly. McKnight Medical Communications, Inc.

Today's OR Nurse; monthly. Charles B. Slack, Inc.
Topics in Clinical Nursing; quarterly. Aspen Publishers, Inc.
Topics in Emergency Medicine; bimonthly. Aspen Publishers, Inc.
Western Journal of Nursing Research; quarterly. Sage Publications, Inc.
Women and Health: The Journal of Women's Health Care; quarterly. Haworth Press, Inc.

N.B. In addition to the periodicals listed here, most of the State Nurses Associations and some local organizations also publish a newsheet or journal regularly.

Appendix XI
Code for Nurses

1. The nurse provides services with respect for human dignity and the uniqueness of the client, unrestricted by considerations of social or economic status, personal attributes, or the nature of health problems.
2. The nurse safeguards the client's right to privacy by judiciously protecting information of a confidential nature.
3. The nurse acts to safeguard the client and the public when health care and safety are affected by the incompetent, unethical, or illegal practice of any person.
4. The nurse assumes responsibility and accountability for individual nursing judgments and actions.
5. The nurse maintains competence in nursing.
6. The nurse exercises informed judgment and uses individual competence and qualifications as criteria in seeking consultation, accepting responsibilities, and delegating nursing activities to others.
7. The nurse participates in activities that contribute to the ongoing development of the profession's body of knowledge.

8. The nurse participates in the profession's efforts to implement and improve standards of nursing.

9. The nurse participates in the profession's efforts to establish and maintain conditions of employment conducive to high quality nursing care.

10. The nurse participates in the profession's effort to protect the public from misinformation and misrepresentation and to maintain the integrity of nursing.

11. The nurse collaborates with members of the health professions and other citizens in promoting community and national efforts to meet the health needs of the public.

A Code for Nurses was adopted by the American Nurses' Association in 1950 and has been revised several times. Information about the Code along with interpretive statements about the elements in it may be found in the publication *Code for Nurses with Interpretive Statements,* which is available from the American Nurses' Association, 2420 Pershing Road, Kansas City, Missouri 64108.

Appendix XII
The Nightingale Pledge

I solemnly pledge myself before God and in the presence of this Assembly:
To pass my life in purity and to practice my profession faithfully.
I will abstain from whatever is deleterious and mischievous, and will not take or knowingly administer any harmful drug.
I will do all in my power to maintain and elevate the standard of my profession, and will hold in confidence all personal matters committed to my keeping, and all family affairs coming to my knowledge in the practice of my profession.
With loyalty will I endeavor to aid the physician in his work, and devote myself to the welfare of those committed to my care.

This pledge was formulated in 1893 by a committee, of which Lystra E. Gretter, R.N. was chairman at the Farrand Training School for Nurses at the Harper Hospital in Detroit, Michigan and was revised in 1935. It is often repeated at graduation exercises in schools of nursing.